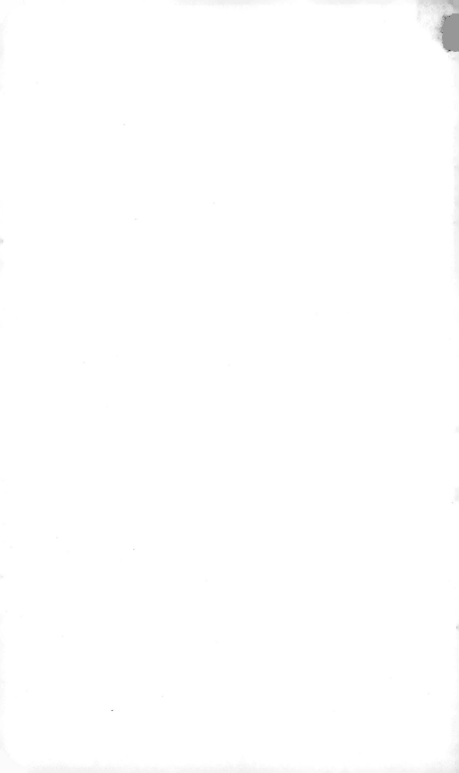

HANDBOOK OF
NURSING
PROCEDURES

SPRINGHOUSE

Springhouse, Pennsylvania

STAFF

Publisher
Judith A. Schilling McCann, RN, MSN

Editorial Director
David Moreau

Clinical Manager
Joan M. Robinson, RN, MSN, CCRN

Editors
Cynthia Breuninger, Stacey Follin,
Julie Munden, Carol Munson, Pat Wittig

Clinical Project Manager
Collette Bishop Hendler, RN, CCRN

Clinical Editors
Kate McGovern, RN, BSN, CCRN;
Beverly Ann Tscheschlog, RN

Copy Editors
Jaime Stockslager (supervisor),
Priscilla Dewitt, Heather Ditch,
Kimberly A.J. Johnson, Marcia Ryan,
Pamela Wingrod

Associate Design Director
Arlene Putterman

Designers
Debra Moloshok (book design and
project manager), Joseph John Clark,
Donna S. Morris

Projects Coordinator
Liz Schaeffer

Electronic Production Services
Diane Paluba (manager), Joyce Rossi Biletz

Manufacturing
Patricia K. Dorshaw (manager),
Otto Mezei (book production manager)

Editorial Assistants
Beverly Lane, Beth Janae Orr, Elfriede Young

Indexer
Manjit K. Sahai

Printed in the United States of America.
HBNP - D
03 02 01   10 9 8 7 6 5 4 3 2

Library of Congress Cataloging-in-Publication Data
Handbook of nursing procedures.
   p. ; cm.
   Includes bibliographical references and index.
   ISBN 1-58255-139-1 (alk. paper)
   1. Nursing — Handbooks, manuals, etc. I.
Springhouse Corporation.
   [DNLM: 1. Nursing Care — Handbooks. 2. Nursing
Process — Handbooks. WY 49 H23574 2001]
   RT51 .H365 2001
   610.73 — dc21   00-068776

CONTENTS

Contributors   iv

Foreword   v

Nursing procedures (in alphabetical order)   **1**

Appendix: Alternative and complementary therapies   936

Selected references   944

Index   946

Contributors

Susan E. Appling, RN, MS, CRNP
Assistant Professor
Johns Hopkins University School of Nursing
Baltimore

Deborah Becker, RN, MSN, CRNP, CS,
CCRN
Assistant Program Director
Adult Critical Care Nurse Practitioner Program
University of Pennsylvania School of Nursing
Philadelphia

Darlene Nebel Cantu, RN,C, MSN
Director
Baptist Health System School of Professional
  Nursing
San Antonio, Tex.
Adjunct Faculty
San Antonio College

Janice T. Chussil, RN,C, MSN, ANP
Nurse Practitioner
Dermatology Associates
Portland, Ore.

Jean Sheerin Coffey, RN, MS, PNP
Unit Leader — Pediatrics
Children's Hospital at Dartmouth
Dartmouth Hitchcock Medical Center
Lebanon, N.H.

Colleen M. Fries, RN, CRNP, MSN, CCRN
Family Nurse Practitioner
Private Practice
Voorhees, N.J.

Rebecca Crews Gruener, RN, MS
Associate Professor of Nursing
Louisiana State University at Alexandria

Sandra Hamilton, RN, MEd, CRNI
Western Director of Pharmacy Nursing Services
Vencare Pharmacy
Boise, Idaho

Dr. Joyce Lyne Heise, MSN, EdD
Associate Professor of Nursing
Kent State University
East Liverpool, Ohio

Lucy J. Hood, RN, DNSc
Associate Professor
Saint Luke's College
Kansas City, Mo.

Mary Ellen Kelly, RN, BSN
Director of Staff Development
Infection Control Coordinator
John L. Montgomery Care Center
Freehold, N.J.

Susan M. Leininger, RN, MSN
Advanced Practice Nurse
Allegheny General Hospital
Pittsburgh

Catherine Todd Magel, RN,C, EdD
Assistant Professor
Villanova (Pa.) University College of Nursing

Donna Nielsen, RN, MSN, CEN, CCRN,
MICN
Nursing Instructor
Pasadena (Calif.) City College

Ruthie Robinson, RN, MSN, CCRN, CEN
Instructor
Lamar University
Beaumont, Tex.

Lisa Salamon, RN,C, MSN, CNS
Clinical Nurse Specialist
The Greens Adult Living Community
Lyndhurst, Ohio

Cynthia C. Small, RN, MSN
Nursing Instructor
Lake Michigan College
Benton Harbor, Mich.

LeeAnne B. Tomasko, MS, APRN, FNP
Associate Director Liver Center
Gastroenterology Center of Connecticut
Hamden, Conn.

FOREWORD

The 21st century has arrived and the nursing profession continues to keep pace with a market-driven health care system — one that requires increasingly complex nursing care while stressing cost containment. Nurses must be prepared to provide quality care efficiently and effectively and meet the needs of patients, families, and communities across all settings and at all levels of care — including early detection, treatment, prevention and wellness, and rehabilitation.

A quick, easy-to-use reference that provides comprehensive coverage of health care procedures is essential for both students and nurses as they strive to meet the diverse needs of their patients as well as monitor and evaluate the care given by nursing assistants.

Handbook of Nursing Procedures is such a reference. With over 260 procedures arranged alphabetically, a full range of health care technologies from simple to complex are covered using a consistent format. Among the complex procedures included are transcranial Doppler monitoring and PAP and PAWP monitoring as well as more basic procedures, such as nasogastric and airway insertions.

Each procedure includes a thorough description, an equipment list, necessary preparatory steps, implementation steps with accompanying rationales, complications, important nursing considerations, and documentation essentials. Students and new graduates will find this format — complete with sidebars, drawings, photographs, and charts to help illustrate procedural steps and clarify equipment function — particularly useful. Throughout the handbook are several helpful logos that alert the reader to valuable information. *Technology update* identifies and explains the latest equipment, while *Troubleshooting* highlights strategies to prevent and solve equipment problems. For the student, *Better charting* presents illustrations and advice on proper documentation of procedures. Specific insights, cautions, and nursing considerations regarding procedures are highlighted by *Nursing alerts,* and *Age alerts* focus attention on procedural alterations necessary for specific patient age-groups.

Finally, an appendix featuring alternative and complementary therapies makes this reference unique among nursing procedure handbooks. It's an essential reference for any nursing library or personal collection and is useful to experienced and novice nurses and students.

Susan E. Appling, RN, MS, CRNP
Assistant Professor
Johns Hopkins University
School of Nursing
Baltimore

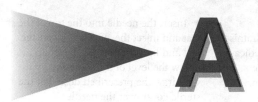

ADMIXTURE OF DRUGS IN A SYRINGE

Combining two drugs in one syringe avoids the discomfort of two injections. Usually, drugs can be mixed in a syringe in one of four ways. They may be combined from two multidose vials (for example, regular and long-acting insulin), from one multidose vial and one ampule, from two ampules, or from a cartridge-injection system combined with either a multidose vial or an ampule.

Such combinations are contraindicated when the drugs aren't compatible and when the combined doses exceed the amount of solution that can be absorbed from a single injection site.

Key nursing diagnoses and patient outcomes
Risk for infection related to improper technique
The patient will:
▶ maintain a normal body temperature
▶ show no signs of infection at the injection site
▶ exhibit a normal white blood cell count and differential.

Equipment
Prescribed medications • patient's medication record and chart • alcohol pad

---

Cartridge-injection system

A cartridge-injection system, such as Tubex or Carpuject, is a convenient, easy-to-use method of injection that facilitates accuracy and sterility. The device consists of a plastic cartridge-holder syringe and a prefilled medication cartridge with a needle attached.

The medication in the cartridge is premixed and premeasured, which saves time and helps ensure an exact dose. The medication remains sealed in the cartridge and sterile until the injection is administered to the patient.

The disadvantage of this system is that not all drugs are available in cartridge form. However, compatible drugs can be added to partially filled cartridges.

• syringe and needle • safety needle
• gauze pad • optional: cartridge-injection system and filter needle

The type and size of the syringe and needle depend on the prescribed medications, patient's body build, and route of administration. Medications that come in prefilled cartridges require a cartridge-injection system. (See *Cartridge-injection system*.)

Implementation

► Verify that the drugs to be administered agree with the patient's medication record and the doctor's orders.
► Calculate the dose to be given.
► Wash your hands.

Mixing drugs from two multidose vials

► Using an alcohol pad, wipe the rubber stopper on the first vial. *This decreases the risk of contaminating the medication as you insert the needle into the vial.*
► Pull back the syringe plunger until the volume of air drawn into the syringe equals the volume to be withdrawn from the drug vial.
► Without inverting the vial, insert the needle into the top of the vial, making sure that the needle's bevel tip doesn't touch the solution. Inject the air into the vial and withdraw the needle. *This replaces air in the vial, thus preventing creation of a partial vacuum on withdrawal of the drug.*
► Repeat the steps above for the second vial. Then, after injecting the air into the second vial, invert the vial, withdraw the prescribed dose, and then withdraw the needle.
► Wipe the rubber stopper of the first vial again and insert the needle, taking care not to depress the plunger. Invert the vial, withdraw the prescribed dose, and then withdraw the needle.

Mixing drugs from a multidose vial and an ampule

► Using an alcohol pad, clean the vial's rubber stopper.
► Pull back on the syringe plunger until the volume of air drawn into the syringe equals the volume to be withdrawn from the drug vial.

► Insert the needle into the top of the vial and inject the air. Then invert the vial and keep the needle's bevel tip below the level of the solution as you withdraw the prescribed dose. Put the sterile cover over the needle.
► Wrap a sterile gauze pad or an alcohol pad around the ampule's neck *to protect yourself from injury in case the glass splinters.* Break open the ampule, directing the force away from you.
► If desired, switch to the filter needle at this point *to filter out any glass splinters.*
► Insert the needle into the ampule. Be careful not to touch the outside of the ampule with the needle. Draw the correct dose into the syringe.
► If you switched to the filter needle, change back to a safety needle to administer the injection.

Mixing drugs from two ampules

► An opened ampule doesn't contain a vacuum. To mix drugs from two ampules in a syringe, calculate the prescribed doses and open both ampules, using aseptic technique. If desired, use a filter needle to draw up the drugs. Then change to a safety needle to administer them.

Special considerations

► Insert a needle through the vial's rubber stopper at a slight angle, bevel up, and exert slight lateral pressure. *By using this method, you won't cut a piece of rubber out of the stopper, which can then be pushed into the vial.*
► When mixing drugs from multidose vials, be careful not to contaminate one drug with the other. Ideally, the needle should be changed after drawing the first medication into the syringe.

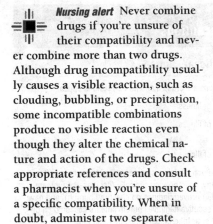 ***Nursing alert*** Never combine drugs if you're unsure of their compatibility and never combine more than two drugs. Although drug incompatibility usually causes a visible reaction, such as clouding, bubbling, or precipitation, some incompatible combinations produce no visible reaction even though they alter the chemical nature and action of the drugs. Check appropriate references and consult a pharmacist when you're unsure of a specific compatibility. When in doubt, administer two separate injections.

▶ Some medications are compatible for only a brief time after being combined and should be administered within 10 minutes after mixing. After this time, environmental factors, such as temperature, exposure to light, and humidity, may alter compatibility.

▶ *To reduce the risk of contamination,* most facilities dispense parenteral medications in single-dose vials. Insulin is one of the few drugs still packaged in multidose vials. Be careful when mixing regular and long-acting insulin. Draw up the regular insulin first *to avoid contamination by the long-acting suspension.* (If a minute amount of the regular insulin is accidentally mixed with the long-acting insulin, it won't appreciably change the effect of the long-acting insulin.) Check your facility's policy before mixing insulins.

▶ When you combine a cartridge-injection system and a multidose vial, use a separate needle and syringe to inject air into the multidose vial. *This prevents contamination of the multidose vial by the cartridge-injection system.*

Documentation
Record the drugs administered, injection site, and time of administration. Document adverse drug effects or other pertinent information.

Airborne Precautions

Airborne precautions, used in addition to standard precautions, prevent the spread of infectious diseases transmitted by airborne pathogens that are breathed, sneezed, or coughed into the environment. (See *Diseases requiring airborne precautions,* page 4.) This precaution category includes the former categories of acid-fast bacillus isolation and respiratory isolation.

Effective airborne precautions require a negative-pressure room with the door kept closed to maintain the proper air pressure balance between the isolation room and the adjoining hallway or corridor. An anteroom is preferred. The negative air pressure must be monitored, and the air is either vented directly to the outside of the building or filtered through high-efficiency particulate air (HEPA) filtration before recirculation.

Respiratory protection must be worn by all persons who enter the room. Such protection is provided by a disposable respirator (such as an N95 respirator or HEPA respirator) or a reusable respirator (such as a HEPA respirator or a powered air-purifying respirator [PAPR]). Regardless of the type of respirator used, the health care worker must ensure proper fit to the face each time she wears the respirator. If the patient must leave the room for an essential procedure, he should wear

Diseases requiring airborne precautions

Disease	Precautionary period
Chickenpox (varicella)	Until lesions are crusted and no new lesions appear
Herpes zoster (disseminated)	Duration of illness
Herpes zoster (localized in immunocompromised patient)	Duration of illness
Measles (rubeola)	Duration of illness
Tuberculosis (pulmonary or laryngeal, confirmed or suspected)	Depends upon clinical response; patient must be on effective therapy, be improving clinically (decreased cough and fever and improved findings on chest radiograph), and have three consecutive negative sputum smears collected on different days, or tuberculosis must be ruled out

a surgical mask to cover his nose and mouth while out of the room.

Key nursing diagnoses and patient outcomes
Risk for infection related to external factors
The patient will:
► maintain a normal body temperature
► state factors that put him at risk for infection
► identify signs and symptoms of infection.

Equipment
Respirators (either disposable N95 or HEPA respirators or reusable HEPA respirators or PAPRs) • surgical masks • isolation door card • other personal protective equipment as needed for standard precautions

Gather any additional supplies for patient care, such as a thermometer, stethoscope, and blood pressure cuff.

Preparation of equipment
Keep all airborne precaution supplies outside the patient's room in a cart or anteroom.

Implementation
► Situate the patient in a negative-pressure room with the door closed. If possible, the room should have an anteroom. The negative pressure should be monitored. If necessary, two patients with the same infection may share a room. Explain isolation precautions to the patient and the patient's family.
► Keep the patient's door (and the anteroom door) closed at all times *to maintain the negative pressure and contain the airborne pathogens.* Put the airborne precautions sign on the door to notify anyone entering the room.
► Pick up your respirator and put it on according to the manufacturer's directions. Adjust the straps for a firm but comfortable fit. Check the fit. (See *Respirator seal check.*)

▶ Instruct the patient to cover his nose and mouth with a facial tissue while coughing or sneezing.

▶ Tape an impervious bag to the patient's bedside *so the patient can dispose of facial tissues correctly.*

▶ Make sure that all visitors wear respiratory protection while in the patient's room.

▶ Limit the patient's movement from the room. If he must leave the room for essential procedures, make sure he wears a surgical mask over his nose and mouth. Notify the receiving department or area of the patient's isolation precautions *so that the precautions will be maintained and the patient can be returned to the room promptly.*

Special considerations

▶ Before leaving the room, remove gloves (if worn) and wash your hands. Remove your respirator outside the patient's room after closing the door.

▶ Depending on the type of respirator and recommendations from the manufacturer, follow your facility's policy and either discard your respirator or store it until the next use. If your respirator is to be stored until the next use, store it in a dry, well-ventilated place (not a plastic bag) to prevent microbial growth. Nondisposable respirators must be cleaned according to the manufacturer's recommendations.

Documentation

Record the need for airborne precautions on the nursing plan of care and as otherwise indicated by your facility. Document initiation and maintenance of the precautions, the patient's tolerance of the procedure, and any patient or family teaching. Also document

Respirator seal check

Before using a respirator, always check the respirator seal. To do this, place both of your hands over the respirator and exhale. If air leaks around your nose, adjust the nosepiece. If air leaks at the respirator's edges, adjust the straps along the side of your head. Recheck respirator fit after this adjustment.

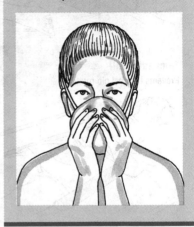

the date airborne precautions were discontinued.

ALIGNMENT AND PRESSURE-REDUCING DEVICE APPLICATION

Various assistive devices can be used to maintain correct body positioning and to help prevent complications that commonly arise when a patient must be on prolonged bed rest. These devices include cradle boots to protect the heels and help prevent skin breakdown, footdrop, and external hip rotation; abduction pillows to help prevent

Common preventive devices

Cradle boot
Prevents footdrop, skin breakdown, and external hip rotation

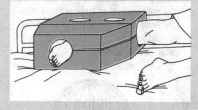

Abduction pillow
Prevents internal hip rotation

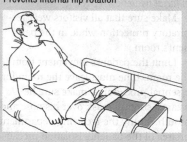

Trochanter roll
Prevents external hip rotation

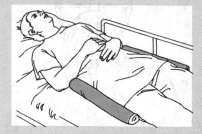

Hand roll
Prevents hand contractures

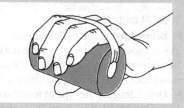

internal hip rotation after femoral fracture, hip fracture, or surgery; trochanter rolls to help prevent external hip rotation; and hand rolls to help prevent hand contractures.

Several of these devices — cradle boots, trochanter rolls, and hand rolls — are especially useful when caring for patients who have a loss of sensation, mobility, or consciousness.

Key nursing diagnoses and patient outcomes
Impaired physical mobility related to prolonged bed rest
The patient will:

▶ maintain muscle strength and joint range of motion
▶ show no evidence of complications, such as contractures, venous stasis, thrombus formation, or skin breakdown.

Risk for impaired skin integrity related to prolonged bed rest
The patient will:
▶ experience no skin breakdown
▶ maintain muscle strength and joint range of motion
▶ maintain adequate skin circulation.

Equipment

Cradle boots or substitute • abduction pillow • trochanter rolls • hand rolls (see *Common preventive devices*)

Cradle boots are made of sponge rubber and have space cut out to enclose the ankle and foot. Other commercial boots are available, but not all help to prevent external hip rotation. Footboards with antirotation blocks help prevent footdrop and external hip rotation but don't prevent heel pressure. High-topped sneakers may be used to help prevent footdrop, but they don't prevent external hip rotation or heel pressure.

The abduction pillow is a wedge-shaped piece of sponge rubber with lateral indentations for the patient's thighs. Its straps wrap around the thighs to maintain correct positioning. Although a properly shaped bed pillow may temporarily substitute for the commercial abduction pillow, it's difficult to apply and fails to maintain the correct lateral alignment.

The commercial trochanter roll is made of sponge rubber, but you can also improvise one from a rolled blanket or towel. The hand roll, available in hard and soft materials, is held in place by fixed or adjustable straps. It can be improvised from a rolled washcloth secured with roller gauze and adhesive tape.

Preparation of equipment

If you're using a device that is available in different sizes, select the appropriate size for the patient.

Implementation

► Explain the purpose and steps of the procedure to the patient.

Applying a cradle boot

► Open the slit on the superior surface of the boot. Then place the patient's heel in the circular cutout area. If the patient is positioned laterally, you may apply the boot only to the bottom foot and support the flexed top foot with a pillow.
► If appropriate, insert the other heel in the second boot.
► Position the patient's legs properly *to prevent strain on hip ligaments and pressure on bony prominences.*

Applying an abduction pillow

► Place the pillow between the supine patient's legs. Slide it toward the groin so that it touches the legs all along their lengths.
► Place the upper part of both legs in the pillow's lateral indentations and secure the straps *to prevent the pillow from slipping.*

Applying a trochanter roll

► Position one roll along the outside of the thigh, from the iliac crest to mid-thigh. Then place another roll along the other thigh. Make sure neither roll extends as far as the knee *to avoid peroneal nerve compression and palsy, which can lead to footdrop.*
► If you've fashioned trochanter rolls from a towel, leave several inches unrolled and tuck this under the patient's thigh *to hold the device in place and maintain the patient's position.*

Applying a hand roll

► Place one roll in the patient's hand to maintain the neutral position. Then secure the strap, if present, or apply roller gauze and secure with hypoallergenic or adhesive tape.
► Place another roll in the other hand.

Special considerations

Remember that the use of assistive devices doesn't preclude regularly scheduled patient positioning, range-of-motion exercises, and skin care.

Home care

Explain the use of appropriate devices to the patient and caregiver. Demonstrate how to use each device, emphasizing proper alignment of extremities, and have the patient or caregiver give a return demonstration so you can check for proper technique. Emphasize measures needed to prevent pressure ulcers.

Complications

Contractures and pressure ulcers may occur with the use of a hand roll and possibly with other assistive devices. To avoid these problems, remove a soft hand roll every 4 hours (every 2 hours if the patient has hand spasticity); remove a hard hand roll every 2 hours.

Documentation

Record the use of these devices in the patient's chart and the nursing plan of care, and indicate assessment for complications. Reevaluate your patient care goals as needed.

AMBULATION, PROGRESSIVE

After surgery or a period of bed rest, patients must begin the gradual return to full ambulation. When it's begun promptly and properly, this process — called progressive ambulation — thwarts many of the complications of prolonged inactivity.

Complications prevented by early progressive ambulation include respiratory stasis and hypostatic pneumonia; circulatory stasis, thrombophlebitis, and emboli; urine retention, urinary tract infection, urinary stasis, and calculus formation; abdominal distention, constipation, and decreased appetite; and sensory deprivation. Progressive ambulation also helps restore the patient's sense of equilibrium and enhances his self-confidence and self-image.

Progressive ambulation begins with dangling the patient's feet over the edge of the bed and progresses to seating him in an armchair or a wheelchair, walking around the room with him, and then walking with him in the halls until he can walk by himself. The patient's progress depends on his physical condition and his tolerance. Successful return to full ambulation requires correct body mechanics, careful patient observation, and open communication between patient, doctor, and nurse.

Key nursing diagnoses and patient outcomes

Impaired physical mobility related to prolonged bed rest
The patient will:
▶ display increased mobility
▶ show no complications of immobility, such as contractures, venous stasis, thrombus formation, or skin breakdown.

Risk for injury related to motor deficits
The patient will:
▶ identify factors that increase the potential for injury
▶ assist in identifying and applying safety measures to prevent injury.

Helping the patient regain mobility

Dangling legs
To help the patient support himself in a dangling position, move an overbed table in front of him and place a pillow on it.

Sitting
Seat the patient in a chair with armrests and a straight back, with his lower back against the rear of the chair, feet flat on the floor, hips and knees at right angles, and upper body straight. Rest his forearms on the armrests.

Walking
Provide a path unimpeded by equipment and other objects and avoid overexertion. If necessary, hold the patient so you can control his upper and lower body and any lateral movements.

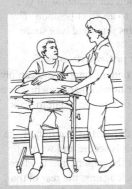

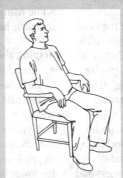

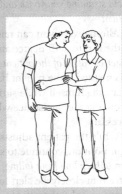

Equipment
Robe • chair or wheelchair • slippers for sitting, hard-soled shoes for walking • assistive device (such as a cane, crutches, or a walker), if necessary

Implementation
▶ If the patient requires an assistive device, the physical therapist usually selects the appropriate one and teaches its use.
▶ Check the patient's history, diagnosis, and therapeutic regimen. Ask him whether he's in pain or weak; if necessary, give an analgesic and wait 30 to 60 minutes for it to take effect before trying ambulation. Remember that a medicated patient may develop hypotension, dizziness, or drowsiness.
▶ Explain the goal of ambulation. (See *Helping the patient regain mobility.*) Provide encouragement *because he may be hesitant or fearful;* reassure him that he need not attempt more than he can reasonably do. If he fears pain from an incision, show him how to support the incision by placing a hand beside or gently over the dressing site or splint the incision for him.
▶ Remove equipment or other objects *to provide a clear path and prevent falls.*
▶ Lock the wheels on the bed or chair, if appropriate.

Dangling the patient's legs

▶ Position the bed horizontally and the patient laterally, facing you. Move his legs over the side of the bed and grasp his shoulders, standing with your feet apart *so you have a wide base of support.* Ask him to help by pushing up from the bed with his arms. Then shift your weight from the foot closest to his head to the other foot as you steadily raise him to the sitting position. Pull with your whole body, not just your arms, *to avoid straining your back and jostling the patient.*

Alternatively, you can raise the head of the bed to a 45-degree angle *to allow easier elevation of the patient.* Don't use this method if the patient has trouble balancing himself while sitting. Ask a coworker for assistance whenever necessary.

▶ While the patient adjusts to an upright position, continue to stand facing him *to keep him from falling,* and observe him closely. Be alert for signs and symptoms of orthostatic hypotension, such as fainting, dizziness, and complaints of blurred vision. If desired, check the patient's pulse rate and blood pressure. If the pulse rate increases more than 20 beats/minute, allow the patient to rest before progressing slowly.

Helping the patient stand

▶ After the patient can dangle his legs and support his weight on them, have him attempt the standing position. Help the patient put on a robe and slippers or shoes. Don't allow a robe, a drainage tube, or anything else to dangle around the patient's feet.

▶ If the patient is alert and fairly strong, place his feet flat on the floor and allow him to stand by himself. As he stands, place one hand under his axilla and the other hand around his waist *to prevent falls.* Help him stand fully erect. Encourage him to look forward and not at the floor *to help maintain his balance.*

▶ If the patient needs help standing up, face him and position your knees at either side of his. Bend your knees, put your arms around his waist, and instruct him to push up from the bed with his arms. Then straighten your knees and pull the patient with you while rising to an erect position. *This technique helps you avoid back strain.*

Helping the patient sit or walk

▶ After the patient stands, you can pivot and lower him into an armchair or a wheelchair, or you can begin to walk with him.

▶ If you've decided to seat him, make sure the chair is secure and won't slip as you lower the patient into it. Place his lower back against the rear of the chair and his feet flat on the floor. Position his hips and knees at right angles and keep his upper body straight. Then flex his elbows and place his forearms on the arms of the chair.

▶ If the patient can walk safely only with your assistance, stand behind him, placing one hand under his axilla and the other hand around his waist. If the patient has weakness or paralysis on one side, stand on the affected side and stabilize him by putting one arm around his waist.

▶ If necessary, ask a coworker to help you. Stand on opposite sides of the patient and place one hand under his arm or on his elbow.

▶ Give the patient verbal and tactile cues *to encourage him.* Stay close to a railed wall or another supportive structure and, if necessary, allow the patient to rest in a chair before attempting to walk back to his room. If he can't walk back, tell him to remain seated while you summon assistance or obtain a wheelchair. Don't leave the patient unattended if you have any reason to think he may fall. If you can't find a chair nearby, have the patient lean against the wall and call for assistance as you help support him. If necessary, steady him as he slides down the wall to sit on the floor.

Special considerations
▶ Patients on medications such as beta-adrenergic blockers and vasodilators may be subject to episodes of bradycardia and hypotension.
▶ If early ambulation is impossible, encourage bed exercises. Don't let the use of catheters and infusion bottles discourage ambulation; secure these devices so they're easily portable and check dressings and tubes carefully afterward *for proper position and changes in drainage.* If appropriate, measure pulse, respiratory rate, and blood pressure. When leaving the patient sitting up in a chair, make certain he has a call button or signal device. Restrain a confused patient.
▶ If the patient begins to fall, try to break his fall by easing him to the bed, chair, or floor, making sure he doesn't strike his head. Then summon help. Don't leave the patient alone — he needs your comfort and reassurance.
▶ If the patient experiences dyspnea, diaphoresis, or orthostatic hypotension, stabilize his position and take vital signs. Place him in semi-Fowler's position *to facilitate breathing.* If his condition doesn't improve rapidly, notify the doctor.

Documentation
Record the type of transfer and assistance needed; the duration of sitting, standing, or walking; the distance walked, if appropriate; the patient's response to ambulation; and any significant changes in blood pressure, pulse, and respiration.

AMNIOCENTESIS

A needle aspiration of amniotic fluid for laboratory analysis, amniocentesis is usually performed between 14 and 20 weeks' gestation. This procedure can detect neural tube and chromosomal defects as well as certain metabolic and other disorders. The procedure also can identify the sex of the fetus and assist in assessing fetal health. When performed in the final trimester, amniocentesis helps to evaluate fetal lung maturity and detect Rh hemolytic disease.

Indications for amniocentesis include maternal age over 35 (associated with Down syndrome), a family history of neural tube or chromosomal defects, or inborn errors of metabolism. Another test, chorionic villi sampling, may also detect fetal disorders. (See *Understanding chorionic villi sampling,* page 12.) Either procedure may be performed in a labor and delivery suite, in the ultrasound department, or in a doctor's office.

Contraindications for amniocentesis include an anterior uterine wall completely covered by the placenta and insufficient amniotic fluid. If the mother is infected with the human immunodeficiency virus, the risks of this procedure must be weighed against its expected benefits.

Understanding chorionic villi sampling

Laboratory analysis of chorionic villi samples can detect genetic, metabolic, and blood disorders — such as Down syndrome, Duchenne's muscular dystrophy, sickle cell anemia, alpha (and some beta) thalassemia, and phenylketonuria. Performed at 10 to 12 weeks' gestation, the procedure can yield results in just a few days.

To obtain the tissue samples, the doctor typically uses ultrasound or endoscopic imaging to guide a plastic catheter through the cervical canal into the uterus (as shown). He aspirates a small portion of chorionic tissue from the fetus, taking care not to contaminate the sample with maternal tissue.

Before the test, make sure that the patient has given her written consent, provide emotional support, and answer any questions.

Arrange for ordered blood studies. Instruct the patient to drink 1 qt (1 L) of water 30 minutes before the test *because a full bladder allows a better view of the uterus.* Also, Rh-negative women should receive RhoGAM beforehand to reduce the risk of isoimmunization.

Assess vital signs before, during, and after the procedure. Watch for vaginal bleeding.

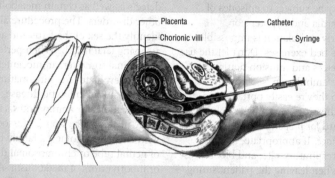

Placenta — Chorionic villi — Catheter — Syringe

Key nursing diagnoses and patient outcomes

Anxiety related to amniocentesis
The patient will:
▶ express feelings of anxiety
▶ make use of available emotional support.

Deficient knowledge related to amniocentesis
The patient will:
▶ learn why the procedure is necessary and how it's performed

▶ recognize that increased knowledge will help her cope with the procedure.

Equipment
Hospital gown • two sets of sterile gloves, sterile gowns, and masks • stethoscope • Ultrasound stethoscope and other appropriate ultrasound equipment • fetoscope or electronic fetal monitor • antiseptic solution with sterile container • local anesthetic • alcohol • 10-ml syringe • sterile 20G or 22G 4" spinal needle with stylet • 22G or 25G needle • sterile 20-ml glass sy-

ringe • clean amber glass specimen container for Rh sensitization and lecithin-sphingomyelin (L/S) ratio tests • three sterile, glass specimen tubes (for genetic tests) • laboratory request forms • adhesive bandage • optional: towel

Preassembled amniocentesis trays are available.

Preparation of equipment

If you don't have an amber specimen container, cover the outside of a clean test tube or glass container with adhesive tape or aluminum foil. Protecting aspirated amniotic fluid from light prevents the breakdown of such pigments as bilirubin. Properly label all specimen containers or tubes.

Implementation

▶ Reinforce the doctor's explanation of the procedure. Confirm that she understands the risk of complications. Emphasize that the doctor may need to repeat the procedure and that amniotic fluid analysis can't detect all birth defects.
▶ Make sure that the doctor has obtained the patient's signed informed consent form.
▶ *To reduce the risk of bladder puncture,* ensure that the patient voids before the procedure if the pregnancy exceeds 20 weeks (before 20 weeks, a full bladder may help to hold the uterus steady).
▶ Provide privacy and instruct the patient to put on a hospital gown. Assist her to a supine position.
▶ If the patient is in her third trimester, place a rolled towel under her right hip. Obtain baseline maternal vital signs.

▶ Next, determine the baseline fetal heart rate (FHR) with the ultrasound stethoscope or the fetoscope.
▶ Instruct the patient to fold her hands on her chest or rest her hands behind her head. Tell her to remain still.
▶ The doctor will use ultrasonography to locate the fetus and placenta. After he identifies an amniotic fluid pocket, he can determine the appropriate needle-insertion depth. Next, he'll put on the sterile gown, sterile gloves, and mask and clean the skin with an antiseptic solution.
▶ If the patient is receiving a local anesthetic, clean the diaphragm of the multidose vial of anesthetic solution with alcohol. Provide a 10-ml syringe and a 22G or 25G needle. Then invert the bottle *to allow the doctor to withdraw the anesthetic.*
▶ Scrub your hands and put on a sterile gown, sterile gloves, and mask *to assist the doctor with amniocentesis, a sterile procedure.*
▶ After the anesthetic takes effect, the doctor, guided by ultrasonographic imaging, will advance the 20G needle with a stylet through the abdomen and uterine wall into the amniotic sac. Then he'll remove the stylet. When a drop of amniotic fluid appears, he'll attach the 20-ml glass syringe to the needle and aspirate the fluid.
▶ If the patient is having genetic studies, open the sterile glass specimen tubes. After the doctor transfers amniotic fluid to the tubes, use aseptic technique when closing the tubes *to avoid contamination, which can yield aberrant test results.*
▶ If the patient is having Rh sensitization or L/S ratio tests, open the amber or covered specimen container so the doctor can transfer the amniotic fluid.

Close the container at once *to protect the fluid from light, which may cause pigments in the fluid, such as bilirubin, to break down and skew test results.*

▶ When the doctor withdraws the needle, place an adhesive bandage over the insertion site.

▶ Complete the laboratory request forms and send the specimens to the laboratory immediately. *Speedy transport is important because if the amniotic fluid contains blood or meconium, immediate centrifugation can preserve the specimen for analysis.*

▶ If the patient is in the final trimester of pregnancy, direct her to lie on her side *to avoid hypotension from pressure of the gravid uterus on the inferior vena cava.*

▶ Assess maternal vital signs and FHR every 15 minutes for 30 minutes *to detect changes from the baseline values.* FHR changes, such as tachycardia and bradycardia, signal distress. If these signs appear, notify the doctor, and continue to monitor FHR.

▶ Electronically monitor the patient for uterine irritability and the fetus for changes in heart rate pattern. Monitoring should continue for a few hours after the procedure *to allow early intervention if complications occur.* Normally, maternal vital signs should remain stable.

▶ Instruct the patient to report signs and symptoms of complications: a vaginal discharge (fluid or blood), decreased fetal movement, contractions, or fever and chills.

▶ Help the patient dress in preparation for discharge.

Special considerations

▶ Monitor the patient for signs and symptoms of supine hypotension, such as light-headedness, nausea, and diaphoresis.

▶ If the patient will receive a dose of RhoGAM, explain that this passive immunizing agent may help prevent an Rh incompatibility between her and the fetus that would cause antibody formation in her blood. This condition is known as erythroblastosis fetalis (hydrops fetalis or hemolytic disease of the newborn).

▶ Inform the patient, her family, and her support person, as appropriate, that test results should be available in 2 to 4 weeks. Provide emotional support as needed.

Complications

Although amniocentesis is an invasive procedure, it rarely produces maternal or fetal complications. Maternal complications, which affect fewer than 1% of patients, include amniotic fluid embolism, hemorrhage, infection, premature labor, abruptio placentae, placenta or umbilical cord trauma, bladder or intestinal puncture, and Rh isoimmunization. Rare fetal complications include intrauterine fetal death, amnionitis, injury from needle puncture, amniotic fluid leakage, bleeding, spontaneous abortion, and premature birth.

Documentation

Record the doctor's name and the date and time of the procedure. Document baseline maternal vital signs and FHR, and note any changes in baseline data. List the ordered laboratory tests. Note the amount and appearance of the specimen and when it was transported to the laboratory. Note leaking from the insertion site or uterine irritability. Document discharge instructions to the patient and how she tolerated the procedure.

AMNIOTOMY

In amniotomy, the doctor or nurse-midwife uses a sterile amnio-hook to rupture the amniotic membranes. This controversial but common procedure prompts amniotic fluid drainage, which enhances the intensity, frequency, and duration of uterine contractions by reducing uterine volume.

Amniotomy is performed to induce or augment labor when the membranes fail to rupture spontaneously. It helps to expedite labor after dilation begins, and it facilitates insertion of an intrauterine catheter and a spiral electrode for direct fetal monitoring.

Oxytocin infusion may precede amniotomy or follow it by 6 to 8 hours if labor fails to progress. If birth doesn't occur within 24 hours after amniotomy, the doctor may decide to perform a cesarean birth to reduce the risk of infection.

When deciding whether to perform amniotomy, the doctor or nurse-midwife considers such factors as fetal presentation, position, and station; the degree of cervical dilation and effacement; contraction frequency and intensity; the fetus's gestational age; existing complications; and maternal and fetal vital signs.

Amniotomy is contraindicated in high-risk pregnancies, unless more accurate fetal assessment using internal fetal monitoring is necessary. It's also contraindicated when the presenting fetal part is unengaged because of the risk of transverse lie and umbilical cord prolapse.

Key nursing diagnoses and patient outcomes

Risk for fetal injury related to external factors
The patient will:
▶ experience no fetal injury as evidenced by positive fetal heart rate patterns and no prolonged variable decelerations.

Anxiety related to amniotomy
The patient will:
▶ state feelings of anxiety
▶ cope with the procedure without experiencing severe signs and symptoms of anxiety.

Equipment

Povidone-iodine solution • linen-saver pads • soap and water • 4″ × 4″ gauze pads • external electronic fetal monitoring equipment or a fetoscope or ultrasound stethoscope • sterile gloves • sterile amnio-hook

Preparation of equipment

Assemble the equipment at the patient's bedside.

Implementation

▶ Reinforce the doctor or nurse-midwife's explanation of the procedure and answer the patient's questions. Wash your hands and put on sterile gloves.
▶ Clean the perineum with soap and water or 4″ × 4″ gauze pads moistened with povidone-iodine solution.
▶ Place linen-saver pads under the patient and then permit the amniotic fluid to drain on the linen-saver pads. Position the patient with her head elevated about 25 degrees *to tilt the pelvis for easier vaginal access.*
▶ Note the baseline fetal heart rate (FHR) *to evaluate fetal status before and*

Understanding amnioinfusion

Amnioinfusion is the intrapartum administration of warmed saline solution into the uterus via a hollow intrauterine pressure catheter. This procedure increases the fluid around the fetus and cushions the umbilical cord.

Amnioinfusion is used to relieve severe or prolonged variable decelerations caused by umbilical cord compression, particularly in patients with oligohydramnios or premature rupture of membranes. It's also used to dilute and lavage meconium from the uterus and, occasionally, to administer antibiotics.

Assembling the equipment
- Gather the following items:
  - 1,000 ml of normal saline solution, prewarmed to 98.6° F (37° C)
  - intrauterine pressure catheter
  - infusion pump
  - tubing.

Administering the infusion
- Attach the infusion tubing to an infusion pump.
- Help the doctor insert the intrauterine catheter.
- Next, attach the tubing to the catheter.
- As ordered, administer a loading volume — usually 10 ml/minute (600 ml/hour) for 1 hour. Continue to administer the infusion at the ordered rate — usually 60 to 120 ml/hour.

Nursing considerations
- Be aware that the duration of the infusion and the total amount of saline solution infused will depend on the patient's condition and the nature of her problem.
- Make sure that continuous fetal and maternal monitoring are maintained.
- Measure and record intrauterine pressures every 15 to 30 minutes.
- Measure the amount of fluid leaking from the vagina to help prevent polyhydramnios.
- Change the patient's underpads frequently because of constant fluid leakage.
- If variable decelerations persist, notify the doctor immediately.

Minimizing complications
Possible complications of amnioinfusion include uterine overdistension and increased uterine resting tone. Releasing some of the fluid can help relieve these problems.

after amniotomy. Use external fetal monitoring throughout the procedure. Otherwise, use the fetoscope or ultrasound stethoscope before and after the procedure.

▶ Using aseptic technique, open the amnio-hook package. Then, wearing sterile gloves, the doctor or nurse-

midwife removes the amnio-hook from the package.

▶ If ordered, apply pressure to the uterine fundus as the doctor or nurse-midwife inserts the amnio-hook vaginally to the cervical os. *This helps to keep the fetal presenting part engaged and reduces the risk of cord prolapse.* Then, carefully avoiding contact with the fetal presenting part, the doctor or nurse-midwife ruptures the amniotic membrane at the internal os.

▶ Without external electronic fetal monitoring equipment, use a fetoscope or ultrasound stethoscope to evaluate FHR for at least 60 seconds after the membrane ruptures *to detect bradycardia*. Otherwise, check the monitor tracing for large, variable decelerations in FHR that suggest cord compression. If these FHR changes occur, the doctor or nurse-midwife will perform a vaginal examination *to check for cord prolapse*. (See *Understanding amnioinfusion*.)

▶ Clean and dry the perineal area. When necessary, replace the linen-saver pad under the patient's buttocks *to promote comfort and hygiene*.

▶ Inspect the amniotic fluid for meconium, blood, or foul odor. Note the color and measure the amount of fluid.

▶ Take the patient's temperature every 2 hours *to detect infection*. If her temperature rises to 100° F (37.8° C), begin hourly checks. Continue to monitor uterine contractions and labor progress.

Special considerations

During a vaginal examination after amniotomy, maintain strict aseptic technique *to prevent uterine infection*. For the same reason, minimize the number of examinations.

Complications

Umbilical cord prolapse — a life-threatening potential complication of amniotomy — is an emergency requiring immediate cesarean birth to prevent fetal death. It occurs when amniotic fluid, gushing from the ruptured sac, sweeps the cord down through the cervix. The risk of prolapse is higher if the fetal head isn't engaged in the pelvis before the rupture occurs. Intrauterine infection can result from failure to use aseptic technique for amniotomy or from prolonged labor after amniotomy.

Documentation

Record FHR before, and at frequent intervals immediately after, amniotomy (every 5 minutes for 20 minutes and then every 30 minutes). Note any meconium or blood in the amniotic fluid. Measure the amount of fluid and note whether the fluid has an odor. Record maternal temperature every 2 hours and labor progress as appropriate.

ANTIEMBOLISM STOCKING APPLICATION

Elastic antiembolism stockings help prevent deep vein thrombosis (DVT) and pulmonary embolism by compressing superficial leg veins. This compression increases venous return by forcing blood into the deep venous system rather than allowing it to pool in the legs and form clots.

Antiembolism stockings can provide equal pressure over the entire leg or a graded pressure that is greatest at the ankle and decreases over the length of the leg. Usually indicated for postoperative, bedridden, elderly, or other patients at risk for DVT, these stockings shouldn't be used on patients with dermatoses or open skin lesions, gangrene, severe arteriosclerosis or other ischemic vascular diseases, pulmonary or any massive edema, recent vein ligation, or vascular or skin grafts. For patients with chronic venous problems, intermittent pneumatic compression stockings may be ordered during surgery and after surgery.

Key nursing diagnoses and patient outcomes

Impaired physical mobility related to (specify)
The patient will:
▶ show no evidence of complications, such as venous stasis and thrombus formation
▶ carry out a mobility regimen
▶ quickly achieve highest level of mobility to avoid complications.

Risk for peripheral neurovascular dysfunction related to immobility
The patient will:
▶ maintain circulation in the extremities
▶ demonstrate correct body-positioning techniques
▶ have no symptoms of neurovascular compromise.

Equipment

Tape measure • antiembolism stockings of correct size and length • talcum powder

Preparation of equipment

Before applying a knee-length stocking, measure the circumference of the patient's calf at its widest point and the leg length from the bottom of the heel to the back of the knee. (See *Measuring for antiembolism stockings.*)

Before applying a thigh-length stocking, measure the circumference of the calf and thigh at their widest points and the leg length from the bottom of the heel to the gluteal fold.

Before applying a waist-length stocking, measure the circumference of the calf and thigh at their widest points and the leg length from the bottom of the heel along the side to the waist.

Obtain the correct size stocking according to the manufacturer's specifications. If the patient's measurements are outside the range indicated by the manufacturer or if his legs are deformed or edematous, ask the doctor if he wants to order custom-made stockings.

Implementation

▶ Check the doctor's order, and assess the patient's condition. If his legs are cold or cyanotic, notify the doctor before proceeding.
▶ Explain the procedure to the patient, provide privacy, and wash your hands thoroughly.
▶ Have the patient lie down. Then dust his ankle with talcum powder *to ease application.*

Applying a knee-length stocking

▶ Insert your hand into the stocking from the top and grasp the heel pocket from the inside. Holding the heel, turn the stocking inside out so that the foot is inside the stocking leg. *This method allows easier application than gathering the entire stocking and working it up over the foot and ankle.*
▶ With the heel pocket down, hook the index and middle fingers of both your hands into the foot section. Facing the patient, ease the stocking over the toes, stretching it sideways as you move it up the foot.
▶ Support the patient's ankle with one hand and use the other hand to pull the heel pocket under the heel. Then center the heel in the pocket.
▶ Gather the loose portion of the stocking at the toe and pull only this section over the heel. Gather the loose material at the ankle and slide the rest of the stocking up over the heel with short pulls, alternating front and back.

Measuring for antiembolism stockings

Measure the patient carefully to ensure that his antiembolism stockings provide enough compression for adequate venous return.

To choose the correct knee-length stocking, measure the circumference of the calf at its widest point (top left) and the leg length from the bottom of the heel to the back of the knee (bottom left).

To choose a thigh-length stocking, measure the calf as for a knee-length stocking and the thigh at its widest point (top right). Then measure leg length from the bottom of the heel to the gluteal fold (bottom right).

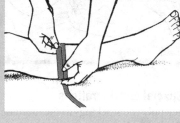
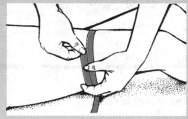
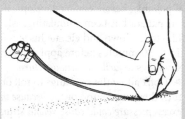
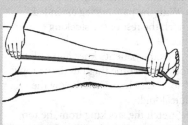

(See *Applying antiembolism stockings: Three key steps,* page 20.)
▶ Insert your index and middle fingers into the gathered stocking at the ankle and ease the fabric up the leg to the knee.
▶ Supporting the patient's ankle with one hand, use your other hand to stretch the stocking toward the knee, front and back, *to distribute the material evenly.* The stocking top should be 1″ to 2″ (2.5 to 5 cm) below the bottom of the patella.

▶ Gently snap the fabric around the ankle *to ensure a tight fit and eliminate gaps that could reduce pressure.*
▶ Adjust the foot section for fabric smoothness and toe comfort by tugging on the toe section. Properly position the toe window, if any.
▶ Repeat the procedure for the second stocking, if ordered.

Applying a thigh-length stocking
▶ Follow the procedure for applying a knee-length stocking, taking care to

Applying antiembolism stockings: Three key steps

Gather the loose part of the stocking at the toes and pull this portion toward the heel.

Then gather the loose part of the stocking and bring it over the heel with short, alternating front and back pulls.

Insert the index and middle fingers into the gathered part of the stocking at the ankle and ease it upward by rocking it slightly up and down.

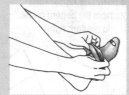 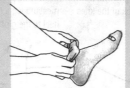 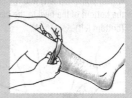

distribute the fabric evenly below the knee before continuing the procedure.

▶ With the patient's leg extended, stretch the rest of the stocking over the knee.

▶ Flex the patient's knee and pull the stocking over the thigh until the top is 1″ to 3″ (2.5 to 7.5 cm) below the gluteal fold.

▶ Stretch the stocking from the top, front and back, *to distribute the fabric evenly over the thigh.*

▶ Gently snap the fabric behind the knee *to eliminate gaps that could reduce pressure.*

Applying a waist-length stocking

▶ Follow the procedure for applying knee-length and thigh-length stockings and extend the stocking top to the gluteal fold.

▶ Fit the patient with the adjustable belt that accompanies the stockings. Make sure that the waistband and the fabric don't interfere with any incision, drainage tube, catheter, or other device.

Special considerations

▶ Apply the stockings in the morning, if possible, before edema develops. If the patient has been ambulating, ask him to lie down and elevate his legs for 15 to 30 minutes before applying the stockings *to facilitate venous return.*

▶ Don't allow the stockings to roll or turn down at the top or toe *because the excess pressure could cause venous strangulation.* Have the patient wear the stockings in bed and during ambulation *to provide continuous protection against thrombosis.*

▶ Check the patient's toes at least once every 4 hours—more often in the patient with a faint pulse or edema. Note skin color and temperature, sensation, swelling, and ability to move. If complications occur, remove the stockings and notify the doctor immediately.

▶ Be alert for an allergic reaction because some patients can't tolerate the sizing in new stockings. Laundering the stockings before applying them reduces the risk of an allergic reaction to sizing. Remove the stockings at least once daily *to bathe the skin and observe for irritation and breakdown.*

▶ Using warm water and mild soap, wash the stockings when soiled. Keep a second pair handy *for the patient to wear while the other pair is being laundered.*

Home care

If the patient will require antiembolism stockings after discharge, teach him or a family member how to apply them correctly and explain why he needs to wear them. Instruct the patient or family member to care for the stockings properly and to replace them when they lose elasticity.

Complications

Obstruction of arterial blood flow — characterized by cold and bluish toes, dusky toenail beds, decreased or absent pedal pulses, and leg pain or cramps — can result from application of antiembolism stockings. Less serious complications, such as an allergic reaction and skin irritation, can also occur.

Documentation

Record the date and time of stocking application and removal, stocking length and size, condition of the leg before and after treatment, condition of the toes during treatment, any complications, and the patient's tolerance of the treatment.

Apgar scoring

Named after its developer, Virginia Apgar, the Apgar score quantifies the neonatal heart rate, respiratory effort, muscle tone, reflexes, and color. Each category is assessed 1 minute after birth and again 5 minutes later. Scores in each category range from 0 to 2. The highest possible score is 10 — the greatest possible sum of the five categories.

The evaluation at 1 minute indicates the neonate's initial adaptation to extrauterine life. The evaluation at 5 minutes gives a clearer picture of overall status.

If the neonate doesn't breathe or his heart rate is less than 100 beats/minute immediately after delivery, call for help and begin resuscitation at once. Don't wait for a 1-minute Apgar test score.

Key nursing diagnoses and patient outcomes

Delayed growth and development related to (specify)

Family members will:

▶ express realistic expectations for the neonate's growth

▶ demonstrate an understanding of the neonate's needs.

Equipment

Apgar score sheet or neonatal assessment sheet • stethoscope • clock with second hand or Apgar timers • gloves (See *Recording the Apgar score,* page 22.)

Preparation of equipment

If you use Apgar timers, make sure both timers are on at the instant of birth.

Implementation

▶ Note the exact time of delivery. Wear gloves *for protection from blood and body fluids.* Dry the neonate *to prevent heat loss.*

▶ Place the neonate in a 15-degree Trendelenburg position *to promote mucus drainage.* Then position his head

Recording the Apgar score

Use this chart to record the neonatal Apgar score at 1 minute and 5 minutes after birth. For each category listed, assign a score of 0 to 2, as shown. A total score of 7 to 10 indicates good condition; 4 to 6, fair condition (the infant may have moderate central nervous system depression, muscle flaccidity, cyanosis, and poor respirations); 0 to 3, danger (the infant needs immediate resuscitation as ordered).

Sign	Apgar score		
	0	1	2
Heart rate	Absent	Less than 100 beats/minute (slow)	More than 100 beats/minute
Respiratory effort	Absent	Slow, irregular	Good crying
Muscle tone	Flaccid	Some flexion and resistance to extension of extremities	Active motion
Reflex irritability	No response	Grimace or weak cry	Vigorous cry
Color	Pallor, cyanosis	Pink body, blue extremities	Completely pink

with the nose slightly tilted upward *to straighten the airway.*

▶ Assess the neonate's respiratory efforts. If necessary, supply stimulation by rubbing his back or gently flicking his foot.

▶ If the neonate exhibits abnormal respiratory responses, begin neonatal resuscitation according to the guidelines of the American Heart Association and the American Academy of Pediatrics. Then use the Apgar score to judge the progress and success of resuscitation efforts. If resuscitation efforts prove futile, you'll need to implement measures for dealing with stillbirth. (See *Dealing with a stillbirth.*)

▶ If the neonate exhibits normal responses, assign the Apgar score at 1 minute after birth.

▶ Repeat the evaluation at 5 minutes after birth and record the score.

Assessing neonatal heart rate

▶ Using a stethoscope, listen to the heartbeat for 30 seconds and record the rate. To obtain beats per minute, double the rate. Alternatively, palpate the umbilical cord where it joins the abdomen, monitor pulsations for 6 seconds, and multiply by 10 to obtain beats per minute. Assign a 0 for no heart rate, a 1 for a rate under 100 beats/minute, and a 2 for a rate greater than 100 beats/minute.

Assessing respiratory effort

▶ Count unassisted respirations for 60 seconds, noting quality and regularity (a normal rate is 30 to 50 respirations/minute). Assign a 0 for no respirations; a 1 for slow, irregular, shallow, or gasping respirations; and a 2 for regular respirations and vigorous crying.

Assessing muscle tone

▶ Observe the extremities for flexion and resistance to extension. This can be done by extending the limbs and observing their rapid return to flexion—the neonate's normal state. Assign a 0 for flaccid muscle tone; a 1 for some flexion and resistance to extension; and a 2 for normal flexion of elbows, knees, and hips, with good resistance to extension.

Assessing reflex irritability

▶ Observe the neonate's response to nasal suctioning or to flicking the sole of his foot. Assign a 0 for no response, a 1 for a grimace or weak cry, and a 2 for a vigorous cry.

Assessing color

▶ Observe skin color, especially at the extremities. Assign a 0 for complete pallor and cyanosis, a 1 for a pink body with blue extremities (acrocyanosis), and a 2 for a completely pink body.
▶ To assess color in a dark-skinned neonate, inspect the oral mucous membranes and conjunctiva, the lips, the palms, and the soles.

Special considerations

▶ If the patient and her support person don't know about the Apgar score, discuss it with them during early labor, when they will be more receptive to new knowledge. *To prevent confusion or misunderstanding at delivery,* explain to them what will occur and why. Add that this is a routine procedure.
▶ If the neonate requires emergency care, make sure that a member of the delivery team offers appropriate support.
▶ Closely observe the neonate whose mother receives heavy sedation just be-

---

Dealing with a stillbirth

If a fetus that is mature enough to survive extrauterine life dies before or during delivery, the event is called a stillbirth and the fetus, a stillborn. Features of maturity include a gestational age of 16 weeks or more and a length of 6¼″ (15.9 cm) or more. Delivery of a less-mature fetus is called a spontaneous abortion.

Nursing interventions

In addition to measuring, weighing, identifying, and preparing the stillborn for the morgue, you'll need to provide emotional support to the parents. They'll need comfort and care whether or not they expected the stillbirth.

If the parents expected the stillbirth, help them continue working through their grief—especially if they've delayed grieving while waiting for delivery. If the parents didn't expect the stillbirth, help them express their anger and relieve their grief in positive ways. Refer them to appropriate support groups.

Offer bereaved parents the opportunity to hold the stillborn. If possible, provide a photograph, identification bracelet, or another memento. If they refuse these mementos, file them with the chart so that the parents can obtain them later if desired.

---

fore delivery. Even if he has a high Apgar score at birth, he may exhibit secondary effects of sedation in the nursery. Be alert for respiratory depression or unresponsiveness.

Documentation

Record the Apgar score on the Apgar score sheet or the neonatal assessment sheet required by your facility. Be sure to indicate the total score and the signs for which points were deducted *to guide postnatal care.*

APNEA MONITORING

By signalling when the breathing rate falls dangerously low, apnea monitors can save a neonate who is vulnerable to apnea. These monitors may be used for vulnerable neonates, such as those born prematurely; those who have survived a life-threatening medical emergency; and those with neurologic disorders, neonatal respiratory distress syndrome, bronchopulmonary dysplasia, congenital heart disease with heart failure, a tracheostomy, a history of sleep-induced apnea, a family history of sudden infant death syndrome, or acute drug withdrawal.

Two types of monitors are used most commonly. The thoracic impedance monitor uses chest electrodes to detect conduction changes caused by respirations. The newest models have alarm systems and memories that record cardiorespiratory patterns. The apnea mattress monitor, or underpad monitor, relies on a transducer connected to a pressure-sensitive pad, which detects pressure changes resulting from altered chest movements.

To guard against potentially life-threatening apneic episodes in vulnerable neonates, monitoring begins in the facility (or birthing center) and continues at home. Parents need to learn how to operate the monitor, what actions to take when the alarm sounds, and how to revive an infant with cardiopulmonary resuscitation (CPR). Crucial steps for correctly using a monitor include testing the alarm system, positioning the sensor properly, and setting the controls correctly. (See *Using a home apnea monitor.*)

Key nursing diagnoses and patient outcomes

Deficient parenting related to compromised neonatal health
The parents will:
▶ communicate feelings regarding the neonate's condition
▶ become involved in planning the neonate's care
▶ express feelings of having greater control over their situation.

Deficient knowledge related to apnea monitoring
Family members will:
▶ set realistic learning goals for developing competence in caring for the neonate
▶ express an understanding of apnea monitoring
▶ demonstrate an ability to use the apnea monitor correctly
▶ contact appropriate resources when necessary.

Equipment

Monitor unit • electrodes • leadwires • electrode belt • conduction gel, if needed • pressure transducer pad, if using apnea mattress • stable surface for monitor placement

Prepackaged and pretreated disposable electrodes are available.

Implementation

▶ Explain the procedure to the parents, as appropriate, and wash your hands.
▶ Plug the monitor's power cord into a grounded wall outlet. Attach the leadwires to the electrodes and attach the electrodes to the belt. If appropriate,

Using a home apnea monitor

If a neonate in your care will require the use of a home apnea monitor, you'll need to prepare his parents to operate the equipment safely, correctly, and confidently. First, review the neonate's breathing problem with his parents. Explain that the monitor will warn them of breathing or heart rate changes.

Then offer the following guidelines:

■ Advise the parents to prepare their home and family for the equipment, for instance, by providing a sturdy, flat surface for the monitor and by posting emergency telephone numbers (doctor, nurse, equipment supplier, and ambulance) accessibly.

■ Teach other responsible family members how to use the monitor safely. Suggest that older siblings, grandparents, babysitters, and other caregivers learn cardiopulmonary resuscitation (CPR).

■ Instruct the parents to notify local service authorities — police, ambulance service, telephone company, and electric company — if their neonate uses an apnea monitor *so that alternative power can be supplied if a failure occurs.*

■ Explain to the parents how a monitor with electrodes works. Advise them to make sure the respiration indicator goes on each time the neonate breathes. If it doesn't, describe troubleshooting techniques, such as moving the electrodes slightly. Tell them to try this technique several times.

■ Show the parents how to respond to either the apnea or bradycardia alarm. Direct them to check the color of the neonate's oral tissues. If the tissues appear bluish and the neonate isn't breathing, tell them to call loudly and touch him — gently at first, then more urgently as needed. Tell them to stop short of shaking him. If he doesn't respond, urge them to begin CPR.

■ Also advise the parents to keep the operator's manual attached to or beside the monitor and to consult it as needed. Explain that an activated loose-lead alarm, for example, may indicate a dirty electrode, a loose electrode patch, a loose belt, or a disconnected or malfunctioning wire or monitor.

---

apply conduction gel to the electrodes. (Or apply gel to the neonate's chest, place the electrodes on top of the gel, and attach the electrodes to the leadwires. Then secure the belt.)

▶ To hold the electrodes securely in position, wrap the belt snugly but not restrictively around the neonate's chest at the point of greatest movement — optimally at the right and left midaxillary line about ³⁄₄″ (2 cm) below the axilla. Be sure to position the leadwires according to the manufacturer's instructions.

▶ Follow the color code to connect the leadwires to the patient cable. Then connect the cable to the proper jack at the rear of the monitoring unit.

▶ Turn the sensitivity controls to maximum *to facilitate tuning when adjusting the system.*

▶ Set the alarms according to recommendations so that an apneic period lasting for a specified time activates the signal.

▶ Turn on the monitor. If the monitor has two alarms — one to signal apnea, one to signal bradycardia — both will sound until you adjust the monitor and reset the alarms according to the manufacturer's instructions.

▶ Adjust the sensitivity controls until the indicator lights blink with each breath and heartbeat.

▶ If you use an apnea mattress, assemble the monitor and pressure transducer pad according to the manufacturer's directions.

▶ Plug the monitor into a grounded wall outlet. Then plug the cable of the transducer pad into the monitor.

▶ Touch the pad to make sure it works. Watch for the monitor's respiration light to blink.

▶ Follow the manufacturer's instructions for pad placement.

▶ If you have difficulty obtaining a signal, place a foam rubber pad under the mattress and sandwich the transducer pad between the foam pad and the mattress.

▶ If you hear the apnea or bradycardia alarm during monitoring, immediately check the neonate's respirations and color but don't touch or disturb him until you confirm apnea.

▶ If he's still breathing and his color is good, readjust the sensitivity controls or reposition the electrodes, if necessary.

▶ If he isn't breathing, but his color looks normal, wait 10 seconds to see if he starts breathing spontaneously. If he isn't breathing and he appears pale, dusky, or blue, immediately try to stimulate breathing in these ways: Sequentially, place your hand on the neonate's back, rub him gently, or flick his soles gently. If he doesn't begin to breathe immediately, start CPR.

Special considerations

▶ *To ensure accurate operation,* don't put the monitor on top of any other electrical device. Make sure it's on a level surface and can't be bumped easily.

▶ Avoid applying lotions, oils, or powders to the neonate's chest, *where they could cause the electrode belt to slip.* Periodically check the alarm by disconnecting the sensor plug. Then listen for the alarm to sound after the preset time delay.

Complications

An apneic episode resulting from upper airway obstruction may not trigger the alarm if the neonate continues to make respiratory efforts without gas exchange. However, the monitor's bradycardia alarm may be triggered by the decreased heart rate resulting from the vagal stimulation (which accompanies obstruction).

If you're using a thoracic impedance monitor without a bradycardia alarm, you may interpret bradycardia during apnea as shallow breathing. That can happen because this type of monitor fails to distinguish between respiratory movement and the large cardiac stroke volume associated with bradycardia. In this case, the alarm won't sound until the heart rate drops below the apnea limit.

Documentation

Record all alarm incidents. Document the time and duration of apnea. Describe the neonate's color, the stimulation measures implemented, and any other pertinent information.

ARTERIAL PRESSURE MONITORING

Direct arterial pressure monitoring permits continuous measurement of systolic, diastolic, and mean pressures and allows arterial blood sampling. Because direct measurement reflects systemic vascular resistance as well as blood flow, it's generally more accurate than indirect methods (such as palpation and auscultation of Korotkoff's, or audible pulse, sounds), which are based on blood flow.

Direct monitoring is indicated when highly accurate or frequent blood pressure measurements are required — for example, in patients with low cardiac output and high systemic vascular resistance. Also, it may be used for patients who are receiving titrated doses of vasoactive drugs or who need frequent blood sampling.

Indirect monitoring, which carries few associated risks, is commonly performed by applying pressure to an artery (such as by inflating a blood pressure cuff around the arm) to decrease blood flow. As pressure is released, flow resumes and can be palpated or auscultated. Korotkoff's sounds presumably result from a combination of blood flow and arterial wall vibrations; with reduced flow, these vibrations may be less pronounced.

Key nursing diagnoses and patient outcomes

Decreased cardiac output related to reduced stroke volume as a result of (specify)
The patient will:
▶ maintain hemodynamic stability: pulse not less than (specify) and not greater than (specify); blood pressure not less than (specify) and not greater than (specify)
▶ have no complaints of chest pain
▶ have adequate cardiac output.

Risk for infection related to arterial line
The patient will:
▶ maintain a normal body temperature

▶ have no evidence of infection (redness, swelling, purulent drainage) at the insertion site
▶ have a normal white blood cell count and differential.

Equipment
For catheter insertion
Gloves • sterile gown • mask • protective eyewear • sterile gloves • 16G to 20G catheter (type and length depend on the insertion site, patient's size, and other anticipated uses of the line) • preassembled preparation kit (if available) • sterile drapes • sheet protector • prepared pressure transducer system • ordered local anesthetic • sutures • syringe and 21G to 25G 1″ needle • I.V. pole • tubing and medication labels • site care kit (containing sterile dressing and hypoallergenic tape) • arm board and soft wrist restraint (for a femoral site, an ankle restraint) • optional: shaving kit (for femoral artery insertion)

For blood sample collection
If an open system is in place: gloves • gown • mask • sterile 4″ × 4″ gauze pads • protective eyewear • sheet protector • 500-ml I.V. bag • 5- or 10-ml syringe for discard sample • syringes of appropriate size and number for ordered laboratory tests • laboratory request forms and labels • needleless device (depending on your facility's policy) • specimen tubes
If a closed system is in place: gloves • gown • mask • protective eyewear • syringes of appropriate size and number for ordered laboratory tests • laboratory request forms and labels • alcohol pad • blood transfer unit • specimen tubes

For arterial line tubing changes

Gloves • gown • mask • protective eyewear • sheet protector • preassembled arterial pressure tubing with flush device and disposable pressure transducer • sterile gloves • 500-ml bag of I.V. flush solution (such as dextrose 5% in water or normal saline solution) • 500 or 1,000 units of heparin • syringe and 21G to 25G 1" needle • alcohol pad • medication label • pressure bag • site care kit • tubing labels

For arterial catheter removal

Gloves • mask • gown • protective eyewear • two sterile 4" × 4" gauze pads • sheet protector • sterile suture removal set • dressing • hypoallergenic tape

For femoral line removal

Additional sterile 4" × 4" gauze pads • small sandbag (which you may wrap in a towel or place in a pillowcase) • adhesive bandage

For a catheter-tip culture

Sterile scissors • sterile container

Preparation of equipment

Before setting up and priming the monitoring system, wash your hands thoroughly. Maintain asepsis by wearing personal protective equipment throughout preparation. (For instructions on setting up and priming the monitoring system, see "Transducer system setup," page 854.)

When you've completed the equipment preparation, set the alarms on the bedside monitor according to your facility's policy.

Implementation

▶ Explain the procedure to the patient and his family, including the purpose of arterial pressure monitoring and the anticipated duration of catheter placement. Make sure the patient signs a consent form. If he's unable to sign, ask a responsible family member to give written consent.

▶ Check the patient's history for an allergy or a hypersensitivity to iodine or the ordered local anesthetic.

▶ Maintain asepsis by wearing personal protective equipment throughout all procedures described below.

▶ Position the patient for easy access to the catheter insertion site. Place a sheet protector under the site.

▶ If the catheter will be inserted into the radial artery, perform Allen's test *to assess collateral circulation in the hand.* (See "Arterial puncture for blood gas analysis," page 33.)

Inserting an arterial catheter

▶ Using a preassembled preparation kit, the doctor prepares and anesthetizes the insertion site. He covers the surrounding area with sterile drapes. The catheter is then inserted into the artery and attached to the fluid-filled pressure tubing.

▶ While the doctor holds the catheter in place, activate the fast-flush release *to flush blood from the catheter.* After each fast-flush operation, observe the drip chamber *to verify that the continuous flush rate is as desired.* A waveform should appear on the bedside monitor.

▶ The doctor may suture the catheter in place, or you may secure it with hypoallergenic tape. Cover the insertion site with a dressing as specified by facility policy.

▶ Immobilize the insertion site. With a radial or brachial site, use an arm board and soft wrist restraint (if the patient's condition so requires). With a femoral site, assess the need for an ankle restraint and maintain the patient on bed rest, with the head of the bed raised no more than 15 to 30 degrees, *to prevent the catheter from kinking.* Level the zeroing stopcock of the transducer with the phlebostatic axis. Then zero the system to atmospheric pressure.

▶ Activate monitor alarms as appropriate.

Obtaining a blood sample from an open system

▶ Assemble the equipment, taking care not to contaminate the dead-end cap, stopcock, and syringes. Turn off or temporarily silence the monitor alarms, depending on your facility's policy. (However, some facilities require that alarms be left on.)

▶ Locate the stopcock nearest the patient. Open a sterile 4″ × 4″ gauze pad. Remove the dead-end cap from the stopcock, and place it on the gauze pad.

▶ Insert the syringe for the discard sample into the stopcock. (This sample is discarded because it's diluted with flush solution.) Follow your facility's policy on how much discard blood to collect. In most cases, you'll withdraw 5 to 10 ml through a 5- or 10-ml syringe.

▶ Next, turn the stopcock off to the flush solution. Slowly retract the syringe to withdraw the discard sample. If you feel resistance, reposition the affected extremity and check the insertion site for obvious problems (such as catheter kinking). After correcting the problem, resume blood withdrawal. Then turn the stopcock halfway back to the open position to close the system in all directions.

▶ Remove the discard syringe, and dispose of the blood in the syringe, observing standard precautions.

▶ Place the syringe for the laboratory sample in the stopcock, turn the stopcock off to the flush solution, and slowly withdraw the required amount of blood. For each additional sample required, repeat this procedure. If the doctor has ordered coagulation tests, obtain blood for this sample from the final syringe *to prevent dilution from the flush device.*

▶ After you've obtained blood for the final sample, turn the stopcock off to the syringe and remove the syringe. Activate the fast-flush release *to clear the tubing.* Then turn off the stopcock to the patient and repeat the fast flush *to clear the stopcock port.*

▶ Turn the stopcock off to the stopcock port, and replace the dead-end cap. Reactivate the monitor alarms. Attach the needleless device to the filled syringes and transfer the blood samples to the appropriate specimen tubes, labeling them according to facility policy. Send all samples to the laboratory with appropriate documentation.

▶ Check the monitor for return of the arterial waveform and pressure reading. (See *Understanding the arterial waveform,* page 30.)

Obtaining a blood sample from a closed system

▶ Assemble the equipment, maintaining aseptic technique. Locate the closed-system reservoir and blood sampling site. Deactivate or temporarily silence monitor alarms. (However, some facilities require that alarms be left on.)

▶ Clean the sampling site with an alcohol pad.

Understanding the arterial waveform

Normal arterial blood pressure produces a characteristic waveform, representing ventricular systole and diastole. The waveform has five distinct components: the anacrotic limb, systolic peak, dicrotic limb, dicrotic notch, and end diastole.

The anacrotic limb marks the waveform's initial upstroke, which results as blood is rapidly ejected from the ventricle through the open aortic valve into the aorta. The rapid ejection causes a sharp rise in arterial pressure, which appears as the waveform's highest point. This is called the systolic peak.

As blood continues into the peripheral vessels, arterial pressure falls, and the waveform begins a downward trend. This part is called the dicrotic limb. Arterial pressure usually will continue to fall until pressure in the ventricle is less than pressure in the aortic root. When this occurs, the aortic valve closes. This event appears as a small notch (the dicrotic notch) on the waveform's downside. When the aortic valve closes, diastole begins, progressing until the aortic root pressure gradually descends to its lowest point. On the waveform, this is known as end diastole.

Normal arterial waveform

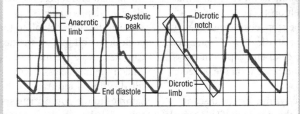

Holding the reservoir upright, grasp the flexures and slowly fill the reservoir with blood over 3 to 5 seconds (this blood serves as discard blood). If you feel resistance, reposition the affected extremity and check the catheter site for obvious problems (such as kinking). Then resume blood withdrawal.

Turn the one-way valve off to the reservoir by turning the handle perpendicular to the tubing. Using a syringe with attached cannula, insert the cannula into the sampling site. (Make sure the plunger is depressed to the bottom of the syringe barrel.) Slowly fill the syringe. Then grasp the cannula near the sampling site, and remove the syringe and cannula as one unit. Repeat the procedure as needed to fill the required number of syringes. If the doctor has ordered coagulation tests, obtain blood for those tests from the final syringe *to prevent dilution from the flush solution.*

After filling the syringes, turn the one-way valve to its original position, parallel to the tubing. Now smoothly and evenly push down on the plunger until the flexures lock in place in the fully closed position and all fluid has been reinfused. The fluid should be reinfused over a 3- to 5-second period. Then activate the fast-flush release to clear blood from the tubing and reservoir.

▶ Clean the sampling site with an alcohol pad. Reactivate the monitor alarms. Using the blood transfer unit, transfer blood samples to the appropriate specimen tubes, labeling them according to facility policy. Send all samples to the laboratory with appropriate documentation.

Changing arterial line tubing

▶ Wash your hands and follow standard precautions. Assemble the new pressure monitoring system.

▶ Consult your facility's policy and procedure manual to determine how much tubing length to change.

▶ Inflate the pressure bag to 300 mm Hg and check for air leaks. Then release the pressure.

▶ Prepare the I.V. flush solution, and prime the pressure tubing and transducer system. At this time, add medication and tubing labels. Apply 300 mm Hg of pressure to the system. Then hang the I.V. bag on a pole.

▶ Place the sheet protector under the affected extremity. Remove the dressing from the catheter insertion site, taking care not to dislodge the catheter or cause vessel trauma. Turn off or temporarily silence the monitor alarms. (However, some facilities require that alarms be left on.)

▶ Turn off the flow clamp of the tubing segment that you'll change. Disconnect the tubing from the catheter hub, taking care not to dislodge the catheter. Immediately insert new tubing into the catheter hub. Secure the tubing and then activate the fast-flush release to clear it.

▶ Reactivate the monitor alarms. Apply an appropriate dressing.

▶ Level the zeroing stopcock of the transducer with the phlebostatic axis, and zero the system to atmospheric pressure.

Removing an arterial line

▶ Consult facility policy to determine whether you're permitted to perform this procedure.

▶ Explain the procedure to the patient.

▶ Assemble all equipment. Wash your hands. Observe standard precautions, including wearing personal protective equipment, for this procedure.

▶ Record the patient's systolic, diastolic, and mean blood pressures. If a manual, indirect blood pressure hasn't been assessed recently, obtain one now *to establish a new baseline.*

▶ Turn off the monitor alarms. Then turn off the flow clamp to the flush solution.

▶ Carefully remove the dressing over the insertion site. Remove any sutures using the suture removal kit and then carefully check that all sutures have been removed.

▶ Withdraw the catheter using a gentle, steady motion. Keep the catheter parallel to the artery during withdrawal *to reduce the risk of traumatic injury.*

▶ Immediately after withdrawing the catheter, apply pressure to the site with a sterile 4″ × 4″ gauze pad. Maintain pressure for at least 10 minutes (longer if bleeding or oozing persists). Apply additional pressure to a femoral site or if the patient has coagulopathy or is receiving anticoagulants.

▶ Cover the site with an appropriate dressing and secure the dressing with tape. If stipulated by facility policy, make a pressure dressing for a femoral site by folding in half four sterile 4″ × 4″ gauze pads, and apply the dressing.

Recognizing abnormal waveforms

Understanding a normal arterial waveform is relatively straightforward. An abnormal waveform, however, is more difficult to decipher. Abnormal patterns and markings may provide important diagnostic clues to the patient's cardiovascular status, or they may simply signal trouble in the monitor. Use this chart to help you recognize and resolve waveform abnormalities.

Abnormality	Possible causes	Nursing interventions
Alternating high and low waves in a regular pattern 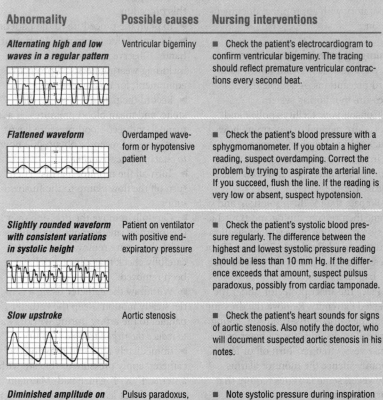	Ventricular bigeminy	■ Check the patient's electrocardiogram to confirm ventricular bigeminy. The tracing should reflect premature ventricular contractions every second beat.
Flattened waveform	Overdamped waveform or hypotensive patient	■ Check the patient's blood pressure with a sphygmomanometer. If you obtain a higher reading, suspect overdamping. Correct the problem by trying to aspirate the arterial line. If you succeed, flush the line. If the reading is very low or absent, suspect hypotension.
Slightly rounded waveform with consistent variations in systolic height	Patient on ventilator with positive end-expiratory pressure	■ Check the patient's systolic blood pressure regularly. The difference between the highest and lowest systolic pressure reading should be less than 10 mm Hg. If the difference exceeds that amount, suspect pulsus paradoxus, possibly from cardiac tamponade.
Slow upstroke	Aortic stenosis	■ Check the patient's heart sounds for signs of aortic stenosis. Also notify the doctor, who will document suspected aortic stenosis in his notes.
Diminished amplitude on inspiration 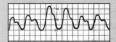	Pulsus paradoxus, possibly from cardiac tamponade, constrictive pericarditis, or lung disease	■ Note systolic pressure during inspiration and expiration. If inspiratory pressure is at least 10 mm Hg less than expiratory pressure, call the doctor. ■ If you're also monitoring pulmonary artery pressure, observe for a diastolic plateau. This occurs when the mean central venous pressure (right atrial pressure), mean pulmonary artery pressure, and mean pulmonary artery wedge pressure are within 5 mm Hg of one another.

Cover the dressing with a tight adhesive bandage; then cover the bandage with a sandbag. Maintain the patient on bed rest for 6 hours with the sandbag in place.

▶ If the doctor has ordered a culture of the catheter tip (to diagnose a suspected infection), gently place the catheter tip on a 4″ × 4″ sterile gauze pad. When the bleeding is under control, hold the catheter over the sterile container. Using sterile scissors, cut the tip *so it falls into the sterile container.* Label the specimen and send it to the laboratory.

▶ Observe the site for bleeding. Assess circulation in the extremity distal to the site by evaluating color, pulses, and sensation. Repeat this assessment every 15 minutes for the first 4 hours, every 30 minutes for the next 2 hours, then hourly for the next 6 hours.

Special considerations

▶ Observing the pressure waveform on the monitor can enhance assessment of arterial pressure. An abnormal waveform may reflect an arrhythmia (such as atrial fibrillation) or other cardiovascular problems, such as aortic stenosis, aortic insufficiency, pulsus alternans, or pulsus paradoxus. (See *Recognizing abnormal waveforms.*)

▶ Change the pressure tubing every 2 to 3 days, according to facility policy. Change the dressing at the catheter site at intervals specified by facility policy. Regularly assess the site for signs of infection, such as redness and swelling. Notify the doctor immediately if you note any such signs.

▶ Be aware that erroneous pressure readings may result from a catheter that is clotted or positional, loose connections, an addition of extra stopcocks or extension tubing, inadvertent entry of

air into the system, or improper calibration, leveling, or zeroing of the monitoring system. If the catheter lumen clots, the flush system may be improperly pressurized. Regularly assess the amount of flush solution in the I.V. bag and maintain 300 mm Hg of pressure in the pressure bag.

Complications

Direct arterial pressure monitoring can cause such complications as arterial bleeding, infection, air embolism, arterial spasm, or thrombosis.

Documentation

Document the date of system setup *so that all caregivers will know when to change the components.* Document systolic, diastolic, and mean pressure readings as well. Record circulation in the extremity distal to the site by assessing color, pulses, and sensation. Carefully document the amount of flush solution infused to avoid hypervolemia and volume overload, and to ensure accurate assessment of the patient's fluid status.

Make sure the position of the patient is documented when each blood pressure reading is obtained. This is important for determining trends.

ARTERIAL PUNCTURE FOR BLOOD GAS ANALYSIS

Obtaining an arterial blood sample requires percutaneous puncture of the brachial, radial, or femoral artery or withdrawal of a sample from an arterial line. Once collected, the sample can be analyzed to determine arterial blood gas (ABG) values.

Performing Allen's test

Rest the patient's arm on the mattress or bedside stand, and support his wrist with a rolled towel. Have him clench his fist. Then, using your index and middle fingers, press on the radial and ulnar arteries. Hold this position for a few seconds.	Without removing your fingers from the patient's arteries, ask him to unclench his fist and hold his hand in a relaxed position. The palm will be blanched because pressure from your fingers has impaired the normal blood flow.	Release pressure on the patient's ulnar artery. If the hand becomes flushed, which indicates blood filling the vessels, you can safely proceed with the radial artery puncture. If the hand doesn't flush, perform the test on the other arm.

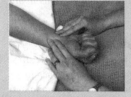 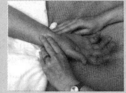 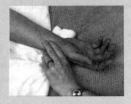

ABG analysis evaluates ventilation by measuring blood pH and the partial pressures of arterial oxygen (Pa_{O_2}) and carbon dioxide (Pa_{CO_2}). Blood pH measurement reveals the blood's acid-base balance. Pa_{O_2} indicates the amount of oxygen that the lungs deliver to the blood, and Pa_{CO_2} indicates the lungs' capacity to eliminate carbon dioxide. ABG samples can also be analyzed for oxygen content and saturation and for bicarbonate values.

Typically, ABG analysis is ordered for patients who have chronic obstructive pulmonary disease, pulmonary edema, acute respiratory distress syndrome, myocardial infarction, or pneumonia. It's also performed during episodes of shock and after coronary artery bypass surgery, resuscitation from cardiac arrest, changes in respiratory therapy or status, and prolonged anesthesia.

Most ABG samples can be collected by a respiratory technician or specially trained nurse. Collection from the femoral artery, however, is usually performed by a doctor. Before attempting a radial puncture, Allen's test should be performed. (See *Performing Allen's test*.)

Key nursing diagnoses and patient outcomes

Ineffective breathing pattern related to (specify)
The patient will:
▶ attain baseline ABG levels
▶ maintain baseline breath sounds
▶ express a feeling of comfort in maintaining air exchange
▶ achieve an acceptable baseline respiratory rate.

Ineffective airway clearance related to (specify)
The patient will:
▶ breathe spontaneously after the obstruction is removed or resolved
▶ maintain baseline respiratory rate

▶ attain baseline ABG levels
▶ maintain baseline breath sounds.

Impaired gas exchange related to (specify)
The patient will:
▶ attain baseline ABG levels
▶ maintain baseline breath sounds
▶ express a feeling of comfort in maintaining air exchange.

Equipment
10-ml glass syringe or plastic luer-lock syringe specially made for drawing blood for ABG analysis • 1-ml ampule of aqueous heparin (1:1,000) • 20G 1¼" needle • 22G 1" needle • gloves • alcohol or povidone-iodine pad • two 2" × 2" gauze pads • rubber cap for syringe hub or rubber stopper for needle • ice-filled plastic bag • label • laboratory request form • adhesive bandage • optional: 1% lidocaine solution

Many health care facilities use a commercial ABG kit that contains all the equipment listed above (except the adhesive bandage and ice). If your facility doesn't use such a kit, obtain a sterile syringe specially made for drawing blood for ABG values and use a clean emesis basin filled with ice instead of the plastic bag to transport the sample to the laboratory.

Preparation of equipment
Prepare the collected equipment before entering the patient's room. Wash your hands thoroughly; then open the ABG kit and remove the sample label and the plastic bag. Record on the label the patient's name and room number, date and collection time, and doctor's name. Fill the plastic bag with ice and set it aside.

If the syringe isn't heparinized, you'll need to do so. To heparinize the sy-

ringe, first attach the 20G needle to the syringe. Then open the ampule of heparin. Draw all the heparin into the syringe *to prevent the sample from clotting.* Hold the syringe upright, and pull the plunger back slowly to about the 7-ml mark. Rotate the barrel while pulling the plunger back *to allow the heparin to coat the inside surface of the syringe.* Then slowly force the heparin toward the hub of the syringe and expel all but about 0.1 ml of the heparin.

To heparinize the needle, first replace the 20G needle with the 22G needle. Then hold the syringe upright, tilt it slightly, and eject the remaining heparin. *Excess heparin in the syringe alters blood pH and Pao$_2$ values.*

Implementation
▶ Tell the patient you need to collect an arterial blood sample and explain the procedure *to help ease anxiety and promote cooperation.* Tell him that the needle stick will cause some discomfort but that he must remain still during the procedure.
▶ After washing your hands and putting on gloves, place a rolled towel under the patient's wrist *for support.* Locate the artery and palpate it for a strong pulse.
▶ Clean the puncture site with an alcohol or a povidone-iodine pad. Don't wipe off the povidone-iodine with alcohol.
▶ Using a circular motion, clean the area, starting in the center of the site and spiraling outward. If you use alcohol, apply it with friction for 30 seconds or until the final sponge comes away clean. Allow the skin to dry.
▶ Palpate the artery with the index and middle fingers of one hand while hold-

Arterial puncture technique

The angle of needle penetration in arterial blood gas sampling depends on which artery will be sampled. For the radial artery, which is used most often, the needle should enter bevel-up at a 30- to 45-degree angle over the radial artery.

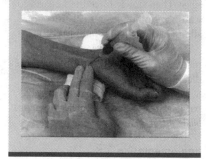

ing the syringe over the puncture site with the other hand.
▶ Hold the needle bevel up at a 30- to 45-degree angle. When puncturing the brachial artery, hold the needle at a 60-degree angle. (See *Arterial puncture technique.*)
▶ Puncture the skin and arterial wall in one motion, following the path of the artery.
▶ Watch for blood backflow in the syringe. Don't pull back on the plunger *because arterial blood should enter the syringe automatically.* Fill the syringe to the 5-ml mark.
▶ Withdraw the needle and then press a gauze pad firmly over the puncture site until the bleeding stops—at least 5 minutes. If the patient is receiving anticoagulant therapy or has a blood dyscrasia, apply pressure for 10 to 15 minutes; if necessary, ask a coworker to hold the gauze pad in place while you prepare the sample for transport to the

laboratory. Don't ask the patient to hold the pad. *If he fails to apply sufficient pressure, a large, painful hematoma may form, hindering future arterial punctures at that site.*
▶ Check the syringe for air bubbles. If any appear, remove them by holding the syringe upright and slowly ejecting some of the blood onto a 2″ × 2″ gauze pad.
▶ Insert the needle into a rubber stopper. *This prevents the sample from leaking and keeps air out of the syringe.*
▶ Put the labeled sample in the ice-filled plastic bag or emesis basin. Attach a properly completed laboratory request form and send the sample to the laboratory immediately.
▶ When bleeding stops, apply a small adhesive bandage to the site.
▶ Monitor the patient's vital signs, and observe for signs of circulatory impairment, such as swelling, discoloration, pain, numbness, or tingling in the arm or leg. Watch for bleeding at the puncture site.

Special considerations

▶ If the patient is receiving oxygen, make sure that his therapy has been in progress for at least 15 minutes before collecting an arterial blood sample.
▶ Unless ordered, don't turn off existing oxygen therapy before collecting arterial blood samples. Be sure to indicate on the laboratory request slip the amount and type of oxygen therapy the patient is receiving.
▶ If the patient isn't receiving oxygen, indicate that he's breathing room air.
▶ If the patient has just received a nebulizer treatment, wait about 20 minutes before collecting the sample.
▶ If necessary, you can anesthetize the puncture site with 1% lidocaine solu-

tion. Consider such use of lidocaine carefully *because it delays the procedure, the patient may be allergic to the drug, or the resulting vasoconstriction may prevent successful puncture.*

▶ When filling out a laboratory request form for ABG analysis, include the following information *to help the laboratory staff calibrate the equipment and evaluate results correctly:* the patient's current temperature, most recent hemoglobin level, current respiratory rate and, if the patient is on a ventilator, fraction of inspired oxygen and tidal volume.

Complications

If you use too much force when attempting to puncture the artery, the needle may touch the periosteum of the bone, causing the patient considerable pain, or you may advance the needle through the opposite wall of the artery. If this happens, slowly pull the needle back a short distance and check to see if you obtain a blood return. If blood still fails to enter the syringe, withdraw the needle completely and start with a fresh heparinized needle. Don't make more than two attempts to withdraw blood from the same site. *Probing the artery may injure it and the radial nerve. Also, hemolysis will alter test results.*

If arterial spasm occurs, blood won't flow into the syringe and you won't be able to collect the sample. If this happens, replace the needle with a smaller one and try the puncture again. *A smaller-bore needle is less likely to cause arterial spasm.*

Documentation

Record the results of Allen's test, the time the sample was drawn, the patient's temperature, the site of the arterial puncture, the amount of time that

Better charting

Documenting blood withdrawal for ABG analysis

When you must obtain blood for arterial blood gas (ABG) analysis, keep careful records of the following:
■ the patient's vital signs and temperature
■ the arterial puncture site
■ the results of Allen's test
■ any indication of circulatory impairment, such as swelling, discoloration, pain, numbness or tingling in the bandaged arm or leg, and bleeding at the puncture site.

Also be sure to document the time that the blood sample was drawn, the length of time pressure was applied to the site to control bleeding and, if appropriate, the type and amount of oxygen therapy that the patient received (as shown here).

1/16/01	1010	Blood drawn from Ⓡ radial
		artery s̄ + Allen's test c̄ brisk
		capillary refill. Pressure
		applied to site for 5 min. and
		pressure drsg. applied. No
		bleeding, hematoma, or swelling
		noted. Hand pink, warm c̄
		2-sec capillary refill. Sample
		for ABGs placed on ice and
		taken to lab. Pt. on 40% CAM.
		T 99.2° F. Hgb 10.2.
		Pat Natting RN

Filling out a laboratory request form

When filling out a laboratory request form for ABG analysis, be sure to include information for laboratory records, including:
■ the patient's current temperature and respiratory rate
■ his most recent hemoglobin level
■ the fraction of inspired oxygen and tidal volume, if he's on mechanical ventilation.

pressure was applied to the site to control bleeding, and the type and amount of oxygen therapy the patient was receiving. (See *Documenting blood withdrawal for ABG analysis,* page 37.)

ARTERIOVENOUS SHUNT CARE

An arteriovenous (AV) shunt consists of two segments of tubing joined (in a U-shape) to divert blood from an artery to a vein. Inserted surgically, usually in a forearm or (rarely) an ankle, the AV shunt provides access to the circulatory system for hemodialysis. After insertion, the shunt requires regular assessment for patency and examination of the surrounding skin for signs of infection.

AV shunt care also includes aseptically cleaning the arterial and venous exit sites, applying antiseptic ointment, and dressing the sites with sterile bandages. When done just before hemodialysis, this procedure prolongs the life of the shunt, helps prevent infection, and allows early detection of clotting. Shunt site care is done more often if the dressing becomes wet or nonocclusive.

Key nursing diagnoses and patient outcomes

Ineffective tissue perfusion (renal) related to decreased cellular exchange
The patient will:
▶ have blood urea nitrogen, creatinine, electrolyte, hemoglobin, and hematocrit levels that remain comparable to baseline levels
▶ not have a weight fluctuation.

Risk for infection related to AV shunt
The patient will:
▶ remain free from signs of infection (pain, redness, swelling, and purulent drainage) at the shunt site
▶ maintain a normal body temperature.

Equipment

Drape • stethoscope • sterile gloves • sterile 4″ × 4″ gauze pads • sterile cotton-tipped applicators • antiseptic (usually povidone-iodine solution) • bulldog clamps • plasticized or hypoallergenic tape • optional: swab specimen kit, prescribed antimicrobial ointment (usually povidone-iodine), sterile elastic gauze bandage, 2″ × 2″ gauze pads, hydrogen peroxide

Kits containing all the necessary equipment can be prepackaged and stored for use.

Implementation

▶ Explain the procedure to the patient. Provide privacy and wash your hands.
▶ Place the drape on a stable surface, such as a bedside table, *to reduce the risk of traumatic injury to the shunt site.* Then place the shunted extremity on the draped surface.
▶ Remove the two bulldog clamps from the elastic gauze bandage and unwrap the bandage from the shunt area.
▶ Carefully remove the gauze dressing covering the shunt and the 4″ × 4″ gauze pad under the shunt.
▶ Assess the arterial and venous exit sites for signs of infection, such as erythema, swelling, excessive tenderness, or drainage. Obtain a swab specimen of any purulent drainage and notify the doctor immediately of any signs of infection.

▶ Check blood flow through the shunt by inspecting the color of the blood and comparing the warmth of the shunt with that of the surrounding skin. The blood should be bright red; the shunt should feel as warm as the skin.

ᏆᏞᎥ **Nursing alert** If the blood is
≡■≡ **dark purple or black and the**
ᏆᏞᎥ **temperature of the shunt is lower than the surrounding skin, clotting has occurred. Notify the doctor immediately.**

▶ Use the stethoscope to auscultate the shunt between the arterial and venous exit sites. A bruit confirms normal blood flow. Palpate the shunt for a thrill (by lightly placing fingertips over the access site and feeling for vibration), which also indicates normal blood flow. Don't use a Doppler device to auscultate *because it will detect peripheral blood flow as well as shunt-related sounds.*

▶ Open a few packages of 4″ × 4″ gauze pads and cotton-tipped applicators, and soak them with the antiseptic. Put on the sterile gloves.

▶ Using a soaked 4″ × 4″ gauze pad, start cleaning the skin at one of the exit sites. Wipe away from the site *to remove bacteria and reduce the chance of contaminating the shunt.*

▶ Use the soaked cotton-tipped applicators to remove any crusted material from the exit site *because the encrustations provide a medium for bacterial growth.*

▶ Clean the other exit site, using fresh, soaked 4″ × 4″ gauze pads and cotton-tipped applicators.

▶ Clean the rest of the skin that was covered by the gauze dressing with fresh, soaked 4″ × 4″ gauze pads.

▶ If ordered, apply antimicrobial ointment to the exit sites *to help prevent infection.*

▶ Place a dry, sterile 4″ × 4″ gauze pad under the shunt. *This prevents the shunt from contacting the skin, which could cause skin irritation and breakdown.*

▶ Cover the exit sites with a dry, sterile 4″ × 4″ gauze pad, and tape the pad securely *to keep the exit sites clean and protected.*

▶ For routine daily care, wrap the shunt with an elastic gauze bandage. Leave a small portion of the shunt cannula exposed *so the patient can check for patency without removing the dressing.*

▶ Place the bulldog clamps on the edge of the elastic gauze bandage *so that the patient can use them quickly to stop hemorrhage in case the shunt separates.*

▶ For care before hemodialysis, don't re-dress the shunt, but keep the bulldog clamps readily accessible.

Special considerations

ᏆᏞᎥ **Nursing alert** Make sure the
≡■≡ **AV junction of the shunt is**
ᏆᏞᎥ **secured with plasticized or hypoallergenic tape. *This prevents separation of the two halves of the shunt, minimizing the risk of hemorrhage.***

▶ Blood pressure measurement and venipuncture should be avoided in the affected arm *to prevent shunt occlusion.*

▶ Always handle the shunt and dressings carefully. Don't use scissors or other sharp instruments to remove the dressing *because you may accidentally cut the shunt.* Never remove the tape securing the AV junction during dressing changes.

▶ When cleaning the shunt exit sites, use each 4″ × 4″ gauze pad only once and avoid wiping any area more than once *to minimize the risk of contamination.* When re-dressing the site, make sure that the tape doesn't kink or occlude the shunt. If the exit sites are heavily encrusted, place a 2″ × 2″ hydrogen peroxide–soaked gauze pad on the area for about 1 hour *to loosen the crust.* Make sure the patient isn't allergic to iodine before using povidone-iodine solution or ointment.

Home care

Ask the patient how he cares for the shunt at home. Then teach proper home care, if necessary.

Documentation

Record that shunt care was administered, the condition of the shunt and surrounding skin, any ointment used, and any instructions given to the patient.

ARTHROPLASTY CARE

Care of the patient after arthroplasty — surgical replacement of all or part of a joint — helps restore mobility and normal use of the affected extremity. Arthroplasty care includes maintaining alignment of the affected joint, assisting with exercises, and providing routine postoperative care. An equally important nursing responsibility is teaching safe mobility while performing activities of daily living, home care, and exercises that may continue for several years, depending on the type of arthroplasty performed and the patient's condition.

Two of the most commonly replaced joints are the hip and knee. Hip replacement may be total, replacing the femoral head and acetabulum, or par-

tial, replacing only one joint component. (See *Total hip replacement.*)

Knee replacement may also be partial, replacing either the medial or lateral compartment of the knee joint, or total, replacing the entire knee joint. Total knee replacement is commonly used to treat severe pain, joint contractures, and deterioration of joint surfaces — all conditions that prohibit full extension or flexion.

Nursing care after these operations — as well as care after less common surgical procedures (such as shoulder, elbow, wrist, ankle, or finger joint replacement) — requires similar skills.

Key nursing diagnoses and patient outcomes

Risk for perioperative positioning injury related to surgery

Total hip replacement

To form a totally artificial hip (such as the McKee-Farrar total hip replacement shown below), the surgeon cements a femoral head prosthesis in place to articulate with a studded cup, which he then cements into the deepened acetabulum. He may avoid using cement by implanting a prosthesis with a porous coating that promotes bony ingrowth.

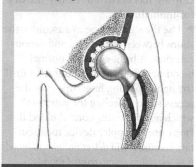

The patient will:
▶ show no evidence of neurologic, musculoskeletal, or vascular compromise
▶ maintain adequate cardiac output
▶ maintain effective gas exchange.

Acute pain related to surgery
The patient will:
▶ identify pain characteristics
▶ articulate factors that intensify pain and modify behavior accordingly
▶ express a feeling of comfort and relief from pain
▶ state and carry out appropriate interventions for pain relief.

Risk for infection related to surgical procedure
The patient will:
▶ maintain a normal body temperature
▶ maintain a normal white blood cell count and differential
▶ remain free from all signs and symptoms of infection.

Equipment

Balkan frame with trapeze • comfort device (such as static air mattress overlay, low-air-loss bed, or sheepskin) • bed sheets • incentive spirometer • continuous passive motion (CPM) machine (total knee replacement) • elastic stocking • sterile dressings • hypoallergenic tape • ice bag • skin lotion • warm water • crutches or walker • pain medications • closed-wound drainage system • I.V. antibiotics • pillow • optional: abduction splint, anticoagulants

After total knee replacement, a knee immobilizer may be applied in the operating room, or the leg may be placed in CPM.

Preparation of equipment

After the patient goes to the operating room, make a Balkan frame with a trapeze on his bed frame. *This will allow him some mobility after the operation.* Then make the bed, using a comfort device and clean sheets. Have the bed taken to the operating room. *This enables immediate placement of the patient on his hospital bed after surgery and eliminates the need for an additional move from his recovery room bed.*

Implementation

▶ Check vital signs every 30 minutes until they stabilize, then every 2 to 4 hours and routinely thereafter, according to facility protocol. Report any changes in vital signs *because they may indicate infection and hemorrhage.*
▶ Encourage the patient to perform deep-breathing and coughing exercises. Assist with incentive spirometry as ordered *to prevent respiratory complications.*
▶ Assess neurovascular status every 2 hours for the first 48 hours and then every 4 hours for signs of complications. Check the affected leg for color, temperature, toe movement, sensation, edema, capillary filling, and pedal pulse. Investigate any complaints of pain, burning, numbness, or tingling.
▶ Apply the elastic stocking to the unaffected leg as ordered *to promote venous return and prevent phlebitis and pulmonary emboli.* Once every 8 hours, remove the stocking, inspect the leg for pressure ulcers, and reapply it.
▶ Administer pain medications as ordered.
▶ Administer I.V. antibiotics as ordered for at least 48 hours after surgery *to minimize the risk of wound infection.*
▶ Administer anticoagulant therapy as ordered *to minimize the risk of throm-*

bophlebitis and embolus formation. Observe for bleeding. Also observe the leg for symptoms of phlebitis, such as warmth, swelling, tenderness, redness, and a positive Homans' sign.

▶ Check dressings for excessive bleeding. Circle any drainage on the dressing and mark it with your initials, the date, and the time. As needed, apply more sterile dressings, using hypoallergenic tape. Report excessive bleeding to the doctor.

▶ Observe the closed-wound drainage system for discharge color. *Proper drainage prevents hematoma. Purulent discharge and fever may indicate infection.* Empty and measure drainage as ordered using aseptic technique *to prevent infection.* (For more information, see "Closed-wound drain management," page 168.)

▶ Monitor fluid intake and output every shift; include wound drainage in the output measurement.

▶ Apply an ice bag as ordered to the affected site for the first 48 hours *to reduce swelling, relieve pain, and control bleeding.*

▶ Reposition the patient every 2 hours. *These position changes enhance comfort, prevent pressure ulcers, and help prevent respiratory complications.*

▶ Help the patient use the trapeze to lift himself every 2 hours. Then provide skin care for the back and buttocks, using warm water and lotion, as indicated.

▶ Instruct the patient to perform muscle-strengthening exercises for affected and unaffected extremities as ordered *to help maintain muscle strength and range of motion and to help prevent phlebitis.*

▶ Before ambulation, give a mild analgesic as ordered *because movement is very painful.* Encourage the patient during exercise.

▶ Help the patient with progressive ambulation, using adjustable crutches or a walker when needed.

After hip arthroplasty

▶ Keep the affected leg in abduction and in the neutral position *to stabilize the hip and keep the cup and femur head in the acetabulum.* Place a pillow between the patient's legs *to maintain hip abduction.*

▶ If the patient desires it, elevate the head of the bed 45 degrees for comfort. (Some doctors permit a 60-degree elevation.) Keep it elevated no more than 30 minutes at a time *to prevent excessive hip flexion.*

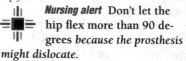 **Nursing alert** Don't let the hip flex more than 90 degrees *because the prosthesis might dislocate.*

▶ Keep the patient in the supine position, with the affected hip in full extension, for 1 hour three times per day and at night. *This will help prevent hip flexion contracture.*

▶ On the day after surgery, have the patient begin plantar flexion and dorsiflexion exercises of the foot on the affected leg. When ordered, instruct him to begin quadriceps exercises. Progressive ambulation protocols vary. Most patients are permitted to begin transfer and progressive ambulation with assistive devices on the first day.

After total knee replacement

▶ Keep the knee immobilized in full extension immediately after surgery. Many hospitals start CPM in the recovery room.

▶ Elevate the affected leg as ordered *to reduce swelling.*

▶ Tell the patient to begin quadriceps exercises and straight leg-raising when ordered (usually on the first postoperative day). Encourage flexion-extension exercises when ordered (usually after the first dressing change).

▶ If the doctor orders use of the CPM machine, he will adjust the machine daily *to gradually increase the degree of flexion of the affected leg.* Typically, patients can dangle their feet on the first day after surgery and begin ambulation with partial weight-bearing as tolerated (cemented knee) or toe-touch ambulation only (uncemented knee) by the second day. The patient may need to wear a knee immobilizer for support when walking; otherwise, he should be in CPM for most of the day and night or during waking hours only. Check your facility's protocol.

Special considerations

▶ Before surgery, explain the procedure to the patient. Emphasize that frequent assessment — including the monitoring of vital signs, neurovascular integrity, and wound drainage — is normal after the operation.

▶ Inform the patient that he'll receive I.V. antibiotics for about 2 days. Also be sure he understands that he'll receive medication around the clock for pain control. Explain the need for immobilizing the affected leg and exercising the unaffected one.

▶ Before discharge, instruct the patient regarding home care and exercises.

Complications

Immobility after arthroplasty may result in such complications as pulmonary embolism, pneumonia, phlebitis, paralytic ileus, urine retention, and bowel impaction. A deep wound or infection at the prosthesis site is a serious complication that may force removal of the prosthesis. Dislocation of a total hip prosthesis may occur after violent hip flexion or adduction or during internal rotation. Signs and symptoms of dislocation include inability to rotate the hip or bear weight, shortening of the leg, and increased pain.

Fat embolism, a potentially fatal complication resulting from release of fat molecules in response to increased intermedullary canal pressure from the prosthesis, may develop within 72 hours after surgery. Watch for such signs and symptoms as apprehension, diaphoresis, fever, dyspnea, pulmonary effusion, tachycardia, cyanosis, seizures, decreased level of consciousness, and a petechial rash on the chest and shoulders.

Documentation

Record the patient's neurovascular status. Describe the patient's position (especially the position of the affected leg), skin care and condition, respiratory care and condition, and the use of elastic stockings. Document all exercises performed and their effect; also record ambulatory efforts and the type of support used.

On the appropriate flowchart, record vital signs and fluid intake and output. Record discharge instructions and how well the patient seems to understand them.

AUTOMATED EXTERNAL DEFIBRILLATION

Automated external defibrillators (AEDs) are commonly used today to meet the need for early defibrillation, which is currently considered the most effective treatment for ventricular fibrillation. Some facilities now require an AED in every noncritical care unit. Their use is also becoming common in such public places as shopping malls, sports stadiums, and airplanes. Instruction in using the AED is already required as part of Basic Life Support (BLS) and Advanced Cardiac Life Support (ACLS) training.

AEDs are being used increasingly to provide early defibrillation — even when no health care provider is present. The AED interprets the victim's cardiac rhythm and gives the operator step-by-step directions on how to proceed if defibrillation is indicated. Most AEDs have a "quick-look" feature that allows visualization of the rhythm with the paddles before electrodes are connected.

The AED is equipped with a microcomputer that senses and analyzes a patient's heart rhythm at the push of a button. Then it audibly or visually prompts you to deliver a shock. AED models all have the same basic function but offer different operating options. For example, all AEDs communicate directions through messages on a display screen, give voice commands, or do both. Some AEDs simultaneously display a patient's heart rhythm.

All devices record your interactions with the patient during defibrillation, either on a cassette tape or in a solid-state memory module. Some AEDs have an integral printer for immediate event documentation. Facility policy determines who is responsible for reviewing all AED interactions; the patient's doctor always has that option. Local and state regulations govern who

is responsible for collecting AED case data for reporting purposes.

Key nursing diagnoses and patient outcomes

Decreased cardiac output related to reduced myocardial perfusion
The patient will:
▶ maintain hemodynamic stability: pulse not less than (specify) and not greater than (specify); blood pressure not less than (specify) and not greater than (specify)
▶ experience no arrhythmias
▶ maintain adequate cardiac output.

Ineffective tissue perfusion (cardiopulmonary) related to decreased cellular exchange
The patient will:
▶ attain hemodynamic stability: pulse not less than (specify) and not greater than (specify); blood pressure not less than (specify) and not greater than (specify)
▶ maintain adequate cardiac output
▶ experience no arrhythmias.

Equipment
AED • two prepackaged electrodes

Implementation
▶ After discovering that your patient is unresponsive to your questions, pulseless, and apneic, follow BLS and ACLS protocols. Then ask a colleague to bring the AED into the patient's room and set it up before the code team arrives.
▶ Open the foil packets containing the two electrode pads. Attach the white electrode cable connector to one pad and the red electrode cable connector to the other. The electrode pads aren't site specific.
▶ Expose the patient's chest. Remove the plastic backing film from the elec-

trode pads, and place the electrode pad attached to the white cable connector on the right upper portion of the patient's chest, just beneath his clavicle.

▶ Place the pad attached to the red cable connector to the left of the heart's apex. To help remember where to place the pads, think "white, right; red, ribs." (Placement for both electrode pads is the same as for manual defibrillation or cardioversion.)

▶ Firmly press the device's ON button, and wait while the machine performs a brief self-test. Most AEDs signal their readiness by a computerized voice that says "Stand clear" or by emitting a series of loud beeps. (If the AED isn't functioning properly, it will convey the message "Don't use the AED. Remove and continue CPR.") Remember to report any AED malfunctions in accordance with your facility's procedure.

▶ Now the machine is ready to analyze the patient's heart rhythm. Ask everyone to stand clear and press the ANALYZE button when prompted by the machine. Be careful not to touch or move the patient while the AED is in analysis mode. (If you get the message "Check electrodes," make sure the electrodes are correctly placed and the patient cable is securely attached; then press the ANALYZE button again.)

▶ In 15 to 30 seconds, the AED will analyze the patient's rhythm. When the patient needs a shock, the AED will display a "Stand clear" message and emit a beep that changes into a steady tone as it's charging.

▶ When an AED is fully charged and ready to deliver a shock, it will prompt you to press the SHOCK button. (Some fully automatic AED models automatically deliver a shock within 15 seconds after analyzing the patient's rhythm. If a

shock isn't needed, the AED will display "No shock indicated" and prompt you to "Check patient.")

▶ Make sure that no one is touching the patient or his bed and call out "Stand clear." Then press the SHOCK button on the AED. Most AEDs are ready to deliver a shock within 15 seconds.

▶ After the first shock, the AED will automatically reanalyze the patient's heart rhythm. If no additional shock is needed, the machine will prompt you to check the patient. However, if the patient is still in ventricular fibrillation, the AED will automatically begin recharging at a higher joule level to prepare for a second shock. Repeat the steps you performed before delivering a shock to the patient. According to the AED algorithm, the patient can receive up to three shocks at increasing joule levels (200, 200 to 300, and 360 joules).

▶ If the patient is still in ventricular fibrillation after three shocks, resume CPR for 1 minute. Then press the ANALYZE button on the AED to identify the heart rhythm. If the patient is still in ventricular fibrillation, continue the algorithm sequence until the code team leader arrives.

Special considerations

▶ Defibrillators vary from one manufacturer to the next, so be sure to familiarize yourself with your facility's equipment.

▶ Defibrillator operation should be checked at least every 8 hours and after each use.

Complications

Defibrillation can cause accidental electric shock to those providing care.

Better charting

Code reporting with the AED

All automated external defibrillator (AED) devices record your interactions with the patient during defibrillation, either on a cassette tape or in a solid-state memory module. Some AEDs have an integral printer for immediate event documentation. Facility policy defines who is responsible for reviewing all AED interactions; the patient's doctor always has that option. Local and state regulations govern who is responsible for collecting AED data for reporting purposes. After using an AED, give a synopsis to the code team leader.

What to report
Remember to report the following:
- the patient's name, age, medical history, and reason for seeking care
- the time you found the patient in cardiac arrest
- the time you began cardiopulmonary resuscitation
- the time you applied the AED
- how many shocks the patient received
- when the patient regained a pulse at any point
- what postarrest care was given, if any
- physical assessment findings.
    Later, be sure to document the code on the appropriate form.

rhythm strip with code data. Follow your facility's policy for analyzing and storing code data. (See *Code reporting with the AED*.) Be sure to document the code on the appropriate form.

Using an insufficient amount of conduction medium can lead to skin burns.

Documentation
After the code, remove and transcribe the AED's computer memory module or tape, or prompt the AED to print a

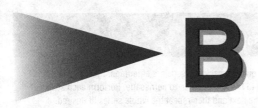

Back care

Regular bathing and massage of the neck, back, buttocks, and upper arms promotes patient relaxation and allows assessment of skin condition. Particularly important for the bedridden patient, massage causes cutaneous vasodilation, helping to prevent pressure ulcers caused by prolonged pressure on bony prominences or by perspiration. Gentle back massage can be performed after myocardial infarction but may be contraindicated in patients with rib fractures, surgical incisions, or other recent traumatic injury to the back.

Key nursing diagnoses and patient outcomes

Risk for impaired skin integrity related to bed rest
The patient will:
▶ exhibit no signs of skin breakdown
▶ show normal skin turgor
▶ perform routine skin care.

Equipment

Basin • soap • bath blanket • bath towel • washcloth • back lotion with lanolin base • gloves, if the patient has open lesions or has been incontinent • optional: talcum powder

Preparation of equipment

Fill the basin two-thirds full with warm water. Place the lotion bottle in the basin to warm it. *Application of warmed lotion prevents chilling or startling the patient, thereby reducing muscle tension and vasoconstriction.*

Implementation

▶ Assemble the equipment at the patient's bedside.
▶ Explain the procedure to the patient and provide privacy. Ask him to tell you if you're applying too much or too little pressure.
▶ Adjust the bed to a comfortable working height and lower the head of the bed, if allowed. Wash your hands and put on gloves, if applicable.
▶ Place the patient in the prone position, if possible, or on his side. Position him along the edge of the bed nearest you *to prevent back strain.*
▶ Untie the patient's gown and expose his back, shoulders, and buttocks. Then drape the patient with a bath blanket *to prevent chills and minimize exposure.* Place a bath towel next to or under the patient's side *to protect bed linens from moisture.*
▶ Fold the washcloth around your hand to form a mitt. *This prevents the loose ends of the cloth from dripping water*

How to give a back massage

Three strokes used commonly when giving a back massage are effleurage, friction, and petrissage. Start with effleurage and go on to friction and then to petrissage. Perform each stroke at least six times before moving on to the next and then repeat the whole series, if desired.

When performing effleurage and friction, keep your hands parallel to the vertebrae to avoid tickling the patient. For all three strokes, maintain a regular rhythm and steady contact with the patient's back *to help him relax.*

Effleurage
Using your palm, stroke from the buttocks up to the shoulders, over the upper arms, and back to the buttocks. Use slightly less pressure on the downward strokes.

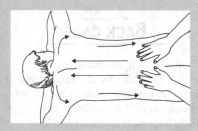

Friction
Use circular thumb strokes to move from buttocks to shoulders; then, using a smooth stroke, return to the buttocks.

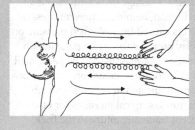

Petrissage
Using your thumb to oppose your fingers, knead and stroke half the back and upper arms, starting at the buttocks and moving toward the shoulder. Then knead and stroke the other half of the back, rhythmically alternating your hands.

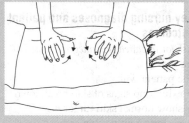

onto the patient and keeps the cloth warm longer. Then work up a lather with soap.

▶ Using long, firm strokes, bathe the patient's back, beginning at the neck and shoulders and moving downward to the buttocks. Rinse and dry well *because moisture trapped between the buttocks can cause chafing and predispose the patient to formation of pressure ulcers.* While giving back care, closely examine the patient's skin, especially the bony prominences of the shoulders, the scapulae, and the coccyx, for redness or abrasions.

▶ Remove the warmed lotion bottle from the basin and pour a small amount of lotion into your palm. Rub your hands together *to distribute the lotion*. Then apply the lotion to the patient's back, using long, firm strokes. *The lotion reduces friction, making back massage easier.*

▶ Massage the patient's back, beginning at the base of the spine and moving upward to the shoulders. For a relaxing effect, massage slowly; for a stimulating effect, massage quickly. Alternate the three basic strokes: effleurage, friction, and petrissage. (See *How to give a back massage.*) Add lotion as needed, keeping one hand on the patient's back *to avoid interrupting the massage*.

▶ Compress, squeeze, and lift the trapezius muscle *to help relax the patient*.

▶ Finish the massage by using long, firm strokes and blot any excess lotion from the patient's back with a towel. Then retie the patient's gown and straighten or change the bed linens as necessary.

▶ Return the bed to its original position and make the patient comfortable. Empty and clean the basin. Dispose of gloves, if used, and return equipment to the appropriate storage area.

Special considerations

▶ Before giving back care, assess the patient's body structure and skin condition and tailor the duration and intensity of the massage accordingly. If you're giving back care at bedtime, have the patient ready for bed beforehand *so the massage can help him fall asleep*.

▶ Use separate lotion for each patient *to prevent cross-contamination*. If the patient has oily skin, substitute a talcum powder or lotion of the patient's choice. However, don't use powder if the patient has an endotracheal or tracheal tube in place *to avoid aspiration*. Also, avoid using powder and lotion together *because this may lead to skin maceration*.

▶ When massaging the patient's back, stand with one foot slightly forward and your knees slightly bent *to allow effective use of your arm and shoulder muscles*.

▶ Give special attention to bony prominences *because these areas are disposed to formation of pressure ulcers*. Don't massage the patient's legs unless ordered *because reddened legs can signal clot formation, and massage can dislodge the clot, causing an embolus*. Develop a turning schedule and give back care at each position change.

Documentation

Chart back care on the flowchart. Record redness, abrasion, or change in skin condition in your notes.

BED-MAKING

For the bedridden patient, daily linen changes promote comfort and help prevent skin breakdown and nosocomial infection. Such changes necessitate the use of side rails to prevent the patient from rolling out of bed and, depending on the patient's condition, the use of a turning sheet to move him from side to side.

Making an occupied bed may require more than one person. It also entails loosening the bottom sheet on one side and fanfolding it to the center of

Making a traction bed

For a patient in traction, obtain help from a coworker to make the bed. Work from head to toe to minimize the risk of traction misalignment.

Preparation
■ Wash your hands. Put on gloves, if necessary. Bring clean linen and arrange it in the order of use on the bedside stand or a chair.
■ Explain the procedure, provide privacy, and remove unnecessary furniture.

Changing the linens
■ Lower both side rails. Stand near the headboard, opposite your coworker.
■ Gently pull the mattress to the head of the bed. Avoid sudden movements *because they can misalign traction and cause patient discomfort.*
■ Remove the pillow from the bed. Loosen the bottom linens and roll them from the headboard toward the patient's head. Then remove the soiled pillowcase and replace it with a clean one.

■ Fold a clean bottom sheet crosswise and place the sheet across the head of the bed. Tell the patient to raise her head and upper shoulders by grasping the trapeze above the bed (as shown below). With your coworker, quickly fanfold the bottom sheet from the head of the bed under the patient's shoulders, so that it meets the soiled linen. If a fitted sheet isn't available tuck at least 12″ (30.5 cm) of the bottom sheet under the head of the mattress. Miter the corners and tuck in the sides.

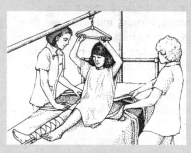

the mattress instead of loosening the bottom sheet on both sides and removing it, as in an unoccupied bed. Also, the foundation of the bed must be made before the top sheet is applied instead of the foundation and top being made on one side before being completed on the other side. (See *Making a traction bed.*)

Key nursing diagnoses and patient outcomes
Risk for impaired skin integrity related to immobility
The patient will:
▶ remain free from skin breakdown
▶ show normal skin turgor
▶ communicate an understanding of skin protection measures.

Equipment
Two sheets (one fitted, if available) • pillowcase • one or two drawsheets • spread • one or two bath blankets • gloves • sheepskin or other comfort-enhancing device as needed • optional: laundry bag and linen-saver pad

Preparation of equipment
Obtain clean linen and make sure it's folded properly as for an unoccupied bed.

- Tell the patient to raise her buttocks by grasping the trapeze. As a team, move toward the foot of the bed and, in one movement, quickly and carefully roll soiled linens and clean linens under the patient.
- Instruct the patient to release the trapeze and to rest. Place a pillow under her head *for comfort.*
- If allowed, remove any pillows from under the patient's extremity. If pillow removal is contraindicated, continue to move linens toward the foot of the bed and under the patient's legs and traction while your coworker lifts the pillows and supports the patient's extremity.
- Put soiled linens in a laundry bag or pillowcase.
- Tuck the remaining loose linens securely under the mattress. To ensure a tight-fitting bottom sheet, have the patient raise herself off the bed by simultaneously grasping the trapeze and raising her buttocks while you pull the sheet tight. As needed, place a drawsheet, linen-saver pad, or sheepskin under her. Complete the bed-making alone.
- If the bottom sheet doesn't cover the foot of the mattress, cover it with a drawsheet. Miter its corners and tuck in the sides.
- Replace the pillows under the patient's extremity, then cover her with a clean top sheet. Fold over the top hem of the sheet approximately 8″ (20 cm). If one or both legs are in traction, fit the lower end of the sheet loosely over the traction apparatus; don't press on the traction ropes. To secure the sheet, tuck in the corner opposite the traction under the foot of the bed and miter the corner. Neatly tuck in the lower corner of the sheet on the traction side to expose the leg and foot.
- If the traction equipment exposes the patient's sides, cover her with a drawsheet — not a full sheet or spread.
- Lower the bed but don't allow the traction weights to touch the floor. Raise the side rails to prevent falls. If allowed, leave one side rail down so the patient can reach the bedside stand.

Implementation

▶ Wash your hands, put on gloves, and bring clean linen to the patient's room.

▶ Identify the patient and tell him you'll be changing his bed linens. Explain how he can help if he's able, adjusting the plan according to his abilities and needs. Provide privacy.

▶ Move any furniture away from the bed *to ensure ample working space.*

▶ Raise the side rail on the far side of the bed *to prevent falls.* Adjust the bed to a comfortable working height *to prevent back strain.*

▶ If allowed, lower the head of the bed *to ensure tight-fitting, wrinkle-free linens.*

▶ When stripping the bed, watch for belongings among the linens.

▶ Cover the patient with a bath blanket *to avoid exposure and provide warmth and privacy.* Then fanfold the top sheet and spread from beneath the bath blanket and bring them back over the blanket. Loosen the top linens at the foot of the bed and remove them separately. If reusing the top linens, fold each piece and hang it over the back of the chair. Otherwise, place it in the laundry bag. *To avoid dispersing microorganisms,* don't fan the linens, hold them against your clothing, or place them on the floor.

► If the mattress slides down when the head of the bed is raised, pull it up again. *Adjusting the mattress after the bed is made loosens the linens.* If the patient is able, ask him to grasp the head of the bed and pull with you; otherwise, ask a coworker to help you.

► Roll the patient to the far side of the bed and turn the pillow lengthwise under his head *to support his neck.* Ask him to help (if he can) by grasping the far side rail as he turns *so that he's positioned at the far side of the bed.*

► Loosen the soiled bottom linens on the side of the bed nearest you. Then roll the linens toward the patient's back in the middle of the bed.

► Place a clean bottom sheet on the bed, with its center fold in the middle of the mattress. For a fitted sheet, secure the top and bottom corners over the side of the mattress nearest you. For a flat sheet, place its end even with the foot of the mattress. Miter the top corner as you would for an unoccupied bed *to keep linens firmly tucked under the mattress, preventing wrinkling.*

► Fanfold the remaining clean bottom sheet toward the patient and place the drawsheet, if needed, about 15″ (38 cm) from the top of the bed, with its center fold in the middle of the mattress. Tuck in the entire edge of the drawsheet on the side nearest you. Fanfold the remaining drawsheet toward the patient.

► If necessary, position a linen-saver pad on the drawsheet *to absorb excretions or surgical drainage* and fanfold it toward the patient.

► Raise the other side rail and roll the patient to the clean side of the bed.

► Move to the unfinished side of the bed and lower the side rail nearest you. Then loosen and remove the soiled bottom linens separately and place them in the laundry bag.

► Pull the clean bottom sheet taut. Secure the fitted sheet, or place the end of a flat sheet even with the foot of the bed, and miter the top corner. Pull the drawsheet taut and tuck it in. Unfold and smooth the linen-saver pad, if used.

► Assist the patient to the supine position if his condition permits.

► Remove the soiled pillowcase and place it in the laundry bag. Then slip the pillow into a clean pillowcase, tucking its corners well into the case *to ensure a smooth fit.* Place the pillow beneath the patient's head, with its seam toward the top of the bed *to prevent it from rubbing against the patient's neck, causing irritation.* Place the pillow's open edge away from the door *to give the bed a finished appearance.*

► Unfold the clean top sheet over the patient with the rough side of the hem facing away from the bed *to avoid irritating the patient's skin.* Allow enough sheet to form a cuff over the spread.

► Remove the bath blanket from beneath the sheet and center the spread over the top sheet.

► Make a 3″ (7.6-cm) toe pleat, or vertical tuck, in the top linens *to allow room for the patient's feet and to prevent pressure that can cause discomfort, skin breakdown, and footdrop.*

► Tuck the top sheet and spread under the foot of the bed and miter the bottom corners. Fold the top sheet over the spread *to give the bed a finished appearance.*

▶ Raise the head of the bed to a comfortable position, make sure both side rails are raised, and then lower the bed and lock its wheels *to ensure the patient's safety.* Assess the patient's body alignment.

▶ Place the call button within the patient's easy reach. Remove the laundry bag from the room.

▶ Remove and discard gloves and wash your hands *to prevent the spread of nosocomial infections.*

Special considerations

▶ Use a fitted sheet, when available, *because a flat sheet slips out from under the mattress easily, especially if the mattress is plastic-coated.*

▶ Prevent the patient from sliding down in bed by tucking a tightly rolled pillow under the top linens at the foot of the bed.

▶ For the diaphoretic or bedridden patient, fold a bath blanket in half lengthwise and place it between the bottom sheet and the plastic mattress cover; *the blanket acts as a cushion and helps absorb moisture.* To help prevent sheet burns on *the heels and bony prominences,* center a bath blanket or sheepskin over the bottom sheet and tuck the blanket under the mattress.

▶ If the patient can't help you move or turn him, devise a turning sheet *to facilitate bed making and repositioning.* To do this, first fold a drawsheet or bath blanket and place it under the patient's buttocks. Make sure the sheet extends from the shoulders to the knees *so that it supports most of the patient's weight.* Roll the sides of the sheet to form handles. Next, ask a coworker to help you lift and move the patient. With one person holding each side of the sheet, you

can move the patient without wrinkling the bottom linens. If you can't get help and must turn the patient yourself, stand at the side of the bed. Turn the patient toward the rail and, if he's able, ask him to grasp the opposite rolled edge of the turning sheet. Pull the rolled edge carefully toward you and turn the patient.

Documentation

Although linen changes aren't usually documented, record their dates and times in your notes for patients with incontinence, excessive wound drainage, pressure ulcers, or diaphoresis.

BEDPAN AND URINAL USE

A bedpan and urinal permit elimination by the bedridden patient and accurate observation and measurement of urine and stool by the nurse. A bedpan is used by the female patient for defecation and urination and by the male patient for defecation; a urinal is used by the male patient for urination. Either device should be offered frequently — before meals, visiting hours, morning and evening care, and any treatments or procedures. Whenever possible, allow the patient privacy.

Key nursing diagnoses and patient outcomes

Risk for constipation related to immobility
The patient will:

▶ move bowels every (specify) day(s) without laxative or enema

▶ maintain normal bowel elimination pattern

▶ state an understanding of factors that cause constipation.

Impaired urinary elimination related to immobility
The patient will:
▶ maintain fluid balance (intake will equal output)
▶ voice increased comfort.

Equipment
Bedpan, fracture pan, or urinal with cover • toilet tissue • two washcloths • soap • gloves • towel • linen-saver pad • bath blanket • pillow • optional: air freshener and talcum powder

Available in adult and pediatric sizes, the bedpan may be disposable or reusable (the latter can be sterilized). The fracture pan, a type of bedpan, is used when spinal injuries, body or leg casts, or other conditions prohibit or restrict turning the patient. Like the bedpan, the urinal may be disposable or reusable.

Preparation of equipment
Obtain the appropriate bedpan or urinal. If you're using a metal bedpan, warm it under running water *to avoid startling the patient and stimulating muscle contraction, which hinders elimination.* Dry the bedpan thoroughly and test its temperature *because metal retains heat.* If necessary, sprinkle talcum powder on the edge of the bedpan *to reduce friction during placement and removal.* For a thin patient, place a linen-saver pad at the edge of the bedpan or use a fracture pan *to minimize pressure on the coccyx.*

Implementation
▶ If the patient's condition permits, provide privacy. Put on gloves *to prevent contact with body fluids and to comply with standard precautions.*

Placing a bedpan
▶ If allowed, elevate the head of the bed slightly *to prevent hyperextension of the spine when the patient raises the buttocks.*
▶ Rest the bedpan on the edge of the bed. Then, turn down the corner of the top linens and draw up the patient's gown. Ask him to raise the buttocks by flexing his knees and pushing down on his heels. While supporting the patient's lower back with one hand, center the curved, smooth edge of the bedpan beneath the buttocks.
▶ If the patient can't raise his buttocks, lower the head of the bed to the horizontal position and help the patient roll onto one side, with buttocks toward you. Position the bedpan properly against the buttocks, then help the patient roll back onto the bedpan. When the patient is positioned comfortably, raise the head of the bed as indicated.
▶ After positioning the bedpan, elevate the head of the bed further, if allowed, until the patient is sitting erect. *This position, like the normal elimination posture, aids in defecation and urination.* (For information on another device that permits normal elimination posture, see *Using a commode.*)
▶ If elevation of the head of the bed is contraindicated, tuck a small pillow or folded bath blanket under the patient's back *to cushion the sacrum against the edge of the bedpan and support the lumbar region.*
▶ If the patient can be left alone, place the bed in a low position and raise the side rails *to ensure his safety.* Place toilet tissue and the call button within the patient's reach and instruct him to push the button after elimination. If the patient is weak or disoriented, remain with him.

▶ Before removing the bedpan, lower the head of the bed slightly. Then ask the patient to raise his buttocks off the bed. Support the lower back with one hand and gently remove the bedpan with the other *to avoid skin injury caused by friction.* If the patient can't raise his buttocks, ask him to roll off the pan while you assist with one hand. Hold the pan firmly with the other hand *to avoid spills.* Cover the bedpan and place it on the chair.

▶ Help clean the anal and perineal area as necessary *to prevent irritation and infection.* Turn the patient on his side, wipe carefully with toilet tissue, clean the area with a damp washcloth and soap, and dry well with a towel. Clean a female patient from front to back *to avoid introducing rectal contaminants into the vaginal or urethral openings.*

Placing a urinal

▶ Lift the corner of the top linens, hand the urinal to the patient, and allow him to position it.

▶ If the patient can't position the urinal himself, spread his legs slightly and hold the urinal in place to prevent spills.

▶ After the patient voids, carefully withdraw the urinal.

After the use of a bedpan or urinal

▶ Give the patient a clean, damp, warm washcloth for his hands. Check the bed linens for wetness or soiling, and straighten or change them if needed. Make the patient comfortable. Place the bed in the low position and raise the side rails.

▶ Take the bedpan or urinal to the bathroom. Observe the color, odor, amount, and consistency of its contents. If ordered, measure urine output

Using a commode

An alternative to a bedpan, a commode is a portable chair made of wood, plastic, or metal with a large opening in the center of the seat. It may have a bedpan or bucket that slides underneath the opening, or it may slide directly over the toilet, adding height to the standard toilet seat. Unlike a bedpan, a commode allows the patient to assume his normal elimination posture, which aids in defecation.

Before the patient uses it, inspect the commode's condition and make sure it is clean. Roll or carry the commode to the patient's room. Place it parallel and as close as possible to the patient's bed and secure its brakes or wheel locks. If necessary, block its wheels with sandbags. Assist the patient onto the commode, provide toilet tissue, and place the call button within his reach. Instruct the patient to push the call button when finished.

If necessary, assist the patient with cleaning. Help the patient into bed and make the patient comfortable. Offer the patient soap, water, and a towel to wash his hands. Then close the lid of the commode or cover the bucket. Roll the commode or carry the bucket to the bathroom. If ordered, observe and measure the contents before disposal. Rinse and clean the bucket and then spray or wipe the bucket and commode seat with disinfectant. Use an air freshener if appropriate.

or liquid stool or obtain a specimen for laboratory analysis.

▶ Empty the bedpan or urinal into the toilet. Rinse with cold water and clean it thoroughly, using a disinfectant solution. Dry and return it to the patient's bedside stand.

▶ Use an air freshener, if necessary, *to eliminate offensive odors and minimize embarrassment.*

▶ Remove gloves and wash your hands.

Special considerations

▶ Explain to the patient that drug treatment and changes in his environment, diet, and activities may disrupt his usual elimination schedule. Try to anticipate elimination needs and offer the bedpan or urinal frequently *to help reduce embarrassment and minimize the risk of incontinence.*

▶ Avoid placing a bedpan or urinal on top of the bedside stand or overbed table *to avoid contamination of clean equipment and food trays.* Similarly, avoid placing it on the floor *to prevent the spread of microorganisms from the floor to the patient's bed linens when the device is used.*

▶ If the patient feels pain during turning or feels uncomfortable on a standard bedpan, use a fracture pan. Unlike the standard bedpan, the fracture pan is slipped under the buttocks from the front rather than the side. Because it's shallower than the standard bedpan, you need only lift the patient slightly to position it. If the patient is obese or otherwise difficult to lift, ask a coworker to help you.

▶ If the patient has an indwelling urinary catheter in place, carefully position and remove the bedpan *to avoid tension on the catheter, which could dislodge it or irritate the urethra.* After the patient defecates, wipe, clean, and dry the anal region, taking care to avoid catheter contamination. If necessary, clean the urinary meatus with povidone-iodine solution.

▶ Avoid leaving the urinal, fracture pan, or bed pan in place for extended periods *to prevent skin breakdown.*

Documentation

Record the time, date, and type of elimination on the flowchart and the amount of urine output or liquid stool on the intake and output record as needed. In your notes, document the amount, color, clarity, and odor of the urine or stool and the presence of blood, pus, or other abnormal characteristics in urine or stool. Document the condition of the perineum.

BEDSIDE BLOOD GLUCOSE AND HEMOGLOBIN TESTING

Increasingly, nurses are monitoring blood glucose and hemoglobin (Hb) levels at the patient's bedside. The fast, accurate results obtained this way allow immediate intervention, if necessary. By contrast, blood samples obtained from traditional monitoring methods must be sent to the laboratory for interpretation. A blood sample that sits at room temperature for an hour may undergo glycolysis, which reduces glucose concentration by 3% to 30%, leading to inaccurate test results.

Numerous testing systems are available for bedside monitoring. Bedside systems are also convenient for the patient's home use.

HemoCue, a widely used system, gives accurate results without having to pipette, dispense, or mix blood and reagents to obtain readings. Thus, it eliminates the risk of leakage, broken tubes, and splattered blood. A plastic,

How to use a bedside blood glucose and hemoglobin monitor

Monitoring blood glucose and hemoglobin levels at the patient's bedside is a straightforward procedure. A photometer, such as the HemoCue analyzer featured here, relies on capillary action to draw blood into a disposable microcuvette.

This method of obtaining blood minimizes a health care worker's exposure to the patient's blood and decreases the risk of cross-contamination. Follow the three steps shown here when using the HemoCue system.

After you pierce the skin, the microcuvette draws blood automatically.	Next, place the microcuvette in the photometer.	The photometer screen displays the blood glucose and hemoglobin levels.

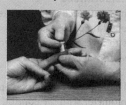 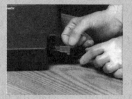 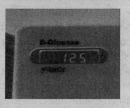

disposable microcuvette functions as a combination pipette, test tube, and measuring vessel. It contains a reagent that produces a precise chemical reaction as soon as it contacts blood. The photometer is powered by a battery or an AC adapter. One model is calibrated at the factory and seldom needs to be recalibrated, returning to zero between tests. Use the control cuvette included with each system to test photometer function. (See *How to use a bedside blood glucose and hemoglobin monitor.*)

Normal glucose values range from 70 to 100 mg/dl. An above-normal glucose level (hyperglycemia) may indicate diabetes mellitus or the use of steroid drugs. A below-normal glucose level may indicate overly rapid glucose use, which may occur with strenuous exercise or infection, resulting in tissues receiving insufficient glucose.

Normal Hb values range from 12.5 to 15 g/dl. A below-normal Hb value may indicate anemia, recent hemorrhage, or fluid retention, causing hemodilution. An elevated Hb value suggests hemoconcentration from polycythemia or dehydration.

Key nursing diagnoses and patient outcomes

Deficient knowledge related to lack of exposure to the procedure
The patient will:
▶ verbalize an understanding of the need for the procedure.

Anxiety related to lack of exposure to the procedure
The patient will:
▶ verbalize feelings of anxiety related to the procedure.

Equipment

Microcuvette • photometer • gloves • alcohol pad • gauze pads

Implementation

▶ Take the equipment to the patient's bedside and explain the test purpose to the patient. Tell him that he'll feel a pinprick in his finger during blood sampling.

▶ Plug the AC adapter into the photometer power inlet. Plug the other end of the adapter into the wall outlet.

▶ Turn the photometer on. If it hasn't been used recently, insert the control cuvette *to make sure that the photometer is working properly.*

▶ Wash your hands and put on gloves.

▶ Select an appropriate puncture site. You'll usually use a fingertip or an earlobe for an adult. The middle and fourth fingers are the best choices. The second finger is usually the most sensitive, and the thumb may have thickened skin or calluses. Blood should circulate freely in the finger from which you're collecting blood, so avoid using a ring-bearing finger.

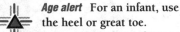 **Age alert** For an infant, use the heel or great toe.

▶ Keep the patient's finger straight and ask him to relax it. Holding his finger between the thumb and index finger of your nondominant hand, gently rock the patient's finger as you move your fingers from his top knuckle to his fingertip. *This causes blood to flow to the sampling point.*

▶ Use an alcohol pad to clean the puncture site, wiping in a circular motion from the center of the site outward. Dry the site thoroughly with a gauze pad.

▶ Pierce the skin quickly and sharply with the microcuvette, which automatically collects about 5 µl of blood.

▶ Place the microcuvette into the photometer. Results will appear on the photometer screen within 40 seconds to 4 minutes.

▶ Place a gauze pad over the puncture site until the bleeding stops.

▶ Dispose of the microcuvette according to your facility's policy. Take off your gloves and wash your hands. Notify the doctor if the test result is outside the expected parameters.

Special considerations

▶ Before using a microcuvette, note its expiration date. Microcuvettes can be stored for up to 2 years; however, after the microcuvette vial is opened, the shelf life is 90 days.

▶ Before collecting a blood sample, operate the photometer with the control cuvette to check for proper function. *To ensure an adequate blood sample,* don't use a cold, cyanotic, or swollen area as the puncture site.

Documentation

Document the values obtained from the photometer as well as the date and time of the test and any interventions performed.

BEDSIDE SPIROMETRY

Bedside spirometry measures forced vital capacity (FVC) and forced expiratory volume (FEV), allowing calculation of other pulmonary function indices such as timed forced expiratory flow rate. Depending on the type of spirometer used, bedside spirometry can also directly measure vital capacity and tidal volume. (See *Digital bedside spirometer.*)

Bedside spirometry aids in diagnosing pulmonary dysfunction before it appears on an X-ray or physical examination, evaluating its severity and determining the patient's response to therapy. Allowing assessment of the relationship of flow rate to vital capacity helps distinguish between obstructive and restrictive pulmonary disease. It's also useful for evaluating preoperative anesthesia risk. Because the required breathing patterns can aggravate conditions such as bronchospasm, use of the bedside spirometer requires a review of the patient's history and close observation during testing.

Key nursing diagnoses and patient outcomes

Ineffective breathing pattern related to (specify)
The patient will:
▶ report discomfort while breathing
▶ achieve maximum lung expansion with adequate ventilation.

Impaired gas exchange related to altered oxygen supply
The patient will:
▶ maintain a respiratory rate within 5 breaths/minute of baseline
▶ express a feeling of comfort in maintaining air exchange
▶ have normal breath sounds.

Equipment

Spirometer • disposable mouthpiece • breathing tube, if required • spirographic chart, if required • chart and pen, if required • optional: vital capacity predicted-values table and noseclips

Preparation of equipment

Review the manufacturer's instructions for assembly and use of the spirometer. If necessary, firmly insert the breathing tube *to ensure a tight connection.* If the

Digital bedside spirometer

Various models of bedside spirometers are commercially available. The instrument shown below has a digital readout. Other models display results on an individual chart record or on a roll of chart paper.

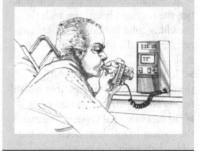

tube comes preconnected, check the seals for tightness and the tubing for leaks.

Check the operation of the recording mechanism and insert a chart and pen, if necessary. Insert the disposable mouthpiece and make sure it's tightly sealed.

Implementation

▶ Explain the procedure to the patient. Emphasize that his cooperation is essential *to ensure accurate results.*
▶ Instruct the patient to remove or loosen any constricting clothing, such as a bra, *to prevent alteration of test results from restricted thoracic expansion and abdominal mobility.*
▶ Instruct the patient to void *to prevent abdominal discomfort.*
▶ Don't perform pulmonary function tests immediately after a large meal *because the patient will experience abdominal discomfort.*

▶ If the patient wears dentures that fit poorly, remove them *to prevent incomplete closure of his mouth, which could allow air to leak around the mouthpiece.* If his dentures fit well, leave them in place *to promote a tight seal.*

▶ Plug in the spirometer and set the baseline time.

▶ If desired, allow the patient to practice the required breathing with the breathing tube unhooked. After practice, replace the tube and check the seal.

▶ Tell the patient not to breathe through his nose. If the patient has difficulty complying, apply noseclips.

▶ To measure vital capacity, instruct the patient to inhale as deeply as possible; then insert the mouthpiece so that his lips are sealed tightly around it *to prevent air leakage and to ensure an accurate digital readout or spirogram recording.*

▶ Tell him to exhale completely. Then remove the mouthpiece *to avoid recording his next inspiration.*

▶ Allow the patient to rest and repeat the procedure twice.

▶ To measure FEV and FVC, repeat this procedure with the chart or timer on but instruct the patient to exhale as quickly and completely as possible. Tell him when to start and turn on the recorder or timer at the same time.

▶ Allow the patient to rest and repeat the procedure twice.

▶ After completing the procedure, discard the mouthpiece, remove the spirographic chart, and follow the manufacturer's instructions for cleaning and sterilizing.

Special considerations

▶ Encourage the patient during the test; *this may help him to exhale more*

forcefully, which can be significant. If the patient coughs during expiration, wait until coughing subsides before repeating the measurement.

▶ Read the vital capacity directly from the readout or spirogram chart. The FVC is the highest volume recorded on the curve. Of the three trials, accept the highest recorded exhalation as the vital capacity result.

▶ To determine the percentage of predicted vital capacity, first determine the patient's predicted value from the vital capacity predicted-values table; then calculate the percentage by using the following formula:

$$\frac{\text{observed vital capacity} \times 100}{\text{predicted vital capacity}}$$

$$= \% \text{ predicted vital capacity}$$

▶ To determine the FEV for a specified time, mark the point on the spirogram where it crosses the desired time, and draw a straight line from this point to the side of the chart, which indicates volume in liters. This measurement is usually calculated for 1, 2, and 3 seconds and reported as a percentage of vital capacity. A healthy patient will have exhaled 75%, 85%, and 95%, respectively, of his FVC. Calculate this percentage by using the following formula:

$$\frac{\text{observed FEV} \times 100}{\text{predicted vital capacity}}$$

$$= \% \text{ vital capacity}$$

Complications

Forced exhalation can cause dizziness or light-headedness, precipitate or worsen bronchospasm, rapidly increase exhaustion (possibly to where the patient will require mechanical support), and increase air trapping in the emphysemic patient.

Documentation
Record the date and time of the procedure; the observed and calculated values, including FEV at 1, 2, and 3 seconds; any complications and the nursing action taken; and the patient's tolerance of the procedure.

BLADDER ULTRASONOGRAPHY

Urine retention, a potentially life-threatening condition, may result from neurologic or psychological disorders or from the obstruction of urine flow. Medications, such as anticholinergics, antihistamines, and antidepressants, may also cause urine retention. Traditionally, the amount of urine retained in the bladder was measured by urinary catheterization, placing the patient at risk for infection. Noninvasive bladder ultrasonography provides an assessment of bladder volume while lowering the risk of urinary tract infection.

Key nursing diagnoses and patient outcomes
Impaired urinary elimination related to urine retention
The patient will:
▶ maintain fluid balance (intake will equal output)
▶ voice increased comfort
▶ voice an understanding of treatment.

Equipment
BladderScan unit with scanhead • ultrasonic transmission gel • alcohol pads • washcloth • gloves

Implementation
▶ Bring the BladderScan unit to the bedside. Explain the procedure to the patient *to help reduce the patient's anxiety*. Wash your hands.
▶ Provide privacy. If this is a postvoiding scan, ask the patient to void; assist him; if necessary. Position the patient in a supine position.
▶ Put on gloves and clean the rounded end of the scanhead with an alcohol pad.
▶ Expose the patient's suprapubic area.
▶ Turn on the BladderScan by pressing the button (designated by a dot within a circle) on the far left and then press SCAN.
▶ Place ultrasonic gel on the scanhead *to promote an airtight seal and optimal sound-wave transmission*.
▶ Tell the patient that the gel will feel cold when placed on the abdomen. Locate the symphysis pubis and place the scanhead about 1″ (2.5 cm) above the symphysis pubis.
▶ Locate the icon (a rough figure of a patient) on the probe and make sure the head of the icon points toward the head of the patient.
▶ Press the scanhead button marked with a sound-wave pattern to activate the scan. Hold the scanhead steady until you hear the beep.
▶ Look at the aiming icon and screen, which displays the bladder position and volume. Reposition the probe and scan until the bladder is centered in the aiming screen. The largest measurement will be saved.
▶ Press DONE when finished.
▶ The BladderScan will display the measured urine volume and the longitudinal and horizontal axis scans.
▶ Press PRINT to obtain a hard copy of your results.

▶ Turn off the BladderScan. Use an alcohol pad to clean the gel off the scanhead.

▶ Using a washcloth, remove the gel from the patient's skin.

▶ Remove your gloves and wash your hands.

Documentation

Write the patient's name, the date, and the time on the printout and attach it to the patient's medical record. Also document the procedure and urine volume as well as any treatment in the patient's medical record.

BLOOD CULTURE

Normally bacteria-free, blood is susceptible to infection through infusion lines as well as from thrombophlebitis, infected shunts, and bacterial endocarditis due to prosthetic heart valve replacements. Bacteria may also invade the vascular system from local tissue infections through the lymphatic system and the thoracic duct.

Blood cultures are performed to detect bacterial invasion (bacteremia) and the systemic spread of such an infection (septicemia) through the bloodstream. In this procedure, a laboratory technician, doctor, or nurse collects a venous blood sample by venipuncture at the patient's bedside and then transfers it into two bottles, one containing an anaerobic medium and the other, an aerobic medium. The bottles are incubated, encouraging any organisms that are present in the sample to grow in the media. Blood cultures identify 67% of pathogens within 24 hours and up to 90% within 72 hours. Although some authorities consider the timing of culture collections debatable and possibly

irrelevant, others advocate drawing three blood samples at least 1 hour apart. The first of these should be collected at the earliest sign of suspected bacteremia or septicemia. To check for suspected bacterial endocarditis, collect three or four samples at 5- to 30-minute intervals before starting antibiotic therapy.

Key nursing diagnoses and patient outcomes

Risk for infection related to (specify)
The patient will:
▶ maintain a normal body temperature
▶ have no pathogens in blood cultures
▶ have a normal white blood cell count and differential.

Equipment

Tourniquet • gloves • alcohol or povidone-iodine pads • 10-ml syringe for an adult; 6-ml syringe for a child • three or four 20G 1″ needles • two or three blood culture bottles (50-ml bottles for adults, 20-ml bottles for infants and children) with sodium polyethanol sulfonate added (one aerobic bottle containing a suitable medium, such as Trypticase soy broth with 10% carbon dioxide atmosphere; one anaerobic bottle with prereduced medium; and, possibly, one hyperosmotic bottle with 10% sucrose medium) • laboratory request form • 2″ × 2″ gauze pads • small adhesive bandages • labels

Preparation of equipment

Check the expiration dates on the culture bottles and replace outdated bottles.

Implementation

▶ Tell the patient that you need to collect a series of blood samples to check for infection. Explain the procedure *to ease his anxiety and promote cooperation.* Explain that the procedure usually requires three blood samples collected at different times.

▶ Wash your hands and put on gloves.

▶ Tie a tourniquet 2″ (5 cm) proximal to the area chosen.

▶ Clean the venipuncture site with an alcohol or a povidone-iodine pad. Don't wipe off the povidone-iodine with alcohol *because alcohol cancels the effect of povidone-iodine.* Start at the site and work outward in a circular motion. Wait 30 to 60 seconds for the skin to dry.

▶ Perform a venipuncture, drawing 10 ml of blood from an adult.

▶ Remove the tourniquet. Apply pressure to the venipuncture site using a 2″ × 2″ dressing. Then cover the site with a small adhesive bandage.

Age alert **Draw only 2 to 6 ml of blood from a child.**

▶ Wipe the diaphragm tops of the culture bottles with a povidone-iodine pad, and change the needle on the syringe used to draw the blood.

▶ Inject 5 ml of blood into each 50-ml bottle or 2 ml into each 20-ml pediatric culture bottle. (Bottle size may vary according to the facility's protocol, but the sample dilution should always be 1:10.)

▶ Label the culture bottles with the patient's name and room number, doctor's name, and date and time of collection. Indicate the suspected diagnosis and the patient's temperature and note on the laboratory request form any recent antibiotic therapy. Send the samples to the laboratory immediately.

▶ Discard syringes, needles, and gloves in the appropriate containers.

Special considerations

▶ Obtain each set of cultures from a different site.

▶ Avoid using existing blood lines for cultures unless the sample is drawn when the line is inserted or catheter sepsis is suspected.

Complications

The most common complication of venipuncture is formation of a hematoma. If a hematoma develops, apply warm soaks to the site.

Documentation

Record the date and time of blood sample collection, name of the test, amount of blood collected, number of bottles used, patient's temperature, and adverse reactions to the procedure.

BLOOD GLUCOSE TESTS

Rapid, easy-to-perform reagent strip tests (such as Glucostix, Chemstrip bG, and Multistix) use a drop of capillary blood obtained by fingerstick, heelstick, or earlobe puncture as a sample. These tests can detect or monitor elevated blood glucose levels in patients with diabetes, screen for diabetes mellitus and neonatal hypoglycemia, and help distinguish diabetic coma from nondiabetic coma. They can be performed in the facility, the doctor's office, or the patient's home.

In blood glucose tests, a reagent patch on the tip of a handheld plastic strip changes color in response to the amount of glucose in the blood sample. Comparing the color change with a standardized color chart provides a semiquantitative measurement of blood glucose levels; inserting the strip in a portable blood glucose meter (such as Accu-Chek Easy and One Touch) provides quantitative measurements that compare in accuracy with other laboratory tests. Some meters store successive test results electronically to help determine glucose patterns.

Key nursing diagnoses and patient outcomes

Deficient knowledge related to lack of exposure to blood glucose testing
The patient will:
▶ verbalize an understanding of the procedure
▶ demonstrate the correct procedure for blood glucose testing
▶ identify parameters for reporting results to the health care provider.

Health seeking behaviors related to elevated blood glucose levels
The patient will:
▶ identify risk factors for elevated blood glucose levels
▶ verbalize the effects of elevated blood glucose levels
▶ state measures to increase control over blood glucose levels.

Equipment

Reagent strips • gloves • portable blood glucose meter, if available • alcohol pads • gauze pads • disposable lancets or mechanical blood-letting device • small adhesive bandage • watch or clock with a second hand

Implementation

▶ Explain the procedure to the patient or the child's parents.
▶ Next, select the puncture site — usually the fingertip or earlobe for an adult or a child.

 Age alert Select the heel or great toe for an infant.

▶ Wash your hands and put on gloves.

▶ If necessary, dilate the capillaries by applying warm, moist compresses to the area for about 10 minutes.
▶ Wipe the puncture site with an alcohol pad and dry it thoroughly with a gauze pad.
▶ To collect a sample from the fingertip with a disposable lancet (smaller than 2 mm), position the lancet on the side of the patient's fingertip, perpendicular to the lines of the fingerprints. Pierce the skin sharply and quickly *to minimize the patient's anxiety and pain and to increase blood flow.* Alternatively, you can use a mechanical blood-letting device such as an Autolet, which uses a spring-loaded lancet.
▶ After puncturing the fingertip, don't squeeze the puncture site *to avoid diluting the sample with tissue fluid.*
▶ Touch a drop of blood to the reagent patch on the strip; make sure you cover the entire patch.
▶ After collecting the blood sample, briefly apply pressure to the puncture site *to prevent painful extravasation of blood into subcutaneous tissues.* Ask the adult patient to hold a gauze pad firmly over the puncture site until bleeding stops.
▶ Make sure you leave the blood on the strip for exactly 60 seconds.
▶ Compare the color change on the strip with the standardized color chart on the product container. If you're using a blood glucose meter, follow the manufacturer's instructions. Meter designs vary, but they all analyze a drop of blood placed on a reagent strip that comes with the unit and provide a digital display of the resulting glucose level.
▶ After bleeding has stopped, you may apply a small adhesive bandage to the puncture site.

Oral and I.V. glucose tolerance tests

For monitoring trends in glucose metabolism, these two tests may offer benefits over blood testing with reagent strips.

Oral glucose tolerance test

The most sensitive test for detecting borderline diabetes mellitus, the oral glucose tolerance test (OGTT) measures carbohydrate metabolism after ingestion of a challenge dose of glucose. The body absorbs this dose rapidly, causing plasma glucose levels to rise and peak within 30 minutes to 1 hour. The pancreas responds by secreting insulin, causing glucose levels to return to normal within 2 to 3 hours. During this period, plasma and urine glucose levels are monitored to assess insulin secretion and the body's ability to metabolize glucose.

Although you may not collect the blood and urine specimens (usually five of each) required for this test, you are responsible for preparing the patient for the test and monitoring his physical condition during the test.

Begin by explaining the OGTT to the patient. Then tell him to maintain a high-carbohydrate diet for 3 days and to fast for 10 to 16 hours before the test as ordered. The patient must not smoke, drink coffee or alcohol, or exercise strenuously for 8 hours before the test or during the test. Inform him that he'll then receive a challenge dose of 100 g of carbohydrate (usually a sweetened carbonated beverage or gelatin).

Tell the patient who will perform the venipunctures and when and that he may feel slight discomfort from the needle punctures and the pressure of the tourniquet. Reassure him that collecting each blood sample usually takes less than 3 minutes. As ordered, withhold drugs that may affect test results. Remind him not to discard the first urine specimen voided after waking.

During the test period, watch for signs and symptoms of hypoglycemia — weakness, restlessness, nervousness, hunger, and sweating — and report them to the doctor immediately. Encourage the patient to drink plenty of water to promote adequate urine excretion. Provide a bedpan, urinal, or specimen container when necessary.

I.V. glucose tolerance test

The I.V. glucose tolerance test may be chosen for patients who are unable to absorb an oral dose of glucose, for example, those with malabsorption disorders and short-bowel syndrome or those who have had a gastrectomy. This test measures blood glucose after an I.V. infusion of 50% glucose over 3 to 4 minutes. Blood samples are then collected after 30 minutes, 1 hour, 2 hours, and 3 hours. After an immediate glucose peak of 300 to 400 mg/dl (accompanied by glycosuria), the normal glucose curve falls steadily, reaching fasting levels within 1 to 1¼ hours. Failure to achieve fasting glucose levels within 2 to 3 hours typically confirms diabetes.

Special considerations

▶ To help detect abnormal glucose metabolism and diagnose diabetes mellitus, the doctor may order other blood glucose tests. (See *Oral and I.V. glucose tolerance tests.*)

▶ Before using reagent strips, check the expiration date on the package and replace outdated strips. Check for special instructions related to the specific reagent. The reagent area of a fresh strip should match the color of the "0" block on the color chart. Protect the strips from light, heat, and moisture.

▶ Before using a blood glucose meter, calibrate it and run it with a control sample *to ensure accurate test results.* Follow the manufacturer's instructions for calibration.

▶ Avoid selecting cold, cyanotic, or swollen puncture sites *to ensure an adequate blood sample.* If you can't obtain a capillary sample, perform venipuncture and place a large drop of venous blood on the reagent strip. If you want to test blood from a refrigerated sample, allow the blood to return to room temperature before testing it.

Home care

If the patient will be using the reagent strip system at home, teach him the proper use of the lancet or Autolet, reagent strips and color chart, and portable blood glucose meter as necessary. Also provide written guidelines.

Documentation

Record the reading from the reagent strip (using a portable blood glucose meter or a color chart) in your notes or on a special flowchart, if available. Also record the time and date of the test.

BODY MECHANICS

Many patient care activities require the nurse to push, pull, lift, and carry. By using proper body mechanics, the nurse can avoid musculoskeletal injury and fatigue and reduce the risk of injuring patients. Correct body mechanics can be summed up in three principles, as presented below.

Keep a low center of gravity by flexing the hips and knees instead of bending at the waist. This position distributes weight evenly between the upper and lower body and helps maintain balance.

Create a wide base of support by spreading the feet apart. This tactic provides lateral stability and lowers the body's center of gravity.

Maintain proper body alignment and keep the body's center of gravity directly over the base of support by moving the feet rather than twisting and bending at the waist.

Key nursing diagnoses and patient outcomes

Risk for injury related to improper use of body mechanics
The patient will:
▶ experience no physical injury related to improper body mechanics
▶ verbalize an understanding of proper body mechanics
▶ demonstrate proper use of body mechanics.

Deficient knowledge related to lack of exposure to proper body mechanics
The patient will:
▶ verbalize an understanding of proper body mechanics
▶ demonstrate proper use of body mechanics.

Implementation

Follow the directions below to push, pull, stoop, lift, and carry correctly.

Pushing and pulling correctly

▶ Stand close to the object, and place one foot slightly ahead of the other, as in a walking position. Tighten the leg muscles and set the pelvis by simultaneously contracting the abdominal and gluteal muscles.
▶ To push, place your hands on the object and flex your elbows. Lean into the object by shifting weight from the

back leg to the front leg and apply smooth, continuous pressure.
▶ To pull, grasp the object and flex your elbows. Lean away from the object by shifting weight from the front leg to the back leg. Pull smoothly, avoiding sudden, jerky movements.
▶ After you've started to move the object, keep it in motion; *stopping and starting uses more energy.*

Stooping correctly
▶ Stand with your feet 10" to 12" (25 to 30 cm) apart and one foot slightly ahead of the other *to widen the base of support.*
▶ Lower yourself by flexing your knees and place more weight on the front foot than on the back foot. Keep the upper body straight by not bending at the waist.
▶ To stand up again, straighten the knees and keep the back straight.

Lifting and carrying correctly
▶ Assume the stooping position directly in front of the object *to minimize back flexion and to avoid spinal rotation when lifting.*
▶ Grasp the object and tighten your abdominal muscles.
▶ Stand up by straightening the knees, using the leg and hip muscles. Always keep your back straight *to maintain a fixed center of gravity.*
▶ Carry the object close to your body at waist height — near the body's center of gravity — *to avoid straining the back muscles.*

Special considerations
▶ Wear shoes with low heels, flexible nonslip soles, and closed backs *to promote correct body alignment, facilitate*

proper body mechanics, and prevent accidents.
▶ When possible, pull rather than push an object *because the elbow flexors are stronger than the extensors.*
▶ When doing heavy lifting or moving, remember to use assistive or mechanical devices, if available, or obtain assistance from coworkers; know your limitations and use sound judgment.

BONE MARROW ASPIRATION AND BIOPSY

A specimen of bone marrow — the major site of blood cell formation — may be obtained by aspiration or needle biopsy. The procedure allows evaluation of overall blood composition by studying blood elements and precursor cells as well as abnormal or malignant cells. Aspiration removes cells through a needle inserted into the marrow cavity of the bone; a biopsy removes a small, solid core of marrow tissue through the needle. Both procedures are usually performed by a doctor, but some facilities authorize specially trained chemotherapy nurses or nurse clinicians to perform them with an assistant.

Aspirates aid in diagnosing various disorders and cancers, such as oat cell carcinoma, leukemia, and lymphomas such as Hodgkin's disease. Biopsies are often performed simultaneously to stage the disease and monitor response to treatment.

Key nursing diagnoses and patient outcomes
Anxiety related to situational crisis
The patient will:

► identify factors that elicit anxious behaviors

► discuss activities that tend to decrease anxious behaviors

► cope with current medical situation (specify) without experiencing severe signs or symptoms of anxiety (specify for individual).

Disturbed body image related to potential medical treatments
The patient will:

► express positive feelings about self

► acknowledge change in body image.

Equipment

For aspiration

Prepackaged bone marrow set, which includes povidone-iodine pads • two sterile drapes (one fenestrated, one plain) • ten 4″ × 4″ sterile gauze pads • ten 2″ × 2″ sterile gauze pads • two 12-ml syringes • 22G 1″ or 2″ needle • scalpel • sedative • specimen containers • bone marrow needle • 70% isopropyl alcohol • 1% lidocaine (unopened bottle) • 26G or 27G ½″ to ⅝″ needle • adhesive tape • sterile gloves • glass slides and coverglass • labels

For biopsy

All equipment listed above • Vim-Silverman, Jamshidi, Illinois sternal, or Westerman-Jensen needle • Zenker's fixative

Implementation

► Tell the patient that the doctor will collect a bone marrow specimen and explain the procedure *to ease his anxiety and ensure cooperation.* Make sure the patient or a responsible family member understands the procedure and signs a consent form obtained by the doctor.

► Inform the patient that the procedure normally takes 5 to 10 minutes, that test results usually are available in 1 day, and that more than one marrow specimen may be required.

► Check the patient's history for hypersensitivity to the local anesthetic. Tell him which bone — sternum or posterior superior or anterior iliac crest — will be sampled. Inform him that he will receive a local anesthetic and will feel heavy pressure from insertion of the biopsy or aspiration needle as well as a brief, pulling sensation. Tell him that the doctor may make a small incision to avoid tearing the skin.

► If the patient has osteoporosis, tell him that the needle pressure may be minimal; if he has osteopetrosis, inform him that a drill may be needed.

► Provide a sedative as ordered before the test.

► Position the patient according to the selected puncture site. (See *Common sites for bone marrow aspiration and biopsy.*)

► Using sterile technique, the puncture site is cleaned with povidone-iodine pads and allowed to dry; then the area is draped.

► To anesthetize the site, the doctor infiltrates it with 1% lidocaine, using a 26G or 27G ½″ to ⅝″ needle *to inject a small amount intradermally* and then a larger 22G 1″ to 2″ needle *to anesthetize the tissue down to the bone.*

► When the needle tip reaches the bone, the doctor anesthetizes the periosteum by injecting a small amount of lidocaine in a circular area about ¾″ (2 cm) in diameter. The needle should be withdrawn from the periosteum after each injection.

► After allowing about 1 minute for the lidocaine to take effect, a scalpel

Common sites for bone marrow aspiration and biopsy

The posterior iliac crest is the preferred site for bone marrow aspiration because no vital organs or vessels are nearby. The patient is placed either in the lateral position with one leg flexed or in the prone position.

For aspiration or biopsy from the anterior iliac crest, the patient is placed in the supine or side-lying position. This site is used with patients who can't lie prone because of severe abdominal distention.

Aspiration from the sternum involves the greatest risk but may be used because this site is near the surface, the cortical bone is thin, and the marrow cavity contains numerous cells and relatively little fat or supporting bone. This site is seldom used for biopsy.

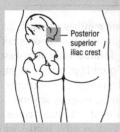
Posterior superior iliac crest

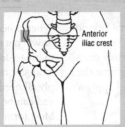
Anterior iliac crest

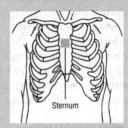
Sternum

may be used to make a small stab incision in the patient's skin to accommodate the bone marrow needle. *This technique avoids pushing skin into the bone marrow and also helps avoid unnecessary skin tearing to help reduce the risk of infection.*

Bone marrow aspiration
▶ The doctor inserts the bone marrow needle and lodges it firmly in the bone cortex. If the patient feels sharp pain instead of pressure when the needle first touches bone, the needle was probably inserted outside the anesthetized area. If this happens, the needle should be withdrawn slightly and moved to the anesthetized area.
▶ The needle is advanced by applying an even, downward force with the heel of the hand or the palm, while twisting

it back and forth slightly. A crackling sensation means that the needle has entered the marrow cavity.
▶ Next, the doctor removes the inner cannula, attaches the syringe to the needle, aspirates the required specimen, and withdraws the needle. The specimen is placed on glass slides and covered with the coverglass. Label the specimen with the patient's name and the date.
▶ Put on gloves and apply pressure to the aspiration site with a gauze pad for 5 minutes *to control bleeding* while an assistant prepares the marrow slides. Clean the area with alcohol *to remove the povidone-iodine,* dry the skin thoroughly with a 4″ × 4″ gauze pad, and apply a sterile pressure dressing.

Bone marrow biopsy

▶ The doctor inserts the biopsy needle into the periosteum and advances it steadily until the outer needle passes into the marrow cavity.

▶ The biopsy needle is directed into the marrow cavity by alternately rotating the inner needle clockwise and counterclockwise. Then a plug of tissue is removed, the needle assembly is withdrawn, and the marrow specimen is expelled into a properly labeled specimen bottle containing Zenker's fixative or formaldehyde.

▶ Put on gloves, clean the area around the biopsy site with alcohol *to remove the povidone-iodine solution,* firmly press a sterile 2″ × 2″ gauze pad against the incision *to control bleeding,* and apply a sterile pressure dressing.

Special considerations

▶ Faulty needle placement may yield too little aspirate. If no specimen is produced, the needle must be withdrawn from the bone (but not from the overlying soft tissue), the stylet replaced, and the needle inserted into a second site within the anesthetized field.

▶ Bone marrow specimens shouldn't be collected from irradiated areas *because radiation may have altered or destroyed the marrow.*

Complications

Bleeding and infection are potentially life-threatening complications of aspiration or biopsy at any site.

Complications of sternal needle puncture are uncommon but include puncture of the heart and major vessels, causing severe hemorrhage; puncture of the mediastinum, causing mediastinitis or pneumomediastinum; and

puncture of the lung, causing pneumothorax.

If a hematoma occurs around the puncture site, apply warm soaks. Give analgesics for site pain or tenderness.

Documentation

Chart the time, date, location, and patient's tolerance of the procedure and the specimen obtained.

BOTTLE-FEEDING

When a neonate requires a special diet or when a mother can't or chooses not to breast-feed, formula is the next-best food source. Formula preparations supply all needed vitamins and nutrients and can be administered by anyone. Most formulas used in facilities come ready-to-feed in disposable bottles with disposable nipples. Some formulas and equipment, however, may require advance preparation, such as mixing and sterilization. The American Academy of Pediatrics (AAP) recommends the use of commercially prepared formula over animal milks or homemade preparations for the infant's first year.

Because formulas must be sterile, they're prepared either by the aseptic method (in which all articles used in formula preparation are sterilized before mixing) or by the terminal heat method (in which the formula is prepared with clean technique and then sterilized using a home sterilizer). In the United States, some pediatricians recommend clean technique and tap water for formulas because water supplies are clean and safe in most areas.

A normal neonate takes 15 to 20 minutes to consume a 1 to 1½-oz (30-

to 45-ml) portion of formula and usually feeds every 3 to 4 hours.

Key nursing diagnoses and patient outcomes

Deficient knowledge related to performing bottle-feeding
The neonate's parents will:
► express increased confidence to perform appropriate feeding techniques
► set realistic learning goals for developing bottle-feeding competence
► report that the neonate gains adequate weight.

Anxiety related to difficulty with bottle-feeding
The neonate's parents will:
► express feelings of anxiety
► identify causes of anxiety
► use emotional support
► verbalize a decrease in feelings of anxiety.

Equipment

Commercially prepared formula or ingredients • bottle, nipple, and cap • tissue or cloth • gown

Preparation of equipment

If you're using commercially prepared formula, uncap the formula bottle and make sure the seal wasn't previously broken *to ensure sterility and freshness.* Then screw on the nipple and cap. Keep the protective sterile cap over the nipple until the neonate is ready to feed. If you're preparing formula, follow the manufacturer's instructions or the doctor's prescription. Administer the formula at room temperature or slightly warmer.

Implementation

► Wash your hands.

► Invert the bottle and shake some formula on your wrist *to test the patency of the nipple hole and the formula's temperature.* The nipple hole should allow formula to drip freely but not to stream out. *If the hole is too large, the neonate may aspirate formula; if it's too small, the extra sucking effort he expends may tire him before he can empty the bottle.*

► Sit comfortably in a semi-reclining position and cradle the neonate in one arm to support his head and back. *This position allows swallowed air to rise to the top of the stomach where it's more easily expelled.* If he can't be held, sit by him and elevate his head and shoulders slightly.

► Place the nipple in the neonate's mouth while making sure the tongue is down, but don't insert it so far that it stimulates the gag reflex. He should begin to suck, pulling in as much nipple as is comfortable. If he doesn't start to suck, stroke him under the chin or on his cheek, or touch his lips with the nipple *to stimulate his sucking reflex.*

► As the neonate feeds, tilt the bottle upward *to keep the nipple filled with formula and to prevent him from swallowing air.* Watch for a steady stream of bubbles in the bottle. This indicates proper venting and flow of formula. If the neonate pushes out the nipple with his tongue, reinsert the nipple. *Expelling the nipple is a normal reflex. It doesn't necessarily mean that the neonate is full.*

► Always hold the bottle for a neonate. If left to feed himself, he may aspirate formula or swallow air if the bottle tilts or empties. *Experts link bottle propping with an increased incidence of otitis media and dental caries in older infants.*

► Burp the neonate after each ½ oz of formula *because he'll typically swallow some air even when fed correctly.* Hold the neonate upright in a slightly forward position, supporting his head and chest with one hand. Or, position a clean cloth *to protect your clothing,* and hold the neonate upright over your shoulder or place him face down across your lap. *The change in position helps the gas to rise or "bring up the bubble."* In either case, rub or gently pat his back until he expels the air.

▶ After you finish feeding and burping the neonate, place him on his back as recommended by the AAP. Neonates are prone to regurgitation because of an immature cardiac sphincter. *Positioning on the back has been demonstrated to reduce the incidence of sudden infant death syndrome.*

▶ Discard any remaining formula, and properly dispose of all equipment.

Special considerations

▶ Change feeding duration by changing the size of the nipple or the nipple hole; *the neonate tires if he feeds too long, and his sucking needs aren't met if he doesn't feed long enough.*

▶ Be sure to note how much formula is in the bottle before and after the feeding. Use the calibrations along the side of the container to calculate the amount of formula consumed.

▶ Be alert for aspiration in the neonate who has a diminished sucking or swallowing reflex and who may have difficulty feeding. Also take appropriate measures according to facility policy to feed the neonate with cleft lip and palate.

▶ Teach parents how to properly prepare and (if required) sterilize formula, bottles, and nipples, and how to feed and burp the neonate. Although most hospitals have a feeding schedule, advise the mother that she may switch to a more flexible demand-feeding schedule when at home. Forewarn her that

the neonate may not feed well on his 1st day home because of the new activity and environment. Inform parents about the forms of formula available (ready-to-feed, concentrate, powders) *so that they can choose the most convenient form.*

▶ Prepare parents to expect the neonate to regurgitate formula. Explain that regurgitation (merely an overflow that typically follows feeding) shouldn't be confused with vomiting (a more complete emptying of the stomach accompanied by symptoms not associated with feeding).

Complications

Bottle-propping may allow the nipple to block the airway, causing suffocation; it may also lead to otitis media or dental caries. Lung infection or death may follow aspiration of regurgitated formula.

Documentation

Record the time of the feeding, the amount of formula consumed, how well the neonate fed, and whether he appeared satisfied. Note any regurgitation or vomiting. If the mother feeds the neonate, observe and describe their interactions. Document any patient teaching.

BREAST-FEEDING ASSISTANCE

Breast-feeding is the safest, simplest, and least expensive way to provide complete infant nourishment. Components of successful and satisfying breast-feeding include proper breast care, normal milk flow, and a comfortably positioned mother and infant.

Breast-feeding is contraindicated for a mother with a severe chronic condition, such as active tuberculosis, human immunodeficiency virus infection, or hepatitis.

Key nursing diagnoses and patient outcomes

Effective breast-feeding
The mother will:
▶ breast-feed the infant successfully and experience satisfaction with breast-feeding
▶ satisfactorily feed the infant on both breasts
▶ see the infant grow and develop normally.

Ineffective breast-feeding related to limited maternal experience
The mother will:
▶ express an understanding of breast-feeding techniques and practices
▶ display decreased anxiety
▶ successfully breast-feed.

Equipment

Nursing or support bra • pillow • protective cover, such as cloth diaper or small towel • optional: commercially available breast pads without plastic liners, or pads made from sanitary napkins, gauze, cloth diapers, or cotton handkerchiefs; instructional materials

Implementation

▶ Explain the procedure to the mother and provide privacy.
▶ Encourage the mother to drink a beverage before and during or after breast-feeding. *This ensures adequate fluid intake, which helps to maintain milk production.*
▶ Encourage the mother to attend to personal needs and to change the infant's wet or soiled diaper before breast-feeding begins *to avoid interruptions during feeding time.*
▶ Wash your hands and instruct the mother to wash hers.
▶ Help the mother find a comfortable position, for example, the cradle or side-lying position, *to promote the let-down reflex.* (See *Breast-feeding positions,* page 74.)
▶ Have her expose one breast and rest the nape of the infant's neck in the crook of her arm, supporting his back with her forearm.
▶ Urge the mother to relax during breast-feeding *because relaxation also promotes the letdown reflex.* Inform her that she may feel a tingling sensation when it occurs and that milk may drip or spray from her breasts. Tell her the reflex may also be initiated by hearing the infant's cry.
▶ Guiding the mother's free hand, have her place her thumb on top of the exposed breast's areola and her first two fingers beneath it, forming a "C" with her hand. Turn the infant so that he faces the breast.
▶ Tell the mother to stroke the infant's cheek located nearest to her exposed breast or the infant's mouth with the nipple. *This stimulates the rooting instinct.* Emphasize that she shouldn't touch the infant's other cheek *because he may turn his head toward the touch and away from the breast.*
▶ When the infant opens his mouth and roots for the nipple, instruct the mother to insert the nipple and as much of the areola as possible into his mouth. *This helps him to exert sufficient pressure with his lips, gums, and cheek muscles on the milk sinuses below the areola.*
▶ Check for occlusion of the infant's nostrils by the mother's breast. If this

Breast-feeding positions

Ordinarily, a maternity patient chooses a breast-feeding position that is comfortable and efficient. If the patient experiences discomfort in one position, she can choose another. In fact, by changing positions periodically, she can alter the infant's grasp on the nipple and thereby avoid contact friction on the same area. As appropriate, suggest the following typical breast-feeding positions.

Cradle position
The cradle position is the most common position for breast-feeding. The mother sits in a comfortable chair and cradles the infant's head in the crook of her arm. If desired, she can support her elbow with pillows *to minimize tension and fatigue.* She can also tuck the infant's lower arm alongside her body *so it stays out of the way.* The infant's mouth should remain even with the nipple, and his stomach should face and touch the mother's stomach.

Side-lying position
The mother may choose the side-lying position for breast-feeding at night or during recovery from a cesarean section. She lies on her side with her stomach facing the infant's and the infant's head near her breast, and as the infant's mouth opens, she pulls him toward the nipple.

Football position
Often selected by a mother with large breasts or one who has had a cesarean section, the football position is also useful for feeding twins or infants who are small or premature. The mother sits in a comfortable chair with a pillow under her arm on the nursing side. She places her hand under the infant's head and brings it close to the breast while placing the fingers of her other hand above and below the nipple. As the infant's mouth opens, she pulls his head close to her breast.

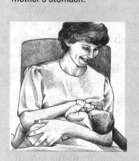
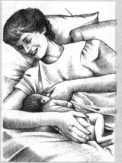
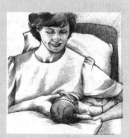

happens, reposition the infant to give him room to breathe.

▶ Suggest that the mother begin nursing the infant for 15 minutes on each breast.

▶ To alternate breasts, instruct the mother to slip a finger into the side of the infant's mouth *to break the seal* and move him to the other breast.

▶ *To burp the infant,* show the mother how to hold the infant in an upright forward-tilting position with one hand supporting his chest and chin. Tell her to gently pat or rub the infant's back *to*

Breast care for new mothers

A mother who plans to breast-feed her infant should prepare her breasts as directed by her doctor. After the infant's birth, she'll need to maintain breast tissue integrity. Although postpartum care varies for breast-feeding and non-breast-feeding mothers, both may benefit from the following guidelines.

For the breast-feeding mother
- Instruct the mother to wash her areolae and nipples with water, without soap or a washcloth, *to avoid washing away the natural oils and keratin.*
- Advise the mother with sore or irritated nipples to apply ice compresses just before breast-feeding. *This numbs and firms the nipples, making them less sensitive and easier for the infant to grasp.*
- Suggest that lubricating the nipple with a few drops of expressed breast milk before feeding may help prevent tenderness.
- Recommend placing breast pads over the nipples to collect colostrum or milk, which commonly leaks during the first few breast-feeding weeks. Advise replacing pads often *to guard against infection.*
- Inform the mother that breast milk comes in 2 to 5 days after delivery and is accompanied by a slight temperature elevation and breast changes—increased size, warmth, and firmness.

- Tell the mother that a well-fitting support bra may help control engorgement.
- Advise the mother with engorged breasts to apply warm compresses, massage the breasts, take a warm shower, or express some milk before feeding. *This dilates the milk ducts, promotes letdown, and makes the nipples more pliable.*

For the non-breast-feeding mother
- Instruct the mother to clean her breasts using the same technique as the breast-feeding mother. Add that she may use soap.
- Advise her to wear a support bra *to help minimize engorgement and to decrease nipple stimulation.*
- Advise her to avoid stimulating the nipples or manually expressing her milk *to minimize further milk production.* Instead, provide pain medication, as ordered, ice packs, or a breast binder.

expel any ingested air. Help her place a protective cover, such as a cloth diaper, under the infant's chin.

▶ Instruct the mother to feed the infant at the other breast. If she wishes and if the infant remains awake, she may nurse him longer. *A demand-feeding routine, in which the infant feeds according to his hunger and desire, establishes an abundant, steady milk supply appropriate for the infant's requirements (the more the infant needs, the more milk the mother produces). What's more, frequent*

nursing satisfies the infant's need to suck. It also promotes bonding.

▶ When the mother finishes breast-feeding, have her place the infant on his back. However, if the mother wishes to hold the infant longer, encourage her to do so. *Touching enhances bonding.*

▶ Instruct the mother to air-dry her nipples for 15 minutes after she finishes feeding and give her additional breast-care instructions as necessary. (See *Breast care for new mothers.*)

▶ Encourage the mother's breast-feeding efforts. To boost these efforts, urge her to eat balanced meals, to drink at least eight 8-oz glasses of fluid daily, and to nap daily for at least the first 2 weeks after giving birth. Answer her questions about breast-feeding and provide instructional materials if available. Before she goes home, inform her about local breast-feeding and parenting support groups such as La Leche League International.

▶ Observe the mother for breast engorgement. If traditional relief measures fail to trigger the letdown reflex, administer an analgesic to relieve discomfort. Also notify the doctor.

▶ Instruct the patient to report signs of mastitis — a red, tender, or warm breast and fever — which may occur after discharge.

Special considerations

▶ Instruct the mother to use the side-lying position for breast-feeding on the delivery table. *This reduces discomfort from pressure on the episiotomy (if she had one).* Or, you can adjust the table so that she can sit up. Because the mother will probably be exhausted from delivery or drowsy from medication, stay with her during this time.

▶ Inform the mother that infants routinely lose weight (several ounces) during the first days of life. Advise her that colostrum, her first milk, is yellow, rich in protein and antibodies, and secreted in small amounts. Her true milk, which is thin and bluish, won't appear for several days.

▶ Advise a mother who's breast-feeding twins that using the football position allows her to feed both infants at once. Instruct her to alternate breasts and infants at each feeding. If the mother

prefers to nurse one infant at a time, make sure the nursery and the mother both keep track of which infant came first during each feeding.

▶ Reassure her that there is no standard schedule for breast-feeding and that developing a comfortable breast-feeding routine takes time.

▶ Tell her to expect uterine cramping during breast-feeding until her uterus returns to its original size. *These contractions result from released oxytocin, a natural hormone that prompts the uterus to return to its prepregnancy state.* Oxytocin also initiates the letdown reflex, thereby allowing the milk to flow from the alveoli into the ducts.

▶ If the infant shows little interest in breast-feeding, reassure the mother that he may need several days to learn and to adjust. If the infant is sleepy, encourage the mother to offer the breast frequently but to refrain from forcing him to nurse. Instead, advise her to try rubbing the infant's feet, unwrapping his blanket, changing his diaper, changing her position or the infant's position, and manually expressing milk and then allowing the infant to suckle. *A balky infant may suck eagerly if milk is already flowing.*

▶ If the infant fails to nurse sufficiently and dehydration seems likely, have the mother give him expressed milk through a medicine dropper or small syringe. Instruct her to avoid frequent feeding with a bottle *because the infant may become used to the artificial nipple and subsequently reject the mother's.*

▶ Advise the mother to start breast-feeding with the breast she used last at the previous feeding *to help avoid breast engorgement.* Suggest attaching a safety pin to the bra strap supporting the breast she last used to serve as a reminder.

Complications

Breast engorgement may result from venous and lymphatic stasis and alveolar milk accumulation. Mastitis occurs postpartum in about 1% of mothers. It usually results from a pathogen that passes from the infant's nose or pharynx into breast tissue through a cracked or fissured nipple.

Documentation

After helping the mother breast-feed, note the areas in which she needs further instruction and help. Document patient teaching. Also document the time of feeding on each breast, the infant's suckling ability, the difficulty in arousing the infant, the positions of feeding, and an assessment of the mother's nipples.

BREAST PUMP USE

By creating suction, manual and electric breast pumps stimulate lactation. Indicated for a mother who wants to maintain milk production while she and her infant are separated or while illness temporarily incapacitates one or the other, or both, a breast pump also can relieve engorgement or collect milk for a premature infant with a weak sucking reflex.

The mother can also use a pump to reduce pressure on sore or cracked nipples or to reestablish her milk supply if a weaned infant becomes allergic to formula. Or, she can use it to collect milk from inverted nipples or to express milk mechanically when she can't express milk by hand or with a manual pump. Electric pumps are more effective and efficient than manual pumps. (See *Comparing breast pumps,* page 78.)

Key nursing diagnoses and patient outcomes

Deficient knowledge related to breast pump use
The neonate's mother will:
▶ verbalize an understanding of breast pump use
▶ demonstrate breast pump use
▶ express increased comfort with breast pump use.

Equipment

Manual cylinder or electric breast pump • sterile collection bag or bottle (to store milk if desired) • pillows • optional: warm compresses

An electric breast pump should come with a sterile, single-use accessory kit, which many pump manufacturers supply. The kit contains shields, milk cups, an overflow bottle, and tubing. These parts can be washed with soap and water and then sterilized for repeated use.

Preparation of equipment

Assemble the breast pump according to the manufacturer's instructions. If milk will be stored or frozen, thoroughly clean any removable parts that the milk will touch.

Implementation

▶ Explain the procedure to the patient.
▶ Give her time to attend to personal needs first *so she won't have to interrupt the procedure for this purpose.* Also, advise her to wash her hands.
▶ Instruct the patient to drink a beverage before and after breast pumping.

Comparing breast pumps

Breast pumps are available in battery-operated, electric, and hand-operated models. The pump that is best for your patient depends on such factors as the pump's purpose and the patient's situation. A description of common pumps and their features follows.

Battery-powered pump

Having a battery-powered motor, this pump can be operated with one hand. Easy to clean, it's a good choice for mothers who work outside the home or who need a breast pump only for short-term use.

Electric pump

Usually used in facilities, this gentle, efficient pump plugs into an electrical outlet and can be operated with one hand. It's available as a small 2-lb (0.9-kg) model or as a larger model about the size of a small sewing machine. Inform your patient that the larger model can be rented from a pharmacy or medical supply company.

Cylinder pump

This pump operates with two plastic cylinders, one inside the other, that create gentle suction as the outer cylinder is moved back and forth. Because two hands are needed to operate this pump, it may be tiring to use. However, it's easily cleaned and portable, and thus relatively efficient for short-term or intermittent use.

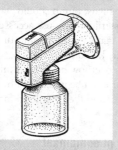
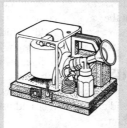
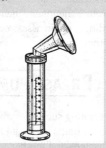

This ensures sufficient fluid intake to maintain adequate milk production.
▶ Help the patient to assume a comfortable position and to relax. Offer pillows for support. Provide privacy and instruct her to uncover her breast completely *to prevent lint and dirt from entering the milk-collection container.*
▶ If the patient's breasts are engorged, have her apply warm compresses for 5 minutes or take a warm shower *to dilate the milk ducts and stimulate the letdown reflex.*

▶ To help trigger the release of milk-producing hormones, instruct the patient to use her thumb and forefinger to stimulate the nipple and areola for 1 to 2 minutes.

Using a manual cylinder pump

▶ Instruct the patient to place the flange or shield against her breast with the nipple in the center of the device. Then tell her to move the outer cylinder of the pump toward the breast and then away from the breast, using a pistonlike motion, to draw the milk from the breast. Have her pump each breast in this manner until no milk flows.

▶ If the milk will be stored or frozen, direct the patient to fill a sterile plastic bottle with the milk from the cylinder. If the infant will drink the milk directly, instruct the patient to attach a rubber nipple to the cylinder.

Using a battery-powered or electric breast pump

▶ Unless the pump is battery-powered, make sure the pump has a three-pronged plug to ground it *to prevent electric shock.*

▶ Instruct the patient to set the suction regulator on low. Tell her to hold the collection unit upright *to prevent milk from being sucked into the machine.* Have her center her nipple in the shield, which she'll place against the breast.

▶ Direct her to activate the machine and adjust the suction regulator to achieve a comfortable pressure. Have her check the operator's manual to determine the pressure setting at which the pump functions most efficiently.

▶ Instruct her to pump each breast for 5 to 8 minutes or until the spray grows scant. Then pump each breast again for 3 to 5 minutes and then again for 2 to 3 minutes. (Usually, 8 oz can be pumped within 15 to 30 minutes.)

▶ Tell the patient to remove the shield from the breast by inserting a finger between the breast and the shield *to break the vacuum seal.* Then she should return the suction regulator to the low setting and turn off the machine.

▶ If the milk will be stored or frozen, pour it from the collection unit into a sterile container. (If it's to be frozen, place it in the freezer immediately.)

▶ If the infant will drink the milk directly, pour it into a sterile plastic bottle.

▶ Label the collected milk with the date, the time of collection, and the amount. Also, be sure the label contains the infant's name if applicable.

Concluding the procedure

▶ Instruct the patient to air-dry her nipples for about 15 minutes.

▶ Instruct her to disassemble the removable parts of the pump and wash them according to the manufacturer's directions.

Special considerations

▶ Provide emotional support *to alleviate the mother's distress related to the infant's absence at feeding time.*

▶ Be sure to use a sterile plastic (not glass) collection bottle for the milk *because antibodies in the breast milk will adhere to a glass bottle.*

▶ If the patient will use a breast pump for some time, have her pump her breasts every 2 to 3 hours *because neonates nurse 8 to 12 times every 24 hours.* Remind her to pump her breasts at night *because the breasts need round-the-clock stimulation to produce an adequate supply of milk.*

▶ Once the milk supply is established, some mothers may need to pump once nightly. Others find that they can sleep for 6 hours and still maintain the milk supply.

▶ Breast milk can be stored in the refrigerator for 48 hours and in the freezer at 0° F (− 17.8° C) for up to 6 months.

Complications

Common complications include nipple injury from suction and contaminated milk from improperly cleaned equipment or incorrect storage.

Documentation

Record the duration that the patient pumped each breast, the amount of milk collected, and the patient's tolerance of the procedure.

BRYANT'S TRACTION

Also called vertical suspension, Bryant's traction is used primarily to reduce developmental hip dislocations in children. With the patient lying supine in a bed or crib, the traction extends the legs vertically at a 90-degree angle to the body. Even if the disorder affects only one leg, the patient will have traction applied to both legs to prevent hip rotation and to ensure equal stress on the legs and even, bilateral bone growth.

Bryant's traction continues for 2 to 4 weeks. Afterward, the patient may be immobilized in a hip spica cast. (See "Hip spica cast care," page 392.) Usually chosen for children under age 2 who weigh 25 to 30 lb (11.5 to 14 kg), Bryant's traction is contraindicated for heavier children because the risk of positional hypertension rises with increased weight.

Key nursing diagnoses and patient outcomes

Impaired physical mobility related to neuromuscular impairment
The patient will:
▶ maintain muscle strength and joint range of motion
▶ show no evidence of complications, such as contractures, venous stasis,

thrombus formation, and skin breakdown.

Equipment

Traction setup (supplied by the orthopedic department) • moleskin traction straps • elastic bandages • foam rubber padding • cotton balls • compound benzoin tincture • adhesive tape • jacket restraint • optional: safety razor, cotton batting, convoluted foam mattress, and sheepskin pad

Preparation of equipment

Assist the doctor and orthopedic technician with measuring and cutting the moleskin straps and with assembling the traction equipment.

Implementation

▶ Thoroughly explain the purpose and function of the traction *to enhance learning and alleviate patient and family anxiety.* If possible, use visual aids to illustrate your teaching. Keep a diagram handy for parents and a doll in traction for the patient.
▶ Ask the parents whether their child is sensitive or allergic to rubber or to adhesive tape.
▶ If the patient has hairy legs, shave or clip the hair with a safety razor *to ensure good contact between the moleskin traction straps and the skin.* Use soap, warm water, and long, downward strokes *to minimize nicking.*
▶ Use cotton balls to apply the compound benzoin tincture, if ordered, to the patient's legs *to protect the skin.*
▶ Assist the doctor or orthopedic technician with placing foam rubber padding and moleskin traction straps against the patient's legs and securing the straps with elastic bandages from foot to thigh. Secure the elastic ban-

Maintaining body alignment and traction

Keeping the patient's body in the correct position with Bryant's traction requires precision and continual supervision and adjustment.

At the same time that the traction apparatus holds the patient's legs perpendicular to the mattress, you'll need to ensure that the patient's buttocks stay slightly elevated *to provide countertraction* and that his shoulders stay flat and in the same position on the mattress *to maintain body alignment.*

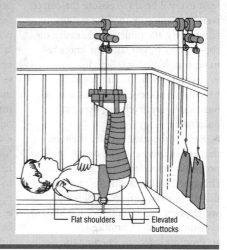

Flat shoulders   Elevated buttocks

---

dages with adhesive tape. If the patient is allergic to rubber or to adhesive tape, wrap the legs in cotton batting before applying the straps.

▶ If necessary to keep the patient positioned properly, apply a jacket restraint *to keep the weights from pulling the patient forward and altering the tractional force.*

▶ Carefully monitor the circulatory status of the patient's legs 15 minutes and 30 minutes after applying initial traction. Then check circulatory status every 4 hours *to detect any impairment caused by traction.* Assess capillary refill, skin color, sensation, movement, temperature, peripheral pulses, and bandage tightness. If you detect circulatory compromise, loosen the elastic bandages and notify the patient's doctor.

▶ Take care to position the elastic bandages precisely. Unless contraindicated, periodically remove the bandages from the unaffected leg *to assess circulation and provide skin care.* When doing so,

have another person hold the traction straps in place *to prevent slipping.* Don't unwrap the affected leg unless ordered to do so by the patient's doctor.

▶ Check the patient's position regularly *to ensure optimum traction.* Be sure to raise the patient's buttocks high enough off the mattress to allow one hand to slide between the skin and the mattress. Avoid raising the buttocks too high, though, *because this may reduce the effectiveness of traction.*

▶ Try marking the bed sheet with an "X" at the correct shoulder position *as a guide to correct body alignment.* Near the patient's bed, post an illustration of the correct alignment *to guide other nurses and caregivers.* (See *Maintaining body alignment and traction.*)

▶ Provide skin care every 4 hours, focusing especially on the back, buttocks, and elbows — *the areas most prone to breakdown.* Place a convoluted foam mattress or a sheepskin pad, or both, beneath the patient *to help prevent or alleviate skin problems.*

▶ Inspect the traction apparatus at least every 2 hours to ensure the correct weight. Make sure that the weights hang freely, the pulleys glide easily, the ropes aren't frayed, and the knots remain snugly tied and taped.

▶ Encourage the patient to take deep breaths at least every 2 hours *to minimize his risk of developing hypostatic pneumonia.*

▶ Review the patient's diet *to ensure that he consumes enough fiber and fluid to prevent constipation and urinary stasis.* (Infants should consume about 130 ml of fluid for each kilogram of body weight every 24 hours; toddlers should consume about 115 ml/kg.)

▶ Promote safety by keeping the side rails raised on the patient's bed whenever you aren't at the bedside.

Special considerations

▶ *To promote regular deep breathing and guard against pneumonia,* allow the patient to blow a horn, whistle, pinwheel, or bubbles heartily or encourage him to sing. *This promotes lung expansion and enjoyment at the same time.*

▶ *Because a child can't always tell you that he's in pain,* carefully observe his behavior, facial expression, and cry to judge discomfort levels. In addition to needing an analgesic or sedative, the patient may need an antispasmodic medication *to relieve irritable muscles and prevent muscle spasms.*

▶ *To foster development, diversion, and mobility,* provide age-appropriate games and activities as permitted within the confines of traction. For infants, this can include mobiles, music boxes, and rattles. Toddlers may enjoy puppets,

large-pieced puzzles, and dolls. Involve the family in their child's care and recreational activities *to increase the patient's sense of security and to minimize the family's sense of anxiety.* If facility policy permits, consider moving the infant's crib to the playroom *so that he can be around other children.*

▶ Eating and drinking are difficult and inconvenient for the patient in Bryant's traction *because of the head-down position. To facilitate digestion and encourage eating*—especially if the patient refuses food—place a small pillow under his head at mealtime. If possible, allow him to choose his own foods and encourage his family to bring food from home.

▶ *To minimize patient movement,* change bed linens every other day unless the linens get wet or soiled. Keep sheets taut and wrinkle-free *to help prevent skin breakdown.*

Complications

Although generally safe, Bryant's traction may lead to pneumonia from restricted lung expansion resulting from the head-down position. Skin necrosis may result from bandages wrapped too tightly. Other complications include urinary stasis and constipation.

Documentation

Record the date and time that traction was applied, the amount of weight applied, and the patient's circulatory status, skin condition, and position. Note whether weights hang freely. Document changes in the patient's status and describe the patient's and family's responses to the traction. Also note the patient's and family's responses to any patient teaching.

BUCCAL, SUBLINGUAL, AND TRANSLINGUAL DRUGS

Certain drugs are given buccally, sublingually, or translingually to prevent their destruction or transformation in the stomach or small intestine. These drugs act quickly because the oral mucosa's thin epithelium and abundant vasculature allow direct absorption into the bloodstream.

Drugs given buccally include nitroglycerin and methyltestosterone; drugs given sublingually include ergotamine tartrate, isosorbide dinitrate, and nitroglycerin. Translingual drugs, which are sprayed onto the tongue, include nitrate preparations for patients with chronic angina.

Key nursing diagnoses and patient outcomes

Deficient knowledge related to lack of exposure to the procedure
The patient will:
▶ demonstrate proficiency in self-administration of buccal, sublingual, or translingual drugs.

Risk for injury related to improper technique
The patient will:
▶ identify factors that increase the risk for injury
▶ assist in identifying and applying safety measures to prevent injury.

Equipment

Patient's medication record and chart • prescribed medication • medication cup

Implementation

▶ Verify the order on the patient's medication record by checking it against the doctor's order on his chart.
▶ Wash your hands with warm water and soap. Explain the procedure to the patient if he's never taken a drug buccally, sublingually, or translingually before.
▶ Check the label on the medication before administering it to make sure you'll be giving the prescribed medication. Verify the expiration date, especially that of nitroglycerin.
▶ Confirm the patient's identity by asking his name and checking the name, room number, and bed number on his wristband.

Buccal and sublingual administration

▶ For buccal administration, place the tablet in the buccal pouch, between the cheek and gum. For sublingual administration, place the tablet under the patient's tongue. (See *Placing drugs in the oral mucosa*, page 84.)
▶ Instruct the patient to keep the medication in place until it dissolves completely *to ensure absorption*.
▶ Caution him against chewing the tablet or touching it with his tongue *to prevent accidental swallowing*.
▶ Tell him not to smoke before the drug has dissolved because nicotine's vasoconstrictive effects slow absorption.

Translingual administration

▶ To administer a translingual drug, tell the patient to hold the medication canister vertically, with the valve head at the top and the spray orifice as close to his mouth as possible.

Placing drugs in the oral mucosa

Buccal and sublingual administration routes allow some drugs, such as nitroglycerin and methyltestosterone, to enter the bloodstream rapidly without being degraded in the GI tract. To give a drug buccally, insert it between the patient's cheek and teeth (as shown below). Ask him to close his mouth and hold the tablet against his cheek until the tablet is absorbed.

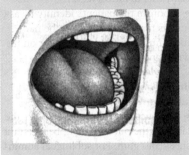

To give a drug sublingually, place it under the patient's tongue (as shown below), and ask him to leave it there until it's dissolved.

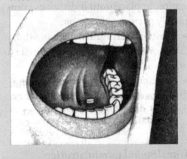

▶ Instruct him to spray the dose onto his tongue by pressing the button firmly.
▶ Remind the patient using a translingual aerosol form that he shouldn't inhale the spray but should release it under his tongue. Also tell him to wait about 10 seconds before swallowing.

Special considerations
▶ Don't give liquids to a patient who is receiving buccal medication because some buccal tablets can take up to 1 hour to be absorbed. Tell the patient not to rinse his mouth until the tablet has been absorbed.
▶ Tell the angina patient to wet the nitroglycerin tablet with saliva and to keep it under his tongue until it has been fully absorbed.

Complications
Some buccal medications may irritate the mucosa. Alternate sides of the mouth for repeat doses *to prevent continuous irritation of the same site.* Sublingual medications—such as nitroglycerin—may cause a tingling sensation under the tongue. If the patient finds this annoying, try placing the drug in the buccal pouch instead.

Documentation
Record the medication administered, dose, date and time, and patient's reaction, if any.

BURN CARE

The goals of burn care are to maintain the patient's physiologic stability, to repair skin integrity, to prevent infection, and to promote maximal functioning and psychosocial health. Competent care immediately after a burn occurs can dramatically improve the success of overall treatment. (See *Burn care at the scene.*)

Burn care at the scene

By acting promptly when a burn injury occurs, you can improve a patient's chance of uncomplicated recovery. Emergency care at the scene should include steps to stop the burn from worsening; assessment of the patient's airway, breathing, and circulation (ABCs); a call for help from an emergency medical team; and emotional and physiologic support for the patient.

Stop the burning process

■ If the victim is on fire, tell him to fall to the ground and roll to put out the flames. (*If he panics and runs, air will fuel the flames, worsening the burn and increasing the risk of inhalation injury.*) Or, if you can, wrap the victim in a blanket or other large covering *to smother the flames and protect the burned area from dirt.* Keep his head outside the blanket *so that he doesn't breathe toxic fumes.* As soon as the flames are out, unwrap the patient *so that the heat can dissipate.*

■ Cool the burned area with any nonflammable liquid. *This decreases pain and stops the burn from growing deeper or larger.*

■ If possible, remove any potential sources of heat, such as jewelry, belt buckles, and some types of clothing. *Besides adding to the burning process, these items may cause constriction as edema develops.* If the patient's clothing adheres to his skin, don't try to remove it. Rather, cut around it.

■ Cover the wound with a tablecloth, sheet, or other smooth, nonfuzzy material.

Assess the damage

■ Assess the patient's ABCs, and perform cardiopulmonary resuscitation, if necessary. Then check for other serious injuries, such as fractures, spinal cord injury, lacerations, blunt trauma, and head contusions.

■ Estimate the extent and depth of the burns. If flames caused the burns and the injury occurred in a closed space, assess for signs of inhalation injury: singed nasal hairs, burns on the face or mouth, soot-stained sputum, coughing or hoarseness, wheezing, or respiratory distress.

■ Call for help as quickly as possible. Send someone to contact the emergency medical service (EMS).

■ If the patient is conscious and alert, try to get a brief medical history as soon as possible.

■ Reassure the patient that help is on the way. Provide emotional support by staying with him, answering questions, and explaining what is being done for him.

■ When help arrives, give the EMS a report on the patient's status.

Burn severity is determined by the depth and extent of the burn and the presence of other factors, such as age, complications, and coexisting illnesses. (See *Estimating burn surfaces in adults and children,* pages 86 and 87, and *Evaluating burn severity,* page 88.)

To promote stability, you'll need to carefully monitor your patient's respiratory status, especially if he has suffered smoke inhalation. Be aware that a patient with burns involving more than 20% of his total body surface area usually needs fluid resuscitation, which aims to support the body's compensatory mechanisms without overwhelming them. Expect to give fluids (such as lactated Ringer's solution) to keep the patient's urine output at 30 to 50 ml/hour, and expect to monitor blood pressure and heart rate. You'll also need to control body temperature because skin loss interferes with temperature regulation. Use warm fluids, heat lamps, and hy-

Estimating burn surfaces in adults and children

You need to use different formulas to compute burned body surface area (BSA) in adults and children because the proportion of BSA varies with growth.

Rule of Nines

You can quickly estimate the extent of an adult patient's burn by using the Rule of Nines. This method quantifies BSA in percentages either in fractions of nine or in multiples of nine. To use this method, mentally assess your patient's burns by the body chart shown below. Add the corresponding percentages for each body section burned. Use the total—a rough estimate of burn extent—to calculate initial fluid replacement needs.

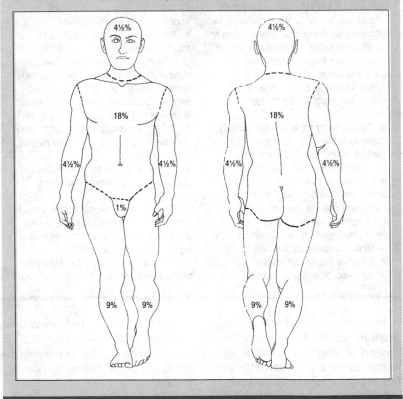

perthermia blankets, as appropriate, to keep the patient's temperature above 97° F (36.1° C), if possible. Additionally, you'll frequently review such laboratory values as serum electrolyte levels to detect early changes in the patient's condition.

Infection can increase wound depth, cause rejection of skin grafts, slow healing, worsen pain, prolong hospitaliza-

Estimating burn surfaces in adults and children *(continued)*

Lund and Browder chart

The Rule of Nines isn't accurate for infants and children because their body shapes differ from those of adults. An infant's head, for example, accounts for about 17% of his total BSA, compared with 7% for an adult. Instead, use the Lund and Browder chart shown here.

Percentage of burned body surface by age

	At birth	0 to 1 yr	1 to 4 yr	5 to 9 yr	10 to 15 yr	Adult
A: Half of head	9½%	8½%	6½%	5½%	4½%	3½%
B: Half of thigh	2¾%	3¼%	4%	4¼%	4½%	4¾%
C: Half of leg	2½%	2½%	2¾%	3%	3¼%	3½%

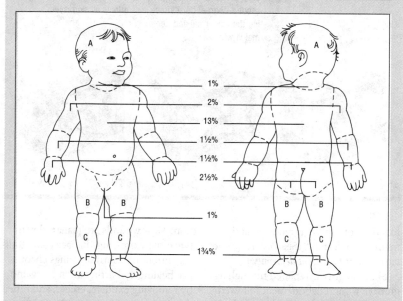

1%
2%
13%
1½%
1½%
2½%
1%
1¾%

tion, and even lead to death. To help prevent infection, use strict aseptic technique during care, dress the burn site as ordered, monitor and rotate I.V. lines regularly, and carefully assess the burn extent, body system function, and the patient's emotional status.

Other interventions, such as careful positioning and regular exercise for burned extremities, help maintain joint

Evaluating burn severity

To judge a burn's severity, assess its depth and extent as well as the presence of other factors.

Superficial partial-thickness (first-degree) burn

Does the burned area appear pink or red with minimal edema? Is the area sensitive to touch and temperature changes? If so, your patient most likely has a superficial partial-thickness, or first-degree, burn affecting only the epidermal skin layer.

Deep partial-thickness (second-degree) burn

Does the burned area appear pink or red, with a mottled appearance? Do red areas blanch when you touch them? Does the skin have large, thick-walled blisters with subcutaneous edema? Does touching the burn cause severe pain? Is the hair still present? If so, the person most likely has a deep partial-thickness, or second-degree, burn affecting the epidermal and dermal layers.

Full-thickness (third-degree) burn

Does the burned area appear red, waxy white, brown, or black? Does red skin remain red with no blanching when you touch it? Is the skin leathery with extensive subcutaneous edema? Is the skin insensitive to touch? Does the hair fall out easily? If so, your patient most likely has a full-thickness, or third-degree, burn that affects all skin layers.

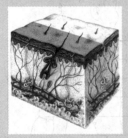 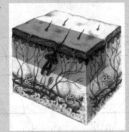 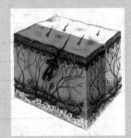

function, prevent contractures, and minimize deformity. (See *Positioning the burn patient to prevent deformity.*)

Skin integrity is repaired through aggressive wound debridement followed by maintenance of a clean wound bed until the wound heals or is covered with a skin graft. Full-thickness burns and some deep partial-thickness burns must be debrided and grafted in the operating room. Surgery takes place as soon as possible after fluid resuscitation. Most wounds are managed with twice-daily dressing changes using topical antibiotics. Burn dressings encourage healing by barring germ entry and by removing exudate, eschar, and other debris that host infection. After thorough wound cleaning, topical antibacterial agents are applied and the wound is covered with absorptive, coarse-mesh gauze. Roller gauze typically tops the dressing and is secured with elastic netting or tape.

Positioning the burn patient to prevent deformity

For each of the potential deformities listed below, you can use the corresponding positioning and interventions to help prevent the deformity.

Burned area	Potential deformity	Preventive positioning	Nursing interventions
Neck	■ Flexion contraction of neck	■ Extension	■ Remove pillow from bed.
	■ Extensor contraction of neck	■ Prone with head slightly elevated	■ Place pillow or rolled towel under upper chest to flex cervical spine, or apply cervical collar.
Axilla	■ Adduction and internal rotation	■ Shoulder joint in external rotation and 100- to 103-degree abduction	■ Use an I.V. pole, bedside table, or sling to suspend arm.
	■ Adduction and external rotation	■ Shoulder in forward flexion and 100- to 130-degree abduction	■ Use an I.V. pole, bedside table, or sling to suspend arm.
Pectoral region	■ Shoulder protraction	■ Shoulders abducted and externally rotated	■ Remove pillow from bed.
Chest or abdomen	■ Kyphosis	■ Same as for pectoral region, with hips neutral (not flexed)	■ Use no pillow under head or legs.
Lateral trunk	■ Scoliosis	■ Supine; affected arm abducted	■ Put pillows or blanket roll at sides.
Elbow	■ Flexion and pronation	■ Arm extended and supinated	■ Use an elbow splint, arm board, or bedside table.
Wrist	■ Flexion	■ Splint in 15-degree extension	■ Apply a hand splint.
	■ Extension	■ Splint in 15-degree flexion	■ Apply a hand splint.
Fingers	■ Adhesions of the extensor tendons; loss of plantar grip	■ Metacarpophalangeal joints in maximum flexion; interphalangeal joints in slight flexion; thumb in maximum abduction	■ Apply a hand splint; wrap fingers separately.
Hip	■ Internal rotation, flexion, and adduction; possibly joint subluxation if contracture is severe	■ Neutral rotation and abduction; extension by prone position	■ Put a pillow under buttocks (if supine) or use trochanter rolls or knee or long leg splints.

(continued)

Positioning the burn patient to prevent deformity (continued)

Burned area	Potential deformity	Preventive positioning	Nursing interventions
Knee	■ Flexion	■ Extension	■ Use a knee splint with no pillows under legs.
Ankle	■ Plantar flexion if foot muscles are weak or their tendons are divided	■ 90-degree dorsiflexion	■ Use a footboard or ankle splint.

Key nursing diagnoses and patient outcomes

Acute pain related to burn injury
The patient will:
▶ identify pain characteristics
▶ articulate factors that intensify pain
▶ express increased comfort and relief of pain.

Risk for injury related to burn injury
The patient will:
▶ have wounds that remain free from signs of infection (purulent drainage)
▶ have a normal body temperature
▶ have a normal white blood cell count and differential.
Impaired skin integrity related to burn injury
The patient will:
▶ verbalize an understanding of the skin care regimen
▶ demonstrate the skin care regimen
▶ express feelings about changed body image.

Equipment

Normal saline solution • sterile bowl • sterile blunt scissors • sterile tissue forceps • ordered topical medication • burn gauze • roller gauze • fine-mesh gauze • elastic gauze • elastic netting or tape • cotton-tipped applicators • ordered pain medication • three pairs of sterile gloves • sterile gown • mask • surgical cap • heat lamps • impervious plastic trash bag • cotton bath blanket • 4″ × 4″ gauze pads

A sterile field is required, and all equipment and supplies used in the dressing should be sterile.

Preparation of equipment

Warm normal saline solution by immersing unopened bottles in warm water. Assemble equipment on the dressing table. Make sure the treatment area has adequate light *to allow accurate wound assessment*. Open equipment packages using aseptic technique. Arrange supplies on a sterile field in order of use.

To prevent cross-contamination, plan to dress the cleanest areas first and the dirtiest or most contaminated areas last. *To help prevent excessive pain or cross-contamination*, you may need to perform the dressing in stages to avoid exposing all wounds at the same time.

Implementation

▶ Administer the ordered pain medication about 20 minutes before beginning

wound care *to maximize patient comfort and cooperation.*
► Explain the procedure to the patient and provide privacy.
► Turn on overhead heat lamps *to keep the patient warm.* Make sure that they don't overheat the patient.
► Pour warmed normal saline solution into the sterile bowl in the sterile field.
► Wash your hands.

Removing a dressing without hydrotherapy
► Put on a gown, a mask, and sterile gloves.
► Remove dressing layers down to the innermost layer by cutting the outer dressings with sterile blunt scissors. Lay open these dressings.
► If the inner layer appears dry, soak it with warm normal saline solution *to ease removal.*
► Remove the inner dressing with sterile tissue forceps or your sterile gloved hand.
► *Because soiled dressings harbor infectious microorganisms,* dispose of the dressings carefully in the impervious plastic trash bag according to facility policy. Dispose of your gloves and wash your hands.
► Put on a new pair of sterile gloves. Using gauze pads moistened with normal saline solution, gently remove any exudate and old topical medication.
► Carefully remove all loose eschar with sterile forceps and scissors, if ordered. (See "Mechanical debridement," page 511.)
► Assess wound condition. The wound should appear clean, with no debris, loose tissue, purulence, inflammation, or darkened margins.
► Before applying a new dressing, remove your gown, gloves, and mask.

Discard them properly, and put on a clean mask, surgical cap, gown, and sterile gloves.

Applying a wet dressing
► Soak fine-mesh gauze and the elastic gauze dressing in a large sterile basin containing the ordered solution (for example, silver nitrate).
► Wring out the fine-mesh gauze until it's moist but not dripping and apply it to the wound. Warn the patient that he may feel transient pain when you apply the dressing.
► Wring out the elastic gauze dressing, and position it to hold the fine-mesh gauze in place.
► Roll an elastic gauze dressing over these two dressings *to keep them intact.*
► Cover the patient with a cotton bath blanket *to prevent chills.* Change the blanket if it becomes damp. Use an overhead heat lamp, if necessary.
► Change the dressings frequently as ordered *to keep the wound moist,* especially if you're using silver nitrate. *Silver nitrate becomes ineffective and the silver ions may damage tissue if the dressings become dry.* (To maintain moisture, some protocols call for irrigating the dressing with solution at least every 4 hours through small slits cut into the outer dressing.)

Applying a dry dressing with a topical medication
► Remove old dressings, and clean the wound (as described previously).
► Apply the ordered medication to the wound in a thin layer (about 2 to 4 mm thick) with your sterile gloved hand. Then apply several layers of burn gauze over the wound *to contain the medication but allow exudate to escape.*

▶ Remember to cut the dry dressing to fit only the wound areas; don't cover unburned areas.

▶ Cover the entire dressing with roller gauze and secure it with elastic netting or tape.

Providing arm and leg care

▶ Apply the dressings from the distal to the proximal area *to stimulate circulation and prevent constriction.* Wrap the burn gauze once around the arm or leg so the edges overlap slightly. Continue wrapping in this way until the gauze covers the wound.

▶ Apply a dry roller gauze dressing *to hold the bottom layers in place.* Secure with elastic netting or tape.

Providing hand and foot care

▶ Wrap each finger separately with a single layer of a 4" × 4" gauze pad *to allow the patient to use his hands and to prevent webbing contractures.*

▶ Place the hand in a functional position and secure this position using a dressing. Apply splints, if ordered.

▶ Put gauze between each toe as appropriate *to prevent webbing contractures.*

Providing chest, abdomen, and back care

▶ Apply the ordered medication to the wound in a thin layer. Then cover the entire burned area with sheets of burn gauze.

▶ Wrap the area with roller gauze or apply a specialty vest dressing *to hold the burn gauze in place.*

▶ Secure the dressing with elastic netting or tape. Make sure the dressing doesn't restrict respiratory motion, especially in very young or elderly patients or in those with circumferential injuries.

Providing facial care

▶ If the patient has scalp burns, clip or shave the hair around the burn as ordered. Clip other hair until it's about 2" (5 cm) long *to prevent contamination of burned scalp areas.*

▶ Shave facial hair if it comes in contact with burned areas.

▶ Typically, facial burns are managed with milder topical agents (such as triple antibiotic ointment) and are left open to air. If dressings are required, make sure they don't cover the eyes, nostrils, or mouth.

Providing ear care

▶ Clip or shave the hair around the affected ear.

▶ Remove exudate and crusts with cotton-tipped applicators dipped in normal saline solution.

▶ Place a layer of 4" × 4" gauze behind the auricle *to prevent webbing.*

▶ Apply the ordered medication to 4" × 4" gauze pads and place the pads over the burned area. Before securing the dressing with a roller bandage, position the patient's ears normally *to avoid damaging the auricular cartilage.*

▶ Assess the patient's hearing ability.

Providing eye care

▶ Clean the area around the eyes and eyelids with a cotton-tipped applicator and normal saline solution every 4 to 6 hours, or as needed, *to remove crusts and drainage.*

▶ Administer ordered eye ointments or eyedrops.

▶ If the eyes can't be closed, apply lubricating ointments or drops as ordered.

▶ Be sure to close the patient's eyes before applying eye pads *to prevent corneal abrasion.* Don't apply any topical oint-

Successful burn care after discharge

You can help the patient make a successful transition from hospital to home by encouraging him to follow the wound care and self-care guidelines below.

Wound care

Instruct the patient or family member to follow this procedure when changing dressings:
- Clean the bathtub, shower, or washbasin thoroughly; then assemble the required equipment (topical medication, if ordered, and dressing supplies). Open the supplies aseptically on a clean surface.
- Wash your hands. Remove the old dressing and discard it.
- Using a clean washcloth and mild soap and water, wash the wound to remove all the old medication. Try to remove any loose skin too. Then pat the skin dry with a clean towel.
- Check the burned area for signs of infection: redness, heat, foul odor, increased pain, and difficulty moving the area. If any of these signs is present, notify the doctor after completing the dressing change.
- Wash your hands. If ordered, apply a thin layer of topical medication to the burned area.
- Cover the burned area with thin layers of gauze and wrap it with a roller gauze. Finally, secure the dressing with tape or elastic netting.

Self-care

To enhance healing, instruct the patient to eat well-balanced meals with adequate carbohydrates and proteins, to eat between-meal snacks, and to include at least one protein source in each meal and snack. Tell him to avoid tobacco, alcohol, and caffeine because they constrict peripheral blood flow.

Advise the patient to wash new skin with mild soap and water. *To prevent excessive skin dryness,* instruct him to use a lubricating lotion and to avoid lotions containing alcohol or perfume. Caution the patient to avoid bumping or scratching regenerated skin tissue.

Recommend nonrestrictive, nonabrasive clothing, which should be laundered in a mild detergent. Advise the patient to wear protective clothing during cold weather to prevent frostbite.

Warn the patient not to expose new skin to strong sunlight and to always wear sunscreen with a sun protection factor of 20 or higher. Also, tell him not to expose new skin to irritants, such as paint, solvents, strong detergents, and antiperspirants. Recommend cool baths or ice packs to relieve itching.

To minimize scar formation, the patient may need to wear a pressure garment — usually for 23 hours a day for 6 months to 1 year. Instruct him to remove it only during daily hygiene. Suspect that the garment is too tight if the patient's fingers or toes are cold, numb, or discolored or if the garment's seams and zippers leave deep, red impressions for more than 10 minutes after the garment is removed.

---

ments near the eyes without a doctor's order.

Providing nasal care

▶ Check the nostrils for inhalation injury: inflamed mucosa, singed vibrissae, and soot.

▶ Clean the nostrils with cotton-tipped applicators dipped in normal saline solution. Remove crusts.

▶ Apply the ordered ointments.

▶ If the patient has a nasogastric tube, use tracheostomy ties to secure the tube. Be sure to check ties frequently for tightness resulting from swelling of facial tissue. Clean the area around the tube every 4 to 6 hours.

Special considerations

▶ Thorough assessment and documentation of the wound's appearance are essential *to detect infection and other complications.* A purulent wound or green-gray exudate indicates infection, an overly dry wound suggests dehydration, and a wound with a swollen, red edge suggests cellulitis. Suspect a fungal infection if the wound is white and powdery. Healthy granulation tissue appears clean, pinkish, faintly shiny, and free of exudate.

▶ *Because blisters protect underlying tissue,* leave them intact unless they impede joint motion, become infected, or cause patient discomfort.

▶ Keep in mind that the patient with healing burns has increased nutritional needs. He'll require extra protein and carbohydrates *to accommodate an almost doubled basal metabolism.*

▶ If you must manage a burn with topical medications, exposure to air, and no dressing, watch for such problems as wound adherence to bed linens, poor drainage control, and partial loss of topical medications.

Home care

Begin discharge planning as soon as the patient enters the facility *to help him (and his family) make a smooth transition from facility to home. To encourage therapeutic compliance,* prepare him to expect scarring, teach him wound management and pain control, and urge him to follow the prescribed exercise regimen.

Provide encouragement and emotional support and urge the patient to join a burn survivor support group. Also, teach the family or caregivers how to encourage, support, and provide care for the patient. (See *Successful burn care after discharge,* page 93.)

Complications

Infection is the most common burn complication.

Documentation

Record the date and time of all care provided. Describe wound condition, special dressing-change techniques, topical medications administered, positioning of the burned area, and the patient's tolerance of the procedure.

BURN DRESSING USE, BIOLOGICAL

Biological dressings provide a temporary protective covering for burn wounds and clean granulation tissue. They also temporarily secure fresh skin grafts and protect graft donor sites. In common use are three organic materials (pigskin, cadaver skin, and amniotic membrane) and one synthetic material (Biobrane). (See *Comparing biological dressings.*) In addition to stimulating new skin growth, these dressings act like normal skin: They reduce heat loss, block infection, and minimize fluid, electrolyte, and protein losses.

Amniotic membrane or fresh cadaver skin is usually applied to the patient in the operating room, although it may be applied in a treatment room. Pigskin or Biobrane may be applied in either the operating room or a treatment room. Before applying a biological dressing,

Comparing biological dressings

Type	Description and uses	Nursing considerations
Cadaver (homograft)	■ Obtained at autopsy up to 24 hours after death ■ Applied in the operating room or at the bedside to debrided, untidy wounds ■ Available as fresh cryopreserved homografts in tissue banks nationwide ■ Provides protection, especially to granulation tissue after escharotomy ■ May be used in some patients as a test graft for autografting ■ Covers excised wounds immediately	■ Observe for exudate. ■ Watch for signs of rejection. ■ Keep in mind that the gauze dressing may be removed every 8 hours *to observe the graft.*
Pigskin (heterograft or xenograft)	■ Applied in the operating room or at the bedside ■ Comes fresh or frozen in rolls or sheets ■ Can cover and protect debrided, untidy wounds, mesh autografts, clean (eschar-free) partial-thickness burns, and exposed tendons	■ Reconstitute frozen form with normal saline solution 30 minutes before use. ■ Watch for signs of rejection. ■ Cover with gauze dressing or leave exposed to air as ordered. ■ Note that pigskin dressings are typically changed every 2 to 5 days.
Amniotic membrane (homograft)	■ Available from the obstetric department ■ Must be sterile and come from an uncomplicated birth; must have had serologic tests done ■ Antimicrobials not required if in bacteriostatic condition ■ May be used to protect partial-thickness burns or (temporarily) granulation tissue before autografting ■ Applied by the doctor to clean wounds only	■ Change the membrane every 48 hours. ■ Cover the membrane with a gauze dressing or leave it exposed as ordered. ■ If you apply a gauze dressing, change it every 48 hours.
Biobrane (biosynthetic membrane)	■ Comes in sterile, prepackaged sheets in various sizes and in glove form for hand burns ■ Used to cover donor graft sites, superficial partial-thickness burns, debrided wounds awaiting autograft, and meshed autografts ■ Provides significant pain relief ■ Applied by the nurse	■ Leave the membrane in place for 3 to 14 days, possibly longer. ■ Don't use this dressing for preparing a granulation bed for subsequent autografting.

the caregiver must clean and debride the wound. The frequency of dressing changes depends on the type of wound and the dressing's specific function.

Key nursing diagnoses and patient outcomes

Impaired skin integrity related to external factors
The patient will:
▶ regain skin integrity
▶ communicate an understanding of skin protection measures
▶ demonstrate skill in care of the burn
▶ perform routine skin care.

Risk for infection related to external factors
The patient will:
▶ maintain a normal body temperature
▶ maintain a normal white cell count and differential
▶ remain free from all signs and symptoms of infection.

Equipment

Ordered analgesic • cap • mask • two pairs of sterile gloves • sterile or clean gown • shoe covers • biological dressing • normal saline solution • sterile basin • Xeroflo gauze • sterile forceps • sterile scissors • sterile hemostat • elastic netting

Preparation of equipment

Place the biological dressing in the sterile basin containing sterile normal saline solution (or open the Biobrane package). Using aseptic technique, open the sterile dressing packages. Arrange the equipment on the dressing cart, and keep the cart readily accessible. Make sure the treatment area has adequate light *to allow accurate wound assessment and dressing placement.*

Implementation

▶ If this is the patient's first treatment, explain the procedure *to allay his fears and promote cooperation.* Provide privacy.
▶ If ordered, administer an analgesic to the patient 20 minutes before beginning the procedure or give an analgesic I.V. immediately before the procedure *to increase the patient's comfort and tolerance levels.*
▶ Wash your hands and put on cap, mask, gown, shoe covers, and sterile gloves.
▶ Clean and debride the wound *to reduce bacteria.* Remove and dispose of gloves. Wash your hands and put on a fresh pair of sterile gloves.
▶ Place the dressing directly on the wound surface. Apply pigskin dermal (shiny) side down; apply Biobrane nylon-backed (dull) side down. Roll the dressing directly onto the skin if applicable. Place the dressing strips so that the edges touch but don't overlap. Use sterile forceps, if necessary. Smooth the dressing. Eliminate folds and wrinkles by rolling out the dressing with the hemostat handle, the forceps handle, or your sterile-gloved hand *to cover the wound completely and ensure adherence.*
▶ Use the scissors to trim the dressing around the wound so that the dressing fits the wound without overlapping adjacent areas.
▶ Place Xeroflo gauze directly over an allograft, pigskin graft, or amniotic membrane. Place a few layers of gauze on top *to absorb exudate,* and wrap with a roller gauze dressing. Secure the dressing with tape or elastic netting. During daily dressing changes, the dressing will be removed down to the Xeroflo gauze, and the gauze will be replaced after the Xeroflo is inspected for

drainage, adherence, and signs of infection.

▶ Place a nonadhesive dressing (such as Exu-dry) over the Biobrane *to absorb drainage and provide stability.* Wrap the dressing with a roller gauze dressing, and secure it with tape or elastic netting. During daily dressing changes, the dressing will be removed down to the Biobrane and the site inspected for signs of infection. After the Biobrane adheres (usually in 2 to 3 days), it doesn't need to be covered with a dressing.

▶ Position the patient comfortably, elevating the area if possible. *This reduces edema, which may prevent the biological dressing from adhering.*

Special considerations
Handle the biological dressing as little as possible.

Home care
Instruct the patient or caregiver to assess the site daily for signs of infection, swelling, blisters, drainage, and separation. Make sure the patient knows whom to contact if these complications develop.

Complications
Infection may develop under a biological dressing. Observe the wound carefully during dressing changes for infection signs. If wound drainage appears purulent, remove the dressing, clean the area with normal saline solution or another prescribed cleaning solution as ordered, and apply a fresh biological dressing.

Documentation
Record the time and date of dressing changes. Note areas of application, quality of adherence, and purulent drainage or other infection signs. Also, describe the patient's tolerance of the procedure.

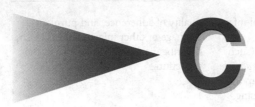

CANE USE

Indicated for the patient with one-sided weakness or injury, occasional loss of balance, or increased joint pressure, a cane provides balance and support for walking and reduces fatigue and strain on weight-bearing joints. Available in various sizes, the cane should extend from the greater trochanter to the floor and have a rubber tip to prevent slipping. Canes are contraindicated for the patient with bilateral weakness; such a patient should use crutches or a walker.

Key nursing diagnoses and patient outcomes

Impaired physical mobility related to pain or discomfort and decreased muscle strength
The patient will:
▶ demonstrate improved physical mobility
▶ ambulate with maximum independence
▶ demonstrate increased activity tolerance.

Impaired walking related to inability to use cane properly
The patient will:
▶ demonstrate proper use of a cane
▶ demonstrate improved ability to maneuver with a cane

▶ remain free from injury related to falls.

Equipment
Rubber-tipped cane • optional: walking belt
   Although wooden canes are available, three types of aluminum canes are used most frequently. The standard aluminum cane (used by the patient who needs only slight assistance with walking) provides the least support; its half-circle handle allows it to be hooked over chairs. The T-handle cane (used by the patient with hand weakness) has a straight-shaped handle with grips and a bent shaft. It provides greater stability than the standard cane. Three- or four-pronged canes are used by the patient with poor balance or one-sided weakness and an inability to hold onto a walker with both hands. The base of these types of canes splits into three or four short, splayed legs and provides greater stability than a standard cane but considerably less than a walker.

Preparation of equipment
Ask the patient to hold the cane on the uninvolved side 4″ to 6″ (10 to 15 cm) from the base of the little toe. If the cane is made of aluminum, adjust its height by pushing in the metal button on the shaft and raising or lowering the shaft; if it's wood, the rubber tip can be

removed and excess length sawed off. At the correct height, the handle of the cane is level with the greater trochanter and allows approximately 15-degree flexion at the elbow. If the cane is too short, the patient will have to drop his shoulder to lean on it; if it's too long, he'll have to raise his shoulder and will have difficulty supporting his weight.

Implementation

▶ Explain the mechanics of cane walking to the patient. Demonstrate the technique; then have the patient return the demonstration. Coordinate practice sessions in the physical therapy department, if necessary.
▶ Tell the patient to hold the cane on the uninvolved side *to promote a reciprocal gait pattern and to distribute weight away from the involved side.*
▶ Instruct the patient to hold the cane close to his body to prevent leaning and to move the cane and the involved leg simultaneously, followed by the uninvolved leg.
▶ Encourage the patient to keep the stride length of each leg and the timing of each step (cadence) equal.

Negotiating stairs

▶ Instruct the patient to always use a railing, if present, when going up or down stairs. Tell him to hold the cane with the other hand or to keep it in the hand grasping the railing. To ascend stairs, the patient should lead with the uninvolved leg and follow with the involved leg; to descend, he should lead with the involved leg and follow with the uninvolved leg. Help the patient remember by telling him to use this mnemonic device: "The good goes up; the bad goes down."

▶ To negotiate stairs without a railing, the patient should use the walking technique to ascend and descend the stairs but should move the cane just before the involved leg. Thus, to ascend stairs, the patient should hold the cane on the uninvolved side, step with the uninvolved leg, advance the cane, and then move the involved leg. To descend, he should hold the cane on the uninvolved side, lead with the cane, advance the involved leg, and then, finally, move the uninvolved leg.

Using a chair

▶ To teach the patient to sit down, stand by his affected side, and tell him to place the backs of his legs against the edge of the seat of the chair. Then tell him to move the cane out from his side and to reach back with both hands to grasp the armrests of the chair. Supporting his weight on the armrests, he can then lower himself onto the seat. While he's seated, he should keep the cane hooked on the armrest or the back of the chair.
▶ To teach the patient to get up, stand by his affected side and tell him to unhook the cane from the chair and hold it in his stronger hand as he grasps the armrests. Then tell him to move his uninvolved foot slightly forward, to lean slightly forward, and to push against the armrests to raise himself upright.
▶ Warn the patient not to lean on the cane when sitting or rising from the chair *to prevent falls.*
▶ Supervise your patient each time he gets in or out of a chair until you're both certain he can do it alone.

Special considerations

To prevent falls during the learning period, guard the patient carefully by standing behind him slightly to his stronger side and putting one foot between his feet and your other foot to the outside of the uninvolved leg. If necessary, use a walking belt.

Complications
A poorly fitted cane can cause the patient to lose his balance and fall.

Documentation
Record the type of cane used, the amount of guarding required, the distance walked, and the patient's understanding and tolerance of cane walking.

CARDIAC MONITORING

Because it allows continuous observation of the heart's electrical activity, cardiac monitoring is used in patients with conduction disturbances and in those at risk for life-threatening arrhythmias. Like other forms of electrocardiography (ECG), cardiac monitoring uses electrodes placed on the patient's chest to transmit electrical signals that are converted into a tracing of cardiac rhythm on an oscilloscope.

Two types of monitoring may be performed: hardwire or telemetry. In hardwire monitoring, the patient is connected to a monitor at the bedside. The rhythm display appears at bedside, but it may also be transmitted to a console at a remote location. Telemetry uses a small transmitter connected to the ambulatory patient to send electrical signals to another location where they're displayed on a monitor screen. Battery-powered and portable, telemetry frees the patient from cumbersome wires and cables and lets him be comfortably mobile and safely isolated from the electri-

cal leakage and accidental shock occasionally associated with hardwire monitoring. Telemetry is especially useful for monitoring arrhythmias that occur during sleep, rest, exercise, or stressful situations. However, unlike hardwire monitoring, telemetry can monitor only heart rate and rhythm.

Regardless of the type, cardiac monitors can display the patient's heart rate and rhythm, produce a printed record of cardiac rhythm, and sound an alarm if the heart rate exceeds or falls below specified limits. Monitors also recognize and count abnormal heartbeats as well as changes. For example, ST-segment monitoring, helps detect myocardial ischemia, electrolyte imbalance, coronary artery spasm, and hypoxic events. The ST segment represents early ventricular repolarization, and any changes in this waveform component reflect alterations in myocardial oxygenation. Any monitoring lead that views an ischemic heart region will reveal ST-segment changes. The monitor's software establishes a template of the patient's normal QRST pattern from the selected leads; then the monitor displays ST-segment changes. Some monitors display such changes continuously, others only on command.

Key nursing diagnoses and patient outcomes
Ineffective tissue perfusion (cardiopulmonary) related to (specify)
The patient will:
▶ attain hemodynamic stability: pulse not less than (specify) beats/minute and not more than (specify) beats/minute; blood pressure not less than (specify) mm Hg and not more than (specify) mm Hg
▶ not exhibit arrhythmias

▶ have a heart rate that remains within prescribed limits while he carries out activities of daily living.

Decreased cardiac output related to (specify)
The patient will:
▶ exhibit no pedal edema
▶ experience a diminished heart workload
▶ maintain adequate cardiac output.

Equipment

Cardiac monitor • leadwires • patient cable • disposable pregelled electrodes (number of electrodes varies from three to five, depending on patient's needs) • alcohol pads • 4″ × 4″ gauze pads • washcloth • optional: shaving supplies

For telemetry
Transmitter • transmitter pouch • telemetry battery pack, leads, and electrodes.

Preparation of equipment

Plug the cardiac monitor into an electrical outlet and turn it on to warm up the unit while you prepare the equipment and the patient. Insert the cable into the appropriate socket in the monitor. Connect the leadwires to the cable. In some systems, the leadwires are permanently secured to the cable. Each leadwire should indicate the location for attachment to the patient: right arm (RA), left arm (LA), right leg (RL), left leg (LL), and ground (C or V). This should appear on the leadwire — if it's permanently connected — or at the connection of the leadwires and cable to the patient. Then connect an electrode to each of the leadwires, carefully checking that each leadwire is in its correct outlet.

For telemetry monitoring, insert a new battery into the transmitter. Be sure to match the poles on the battery with the polar markings on the transmitter case. By pressing the button at the top of the unit, test the battery charge and test the unit to ensure that the battery is operational. If the leadwires aren't permanently affixed to the telemetry unit, attach them securely. If they must be attached individually, be sure to connect each one to the correct outlet.

Implementation

▶ Explain the procedure to the patient, provide privacy, and ask the patient to expose his chest. Wash your hands.
▶ Determine electrode positions on the patient's chest, based on which system and lead you're using. (See *Positioning monitoring leads,* pages 102 and 103.)
▶ If the leadwires and patient cable aren't permanently attached, verify that the electrode placement corresponds to the label on the patient cable.
▶ If necessary, shave an area about 4″ (10 cm) in diameter around each electrode site. Clean the area with an alcohol pad and dry it completely *to remove skin secretions that may interfere with electrode function.* Gently abrade the dried area by rubbing it briskly until it reddens *to remove dead skin cells and to promote better electrical contact with living cells.* (Some electrodes have a small, rough patch for abrading the skin; otherwise, use a dry washcloth or a dry gauze pad.)
▶ Remove the backing from the pregelled electrode. Check the gel for moistness. If the gel is dry, discard it and replace it with a fresh electrode.

Positioning monitoring leads

This chart shows the correct electrode positions for some of the monitoring leads you'll use most often. For each lead, you'll see electrode placement for a five-leadwire system, a three-leadwire system, and a telemetry system.

In the two hardwire systems, the electrode positions for one lead may be identical to the electrode positions for another lead. In this case, you simply change the lead selector switch to the setting that corresponds to the lead you want. In some cases, you'll need to reposition the electrodes.

In the telemetry system, you can create the same lead with two electrodes that you do with three, simply by eliminating the ground electrode.

The illustrations below use these abbreviations: RA, right arm; LA, left arm; RL, right leg; LL, Left leg; C, chest; and G, ground.

Five-leadwire system	Three-leadwire system	Telemetry system

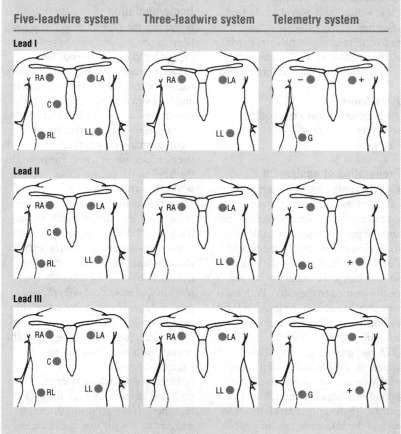

Lead I

Lead II

Lead III

Positioning monitoring leads *(continued)*

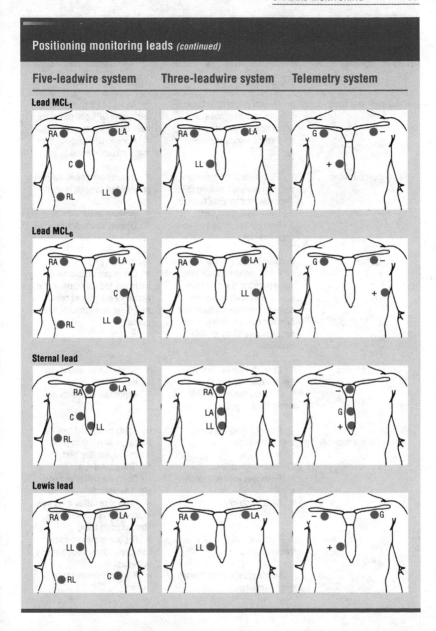

Five-leadwire system	Three-leadwire system	Telemetry system

Lead MCL_1

Lead MCL_6

Sternal lead

Lewis lead

▶ Apply the electrode to the site and press firmly *to ensure a tight seal*. Repeat with the remaining electrodes.

▶ When all the electrodes are in place, check for a tracing on the cardiac mon-

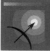

Troubleshooting

Identifying cardiac monitor problems

Problem	Possible causes	Solutions
False–high-rate alarm	■ Monitor interpreting large T waves as QRS complexes, which doubles the rate ■ Skeletal muscle activity	■ Reposition electrodes to lead where QRS complexes are taller than T waves. ■ Place electrodes away from major muscle masses.
False–low-rate alarm	■ Shift in electrical axis from patient movement, making QRS complexes too small to register ■ Low amplitude of QRS ■ Poor contact between electrode and skin	■ Reapply electrodes. Set gain so height of complex is greater than 1 millivolt. ■ Increase gain. ■ Reapply electrodes.
Low amplitude	■ Gain dial set too low ■ Poor contact between skin and electrodes; dried gel; broken or loose leadwires; poor connection between patient and monitor; malfunctioning monitor; physiologic loss of QRS amplitude	■ Increase gain. ■ Check connections on all leadwires and monitoring cable. Replace electrodes as necessary. Reapply electrodes, if required.
Wandering baseline	■ Poor position or contact between electrodes and skin ■ Thoracic movement with respirations	■ Reposition or replace electrodes. ■ Reposition electrodes.
Artifact (waveform interference)	■ Patient having seizures, chills, or anxiety ■ Patient movement ■ Electrodes applied improperly ■ Static electricity ■ Electrical short circuit in leadwires or cable ■ Interference from decreased room humidity	■ Notify doctor and treat patient as ordered. Keep patient warm and reassure him. ■ Help patient relax. ■ Check electrodes and reapply, if necessary. ■ Make sure cables don't have exposed connectors. Change static-causing linens. ■ Replace broken equipment. Use stress loops when applying leadwires. ■ Regulate humidity to 40%.

Identifying cardiac monitor problems *(continued)*

Problem	Possible causes	Solutions
Broken leadwires or cable	■ Stress loops not used on leadwires ■ Cables and leadwires cleaned with alcohol or acetone, causing brittleness	■ Replace leadwires and re-tape them, using stress loops. ■ Clean cable and leadwires with soapy water. Don't allow cable ends to become wet. Replace cable as needed.
60-cycle interference (fuzzy baseline)	■ Electrical interference from other equipment in room ■ Patient's bed improperly grounded	■ Attach all electrical equipment to common ground. Check plugs to make sure prongs aren't loose. ■ Attach bed ground to the room's common ground.
Skin excoriation under electrode	■ Patient allergic to electrode adhesive ■ Electrode on skin too long	■ Remove electrodes and apply hypoallergenic electrodes and hypoallergenic tape. ■ Remove electrode, clean site, and reapply electrode at new site.

itor. Assess the quality of the ECG. (See *Identifying cardiac monitor problems.*)

▶ To verify that each beat is being detected by the monitor, compare the digital heart rate display with your count of the patient's heart rate.

▶ If necessary, use the gain control to adjust the size of the rhythm tracing and use the position control to adjust the waveform position on the recording paper.

▶ Set the upper and lower limits of the heart rate alarm, based on unit policy. Turn the alarm on.

For telemetry monitoring

▶ Wash your hands. Explain the procedure to the patient and provide privacy.

▶ Expose the patient's chest, and select the lead arrangement. Remove the backing from one of the gelled electrodes. Check the gel for moistness. If it's dry, discard the electrode and obtain a new one.

▶ Apply the electrode to the appropriate site by pressing one side of the electrode against the patient's skin, pulling gently, and then pressing the other side against the skin. Press your fingers in a circular motion around the electrode *to fix the gel and stabilize the electrode.* Repeat for each electrode.

▶ Attach an electrode to the end of each leadwire.

▶ Place the transmitter in the pouch. Tie the pouch strings around the patient's neck and waist, making sure that the pouch fits snugly without causing him discomfort. If no pouch is available, place the transmitter in the patient's bathrobe pocket.

▶ Check the patient's waveform for clarity, position, and size. Adjust the gain and baseline as needed. (If necessary, ask the patient to remain resting or sitting in his room while you locate his telemetry monitor at the central station.)

▶ To obtain a rhythm strip, press the RECORD key at the central station. Label the strip with the patient's name and room number, date, and time. Also, identify the rhythm. Place the rhythm strip in the appropriate location in the patient's chart.

Special considerations

▶ Make sure that all electrical equipment and outlets are grounded *to avoid electric shock and interference (artifacts)*. Also, ensure that the patient is clean and dry *to prevent electric shock*.

▶ Avoid opening the electrode packages until just before using *to prevent the gel from drying out*.

▶ Avoid placing the electrodes on bony prominences, hairy locations, areas where defibrillator pads will be placed, or areas for chest compression.

▶ If the patient's skin is very oily, scaly, or diaphoretic, rub the electrode site with a dry 4″ × 4″ gauze pad before applying the electrode *to help reduce interference in the tracing*. Have the patient breathe normally during the procedure. If his respirations distort the recording, ask him to hold his breath briefly *to reduce baseline wander in the tracing*.

▶ Assess skin integrity and reposition the electrodes every 24 hours or as necessary.

▶ If the patient is being monitored by telemetry, show him how the transmitter works. If applicable, show him the button that will produce a recording of his ECG at the central station. Teach him how to push the button whenever he has symptoms. *This causes the central console to print a rhythm strip.* Tell the patient to remove the transmitter if he takes a shower or bath, but stress that he should tell you before removing the unit.

Documentation

Record in your nurse's notes the date and time that monitoring begins and the monitoring lead used. Document a rhythm strip at least every 8 hours and with any changes in the patient's condition (or as stated by your facility's policy). Label the rhythm strip with the patient's name and room number, the date, and the time.

CARDIAC OUTPUT MEASUREMENT

Cardiac output — the amount of blood ejected by the heart — helps evaluate cardiac function. The most widely used method of calculating this measurement is the bolus thermodilution technique. Performed at the patient's bedside, the thermodilution technique is the most practical method of evaluating the cardiac status of critically ill patients and those suspected of having cardiac disease. Other methods include the Fick method and the dye dilution test. (See *Other methods of measuring cardiac output.*)

To measure cardiac output, a quantity of solution colder than the patient's blood is injected into the right atrium via a port on a pulmonary artery (PA) catheter. This indicator solution mixes with the blood as it travels through the right ventricle into the pulmonary

Other methods of measuring cardiac output

In the Fick method (especially useful in detecting low cardiac output levels), the blood's oxygen content is measured before and after it passes through the lungs. First, blood is removed from the pulmonary and the brachial arteries and analyzed for oxygen content. Then, a spirometer measures oxygen consumption—the amount of air entering the lungs each minute. Next, cardiac output (CO) is calculated using this formula:

$$\text{CO (L/minute)} = \frac{\text{oxygen consumption (ml/min)}}{\text{arterial oxygen content} - \text{venous oxygen content (ml/minute)}}$$

In the dye dilution test, a known volume and concentration of dye is injected into the pulmonary artery and measured by simultaneously sampling the amount of dye in the brachial artery. To calculate cardiac output, these values are entered into a formula or plotted into a time and dilution-concentration curve. A computer, similar to the one used for the thermodilution test, performs the computation. Dye dilution measurements are particularly helpful in detecting intracardiac shunts and valvular regurgitation.

artery, and a thermistor on the catheter registers the change in temperature of the flowing blood. A computer then plots the temperature change over time as a curve and calculates flow based on the area under the curve.

Iced or room-temperature injectant may be used. The choice should be based on facility policy as well as the patient's status. The accuracy of the bolus thermodilution technique depends on the computer being able to differentiate the temperature change caused by the injectant in the pulmonary artery and the temperature changes in the pulmonary artery. Because iced injectant is colder than room-temperature injectant, it provides a stronger signal to be detected.

Typically, however, room-temperature injectant is more convenient and provides equally accurate measurements. Iced injectant may be more accurate in patients with high or low cardiac outputs, hypothermic patients, or when smaller volumes of injectant must

be used (3 to 5 ml), as in patients with volume restrictions or in children.

Key nursing diagnoses and patient outcomes

Decreased cardiac output related to reduced stroke volume
The patient will:
▶ maintain hemodynamic stability: pulse not less than (specify) and not greater than (specify); blood pressure not less than (specify) mm Hg and not greater than (specify) mm Hg
▶ exhibit no signs of arrhythmias
▶ not complain of chest pain, dizziness, or syncope.

Ineffective tissue perfusion (cardiopulmonary) related to decreased cellular exchange
The patient will:
▶ maintain adequate cardiac output
▶ have arterial blood gas results within normal limits
▶ have clear breath sounds on auscultation.

Equipment

For the thermodilution method

Thermodilution PA catheter in position • output computer and cables (or a module for the bedside cardiac monitor) • closed or open injectant delivery system • 10-ml syringe • 500-ml bag of dextrose 5% in water or normal saline solution • crushed ice and water (if iced injectant is used)

The newer bedside cardiac monitors measure cardiac output continuously, using either an invasive or a noninvasive method. If your bedside monitor doesn't have this capability, you'll need a free-standing cardiac output computer.

Preparation of equipment

Wash your hands thoroughly, and assemble the equipment at the patient's bedside. Insert the closed injectant system tubing into the 500-ml bag of I.V. solution. Connect the 10-ml syringe to the system tubing and prime the tubing with I.V. solution until it's free of air. Then clamp the tubing. The steps that follow differ, depending on the temperature of the injectant.

Room-temperature injectant closed delivery system

After clamping the tubing, connect the primed system to the stopcock of the proximal injectant lumen of the PA catheter. Next, connect the temperature probe from the cardiac output computer to the closed injectant system's flow-through housing device. Connect the cardiac output computer cable to the thermistor connector on the PA catheter and verify the blood temperature reading. Finally, turn on the cardiac output computer and enter the correct computation constant as provided by the catheter's manufacturer.

The constant is determined by the volume and temperature of the injectant as well as the size and type of catheter.

 Age alert For children, you'll need to adjust the computation constant to reflect a smaller volume and a smaller catheter size.

Iced injectant closed delivery system

After clamping the tubing, place the coiled segment into the Styrofoam container and add crushed ice and water to cover the entire coil. Let the solution cool for 15 to 20 minutes. The rest of the steps are the same as those for the room-temperature injectant closed delivery system.

Implementation

▶ Make sure your patient is in a comfortable position. Tell him not to move during the procedure *because movement can cause an error in measurement.*

▶ Explain to the patient that the procedure will help determine how well his heart is pumping and that he'll feel no discomfort.

For iced injectant closed delivery system

▶ Unclamp the I.V. tubing and withdraw 5 ml of solution into the syringe.

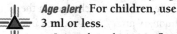 **Age alert** For children, use 3 ml or less.

▶ Inject the solution to flow past the temperature sensor, verifying that the injectant temperature registers between 43° and 54° F (6° and 12° C) on the computer.

▶ Verify the presence of a PA waveform on the cardiac monitor.

▶ Withdraw exactly 10 ml of cooled solution before reclamping the tubing.

▶ Turn the stopcock at the catheter injectant hub to open a fluid path between the injectant lumen of the PA catheter and syringe.

▶ Press the START button on the cardiac output computer or wait for the INJECT message to flash.

▶ Inject the solution smoothly within 4 seconds, making sure it doesn't leak at the connectors.

▶ If available, analyze the contour of the thermodilution washout curve on a strip chart recorder for a rapid upstroke and a gradual, smooth return to baseline.

▶ Wait 1 minute between injections and repeat the procedure until three values are within 10% and 15% of the median value. Compute the average and record the patient's cardiac output.

▶ Return the stopcock to its original position, and make sure the injectant delivery system tubing is clamped.

▶ Verify the presence of a PA waveform on the cardiac monitor.

For room-temperature injectant closed delivery system

▶ Verify the presence of a PA waveform on the cardiac monitor.

▶ Unclamp the I.V. tubing and withdraw exactly 10 ml of solution. Reclamp the tubing.

▶ Turn the stopcock at the catheter injectant hub to open a fluid path between the injectant lumen of the PA catheter and the syringe.

▶ Press the START button on the cardiac output computer or wait for an INJECT message to flash.

▶ Inject the solution smoothly within 4 seconds, making sure it doesn't leak at the connectors.

▶ If available, analyze the contour of the thermodilution washout curve on a strip chart recorder for a rapid upstroke and a gradual, smooth return to the baseline.

▶ Repeat these steps until three values are within 10% and 15% of the median value. Compute the average and record the patient's cardiac output.

▶ Return the stopcock to its original position and make sure the injectant delivery system tubing is clamped.

▶ Verify the presence of a PA waveform on the cardiac monitor.

▶ Discontinue cardiac output measurements when the patient is hemodynamically stable and weaned from his vasoactive and inotropic medications. You can leave the PA catheter inserted for pressure measurements.

▶ Disconnect and discard the injectant delivery system and the I.V. bag. Cover any exposed stopcocks with air-occlusive caps.

▶ Monitor the patient for signs and symptoms of inadequate perfusion, including restlessness, fatigue, changes in level of consciousness, decreased capillary refill time, diminished peripheral pulses, oliguria, and pale, cool skin.

Special considerations

▶ The normal range for cardiac output is 4 to 8 L/minute. The adequacy of a patient's cardiac output is better assessed by calculating his cardiac index (CI), adjusted for his body size.

▶ To calculate the patient's CI, divide his cardiac output by his body surface area (BSA), a function of height and weight. For example, a cardiac output of 4 L/minute might be adequate for a 65″, 120-lb (165-cm, 54-kg) patient (normally a BSA of 1.59 and a CI of 2.5) but would be inadequate for a 74″, 230-lb (188-cm, 104-kg) patient (normally a BSA of 2.26 and a CI of 1.8). The normal CI for adults ranges from 2.5 to 4.2 L/minute/m^2; for pregnant women, 3.5 to 6.5 L/minute/m^2.

Age alert Normal CI for infants and children is 3.5 to 4 L/minute/m². Normal CI for elderly adults is 2 to 2.5 L/minute/m².

▶ Add the fluid volume injected for cardiac output determinations to the patient's total intake. Injectant delivery of 30 ml/hour will contribute 720 ml to the patient's 24-hour intake.
▶ After cardiac output measurement, make sure the clamp on the injectant bag is secured *to prevent inadvertent delivery of the injectant to the patient.*

Documentation
Document your patient's cardiac output, CI, and other hemodynamic values and vital signs at the time of measurement. Note the patient's position during measurement and any other unusual occurrences, such as bradycardia or neurologic changes.

CAST PREPARATION

A cast is a hard mold that encases a body part, usually an extremity, to provide immobilization of bones and surrounding tissue. It can be used to treat injuries (including fractures), correct orthopedic conditions (such as deformities), or promote healing after general or plastic surgery, amputation, or nerve and vascular repair.

Casts may be constructed of plaster, fiberglass, or other synthetic materials. Plaster — a commonly used material — is inexpensive, nontoxic, nonflammable, easy to mold, and rarely causes allergic reactions or skin irritation. However, fiberglass is lighter, stronger, and more resilient than plaster. Because fiberglass dries rapidly, it is more diffi-

cult to mold, but it can bear body weight immediately if needed. (See *Types of cylindrical casts.*)

Typically, a doctor applies a cast and a nurse prepares the patient and the equipment and assists during the procedure. With special preparation, a nurse may apply or change a standard cast, but an orthopedist must reduce the fracture and set the fracture.

Contraindications for casting may include skin diseases, peripheral vascular disease, diabetes mellitus, open or draining wounds, overwhelming edema, and susceptibility to skin irritations. However, these aren't strict contraindications; the doctor must weigh the potential risks and benefits for each patient.

Key nursing diagnoses and patient outcomes
Impaired physical mobility related to fracture
The patient will:
▶ state relief from pain
▶ show no evidence of complications, such as contractures, venous stasis, thrombus formation, or skin breakdown
▶ demonstrate the ability to perform mobility regimen.

Ineffective tissue perfusion (peripheral) related to fracture
The patient will:
▶ have no numbness, tingling, or pain in body parts distal to the cast
▶ have unchanged skin color and temperature
▶ have strong peripheral pulses.

Equipment
Tubular stockinette • casting material • plaster rolls • plaster splints (if neces-

Types of cylindrical casts

Made of plaster, fiberglass, or synthetic material, casts may be applied almost anywhere on the body to support a single finger or the entire body. Common casts are shown here.

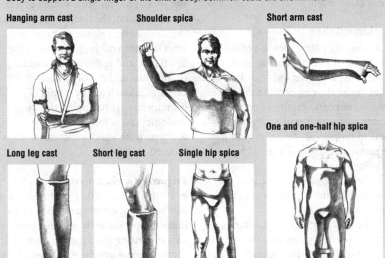

Hanging arm cast

Shoulder spica

Short arm cast

One and one-half hip spica

Long leg cast

Short leg cast

Single hip spica

sary) • bucket of water • sink equipped with plaster trap • linen-saver pad • sheet wadding • sponge or felt padding (if necessary) • pillows or bath blankets • cast scissors, cast saw, and cast spreader (for removing a cast) • optional: rubber gloves, cast stand, moleskin or adhesive tape

Gather the tubular stockinette, cast material, and plaster splints in the appropriate sizes. Tubular stockinettes range from 2″ to 12″ (5 to 30.5 cm) wide; plaster rolls, from 2″ to 6″ (5 to 15 cm) wide; and plaster splints, from 3″ to 6″ (8 to 15 cm) wide. Wear rubber gloves, especially if applying a fiberglass cast.

Preparation of equipment

Gently squeeze the packaged casting material to make sure the envelopes don't have any air leaks. *Humid air penetrating such leaks can cause plaster to become stale, which can make it set too quickly, form lumps, fail to bond with lower layers, or set as a soft, friable mass.* (Baking a stale plaster roll at a medium temperature for 1 hour can make it usable again.)

Follow the manufacturer's directions for water temperature when preparing plaster. Usually, room temperature or slightly warmer water is best *because it allows the cast to set in about 7 minutes without excessive exothermia.* (Cold water retards the rate of setting and may be used to facilitate difficult molding; warm water speeds the rate of setting and raises skin temperature under the cast.) Place all equipment within the doctor's reach.

Implementation

▶ *To allay the patient's fears,* explain the procedure. If plaster is being used, make sure he understands that heat will build under the cast because of a chemical reaction between the water and plaster. Also begin explaining some aspects of proper cast care *to prepare him for patient teaching and to assess his knowledge level.*
▶ Cover the appropriate parts of the patient's bedding and gown with a linen-saver pad.
▶ If the cast is applied to the wrist or arm, remove rings that may interfere with circulation in the fingers.
▶ Assess the condition of the skin in the affected area, noting any redness, contusions, or open wounds. *This will make it easier to evaluate any complaints the patient may have after the cast is applied.*
▶ If the patient has an open wound, prepare him for a local anesthetic if the doctor will administer one. Clean the wound. Assist the doctor as he closes the wound and applies a dressing.
▶ *To establish baseline measurements,* assess neurovascular status. Palpate the distal pulses; assess the color, temperature, and capillary refill of the appropriate fingers or toes; and check neurologic function, including sensation and motion in the affected and unaffected extremities.
▶ Help the doctor position the limb as ordered. (Commonly, the limb is immobilized in the neutral position.)

▶ Support the limb in the prescribed position while the doctor applies the tubular stockinette and sheet wadding. The stockinette should extend beyond the ends of the cast *to pad the edges.* (If the patient has an open wound or a severe contusion, the doctor may not use the stockinette.) He then wraps the limb in sheet wadding, starting at the distal end, and applies extra wadding to the distal and proximal ends of the cast area, as well as any points of prominence. As he applies the sheet wadding, check for wrinkles.
▶ Prepare the various cast materials as ordered.

Preparing a plaster cast
▶ Place a roll of plaster casting on its end in the bucket of water. Be sure to immerse it completely. When air bubbles stop rising from the roll, remove it, gently squeeze out the excess water and hand the casting material to the doctor, who will begin applying it to the extremity. As he applies the first roll, prepare a second roll in the same manner. (Stay at least one roll ahead of the doctor during the procedure.)
▶ After the doctor applies each roll, he'll smooth it to remove wrinkles, spread the plaster into the cloth webbing, and empty air pockets. If he's using plaster splints, he'll apply them in the middle layers of the cast. Before wrapping the last roll, he'll pull the ends of the tubular stockinette over the cast edges *to create padded ends, prevent cast crumbling, and reduce skin irritation.* He'll then use the final roll to keep the ends of the stockinette in place.

Preparing a fiberglass cast
▶ If you're using water-activated fiberglass, immerse the tape rolls in tepid

water for 10 to 15 minutes *to initiate the chemical reaction that causes the cast to harden.* Open one roll at a time. Avoid squeezing out excess water before application.

▶ If you're using light-cured fiberglass, you can unroll the material more slowly. This casting remains soft and malleable until it's exposed to ultraviolet light, *which sets it.*

Completing the cast
▶ As necessary, "petal" the cast's edges *to reduce roughness and to cushion pressure points.* (See *How to petal a cast.*)

▶ Use a cast stand or your palm to support the cast in the therapeutic position until it becomes firm to the touch (usually 6 to 8 minutes) *to prevent indentations in the cast.* Place the cast on a firm smooth surface to continue drying. Place pillows under joints to maintain flexion, if necessary.

▶ *To check circulation in the casted limb,* palpate the distal pulse and assess the color, temperature, and capillary refill of the fingers or toes. Determine neurologic status by asking the patient if he's experiencing paresthesia in the extremity or decreased motion of the extremity's uncovered joints. Assess the unaffected extremity in the same manner and compare findings.

▶ Elevate the limb above heart level with pillows or bath blankets as ordered *to facilitate venous return and reduce edema.*

▶ The doctor will then send the patient for X-rays *to ensure proper positioning.*

▶ Instruct the patient to notify the doctor of any pain, foul odor, drainage, or burning sensation under the cast. (After the cast hardens, the doctor may cut a window in it to inspect the painful or burning area.)

How to petal a cast

Rough cast edges can be cushioned by petaling them with adhesive tape or moleskin. To do this, first cut several 4″ × 2″ (10 × 5 cm) strips. Round off one end of each strip *to keep it from curling.* Then, making sure the rounded end of the strip is on the outside of the cast, tuck the straight end just inside the cast edge.

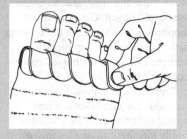

Smooth the moleskin with your finger until you're sure it's secured inside and out. Repeat the procedure, overlapping the moleskin pieces until you've gone all the way around the cast edge.

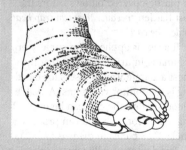

▶ Pour water from the plaster bucket into a sink containing a plaster trap. Don't use a regular sink *because plaster will block the plumbing.*

Special considerations
▶ A fiberglass cast dries immediately after application. A plaster extremity

cast dries in approximately 24 to 48 hours; a plaster spica or body cast, in 48 to 72 hours. During this drying period, the cast must be properly positioned *to prevent a surface depression that could cause pressure areas or dependent edema*. Neurovascular status must be assessed, drainage monitored, and the condition of the cast checked periodically.

▶ After the cast dries completely, it looks white and shiny and no longer feels damp or soft. Care consists of monitoring for changes in the drainage pattern, preventing skin breakdown near the cast, and averting the complications of immobility.

▶ Patient teaching must begin immediately after the cast is applied and should continue until the patient or a family member can care for the cast.

▶ Never use the bed or a table to support the cast as it sets *because molding can result, causing pressure necrosis of underlying tissue*. Also, don't use rubber- or plastic-covered pillows before the cast hardens *because they can trap heat under the cast*.

▶ If a cast is applied after surgery or traumatic injury, remember that the most accurate way to assess for bleeding is to monitor vital signs. A visible blood spot on the cast can be misleading: One drop of blood can produce a circle 3″ (7.6 cm) in diameter.

▶ The doctor usually removes the cast at the appropriate time, with a nurse assisting. (See *Removing a plaster cast.*) Tell the patient that when the cast is removed, his casted limb will appear thinner and flabbier than the uncasted limb. In addition, his skin will appear yellowish or gray from the accumulated dead skin and oils from the glands near the skin surface. Reassure him that with

exercise and good skin care, his limb will return to normal.

Home care

Before the patient goes home, teach him how to care for his cast. Tell him to keep the casted limb elevated above heart level *to minimize swelling*. Raise a casted leg by having the patient lie in a supine position with his leg on top of pillows. Prop a casted arm so that the hand and elbow are higher than the shoulder.

Instruct the patient to call the doctor if he can't move his fingers or toes, if he has numbness or tingling in the affected limb, or if he has symptoms of infection such as fever, unusual pain, or a foul odor from the cast. Advise him to maintain muscle strength by continuing any recommended exercises.

If the cast needs repair (if it loosens, cracks, or breaks) or if the patient has any questions about cast care, advise him to notify his doctor. Warn him not to get the cast wet. *Moisture will weaken or destroy it.* If the doctor approves, have the patient cover the cast with a plastic bag or cast cover for showering or bathing.

Urge the patient not to insert anything (such as a back scratcher or powder) into the cast to relieve itching. *Foreign matter can damage the skin and cause an infection.* Tell him, though, that he can apply alcohol on the skin at the cast edges. Warn the patient not to chip, crush, cut, or otherwise break any area of the cast and not to bear weight on the cast unless instructed to do so by the doctor.

If the patient must use crutches, instruct him to remove throw rugs from the floor and to rearrange furniture *to reduce the risk of tripping and falling*. If

Removing a plaster cast

Typically, a cast is removed when a fracture heals or requires further manipulation. Less common indications include cast damage, a pressure ulcer under the cast, excessive drainage or bleeding, and a constrictive cast.

Explain the procedure to the patient. Tell him he'll feel some heat and vibration as the cast is split with the cast saw. If the patient is a child, tell him that the saw is very noisy but won't cut the skin beneath. Warn the patient that when the padding is cut, he'll see discolored skin and signs of poor muscle tone. Reassure him that you'll stay with him. The illustrations here show how a plaster cast is removed.

The doctor cuts one side of the cast, then the other. As he does so, closely monitor the patient's anxiety level.	Next, the doctor opens the cast pieces with a spreader.	Finally, using cast scissors, the doctor cuts through the cast padding.

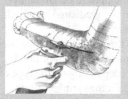 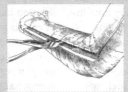 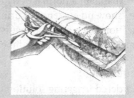

When the cast is removed, provide skin care to remove accumulated dead skin and to begin restoring the extremity's normal appearance.

the patient has a cast on his dominant arm, he may need help with bathing, toileting, eating, and dressing.

Complications

Complications of improper cast application include compartment syndrome, palsy, paresthesia, ischemia, ischemic myositis, pressure necrosis and, eventually, misalignment or nonunion of fractured bones.

Documentation

Record the date and time of cast application and skin condition of the extremity before the cast was applied. Note contusions, redness, or open wounds; results of neurovascular checks, before and after application, for the affected and unaffected extremities; location of any special devices, such as felt pads or plaster splints; and any patient teaching.

CATHETER IRRIGATION, URINARY

To avoid introducing microorganisms into the bladder, the nurse irrigates an indwelling catheter only to remove an obstruction such as a blood clot that develops after bladder, kidney, or prostate surgery.

Key nursing diagnoses and patient outcomes

Impaired urinary elimination related to possible obstruction
The patient will:
▶ maintain fluid balance (intake will equal output)
▶ have few if any complications
▶ describe feelings and concerns regarding the indwelling urinary catheter.

Risk for infection related to presence of the indwelling urinary catheter
The patient will:
▶ have no pathogens appear in cultures
▶ maintain a normal body temperature
▶ show no evidence of urinary tract infection, such as urine that is cloudy, malodorous, or with sediment.

Equipment

Ordered irrigating solution (such as normal saline solution) • sterile graduated receptacle or emesis basin • sterile bulb syringe or 50-ml catheter tip syringe • two alcohol pads • sterile gloves • linen-saver pad • intake-output sheet • optional: basin of warm water
    Commercially packaged kits containing sterile irrigating solution, a graduated receptacle, and a bulb or 50-ml catheter tip syringe are available. If the volume of irrigating solution instilled must be measured, use a graduated syringe instead of a noncalibrated bulb syringe.

Preparation of equipment

Check the expiration date on the irrigating solution. *To prevent vesical spasms during instillation of solution,* warm it to room temperature. If necessary, place the container in a basin of warm water. Never heat the solution on a burner or in a microwave oven. *Hot irrigating solution can injure the patient's bladder.*

Implementation

▶ Wash your hands and assemble the equipment at the bedside. Explain the procedure to the patient and provide privacy.
▶ Place the patient in the dorsal recumbent position. Then place a linen-saver pad under the patient's buttocks *to protect the bed linens.*
▶ Create a sterile field at the patient's bedside by opening the sterile equipment tray or commercial kit. Using aseptic technique, clean the lip of the solution bottle by pouring a small amount into a sink or waste receptacle. Then pour the prescribed amount of solution into the graduated receptacle or emesis basin.
▶ Place the tip of the syringe into the solution. Squeeze the bulb or pull back the plunger (depending on the type of syringe) and fill the syringe with the appropriate amount of solution (usually 30 ml).
▶ Open the package of alcohol pads; then put on sterile gloves. Clean the juncture of the catheter and drainage tube with an alcohol pad *to remove as many bacterial contaminants as possible.*
▶ Disconnect the catheter and drainage tube by twisting them in opposite directions and carefully pulling them apart without creating tension on the catheter. Don't let go of the catheter — hold it in your nondominant hand. Then place the end of the drainage tube on the sterile field, making sure not to contaminate the tube. Keep the end of the drainage tube sterile by placing a sterile gauze over it and securing the gauze with a piece of tape.
▶ Twist the bulb syringe or catheter-tip syringe onto the catheter's distal end.
▶ Squeeze the bulb or slowly push the plunger of the syringe *to instill the irrigating solution through the catheter.* If

necessary, refill the syringe and repeat this step until you've instilled the prescribed amount of irrigating solution.

▶ Remove the syringe and direct the return flow from the catheter into a graduated receptacle or emesis basin. Don't let the catheter end touch the drainage in the receptacle or become contaminated in any other way.

▶ Wipe the end of the drainage tube and catheter with the remaining alcohol pad.

▶ Wait a few seconds until the alcohol evaporates; then reattach the drainage tubing to the catheter.

▶ Dispose of all used supplies properly.

Special considerations

▶ Catheter irrigation requires strict aseptic technique *to prevent bacteria from entering the bladder.* The ends of the catheter and drainage tube and the tip of the syringe must be kept sterile throughout the procedure.

▶ If you encounter any resistance during instillation of the irrigating solution, don't try to force the solution into the bladder. Instead, stop the procedure and notify the doctor. If an indwelling catheter becomes totally obstructed, obtain an order to remove it and replace it with a new one *to prevent bladder distention, acute renal failure, urinary stasis, and subsequent infection.*

▶ The doctor may order a continuous irrigation system. *This decreases the risk of infection by eliminating the need to disconnect the catheter and drainage tube repeatedly.*

▶ Encourage catheterized patients not on restricted fluid intake to increase intake to 3,000 ml per day *to help flush the urinary system and reduce sediment formation. To keep the patient's urine acidic and help prevent calculus formation,* tell the patient to eat foods containing ascorbic acid, including citrus fruits and juices, cranberry juice, and dark green and deep yellow vegetables.

Documentation

Note the amount, color, and consistency of return urine flow and document the patient's tolerance for the procedure. Also note any resistance during instillation of the solution. If the return flow volume is less than the amount of solution instilled, note this on the intake and output balance sheets and in your notes.

CENTRAL VENOUS LINE INSERTION AND REMOVAL

A central venous catheter (CVC) is a sterile catheter made of polyurethane, polyvinyl chloride, or silicone rubber. It's inserted through a large vein such as the subclavian vein or, less commonly, the jugular vein. (See *Central venous catheter pathways,* page 118.)

By providing access to the central veins, central venous (CV) therapy offers several benefits. It allows monitoring of CV pressure, which indicates blood volume or pump efficiency and permits aspiration of blood samples for diagnostic tests. It also allows administration of I.V. fluids (in large amounts if necessary) in emergencies or when decreased peripheral circulation makes peripheral vein access difficult; when prolonged I.V. therapy reduces the number of accessible peripheral veins; when solutions must be diluted (for large fluid volumes or for irritating or hypertonic fluids, such as total parenteral nutrition solutions); and when a patient requires long-term venous access. Because multiple blood samples

Central venous catheter pathways

The illustrations below show several common pathways for central venous catheter (CVC) insertion. Typically, a CVC is inserted in the subclavian vein or in the internal jugular vein. The catheter typically terminates in the superior vena cava. The CVC is tunneled when long-term placement is required.

Insertion: Subclavian vein
Termination: Superior vena cava

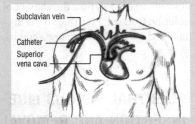

Insertion: Internal jugular vein
Termination: Superior vena cava

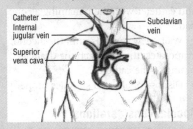

Insertion: Basilic vein (peripheral)
Termination: Superior vena cava

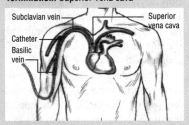

Insertion: Through a subcutaneous tunnel to the subclavian vein (Dacron cuff helps hold catheter in place.)
Termination: Superior vena cava

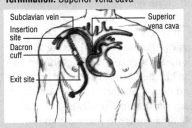

can be drawn through it without repeated venipuncture, the CV line decreases the patient's anxiety and preserves or restores peripheral veins.

A variation of CV therapy, peripheral CV therapy involves the insertion of a catheter into a peripheral vein instead of a central vein, but with the catheter tip still lying in the CV circulation. A peripherally inserted central catheter (PICC) usually enters at the basilic vein and terminates in the superior vena cava. PICCs may be inserted by a specially trained nurse. New catheters have longer needles and smaller lumens, facilitating this procedure. PICCs are commonly used in home I.V. therapy but may also be used with chest injury; chest, neck, or shoulder burns; compromised respiratory function; proximity of a surgical site to the CV line placement site; and if a doctor isn't available to insert a CV line.

CV therapy increases the risk of complications, such as pneumothorax, sepsis, thrombus formation, and vessel and adjacent organ perforation (all life-threatening conditions). Also, the CVC may decrease patient mobility, is difficult to insert, and costs more than a peripheral I.V. catheter.

Removal of a CVC—a sterile procedure—usually is performed by a doctor or nurse either at the end of therapy or at the onset of complications. A peripherally inserted central line may be removed by a specially trained nurse. If the patient may have an infection, the removal procedure includes collection of the catheter tip as a specimen for culture.

Key nursing diagnoses and patient outcomes

Risk for infection related to presence of CVC
The patient will:
▶ have no pathogens appear in cultures
▶ have a temperature that remains within normal limits
▶ show no evidence of infection at the insertion site, such as redness, swelling, or drainage.

Deficient fluid volume related to (specify)
The patient will:
▶ have vital signs remain stable
▶ produce at least 30 ml of urine/hour
▶ have electrolyte levels stay within normal range.

Equipment

For insertion of a CVC
Shave preparation kit, if necessary • sterile gloves and gowns • blanket • linen-saver pad • sterile towel • sterile drape • masks • an alcohol applicator or an applicator that contains povidone-iodine solution or other approved antimicrobial solution • alcohol pads • 10% povidone-iodine pads or other approved antimicrobial solution, such as 70% isopropyl alcohol or tincture of iodine 2% • normal saline solution • antibiotic ointment, if necessary • 3-ml syringe with 25G 1″ needle • 1% or 2% injectable lidocaine • dextrose 5% in water • syringes for blood sample collection • suture material • two 14G or 16G CVCs • I.V. solution with administration set prepared for use • infusion pump or controller, as needed • sterile 4″ × 4″ gauze pads • 1″ adhesive tape • sterile scissors • heparin or normal saline flushes as needed • portable X-ray machine • optional: transparent semipermeable dressing

For flushing a catheter
Normal saline solution or heparin flush solution • alcohol pad • 70% alcohol solution

For changing an injection cap
Alcohol or povidone-iodine pad • injection cap • padded clamp

For removing a CVC
Clean gloves and sterile gloves • sterile suture removal set • alcohol pads • povidone-iodine • sterile 4″ × 4″ gauze • forceps • tape • sterile, plastic adhesive-backed dressing or transparent semipermeable dressing • agar plate or culture tube, if necessary for culture

The type of catheter selected depends on the type of therapy to be used. (See *Guide to central venous catheters,* pages 120 to 123.)

Some facilities have prepared trays containing most of the equipment for catheter insertion.

(*Text continues on page 124.*)

Guide to central venous catheters

Type	Description	Indications
Groshong catheter	■ Silicone rubber ■ About 35″ (90 cm) long ■ Closed end with pressure-sensitive two-way valve ■ Dacron cuff ■ Single or double lumen ■ Tunneled	■ Long-term central venous (CV) access ■ Patient with heparin allergy

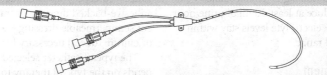

Short-term single-lumen catheter	■ Polyvinyl chloride (PVC) or polyurethane ■ About 8″ (20 cm) long ■ Lumen gauge varies ■ Percutaneously placed	■ Short-term CV access ■ Emergency access ■ Patient who needs only one lumen

Short-term multilumen catheter	■ PVC or polyurethane ■ Two, three, or four lumens exiting at ¾″ (2-cm) intervals ■ Lumen gauges vary ■ Percutaneously placed	■ Short-term CV access ■ Patient with limited insertion sites who requires multiple infusions

Advantages and disadvantages	Nursing considerations
Advantages ■ Less thrombogenic ■ Pressure-sensitive two-way valve eliminates frequent heparin flushes. ■ Dacron cuff anchors catheter and prevents bacterial migration. **Disadvantages** ■ Requires surgical insertion ■ Tears and kinks easily ■ Blunt end makes it difficult to clear substances from its tip.	■ Two surgical sites require dressing after insertion. ■ Handle catheter gently. ■ Check the external portion frequently for kinks and leaks. ■ Repair kit is available. ■ Remember to flush with enough saline solution to clear the catheter, especially after drawing or administering blood.
Advantages ■ Easily inserted at bedside ■ Easily removed ■ Stiffness aids central venous pressure (CVP) monitoring. **Disadvantages** ■ Limited functions ■ PVC is thrombogenic and irritates inner lumen of vessel. ■ Should be changed every 3 to 7 days (frequency may depend on facility's CV line infection rate)	■ Minimize patient movement. ■ Assess frequently for signs of infection and clot formation.
Advantages ■ Same as single-lumen catheter ■ Allows infusion of multiple (even incompatible) solutions through the same catheter **Disadvantages** ■ Same as single-lumen catheter	■ Know gauge and purpose of each lumen. ■ Use the same lumen for the same task.

(continued)

Guide to central venous catheters (continued)

Type	Description	Indications
Hickman catheter	■ Silicone rubber ■ About 35″ (90 cm) long ■ Open end with clamp ■ Dacron cuff 11¾ ″ (30 cm) from hub ■ Single lumen or multilumen ■ Tunneled	■ Long-term CV access ■ Home therapy

Type	Description	Indications
Broviac catheter	■ Identical to Hickman except smaller inner lumen	■ Long-term CV access ■ Patient with small central vessels (pediatric or geriatric)

Type	Description	Indications
Hickman/Broviac catheter	■ Hickman and Broviac catheters combined ■ Tunneled	■ Long-term CV access ■ Patient who needs multiple infusions

Type	Description	Indications
Peripherally inserted central catheter	■ Silicone rubber ■ 20″ (50.8 cm) long ■ Available in 16G, 18G, 20G, and 22G ■ Can be used as midline catheter ■ Percutaneously placed	■ Long-term CV access ■ Patient with poor CV access ■ Patient at risk for fatal complications from CV catheter insertion ■ Patient who needs CV access but is scheduled for or has had head or neck surgery

Advantages and disadvantages

Advantages
- Less thrombogenic
- Dacron cuff prevents excess motion and migration of bacteria.
- Clamps eliminate need for Valsalva's maneuver.

Disadvantages
- Requires surgical insertion
- Open end
- Requires doctor for removal
- Tears and kinks easlly

Advantages
- Smaller lumen

Disadvantages
- Small lumen may limit uses.
- Single lumen

Advantages
- Double-lumen Hickman catheter allows sampling and administration of blood.
- Broviac lumen delivers I.V. fluids, including total parenteral nutrition.

Disadvantages
- Same as Hickman catheter

Advantages
- Peripherally inserted
- Easily inserted at bedside with minimal complications
- May be inserted by a specially trained nurse in some states

Disadvantages
- Catheter may occlude smaller peripheral vessels.
- May be difficult to keep immobile
- Long path to CV circulation

Nursing considerations

- Two surgical sites require dressing after insertion.
- Handle catheter gently.
- Observe frequently for kinks and tears.
- Repair kit is available.
- Clamp catheter with a nonserrated clamp any time it becomes disconnected or opens.

- Check your facility's policy before drawing blood or administering blood or blood products.

- Know the purpose and function of each lumen.
- Label lumens to prevent confusion.

- Check frequently for signs of phlebitis and thrombus formation.
- Insert catheter above the antecubital fossa.
- Basilic vein is preferable to cephalic vein.
- Use arm board, if necessary.
- Length of catheter may alter CVP measurements.

Teaching Valsalva's maneuver

Increased intrathoracic pressure reduces the risk of air embolus during insertion and removal of a central venous catheter. A simple way to achieve this is to ask the patient to perform Valsalva's maneuver: forced exhalation against a closed airway. Instruct the patient to take a deep breath and hold it and then to bear down for 10 seconds. Then tell the patient to exhale and breathe quietly.

Valsalva's maneuver raises intrathoracic pressure from its normal level of 3 to 4 mm Hg to levels of 60 mm Hg or higher. It also slows the pulse rate, decreases the return of blood to the heart, and increases venous pressure.

This maneuver is contraindicated in patients with increased intracranial pressure. It shouldn't be taught to patients who aren't alert or cooperative.

Preparation of equipment

Before insertion of a CV catheter, confirm catheter type and size with the doctor; usually, a 14G or 16G catheter is selected. Set up the I.V. solution and prime the administration set using strict aseptic technique. Attach the line to the infusion pump or controller if ordered. Recheck all connections to make sure they're tight. As ordered, notify the radiology department that a portable X-ray machine will be needed.

Implementation

▶ Wash your hands thoroughly *to prevent the spread of microorganisms.*

Inserting a CVC

▶ Reinforce the doctor's explanation of the procedure and answer the patient's questions. Ensure that the patient has signed a consent form, if necessary, and check his history for hypersensitivity to iodine, latex, or the local anesthetic.

▶ Place the patient in Trendelenburg's position *to dilate the veins and reduce the risk of air embolism.*

▶ For subclavian insertion, place a rolled blanket lengthwise between the shoulders *to increase venous distention.* For jugular insertion, place a rolled blanket under the opposite shoulder *to extend the neck, making anatomic landmarks more visible.* Place a linen-saver pad under the patient *to prevent soiling the bed.*

▶ Turn the patient's head away from the site *to prevent possible contamination from airborne pathogens and to make the site more accessible.* Or, if dictated by facility policy, place a mask on the patient unless this increases his anxiety or is contraindicated because of his respiratory status.

▶ Prepare the insertion site. Make sure the skin is free of hair *because hair can harbor microorganisms.* Infection-control practitioners recommend clipping the hair close to the skin rather than shaving. *Shaving may cause skin irritation and create multiple small open wounds, increasing the risk of infection.* (If the doctor orders that the area be shaved, try shaving it the evening before catheter insertion; *this allows minor skin irritations to heal partially.*) You may also need to wash the skin with soap and water first.

▶ Establish a sterile field on a table, using a sterile towel or the wrapping from the instrument tray.

▶ Put on a mask and sterile gloves and gown and clean the area around the insertion site with an alcohol applicator or an applicator that contains povidone-iodine solution or other approved antimicrobial solution, working in a circular motion outward from the site. If the patient is sensitive to iodine, use alcohol.

▶ After the doctor puts on a sterile mask, a sterile gown, and sterile gloves and drapes the area to create a sterile field, open the packaging of the 3-ml syringe and 25G needle and give the syringe to him using sterile technique.

▶ Wipe the top of the lidocaine vial with an alcohol pad and invert it. The doctor then fills the 3-ml syringe and injects the anesthetic into the site (as shown below).

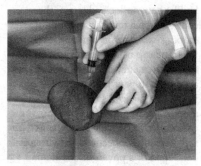

▶ Open the catheter package and give the catheter to the doctor using aseptic technique. The doctor then inserts the catheter.

▶ During this time, prepare the I.V. administration set for immediate attachment to the catheter hub. Ask the patient to perform Valsalva's maneuver while the doctor attaches the I.V. line to the catheter hub. *This increases intrathoracic pressure, reducing the possibility of an air embolus.* (See *Teaching Valsalva's maneuver.*)

▶ After the doctor attaches the I.V. line to the catheter hub, set the flow rate at a keep-vein-open rate to maintain venous access. (Alternatively, the catheter may be capped and flushed with heparin.) The doctor then sutures the catheter in place.

▶ After an X-ray confirms correct catheter placement in the midsuperior vena cava, set the flow rate as ordered.

▶ Use normal saline solution *to remove dried blood that could harbor microorganisms.* Secure the catheter with adhesive tape, and apply a sterile 4″ × 4″ gauze pad. You may also use a transparent semipermeable dressing either alone or placed over the gauze pad (as shown below).

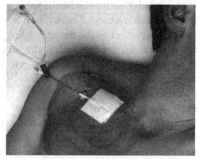

▶ Expect some serosanguineous drainage during the first 24 hours. Label the dressing with the time and date of catheter insertion and catheter length and gauge (as shown below), if not imprinted on the catheter.

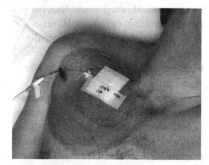

▶ Place the patient in a comfortable position and reassess his status.

Flushing the catheter
▶ *To maintain patency,* flush the catheter routinely according to your

facility's policy. If the system is being maintained as a heparin lock and the infusions are intermittent, the flushing procedure will vary according to policy, the medication administration schedule, and the type of catheter.

▶ All lumens of a multilumen catheter must be flushed regularly. Most facilities use a heparin flush solution available in premixed 10-ml multidose vials. Recommended concentrations vary from 10 to 100 units of heparin per milliliter. Use normal saline solution instead of heparin to maintain patency in two-way valved devices, such as the Groshong type, *because research suggests that heparin isn't always needed to keep the line open.*

▶ The recommended frequency for flushing CVCs varies from once every 12 hours to once weekly.

▶ The recommended amount of flushing solution also varies. Facilities recommend using twice the volume of the capacity of the cannula and the add-on devices if this volume is known. If the volume is unknown, most facilities recommend 3 to 5 ml of solution to flush the catheter, although some facility policies call for as much as 10 ml of solution. Different catheters require different amounts of solution.

▶ To perform the flushing procedure, start by cleaning the cap with an alcohol pad. Allow the cap to dry. If using the needleless system, follow the manufacturer's guidelines.

▶ Access the cap and aspirate *to confirm the patency of the CVC.*

▶ Inject the recommended type and amount of flush solution.

▶ After flushing the catheter, maintain positive pressure by keeping your thumb on the plunger of the syringe while withdrawing the needle. *This pre-*

vents blood backflow and clotting in the line. If flushing a valved catheter, close the clamp just before the last of the flush solution leaves the syringe.

Changing the injection cap

▶ CVCs used for intermittent infusions have needle-free injection caps (short luer-lock devices similar to the heparin lock adapters used for peripheral I.V. infusion therapy). These caps must be luer-lock types *to prevent inadvertent disconnection and an air embolism.* Unlike heparin lock adapters, these caps contain a minimal amount of empty space, so you don't have to preflush the cap before connecting it.

▶ The frequency of cap changes varies according to your facility's policy and how often the cap is used. Use strict aseptic technique when changing the cap.

▶ Clean the connection site with an alcohol pad or a povidone-iodine pad.

▶ Instruct the patient to perform Valsalva's maneuver while you quickly disconnect the old cap and connect the new cap using aseptic technique. If he can't perform this maneuver, use a padded clamp to prevent air from entering the catheter.

Removing a CVC

▶ If you'll be removing the CVC, first check the patient's record for the most recent placement (confirmed by an X-ray) *to trace the catheter's path as it exits the body.* Make sure that assistance is available if a complication (such as uncontrolled bleeding) occurs during catheter removal. (*Some vessels, such as the subclavian vein, can be difficult to compress.*) Before you remove the catheter, explain the procedure to the patient.

► Place the patient in a supine position *to prevent an embolism*.

► Wash your hands and put on clean gloves and a mask.

► Turn off all infusions and prepare a sterile field, using a sterile drape.

► Remove and discard the old dressing and change to sterile gloves.

► Clean the site with an alcohol pad or a gauze pad soaked in povidone-iodine solution. Inspect the site for signs of drainage and inflammation.

► Clip the sutures and, using forceps, remove the catheter in a slow, even motion. Have the patient perform Valsalva's maneuver as the catheter is withdrawn *to prevent an air embolism*.

► Apply pressure with a sterile gauze pad immediately after removing the catheter.

► Apply povidone-iodine ointment to the insertion site *to seal it*. Cover the site with a gauze pad and place a transparent semipermeable dressing over the gauze. Label the dressing with the date and time of the removal and your initials. Keep the site covered for 48 hours.

► Inspect the catheter tip and measure the length of the catheter *to ensure that the catheter has been completely removed*. If you suspect that the catheter hasn't been completely removed, notify the doctor immediately and monitor the patient closely for signs of distress. If you suspect an infection, swab the catheter on a fresh agar plate and send to the laboratory for culture.

► Dispose of the I.V. tubing and equipment properly.

Special considerations

► While you're awaiting chest X-ray confirmation of proper catheter placement, infuse an I.V. solution such as dextrose 5% in water or normal saline solution at a keep-vein-open rate until correct placement is ensured. Or use heparin to flush the line. *Infusing an isotonic solution avoids the risk of vessel wall thrombosis.*

Nursing alert Be alert for such signs of air embolism as sudden onset of pallor, cyanosis, dyspnea, coughing, and tachycardia, progressing to syncope and shock. If any of these signs occur, place the patient on his left side in Trendelenburg's position and notify the doctor.

► After insertion, also watch for signs and symptoms of pneumothorax, such as shortness of breath, uneven chest movement, tachycardia, and chest pain. Notify the doctor immediately if such signs and symptoms appear.

► Change the dressing at least every 48 hours if a gauze dressing is used or every 3 to 7 days if a transparent semipermeable dressing is used, according to your facility's policy, or whenever it becomes moist or soiled. Change the tubing every 48 hours and the solution every 24 hours or according to your facility's policy while the CVC is in place. Dressing, tubing, and solution changes for a CVC should be performed using aseptic technique. (See *Key steps in changing a central venous dressing,* page 128.) Assess the site for signs and symptoms of infection, such as discharge, inflammation, and tenderness.

► *To prevent an air embolism,* close the catheter clamp or have the patient perform Valsalva's maneuver each time the catheter hub is open to air. (A Groshong catheter doesn't require clamping *because it has an internal valve*.)

Key steps in changing a central venous dressing

Expect to change your patient's central venous (CV) dressing every 3 to 7 days. Many facilities specify dressing changes whenever the dressing becomes soiled, moist, or loose. The following illustrations show the key steps you'll perform.

First, put on clean gloves and remove the old dressing by pulling it toward the exit site of a long-term catheter or toward the insertion site of a short-term catheter. *This technique helps you avoid pulling out the line.* Remove and discard your gloves.

Next, put on sterile gloves and clean the skin around the site three times using a new applicator soaked in povidone-iodine solution. Start at the center and move outward, using a circular motion (as shown below).

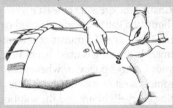

After the solution has dried, cover the site with a dressing, such as a gauze dressing or the transparent semipermeable dressing shown here. Write the time and date on the dressing.

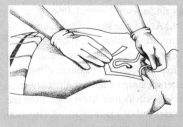

Home care

Long-term use of a CVC allows patients to receive caustic fluids and blood infusions at home. These catheters have a much longer life because they are less thrombogenic and less prone to infection than short-term devices.

A candidate for home therapy must have a family member or friend who can safely and competently administer the I.V. fluids, a backup helper, a suitable home environment, a telephone, transportation, adequate reading skills, and the ability to prepare, handle, store, and dispose of the equipment. The care procedures used in the home are the same as those used in the facility, except that the home therapy patient uses clean instead of aseptic technique.

The overall goal of home therapy is patient safety, so your patient teaching must begin well before discharge. After discharge, a home therapy coordinator will provide follow-up care until the patient or someone close to him can provide catheter care and infusion therapy independently. Many home therapy patients learn to care for the catheter themselves and infuse their own medications and solution.

Complications

Complications can occur at any time during infusion therapy. Traumatic complications such as pneumothorax typically occur on catheter insertion but may not be noticed until after the procedure is completed. Systemic complications such as sepsis typically occur later during infusion therapy. Other complications include phlebitis (especially in peripheral CV therapy), thrombus formation, and air embolism.

Documentation

Record the time and date of insertion, length and location of the catheter, solution infused, doctor's name, and patient's response to the procedure. Document the time of the X-ray, its results, and your notification of the doctor.

Also record the time and date of removal and the type of antimicrobial ointment and dressing applied. Note the condition of the catheter insertion site and collection of a culture specimen.

CENTRAL VENOUS PRESSURE MONITORING

In central venous pressure (CVP) monitoring, the doctor inserts a catheter through a vein and advances it until its tip lies in or near the right atrium. Because no major valves lie at the junction of the superior vena cava and right atrium, pressure at end diastole reflects back to the catheter. When connected to a manometer, the catheter measures CVP, an index of right ventricular function.

CVP monitoring helps to assess cardiac function, to evaluate venous return to the heart, and to indirectly gauge how well the heart is pumping. The central venous (CV) line also provides access to a large vessel for rapid, high-volume fluid administration and allows frequent blood withdrawal for laboratory samples.

CVP monitoring can be done *intermittently or continuously*. The catheter is inserted percutaneously or using a cutdown method. To measure the patient's volume status, a disposable plastic water manometer may be attached between the I.V. line and the central catheter with a three- or four-way stopcock. CVP may also be monitored continuously through a CV catheter that is attached to a pressure transducer. CVP is recorded in centimeters of water (cm H_2O) or millimeters of mercury (mm Hg).

Normal CVP ranges from 5 to 10 cm H_2O. Any condition that alters venous return, circulating blood volume, or cardiac performance may affect CVP. If circulating volume increases (such as with enhanced venous return to the heart), CVP rises. If circulating volume decreases (such as with reduced venous return), CVP drops.

Key nursing diagnoses and patient outcomes

Deficient fluid volume related to compromised circulatory mechanisms
The patient will:
▶ have stable vital signs
▶ produce adequate urine volume
▶ maintain CVP reading between 5 and 10 cm H_2O.

Excessive fluid volume related to compromised regulatory mechanisms
The patient will:
▶ maintain blood pressure not less than (specify) mm Hg and not greater than (specify) mm Hg
▶ maintain fluid intake of not more than (specify) and output of not less than (specify)
▶ maintain a CVP reading between 5 and 10 cm H_2O.

Equipment
For intermittent CVP monitoring
Disposable CVP manometer set • leveling device (such as a rod from a reusable CVP pole holder or a carpenter's level or rule) • additional stopcock (to attach the CVP manometer to the

catheter) • extension tubing (if needed) • I.V. pole • I.V. solution • I.V. drip chamber and tubing

For continuous CVP monitoring
Pressure monitoring kit with disposable pressure transducer • leveling device • bedside pressure module • continuous I.V. flush solution • pressure bag

For withdrawing blood samples through the CV line
Appropriate number of syringes for the ordered tests • 5- or 10-ml syringe for the discard sample (syringe size depends on the tests ordered)

For using an intermittent CV line
Syringe with normal saline solution • syringe with heparin flush solution

For removing a CV catheter
Sterile gloves • suture removal set • sterile gauze pads • povidone-iodine ointment • dressing • tape

Implementation
▶ Gather the necessary equipment. Explain the procedure to the patient *to reduce his anxiety.*
▶ Assist the doctor as he inserts the CV catheter. (The procedure is similar to that used for pulmonary artery pressure monitoring, except that the catheter is advanced only as far as the superior vena cava.)

Obtaining intermittent CVP readings with a water manometer
▶ With the CV line in place, position the patient flat. Align the base of the manometer with the previously determined zero reference point by using a leveling device. Because CVP reflects right atrial pressure, you must align the right atrium (the zero reference point) with the zero mark on the manometer. To find the right atrium, locate the fourth intercostal space at the midaxillary line. Mark the appropriate place on the patient's chest *so that all subsequent recordings will be made using the same location.*
▶ If the patient can't tolerate a flat position, place him in semi-Fowler's position. When the head of the bed is elevated, the phlebostatic axis remains constant but the midaxillary line changes. Use the same degree of elevation for all subsequent measurements.
▶ Attach the water manometer to an I.V. pole or place it next to the patient's chest. Make sure the zero reference point is level with the right atrium. (See *Measuring CVP with a water manometer.*)
▶ Verify that the water manometer is connected to the I.V. tubing. Typically, markings on the manometer range from −2 to 38 cm H_2O. However, manufacturer's markings may differ, so be sure to read the directions before setting up the manometer and obtaining readings.
▶ Turn the stopcock off to the patient and slowly fill the manometer with I.V. solution until the fluid level is 10 to 20 cm H_2O higher than the patient's expected CVP value. Don't overfill the tube *because fluid that spills over the top can become a source of contamination.*
▶ Turn the stopcock off to the I.V. solution and open to the patient. The fluid level in the manometer will drop. When the fluid level comes to rest, it will fluctuate slightly with respirations. Expect it to drop during inspiration and to rise during expiration.
▶ Record CVP at the end of inspiration, when intrathoracic pressure has a negligible effect. Depending on the type of water manometer used, note the val-

Measuring CVP with a water manometer

To ensure accurate central venous pressure (CVP) readings, make sure the manometer base is aligned with the patient's right atrium (the zero reference point). The manometer set usually contains a leveling rod to allow you to determine this quickly.

After adjusting the manometer's position, examine the typical three-way stopcock. By turning it to any position shown at right, you can control the direction of fluid flow. Four-way stopcocks also are available.

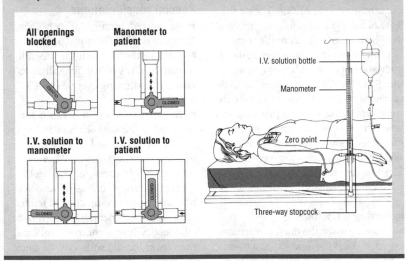

All openings blocked

Manometer to patient

I.V. solution to manometer

I.V. solution to patient

I.V. solution bottle

Manometer

Zero point

Three-way stopcock

---

ue either at the bottom of the meniscus or at the midline of the small floating ball.

▶ After you've obtained the CVP value, turn the stopcock to resume the I.V. infusion. Adjust the I.V. drip rate as required.

▶ Place the patient in a comfortable position.

Obtaining continuous CVP readings with a water manometer

▶ Make sure the stopcock is turned so that the I.V. solution port, CVP column port, and patient port are open. Be aware that with this stopcock position, infusion of the I.V. solution increases

CVP. Therefore, expect higher readings than those taken with the stopcock turned off to the I.V. solution. If the I.V. solution infuses at a constant rate, CVP will change as the patient's condition changes, although the initial reading will be higher. Assess the patient closely for changes.

Obtaining continuous CVP readings with a pressure monitoring system

▶ Make sure the CV line or the proximal lumen of a pulmonary artery catheter is attached to the system. (If the patient has a CV line with multiple lumens, one lumen may be dedicated to continuous CVP monitoring and the other lumens used for fluid administration.)

▶ Set up a pressure transducer system. Connect pressure tubing from the CVP catheter hub to the transducer. Then connect the flush solution container to a flush device.

▶ To obtain values, position the patient flat. If he can't tolerate this position, use semi-Fowler's position. Locate the level of the right atrium by identifying the phlebostatic axis. Zero the transducer, leveling the transducer air-fluid interface stopcock with the right atrium. Read the CVP value from the digital display on the monitor and note the waveform. Make sure the patient is still when the reading is taken *to prevent artifact.* (See *Identifying hemodynamic pressure monitoring problems,* pages 133 to 135.) Be sure to use this position for all subsequent readings.

Removing a CV line

▶ You may assist the doctor in removing a CV line. (In some states, a nurse is permitted to remove the catheter with a doctor's order or when acting under advanced collaborative standards of practice.)

▶ If the head of the bed is elevated, minimize the risk of air embolism during catheter removal — for instance, by placing the patient in Trendelenburg's position, if the line was inserted using a superior approach. If he can't tolerate this, position him flat.

▶ Turn the patient's head to the side opposite the catheter insertion site. The doctor removes the dressing and exposes the insertion site. If sutures are in place, he removes them carefully.

▶ Turn the I.V. solution off.

▶ The doctor pulls the catheter out in a slow, smooth motion and then applies pressure to the insertion site.

▶ Put on sterile gloves. Clean the insertion site, apply povidone-iodine ointment, and cover it with a sterile gauze dressing as ordered. Remove gloves and wash your hands.

▶ Assess the patient for signs of respiratory distress, *which may indicate an air embolism.*

Special considerations

▶ As ordered, arrange for daily chest X-rays *to check catheter placement.*

▶ Care for the insertion site according to your facility's policy. Typically, you'll change the dressing every 24 to 48 hours.

▶ Be sure to wash your hands before performing dressing changes and to use aseptic technique and sterile gloves when re-dressing the site. When removing the old dressing, observe for signs of infection such as redness and note any patient complaints of tenderness. Apply ointment, if directed by facility policy (use is controversial), and then cover the site with a sterile gauze dressing or a clear occlusive dressing.

▶ After the initial CVP reading, reevaluate readings frequently *to establish a baseline for the patient.* Authorities recommend obtaining readings at 15-, 30-, and 60-minute intervals to establish a baseline. If the patient's CVP fluctuates by more than 2 cm H_2O, suspect a change in his clinical status and report this finding to the doctor.

▶ Change the I.V. solution every 24 hours and the I.V. tubing every 48 hours, according to facility policy. Expect the doctor to change the catheter every 72 hours. Label the I.V. solution, tubing, and dressing with the date, the time, and your initials.

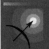

Troubleshooting

Identifying hemodynamic pressure monitoring problems

Problem	Possible causes	Interventions
No waveform	■ Power supply turned off ■ Monitor screen pressure range set too low ■ Loose connection in line ■ Transducer not connected to amplifier ■ Stopcock off to patient ■ Catheter occluded or out of blood vessel	■ Check the power supply. ■ Raise the monitor screen pressure range, if necessary. ■ Rebalance and recalibrate the equipment. ■ Tighten loose connections. ■ Check and tighten the connection. ■ Position the stopcock correctly. ■ Use the fast-flush valve to flush line, or try to aspirate blood from the catheter. If the line remains blocked, notify the doctor and prepare to replace the line.
Drifting waveforms	■ Improper warm-up ■ Electrical cable kinked or compressed ■ Temperature change in room air or I.V. flush solution	■ Allow the monitor and transducer to warm up for 10 to 15 minutes. ■ Place the monitor's cable where it can't be stepped on or compressed. ■ Routinely zero and calibrate the equipment 30 minutes after setting it up. This allows I.V. fluid to warm to room temperature.
Line fails to flush	■ Stopcocks positioned incorrectly ■ Inadequate pressure from pressure bag ■ Kink in pressure tubing ■ Blood clot in catheter	■ Make sure stopcocks are positioned correctly. ■ Make sure the pressure bag gauge reads 300 mm Hg. ■ Check the pressure tubing for kinks. ■ Try to aspirate the clot with a syringe. If the line still won't flush, notify the doctor and prepare to replace the line, if necessary. *Important:* Never use a syringe to flush a hemodynamic line.
Artifact (waveform interference)	■ Patient movement ■ Electrical interference ■ Catheter fling (tip of pulmonary artery catheter moving rapidly in large blood vessel in heart chamber)	■ Wait until the patient is quiet before taking a reading. ■ Make sure electrical equipment is connected and grounded correctly. ■ Notify the doctor, who may try to reposition the catheter.

(continued)

Identifying hemodynamic pressure monitoring problems *(continued)*

Problem	Possible causes	Interventions
False-high readings	■ Transducer balancing port positioned below patient's right atrium	■ Position the balancing port level with the patient's right atrium.
	■ Flush solution flow rate that is too fast	■ Check the flush solution flow rate. Maintain it at 3 to 4 ml/hour.
	■ Air in system	■ Remove air from the lines and the transducer.
	■ Catheter fling (tip of pulmonary artery catheter moving rapidly in large blood vessel or heart chamber)	■ Notify the doctor, who may try to reposition the catheter.
False-low readings	■ Transducer balancing port positioned above right atrium	■ Position the balancing port level with the patient's right atrium.
	■ Transducer imbalance	■ Make sure the transducer's flow system isn't kinked or occluded and rebalance and recalibrate the equipment.
	■ Loose connection	■ Tighten loose connections.
Damped waveform	■ Air bubbles	■ Secure all connections. ■ Remove air from the lines and the transducer. ■ Check for and replace cracked equipment.
	■ Blood clot in catheter	■ Refer to "Line fails to flush" (earlier in this chart).
	■ Blood flashback in line	■ Make sure stopcock positions are correct; tighten loose connections and replace cracked equipment; flush the line with the fast-flush valve; replace the transducer dome, if blood backs up into it.
	■ Incorrect transducer position	■ Make sure the transducer is kept at the level of the right atrium at all times. Improper levels give false-high or false-low pressure readings.
	■ Arterial catheter out of blood vessel or pressed against vessel wall	■ Reposition the catheter if it's against the vessel wall. ■ Try to aspirate blood to confirm proper placement in the vessel. If you can't aspirate blood, notify the doctor and prepare to replace the line. *Note:* Bloody drainage at the insertion site may indicate catheter displacement. Notify the doctor immediately.

Identifying hemodynamic pressure monitoring problems *(continued)*

Problem	Possible causes	Interventions
Pulmonary artery wedge pressure tracing unobtainable	■ Ruptured balloon	■ If you feel no resistance when injecting air, or if you see blood leaking from the balloon inflation lumen, stop injecting air and notify the doctor. If the catheter is left in, label the inflation lumen with a warning not to inflate.
	■ Incorrect amount of air in balloon	■ Deflate the balloon. Check the label on the catheter for correct volume. Reinflate slowly with the correct amount. To avoid rupturing the balloon, never use more than the stated volume.
	■ Catheter malpositioned	■ Notify the doctor. Obtain a chest X-ray.

Complications

Complications of CVP monitoring include pneumothorax (which typically occurs upon catheter insertion), sepsis, thrombus, vessel or adjacent organ puncture, and air embolism.

Documentation

Document all dressing, tubing, and solution changes. Document the patient's tolerance of the procedure, the date and time of catheter removal, and the type of dressing applied. Note the condition of the catheter insertion site and whether a culture specimen was collected. Note any complications and actions taken.

CEREBRAL BLOOD FLOW MONITORING

Traditionally, caregivers have estimated cerebral blood flow (CBF) in neurologically compromised patients by calculating cerebral perfusion pressure. However, modern technology permits continuous regional blood flow monitoring at the bedside.

A sensor placed on the cerebral cortex calculates CBF in the capillary bed by thermal diffusion. Thermistors within the sensor detect the temperature differential between two metallic plates — one heated, one neutral. This differential is inversely proportional to CBF: As the differential decreases, CBF increases — and vice versa. This monitoring technique reveals important information about the effects of interventions on CBF. It also yields continuous real-time values for CBF, which are essential in conditions in which compromised blood flow may put the patient at risk for complications, such as ischemia and infarction.

CBF monitoring is indicated whenever CBF alterations are anticipated. It's used most commonly in patients with subarachnoid hemorrhage (in which a vasospasm may restrict blood flow),

CBF monitoring system

To monitor cerebral blood flow (CBF) at the patient's bedside, you may use a monitor such as the one shown below. This monitor has a digital display; some also display waveforms. The CBF sensor, placed in the cerebral cortex, measures cortical blood flow continuously.

Bedside CBF monitor

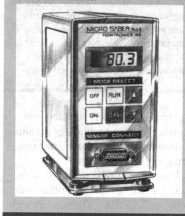

trauma associated with high intracranial pressure, or vascular tumors.

Key nursing diagnoses and patient outcomes

Ineffective tissue perfusion (cerebral) related to decreased cellular exchange
The patient will:
▶ maintain or improve current level of consciousness
▶ maintain intracranial pressure between (specify) mm Hg and (specify) mm Hg
▶ maintain blood pressure high enough to maintain cerebral perfusion pressure but low enough to prevent increased bleeding or cerebral swelling.

Risk for infection related to CBF sensor
The patient will:
▶ remain afebrile
▶ present no pathogen in cultures
▶ have a normal white blood cell count and differential.

Equipment

CBF monitoring requires a special sensor that attaches to a computer data system or to a small analog monitor that operates on a battery for patient transport. (See *CBF monitoring system.*)

For care of site

Sterile 4″ × 4″ gauze pads • clean gloves • sterile gloves • povidone-iodine solution or ointment • adhesive tape

For removing sensor

Sterile suture removal tray • 1″ adhesive tape • sterile 4″ × 4″ gauze pads • clean gloves • sterile gloves • suture material

Preparation of equipment

Make sure that the patient or a family member is fully informed about the procedures involved in CBF monitoring and obtain a consent form. If the patient will need CBF monitoring after surgery, advise him that a sensor will be in place for about 3 days. Tell the patient that the insertion site will be covered with a dry, sterile dressing. Mention that the sensor may be removed at the bedside.

Setting up the sensor monitor

Depending on the type of system you're using, you may need to verify that a battery has been inserted in the monitor to allow CBF monitoring during patient transport to the intensive care unit.

Inserting a CBF sensor

Typically, the surgeon inserts a cerebral blood flow (CBF) sensor during a craniotomy. He tunnels the sensor toward the craniotomy site and then carefully inserts the metallic plates of the thermistor to make sure that they continuously contact the surface of the cerebral cortex. After closing the dura and replacing the bone flap, he closes the scalp.

Insertion site

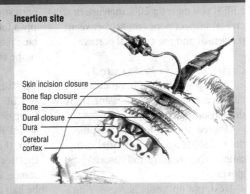

Skin incision closure
Bone flap closure
Bone
Dural closure
Dura
Cerebral cortex

The sensor measures CBF by means of thermistors housed inside it. The thermistors consist of two metallic plates — one heated and one neutral. The sensor detects the temperature difference between the two plates. This difference is inversely proportional to CBF. As CBF increases, the temperature difference decreases — and vice versa.

Sensor

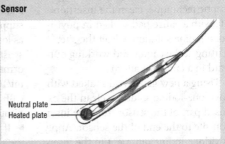

Neutral plate
Heated plate

First, assemble the following equipment at the bedside: a monitor and a sensor cable with an attached sensor. Attach the distal end of the sensor cable (from the patient's head) to the SENSOR CONNECT port on the monitor. When the sensor cable is securely in place, press the ON key to activate the monitor.

Next, calibrate the system by pressing the CAL key. You should see the red light appear on the CAL button. Ideally, you'll begin by calibrating the sensor to 00.0 by pressing the directional arrows. Readouts of plus or minus 0.1 are also acceptable.

Implementation

▶ The surgeon typically inserts the sensor in the operating room during or following a craniotomy. (Occasionally, he may insert it through a burr hole.) He implants the sensor far from major blood vessels and verifies that the metallic plates have good contact with the brain surface. (See *Inserting a CBF sensor.*)

▶ Press the RUN key to display the CBF reading. Observe the monitor's digital display and document the baseline value.

▶ Record the CBF hourly. Be sure to watch for trends and correlate values with the patient's clinical status. Be aware that stimulation or activity may cause a 10% increase or decrease in CBF. If you detect a 20% increase or decrease, suspect poor contact between the sensor and the cerebral cortex.

Caring for the insertion site
▶ Wash your hands. Put on clean gloves, and remove the dressing from the sensor insertion site.
▶ Observe the site for cerebrospinal fluid (CSF) leakage, a potential complication. Then remove and discard your gloves.
▶ Next, put on sterile gloves. Using aseptic technique, clean the insertion site with a gauze pad soaked in povidone-iodine solution. Clean the site, starting at the center and working outward in a circular pattern.
▶ Using a new gauze pad soaked with povidone-iodine solution, clean the exposed part of the sensor from the insertion site to the end of the sensor. Apply povidone-iodine ointment to the insertion site if your facility's policy permits.
▶ Next, place sterile 4″ × 4″ gauze pads over the insertion site to completely cover it. Tape all edges securely *to create an occlusive dressing.*

Removing the sensor
▶ In most cases, the CBF sensor remains in place for about 3 days when used for postoperative monitoring.
▶ Explain the procedure to the patient; then wash your hands. Put on clean gloves, remove the dressing, and dispose of the gloves and dressing properly.
▶ Open the suture removal tray and the package of suture material. The surgeon removes the anchoring sutures

and then gently removes the sensor from the insertion site.
▶ After the surgeon closes the wound with stitches, put on sterile gloves, apply a folded gauze pad to the site, and tape it in place. Observe the condition of the site, including any leakage.

Special considerations
▶ CBF fluctuates with the brain's metabolic demands, ranging from 60 to 90 ml/100 g/minute normally. However, the patient's neurologic condition dictates the acceptable range. For instance, in a patient in a coma, CBF may be half the normal value; in a patient in a barbiturate-induced coma with burst suppression on the EEG, CBF may be as low as 10 ml/100 g/minute. Vasospasm secondary to subarachnoid hemorrhage may result in CBF below 40 ml/100 g/minute. In an awake patient, CBF above 90 ml/100 g/minute may indicate hyperemia.
▶ If you suspect poor contact between the sensor and the cerebral cortex, turn the patient toward the side of the sensor or gently wiggle the catheter back and forth (using a sterile-gloved hand). *To determine whether these maneuvers have improved contact between the sensor and the cortex,* observe the CBF value on the monitor as you perform them.
▶ If your patient has low CBF but no neurologic signs that indicate ischemia, suspect a fluid layer (a small hematoma) between the sensor and the cortex.
▶ As with intracranial pressure monitoring, CBF monitoring may lead to infection. Administer prophylactic antibiotics as ordered and maintain a sterile dressing around the insertion site. CSF leakage, another potential complication, may occur at the sensor insertion site. *To prevent leakage,* the surgeon

usually places an additional suture at the site.

▶ *To reduce the risk of infection,* change the dressing at the insertion site daily.

Documentation

Document cleaning of the site, appearance of the site, and dressing changes. After sensor removal, document any leakage from the site.

CEREBROSPINAL FLUID DRAINAGE

Cerebrospinal fluid (CSF) drainage aims to reduce CSF pressure to the desired level and then to maintain it at that level. Fluid can be withdrawn from the lateral ventricle (ventriculostomy) or the lumbar subarachnoid space, depending on the indication and the desired outcome. Ventricular drainage is used to reduce increased intracranial pressure (ICP), whereas lumbar drainage is used to aid healing of the dura mater. External CSF drainage is used most commonly to manage increased ICP and to facilitate spinal or cerebral dural healing after traumatic injury or surgery. In either case, CSF is drained by a catheter or a ventriculostomy tube in a sterile, closed drainage collection system.

Other therapeutic uses include ICP monitoring via the ventriculostomy; direct instillation of medications, contrast media, or air for diagnostic radiology; and aspiration of CSF for laboratory analysis.

To place the ventricular drain, the doctor inserts a ventricular catheter through a burr hole in the patient's skull. Usually, this is done in the operating room, with the patient receiving a general anesthetic. To place the lumbar subarachnoid drain, the doctor may administer a local spinal anesthetic at bedside or in the operating room. (See *Methods of CSF drainage,* page 140.)

Key nursing diagnoses and patient outcomes

Ineffective tissue perfusion (cerebral) related to decreased cellular exchange
The patient will:
▶ maintain or improve level of consciousness
▶ maintain a balanced intake and output
▶ maintain intracranial pressure between (specify) mm Hg and (specify) mm Hg.

Risk for infection related to presence of CSF drain
The patient will:
▶ remain afebrile
▶ have no pathogens appear in cultures
▶ show no evidence of infection (such as redness, swelling, or drainage) at the insertion site.

Equipment

Overbed table • sterile gloves • sterile cotton-tipped applicators • povidone-iodine solution • alcohol pads • sterile fenestrated drape • 3-ml syringe for local anesthetic • 25G ¾″ needle for injecting anesthetic • local anesthetic (usually 1% lidocaine) • 18G or 20G sterile spinal needle or Tuohy needle • #5 French whistle-tip catheter or ventriculostomy tube • external drainage set (includes drainage tubing and sterile collection bag) • suture material • 4″ × 4″ dressings • paper tape • lamp or another light source • I.V. pole • ventriculostomy tray • twist drill •

Methods of CSF drainage

Cerebrospinal fluid (CSF) drainage aims to control intracranial pressure (ICP) during treatment for traumatic injury or other conditions that cause a rise in ICP. Two commonly used procedures are described below.

Ventricular drain

For a ventricular drain, the doctor makes a burr hole in the patient's skull and inserts the catheter into the ventricle. The distal end of the catheter is connected to a closed drainage system.

Lumbar drain

For a lumbar drain, the doctor inserts a catheter beneath the dura into the L3-L4 interspace. The distal end of the catheter is connected to a sterile, closed drainage system affixed securely to the bed or to an I.V. pole. The drip chamber should be set at the level ordered by the doctor

Closed drainage system

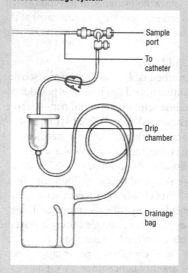

- Sample port
- To catheter
- Drip chamber
- Drainage bag

optional: pain medication (such as an analgesic), and an anti-infective agent (such as an antibiotic)

Preparation of equipment

Open all equipment using sterile technique. Check all packaging for breaks in seals and for expiration dates. After the doctor places the catheter, connect it to the external drainage system tubing. Secure connection points with tape or a connector. Place the collection system, including drip chamber and collection bag, on an I.V. pole.

Implementation

▶ Explain the procedure to the patient and family. Make sure the patient or a responsible family member signs a consent form and document according to policy.
▶ Wash your hands thoroughly.
▶ Perform a baseline neurologic assessment, including vital signs, *to help detect alterations or signs of deterioration.*

Inserting a ventricular drain

▶ Place the patient in the supine position.
▶ Place the equipment tray on the overbed table and unwrap the tray.
▶ Adjust the height of the bed *so that the doctor can perform the procedure comfortably.*
▶ Illuminate the area of the catheter insertion site.
▶ The doctor will clean the insertion site and administer a local anesthetic. He'll put on sterile gloves and drape the insertion site.
▶ To insert the drain, the doctor will request a ventriculostomy tray with a twist drill. After completing the ventriculostomy, he'll connect the drainage system and suture the catheter in place.

He'll then cover the insertion site with a sterile dressing.

Inserting a lumbar subarachnoid drain

▶ Position the patient in a side-lying position with his chin tucked to his chest and knees drawn up to his abdomen, as for a lumbar puncture. Urge him to remain as still as possible during the procedure.
▶ To insert the drain, the doctor attaches a Tuohy needle (or spinal needle) to the whistle-tip catheter. After the doctor removes the needle, he connects the drainage system, sutures or tapes the catheter securely in place, and covers it with a sterile dressing.

Monitoring CSF drainage

▶ Maintain a continuous hourly output of CSF by raising or lowering the drainage system drip chamber. To maintain CSF outflow, the drip chamber should be slightly lower than or at the level of the lumbar drain insertion site. Sometimes you may need to carefully raise or lower the drip chamber to increase or decrease CSF flow. For ventricular drains, ensure that the flow chamber of the ICP monitoring setup remains positioned as ordered.
▶ To drain CSF as ordered, put on gloves, and then turn the main stopcock on to drainage. *This allows CSF to collect in the graduated flow chamber.* Document the time and the amount of CSF obtained. Then turn the stopcock off to drainage. To drain the CSF from this chamber into the drainage bag, release the clamp below the flow chamber. Never empty the drainage bag. Instead, replace it when full using sterile technique.

▶ Check the dressing frequently for drainage, which could indicate CSF leakage.
▶ Check the tubing for patency by watching the CSF drops in the drip chamber.
▶ Observe the CSF for color, clarity, amount, blood, and sediment. CSF specimens for laboratory analysis should be obtained from the collection port attached to the tubing, not from the collection bag.
▶ Change the collection bag when it's full or every 24 hours according to your facility's policy.

Special considerations

▶ Maintaining a continual hourly output of CSF is essential *to prevent overdrainage or underdrainage.* Underdrainage or lack of CSF may reflect kinked tubing, catheter displacement, or a drip chamber placed higher than the catheter insertion site. Overdrainage can occur if the drip chamber is placed too far below the catheter insertion site.
▶ Raising or lowering the head of the bed can affect the CSF flow rate. When changing the patient's position, reposition the drip chamber.
▶ Patients may experience a chronic headache during continuous CSF drainage. Reassure the patient that this isn't unusual; administer analgesics as appropriate.

Complications

Signs and symptoms of excessive CSF drainage include headache, tachycardia, diaphoresis, and nausea. Acute overdrainage may result in collapsed ventricles, tonsillar herniation, and medullary compression.

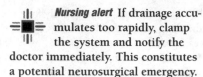 **Nursing alert** If drainage accumulates too rapidly, clamp the system and notify the doctor immediately. This constitutes a potential neurosurgical emergency.

Cessation of drainage may indicate clot formation. If you can't quickly identify the cause of the obstruction, notify the doctor. If drainage is blocked, the patient may develop signs of increased ICP.

Infection may cause meningitis. To prevent this, administer antibiotics as ordered.

Documentation

Record the time and date of the insertion procedure and the patient's response. Record routine vital signs and neurologic assessment findings at least every 4 hours.

Document the color, clarity, and amount of CSF at least every 8 hours. Record hourly and 24-hour CSF output and describe the condition of the dressing.

CERVICAL COLLAR APPLICATION

A cervical collar may be used for an acute injury (such as strained cervical muscles) or a chronic condition (such as arthritis or cervical metastasis). Or it may augment such splinting devices as a spine board to prevent potential cervical spine fracture or spinal cord damage.

Designed to hold the neck straight with the chin slightly elevated and tucked in, the collar immobilizes the cervical spine, decreases muscle spasms, and reduces pain; it also prevents further injury and promotes healing. As symptoms of an acute injury subside, the patient may gradually discontinue wearing the collar, alternating periods of wear with increasing periods of removal, until he no longer needs the collar.

Key nursing diagnoses and patient outcomes

Impaired physical mobility related to cervical injury
The patient will:
▶ state relief from pain
▶ attain highest degree of mobility possible within the confines of the disease
▶ state or demonstrate the mobility regimen.

Acute pain related to cervical injury
The patient will:
▶ obtain pain relief with proper cervical collar placement and minimal analgesia
▶ state satisfaction with the pain-management regimen
▶ cooperate with the pain-management treatment plan.

Equipment

Cervical collar in the appropriate size • optional: cotton (for padding) (see *Types of cervical collars*)

Implementation

▶ Check the patient's neurovascular status before application.
▶ Instruct the patient to position his head slowly to face directly forward.
▶ Place the cervical collar in front of the patient's neck *to ensure that the size is correct.*

▶ Fit the collar snugly around the neck and attach the Velcro fasteners or buckles at the back of the neck.

▶ Check the patient's airway and his neurovascular status *to ensure that the collar isn't too tight.*

Special considerations

▶ For a sprain or a potential cervical spine fracture, make sure the collar isn't too high in front *because this may hyperextend the neck.* In a neck sprain, such hyperextension may cause ligaments to heal in a shortened position. In a potential cervical spine fracture, hyperextension may cause serious neurologic damage.

▶ If the patient complains of pressure, the collar may be too tight. Remove and reapply it. If the patient complains of skin irritation or friction, the collar itself may be irritating him. Apply protective cotton padding between the irritated skin and the collar.

Home care

Teach the patient how to apply the collar and how to do a neurovascular check. Have the patient demonstrate how to apply the collar after you have instructed him. Some collars are complex and the patient (or caregiver) may need to practice if he will be responsible for application. If indicated, advise sleeping without a pillow.

Documentation

Note the type and size of the cervical collar and the time and date of application in your notes. Record the results of neurovascular checks. Document patient comfort, the collar's snugness, and all patient instructions.

Types of cervical collars

Cervical collars are used to support an injured or weakened cervical spine and to maintain alignment during healing.

Made of rigid plastic, the molded cervical collar holds the patient's neck firmly, keeping it straight, with the chin slightly elevated and tucked in.

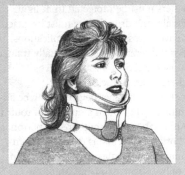

The soft cervical collar, made of spongy foam, provides gentler support and reminds the patient to avoid cervical spine motion.

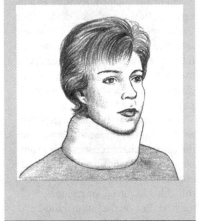

CHEMOTHERAPEUTIC DRUG ADMINISTRATION

Administration of chemotherapeutic drugs requires skills in addition to those used when giving other drugs. For example, some drugs require special equipment or must be given through an unusual route. Others become unstable after a while, and still others must be protected from light. Finally, the drug dosage must be exact to avoid possibly fatal complications. For these reasons, only specially trained nurses and doctors should give chemotherapeutic drugs.

Chemotherapeutic drugs may be administered through a number of routes. Although the I.V. route (using peripheral or central veins) is used most commonly, these drugs may also be given orally, subcutaneously, I.M., intra-arterially, into a body cavity, through a central venous catheter, through an Ommaya reservoir into the spinal canal, or through a device implanted in a vein or subcutaneously such as a patient-controlled analgesia device. (See *Understanding patient-controlled analgesia*.) They may also be administered into an artery, the peritoneal cavity, or the pleural space. (See *Intraperitoneal chemotherapy: An alternative approach*, page 146.)

The administration route depends on the drug's pharmacodynamics and the tumor's characteristics. For example, if a malignant tumor is confined to one area, the drug may be administered through a localized, or regional, method. Regional administration allows delivery of a high drug dose directly to the tumor. This is particularly advantageous because many solid tumors don't respond to drug levels that are safe for systemic administration.

Chemotherapy may be administered to a patient whose cancer is believed to have been eradicated through surgery or radiation therapy. This treatment, known as adjuvant chemotherapy, helps to ensure that no undetectable metastasis exists. A patient may also receive chemotherapy before surgery or radiation therapy. This is called induction chemotherapy (or neoadjuvant or synchronous chemotherapy). Induction chemotherapy helps improve survival rates by shrinking a tumor before surgical excision or radiation therapy.

In general, chemotherapeutic drugs prove more effective when given in higher doses, but their adverse effects often limit the dosage. An exception to this rule is methotrexate. This drug is particularly effective against rapidly growing tumors, but it's also toxic to normal tissues that are growing and dividing rapidly. However, doctors have discovered that they can give a large dose of methotrexate to destroy cancer cells and then, before the drug has had a chance to permanently damage vital organs, give a dose of folinic acid as an antidote. The antidote stops the effects of methotrexate, thus preserving normal tissue.

Key nursing diagnoses and patient outcomes

Acute pain related to cancer or chemotherapy
The patient will:
▶ carry out alternative pain-control measures, such as heat or cold applications
▶ express comfort.

Understanding patient-controlled analgesia

In patient-controlled analgesia (PCA), the patient controls I.V. delivery of an analgesic (usually morphine) by pressing the button on a delivery device. In this way, he receives analgesia at the level he needs and at the time he needs it. The device prevents the patient from accidentally overdosing by imposing a lockout time between doses — usually 6 to 10 minutes. During this interval, the patient won't receive any analgesic, even if he pushes the button.

The device shown below is a reusable, battery-operated peristaltic action pump that delivers a drug dose when the patient presses a call button at the end of a cord.

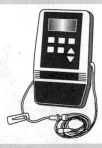

Indications and advantages

Indicated for patients who need parenteral analgesia, PCA therapy is typically given to trauma patients postoperatively and to terminal cancer patients and others with chronic diseases. To receive PCA therapy, a patient must be mentally alert and able to understand and comply with instructions and procedures and have no history of allergy to the analgesic. Patients ineligible for therapy include those with limited respiratory reserve, a history of drug abuse or chronic sedative or tranquilizer use, or a psychiatric disorder. PCA therapy's advantages include:

■ no need for I.M. analgesics
■ pain relief tailored to each patient's size and pain tolerance

■ a sense of control over pain
■ ability to sleep at night with minimal daytime drowsiness
■ lower narcotic use compared with patients not on PCA
■ improved postoperative deep-breathing, coughing, and ambulation.

PCA setup

To set up a PCA system, the doctor's order should include:
■ a loading dose, given by I.V. push at the start of PCA therapy (typically, 2 mg of morphine)
■ the appropriate lockout interval
■ the maintenance dose (basal dose)
■ the amount the patient will receive when he activates the device (typically, 1 mg of morphine)
■ the maximum amount the patient can receive within a specified time (if an adjustable device is used).

Nursing considerations

Because the primary adverse effect of analgesics is respiratory depression, monitor the patient's respiratory rate routinely. Also, check for infiltration into the subcutaneous tissues and for catheter occlusion, which may cause the drug to back up in the primary I.V. tubing. If the analgesic nauseates the patient, you may need to administer an antiemetic drug.

Before the patient starts using the PCA device, teach him how it works. Then have the patient practice with a sample device. Explain that he should take enough analgesic to relieve acute pain but not enough to induce drowsiness.

During therapy, monitor and record the amount of analgesic infused, the patient's respiratory rate, and the patient's assessment of pain relief. If the patient reports insufficient pain relief, notify the doctor.

Intraperitoneal chemotherapy: An alternative approach

Administering chemotherapeutic drugs into the peritoneal cavity has several benefits for patients with malignant ascites or ovarian cancer that has spread to the peritoneum. This technique passes drugs directly to the tumor area in the peritoneal cavity, exposing malignant cells to high concentrations of chemotherapy—up to 1,000 times the amount that could be safely given systemically. What is more, the semipermeable peritoneal membrane permits prolonged exposure of malignant cells to the drug.

Typically, intraperitoneal chemotherapy is performed using a peritoneal dialysis kit, but drugs can also be administered directly to the peritoneal cavity, by way of a Tenckhoff catheter (as shown at right). This method can be performed on an outpatient basis, if necessary; it uses equipment that is readily available on most units with oncology patients.

In this technique, the chemotherapy bag is connected directly to the Tenckhoff catheter with a length of I.V. tubing, the solution is infused, and the catheter and I.V. tubing are clamped. Then the patient is asked to change positions every 10 to 15 minutes for

1 hour to move the solution around in the peritoneal cavity.

After the prescribed dwell time, the chemotherapeutic drugs are drained into an I.V. bag. The patient is encouraged to change positions to facilitate drainage. Then the I.V. tubing and catheter are clamped, the I.V. tubing is removed, and a new intermittent infusion cap is fitted to the catheter. Finally, the catheter is flushed with a syringe of heparin flush solution.

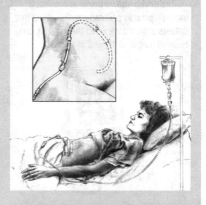

Powerlessness related to treatment
The patient will:
▶ participate in planning care
▶ enumerate treatment factors that he can control
▶ communicate a sense of having gained control.

Equipment

Prescribed drug • gloves • aluminum foil or a brown paper bag (if the drug is photosensitive) • normal saline solution • syringes and needleless adapters • infusion pump or controller • impervious containers labeled CAUTION: BIO-HAZARD

Preparation of equipment

Verify the drug, dosage, and administration route by checking the medication record against the doctor's order. Make sure you know the immediate and delayed adverse effects of the ordered drug. Follow administration guidelines for appropriate procedures in this chapter.

Implementation

▶ Assess the patient's physical condition and review his medical history.
▶ Make sure you understand the drug that needs to be given and by what route and provide the necessary teach-

ing and support to the patient and his family.

▶ Determine the best site to administer the drug. When selecting the site, consider drug compatibilities, frequency of administration, and vesicant potential of the drug. (See *Classifying chemotherapeutic drugs*.) For example, if the doctor has ordered the intermittent administration of a vesicant drug, you can give it either by instilling the drug into the side port of an infusing I.V. line or by direct I.V. push. If the vesicant drug is to be infused continuously, you should administer it only through a central venous line or a vascular access device. On the other hand, nonvesicant agents (including irritants) may be given by direct I.V. push, through the side port of an infusing I.V. line, or as a continuous infusion.

Check your facility's policy before administering a vesicant. *Because vein integrity decreases with time,* some facilities require that vesicants be administered before other drugs. Conversely, *because vesicants increase vein fragility,* some facilities require that vesicants be given after other drugs.

▶ Evaluate your patient's condition, paying particular attention to the results of recent laboratory studies, specifically the complete blood count, blood urea nitrogen level, platelet count, urine creatinine level, and liver function studies.

▶ Determine whether the patient has received chemotherapy before, and note the severity of any adverse effects.

▶ Check his drug history for medications that might interact with chemotherapy. As a rule, you shouldn't mix chemotherapeutic drugs with other medications. If you have questions or concerns about giving the chemothera-

Classifying chemotherapeutic drugs

Irritants
- carmustine
- etoposide
- streptozocin

Vesicants
- dacarbazine
- dactinomycin
- daunorubicin
- doxorubicin
- mechlorethamine
- mitomycin
- mitoxantrone
- plicamycin
- vinblastine
- vincristine

Nonvesicants
- asparaginase
- bleomycin
- carboplatin
- cisplatin
- cyclophosphamide
- cytarabine
- floxuridine
- fluorouracil
- ifosfamide

peutic drug, talk with the doctor or pharmacist before you give it.

▶ Next, double-check the patient's chart for the complete chemotherapy protocol order, including the patient's name, drug's name and dosage, and route, rate, and frequency of administration. See if the drug's dosage depends on certain laboratory values. Be aware that some facilities require two nurses to read the dosage order and to check the drug and amount being administered.

▶ Check to see whether the doctor has ordered an antiemetic, fluids, a diuretic, or electrolyte supplements to be given before, during, or after chemotherapy administration.

▶ Evaluate the patient's and his family's understanding of chemotherapy and make sure the patient or a responsible family member has signed the consent form.

▶ Next, put on gloves. Keep them on through all stages of handling the drug, including preparation, priming the I.V. tubing, and administration.

▶ Before administering the drug, perform a new venipuncture proximal to the old site. Avoid giving chemotherapeutic drugs through an existing I.V. line. To identify an administration site, examine the patient's veins, starting with his hand and proceeding to his forearm.

▶ When an appropriate line is in place, infuse 10 to 20 ml of normal saline solution to test vein patency. Never test vein patency with a chemotherapeutic drug. Next, administer the drug as appropriate: nonvesicants by I.V. push or admixed in a bag of I.V. fluid; vesicants by I.V. push through a piggyback set connected to a rapidly infusing I.V. line.

▶ During I.V. administration, closely monitor the patient for signs of a hypersensitivity reaction or extravasation. Check for adequate blood return after 5 ml of the drug has been infused or according to your facility's guidelines.

▶ After infusion of the medication, infuse 20 ml of normal saline solution. Do this between administrations of different chemotherapeutic drugs and before discontinuing the I.V. line.

▶ Dispose of used needles and syringes carefully. *To prevent aerosol dispersion of*

chemotherapeutic drugs, don't clip needles. Place them intact in an impervious container for incineration. Dispose of I.V. bags, bottles, gloves, and tubing in a properly labeled and covered trash container.

▶ Wash your hands thoroughly with soap and warm water after giving any chemotherapeutic drug, even though you have worn gloves.

Special considerations

▶ Observe the I.V. site frequently for signs of extravasation and an allergic reaction (swelling, redness, urticaria). If you suspect extravasation, stop the infusion immediately. Leave the I.V. catheter in place and notify the doctor. A conservative method for treating extravasation involves aspirating any residual drug from the tubing and I.V. catheter, instilling an I.V. antidote, and then removing the I.V. catheter. Afterward, you may apply heat or cold to the site and elevate the affected limb. (See *Managing extravasation.*)

▶ During infusion, some drugs need protection from direct sunlight *to avoid possible drug breakdown.* If this is the case, cover the vial with a brown paper bag or aluminum foil.

▶ When giving vesicants, avoid sites where damage to underlying tendons or nerves may occur (veins in the antecubital fossa, near the wrist, or in the dorsal surface of the hand).

▶ If you're unable to stay with the patient during the entire infusion, use an infusion pump or controller *to ensure drug delivery within the prescribed time and rate.*

▶ Observe the patient at regular intervals and after treatment for adverse reactions. Monitor his vital signs throughout the infusion *to assess any changes during chemotherapy administration.*

▶ Maintain a list of the types and amounts of drugs the patient has received. This is especially important if he has received drugs that have a cumulative effect and that can be toxic to such organs as the heart and kidneys.

Complications

Common adverse effects of chemotherapy are nausea and vomiting, ranging from mild to debilitating. Another major complication is bone marrow suppression, leading to neutropenia and thrombocytopenia. Other adverse effects include intestinal irritation, stomatitis, pulmonary fibrosis, cardiotoxicity, nephrotoxicity, neurotoxicity, hearing loss, anemia, alopecia, urticaria, radiation recall (if drugs are given with or soon after radiation therapy), anorexia, esophagitis, diarrhea, and constipation.

I.V. administration of chemotherapeutic drugs may also lead to extravasation, causing inflammation, ulceration, necrosis, and loss of vein patency.

Documentation

Record the location and description of the I.V. site before treatment or the presence of blood return during bolus administration. Also record the drugs and dosages administered, sequence of drug administration, needle type and size used, amount and type of flushing solution, and site condition after treatment. Document any adverse reactions, the patient's tolerance of the treatment, and topics discussed with the patient and his family.

Managing extravasation

Extravasation — the infiltration of a vesicant drug into the surrounding tissue — can result from a punctured vein or leakage around a venipuncture site. If vesicant drugs or fluids extravasate, severe local tissue damage may result. This may cause prolonged healing, infection, cosmetic disfigurement, and loss of function and may necessitate multiple debridements and, possibly, amputation.

Extravasation of vesicant drugs requires emergency treatment. Follow your facility's protocol. Essential steps include:

■ Stop the I.V. flow, aspirate the remaining drug in the catheter, and remove the I.V. line, unless you need the needle to infiltrate the antidote.

■ Estimate the amount of extravasated solution and notify the doctor.

■ Instill the appropriate antidote according to your facility's protocol.

■ Elevate the extremity.

■ Record the extravasation site, patient's symptoms, estimated amount of infiltrated solution, and treatment. Include the time you notified the doctor and the doctor's name. Continue documenting the appearance of the site and associated symptoms.

■ Ice is typically applied to all extravasated areas, with the exception of etoposide and vinca alkaloids, for 15 to 20 minutes every 4 to 6 hours for about 3 days. For etoposide and vinca alkaloids, heat is applied.

■ If skin breakdown occurs, apply dressings as ordered.

■ If severe tissue damage occurs, plastic surgery and physical therapy may be needed.

CHEMOTHERAPEUTIC DRUG PREPARATION AND HANDLING

When preparing chemotherapeutic drugs, take extra care, for the patient's safety and for your own. Patients who receive chemotherapeutic drugs risk teratogenic, mutagenic, and carcinogenic effects, but the people who prepare and handle the drugs are at risk as well. Although the danger from handling these drugs hasn't been fully determined, chemotherapeutic drugs can increase the handler's risk of reproductive abnormalities. These drugs also pose environmental threats, and the best method for handling them hasn't been determined.

The Occupational Safety and Health Administration (OSHA) has set certain guidelines for handling chemotherapeutic drugs. Although these guidelines are simply recommendations, adhering to them will help ensure both your safety and that of your environment.

The OSHA guidelines outline two basic requirements. The first is that all health care workers who handle chemotherapeutic drugs must be educated and trained. A key element of such training involves learning how to reduce your exposure when handling the drugs. The second requirement states that the drugs should be prepared in a class II biological safety cabinet.

Key nursing diagnoses and patient outcomes

Acute pain related to cancer or chemotherapy
The patient will:

▶ articulate factors that intensify pain and will modify behavior accordingly
▶ carry out alternative pain-control measures, such as heat or cold applications
▶ express comfort.

Powerlessness related to treatment
The patient will:
▶ participate in planning care
▶ enumerate treatment factors that he can control
▶ communicate a sense of having gained control.

Equipment

Prescribed drug or drugs • patient's medication record and chart • long-sleeved gown • latex surgical gloves • face shield or goggles • eyewash • plastic absorbent pad • alcohol pads • sterile gauze pads • shoe covers • impervious container with the label CAUTION: BIOHAZARD for the disposal of any unused drug or equipment • I.V. solution • diluent (if necessary) • compatibility reference source • medication labels • class II biological safety cabinet • disposable towel • hydrophobic filter or dispensing pin • 18G needle • syringes and needles of various sizes • I.V. tubing with luer-lock fittings • I.V. controller pump (if available)

Have a chemotherapeutic spill kit available. Kit includes water-resistant, nonpermeable, long-sleeved gown with cuffs and back closure • shoe covers • two pairs of gloves (for double gloving) • goggles • mask • disposable dustpan • plastic scraper (for collecting broken glass) • plastic-backed or absorbable towels • container of desiccant powder or granules (to absorb wet contents) • two disposable sponges • puncture-proof, leakproof container labeled BIO-

HAZARD WASTE • container of 70% alcohol for cleaning the spill area.

Implementation

▶ Remember to wash your hands before and after drug preparation and administration.

▶ Prepare the drugs in a class II biological safety cabinet.

▶ Wear protective garments (such as a long-sleeved gown, gloves, a face shield or goggles, and shoe covers) as indicated by your facility's policy. Don't wear the garments outside the preparation area.

▶ Don't eat, drink, smoke, or apply cosmetics in the drug preparation area.

▶ Before you prepare the drug (and after you finish), clean the internal surfaces of the cabinet with 70% alcohol and a disposable towel. Discard the towel in a leakproof chemical waste container.

▶ Cover the work surface with a clean plastic absorbent pad *to minimize contamination by droplets or spills.* Change the pad at the end of the shift or whenever a spill occurs.

▶ Consider all the equipment used in drug preparation as well as any unused drug as hazardous waste. Dispose of them according to your facility's policy.

▶ Place all chemotherapeutic waste products in labeled, leakproof, sealable plastic bags or other appropriate impervious containers.

Special considerations

▶ Prepare the drugs according to current product instructions, paying attention to compatibility, stability, and reconstitution technique. Label the prepared drug with the patient's name, dosage strength, and date and time of preparation.

▶ Take precautions to reduce your exposure to chemotherapeutic drugs. Systemic absorption can occur through ingestion of contaminated materials, skin contact, and inhalation. You can inhale a drug without realizing it, such as while opening a vial, clipping a needle, expelling air from a syringe, or discarding excess drug. You can also absorb a drug from handling contaminated stools or body fluids.

▶ *For maximum protection,* mix all chemotherapeutic drugs in an approved class II biological safety cabinet. Also, prime all I.V. bags that contain chemotherapeutic drugs under the hood. Leave the hood blower on 24 hours a day, 7 days a week.

▶ If a hood isn't available, prepare drugs in a well-ventilated work space, away from heating or cooling vents and other personnel. Vent vials with a hydrophobic filter, or use negative-pressure techniques. Also, use a needle with a hydrophobic filter to remove solution from a vial. To break an ampule, wrap a sterile gauze pad or alcohol pad around the neck of the ampule *to cut the contamination risk.*

▶ Make sure the biological safety cabinet is examined every 6 months or any time the cabinet is moved by a company specifically qualified to perform this work. If the cabinet passes certification, the certifying company will affix a sticker to the cabinet attesting to its approval.

▶ Use only syringes and I.V. sets that have luer-lock fittings. Label all chemotherapeutic drugs with a CHEMOTHERAPY HAZARD label.

▶ Don't clip needles, break syringes, or remove the needles from syringes. Use a gauze pad when removing syringes and needles from I.V. bags of chemo-therapeutic drugs.

▶ Place used syringes and needles in a puncture-proof container, along with other sharp or breakable items.

▶ When mixing chemotherapeutic drugs, wear latex surgical gloves and a gown of low-permeability fabric with a closed front and cuffed long sleeves. When working steadily with chemo-therapeutic drugs, change gloves every 30 minutes. If you spill a drug solution or puncture or tear a glove, remove the gloves at once. Wash your hands before putting on new gloves and anytime you remove your gloves.

▶ If some of the drug comes in contact with your skin, wash the involved area thoroughly with soap (not a germicidal agent) and water. If eye contact occurs, flood the eye with water or an isotonic eyewash for at least 5 minutes while holding the eyelid open. Obtain a medical evaluation as soon as possible after accidental exposure.

▶ If a major spill occurs, use a chemo-therapeutic spill kit to clean the area.

▶ Discard disposable gowns and gloves in an appropriately marked, waterproof receptacle when contaminated or when you leave the work area.

▶ Don't place any food or drinks in the same refrigerator as chemotherapeutic drugs.

▶ Become familiar with drug excretion patterns and take appropriate precautions when handling a chemotherapy patient's body fluids.

▶ Give male patients a urinal with a tight-fitting lid. Wear disposable latex surgical gloves when handling body fluids. Before flushing the toilet, place a waterproof pad over the toilet bowl *to avoid splashing*. Wear gloves and a gown when handling linens soiled with body fluids. Place soiled linens in isolation linen bags designated for separate laundering.

▶ Women who are pregnant, trying to conceive, or breast-feeding should exercise caution when handling chemother-apeutic drugs.

Home care

When teaching your patient about handling chemotherapeutic drugs, discuss appropriate safety measures. If the patient will be receiving chemotherapy at home, teach him how to dispose of contaminated equipment. Tell the patient and his family to wear gloves whenever handling chemotherapy equipment and contaminated linens or gowns. Instruct them to place soiled linens in a separate washable pillowcase and to launder the pillowcase twice, with the soiled linens inside, separately from other linens. When providing home care, empty waste products into the toilet close to the water *to minimize splashing*. Close the lid and flush two or three times.

All materials used for the treatment should be placed in a leakproof container and taken to a designated disposal area. The patient or his family should make arrangements with either a facility or a private company for pickup and proper disposal of contaminated waste.

Complications

Chemotherapeutic drugs may be mutagenic. Chronic exposure to chemother-apeutic drugs may damage the liver or chromosomes. Direct exposure to these drugs may burn and damage the skin.

Documentation

Document each incident of exposure according to your facility's policy.

CHEST PHYSIOTHERAPY

Chest physiotherapy includes postural drainage, chest percussion and vibration, and coughing and deep-breathing exercises. Together, these techniques mobilize and eliminate secretions, reexpand lung tissue, and promote efficient use of respiratory muscles. Of critical importance to the bedridden patient, chest physiotherapy (PT) helps prevent or treat atelectasis and may also help prevent pneumonia, two respiratory complications that can seriously impede recovery.

Postural drainage performed in conjunction with percussion and vibration encourages peripheral pulmonary secretions to empty by gravity into the major bronchi or trachea and is accomplished by sequential repositioning of the patient. Usually, secretions drain best with the patient positioned so that the bronchi are perpendicular to the floor. Lower and middle lobe bronchi usually empty best with the patient in the head-down position; upper lobe bronchi, in the head-up position. (See *Positioning patients for postural drainage*, pages 154 to 156.)

Percussing the chest with cupped hands mechanically dislodges thick, tenacious secretions from the bronchial walls. Vibration can be used with percussion or as an alternative to it in a patient who is frail, in pain, or recovering from thoracic surgery or trauma. A new device called the "vest" offers an alternative to chest physiotherapy. (See *Airway clearance therapy vest.*)

Candidates for chest PT include patients who expectorate large amounts of sputum such as those with bronchiectasis and cystic fibrosis. The procedure

Technology update

Airway clearance therapy vest

A promising advance for those with pulmonary complications is an inflatable vest that is used to clear the patient's airway. A hose connected to an air-pulse generator quickly inflates and deflates the vest, thereby compressing and releasing the patient's chest wall. Such rapid action moves mucus toward the larger airways, where it can be cleared by coughing or suctioning.

This type of airway clearance therapy is commonly called high-frequency chest wall oscillation. Most patients tolerate the therapy well, and it can be self-administered, so compliance is usually high.

The vest can be used for patients with various conditions that affect respiratory function, including cystic fibrosis, bronchiectasis, muscular dystrophy, cerebral palsy, spinal cord injuries, and asthma.

hasn't proved effective in treating patients with status asthmaticus, lobar pneumonia, or acute exacerbations of chronic bronchitis when the patient has scant secretions and is being mechanically ventilated. Chest PT has little value for treating patients with stable, chronic bronchitis.

Contraindications may include active pulmonary bleeding with hemoptysis and the immediate posthemorrhage stage, fractured ribs or an unstable chest wall, lung contusions, pulmonary tuberculosis, untreated pneumothorax, acute asthma or bronchospasm, lung abscess or tumor, bony metastasis, head injury, and recent myocardial infarction.

(Text continues on page 156.)

Positioning patients for postural drainage

The following illustrations show the various postural drainage positions and the areas of the lungs affected by each.

Lower lobes:
Posterior basal segments

Elevate the foot of the bed 30 degrees. Have the patient lie prone with his head lowered. Position pillows under his chest and abdomen. Percuss his lower ribs on both sides of his spine.

Posterior view

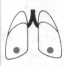
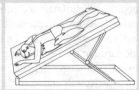

Lower lobes:
Lateral basal segments

Elevate the foot of the bed 30 degrees. Instruct the patient to lie on his abdomen with his head lowered and his upper leg flexed over a pillow for support. Then have him rotate a quarter turn upward. Percuss his lower ribs on the uppermost portion of his lateral chest wall.

Anterior view

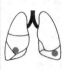
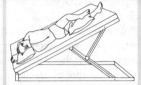

Lower lobes:
Anterior basal segments

Elevate the foot of the bed 30 degrees. Instruct the patient to lie on his side with his head lowered. Then place pillows as shown. Percuss with a slightly cupped hand over his lower ribs just beneath the axilla. If an acutely ill patient has trouble breathing in this position, adjust the bed to an angle he can tolerate. Then begin percussion.

Anterior view

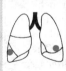
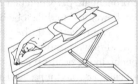

Lower lobes:
Superior segments

With the bed flat, have the patient lie on his abdomen. Place two pillows under his hips. Percuss on both sides of his spine at the lower tip of his scapulae.

Posterior view

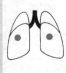
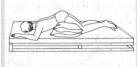

Positioning patients for postural drainage *(continued)*

Right middle lobe: Medial and lateral segments

Elevate the foot of the bed 15 degrees. Have the patient lie on his left side with his head down and his knees flexed. Then have him rotate a quarter turn backward. Place a pillow beneath him. Percuss with your hand moderately cupped over the right nipple. For a woman, cup your hand so that the heel of the hand is under the armpit and your fingers extend forward beneath the breast.

Anterior view

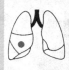
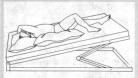

Left upper lobe: Superior and inferior segments, lingular portion

Elevate the foot of the bed 15 degrees. Have the patient lie on his right side with his head down and knees flexed. Then have him rotate a quarter turn backward. Place a pillow behind him, from shoulders to hips. Percuss with your hand moderately cupped over his left nipple. For a woman, cup your hand so that the heel of the hand is beneath the armpit and your fingers extend forward beneath the breast.

Anterior view

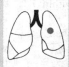
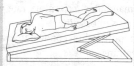

Upper lobes: Anterior segments

Make sure the bed is flat. Have the patient lie on his back with a pillow folded under his knees. Then have him rotate slightly away from the side being drained. Percuss between his clavicle and nipple.

Anterior view

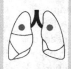
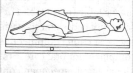

Upper lobes: Apical segments

Keep the bed flat. Have the patient lean back at a 30-degree angle against you and a pillow. Percuss with a cupped hand between his clavicles and the top of each scapula.

Posterior view

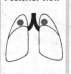
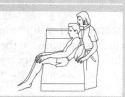

(continued)

Positioning patients for postural drainage *(continued)*

Upper lobes: Posterior segments

Keep the bed flat. Have the patient lean forward over a pillow at a 30-degree angle. Percuss and clap his upper back on each side.

Posterior view

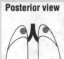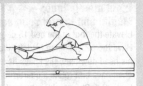

Key nursing diagnoses and patient outcomes

Ineffective breathing pattern related to physical condition
The patient will:
▶ maintain a respiratory rate within 5 breaths of baseline
▶ report feeling comfortable when breathing.

Impaired gas exchange related to altered oxygen supply
The patient will:
▶ cough effectively
▶ expectorate sputum
▶ have normal breath sounds.

Equipment

Stethoscope • pillows • tilt or postural drainage table (if available) or adjustable facility bed • emesis basin • facial tissues • suction equipment as needed • equipment for oral care • trash bag • optional: sterile specimen container, mechanical ventilator, and supplemental oxygen

Preparation of equipment

Gather the equipment at the patient's bedside. Set up suction equipment, if needed, and test its function.

Implementation

▶ Explain the procedure to the patient, provide privacy, and wash your hands.
▶ Auscultate the patient's lungs to determine baseline respiratory status.
▶ Position the patient as ordered. In generalized disease, drainage usually begins with the lower lobes, continues with the middle lobes, and ends with the upper lobes. In localized disease, drainage begins with the affected lobes and then proceeds to the other lobes *to avoid spreading the disease to uninvolved areas.*
▶ Instruct the patient to remain in each position for 10 to 15 minutes. During this time, perform percussion and vibration as ordered. (See *Performing percussion and vibration.*)
▶ After postural drainage, percussion, or vibration, instruct the patient to cough *to remove loosened secretions.* First, tell him to inhale deeply through his nose and then exhale in three short huffs. Then have him inhale deeply again and cough through a slightly open mouth. Three consecutive coughs are highly effective. An effective cough sounds deep, low, and hollow; an ineffective one, high-pitched. Have the patient perform exercises for about 1 minute and then rest for 2 minutes.

Gradually progress to a 10-minute exercise period four times daily.

▶ Provide oral hygiene *because secretions may have a foul taste or a stale odor.*

▶ Auscultate the patient's lungs *to evaluate the effectiveness of therapy.*

Special considerations

▶ For optimal effectiveness and safety, modify chest PT according to the patient's condition. For example, initiate or increase the flow of supplemental oxygen, if indicated. Also, suction the patient who has an ineffective cough reflex. If the patient tires quickly during therapy, shorten the sessions *because fatigue leads to shallow respirations and increased hypoxia.*

▶ Maintain adequate hydration in the patient receiving chest PT *to prevent mucus dehydration and promote easier mobilization.* Avoid performing postural drainage immediately before or within 1½ hours after meals *to avoid nausea and aspiration of food or vomitus.*

▶ *Because chest percussion can induce bronchospasm,* any adjunct treatment (for example, intermittent positive-pressure breathing, aerosol, or nebulizer therapy) should precede chest PT.

▶ Refrain from percussing over the spine, liver, kidneys, or spleen *to avoid injury to the spine or internal organs.* Also avoid performing percussion on bare skin or the female patient's breasts. Percuss over soft clothing (but not over buttons, snaps, or zippers), or place a thin towel over the chest wall. Remember to remove jewelry that might scratch or bruise the patient.

▶ Explain coughing and deep-breathing exercises preoperatively *so that the patient can practice them when he's pain-free and better able to concentrate.* Postoperatively, splint the patient's incision using

Performing percussion and vibration

To perform percussion, instruct the patient to breathe slowly and deeply, using the diaphragm, *to promote relaxation.* Hold your hands in a cupped shape, with fingers flexed and thumbs pressed tightly against your index fingers. Percuss each segment for 1 to 2 minutes by alternating your hands against the patient in a rhythmic manner. Listen for a hollow sound on percussion to verify correct performance of the technique.

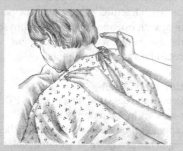

To perform vibration, ask the patient to inhale deeply and then exhale slowly through pursed lips. During exhalation, firmly press your fingers and the palms of your hands against the chest wall. Tense the muscles of your arms and shoulders in an isometric contraction to send fine vibrations through the chest wall. Vibrate during five exhalations over each chest segment.

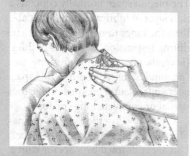

your hands or, if possible, teach the patient to splint it himself *to minimize pain during coughing.*

Complications

During postural drainage in head-down positions, pressure on the diaphragm by abdominal contents can impair respiratory excursion and lead to hypoxia or orthostatic hypotension. The head-down position also may lead to increased intracranial pressure, which precludes the use of chest PT in a patient with acute neurologic impairment. Vigorous percussion or vibration can cause rib fracture, especially in the patient with osteoporosis. In an emphysematous patient with blebs, coughing could lead to pneumothorax.

Documentation

Record the date and time of chest PT; positions for secretion drainage and length of time each is maintained; chest segments percussed or vibrated; color, amount, odor, and viscosity of secretions produced and the presence of any blood; any complications and nursing actions taken; and the patient's tolerance of treatment.

CHEST TUBE INSERTION

The pleural space normally contains a thin layer of lubricating fluid that allows the lungs to move without friction during respiration. An excess of fluid (hemothorax or pleural effusion), air (pneumothorax), or both in this space alters intrapleural pressure and causes partial or complete lung collapse.

Chest tube insertion allows drainage of air or fluid from the pleural space. Usually performed by a doctor with a nurse assisting, this procedure requires sterile technique. The insertion site varies depending on the patient's condition and the doctor's judgment. For pneumothorax, the second intercostal space is the usual site because air rises to the top of the intrapleural space. For hemothorax or pleural effusion, the sixth to eighth intercostal spaces are common sites because fluid settles to the lower levels of the intrapleural space. For removal of air and fluid, a chest tube is inserted into a high and a low site.

After insertion, one or more chest tubes are connected to a thoracic drainage system that removes air, fluid, or both from the pleural space and prevents backflow into that space, thus promoting lung reexpansion. (See "Thoracic drainage," page 799.)

Key nursing diagnoses and patient outcomes

Ineffective breathing pattern related to pain
The patient will:
▶ report ability to breathe more comfortably
▶ achieve comfort without experiencing depressed respirations.

Anxiety related to situational crisis
The patient will:
▶ discuss activities that tend to decrease anxiety
▶ cope with current medical situation without demonstrating severe anxiety.

Equipment

Two pairs of sterile gloves • sterile drape • vial of 1% lidocaine • povidone-iodine solution • 10-ml syringe • alcohol pad • 22G 1″ needle • 25G ⅜″ needle • sterile scalpel (usually with #11 blade) • sterile forceps • two rubber-tipped clamps for each chest tube inserted • sterile 4″ × 4″ gauze pads • two sterile 4″ × 4″ drain dressings (gauze pads with slit) • 3″ or 4″ sturdy, elastic tape • 1″ adhesive tape for connections • chest tube of appropriate size (#16 to #20 French catheter for air or serous fluid; #28 to #40 French catheter for blood, pus, or thick fluid), with or without a trocar • sterile Kelly clamp • suture material (usually 2-0 silk with cutting needle) • thoracic drainage system • sterile drainage tubing, 6″ (15.2 cm) long, and connector • sterile Y-connector (for two chest tubes on the same side) • optional: petroleum gauze

Preparation of equipment

Check the expiration date on the sterile packages and inspect for tears. In a nonemergency situation, make sure that the patient has signed the appropriate consent form. Then assemble all equipment in the patient's room and set up the thoracic drainage system. Place it next to the patient's bed below the chest level to facilitate drainage.

Implementation

▶ Explain the procedure to the patient, provide privacy, and wash your hands.
▶ Record baseline vital signs and respiratory assessment.
▶ Position the patient appropriately. If he has a *pneumothorax,* place him in high Fowler's, semi-Fowler's, or the supine position. The doctor will insert the tube in the anterior chest at the midclavicular line in the second to third intercostal space. If the patient has a *hemothorax,* have him lean over the overbed table or straddle a chair with his arms dangling over the back. The doctor will insert the tube in the

fourth to sixth intercostal space at the midaxillary line. For either pneumothorax or hemothorax, the patient may lie on his unaffected side with arms extended over his head.
▶ When you've positioned the patient properly, place the chest tube tray on the overbed table. Open it using sterile technique.
▶ The doctor puts on sterile gloves and prepares the insertion site by cleaning the area with povidone-iodine solution.
▶ Wipe the rubber stopper of the lidocaine vial with an alcohol pad. Then invert the bottle and hold it for the doctor to withdraw the anesthetic.
▶ After the doctor anesthetizes the site, he makes a small incision and inserts the chest tube. Then he either immediately connects the chest tube to the thoracic drainage system or momentarily clamps the tube close to the patient's chest until he can connect it to the drainage system. He may then secure the tube to the skin with a suture.
▶ As the doctor is inserting the chest tube, reassure the patient and assist the doctor as necessary.
▶ Open the packages containing the 4″ × 4″ drain dressings and gauze pads and put on sterile gloves. Then place two 4″ × 4″ drain dressings around the insertion site, one from the top and the other from the bottom. Place several 4″ × 4″ gauze pads on top of the drain dressings. Tape the dressings, covering them completely.
▶ Tape the chest tube to the patient's chest distal to the insertion site *to help prevent accidental tube dislodgment.*
▶ Tape the junction of the chest tube and the drainage tube *to prevent their separation.*
▶ Coil the drainage tubing, and secure it to the bed linen with tape and a safe-

Removing a chest tube

After the patient's lung has reexpanded, you may assist the doctor in removing the chest tube. To do so, first obtain the patient's vital signs and perform a respiratory assessment. After explaining the procedure to the patient, administer an analgesic as ordered 30 minutes before tube removal. Then follow the steps listed below:

■ Place the patient in semi-Fowler's position or on his unaffected side.

■ Place a linen-saver pad under the affected side *to protect the linen from drainage and to provide a place to put the chest tube after removal.*

■ Put on clean gloves and remove the chest tube dressings, being careful not to dislodge the chest tube. Discard soiled dressings.

■ The doctor puts on sterile gloves, holds the chest tube in place with sterile forceps, and cuts the suture anchoring the tube.

■ Make sure the chest tube is securely clamped and then instruct the patient to perform Valsalva's maneuver by exhaling fully and bearing down. Valsalva's maneuver effectively increases intrathoracic pressure.

■ The doctor holds an airtight dressing, usually petroleum gauze, so that he can cover the insertion site with it immediately after removing the tube. After he removes the tube and covers the insertion site, secure the dressing with tape. Be sure to cover the dressing completely with tape to make it as airtight as possible.

■ Dispose of the chest tube, soiled gloves, and equipment according to your facility's policy.

■ Take vital signs as ordered and assess the depth and quality of the patient's respirations. Assess the patient carefully for signs and symptoms of pneumothorax, subcutaneous emphysema, or infection.

ty pin, leaving enough slack for the patient to move and turn. *These measures prevent the tubing from getting kinked or dropping to the floor, and they help prevent accidental dislodgment of the chest tube.*

▶ Immediately after the drainage system is connected, instruct the patient to take a deep breath, hold it momentarily, and slowly exhale *to assist drainage of the pleural space and lung reexpansion.*

▶ A portable chest X-ray is then done *to check tube position.*

▶ Take the patient's vital signs every 15 minutes for 1 hour, then as his condition indicates. Auscultate his lungs at least every 4 hours following the procedure *to assess air exchange in the affected lung.* Diminished or absent breath sounds indicate that the lung hasn't reexpanded.

Special considerations

▶ If the chest tube comes out, cover the site immediately with 4″ × 4″ gauze pads and tape them in place. Stay with the patient, and monitor his vital signs every 10 minutes. Observe him for signs and symptoms of tension pneumothorax (such as hypotension, distended neck veins, absent breath sounds, tracheal shift, hypoxemia, weak and rapid pulse, dyspnea, tachypnea, diaphoresis, and chest pain). Have another staff member notify the doctor and gather the equipment needed to reinsert the tube.

▶ Place the rubber-tipped clamps at the bedside. If the drainage system cracks, or a tube disconnects, clamp the chest tube momentarily as close to the insertion site as possible. *Because no air or liquid can escape from the pleural space while the tube is clamped,* observe the patient closely for signs and symp-

toms of tension pneumothorax while the clamp is in place.
► Petroleum gauze may be wrapped around the tube at the insertion site *to make an airtight seal.*
► The tube may be clamped with large, smooth, rubber-tipped clamps for several hours before removal. *This allows time to observe the patient for signs of respiratory distress, an indication that air or fluid remains trapped in the pleural space.* A chest tube is usually removed within 7 days of insertion *to prevent infection along the tube tract.* (See *Removing a chest tube.*)

Documentation
Record the date and time of chest tube insertion, the insertion site, drainage system used, presence of drainage and bubbling, vital signs and auscultation findings, any complications, and the nursing action taken.

CIRCUMCISION

Steeped in controversy and history, circumcision (the removal of the penile foreskin) is thought to promote a clean glans and to minimize the risk of phimosis (tightening of the foreskin) in later life. It's also thought to reduce the risk of penile cancer and cervical cancer in sexual partners, although the American Academy of Pediatrics (AAP) has contended since 1971 that no valid medical reason exists for routine circumcision. Currently, the AAP is continuing its studies on the effects of circumcision.

In Judaism, circumcision (known as a *bris*) is a religious rite performed by a *mohel* on the 8th day after birth, when the neonate officially receives his name.

Because most neonates are discharged before this time, a *bris* is rarely performed in a facility.

One method of circumcision involves removing the foreskin by using a Yellen clamp to stabilize the penis. With this device, a cone that fits over the glans provides a cutting surface and protects the glans penis. Another technique uses a plastic circumcision bell (Plastibell) over the glans and a suture tied tightly around the base of the foreskin. This method prevents bleeding. The resultant ischemia causes the foreskin to slough off within 5 to 8 days. This method is thought to be painless because it stretches the foreskin, which inhibits sensory conduction.

Circumcision is contraindicated in neonates who are ill or who have bleeding disorders, ambiguous genitalia, or congenital anomalies of the penis, such as hypospadias or epispadias, *because the foreskin may be needed for later reconstructive surgery.*

Key nursing diagnoses and patient outcomes
Risk for infection related to circumcision
The patient will:
► remain afebrile
► show no evidence of infection at the surgical site.

Equipment
Circumcision tray (contents vary but usually include circumcision clamps, various-sized cones, scalpel, probe, scissors, forceps, sterile basin, sterile towel, and sterile drapes) • povidone-iodine solution • restraining board with arm and leg restraints • sterile gloves • petroleum gauze • sterile 4″ × 4″ gauze pads • optional: sutures, plastic circumcision bell, antimicrobial oint-

ment, topical anesthetic, and overhead warmer

Preparation of equipment
Using a Yellen clamp
Assemble the sterile tray and other equipment in the procedure area. Open the sterile tray and pour povidone-iodine solution into the sterile basin. Using aseptic technique, place sterile 4″ × 4″ gauze pads and petroleum gauze on the sterile tray. Arrange the restraining board and direct adequate light on the area.

Using a plastic circumcision bell
You won't need a circumcision tray, but do assemble sterile gloves, sutures, restraining board, petroleum gauze and, if ordered, antibiotic ointment. A *mohel* usually brings his own equipment.

Implementation
▶ Beforehand, make sure the parents understand the procedure and have signed the proper consent form.
▶ Withhold feeding for at least 1 hour before the procedure *to reduce the possibility of emesis or aspiration, or both.*
▶ Place the neonate on the restraining board, and restrain his arms and legs. Don't leave him unattended.
▶ Assist the doctor as necessary throughout the procedure, and comfort the neonate as needed.

Using a Yellen clamp
▶ After putting on sterile gloves, the doctor will clean the penis and scrotum with povidone-iodine and drape the neonate.
▶ He'll apply a Yellen clamp to the penis, loosen the foreskin, insert the cone under it *to provide a cutting surface and to protect the penis,* and remove the foreskin.
▶ Then he'll cover the wound with sterile petroleum gauze *to prevent infection and control bleeding.*

Using a plastic bell
▶ The doctor will slide the plastic bell device between the foreskin and the glans penis.
▶ Then he'll tie a suture tightly around the foreskin at the coronal edge of the glans. The foreskin distal to the suture will become ischemic and then atrophic. After 5 to 8 days, the foreskin will drop off with the plastic bell attached, leaving a clean, well-healed excision. No special care is required, but watch for swelling, which may indicate infection or interfere with urination.

Providing aftercare
▶ Remove the neonate from the restraining board, and check for bleeding.
▶ Place him in a side-lying position, rather than prone, *to minimize pressure on the excisional area.* Leave him diaperless for 1 to 2 hours *to observe for bleeding and to reduce possible chafing and irritation.*
▶ Show the neonate to his parents *to reassure them that he's all right.*
▶ Once you rediaper the neonate, change his diaper as soon as he voids. If the dressing falls off, clean the wound with warm water *to minimize pain from urine on the circumcised area.* Don't remove the original dressing until it falls off (usually after the first or second voiding).
▶ Check for bleeding every 15 minutes for the 1st hour and then every hour for the next 24 hours. If bleeding occurs, apply pressure with sterile gauze

pads. Notify the doctor if bleeding continues.

▶ Loosely diaper the neonate *to prevent irritation*. At each diaper change, apply ordered antimicrobial ointment, petroleum jelly, or petroleum gauze until the wound appears healed. Avoid leaving the neonate under the radiant warmer after placing petroleum gauze on the penis *because the area might burn.*

▶ Watch for drainage, redness, or swelling. Don't remove the thin, yellow-white exudate that forms over the healing area within 1 to 2 days. *This normal incrustation protects the wound until it heals in 3 to 4 days.*

▶ Don't discharge the neonate until he has voided.

Special considerations

▶ Always be sure to show parents the circumcision before discharge *so they can ask any questions and so you can teach them how to care for the area.*

▶ If the neonate's mother has human immunodeficiency virus (HIV) infection, circumcision will be delayed until the doctor knows the neonate's HIV status. The neonate whose mother has HIV infection has a higher-than-normal risk of infection.

Home care

Inform the mother that the circumcision site may appear yellow in light-skinned neonates and lighter than the surrounding skin in dark-skinned neonates. Tell her that this signifies healing and isn't a cause for concern.

Instruct the mother to observe the circumcision site regularly for pus or bloody discharge, which may indicate delayed healing or infection. If these signs occur, she should notify the doctor.

Tell the mother that the rim of the device used for circumcision may remain in place after discharge from the facility. Reassure her that the rim will fall off harmlessly in 3 or 4 days. If it doesn't fall off after 1 week, tell her to notify the doctor. *A retained rim may lead to infection.*

Complications

After a Yellen clamp procedure, infection and bleeding may occur. The skin of the penile shaft can adhere to the glans, resulting in scarring or fibrous bands. The most severe complications are urethral fistulae and edema. Incomplete amputation of the foreskin can follow application of the plastic circumcision bell.

Documentation

Note the time and date of the circumcision, any parent teaching, and any excessive bleeding.

CLAVICLE STRAP
APPLICATION

Also called a figure-eight strap, a clavicle strap reduces and immobilizes fractures of the clavicle. It does this by elevating, extending, and supporting the shoulders in position for healing, known as the position of attention. A commercially available figure-eight strap or a 4″ elastic bandage may serve as a clavicle strap. This strap is contraindicated for an uncooperative patient.

Key nursing diagnoses and patient outcomes

Impaired physical mobility related to pain or discomfort

Types of clavicle straps

Clavicle straps provide support to the shoulder to help heal a fractured clavicle. These straps are available ready-made. They can also be made from a bandage.

Commercially made clavicle straps have a short back panel and long straps that extend around the patient's shoulders and axillae. They have Velcro pads or buckles on the ends for easy fastening.

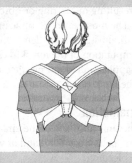

When making a clavicle strap with a wide elastic bandage, start in the middle of the patient's back. After wrapping the bandage around the shoulders, fasten the ends with safety pins.

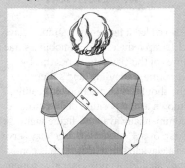

The patient will:
► attain the highest degree of mobility possible within the confines of the disease

► show no evidence of complications, such as contractures or skin breakdown.

Acute pain related to the physical condition
The patient will:
► articulate factors that intensify pain and will modify behavior accordingly
► express a feeling of comfort and relief from pain.

Equipment
Powder or cornstarch • figure-eight clavicle strap or 4″ elastic bandage • safety pins, if necessary • tape • cotton batting or padding • marking pen • analgesics as ordered • optional: scissors

Implementation
► Explain the procedure to the patient and provide privacy.
► Help the patient take off his shirt or cut off the shirt if movement is too painful.
► Assess neurovascular integrity by palpating skin temperature; noting the color of the hand and fingers; palpating the radial, ulnar, and brachial pulses bilaterally; and then comparing the affected side with the unaffected side. Ask the patient about any numbness or tingling distal to the injury and assess his motor function.
► Determine the patient's degree of comfort and administer analgesics as ordered.
► Demonstrate how to assume the position of attention. Instruct the patient to sit upright and assume this position gradually *to minimize pain.*
► Gently apply powder as appropriate to the axillae and shoulder area *to reduce friction from the clavicle strap.* You

can use cornstarch if the patient is allergic to powder.

Applying a figure-eight strap

▶ Place the apex of the triangle between the scapulae and drape the straps over the shoulders. Bring the strap with the Velcro or buckle end under one axilla and through the loop; then pull the other strap under the other axilla and through the loop. (See *Types of clavicle straps.*)

▶ Gently adjust the straps so they support the shoulders in the position of attention.

▶ Bring the straps back under the axillae toward the anterior chest, making sure that they maintain the position of attention.

Applying a 4″ elastic bandage

▶ Roll both ends of the elastic bandage toward the middle, leaving between 12″ and 18″ (30.5 to 46 cm) unrolled.

▶ Place the unrolled portion diagonally across the patient's back, from right shoulder to left axilla.

▶ Bring the lower end of the bandage under the left axilla and back over the left shoulder; loop the upper end over the right shoulder and under the axilla.

▶ Pull the two ends together at the center of the back *so that the bandage supports the position of attention.*

Completing a figure-eight strap or elastic bandage

▶ Secure the ends using safety pins, Velcro pads, or a buckle, depending on the equipment. Make sure a buckle or any sharp edges face away from the skin. Tape the secured ends to the underlying strap or bandage.

▶ Place cotton batting or padding under the straps, as well as under the buckle or pins, *to avoid skin irritation.*

▶ Use a pen to mark the strap at the site of the loop of the figure-eight strap or the site where the elastic bandage crosses on the patient's back. *If the strap loosens, this mark helps you tighten it to the original position.*

▶ Assess neurovascular integrity, *which may be impaired by a strap that is too tight.* If neurovascular integrity is compromised when the strap is correctly applied, notify the doctor. *He may want to change the treatment.*

Special considerations

▶ If possible, perform the procedure with the patient standing. However, this may not be feasible because the pain from the fracture can cause syncope. If the patient can't stand, have him sit upright.

▶ An adult with a clavicle strap made from an elastic bandage may require a triangular sling *to help support the weight of the arm, enhance immobilization, and reduce pain.* (See "Triangular sling application," page 880.) For a small child or a confused adult, a well-molded plaster jacket is needed to ensure immobilization. *Inadequate immobilization can cause improper healing.*

▶ Instruct the patient not to remove the clavicle strap. Explain that, with help, he can maintain proper hygiene by lifting segments of the strap to remove the cotton and by washing and powdering the skin daily. Explain that fresh cotton should be applied after cleaning.

▶ For a hospitalized patient, monitor the position of the strap by checking the pen markings every 8 hours. Also assess neurovascular integrity. Teach the outpatient how to assess his own neurovascular integrity and to recognize symptoms to report promptly to the doctor.

▶ Clavicle straps are typically worn for 4 to 8 weeks.

Documentation

In the appropriate section of the emergency department sheet or in your notes, record the date and time of strap application, type of clavicle strap, use of powder and padding, bilateral neurovascular integrity before and after the procedure, and instructions to the patient.

CLINITRON THERAPY BED USE

Originally designed for managing burns, the Clinitron therapy bed is now used for patients with various debilities. By allowing harmless contact between the bed's surface and grafted sites, the bed promotes comfort and healing.

The bed is actually a large tub that supports the patient on a thick layer of silicone-coated microspheres of lime glass. (See *A look at the Clinitron therapy bed.*) A monofilament polyester filter sheet covers the microsphere-filled tub. Warmed air, propelled by a blower beneath the bed, passes through it. The resulting fluidlike surface reduces pressure on the skin to avoid obstructing capillary blood flow, thereby helping to prevent pressure ulcers and to promote wound healing. The bed's air temperature can be adjusted to help control hypothermia and hyperthermia.

The Clinitron therapy bed is contraindicated for patients with an unsta-

ble spine. It may also be contraindicated for the patient unable to mobilize and expel pulmonary secretions because the lack of back support impairs productive coughing. Operation of the Clinitron therapy bed is complex and requires special training.

Key nursing diagnoses and patient outcomes

Risk for imbalanced body temperature related to the patient's condition
The patient will:
▶ have skin that remains warm and dry
▶ maintain a normal body temperature.

Impaired physical mobility related to limitations imposed by the device
The patient will:
▶ attain the highest degree of mobility possible within the confines of the disease
▶ show no evidence of skin breakdown.

Equipment

Clinitron therapy bed with microspheres (about 1,650 lb [750 kg]) • filter sheet • six aluminum rails (for restraining and sealing filter sheet) • flat sheet • elastic cord

Preparation of equipment

Normally, a manufacturer's representative or a trained staff member prepares the bed for use. If you must help with the preparation, make sure the microspheres reach to within ½″ (1.3 cm) of the top of the tank. Then position the filter sheet on the bed with its printed side facing up. Match the holes in the sheet to the holes in the edge of the bed's frame. Place the aluminum rails

A look at the Clinitron therapy bed

The Clinitron therapy bed is a large tub filled with microspheres that are suspended by air pressure and give the patient fluidlike support. The bed provides the advantages of flotation without the disadvantages of instability, patient positioning difficulties, and immobility.

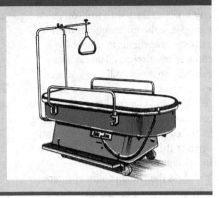

on the frame, with the studs in the proper holes. Depress the rails firmly, and secure them by tightening the knurled knobs to seal the filter sheet. Place a flat sheet over the filter sheet and secure it with the elastic cord. Turn on the air current *to activate the microspheres and to ensure that the bed is working properly;* then turn it off.

Implementation

▶ Explain and, if possible, demonstrate the operation of the Clinitron therapy bed. Tell the patient the reason for its use and that he'll feel as though he's floating.
▶ With the help of three or more coworkers, transfer the patient to the bed using a lift sheet.
▶ Turn on the air pressure to activate the bed.
▶ Adjust the air temperature as necessary. *Because the bed usually operates within 10° to 12° F (5.5° to 6.7° C) of ambient air temperature,* set the room temperature to 75° F (24° C). If microsphere temperature reaches 105° F (40.6° C), the bed automatically shuts

off. It restarts automatically after 30 minutes.

Special considerations

▶ Monitor fluid and electrolyte status *because the Clinitron therapy bed increases evaporative water loss.* Because of this drying effect, always cover a mesh graft for the first 2 to 8 days as ordered. If the patient has excessive upper respiratory tract dryness, use a humidifier and mask as ordered. Encourage coughing and deep breathing. After prolonged use of a Clinitron bed, watch for hypocalcemia and hypophosphatemia.
▶ To position a bedpan, roll the patient away from you, place the bedpan on the flat sheet, and push it into the microspheres. Then reposition the patient. To remove the bedpan, hold it steady and roll the patient away from you. Turn off the air pressure and remove the bedpan. Then turn the air on and reposition the patient.
▶ Don't wear a watch when handling the microspheres *because they can damage the mechanism.* Don't secure the filter sheet with pins or clamps, *which*

may puncture the sheet and release microspheres. Take care to avoid puncturing the bed when giving injections. Repair any holes or tears with iron-on patching tape. Sieve the microspheres monthly or between patients *to remove any clumped microspheres.* Handle them carefully to avoid spills; *spilled microspheres may cause falls.* Treat a soiled filter sheet and clumped microspheres as contaminated items; handle according to policy. Change the filter sheet and operate the unit unoccupied for 24 hours between patients.

▶ Assess the patient's skin and reposition him every 2 hours. Specialty beds don't end the need for frequent assessment and position changes.

Documentation

Record the duration of therapy and the patient's response to it. Document the condition of the patient's skin, pressure ulcers, and other wounds.

CLOSED-WOUND DRAIN MANAGEMENT

Typically inserted during surgery in anticipation of substantial postoperative drainage, a closed-wound drain promotes healing and prevents swelling by suctioning the serosanguineous fluid that accumulates at the wound site. By removing this fluid, the closed-wound drain helps reduce the risk of infection and skin breakdown as well as the number of dressing changes. Hemovac and Jackson-Pratt closed drainage systems are used most commonly.

A closed-wound drain consists of perforated tubing connected to a portable vacuum unit. The distal end of the tubing lies within the wound and usually leaves the body from a site other than the primary suture line to preserve the integrity of the surgical wound. The tubing exit site is treated as an additional surgical wound; the drain is usually sutured to the skin.

If the wound produces heavy drainage, the closed-wound drain may be left in place for longer than 1 week. Drainage must be emptied and measured frequently to maintain maximum suction and prevent strain on the suture line.

Key nursing diagnoses and patient outcomes

Impaired skin integrity related to presence of the drain
The patient will:
▶ exhibit a wound that is healing properly
▶ have few if any complications.

Risk for infection related to the surgical incision
The patient will:
▶ exhibit normal vital signs, body temperature, and laboratory values
▶ have no signs or symptoms of infection at the incision site.

Equipment

Graduated biohazard cylinder • sterile laboratory container, if needed • alcohol pads • gloves • gown • face shield • trash bag • sterile gauze pads • antiseptic cleaning agent • prepackaged povidone-iodine swabs • optional: label

Implementation

▶ Check the doctor's order and assess the patient's condition.
▶ Explain the procedure to the patient, provide privacy, and wash your hands.

Using a closed-wound drainage system

The portable closed-wound drainage system draws drainage from a wound site, such as the chest wall postmastectomy (shown at left), by means of a Y-tube. To empty the drainage, remove the plug and empty it into a graduated cylinder. To reestablish suction, compress the drainage unit against a firm surface to expel air and, while holding it down, replace the plug with your other hand (as shown in the center). The same principle is used for the Jackson-Pratt bulb drain (shown at right).

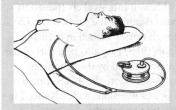 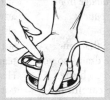 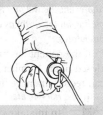

▶ Unclip the vacuum unit from the patient's bed or gown.

▶ Using aseptic technique, release the vacuum by removing the spout plug on the collection chamber. The container expands completely as it draws in air.

▶ Empty the unit's contents into a graduated biohazard cylinder, and note the amount and appearance of the drainage. If diagnostic tests will be performed on the fluid specimen, pour the drainage directly into a sterile laboratory container, note the amount and appearance, label the specimen, and send it to the laboratory.

▶ Maintaining aseptic technique, use an alcohol pad to clean the unit's spout and plug.

▶ *To reestablish the vacuum that creates the drain's suction power,* fully compress the vacuum unit. With one hand holding the unit compressed to maintain the vacuum, replace the spout plug with your other hand. (See *Using a closed-wound drainage system.*)

▶ Check the patency of the equipment. Make sure the tubing is free of twists, kinks, and leaks *because the drainage system must be airtight to work properly.* The vacuum unit should remain compressed when you release manual pressure; rapid reinflation indicates an air leak. If this occurs, recompress the unit and make sure the spout plug is secure.

▶ Secure the vacuum unit to the patient's gown. Fasten it below wound level *to promote drainage.* Don't apply tension on drainage tubing when fastening the unit to prevent possible dislodgment. Remove and discard your gloves and wash your hands thoroughly.

▶ Observe the sutures that secure the drain to the patient's skin; look for signs of pulling or tearing and for swelling or infection of surrounding skin. Gently clean the sutures with sterile gauze pads soaked in an antiseptic cleaning agent or with a povidone-iodine swab.

▶ Properly dispose of drainage, solutions, and trash bag and clean or dispose of soiled equipment and supplies according to facility policy.

Special considerations

▶ Empty the drain and measure its contents once during each shift if drainage has accumulated, more often if drainage is excessive. *Removing excess drainage maintains maximum suction and avoids straining the drain's suture line.*

▶ Empty the drain and measure its contents before the patient ambulates *to prevent the weight of drainage from pulling on the drain as the patient ambulates.*

▶ If the patient has more than one closed drain, number the drains so you can record drainage from each site.

Nursing alert Be careful not to mistake chest tubes for closed-wound drains *because the vacuum of a chest tube should never be released.*

Complications

Occlusion of the tubing by fibrin, clots, or other particles can reduce or obstruct drainage.

Documentation

Record the date and time you empty the drain, appearance of the drain site and presence of swelling or signs of infection, equipment malfunction and consequent nursing action, and patient's tolerance of the treatment. On the intake and output sheet, record drainage color, consistency, type, and amount. If the patient has more than one closed-wound drain, number the drains and record the information above separately for each drainage site.

CODE MANAGEMENT

The goals of any code are to restore the patient's spontaneous heartbeat and respirations and to prevent hypoxic damage to the brain and other vital organs. Fulfilling these goals requires a team approach. Ideally, the team should consist of health care workers trained in advanced cardiac life support (ACLS), although nurses trained in basic life support (BLS) may also be a part of the team. Sponsored by the American Heart Association, the ACLS course incorporates BLS skills with advanced resuscitation techniques.

In most health care facilities, ACLS-trained nurses provide the first resuscitative efforts to cardiac arrest patients, often administering cardiac medications and performing defibrillation before the doctor's arrival. Because ventricular fibrillation commonly precedes sudden cardiac arrest, initial resuscitative efforts focus on rapid recognition of arrhythmias and, when indicated, defibrillation. If monitoring equipment isn't available, you should simply perform BLS measures. Of course, the scope of your responsibilities in any situation depends on your facility's policies and procedures and your state's nurse practice act.

A code may be called for patients with absent pulse, apnea, ventricular fibrillation, ventricular tachycardia, or asystole.

Key nursing diagnoses and patient outcomes

Ineffective tissue perfusion (cardiopulmonary) related to cardiac arrest
The patient will:

▶ attain hemodynamic stability: pulse not less than (specify) beats/minute and not greater than (specify) beats/minute; blood pressure not less than (specify) mm Hg and not greater than (specify) mm Hg
▶ maintain cardiac output
▶ suffer no complications from CPR.

Impaired spontaneous ventilation related to (specify)
The patient will:
▶ have normal arterial blood gas levels
▶ have a breathing pattern that returns to baseline.

Equipment

Oral, nasal, and endotracheal (ET) airways • one-way valve masks • oxygen source • oxygen flowmeter • intubation supplies • handheld resuscitation bag • suction supplies • nasogastric (NG) tube • goggles, masks, and gloves • cardiac arrest board • peripheral I.V. supplies, including 14G and 18G peripheral I.V. catheters • central I.V. supplies, including an 18G thin-wall catheter, a 6-cm needle catheter, and a 16G 15- to 20-cm catheter • I.V. administration sets (including microdrip and minidrip) • I.V. fluids, including dextrose 5% in water (D_5W), normal saline solution, and lactated Ringer's solution • electrocardiogram (ECG) monitor and leads • cardioverter-defibrillator • conductive medium • cardiac drugs, including adenosine, amiodarone, atropine, calcium chloride, dobutamine, dopamine, epinephrine, isoproterenol, lidocaine, procainamide, and vasopressin • optional: transthoracic pacemaker, percutaneous transvenous pacer, cricothyrotomy kit, and end-tidal carbon dioxide detector

Preparation of equipment

Because effective emergency care depends on reliable and accessible equipment, the equipment, as well as the personnel, must be ready for a code at any time. (See *Organizing your crash cart,* page 172.) You also should be familiar with the cardiac drugs you may have to administer. (See *Common emergency cardiac drugs,* pages 173 to 175.)

Always be aware of your patient's code status as defined by the doctor's orders, the patient's advance directives, and family wishes. If the doctor has ordered a "no code," make sure that he has written and signed the order. If possible, have the patient or a responsible family member co-sign the order.

In some cases, you may need to consider whether the family wishes to be present during a code. If they do want to be present, and if a nurse or clergyman can remain with them, consider allowing them to remain during the code.

Implementation

▶ If you're the first to arrive at the site of a code, assess the patient's level of consciousness (LOC), airway, breathing, and circulation, and then begin cardiopulmonary resuscitation (CPR). Use a pocket mask, if available, to ventilate the patient.
▶ Call for help. When a second BLS provider arrives, have that person call a code and retrieve the emergency equipment.
▶ When the emergency equipment arrives, have the second BLS provider place the cardiac arrest board under the patient and then assist with two-rescuer CPR. Meanwhile, have the nurse assigned to the patient relate the patient's

Organizing your crash cart

When responding to a code, you can't waste time searching the drawers of your crash cart for the equipment you need. One way to make sure you know the precise location of everything is to follow the ABCD plan to an organized crash cart. Label the crash cart drawers with the letters A, B, C, and D and fill them as follows.

A: Airway control drawer

This drawer should contain all of the equipment necessary for maintaining a patient's airway, including oral, nasal, and endotracheal airways; an intubation tray containing a laryngoscope and blades; an extra laryngoscope; lidocaine ointment; tape; a 10-ml syringe to inflate the endotracheal balloon; extra batteries and light bulbs; and suction devices.

B: Breathing drawer

This drawer should contain all of the equipment needed to support the patient's ventilation and oxygenation. Oxygenation is maintained with nasal cannulas, face masks, and Venturi masks. Ventilation is supported by maintaining gastric compression with nasogastric tubes.

C: Circulation drawer

In this drawer, place anything needed to start a central or peripheral I.V. line, such as catheters, tubing, start kits, pump tubing, and 250-ml or 500-ml bags of I.V. solutions (dextrose 5% in water and normal saline solution).

D: Drug drawer

This drawer should contain all medications needed for advanced cardiac life support.

medical history and describe the events leading to cardiac arrest.

► A third person, either a nurse certified in BLS or a respiratory therapist, will then attach the handheld resuscitation bag to the oxygen source and begin to ventilate the patient with 100% oxygen.

► When the ACLS-trained nurse arrives, she'll expose the patient's chest and apply defibrillator pads. She'll then apply the paddles to the patient's chest to obtain a "quick look" at the patient's cardiac rhythm. If the patient is in ventricular fibrillation, ACLS protocol calls for defibrillation as soon as possible with 200 joules. If defibrillation is unsuccessful, the nurse should defibrillate next using 200 to 300 joules and then using 360 joules, if necessary. The ACLS-trained nurse will act as code leader until the doctor arrives.

► If not already in place, apply ECG electrodes and attach the patient to the defibrillator's cardiac monitor. Avoid placing electrodes on bony prominences or hairy areas. Also avoid the areas where the defibrillator pads will be placed and where chest compressions will be given.

► As CPR continues, you or an ACLS-trained nurse will then start two peripheral I.V. lines with large-bore I.V. catheters. Be sure to use only a large vein, such as the antecubital vein, *to allow for rapid fluid administration and to prevent drug extravasation.*

► As soon as the I.V. catheter is in place, begin an infusion of normal saline solution or lactated Ringer's solution *to help prevent circulatory collapse.* D_5W continues to be acceptable but the latest ACLS guidelines encourage the use of normal saline solution or lactat-

Common emergency cardiac drugs

You may be called on to administer a variety of cardiac drugs during a code. The following chart lists the most commonly used emergency cardiac drugs, along with their actions, indications, and dosage.

Drug	Actions	Indications	Usual adult dosage
adenosine (Adenocard)	■ Slows conduction through atrioventricular (AV) node; may interrupt reentry through AV node ■ Shortens duration of atrial action potential during supraventricular tachycardia	■ Supraventricular tachycardia, including those associated with accessory bypass tracts (Wolff-Parkinson-White syndrome)	■ 6 mg I.V. push over 1 to 3 seconds initially; may be increased to 12 mg if conversion hasn't occurred within 1 to 2 minutes. Each dose should quickly be followed by a 20-ml saline flush. ■ *Caution:* Slower-than-recommended administration decreases drug's effectiveness.
amiodarone	■ Thought to prolong the refractory period and action potential duration	■ Supraventricular tachycardia ■ Persistent VT or VF	■ 150 mg over 10 minutes, followed by 1 mg/minute infusion for 6 hours, and then 0.5 mg/minute. ■ *Caution:* Amiodarone may cause hypotension and bradycardia, which can be prevented by slowing the infusion rate.
atropine	■ Accelerates AV conduction and heart rate by blocking vagal nerve	■ Symptomatic bradycardia ■ Asystole ■ AV block ■ pulseless electrical activity (slow rate)	■ 0.5 to 1 mg I.V. push (for asystole, 1 mg); repeated every 3 to 5 minutes until heart rate exceeds 60 beats/minute (up to 3 mg total)
dobutamine (Dobutrex)	■ Increases myocardial contractility without raising oxygen demand	■ Heart failure ■ Cardiogenic shock	■ 2 to 20 mcg/kg/minute by continuous I.V. infusion. Dilute 2 to 4 ampules (250 mg/ampule) in 250 ml of D5W or normal saline solution.
dopamine (Intropin)	■ Produces inotropic effect, increasing cardiac output, blood pressure, and renal perfusion	■ Hypotension (except when caused by hypovolemia)	■ Continuous I.V. infusion at 1 to 5 mcg/kg/minute initially; can be increased to 20 mcg/kg/minute, as needed (*Note:* Always dilute and give I.V. drip, never I.V. push.) ■ *Caution:* Don't administer in same I.V. line with alkaline solution.

(continued)

Common emergency cardiac drugs (continued)

Drug	Actions	Indications	Usual adult dosage
epinephrine (Adrenalin)	■ Increases heart rate, peripheral resistance, and blood flow to heart (enhancing myocardial and cerebral oxygenation) ■ Strengthens myocardial contractility ■ Increases coronary perfusion pressure during cardiopulmonary resuscitation	■ VF ■ Pulseless VT ■ Pulseless electrical activity ■ Asystole ■ Hypotension (secondary agent)	■ 10 ml of 1:10,000 solution (1 mg) I.V. push initially; may be repeated every 3 to 5 minutes, as needed (After each dose, flush with 20 ml of I.V. fluid, if administered peripherally.) ■ 2 to 2½ times the I.V. dose endotracheally if no I.V. line is available (*Note:* 1:1,000 solution contains 1 mg/ml, so it must be diluted in 9 ml of normal saline solution to provide 1 mg/10 ml.) ■ For hypotension, 1 mg/500 ml of D_5W by continuous infusion, starting at 1 mcg/minute and titrated to desired effect (2 to 10 mcg/minute) ■ *Caution:* Don't administer in same I.V. line with alkaline solutions. ■ Many reports have shown that doses of 10 mg I.V. or more are needed to achieve resuscitation.
isoproterenol hydrochloride (Isuprel)	■ Enhances automaticity and accelerates conduction ■ Increases heart rate and cardiac contractility, but exacerbates ischemia and arrhythmias in patients with ischemic heart disease	■ Indicated only for temporary control of severe bradycardia unresponsive to atropine (while awaiting pacemaker insertion) ■ Not indicated for cardiac arrest	■ Start I.V. drip of 1 mg in 500 ml of D_5W at 2 mcg/minute; titrate to produce heart rate of 60 beats/minute or systolic blood pressure greater than 90 mm Hg (2 to 10 mcg/minute) ■ *Caution:* Don't give I.V. push or mix with another drug.
lidocaine (Xylocaine)	■ Depresses automaticity and conduction of ectopic impulses in ventricles, especially in ischemic tissue ■ Raises fibrillation threshold, especially in an ischemic heart	■ Frequent premature ventricular contractions (PVCs) ■ VT ■ VF	■ 1 to 1.5 mg/kg (usually 50 to 75 mg) I.V. push initially; may be followed by 0.5 to 0.75 mg/kg bolus dose every 5 to 10 minutes up to total of 3 mg/kg ■ Continuous I.V. infusion of 2 g/500 ml of D_5W at 1 to 4 mg/minute to prevent recurrence of lethal arrhythmias; reduced by 50% after 24 hours

Common emergency cardiac drugs *(continued)*

Drug	Actions	Indications	Usual adult dosage
magnesium sulfate	■ Mechanism of action is unclear but drug may help in cardiac arrest associated with refractory VT or VF	■ Cardiac arrest associated with refractory VT or VF	■ For life-threatening arrhythmias, 1 to 2 g I.V. in 100 ml of D_5W over 1 to 2 minutes ■ In a nonemergency situation, I.V. infusion of 0.5 to 1g/hour for up to 24 hours ■ *Caution:* If hypotension develops, slow or stop infusion.
procainamide hydrochloride (Pronestyl)	■ Depresses automaticity and conduction ■ Prolongs refraction in the atria and ventricles	■ Suppresses PVCs and VT unresponsive to lidocaine	■ 20 mg/minute I.V. infusion up to a total of 17 mg/kg, followed by maintenance dose of 1 to 4 mg/minute by I.V. infusion
vasopressin	■ Causes peripheral vasoconstriction	■ Refractory VF	■ 40 U I.V. single dose, 1 time only
verapamil (Isoptin)	■ Slows conduction through AV node ■ Causes vasodilation ■ Produces negative inotropic effect on heart, depressing myocardial contractility	■ Paroxysmal supraventricular tachycardia (PSVT) with narrow QRS complex and rate control in atrial fibrillation	■ 2.5 to 5 mg I.V. push over 2 minutes initially; may be increased to 5 to 10 mg and repeated in 15 to 30 minutes to maximum dose of 30 mg if PSVT persists and patient demonstrates no adverse reaction to initial dose

ed Ringer's solution *because D_5W can produce hyperglycemic effects during a cardiac arrest.*

▶ While one nurse starts the I.V. lines, the other nurse will set up portable or wall suction equipment and suction the patient's oral secretions as necessary *to maintain an open airway.*

▶ The ACLS-trained nurse will then prepare and administer emergency cardiac drugs as needed. (See *Treating lethal arrhythmias,* page 176.) Keep in mind that drugs administered through a central line reach the myocardium more quickly than those administered through a peripheral line.

▶ If the patient doesn't have an accessible I.V. line, you may administer such medications as epinephrine, lidocaine, and atropine through an ET tube. To do so, dilute the drugs in 10 ml of normal saline solution or sterile water and then

Treating lethal arrhythmias

The American Heart Association's advanced cardiac life support (ACLS) course outlines specific protocol for treating life-threatening arrhythmias. The ACLS course defines a lethal arrhythmia as having the following characteristics:

- ventricular rhythm rapid and chaotic, indicating varying degrees of depolarization and repolarization; QRS complexes not identifiable
- patient unconscious at onset
- absent pulses, heart sounds, and blood pressure
- dilated pupils
- rapid development of cyanosis.

The flowchart at right outlines the steps an ACLS-certified nurse should take to treat such potentially lethal arrhythmias as ventricular fibrillation and pulseless ventricular tachycardia. Even if you aren't certified in ACLS, the chart will help you know what to expect in such an emergency.

Establish responsiveness.
▼
Check pulse. If no pulse then:
▼
Perform CPR until a defibrillator is available.
▼
Check rhythm. If ventricular fibrillation or tachycardia appears, then:
▼
Defibrillate using 200 joules.
▼
Defibrillate using 200 to 300 joules.
▼
Defibrillate using 360 joules.
▼
If ventricular fibrillation or tachycardia persists, then:
▼
Continue CPR.
▼
Intubate as soon as possible.
▼
Establish I.V. access.
▼
Administer epinephrine, 1:10,000, 1 mg I.V. push every 3 to 5 minutes or vasopressin, 40 units I.V. single dose.
▼
Defibrillate using 360 joules, within 30 to 60 seconds.
▼
Administer amiodarone, 150 mg I.V. push over 10 minutes
May consider lidocaine, magnesium (if patient is in a hypomagnesemic state), or procainamide for recurrent ventricular fibrillation.
▼
Defibrillate using 360 joules.
▼
Administer a second dose of amiodarone, over 10 minutes (may repeat every 10 to 15 minutes; maximum total dose in 24 hours is 2.2 g).
▼
Defibrillate using 360 joules.
▼
Consider sodium bicarbonate.
▼
Defibrillate using 360 joules.

instill them into the patient's ET tube. Afterward, ventilate the patient manually *to improve absorption by distributing the drug throughout the bronchial tree.*

▶ The ACLS-trained nurse will also prepare for, and assist with, ET intubation. During intubation attempts, take care not to interrupt CPR for longer than 30 seconds.

▶ Suction the patient as needed. After the patient has been intubated, assess his breath sounds *to ensure proper tube placement.* If the patient has diminished or absent breath sounds over the left lung field, the doctor will pull back the ET tube slightly and reassess. When the tube is correctly positioned, tape it securely. *To serve as a reference,* mark the point on the tube that is level with the patient's lips.

▶ Throughout the code, check the patient's carotid or femoral pulses before and after each defibrillation. Also check the pulses frequently during the code *to evaluate the effectiveness of cardiac compressions.*

▶ Meanwhile, other members of the code team should keep a written record of the events. Other duties include prompting participants about when to perform certain activities (such as when to check a pulse or take vital signs), overseeing the effectiveness of CPR, and keeping track of the time between therapies. Each team member should know what each participant's role is *to prevent duplicating effort.* Finally, someone from the team should make sure that the primary nurse's other patients are reassigned to another nurse.

▶ If the family is present during the code, have someone, such as a clergy member or social worker, remain with them. Be sure to keep the family regularly informed of the patient's status.

▶ If the family isn't at the facility, contact them as soon as possible. Encourage them not to drive to the facility but offer to call someone who can give them a ride.

Special considerations

▶ When the patient's condition has stabilized, assess his LOC, breath sounds, heart sounds, peripheral perfusion, bowel sounds, and urine output. Measure his vital signs every 15 minutes and monitor his cardiac rhythm continuously.

▶ Make sure the patient receives an adequate supply of oxygen, whether through a mask or a ventilator.

▶ Check the infusion rates of all I.V. fluids and use infusion pumps to deliver vasoactive drugs. *To evaluate the effectiveness of fluid therapy,* insert an indwelling catheter if the patient doesn't already have one. Also insert an NG tube *to relieve or prevent gastric distention.*

▶ If appropriate, reassure the patient and explain what is happening. Allow the patient's family to visit as soon as possible. If the patient dies, notify the family and allow them to see the patient as soon as possible.

▶ *To make sure your code team performs optimally,* schedule a time to review the code.

Complications

Even when performed correctly, CPR can cause fractured ribs, liver laceration, lung puncture, and gastric distention. Defibrillation can cause electric shock, and emergency intubation can result in esophageal or tracheal laceration, subcutaneous emphysema, or accidental right mainstem bronchus intubation. (Decreased or absent breath sounds on the left side of the chest and normal breath sounds on the right may signal accidental right mainstem bronchus intubation.)

Documentation

During the code, document the events in as much detail as possible. Note whether the arrest was witnessed or unwitnessed, the time of the arrest, the time CPR was begun, the time the ACLS-trained nurse arrived, and the total resuscitation time. Also document the number of defibrillations, the times they were performed, the joule level, the patient's cardiac rhythm before and after the defibrillation, and whether or not the patient had a pulse.

Document all drug therapy, including dosages, routes of administration, and patient response. You'll also want to record all procedures, such as peripheral and central line insertion, pacemaker insertion, and ET tube insertion, as well as the time they were performed and the patient's tolerance of the procedures. Also keep track of all arterial blood gas results.

Record whether the patient is transferred to another unit or facility along with his condition at the time of transfer and whether or not his family was notified. Finally, document any complications and the measures taken to correct them. When your documentation is complete, have the doctor and ACLS nurse review and then sign the document.

COLD APPLICATION

The application of cold constricts blood vessels; inhibits local circulation, suppuration, and tissue metabolism; relieves vascular congestion; slows bacterial activity in infections; reduces body temperature; and may act as a temporary anesthetic during brief, painful procedures. (See *Reducing pain with ice massage.*) Because treatment with cold also relieves inflammation, reduces edema, and slows bleeding, it may provide effective initial treatment after eye injuries, strains, sprains, bruises, muscle spasms, and burns. Cold doesn't reduce preexisting edema however, because it inhibits reabsorption of excess fluid.

Cold may be applied in dry or moist forms, but ice shouldn't be placed directly on a patient's skin because it may further damage tissue. Moist application is more penetrating than dry because moisture facilitates conduction. Devices for applying cold include an ice bag or collar, K pad (which can produce cold or heat), and chemical cold packs and ice packs. Devices for applying moist cold include cold compresses for small body areas and cold packs for large areas.

Apply cold treatments cautiously on patients with impaired circulation, on children, and on elderly or arthritic patients because of the risk of ischemic tissue damage.

Key nursing diagnoses and patient outcomes

Risk for injury related to cold application
The patient will:
▶ experience no injury from application of cold

► identify factors that increase potential for injury

► verbalize an understanding of safety measures to prevent injury from application of cold.

Risk for impaired skin integrity related to direct cold application
The patient will:

► experience no skin breakdown

► communicate an understanding of preventive skin measures.

Equipment

Patient thermometer • towel • adhesive tape or roller gauze • gloves, if necessary

For an ice bag or collar

Tap water • ice chips • absorbent, protective cloth covering

For a K pad

Temperature-adjustment key • distilled water • absorbent, protective cloth covering

For a chemical cold pack

Single-use packs are available for applying dry cold. These lightweight plastic packs contain a chemical that turns cold when activated. Reusable, sealed cold packs, filled with an alcohol-based solution, are also available. These packs may be stored frozen until use and, after exterior disinfection, may be refrozen and used again. Other chemical packs are activated by striking, squeezing, or kneading them.

For a cold compress or pack

Basin of ice chips • container of tap water • bath thermometer • compress material (4″ × 4″ gauze pads or washcloths) or pack material (towels or flannel) • linen-saver pad • waterproof covering

Reducing pain with ice massage

Normally, ice should not be applied directly to a patient's skin *because it risks damaging the skin surface and underlying tissues.* However, when carefully performed, ice massage may help patients tolerate brief, painful procedures, such as bone marrow aspiration, catheterization, chest tube removal, injection into joints, lumbar puncture, and suture removal.

Prepare for ice massage by gathering the ice, a porous covering to hold it in (if desired), and a cloth for wiping water from the patient as the ice melts.

Just before the procedure begins, rub the ice over the appropriate area to numb it. Assess the site frequently; stop rubbing immediately if you detect signs of tissue intolerance.

As the procedure begins, rub the ice over a point near but not at the site. This distracts the patient from the procedure itself and gives him another stimulus on which to concentrate.

If the procedure lasts longer than 10 minutes or if you think tissue damage may occur, move the ice to a different site and continue massage.

If you know in advance that the procedure probably will last longer than 10 minutes, massage the site intermittently — 2 minutes of massage alternating with a rest period — until the skin regains its normal color. Alternatively, you can divide the area into several sites and apply ice to each one for several minutes at a time.

Preparation of equipment
Ice bag or collar
Select a device of the correct size, fill it with cold tap water, and check for leaks. Then empty the device and fill it about halfway with crushed ice. *Using small pieces of ice helps the device mold to the patient's body.* Squeeze the device *to expel air that might reduce conduction.* Fasten the cap and wipe any moisture from the outside of the device. Wrap the bag or collar in a cloth covering, and secure the cover with tape or roller gauze. *The protective cover prevents tissue trauma and absorbs condensation.*

K pad
Check the cord for frayed or damaged insulation. Then fill the control unit two-thirds full with distilled water or to the level recommended by the manufacturer. Don't use tap water *because it leaves mineral deposits in the unit.* Check for leaks and then tilt the unit several times *to clear the pad's tubing of air.* Tighten the cap. After ensuring that the hoses between the control unit and pad are free of tangles, place the unit on the bedside table, slightly above the patient *so that gravity can assist water flow.* If the central supply department hasn't preset the temperature, use the temperature-adjustment key to adjust the control unit setting to the lowest temperature. Cover the pad with an absorbent, protective cloth and secure the cover with tape or roller gauze. Plug in the unit and turn it on. Allow the pad to cool for 2 minutes before placing it on the patient.

Chemical cold pack
Select a pack of the appropriate size, and follow the manufacturer's direc-tions (strike, squeeze, or knead) *to activate the cold-producing chemicals.* Make certain that the container hasn't been broken during activation. Wrap the pack in a cloth cover and secure the cover with tape or roller gauze.

Cold compress or pack
Cool a container of tap water by placing it in a basin of ice or by adding ice to the water. Using a bath thermometer for guidance, adjust the water temperature to 59° F (15° C) or as ordered. Immerse the compress or pack material in the water.

Implementation
▶ Check the doctor's order and assess the patient's condition.
▶ Explain the procedure to the patient, provide privacy, and make sure the room is warm and free of drafts. Wash your hands thoroughly.
▶ Record the patient's temperature, pulse, and respirations *to serve as a baseline.*
▶ Expose only the treatment site *to avoid chilling the patient.*

Applying an ice bag or collar, a K pad, or a chemical cold pack
▶ Place the covered cold device on the treatment site and begin timing the application.
▶ Observe the site frequently for signs of tissue intolerance, such as blanching, mottling, cyanosis, maceration, and blisters. Also be alert for shivering and complaints of burning or numbness. If this sign or these symptoms develop, discontinue treatment and notify the doctor.
▶ Refill or replace the cold device as necessary *to maintain the correct temper-*

ature. Change the protective cover if it becomes wet.
▶ Remove the device after the prescribed treatment period (usually 30 minutes).

Applying a cold compress or pack
▶ Place a linen-saver pad under the site.
▶ Remove the compress or pack from the water and wring it out *to prevent dripping.* Apply it to the treatment site and begin timing the application.
▶ Cover the compress or pack with a waterproof covering *to provide insulation and to keep the surrounding area dry.* Secure the covering with tape or roller gauze *to prevent it from slipping.*
▶ Check the application site frequently for signs of tissue intolerance and note complaints of burning or numbness. If these symptoms develop, discontinue treatment and notify the doctor.
▶ Change the compress or pack as needed to maintain the correct temperature. Remove it after the prescribed treatment period (usually 20 minutes).

Concluding all cold applications
▶ Dry the patient's skin and re-dress the treatment site according to the doctor's orders. Then position the patient comfortably and take his temperature, pulse, and respirations *for comparison with baseline.*
▶ Dispose of liquids and soiled materials properly. If the cold treatment will be repeated, clean and store the equipment in the patient's room, out of his reach; otherwise, return it to storage.

Special considerations
▶ Apply cold immediately after an injury to minimize edema. (See *Using cold for a muscle sprain.*) Although colder

Using cold for a muscle sprain

Cold can help relieve pain and reduce edema during the first 24 to 72 hours after a sprain occurs. Tell the patient to apply cold to the area four times daily for 20 to 30 minutes each time.

For each application, instruct the patient to obtain enough crushed ice to cover the painful area, place it in a plastic bag, and place the bag inside a pillowcase or large piece of cloth (as shown below).

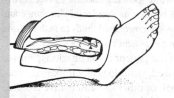

For later applications, the patient may want to fill a paper cup with water, stand a tongue blade in the cup, and place it in the freezer. After the water freezes, he can peel the paper off the ice and hold it with the protruding handle. If he chooses this method, tell him to first cover the area with a cloth. Applying ice directly to the skin can cause frostbite or cold shock.

Instruct the patient to rub the ice over the painful area for the specified treatment time. Warn him that although ice eases pain in a joint that has begun to stiffen, he shouldn't let the analgesic effect encourage overuse of the joint.

After 24 to 72 hours, when heat and swelling have subsided or when cold no longer helps, the patient should switch to heat application.

temperatures can be tolerated for a longer time when the treatment site is small, don't continue any application for longer than 1 hour *to avoid reflex vasodilation.* The application of temperatures below 59° F (15° C) also causes local reflex vasodilation.

▶ Use sterile technique when applying cold to an open wound or to a lesion that may open during treatment. Also maintain sterile technique during eye treatment, with separate sterile equipment for each eye to prevent cross-contamination.

▶ Avoid securing cooling devices with pins *because an accidental puncture could allow extremely cold fluids to leak out and burn the patient's skin.*

▶ If the patient is unconscious, anesthetized, neurologically impaired, irrational, or otherwise insensitive to cold, stay with him throughout the treatment and check the application site frequently for complications.

▶ Warn the patient against placing ice directly on his skin *because the extreme cold can cause burns.*

Complications
Hemoconcentration may cause thrombi. Intense cold may cause pain, burning, or numbness.

Documentation
Record the time, date, and duration of cold application; type of device used (ice bag or collar, K pad, or chemical cold pack); site of application; temperature or temperature setting; patient's temperature, pulse, and respirations before and after application; skin appearance before, during, and after application; signs or symptoms of complications; and the patient's tolerance of treatment.

Colostomy and Ileostomy Care

A patient with an ascending or transverse colostomy or an ileostomy must wear an external pouch to collect emerging fecal matter, which will be watery or pasty. Besides collecting waste matter, the pouch helps to control odor and protect the stoma and peristomal skin. Most disposable pouching systems can be used for 2 to 7 days; some models last even longer.

All pouching systems need to be changed immediately if a leak develops, and every pouch must be emptied when it's one-third to one-half full. The patient with an ileostomy may need to empty his pouch four or five times daily.

Naturally, the best time to change the pouching system is when the bowel is least active, usually between 2 and 4 hours after meals. After a few months, most patients can predict the best changing time.

The selection of a pouching system should take into consideration which system provides the best adhesive seal and skin protection for the individual patient. The type of pouch selected also depends on the stoma's location and structure, availability of supplies, wear time, consistency of effluent, personal preference, and finances.

Pouching systems may be drainable or closed-bottomed, disposable or reusable, adhesive-backed, and one-piece or two-piece. (See *Comparing ostomy pouching systems.*)

Comparing ostomy pouching systems

Manufactured in many shapes and sizes, ostomy pouches are fashioned for comfort, safety, and easy application. For example, a disposable closed-end pouch may meet the needs of a patient who irrigates his ostomy, who wants added security, or who wants to discard the pouch after each bowel movement. Another patient may prefer a reusable, drainable pouch. Some commonly available pouches are described below.

Disposable pouches

The patient who must empty his pouch often (because of diarrhea or a new colostomy or ileostomy) may prefer a one-piece, drainable, disposable pouch with a closure clamp attached to a skin barrier (below left).

These transparent or opaque, odor-proof, plastic pouches come with attached adhesive or karaya seals. Some pouches have microporous adhesive or belt tabs. The bottom opening allows for easy draining. This pouch may be used permanently or temporarily, until stoma size stabilizes.

Also disposable and made of transparent or opaque odor-proof plastic, a one-piece disposable closed-end pouch (below right) may come in a kit with adhesive seal, belt tabs, skin barrier, or carbon filter for gas release. A patient with a regular bowel elimination pattern may choose this style for additional security and confidence.

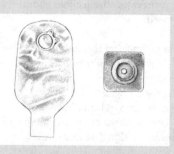

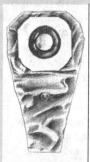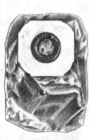

A two-piece disposable drainable pouch with separate skin barrier (top of next column) permits frequent changes and also minimizes skin breakdown. Also made of transparent or opaque odor-proof plastic, this style comes with belt tabs and usually snaps to the skin barrier with a flange mechanism.

Reusable pouches

Typically manufactured from sturdy, opaque, hypoallergenic plastic, the reusable pouch comes with a separate custom-made faceplate and O-ring (as shown below). Some pouches have a pressure valve for releasing gas. The device has a 1- to 2-month life span, depending on how frequently the patient empties the pouch.

Reusable equipment may benefit a patient who needs a firm faceplate or who wishes to minimize cost. However, many reusable ostomy pouches aren't odor-proof.

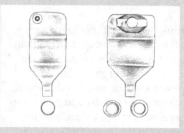

Key nursing diagnoses and patient outcomes

Disturbed body image related to the presence of a colostomy or an ileostomy
The patient will:
▶ acknowledge changes in body image
▶ communicate feelings about changes in body image
▶ express positive feelings about himself.

Risk for impaired skin integrity related to the presence of a colostomy or an ileostomy
The patient will:
▶ experience no skin breakdown
▶ communicate an understanding of preventive skin care measures.

Equipment

Pouching system • stoma measuring guide • stoma paste (if drainage is watery to pasty or stoma secretes excess mucus) • plastic bag • water • washcloth and towel • closure clamp • toilet or bedpan • water or pouch cleaning solution • gloves • facial tissues • optional: ostomy belt, paper tape, mild nonmoisturizing soap, skin shaving equipment, liquid skin sealant, pouch deodorant

Implementation

▶ Provide privacy and emotional support.

Fitting the pouch and skin barrier

▶ For a pouch with an attached skin barrier, measure the stoma with the stoma measuring guide. Select the opening size that matches the stoma.
▶ For an adhesive-backed pouch with a separate skin barrier, measure the stoma with the measuring guide and select the opening that matches the

stoma. Trace the selected size opening onto the paper back of the skin barrier's adhesive side. Cut out the opening. (If the pouch has precut openings, which can be handy for a round stoma, select an opening that is 1/8" larger than the stoma. If the pouch comes without an opening, cut the hole 1/8" wider than the measured tracing.) The cut-to-fit system works best for an irregularly shaped stoma.
▶ For a two-piece pouching system with flanges, see *Applying a skin barrier and pouch.*
▶ Avoid fitting the pouch too tightly *because the stoma has no pain receptors. A constrictive opening could injure the stoma or skin tissue without the patient feeling warning discomfort.* Also avoid cutting the opening too big *because this may expose the skin to fecal matter and moisture.*
▶ The patient with a descending or sigmoid colostomy who has formed stools and whose ostomy doesn't secrete much mucus may choose to wear only a pouch. In this case, make sure the pouch opening closely matches the stoma size.
▶ Between 6 weeks and 1 year after surgery, the stoma will shrink to its permanent size. At that point, pattern-making preparations will be unnecessary unless the patient gains weight, has additional surgery, or injures the stoma.

Applying or changing the pouch

▶ Collect all equipment.
▶ Wash your hands and provide privacy.
▶ Explain the procedure to the patient. As you perform each step, explain what you are doing and why *because the patient will eventually perform the procedure himself.*

Applying a skin barrier and pouch

Fitting a skin barrier and ostomy pouch properly can be done in a few steps. Shown below is a two-piece pouching system with flanges, which is in common use.

Measure the stoma using a measuring guide.

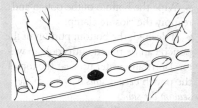

Trace the appropriate circle carefully on the back of the skin barrier.

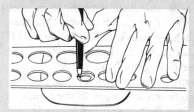

Cut the circular opening in the skin barrier. Bevel the edges to keep them from irritating the patient.

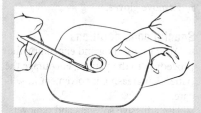

Remove the backing from the skin barrier and moisten it or apply barrier paste as needed along the edge of the circular opening.

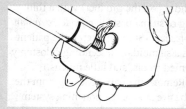

Center the skin barrier over the stoma, adhesive side down, and gently press it to the skin.

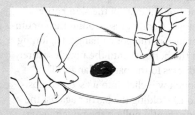

Gently press the pouch opening onto the ring until it snaps into place.

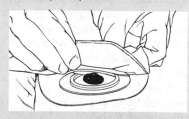

▶ Put on gloves.
▶ Remove and discard the old pouch. Wipe the stoma and peristomal skin gently with a facial tissue.
▶ Carefully wash with mild soap and water and dry the peristomal skin by patting gently. Allow the skin to dry thoroughly. Inspect the peristomal skin and stoma. If necessary, shave surrounding hair (in a direction away from the stoma) *to promote a better seal and*

avoid skin irritation from hair pulling against the adhesive.

▶ If applying a separate skin barrier, peel off the paper backing of the prepared skin barrier, center the barrier over the stoma, and press gently *to ensure adhesion.*

▶ You may want to outline the stoma on the back of the skin barrier (depending on the product) with a thin ring of stoma paste *to provide extra skin protection.* (Skip this step if the patient has a sigmoid or descending colostomy, formed stools, and little mucus.)

▶ Remove the paper backing from the adhesive side of the pouching system and center the pouch opening over the stoma. Press gently to secure.

▶ For a pouching system with flanges, align the lip of the pouch flange with the bottom edge of the skin barrier flange. Gently press around the circumference of the pouch flange, beginning at the bottom, until the pouch securely adheres to the barrier flange. (The pouch will click into its secured position.) Holding the barrier against the skin, gently pull on the pouch *to confirm the seal between flanges.*

▶ Encourage the patient to stay quietly in position for about 5 minutes *to improve adherence. The patient's body warmth also helps to improve adherence and soften a rigid skin barrier.*

▶ Attach an ostomy belt *to further secure the pouch,* if desired. (Some pouches have belt loops, and others have plastic adapters for belts.)

▶ Leave a bit of air in the pouch *to allow drainage to fall to the bottom.*

▶ Apply the closure clamp, if necessary.

▶ If desired, apply paper tape in a picture-frame fashion to the pouch edges *for additional security.*

Emptying the pouch

▶ Put on gloves.

▶ Tilt the bottom of the pouch upward and remove the closure clamp.

▶ Turn up a cuff on the lower end of the pouch and allow it to drain into the toilet or bedpan.

▶ Wipe the bottom of the pouch and reapply the closure clamp.

▶ If desired, the bottom portion of the pouch can be rinsed with cool tap water. Don't aim water up near the top of the pouch *because this may loosen the seal on the skin.*

▶ A two-piece flanged system can also be emptied by unsnapping the pouch. Let the drainage flow into the toilet.

▶ Release flatus through the gas release valve if the pouch has one. Otherwise, release flatus by tilting the pouch bottom upward, releasing the clamp, and expelling the flatus. To release flatus from a flanged system, loosen the seal between the flanges. (Some pouches have gas release valves.)

▶ Never make a pinhole in a pouch to release gas. *This destroys the odor-proof seal.*

▶ Remove gloves.

Special considerations

▶ After performing and explaining the procedure to the patient, encourage the patient's increasing involvement in self-care.

▶ Use adhesive solvents and removers only after patch-testing the patient's skin *because some products may irritate the skin or produce hypersensitivity reactions.* Consider using a liquid skin sealant, if available, *to give skin tissue additional protection from drainage and adhesive irritants.*

▶ Remove the pouching system if the patient reports burning or itching beneath it or purulent drainage around the stoma. Notify the doctor or therapist of any skin irritation, breakdown, rash, or unusual appearance of the stoma or peristomal area.

▶ Use commercial pouch deodorants, if desired. However, most pouches are odor-free, and odor should only be evident when you empty the pouch or if it leaks. Before discharge, suggest that the patient avoid odor-causing foods, such as fish, eggs, onions, and garlic.

▶ If the patient wears a reusable pouching system, suggest that he obtain two or more systems *so that he can wear one while the other dries after cleaning with soap and water or a commercially prepared cleaning solution.*

Complications

Failure to fit the pouch properly over the stoma or improper use of a belt can injure the stoma. Be alert for a possible allergic reaction to adhesives and other ostomy products.

Documentation

Record the date and time of the pouching system change; note the character of drainage, including color, amount, type, and consistency. Also describe the appearance of the stoma and the peristomal skin. Document patient teaching. Describe the teaching content. Record the patient's response to self-care and evaluate his learning progress.

COLOSTOMY IRRIGATION

Irrigation of a colostomy can serve two purposes: It allows a patient with a descending or sigmoid colostomy to regulate bowel function, and it cleans the

large bowel before and after tests, surgery, or other procedures.

Colostomy irrigation may begin as soon as bowel function resumes after surgery. However, most clinicians recommend waiting until bowel movements are more predictable. Initially, the nurse or the patient irrigates the colostomy at the same time every day, recording the amount of output and any spillage between irrigations. Between 4 and 6 weeks may pass before colostomy irrigation establishes a predictable elimination pattern.

Key nursing diagnoses and patient outcomes

Disturbed body image related to the presence of a colostomy or an ileostomy
The patient will:
▶ acknowledge changes in body image
▶ express positive feelings about himself.

Ineffective individual coping related to situational crisis
The patient will:
▶ communicate feelings about the situation
▶ become involved in planning his care.

Equipment

Colostomy irrigation set (contains an irrigation drain or sleeve, an ostomy belt [if needed] to secure the drain or sleeve, water-soluble lubricant, drainage pouch clamp, and irrigation bag with clamp, tubing, and cone tip) • 1,000 ml of tap water irrigant warmed to about 100° F (37.8° C) • normal saline solution (for cleansing enemas) • I.V. pole or wall hook • washcloth and towel • water • ostomy pouching system • linen-saver pad • gloves • optional: bedpan or chair, mild nonmoisturizing soap, rubber band or clip, small dressing or bandage, and stoma cap

Preparation of equipment

Depending on the patient's condition, colostomy irrigation may be performed in bed using a bedpan or in the bathroom using the chair and the toilet.

Set up the irrigation bag with tubing and cone tip. If irrigation will take place with the patient in bed, place the bedpan beside the bed and elevate the head of the bed between 45 and 90 degrees, if allowed. If irrigation will take place in the bathroom, have the patient sit on the toilet or on a chair facing the toilet, whichever he finds more comfortable.

Fill the irrigation bag with warmed tap water (or normal saline solution, if the irrigation is for bowel cleansing). Hang the bag on the I.V. pole or wall hook. The bottom of the bag should be at the patient's shoulder level *to prevent the fluid from entering the bowel too quickly.* Most irrigation sets also have a clamp that regulates the flow rate.

Prime the tubing with irrigant *to prevent air from entering the colon and possibly causing cramps and gas pains.*

Implementation

▶ Explain every step of the procedure to the patient *because he'll probably be irrigating the colostomy himself.*
▶ Provide privacy and wash your hands.
▶ If the patient is in bed, place a linen-saver pad under him *to protect the sheets from soiling.*
▶ Put on gloves.
▶ Remove the ostomy pouch, if the patient uses one.

▶ Place the irrigation sleeve over the stoma. If the sleeve doesn't have an adhesive backing, secure the sleeve with an ostomy belt. If the patient has a two-piece pouching system with flanges, snap off the pouch and save it. Snap on the irrigation sleeve.
▶ Place the open-ended bottom of the irrigation sleeve in the bedpan or toilet *to promote drainage by gravity.* If necessary, cut the sleeve so that it meets the water level inside the bedpan or toilet. *Effluent may splash from a short sleeve or may not drain from a long sleeve.*
▶ Lubricate your gloved small finger with water-soluble lubricant and insert the finger into the stoma. If you're teaching the patient, have him do this *to determine the bowel angle at which to insert the cone safely.* Expect the stoma to tighten when the finger enters the bowel and then to relax in a few seconds.
▶ Lubricate the cone with water-soluble lubricant *to prevent it from irritating the mucosa.*
▶ Insert the cone into the top opening of the irrigation sleeve and then into the stoma. Angle the cone to match the bowel angle. Insert it gently but snugly; never force it in place.
▶ Unclamp the irrigation tubing and allow the water to flow slowly. If you don't have a clamp to control the irrigant's flow rate, pinch the tubing *to control the flow.* The water should enter the colon over 10 to 15 minutes. (If the patient reports cramping, slow or stop the flow, keep the cone in place, and have the patient take a few deep breaths until the cramping stops.) *Cramping during irrigation may result from a bowel that is ready to empty, water that is too cold, a rapid flow rate, or air in the tubing.*

▶ Have the patient remain stationary for 15 or 20 minutes *so that the initial effluent can drain.*

▶ If the patient is ambulatory, he can stay in the bathroom until all effluent empties, or he can clamp the bottom of the drainage sleeve with a rubber band or clip and return to bed. Explain that ambulation and activity stimulate elimination. Suggest that the nonambulatory patient lean forward or massage his abdomen *to stimulate elimination.*

▶ Wait about 45 minutes for the bowel to finish eliminating the irrigant and effluent. Then remove the irrigation sleeve.

▶ If the irrigation was intended to clean the bowel, repeat the procedure with warmed normal saline solution until the return solution appears clear.

▶ Using a washcloth, mild soap, and water, gently clean the area around the stoma. Rinse and dry the area thoroughly with a clean towel.

▶ Inspect the skin and stoma for changes in appearance. Usually dark pink to red, stoma color may change with the patient's status. Notify the doctor of marked stoma color changes *because a pale hue may result from anemia, and substantial darkening suggests a change in blood flow to the stoma.*

▶ Apply a clean pouch. If the patient has a regular bowel elimination pattern, he may prefer a small dressing, bandage, or commercial stoma cap.

▶ Discard a disposable irrigation sleeve. Rinse a reusable irrigation sleeve and hang it to dry along with the irrigation bag, tubing, and cone.

Special considerations
▶ Irrigating a colostomy to establish a regular bowel elimination pattern

doesn't work for all patients. If the bowel continues to move between irrigations, try decreasing the volume of irrigant. *Increasing the irrigant won't help because it serves only to stimulate peristalsis.* Keep a record of results. Also consider irrigating every other day.

▶ Irrigation may help to regulate bowel function in patients with a descending or sigmoid colostomy *because this is the bowel's stool storage area.* However, a patient with an ascending or transverse colostomy won't benefit from irrigation. Also, a patient with a descending or sigmoid colostomy who is missing part of the ascending or transverse colon may not be able to irrigate successfully *because his ostomy may function like an ascending or transverse colostomy.*

▶ If diarrhea develops, discontinue irrigations until stools form again. Keep in mind that irrigation alone won't achieve regularity for the patient. He must also observe a complementary diet and exercise regimen.

▶ If the patient has a strictured stoma that prohibits cone insertion, remove the cone from the irrigation tubing and replace it with a soft silicone catheter. Angle the catheter gently 2″ to 4″ (5 to 10 cm) into the bowel to instill the irrigant. Don't force the catheter into the stoma, and don't insert it further than the recommended length *because you may perforate the bowel.*

Complications
Bowel perforation may result if a catheter is incorrectly inserted into the stoma. Fluid and electrolyte imbalances may result from using too much irrigant.

Documentation

Record the date and time of irrigation and the type and amount of irrigant. Note the stoma's color and the character of drainage, including the drainage color, consistency, and amount. Record any patient teaching. Describe teaching content and patient response to self-care instruction. Evaluate the patient's learning progress.

CONTACT LENS CARE

Illness or emergency treatment may require that you insert or remove and store a patient's contact lenses. Proper handling and lens care techniques help prevent eye injury and infection as well as lens loss or damage. Appropriate lens-handling techniques depend in large part on what type of lenses the patient wears.

All contact lenses float on the corneal tear layer. Rigid lenses typically have a smaller diameter than the cornea; soft lens diameter typically exceeds that of the cornea. Because they're larger and more pliable, soft lenses tend to mold themselves more closely to the eye for a more stable fit than rigid lenses.

Modes of lens wear vary widely. Although most patients remove and clean their lenses daily, some wear lenses overnight or for several days (sometimes up to a month) without removing them for cleaning. Still other patients wear disposable lenses, which means that they replace old lenses with new ones at regular intervals (a few days to a few months), possibly without removing them for cleaning between replacements.

Keep in mind that lenses handled improperly can provide a direct source of contamination to the eye.

Key nursing diagnoses and patient outcomes

Risk for infection related to improper handling of contact lens
The patient will:
▶ remain free from infection
▶ have no signs or symptom of infection, such as redness, irritation, or drainage from the eye.

Equipment

Lens storage case or two small medicine cups and adhesive tape • gloves • patient's equipment for contact lens care, if available • sterile normal saline solution or soaking solution • flashlight, if needed • optional: suction cup

Preparation of equipment

If a commercial lens storage case isn't available, place enough sterile normal saline solution into two small medicine cups to submerge a lens in each one. *To avoid confusing the left and right lenses, which may have different prescriptions,* mark one cup "L" and the other cup "R" and place the corresponding lens in each cup.

Implementation

▶ Tell the patient what you're about to do, wash your hands, and put on gloves *to help prevent ocular infection.*

Inserting rigid lenses

▶ Wet one lens with solution; gently rub it between your thumb and index finger or place it on your palm and rub it with your opposite index finger.

Rinse well with the solution, leaving a small amount in the lens.

▶ Place the lens, convex side down, on the tip of the index finger of your dominant hand.

▶ Instruct the patient to gaze upward slightly. Separate the eyelids with your other thumb and index finger and place the lens directly and gently on the cornea. You need not press it to the eye; the tear film will attract it naturally at the first touch. Using the same procedure, insert the opposite lens.

Inserting soft lenses

▶ To see if the lens is inside out, bend it between your thumb and index finger or fill it with saline or soaking solution. If the lens tends to roll inward or the edge points slightly inward, it's oriented correctly. If the edge points outward or the lens tends to collapse over your fingertip, it's probably inside out and should be reversed.

▶ Wet the lens with fresh normal saline solution and rub it gently between your thumb and index finger, or place it on your palm and rub it with your opposite index finger. Rinse well.

▶ Place the lens, convex side down, on the tip of the index finger of your dominant hand.

▶ Instruct the patient to gaze upward slightly. Separate the eyelids with your other thumb and index finger and place the lens on the sclera, just below the cornea. Then, slide the lens gently upward with your finger until it centers on the cornea. Using the same procedure, insert the opposite lens.

Removing rigid lenses

▶ Before removing a lens, position the patient supine *to prevent the lens from popping out onto the floor, risking loss or damage.*

▶ Place one thumb against the patient's upper eyelid and the other thumb against the lower eyelid. Move the lids toward each other while gently pressing inward against the eye *to trap the lens edge and break the suction.* Extract the lens from the patient's eyelashes. (See *Removing a patient's contact lenses,* page 192.)

▶ Depending on the lens type and thickness, it may pop out when the suction breaks. You may want to try to break the suction with one hand while cupping the other hand below the patient's eye *to catch the lens as it falls.*

▶ Sometimes the lens will pop out on its own if you ask the patient to blink after stretching the corner of the eyelids toward the temporal bone, thus tightening the lid edges against the globe of the eye.

▶ After removal, place the lens in the proper well of the storage case (L or R) with enough of the appropriate storage solution to cover it. Alternatively, place the lens in a labeled medicine cup with solution and secure adhesive tape over the top of the cup *to prevent loss of the lens.*

▶ Remove and care for the opposite lens using the same technique.

Removing soft lenses

▶ Place the patient in the supine position. Using your nondominant hand, raise the patient's upper eyelid and hold it against the orbital rim.

▶ Lightly place the forefinger of your other hand on the lens and move it down onto the sclera below the cornea. Then pinch the lens between your forefinger and thumb; it should pop off.

Removing a patient's contact lenses

Contact lens removal techniques depend largely on the type of lenses the patient wears and how readily they come off the eye. For successful removal of soft and rigid lenses, follow the steps outlined below. If you have trouble removing lenses manually, try using a specially made suction cup.

Soft lenses

With the patient looking up and his upper lid raised, use your dominant index finger to slide the lens onto the lower cornea. Pinch the lens between your index finger and thumb to remove it (as shown below).

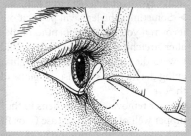

Rigid lenses

Place one thumb on each eyelid and move the lids toward each other, pressing gently against the eyeball. When the lids meet the lens edges, the suction breaks and the lens is released (as shown above right). Catch the lens in your lower hand or remove it from the patient's lashes.

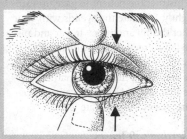

Using a suction cup

Separate the lids with your nondominant hand. Squeeze the suction cup with your dominant hand and place it gently against the lens (as shown below). Open your fingers slightly to create suction between the lens and the cup. Rock the lens gently to remove it.

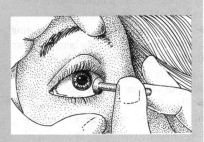

▶ Place the lens in the proper well of the storage case with enough of the appropriate storage solution to cover it. Alternatively, place the lens in a labeled medicine cup with solution and secure adhesive tape over the top of the cup to prevent loss of the lens.

▶ Remove and care for the other lens using the same technique.

Cleaning lenses

▶ Because lens-cleaning steps vary with lens type and with each manufacturer's and doctor's instructions, ask the patient to guide you step-by-step through his normal cleaning routine.

▶ If the patient is unable to tell you how to clean his lenses properly, remember that most lens types require two steps: cleaning and disinfection.

▶ Cleaning involves rubbing the lens with a surfactant solution designed to remove most surface deposits. For some patients, especially those who wear soft lenses, the cleaning step also may include use of an enzyme agent to remove protein deposits against which surfactant cleaners typically are ineffective. Enzyme cleaning involves soaking the lenses overnight in a solution with dissolved special enzyme tablets. For patients who use a storage solution that contains a disinfectant, cleaning with an enzyme agent isn't necessary.

▶ Disinfection, which doesn't require rubbing, may be accomplished through chemical means or by heat. This step aims to rid the lens of infectious organisms.

▶ If you must clean a patient's lenses, use only his own solutions. *This minimizes the risk of allergic reactions to substances included in other solution brands.* Never touch the nozzle opening of a solution bottle to the lens, your fingers, or anything else *to avoid contaminating solution remaining in the bottle.*

Special considerations

▶ If the patient's eyes appear dry or you have trouble moving the lens on the eye, instill several drops of sterile normal saline solution and wait a few minutes before trying again to remove the lens *to prevent corneal damage.* If you still can't remove the lens easily, notify the doctor. Avoid instilling eye medication while the patient is wearing lenses. *The lenses could trap the medication, possibly causing eye irritation or lens damage.*

▶ Don't allow soft lenses, which are 40% to 60% water, to dry out. If they do, soak them in sterile normal saline solution and they may return to their natural shape.

▶ If an unconscious patient is admitted to the emergency department, check for contact lenses by opening each eyelid and searching with a small flashlight. If you detect lenses, remove them immediately *because tears can't circulate freely beneath the lenses with eyelids closed, possibly leading to corneal oxygen depletion or infection.*

▶ Advise contact lens wearers to carry appropriate identification *to speed lens removal and ensure proper care in an emergency.*

▶ If a patient can't provide adequate care for his lenses during hospitalization, encourage him to send them home with a family member. If you aren't sure how to care for the lenses in the interim, store them in sterile normal saline solution until the family member can take them home.

Documentation

Record eye condition before and after removal of lenses; the time of lens insertion, removal, and cleaning; the location of stored lenses; and, if applicable, the removal of lenses from the facility by a family member.

CONTACT PRECAUTIONS

Contact precautions prevent the spread of infectious diseases transmitted by contact with body substances containing the infectious agent or items contaminated with the body substances containing the infectious agent. Contact precautions apply to patients who are infected or colonized (presence of microorganism without clinical signs or symptoms of infection) with epidemio-

Diseases requiring contact precautions

Disease	Precautionary period
Infection or colonization with multidrug-resistant bacteria	Until off antibiotics and culture negative
Clostridium difficile enteric infection	Duration of illness
Escherichia coli disease, in diapered or incontinent patient	Duration of illness
Shigellosis, in diapered or incontinent patient	Duration of illness
Hepatitis A, in diapered or incontinent patient	Duration of illness
Rotavirus infection, in diapered or incontinent patient	Duration of illness
Respiratory syncytial virus infection, in infants and young children	Duration of illness
Parainfluenza virus infection, in diapered or incontinent patient	Duration of illness
Enteroviral infection, in diapered or incontinent patient	Duration of illness
Scabies	Until off antibiotic and two cultures taken at least 24 hours apart are negative
Diphtheria (cutaneous)	Duration of illness
Herpes simplex virus infection (neonatal or mucocutaneous)	Until 24 hours after initiation of effective therapy
Impetigo	Duration of illness
Major (noncontained) abscesses, cellulitis, or pressure ulcers	Until 24 hours after initiation of effective therapy
Pediculosis (lice)	Place infant on precautions during any admission until age 1, unless nasopharyngeal and urine culture are negative for virus after age 3 months
Rubella, congenital syndrome	Until 24 hours after initiation of effective therapy
Staphylococcal furunculosis in infants and young children	Duration of illness
Acute viral (acute hemorrhagic) conjunctivitis	Duration of illness
Viral hemorrhagic infections (Ebola, Lassa, Marburg)	Duration of illness
Zoster (chickenpox, disseminated zoster, or localized zoster in immunodeficient patient)	Until all lesions are crusted
Acquired immunodeficiency syndrome	Until white blood cell count reaches 1,000 µl or more, or according to facility guidelines
Agranulocytosis	Until remission

Diseases requiring contact precautions *(continued)*

Disease	Precautionary period
Burns, extensive noninfected	Until skin surface heals substantially
Dematitis, noninfected vesicular, bullous, or eczematous disease (when severe and extensive)	Until skin surface heals substantially
Immunosuppressive therapy	Until patient's immunity is adequate
Lymphomas and leukemia, especially late stages of Hodgkin's disease or acute leukemia	Until clinical improvement is substantial

logically important organisms that can be transmitted by direct or indirect contact. (See *Diseases requiring contact precautions.*)

Effective contact precautions require a single room and the use of gloves and gowns by anyone having contact with the patient, the patient's support equipment, or items soiled with body substances containing the infectious agent. Thorough hand washing and proper handling and disposal of articles contaminated by the body substance containing the infectious agent are also essential.

Key nursing diagnoses and patient outcomes

Risk for infection related to hospital admission
The patient will:
▶ remain free from all signs and symptoms of infection
▶ state factors that put him at risk for infection
▶ identify signs and symptoms of infection.

Equipment

Gloves • gowns or aprons • masks, if necessary • isolation door card • plastic bags

Gather any additional supplies, such as a thermometer, stethoscope, and blood pressure cuff.

Preparation of equipment

Keep all contact precaution supplies outside the patient's room in a cart or anteroom.

Implementation

▶ Situate the patient in a single room with private toilet facilities and an anteroom if possible. If necessary, two patients with the same infection may share a room. Explain isolation procedures to the patient and his family.
▶ Place a contact precautions card on the door *to notify anyone entering the room.*
▶ Wash your hands before entering and after leaving the patient's room and after removing gloves.
▶ Place any laboratory specimens in impervious, labeled containers, and send them to the laboratory at once. Attach requisition slips to the outside of the container.
▶ Instruct visitors to wear gloves and a gown while visiting the patient and to wash their hands after removing the gown and gloves.

▶ Place all items that have come in contact with the patient in a single impervious bag, and arrange for their disposal or disinfection and sterilization.
▶ Limit the patient's movement from the room. If the patient must be moved, cover any draining wounds with clean dressings. Notify the receiving department or area of the patient's isolation precautions *so that the precautions will be maintained and the patient can be returned to the room promptly.*

Special considerations
▶ Cleaning and disinfection of equipment between patients is essential.
▶ Try to dedicate certain reusable equipment (thermometer, stethoscope, blood pressure cuff) for the patient in contact precautions *to reduce the risk of transmitting infection to other patients.*
▶ Remember to change gloves during patient care as indicated by the procedure or task. Wash your hands after removing gloves and before putting on new gloves.

Documentation
Record the need for contact precautions on the nursing care plan and as otherwise indicated by your facility. Document initiation and maintenance of the precautions, the patient's tolerance of the procedure, and any patient or family teaching. Also document the date contact precautions were discontinued.

CONTINENT ILEOSTOMY CARE

An alternative to a conventional ileostomy, a continent, or pouch, ileostomy (also called a Kock ileostomy or an ileal

pouch) features an internal reservoir fashioned from the terminal ileum. This procedure may be used for a patient who requires proctocolectomy for chronic ulcerative colitis or multiple polyposis. Other patients may have a traditional ileostomy converted to a continent ileostomy. This procedure is contraindicated in Crohn's disease or gross obesity. Patients who need emergency surgery and those who can't care for the pouch are also unlikely to have this procedure.

The length of preoperative hospitalization varies with the patient's condition. Nursing responsibilities include providing bowel preparation, antibiotic therapy, and emotional support. After surgery, nursing responsibilities include ensuring patency of the drainage catheter, assessing GI function, caring for the stoma and peristomal skin, managing pain resulting from surgery and, if necessary, perineal skin care.

Daily patient teaching on pouch intubation and drainage usually begins soon after surgery. Continuous drainage is maintained for about 2 to 6 weeks to allow the suture lines to heal. During this period, a drainage catheter is attached to low intermittent suction. After the suture line heals, the patient learns how to drain the pouch himself.

Key nursing diagnoses and patient outcomes
Deficient knowledge related to lack of exposure to a new procedure
The patient will:
▶ verbalize an understanding of the procedure for continent ileostomy care
▶ demonstrate the correct procedure for continent ileostomy care
▶ verbalize reasons to contact the doctor, nurse, or appropriate caregivers

Understanding pouch construction

Depending on the patient and related factors during intestinal surgery, the doctor may construct a pouch to collect fecal matter internally. To make such a pouch, the doctor loops about 12″ (30 cm) of ileum and sutures the inner sides together.

He opens the loop with a U-shaped cut and seams the inside to create a smooth lining. Then he fashions a nipple or valve between what is becoming the pouch and what will be the stoma. He folds the open ileum over, sews the pouch closed, and fixes the pouch to the abdominal wall.

Because the pouch holds fecal matter in reserve, the patient benefits from not having to change and empty ostomy equipment. Instead, he empties and irrigates the pouch as needed by inserting a catheter though the stoma and into the pouch.

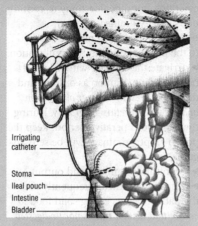

Irrigating catheter

Stoma
Ileal pouch
Intestine
Bladder

Initially after surgery, the nurse performs this procedure until the patient can do it himself.

▶ identify local support groups and appropriate resources for obtaining equipment.

Risk for infection related to an ileostomy pouch
The patient will:
▶ maintain a normal body temperature
▶ maintain proper personal hygiene at the pouch site
▶ show no signs of skin breakdown
▶ identify signs and symptoms of infection.

Equipment
Leg drainage bag • bedside drainage bag • normal saline solution • 50-ml catheter-tip syringe • extra continent ileostomy catheter • 4″ × 4″ × 1″ foam dressing and Montgomery straps • 20-ml syringe with adapter • precut drain dressing • gloves • water-soluble lubricant • graduated container • skin sealant • optional: commercial catheter securing device

Implementation
▶ Nursing interventions for a patient undergoing a continent ileostomy range from standard preoperative and postoperative care to pouch care and patient teaching.

Preoperative care
▶ Reinforce and, if necessary, supplement the doctor's explanation of a continent ileostomy and its implications for the patient. (See *Understanding pouch construction.*)
▶ Assess patient and family attitudes related to the operation and to the forthcoming changes in the patient's body image.
▶ Provide encouragement and support.

Postoperative care

▶ When the patient returns to his room, attach the drainage catheter emerging from the ileostomy to continuous gravity drainage.

▶ A leg drainage bag may be attached to the patient's thigh during ambulation.

▶ Irrigate the catheter with 30 ml of normal saline solution as ordered and needed *to prevent catheter obstruction and allow fluid return by gravity.* During the early postoperative period, keep the pouch empty; drainage will be serosanguineous.

▶ Monitor fluid intake and output.

▶ Check the catheter frequently once the patient begins eating solid food *to ensure that neither mucus nor undigested food particles block it.*

▶ If the patient complains of abdominal cramps, distention, and nausea — signs and symptoms of bowel obstruction — the catheter may be clogged. Gently irrigate with 20 to 30 ml of water or normal saline solution until the catheter drains freely. Then move the catheter slightly or rotate it gently *to help clear the obstruction.* Finally, try milking the catheter. If these measures fail, notify the doctor.

▶ Check the stoma frequently for color, edema, and bleeding. Normally pink to red, a stoma that turns dark red or blue-red may have a compromised blood supply.

▶ To care for the stoma and peristomal skin, put on gloves. Remove the dressing, gently clean the peristomal area with water and pat it dry. Use a skin sealant around the stoma *to prevent skin irritation.*

▶ One way to apply a stoma dressing is to slip a precut drain dressing around the catheter to cover the stoma. Cut a hole slightly larger than the lumen of the catheter in the center of a 4″ × 4″ × 1″ piece of foam. Disconnect the catheter from the drainage bag and insert the distal end of the catheter through the hole in the foam. Slide the foam pad onto the dressing. Secure the foam in place with Montgomery straps. Secure the catheter by wrapping the strap ties around it or by using a commercial catheter securing device. Then reconnect the catheter to the drainage bag. (The surgeon will remove the drainage catheter when he determines that the suture line has healed.)

▶ Assess the peristomal skin for irritation from moisture.

▶ *To reduce discomfort from gas pains,* encourage the patient to ambulate. Also recommend that he avoid swallowing air (to minimize gas pains) by chewing food well, limiting conversation while eating, and not drinking from a straw.

Draining the pouch

▶ Provide privacy, explain the procedure to the patient, and wash your hands.

▶ Put on gloves.

▶ Have the patient with a pouch conversion sit on the toilet *to help him feel more at ease during the procedure.*

▶ Remove the stoma dressing.

▶ Encourage the patient to relax his abdominal muscles *to allow the catheter to slide easily into the pouch.*

▶ Lubricate the tip of the drainage catheter tip with the water-soluble lubricant and insert it in the stoma. Gently push the catheter downward. (The direction of insertion may vary depending on the patient.)

▶ When the catheter reaches the nipple valve of the internal pouch or reservoir (after about 2″ or 2½″ [5 or 6.5 cm]), you'll feel resistance. Instruct the patient to take a deep breath as you exert gentle pressure on the catheter to insert it through the valve. If this fails, have the patient lie supine and rest for a few minutes. Then, with the patient still supine, try to insert the catheter again.

▶ Gently advance the catheter to the suture marking made by the surgeon.

▶ Let the pouch drain completely. This usually takes 5 to 10 minutes. With thick drainage or a clogged catheter, the process may take 30 minutes.

▶ If the tube clogs, irrigate with 30 ml of water or normal saline using the 50-ml catheter-tip syringe. Also, rotate and milk the tube. If these steps fail, remove, rinse, and reinsert the catheter.

▶ Remove the catheter after completing drainage.

▶ Measure output, subtracting the amount of irrigant used.

▶ Rinse the catheter thoroughly with warm water.

▶ Clean the peristomal area and apply a fresh stoma dressing.

Predischarge teaching

▶ Make sure the patient can properly intubate and drain the pouch himself.

▶ Provide the patient with appropriate equipment. If the postoperative drainage catheter is still in place, teach the patient how to care for it properly.

▶ Make sure the patient has a pouch-draining schedule and give him appropriate pamphlets or video instructions on pouch care.

▶ Make sure he feels comfortable calling the doctor, nurse, or appropriate other caregivers with questions or problems.

▶ Tell the patient where to obtain supplies.

▶ Refer the patient to a local ostomy group.

▶ Provide dietary counseling.

Special considerations

▶ Never aspirate fluid from the catheter *because the resulting negative pressure may damage inflamed tissue.*

▶ The first few times you intubate the pouch, the patient may be tense, making insertion difficult. Encourage relaxation. *To shorten drainage time,* have the patient cough, press gently on his abdomen over the pouch, or suddenly tighten his abdominal muscles and then relax them.

▶ Keep an accurate record of intake and output *to ensure fluid and electrolyte balance.* The average daily output should be 1,000 ml. Report inadequate or excessive output (more than 1,400 ml daily).

Complications

Common postoperative complications include obstruction, fistula, pouch perforation, nipple valve dysfunction, abscesses, diarrhea, skin irritation, stenosis of the stoma, and bacterial overgrowth in the pouch.

Documentation

Record the date, time, and all aspects of preoperative and postoperative care: condition of the stoma and peristomal skin, diet, medications, intubations, patient teaching, and discharge planning.

CONTINUOUS AMBULATORY PERITONEAL DIALYSIS

Continuous ambulatory peritoneal dialysis (CAPD) requires insertion of a permanent peritoneal catheter (such as a Tenckhoff catheter) to circulate dialysate in the peritoneal cavity constantly. Inserted under local anesthetic, the catheter is sutured in place and its distal portion tunneled subcutaneously to the skin surface. There it serves as a port for the dialysate, which flows in and out of the peritoneal cavity by gravity. (See *Three major steps of continuous ambulatory peritoneal dialysis*.)

CAPD is used most commonly for patients with end-stage renal disease. CAPD can be a welcome alternative to hemodialysis, because it gives the patient more independence and requires less travel for treatments. It also provides more stable fluid and electrolyte levels than conventional hemodialysis.

Patients or family members can usually learn to perform CAPD after only 2 weeks of training. In addition, because the patient can resume normal daily activities between solution changes, CAPD helps promote independence and a return to a near-normal lifestyle. It also costs less than hemodialysis.

Conditions that may prohibit CAPD include recent abdominal surgery, abdominal adhesions, an infected abdominal wall, diaphragmatic tears, ileus, and respiratory insufficiency.

Key nursing diagnoses and patient outcomes

Risk for infection related to an invasive procedure
The patient will:

▶ have normal vital signs and laboratory values
▶ have no pathogens appear in cultures
▶ show no signs or symptoms of infection at the I.V. insertion site.

Risk for deficient fluid volume related to CAPD
The patient will:
▶ have normal skin color and temperature
▶ exhibit no signs of dehydration
▶ maintain a urine output of at least (specify) ml/hour
▶ have electrolyte values remain within normal range
▶ maintain fluid balance (intake will equal output).

Equipment
To infuse dialysate
Prescribed amount of dialysate (usually in 2-L [2-qt] bags) • heating pad or commercial warmer • three face masks • 42″ connective tubing with drain clamp • six to eight packages of sterile 4″ × 4″ gauze pads • medication, if ordered • povidone-iodine pads • hypoallergenic tape • plastic snap-top container • povidone-iodine solution • sterile basin • container of alcohol • sterile gloves • belt or fabric pouch • two sterile waterproof paper drapes (one fenestrated) • optional: syringes, labeled specimen container

To discontinue dialysis temporarily
Three sterile waterproof paper barriers (two fenestrated) • 4″ × 4″ gauze pads (for cleaning and dressing the catheter) • two face masks • sterile basin • hypoallergenic tape • povidone-iodine solution • sterile gloves • sterile rubber catheter cap

Three major steps of continuous ambulatory peritoneal dialysis

A bag of dialysate is attached to the tube entering the patient's abdominal area so the fluid flows into the peritoneal cavity.

While the dialysate remains in the peritoneal cavity, the patient can roll up the bag, place it under his shirt, and go about his normal activities.

Unrolling the bag and suspending it below the pelvis allows the dialysate to drain from the peritoneal cavity back into the bag.

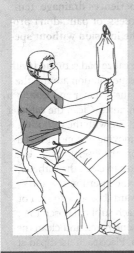 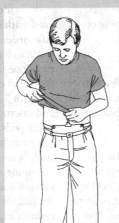 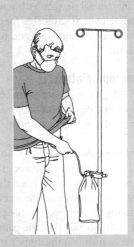

All equipment for infusing the dialysate and discontinuing the procedure must be sterile. Commercially prepared sterile CAPD kits are available.

Preparation of equipment

Check the concentration of the dialysate against the doctor's order. Also check the expiration date and appearance of the solution — it should be clear, not cloudy. Warm the solution to body temperature with a heating pad or a commercial warmer if one is available. Don't warm the solution in a microwave oven *because the temperature is unpredictable.*

To minimize the risk of contaminating the bag's port, leave the dialysate container's wrapper in place. This also keeps the bag dry, which makes examining it for leakage easier after you remove the wrapper.

Wash your hands and put on a surgical mask. Remove the dialysate container from the warming setup, and remove its protective wrapper. Squeeze the bag firmly to check for leaks.

If ordered, use a syringe to add any prescribed medication to the dialysate, using sterile technique *to avoid contamination.* (The ideal approach is to add medication under a laminar flow hood.) Disinfect multiple-dose vials in a 5-minute povidone-iodine soak. Insert the connective tubing into the dialysate container. Open the drain clamp to prime the tube. Then close the clamp.

Place a povidone-iodine pad on the dialysate container's port. Cover the port with a dry gauze pad, and secure the pad with tape. Remove and discard the surgical mask. Tear the tape *so it will be ready to secure the new dressing.* Commercial devices with povidone-iodine pads are available for covering the dialysate container and tubing connection.

Implementation

▶ Weigh the patient *to establish a baseline level.* Weigh him at the same time every day *to help monitor fluid balance.*

Infusing dialysate

▶ Assemble all equipment at the patient's bedside, and explain the procedure to him. Prepare the sterile field by placing a waterproof, sterile paper drape on a dry surface near the patient. Take care to maintain the drape's sterility.

▶ Fill the snap-top container with povidone-iodine solution and place it on the sterile field. Place the basin on the sterile field. Then place four pairs of sterile gauze pads in the sterile basin, and saturate them with the povidone-iodine solution. Drop the remaining gauze pads on the sterile field. Loosen the cap on the alcohol container and place it next to the sterile field.

▶ Put on a clean surgical mask and provide one for the patient.

▶ Carefully remove the dressing covering the peritoneal catheter and discard it. Be careful not to touch the catheter or skin. Check skin integrity at the catheter site and look for signs of infection such as purulent drainage. If drainage is present, obtain a swab speci-

men, put it in a labeled specimen container, and notify the doctor.

▶ Put on the sterile gloves and palpate the insertion site and subcutaneous tunnel route for tenderness or pain. If these symptoms occur, notify the doctor.

Nursing alert If the patient experiences drainage, tenderness, or pain, don't proceed with the infusion without specific orders.

▶ Wrap one gauze pad saturated with povidone-iodine solution around the distal end of the catheter and leave it in place for 5 minutes. Clean the catheter and insertion site with the rest of the gauze pads, moving in concentric circles away from the insertion site. Use straight strokes to clean the catheter, beginning at the insertion site and moving outward. Use a clean area of the pad for each stroke. Loosen the catheter cap one notch and clean the exposed area. Place each used pad at the base of the catheter *to help support it.* After using the third pair of pads, place the fenestrated paper drape around the base of the catheter. Continue cleaning the catheter for another minute with one of the remaining pads soaked with povidone-iodine.

▶ Remove the povidone-iodine pad on the catheter cap, remove the cap, and use the remaining povidone-iodine pad to clean the end of the catheter hub. Attach the connective tubing from the dialysate container to the catheter. Be sure to secure the luer-lock connector tightly.

▶ Open the drain clamp on the dialysate container *to allow solution to enter the peritoneal cavity by gravity* over a period of 5 to 10 minutes. Leave a small amount of fluid in the bag *to make folding it easier.* Close the drain clamp.

▶ Fold the bag and secure it with a belt, or tuck it in the patient's clothing or a small fabric pouch.

▶ After the prescribed dwell time (usually 4 to 6 hours), unfold the bag, open the clamp, and allow peritoneal fluid to drain back into the bag by gravity.

▶ When drainage is complete, attach a new bag of dialysate and repeat the infusion.

▶ Discard used supplies appropriately.

Discontinuing dialysis temporarily

▶ Wash your hands, put on a surgical mask, and provide one for the patient. Explain the procedure to him.

▶ Using sterile gloves, remove and discard the dressing over the peritoneal catheter.

▶ Set up a sterile field next to the patient by covering a clean, dry surface with a waterproof drape. Be sure to maintain the drape's sterility. Place all equipment on the sterile field and place the 4″ × 4″ gauze pads in the basin. Saturate them with the povidone-iodine solution. Open the 4″ × 4″ gauze pads to be used as the dressing and drop them onto the sterile field. Tear pieces of tape as needed.

▶ Tape the dialysate tubing to the side rail of the bed *to keep the catheter and tubing off the patient's abdomen.*

▶ Change to another pair of sterile gloves. Then place one of the fenestrated drapes around the base of the catheter.

▶ Use a pair of povidone-iodine pads to clean about 6″ (15 cm) of the dialysis tubing. Clean for 1 minute, moving in one direction only, away from the catheter. Then clean the catheter, moving from the insertion site to the junction of the catheter and dialysis tubing. Place used pads at the base of the catheter *to prop it up.* Use two more pairs of pads to clean the junction for a total of 3 minutes.

▶ Place the second fenestrated paper drape over the first at the base of the catheter. With the fourth pair of pads, clean the junction of the catheter and 6″ of the dialysate tubing for another minute.

▶ Disconnect the dialysate tubing from the catheter. Pick up the catheter cap and fasten it to the catheter, making sure it fits securely over both notches of the hard plastic catheter tip.

▶ Clean the insertion site and a 2″ (5-cm) radius around it with povidone-iodine pads, working from the insertion site outward. Let the skin air-dry before applying the dressing.

▶ Discard used supplies appropriately.

Special considerations

▶ If inflow and outflow are slow or absent, check the tubing for kinks. You can also try raising the solution or repositioning the patient *to increase the inflow rate.* Repositioning the patient or applying manual pressure to the lateral aspects of the patient's abdomen may also help increase drainage.

Home care

Teach the patient and family how to use sterile technique throughout the procedure, especially for cleaning and dressing changes, *to prevent complications such as peritonitis.* Also teach them the signs and symptoms of peritonitis — cloudy fluid, fever, abdominal pain, and tenderness — and stress the importance of notifying the doctor immediately if such signs or symptoms arise. Also encourage them to call the doctor

Continuous-cycle peritoneal dialysis

Continuous ambulatory peritoneal dialysis is easier for the patient who uses an automated continuous cycler system. When set up, this system runs the dialysis treatment automatically until all the dialysate is infused. The system remains closed throughout the treatment, which cuts the risk of contamination. Continuous-cycle peritoneal dialysis (CCPD) can be performed while the patient is awake or asleep. The system's alarms warn about general system, dialysate, and patient problems.

The cycler can be set to an intermittent or continuous dialysate schedule at home or in a health care facility. The patient typically initiates CCPD at bedtime and undergoes three to seven exchanges depending on individual prescriptions. Upon awakening, the patient infuses the prescribed dialysis volume, disconnects himself from the unit, and carries the dialysate in his peritoneal cavity during the day.

The continuous cycler follows the same aseptic care and maintenance procedures as the manual method.

immediately if redness and drainage occur; these are also signs of infection.

Inform the patient about the advantages of an automated continuous cycler system for home use. (See *Continuous-cycle peritoneal dialysis.*)

Instruct the patient to record his weight and blood pressure daily and to check regularly for swelling of the extremities. Teach him to keep an accurate record of intake and output.

Complications

Peritonitis is the most frequent complication of CAPD. Although treatable, it can permanently scar the peritoneal membrane, decreasing its permeability and reducing the efficiency of dialysis. Untreated peritonitis can cause septicemia and death.

Excessive fluid loss may result from a concentrated (4.25%) dialysate solution, improper or inaccurate monitoring of inflow and outflow, or inadequate oral fluid intake. Excessive fluid retention may result from improper or inaccurate monitoring of inflow and outflow, or excessive salt or oral fluid intake.

Documentation

Record the type and amount of fluid instilled and returned for each exchange, the time and duration of the exchange, and any medications added to the dialysate. Note the color and clarity of the returned exchange fluid and check it for mucus, pus, and blood. Also note any discrepancy in the balance of fluid intake and output, as well as any signs of fluid imbalance, such as weight changes, decreased breath sounds, peripheral edema, ascites, and changes in skin turgor. Record the patient's weight, blood pressure, and pulse rate after his last fluid exchange for the day.

CONTINUOUS ARTERIOVENOUS HEMOFILTRATION

When patients have fluid overload but don't require dialysis, continuous arteriovenous hemofiltration (CAVH) is used for treatment. CAVH filters fluid, solutes, and electrolytes from the patient's blood and infuses a replacement solution.

The hemofilter, composed of about 5,000 hollow fiber capillaries, filters blood at a rate of about 250 ml/minute and is driven by the patient's arterial blood pressure (a systolic blood pressure of 60 mm Hg is adequate for the procedure). Some of the ultrafiltrate collected during CAVH is replaced with a filter replacement fluid (FRF), which can be lactated Ringer's solution or any solution that resembles plasma. Because the amount of fluid removed exceeds the amount replaced, the patient gradually loses fluid (12 to 15 L daily).

CAVH carries a much lower risk of hypotension than conventional hemodialysis because it withdraws fluid more slowly—at about 200 ml/hour. CAVH can be performed in hypotensive patients who require fluid removal, who can't undergo peritoneal dialysis, or whose requirements for parenteral nutrition would make fluid volume control problematic. CAVH reduces the risk of other complications and makes maintaining a stable fluid volume and regulating fluid and electrolyte balance easier.

A similar procedure, continuous arteriovenous hemofiltration and dialysis (CAVH-D), combines hemodialysis with hemofiltration. Like CAVH, it can also be performed in patients with hypotension and fluid overload.

Commonly used to treat patients in acute renal failure, CAVH-D is also used for treating fluid overload that doesn't respond to diuretics and for some electrolyte and acid-base disturbances.

Key nursing diagnoses and patient outcomes

Ineffective tissue perfusion (renal) related to decreased cellular exchange
The patient will:

▶ maintain fluid balance
▶ communicate an understanding of the medical regimen, medications, diet, and activity restrictions.

Excessive fluid volume related to (specify)
The patient will:
▶ have blood pressure, pulse rate, cardiac rhythm, and breath sounds return to baseline within 24 hours
▶ maintain skin integrity
▶ not have a weight fluctuation.

Equipment

CAVH equipment • heparin flush solution • occlusive dressings for catheter insertion sites • sterile gloves • sterile mask • povidone-iodine solution • sterile 4″ × 4″ gauze pads • tape • FRF as ordered • infusion pump

Implementation

▶ Wash your hands. Assemble your equipment at the patient's bedside and explain the procedure to him. (See *CAVH setup,* page 206.)
▶ If necessary, assist with inserting the catheters into the femoral artery and vein, using strict aseptic technique. (In some cases, an internal arteriovenous fistula or external arteriovenous shunt may be used instead of the femoral route.) If ordered, flush both catheters with the heparin flush solution *to prevent clotting.*
▶ Apply occlusive dressings to the insertion sites, and mark the dressings with the date and time. Secure the tubing and connections with tape.
▶ Assess all pulses in the affected leg every hour for the first 4 hours, then every 2 hours afterward.
▶ Weigh the patient, take baseline vital signs, and make sure that all necessary laboratory studies have been done (usually, electrolyte levels, coagulation

CAVH setup

During continuous arteriovenous hemofiltration (CAVH), the patient's arterial blood pressure serves as a natural pump, driving blood through the arterial line. A hemofilter removes water and toxic solutes (ultrafiltrate) from the blood. Replacement fluid is infused into a port on the arterial side; this same port can be used to infuse heparin. The venous line carries the replacement fluid, along with purified blood, to the patient.

This illustration shows one of several CAVH setups.

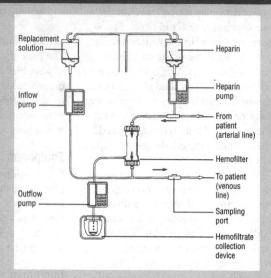

factors, complete blood count, blood urea nitrogen, and creatinine studies). Monitor the patient's weight and vital signs hourly.

▶ Put on the sterile gloves and mask. Prepare the connection sites by cleaning them with gauze pads soaked in povidone-iodine solution; then connect them to the exit port of each catheter.

▶ Connect the arterial and venous lines to the hemofilter. Use aseptic technique.

▶ Turn on the hemofilter and monitor the blood flow rate through the circuit. The flow rate is usually kept between 500 and 900 ml/hour.

▶ Inspect the ultrafiltrate during the procedure. It should remain clear yellow, with no gross blood. Pink-tinged or bloody ultrafiltrate may signal a membrane leak in the hemofilter, *which permits bacterial contamination.* If a leak

occurs, notify the doctor so he can have the hemofilter replaced.

▶ Assess the affected leg for signs of obstructed blood flow, such as coolness, pallor, and weak pulse. Check the groin area on the affected side for signs of hematoma. Also ask the patient if he has pain at the insertion sites.

▶ Calculate the amount of FRF every hour, or as ordered, according to policy. Then infuse the prescribed amount and type of FRF through the infusion pump into the arterial side of the circuit.

Special considerations

▶ *Because blood flows through an extracorporeal circuit during CAVH, the blood in the hemofilter may need to be anticoagulated. To do this, infuse heparin in low doses (usually starting at 500 units/ hour) into an infusion port on the arterial side of the setup. Then measure* thrombin clotting time or the activated clotting time (ACT). *This ensures that the circuit, not the patient, is anticoagulated.* A normal ACT is 100 seconds; during CAVH, keep it between 100 and 300 seconds, depending on the patient's clotting times. If the ACT is too high or too low, the doctor will adjust the heparin dose accordingly.

▶ Another way to prevent clotting in the hemofilter is not to infuse medications or blood through the venous line. Run infusions through another line if possible.

▶ A third way to help prevent clots in the hemofilter, and also to prevent kinks in the catheter, is to make sure the patient doesn't bend the affected leg more than 30 degrees at the hip.

▶ *To prevent infection,* perform skin care at the catheter insertion sites every 48 hours, using aseptic technique. Cover the sites with an occlusive dressing.

▶ If the ultrafiltrate flow rate decreases, raise the bed *to increase the distance between the collection device and the hemofilter.* Lower the bed *to decrease the flow rate.* (Clamping the ultrafiltrate line is contraindicated with some types of hemofilters *because pressure may build up in the filter, clotting it and collapsing the blood compartment.*)

Complications

Possible complications include bleeding, hemorrhage, hemofilter occlusion, infection, and thrombosis.

Documentation

Record the time the treatment began and ended, fluid balance information, times of dressing changes, complications, medications given, and the patient's tolerance.

CONTINUOUS BLADDER IRRIGATION

Continuous bladder irrigation can help prevent urinary tract obstruction by flushing out small blood clots that form after prostate or bladder surgery. It may also be used to treat an irritated, inflamed, or infected bladder lining.

This procedure requires placement of a triple-lumen catheter. One lumen controls balloon inflation, one allows irrigant inflow, and one allows irrigant outflow. The continuous flow of irrigating solution through the bladder also creates a mild tamponade that may help prevent venous hemorrhage. (See *Setup for continuous bladder irrigation,* page 208.) Although the patient typically receives the catheter while he's in the operating room after prostate or bladder surgery, he may have it inserted at bedside if he isn't a surgical patient.

Key nursing diagnoses and patient outcomes

Impaired urinary elimination related to neuromuscular impairment
The patient will:
▶ voice increased comfort
▶ maintain fluid balance (intake will equal output)
▶ discuss the impact of a urologic disorder on himself and others.

Urinary retention related to neuromuscular impairment
The patient will:
▶ voice an understanding of treatment
▶ have few if any complications.

Equipment

One 4,000-ml container or two 2,000-ml containers of irrigating solution

Setup for continuous bladder irrigation

In continuous bladder irrigation, a triple-lumen catheter allows irrigating solution to flow into the bladder through one lumen and flow out through another, as shown in the inset. The third lumen is used to inflate the balloon that holds the catheter in place.

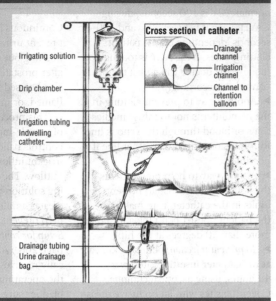

Irrigating solution

Drip chamber

Clamp
Irrigation tubing
Indwelling catheter

Cross section of catheter

Drainage channel
Irrigation channel
Channel to retention balloon

Drainage tubing
Urine drainage bag

(usually normal saline solution) or the prescribed amount of medicated solution • Y-type tubing made specifically for bladder irrigation • alcohol or povidone-iodine pad

Normal saline solution is usually prescribed for bladder irrigation after prostate or bladder surgery. Large volumes of irrigating solution are usually required during the first 24 to 48 hours after surgery. This explains the use of Y-type tubing, which allows immediate irrigation with reserve solution.

Preparation of equipment

Before starting continuous bladder irrigation, double-check the irrigating solution against the doctor's order. If the solution contains an antibiotic, check the patient's chart *to make sure he isn't allergic to the drug.* Unless specified oth-

erwise, the patient should remain on bed rest throughout continuous bladder irrigation.

Implementation

▶ Wash your hands. Assemble all equipment at the patient's bedside. Explain the procedure and provide privacy.

▶ Insert the spike of the Y-type tubing into the container of irrigating solution. (If you have a two-container system, insert one spike into each container.)

▶ Squeeze the drip chamber on the spike of the tubing.

▶ Open the flow clamp and flush the tubing *to remove air, which could cause bladder distention.* Then close the clamp.

▶ To begin, hang the bag of irrigating solution on the I.V. pole.

▶ Clean the opening to the inflow lumen of the catheter with the alcohol or povidone-iodine pad.

▶ Insert the distal end of the Y-type tubing securely into the inflow lumen (third port) of the catheter.

▶ Make sure the catheter's outflow lumen is securely attached to the drainage bag tubing.

▶ Open the flow clamp under the container of irrigating solution and set the drip rate as ordered.

▶ *To prevent air from entering the system,* don't let the primary container empty completely before replacing it.

▶ If you have a two-container system, simultaneously close the flow clamp under the nearly empty container and open the flow clamp under the reserve container. *This prevents reflux of irrigating solution from the reserve container into the nearly empty one.* Hang a new reserve container on the I.V. pole and insert the tubing, maintaining asepsis.

▶ Empty the drainage bag about every 4 hours, or as often as needed. Use sterile technique *to avoid the risk of contamination.*

▶ Monitor vital signs at least every 4 hours during irrigation; increase the frequency if the patient becomes unstable.

Special considerations

▶ Check the inflow and outflow lines periodically for kinks *to make sure the solution is running freely.* If the solution flows rapidly, check the lines frequently.

▶ Measure the outflow volume accurately. It should, allowing for urine production, exceed inflow volume. If inflow volume exceeds outflow volume postoperatively, suspect bladder rupture at the suture lines or renal damage, and notify the doctor immediately.

▶ Also assess outflow for changes in appearance and for blood clots, especially if irrigation is being performed postoperatively to control bleeding. If drainage is bright red, irrigating solution should usually be infused rapidly *with the clamp wide open* until drainage clears. Notify the doctor at once if you suspect hemorrhage. If drainage is clear, the solution is usually given at a rate of 40 to 60 drops/minute. The doctor typically specifies the rate for antibiotic solutions.

▶ Encourage oral fluid intake of 2 to 3 L/day unless contraindicated by another medical condition.

Complications

Interruptions in a continuous irrigation system can predispose the patient to infection. Obstruction in the catheter's outflow lumen can cause bladder distention.

Documentation

Each time you finish a container of solution, record the date, time, and amount of fluid given on the intake and output record. Also record the time and amount of fluid each time you empty the drainage bag. Note the appearance of the drainage and any complaints the patient has.

CREDÉ'S MANEUVER

When lower motor neuron damage impairs the voiding reflex, the bladder may become flaccid or areflexic. Because the bladder fails to contract properly, urine collects inside it, causing distention. Credé's maneuver — application of manual pressure over the lower abdomen — promotes complete

Performing Credé's maneuver

Credé's maneuver is performed by applying manual pressure over the lower abdomen as shown below. This procedure promotes complete emptying of the bladder in patients with lower motor neuron damage that impairs the voiding reflex.

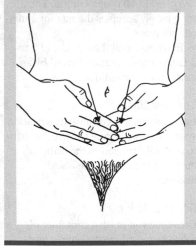

emptying of the bladder. After appropriate instruction, the patient can perform the maneuver himself, unless he can't reach his lower abdomen or lacks sufficient strength and dexterity. Even when performed properly, however, Credé's maneuver isn't always successful and doesn't always eliminate the need for catheterization.

Credé's maneuver can't be used after abdominal surgery if the incision isn't completely healed. When a patient uses Credé's maneuver, close monitoring of urine output is necessary to help detect possible infection from accumulation of residual urine.

Key nursing diagnoses and patient outcomes

Impaired urinary elimination related to neuromuscular impairment
The patient will:
▶ voice increased comfort
▶ maintain fluid balance (intake will equal output)
▶ discuss the impact of urologic disorder on himself and others.

Urinary retention related to neuromuscular impairment
The patient will:
▶ voice an understanding of treatment
▶ have few if any complications.

Equipment
Bedpan, urinal, or bedside commode

Implementation
▶ Explain the procedure to the patient and wash your hands.
▶ If allowed, place the patient in Fowler's position and position the bedpan or urinal. Alternatively, if the patient's condition permits, assist him onto the bedside commode.
▶ Place your hands flat on the patient's abdomen just below the umbilicus. Ask the female patient to bend forward from the hips. Then firmly stroke downward toward the bladder about six times *to stimulate the voiding reflex.*
▶ Place one hand on top of the other above the pubic arch. Press firmly inward and downward *to compress the bladder and expel residual urine.* (See *Performing Credé's maneuver.*)

Patient teaching
▶ Explain to the patient that Credé's maneuver is a simple exercise that can be done at home. Tell the patient that he can start a stream of urine from his

bladder by performing this easy-to-do maneuver. Tell the male patient to void directly into the toilet from a standing position if possible. The female patient should sit on the toilet as she normally would.

▶ Show the female patient how to lean forward, bending at the hips, to increase pressure on the bladder.

▶ Have the patient place one hand on top of the other in a return demonstration. Explain that the stroking movement compresses the bladder and expels urine.

Special considerations

▶ Some facilities require a doctor's order for performing Credé's maneuver. This procedure shouldn't be performed on patients with normal bladder tone or bladder spasms.

▶ After the patient has learned the procedure and can use it successfully, measuring the expelled urine may not be necessary. The patient may then use the maneuver to void directly into the toilet.

Documentation

Record the date and time of the procedure, the amount of urine expelled, and the patient's tolerance of the procedure.

CRICOTHYROTOMY

When endotracheal intubation or a tracheotomy can't be performed quickly to establish an airway, an emergency cricothyrotomy may be necessary. Performed rarely, this procedure involves puncturing the trachea through the cricothyroid membrane.

Usually, your role will be to assist a doctor with this procedure. However, if a doctor isn't available and the patient is likely to die before he can be intubated, you may have to perform the procedure yourself. Ideally, cricothyrotomy is performed using sterile technique but, in an emergency, this may not be possible.

Key nursing diagnoses and patient outcomes

Impaired spontaneous ventilation related to possible obstruction
The patient will:
▶ have normal arterial blood gas levels
▶ have a breathing pattern that returns to baseline.

Ineffective breathing pattern related to an inability to maintain adequate rate and depth of respirations
The patient will:
▶ demonstrate an adequate breathing pattern
▶ demonstrate an oxygen saturation above 95%
▶ exhibit a normal respiratory rate.

Equipment

For scalpel or needle cricothyrotomy
Sterile gloves • povidone-iodine solution • sterile 4″ × 4″ gauze pads • dilator • tape • oxygen source

For scalpel cricothyrotomy
Scalpel #6 or smaller tracheostomy tube (if available) • handheld resuscitation bag or T tube and wide-bore oxygen tubing

For needle cricothyrotomy
14G (or larger) through-the-needle or over-the-needle catheter • 10-ml syringe • tape • I.V. extension tubing • hand-operated release valve or pressure-regulating adjustment valve

Performing an emergency cricothyrotomy

To perform this procedure, first put on sterile gloves and clean the patient's neck with a gauze pad soaked in povidone-iodine solution. To reduce the risk of contamination, use a circular motion, working outward from the incision site.

■ Locate the precise insertion site by sliding your thumb and fingers down to the thyroid gland. You'll know you've located its outer borders when the space between your fingers and thumb widens.

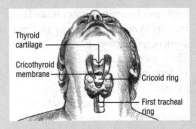

Thyroid cartilage
Cricothyroid membrane
Cricoid ring
First tracheal ring

■ Move your finger across the center of the gland, over the anterior edge of the cricoid ring.

Using a scalpel
■ Make a horizontal incision, less than ½" (1.3 cm) long, in the cricothyroid membrane just above the cricoid ring.
■ Insert a dilator to prevent tissue from closing around the incision. If a dilator isn't available, insert the handle of the scalpel and rotate it 90 degrees (as shown below).

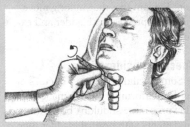

■ If a small tracheostomy tube (#6 or smaller) is available, insert it into the opening and secure it to help maintain a patent airway. If a tracheostomy tube isn't available, tape the dilator or scalpel handle in place until a tracheostomy tube is available.
■ If the patient can breathe spontaneously, attach a humidified oxygen source to the

Implementation
▶ Have someone collect the necessary equipment while you hyperextend the patient's neck *to expose the area of the incision site.*
▶ Have someone hold the patient's head in the correct position while you perform the procedure. (See *Performing an emergency cricothyrotomy.*)

Special considerations
▶ Immediately after the procedure, check for bleeding at the insertion site, subcutaneous emphysema or inade-

quate ventilation, and tracheal or vocal cord damage.

 Age alert Scalpel cricothyrotomy isn't recommended for children under age 12 *because it could damage the cricoid cartilage* — the only circumferential support to the upper trachea.

Complications
Hemorrhage, perforation of the thyroid or esophagus, and subcutaneous or mediastinal emphysema may occur from

tracheostomy tube with a T tube; if he can't, attach a handheld resuscitation bag. You'll need to inflate the cuff of the tracheostomy tube with a syringe to provide positive-pressure ventilation.

■ Auscultate bilaterally for breath sounds, and take the patient's vital signs.

■ Dispose of the gloves properly and wash your hands.

Using a needle

■ Attach a 10-ml syringe to a 14G (or larger) through-the-needle or over-the-needle catheter. Then insert the catheter into the cricothyroid membrane just above the cricoid ring.

■ Direct the catheter downward to the trachea at a 45-degree angle (as shown) to avoid damaging the vocal cords. Maintain negative pressure by pulling back the syringe plunger as you advance the catheter. You'll know the catheter has entered the trachea when air enters the syringe.

■ When the catheter reaches the trachea, advance it and remove the needle and syringe. Tape the catheter in place.

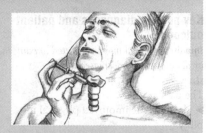

■ Attach the catheter hub to one end of the I.V. extension tubing. At the other end, attach a hand-operated release valve or a pressure-regulating adjustment valve. Connect the entire assembly to an oxygen source.

■ Press the release valve to introduce oxygen into the trachea and inflate the lungs. When you can see that they're inflated, release the valve to allow passive exhalation. Adjust the pressure-regulating valve to the minimum pressure needed for adequate lung inflation.

■ Auscultate bilaterally for breath sounds and take the patient's vital signs.

■ Dispose of the gloves properly and wash your hands.

---

this procedure. Infection may also occur several days after the procedure.

Documentation

Your documentation of the procedure should include the date, time, and circumstances requiring the procedure and the patient's vital signs. Note whether the patient initiated spontaneous respirations after the procedure.

Record how much and by what method oxygen was delivered. Also document any procedures that were performed after the airway was estab-

lished — for example, endotracheal intubation.

CRUTCH USE

Crutches remove weight from one or both legs, enabling the patient to support himself with his hands and arms. Typically prescribed for a patient with lower-extremity injury or weakness, crutches require balance, stamina, and upper-body strength for successful use. Crutch selection and walking gait depend on the patient's condition. A patient who can't use crutches may be able to use a walker.

Key nursing diagnoses and patient outcomes

Impaired physical mobility related to pain or discomfort and decreased muscle strength
The patient will:
▶ demonstrate improved physical mobility
▶ ambulate with maximum independence
▶ demonstrate increased activity tolerance

Impaired walking related to an inability to use crutches properly
The patient will:
▶ demonstrate proper use of crutches
▶ demonstrate improved ability to maneuver with crutches
▶ remain free from injury related to falls.

Equipment

Crutches with axillary pads, handgrips, and rubber suction tips • optional: walking belt

Three types of crutches are commonly used. Standard aluminum or wooden crutches are used by the patient with a sprain, strain, or cast. They require stamina and upper-body strength. Aluminum forearm crutches are used by the paraplegic or other patient using the swing-through gait. They have a collar that fits around the forearm and a horizontal handgrip that provides support. Platform crutches are used by the arthritic patient who has an upper-extremity deficit that prevents weight bearing

through the wrist. They provide padded surfaces for the upper extremities.

Preparation of equipment

After choosing the appropriate crutches, adjust their height with the patient standing or, if necessary, recumbent. (See *Fitting a patient for a crutch.*)

Implementation

▶ Consult with the patient's doctor and physical therapist *to coordinate rehabilitation orders and teaching.*
▶ Describe the gait you will teach and the reason for your choice. Then demonstrate the gait as necessary. Have the patient give a return demonstration.
▶ Place a walking belt around the patient's waist, if necessary, *to help prevent falls.* Tell the patient to position the crutches and to shift his weight from side to side. Then place him in front of a full-length mirror *to facilitate learning and coordination.*
▶ Teach the four-point gait to the patient who can bear weight on both legs. Although this is the safest gait *because three points are always in contact with the floor,* it requires greater coordination than others *because of its constant shifting of weight.* Use this sequence: right crutch, left foot, left crutch, right foot. Suggest counting to help develop rhythm and make sure each short step is of equal length. If the patient gains proficiency at this gait, teach him the faster two-point gait.
▶ Teach the two-point gait to the patient with weak legs but good coordination and arm strength. This is the most natural crutch-walking gait *because it mimics walking, with alternating swings of the arms and legs.* Instruct the patient to advance the right crutch and left foot

simultaneously, followed by the left crutch and right foot.

▶ Teach the three-point gait to the patient who can bear only partial or no weight on one leg. Instruct him to advance both crutches 6″ to 8″ (15 to 20 cm) along with the involved leg. Then tell him to bring the uninvolved leg forward and to bear the bulk of his weight on the crutches but some of it on the involved leg, if possible. Stress the importance of taking steps of equal length and duration with no pauses.

▶ Teach the swing-to or swing-through gaits — the fastest ones — to the patient with complete paralysis of the hips and legs. Instruct him to advance both crutches simultaneously and to swing the legs parallel to (swing-to) or beyond the crutches (swing-through).

▶ To teach the patient who uses crutches to get up from a chair, tell him to hold both crutches in one hand, with the tips resting firmly on the floor. Then instruct him to push up from the chair with his free hand, supporting himself with the crutches.

▶ To sit down, the patient reverses the process: Tell him to support himself with the crutches in one hand and to lower himself with the other.

▶ To teach the patient to ascend stairs using the three-point gait, tell him to lead with the uninvolved leg and to follow with both the crutches and the involved leg. To descend stairs, he should lead with the crutches and the involved leg and follow with the good leg. He may find it helpful to remember "The good goes up; the bad goes down."

Special considerations
Encourage arm- and shoulder-strengthening exercises to prepare the patient

Fitting a patient for a crutch

Position the crutch so that it extends from a point 4″ to 6″ (10 to 15 cm) to the side and 4″ to 6″ in front of the patient's feet to 1½″ to 2″ (4 to 5 cm) below the axillae (about the width of two fingers). Then adjust the handgrips so that the patient's elbows are flexed at a 15-degree angle when he's standing with the crutches in the resting position.

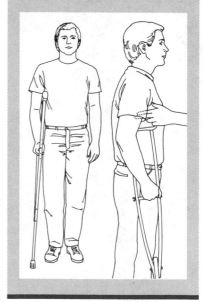

for crutch walking. If possible, teach two techniques — one fast and one slow — *so the patient can alternate between them to prevent excessive muscle fatigue and can adjust more easily to various walking conditions.*

Complications
When used with chronic conditions, the swing-to and swing-through gaits can lead to atrophy of the hips and legs

if appropriate therapeutic exercises aren't performed routinely. Warn the patient against habitually leaning on his crutches *because prolonged pressure on the axillae can damage the brachial nerves, causing brachial nerve palsy.*

Documentation

Record the type of gait the patient used, the amount of assistance required, the distance walked, and the patient's tolerance of the crutches and gait.

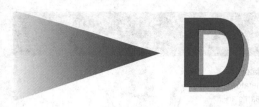

DEFIBRILLATION

The standard treatment for ventricular fibrillation, defibrillation involves using electrode paddles to direct an electric current through the patient's heart. The current causes the myocardium to depolarize, which in turn encourages the sinoatrial node to resume control of the heart's electrical activity. The electrode paddles delivering the current may be placed on the patient's chest or, during cardiac surgery, directly on the myocardium.

Because ventricular fibrillation leads to death if not corrected, the success of defibrillation depends on early recognition and quick treatment of this arrhythmia. In addition to treating ventricular fibrillation, defibrillation may also be used to treat ventricular tachycardia that doesn't produce a pulse.

A patient with a history of ventricular fibrillation may be a candidate for an implantable cardioverter-defibrillator, a sophisticated device that automatically discharges an electric current when it senses a ventricular tachyarrhythmia. (See *Understanding the ICD,* page 218.)

Key nursing diagnoses and patient outcomes

Anxiety related to threat of death
The patient will:
▶ identify the cause of the anxiety

▶ cope with anxiety by being involved in decisions about care.

Decreased cardiac output related to reduced stroke volume as a result of electrophysiologic problems
The patient will:
▶ have no arrhythmias
▶ remain hemodynamically stable as evidenced by pulse not less than (specify) and not more than (specify); blood pressure not less than (specify) mm Hg and not greater than (specify) mm Hg.

Equipment

Defibrillator • external paddles • internal paddles (sterilized for cardiac surgery) • conductive medium pads • electrocardiogram (ECG) monitor with recorder • oxygen therapy equipment • handheld resuscitation bag • airway equipment • emergency pacing equipment • emergency cardiac medications

Implementation

▶ Assess the patient *to determine if he lacks a pulse.* Call for help and perform cardiopulmonary resuscitation (CPR) until the defibrillator and other emergency equipment arrive.
▶ If the defibrillator has "quick-look" capability, place the paddles on the patient's chest *to quickly view his cardiac rhythm.* Otherwise, connect the moni-

Understanding the ICD

The implantable cardioverter-defibrillator (ICD) has a programmable pulse generator and lead system that monitors the heart's activity, detects ventricular bradyarrhythmias and tachyarrhythmias, and responds with appropriate therapies. The range of therapies includes antitachycardia and bradycardia pacing, cardioversion, and defibrillation. Newer defibrillators also have the ability to pace the atrium and the ventricle.

Implantation of the ICD is similar to that of a permanent pacemaker. The cardiologist positions the lead (or leads) transvenously in the endocardium of the right ventricle (and in the right atrium, if both chambers require pacing). The lead connects to a generator box, which is implanted in the right or left upper chest near the clavicle.

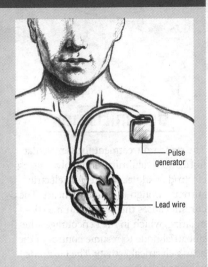

Pulse generator

Lead wire

toring leads of the defibrillator to the patient and assess his cardiac rhythm.

▶ Expose the patient's chest and apply conductive pads at the paddle placement positions. For anterolateral placement, place one paddle to the right of the upper sternum, just below the right clavicle, and the other over the fifth or sixth intercostal space at the left anterior axillary line. For anteroposterior placement, place the anterior paddle directly over the heart at the precordium, to the left of the lower sternal border. Place the flat posterior paddle under the patient's body beneath the heart and immediately below the scapulae (but not under the vertebral column).

▶ Turn on the defibrillator and, if performing external defibrillation, set the energy level for 200 joules for an adult patient.

▶ Charge the paddles by pressing the charge buttons, which are located ei-

ther on the machine or on the paddles themselves.

▶ Place the paddles over the conductive pads and press firmly against the patient's chest, using 25 lb (11.3 kg) of pressure.

▶ Reassess the patient's cardiac rhythm.

▶ If the patient remains in ventricular fibrillation or pulseless ventricular tachycardia, instruct all personnel to stand clear of the patient and the bed.

▶ Discharge the current by pressing both paddle charge buttons simultaneously.

▶ Leaving the paddles in position on the patient's chest, reassess the patient's cardiac rhythm and have someone else assess the pulse.

▶ If necessary, prepare to defibrillate a second time. Instruct someone to reset the energy level on the defibrillator to 200 to 300 joules. Announce that you're preparing to defibrillate and follow the procedure described above.

▶ Reassess the patient. If defibrillation is again necessary, instruct someone to reset the energy level to 360 joules. Then follow the same procedure as before.

▶ Perform the three countershocks in rapid succession, reassessing the patient's rhythm before each defibrillation.

▶ If the patient still has no pulse after three initial defibrillations, resume CPR, give supplemental oxygen, and begin administering appropriate medications such as epinephrine. Also consider possible causes for failure of the patient's rhythm to convert, such as acidosis and hypoxia.

▶ If defibrillation restores a normal rhythm, check the patient's central and peripheral pulses and obtain a blood pressure reading, heart rate, and respiratory rate. Assess the patient's level of consciousness, cardiac rhythm, breath sounds, skin color, and urine output. Obtain baseline arterial blood gas levels and a 12-lead ECG. Provide supplemental oxygen, ventilation, and medications as needed. Check the patient's chest for electrical burns and treat them as ordered with corticosteroid or lanolin-based creams. Also prepare the defibrillator for immediate reuse.

Special considerations

▶ Defibrillators vary from one manufacturer to the next, so familiarize yourself with your facility's equipment. Defibrillator operation should be checked at least every 8 hours and after each use.

▶ Defibrillation can be affected by several factors, including paddle size and placement, condition of the patient's myocardium, duration of the arrhyth-

mia, chest resistance, and the number of countershocks.

Complications

Defibrillation can cause accidental electric shock to those providing care. Use of an insufficient amount of conductive medium can lead to skin burns.

Documentation

Document the procedure, including the patient's ECG rhythms before and after defibrillation; the number of times defibrillation was performed; the voltage used during each attempt; whether a pulse returned; the dosage, route, and time of drug administration; whether CPR was used; how the airway was maintained; and the patient's outcome.

DOPPLER USE

More sensitive than palpation for determining pulse rate, the Doppler ultrasound blood flow detector is especially useful when a pulse is faint or weak. Unlike palpation, which detects arterial wall expansion and retraction, this instrument detects the motion of red blood cells (RBCs).

Key nursing diagnoses and patient outcomes

Ineffective tissue perfusion (peripheral) related to (specify)
The patient will:

▶ express a feeling of comfort or absence of pain at rest

▶ have strong peripheral pulses

▶ maintain normal skin color and temperature

▶ have no evidence of pressure ulcers

▶ maintain tissue perfusion and cellular oxygenation.

Decreased cardiac output related to reduced stroke volume

The patient will:

▶ attain hemodynamic stability as evidenced by a pulse not less than (specify) beats/minute and not greater than (specify) beats/minute; blood pressure not less than (specify) mm Hg and not greater than (specify) mm Hg

▶ have warm and dry skin

▶ have a diminished cardiac workload

▶ maintain adequate cardiac output.

Equipment

Doppler ultrasound blood flow detector • coupling or transmission gel • soft cloth • antiseptic solution or soapy water

Implementation

▶ Apply a small amount of coupling gel or transmission gel (not water soluble lubricant) to the ultrasound probe.

▶ Position the probe on the skin directly over the selected artery.

▶ When using a Doppler model with a speaker, turn the instrument on and, moving counter-clockwise, set the volume control to the lowest setting. If your model doesn't have a speaker, plug in the earphones and slowly raise the volume. The Doppler ultrasound stethoscope is basically a stethoscope fitted with an audio unit, volume control, and transducer, which amplifies the movement of RBCs.

▶ To obtain the best signals with either device, tilt the probe 45 degrees from the artery, making sure to put gel between the skin and the probe. Slowly move the probe in a circular motion to locate the center of the artery and the Doppler signal — a hissing noise at the heartbeat.

▶ Avoid moving the probe rapidly *because it distorts the signal.*

▶ Count the signals for 60 seconds to determine the pulse rate.

▶ After you've measured the pulse rate, clean the probe with a soft cloth soaked in antiseptic solution or soapy water. Don't immerse the probe or bump it against a hard surface.

Documentation

Record the location and quality of the pulse as well as the pulse rate and time of measurement.

DROPLET PRECAUTIONS

Droplet precautions prevent the spread of infectious diseases (including some diseases formerly included in respiratory isolation) that are transmitted when nasal or oral secretions from the infected patient come in contact with the mucous membranes of the susceptible host. The droplets of moisture, which arise from coughing or sneezing, are heavy and generally fall to the ground within 3′ (0.9 m); the organisms that the droplets contain don't become airborne or suspended in the air. (See *Diseases requiring droplet precautions.*)

Effective droplet precautions require a single room (not necessarily a negative-pressure room), and the door doesn't need to be closed. Persons having direct contact with and those who will be within 3′ of the patient should wear a surgical mask covering the nose and mouth.

When handling infants or young children who require droplet precautions, you may also need to wear gloves and a gown to prevent soiling of clothing with nasal and oral secretions.

Diseases requiring droplet precautions

Disease	Precautionary period
Invasive *Haemophilus influenzae* type b disease, including meningitis, pneumonia, and sepsis	Until 24 hours after initiation of effective therapy
Invasive *Neisseria meningitidis* disease, including meningitis, pneumonia, epiglottiditis, and sepsis	Until 24 hours after initiation of effective therapy
Diphtheria (pharyngeal)	Until off antibiotics and two cultures taken at least 24 hours apart are negative
Mycoplasma pneumoniae infection	Duration of illness
Pertussis	Until 5 days after initiation of effective therapy
Pneumonic plague	Until 72 hours after initiation of effective therapy
Streptococcal pharyngitis, pneumonia, or scarlet fever in infants and young children	Until 24 hours after initiation of effective therapy
Adenovirus infection in infants and young children	Duration of illness
Influenza	Duration of illness
Mumps	For 9 days after onset of swelling
Human parvovirus B19	Duration of hospitalization when chronic disease occurs in an immunodeficient patient; 7 days for patients with transient aplastic crisis or red-cell crisis
Rubella (German measles)	Until 7 days after onset of rash

Key nursing diagnoses and patient outcomes

Risk for infection related to external factors
The patient will:
▶ have no pathogens appear in culture
▶ show no evidence of signs and symptoms of infection
▶ remain afebrile.

Deficient knowledge related to lack of exposure to the droplet precautions procedure

The patient will:
▶ state or demonstrate an understanding of the need for the procedure
▶ recognize that increased knowledge will help him better cope with the procedure.

Equipment

Masks • gowns and gloves, if necessary • plastic bags • droplet precautions door card

Gather any additional supplies needed for routine patient care, such as a thermometer, stethoscope, and blood pressure cuff.

Preparation of equipment

Keep all droplet precaution supplies outside the patient's room in a cart or anteroom.

Implementation

▶ Place the patient in a single room with private toilet facilities and an anteroom, if possible. If necessary, two patients with the same infection may share a room. Explain isolation procedures to the patient and his family.
▶ Put a droplet precautions card on the door *to notify anyone entering the room.*
▶ Wash your hands before entering and after leaving the room and during patient care as indicated.
▶ Pick up your mask by the top strings, adjust it around your nose and mouth, and tie the strings for a comfortable fit. If the mask has a flexible metal nose strip, adjust it to fit firmly but comfortably.
▶ Instruct the patient to cover his nose and mouth with a facial tissue while coughing or sneezing.
▶ Tape a plastic bag to the patient's bedside *so that the patient can dispose of facial tissues correctly.*
▶ Make sure all visitors wear masks when they're within 3′ (0.9 m) of the patient and, if necessary, wear gowns and gloves.
▶ If the patient must leave the room for essential procedures, make sure he wears a surgical mask over his nose and mouth. Notify the receiving department or area of the patient's isolation precautions *so that the precautions will be main-* *tained and the patient can be returned to the room promptly.*

Special considerations

▶ Before removing your mask, remove your gloves (if worn) and wash your hands.
▶ Untie the strings and dispose of the mask, handling it only by the strings.

Documentation

Record the need for droplet precautions on the nursing plan of care and as otherwise indicated by your facility.

Document initiation and maintenance of the precautions, the patient's tolerance of the procedure, and any patient or family teaching. Also document the date droplet precautions were discontinued.

DRUG ADMINISTRATION IN CHILDREN

Because a child responds to drugs more rapidly and unpredictably than an adult, pediatric drug administration requires special care. Such factors as age, weight, body surface area, and drug form and route may dramatically affect a child's response to a drug. For example, because of his thin epithelium, a neonate or an infant absorbs topical medications much faster than an older child does.

Certain disorders also affect a child's response to medication. For example, gastroenteritis increases gastric motility, which in turn impairs absorption of certain oral medications. Liver or kidney disorders can hinder the metabolism of some medications.

Usual drug administration techniques may need adjustment to account for the child's age, size, and developmental level. A tablet for a young child, for example, may be crushed and mixed with a liquid for oral administration. In addition, the injection site and needle size will vary depending on the child's age and physical development.

Key nursing diagnoses and patient outcomes

Risk for injury related to improper technique
The patient will:
▶ remain free from injury
▶ identify factors that increase risk for injury
▶ assist in identifying and applying safety measures to prevent injury.

Equipment

For oral medications
Prescribed medication • plastic disposable syringe, plastic medicine dropper, or spoon • medication cup • water, syrup, or jelly (for tablets) • optional: fruit juice

For injectable medications
Prescribed medication • appropriately sized syringe and needle • alcohol pads or povidone-iodine solution • gloves • gauze pad • adhesive bandage • optional: cold compress, eutectic mixture of local anesthetic (EMLA), and transparent occlusive dressing

Preparation of equipment
Check the doctor's order for the prescribed drug, dosage, and route. Compare the order with the drug label, check the drug expiration date, and review the patient's chart for drug allergies.

Carefully calculate the dosage, if necessary, and have another nurse verify it. Typically, you'll double-check dosages for potentially hazardous or lethal drugs, such as insulin, heparin, digoxin, epinephrine, and narcotics. Check your facility's policy *to learn which drugs must be calculated and checked by two nurses.*

For giving an injection, select the appropriate needle. Typically, for I.M. injections in infants, you'll use a 25G ¾″ needle and, in older children, a 23G 1″ needle. For subcutaneous injections, select a ¾″ or ½″ needle and, for intradermal medications, a 27G ½″ needle. To administer viscous medications, select a larger-gauge needle.

Implementation
▶ Assess the child's condition *to determine the need for the medication and the effectiveness of previous therapy.*
▶ Carefully observe the child for a rash, pruritus, cough, or other signs of an adverse reaction to a previously administered drug.
▶ Identify the child by comparing the name on his wristband with that on the medication card. If the child can talk and respond, ask him his name.
▶ Explain the procedure to the child and his parents. Use terms the child can understand. Give the child choices, if possible; for example, ask the child if he wants the medication mixed with chocolate or strawberry syrup.
▶ Provide privacy, especially for an older child.

Giving oral medication to an infant
▶ Use either a plastic syringe without a needle or a drug-specific medicine dropper to measure the dose. If the medication comes in tablet form, first

Giving oral medication to an infant

Use a dropper or syringe without a needle to administer an oral medication to an infant. Place the dropper or syringe at the corner of the infant's mouth so the medication will run into the pocket between the infant's cheek and gum. *This keeps him from spitting it out and reduces the risk of aspiration.*

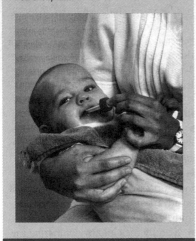

crush the tablet (if appropriate) and mix it with water or syrup. Then draw the mixture into the syringe or dropper.
▶ Pick up the infant, raising his head and shoulders or turning his head to one side *to prevent aspiration.* Hold the infant close to your body *to help restrain him.*
▶ Using your thumb, press down on the infant's chin *to open his mouth.*
▶ Slide the syringe or medicine dropper into the infant's mouth alongside his tongue. (See *Giving oral medication to an infant.*) Release the medication slowly *to let the infant swallow and to prevent choking.* If appropriate, allow

him to suck on the syringe as you expel the medication.
▶ If not contraindicated, give fruit juice after giving medication.
▶ Place a particularly small or inactive infant on his side or back as recommended by the American Academy of Pediatrics *to decrease the risk of sudden infant death syndrome.* Allow an active infant to assume a position that is comfortable for him; avoid forcing him into a side-lying position *to prevent agitation.*

Giving oral medication to a toddler
▶ Use a plastic, disposable syringe or dropper to measure liquid medication. Then transfer the fluid to a medication cup.
▶ Elevate the toddler's head and shoulders *to prevent aspiration.*
▶ If possible, ask him to help hold the cup *to enlist his cooperation.* Otherwise, hold the cup to the toddler's lips or use a syringe or a spoon to administer the liquid. Make sure that the toddler ingests all of the medication.
▶ If the medication is in tablet form, first crush the tablet, if appropriate, and mix it with water, syrup, or jelly. Use a spoon, syringe, or dropper to administer the medication. (See *Drugs that shouldn't be crushed.*)

Giving oral medication to an older child
▶ If possible, let the child choose both the liquid medication mixer and a beverage to drink after taking the medication.
▶ If appropriate, allow him to choose where he'll take the medication, for example, sitting in bed or sitting on a parent's lap.
▶ If the medication comes in tablet or capsule form and if the child is old

Drugs that shouldn't be crushed

When administering medication to infants and children, remember that not all pills can be crushed for easier administration. Avoid crushing the following drugs for the reason noted beside them:

Acutrim (slow release)

Aerolate Sr., Jr., III (slow release)

Aller-Chlor (slow release)

Allerest Maximum Strength 12 Hour (slow release)

Atrohist LA, Sprinkle (slow release)

Azulfidine EN-Tabs (enteric coated)

Bisco-Lax (enteric coated)

Breonesin (liquid filled)

Bromfed (slow release)

Bromfed PD (slow release)

Bromophen T.D. (slow release)

Bromphen (slow release)

Cardizem CD, SR (slow release)

Ceftin (taste)

Cerespan (slow release)

Charcoal Plus (enteric coated)

Chloral hydrate (liquid within a capsule, taste)

Chlor-Trimeton Repetabs (slow release)

Choledyl (enteric coated)

Choledyl SA (slow release)

Cipro (taste)

Colace (liquid within a capsule, taste)

Compazine Spansule (slow release)

Congess SR, JR (slow release)

Control (slow release)

Cotazym-S (enteric coated)

Creon (enteric coated)

Dallergy (slow release)

Dallergy-D (slow release)

Dallergy-JR (slow release)

Deconamine SR (slow release)

Deconsal Sprinkle (slow release)

Dehist (slow release)

Depakene (slow release, mucous membrane irritant)

Depakote (enteric coated)

Desoxyn Gradumet (slow release)

Dexedrine Spansule (slow release)

Diamox Sequels (slow release)

Dimetane Extentabs (slow release)

Dimetapp Extentabs (slow release)

Disobrom (slow release)

Donnatal Extentabs (slow release)

Drisdol (liquid filled)

Drixoral (slow release)

Drixoral Allergy Sinus (slow release)

Drize (slow release)

Dulcolax (enteric coated)

Easprin (enteric coated)

Ecotrin (enteric coated)

Ecotrin Maximum Strength (enteric coated)

E.E.S. 400 Filmtab (enteric coated)

Elixophyllin SR (slow release)

E-Mycin (enteric coated)

Entex LA (slow release)

Entozyme (enteric coated)

Equanil (taste)

Ergostat (sublingual)

ERYC (enteric coated)

Ery-Tab (enteric coated)

Erythrocin Stearate (enteric coated)

Erythromycin Base (enteric coated)

Eskalith CR (slow release)

Extendryl SR, JR (slow release)

Fedahist Gyrocaps, Timecaps (slow release)

Feosol (enteric coated)

Feratab (enteric coated)

Fergon (slow release)

Fero-Grad-500 (slow release)

Fero-Gradumet (slow release)

(continued)

Drugs that shouldn't be crushed *(continued)*

Ferralet Slow Release (slow release)

Ferralyn Lanacaps (slow release)

Ferro-Sequels (slow release)

Feverall Sprinkle Caps, Children's (taste)

Fumatinic (slow release)

Genabid (slow release)

Geocillin (taste)

Gris-PEG (crushing may cause precipitation of larger particles)

Guaifed (slow release)

Guaifed-PD (slow release)

Humibid Sprinkle, DM, DM Sprinkle, L.A. (slow release)

Hytakerol (liquid filled)

Iberet (slow release)

Iberet-500 (slow release)

Ilotycin (enteric coated)

Inderal LA (slow release)

Inderide LA (slow release)

Indocin SR (slow release)

Isordil Sublingual (sublingual)

Isosorbide Dinitrate Sublingual (sublingual)

Kaon-Cl (slow release)

K-Dur (slow release)

Klor-Con (slow release)

Klotrix (slow release)

K-Tab (slow release)

Meprospan (slow release)

Mestinon Timespans (slow release)

Micro-K (slow release)

Micro-K Extencaps (slow release)

Motrin (taste)

MS Contin (slow release)

Naldecon (slow release)

Nico-400 (slow release)

Nolamine (slow release)

Norpace CR (slow release)

Novafed (slow release)

Novafed A (slow release)

Oramorph SR (slow release)

Pancrease (enteric coated)

Pancrease MT (enteric coated)

PCE (slow release)

Perdiem (wax coated)

Phenergan (taste)

Phyllocontin (slow release)

Polaramine Repetabs (slow release)

Procan SR (slow release)

Procardia (delayed absorption)

Pronestyl-SR (slow release)

Proventil Repetabs (slow release)

Prozac (slow release)

Quibron-T/SR Dividose (slow release)

Respbid (slow release)

Ritalin-SR (slow release)

Rondec-TR (slow release)

Slo-bid Gyrocaps (slow release)

Slo-Phyllin GG, Gyrocaps (slow release)

Slow Fe (slow release)

Slow-K (slow release)

Sorbitrate SA (slow release)

Sparine (taste)

Sudafed 12 Hour (slow release)

Teldrin (slow release)

Theobid Duracaps (slow release)

Theochron (slow release)

Theoclear L.A. (slow release)

Theo-Dur (slow release)

Theo-Dur Sprinkle (slow release)

Theolair-SR (slow release)

Theo-Sav (slow release)

Theospan-SR (slow release)

Theo-Time (slow release)

Theo-24 (slow release)

Theovent (slow release)

Theo-X (slow release)

Thorazine Spansule (slow release)

Tranxene-SD (slow release)

Triaminic (slow release)

Triaminic-12 (slow release)

Triaminic TR (slow release)

Trilafon Repetabs (slow release)

Triptone Caplets (slow release)

Uniphyl (slow release)

Valrelease (slow release)

Verelan (slow release)

Voltaren SR (enteric coated)

Wygesic (taste)

Zymase (enteric coated)

enough (between ages 4 and 6), teach him how to swallow solid medication. (If he already knows how to do this, review the procedure with him *for safety's sake.*) Tell him to place the pill on the back of his tongue and to swallow it immediately by drinking water or juice. Focus most of your explanation on the water or juice *to draw the child's attention away from the pill.* Make sure the child drinks enough water or juice *to keep the pill from lodging in his esophagus.* Afterward, look inside the child's mouth *to confirm that he swallowed the pill.*

▶ If the child can't swallow the pill whole, crush it (if appropriate) and mix it with water, syrup, or jelly. Or, after checking with the child's doctor, order the medication in liquid form.

Giving an I.M. injection

▶ Choose an injection site that is appropriate for the child's age and muscle mass. If time allows, place an EMLA cream on the intended skin site at least 1 hour before the procedure. Don't spread the cream or rub it in. Cover with a transparent occlusive dressing.
▶ Immediately before the procedure, remove the dressing and wipe the skin with a gauze pad *to remove the cream.* (See *I.M. injection sites in children,* page 228.)
▶ Position the patient appropriately for the site chosen and locate key landmarks, for example, the posterior superior iliac spine and the greater trochanter. Have someone help you restrain an infant; seek an older child's cooperation before enlisting assistance.
▶ Put on gloves. Clean the injection site with an alcohol or povidone-iodine pad. Wipe outward from the center

with a spiral motion *to avoid contaminating the clean area.*
▶ Grasp the tissue surrounding the site between your index finger and thumb *to immobilize the site and to create a muscle mass for the injection.*
▶ Insert the needle quickly, using a darting motion. If you're using the ventrogluteal site, insert the needle at a 45-degree angle toward the knee.
▶ Aspirate the plunger to ensure that the needle isn't in a blood vessel. If no blood appears, inject the medication slowly *so that the muscle can distend to accommodate the volume.*
▶ Withdraw the needle and gently massage the area with a gauze pad *to stimulate circulation and enhance absorption.*
▶ Provide comfort and praise.

Giving a subcutaneous injection

▶ Select from these possible sites: the middle third of the upper outer arm, the middle third of the upper outer thigh, or the abdomen. You may apply a cold compress or EMLA, as described above, to the injection site *to minimize pain.*
▶ Put on gloves and prepare the injection site with alcohol or povidone-iodine solution according to the patient's needs and your facility's policy.
▶ Pinch the tissue surrounding the site between your index finger and thumb *to ensure injection into the subcutaneous tissue.* Holding the needle at a 45- to 90-degree angle, quickly insert it into the tissue. Release your grasp on the tissue and slowly inject the medication. Remove the needle quickly *to decrease discomfort.* Unless contraindicated, gently massage the area *to facilitate the drug's absorption.*

I.M. injection sites in children

When selecting the best site for a child's I.M. injection, consider the child's age, weight, and muscular development; the amount of subcutaneous fat over the injection site; the type of drug you're administering; and the drug's absorption rate.

Vastus lateralis and rectus femoris

For a child under age 3, you'll typically use the vastus lateralis or rectus femoris muscle for an I.M. injection. Constituting the largest muscle mass in this age-group, the vastus lateralis and rectus femoris have fewer major blood vessels and nerves.

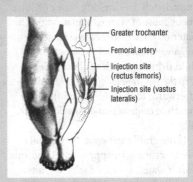

Greater trochanter
Femoral artery
Injection site (rectus femoris)
Injection site (vastus lateralis)

Ventrogluteal and dorsogluteal

For a child who can walk and is over age 3, use the ventrogluteal and dorsogluteal muscles. Like the vastus lateralis, the ventrogluteal site is relatively free of major blood vessels and nerves. Before you select either site, make sure that the child has been walking for at least 1 year to ensure sufficient muscle development.

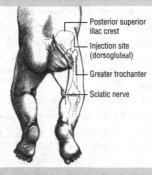

Posterior superior iliac crest
Injection site (dorsogluteal)
Greater trochanter
Sciatic nerve

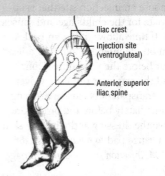

Iliac crest
Injection site (ventrogluteal)
Anterior superior iliac spine

Deltoid

For a child older than 18 months who needs rapid medication results, consider using the deltoid muscle for the injection. Because blood flows faster in the deltoid muscle than in other muscles, drug absorption should be faster. Be careful if you use this site because the deltoid doesn't develop fully until adolescence. In a younger child, it's small and close to the radial nerve, which may be injured during needle insertion.

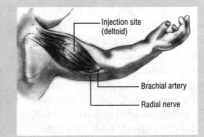

Injection site (deltoid)
Brachial artery
Radial nerve

Giving an intradermal injection

▶ Put on gloves and pull the patient's skin taut (the site of choice is the inner aspect of the forearm).

▶ Insert the needle, bevel up, at a 10- to 15-degree angle just beneath the outer skin layer.

▶ Slowly inject the medication and watch for a bleb to appear. Quickly remove the needle, being careful to maintain the injection angle. If appropriate — for example, if the injection is related to allergy testing — draw a circle around the bleb and avoid massaging the area *to avoid interfering with test results.*

Special considerations

▶ Don't hesitate to consult the parents for tips on successfully giving medication to their child. If possible, have a parent administer a prescribed oral drug while you supervise. However, avoid asking a parent to help with injections *because the child may perceive the parent as a cause of pain.*

▶ Aim for a trusting relationship with the child and his parents *so that you can offer support and promote cooperation even when a medication causes discomfort.* If the child will receive one injection, allow him to choose from the appropriate sites. However, if he'll receive numerous injections, remember that site rotation must follow a set pattern. Allow the child to play with a medication cup or syringe and to pretend to give medication to a doll.

▶ When giving medication to an older child, be honest. Reassure him that distaste or discomfort will be brief. Emphasize that he must remain still *to promote safety and minimize discomfort.* Explain to the child and his parents that an assistant will help the child re-

main still, if necessary. Keep your explanations brief and simple.

▶ *To divert the child's attention,* have him start counting just before the injection and challenge him to try to reach 10 before you finish the injection. If the child cries, don't scold him or allow the parents to scold him. Have one of the parents hold a younger child and praise him for allowing you to give him the injection. You can also apply an adhesive bandage to the injection site *as a form of reward or badge.*

▶ If the prescribed medication comes only in tablet form, consult the pharmacist (or an appropriate drug reference book) *to make sure that crushing the tablet won't invalidate its effectiveness.* Avoid adding medication to a large amount of liquid, such as the child's milk or formula, *because the child may not drink the entire amount, resulting in an inaccurate dose of medication.*

▶ Because infants and toddlers can't tell you what effects they're experiencing from a medication, you must be alert for signs of an adverse reaction. Compile a list of appropriate emergency drugs, calculating the dosages to the patient's weight. Post the list near the patient's bed *for reference in an emergency.*

▶ If you have any doubt about proper medication dosage, always consult the doctor who ordered the drug. Double-check information in a reliable drug reference.

▶ EMLA cream isn't approved for use in infants less than age 1 month.

Home care

Teach the parents about the proper dosage and administration of all prescribed medications. If the parents will administer a liquid medication, advise them to use a commercially available,

Using subcutaneous injectors

Currently available for use by patients at home, subcutaneous injectors feature disposable needles or pressure jets to deliver doses of prescribed medications such as short-acting insulin. Appropriate for use in children, these devices deliver medication safely and accurately. The NovoPen, for instance, has disposable needles and replaceable cartridges. Preci-Jet, Vitajet, and Medi-Jector draw their medications from standard bottles. A pressure jet deposits the drug in subcutaneous tissue.

Although still relatively expensive, these devices are easy to use. For example, studies indicate that jet-injected insulin disperses faster and is absorbed more rapidly *because it avoids the puddling effect common with needle delivery.*

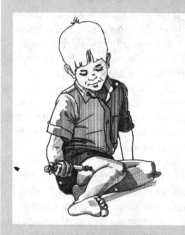

Needle injection

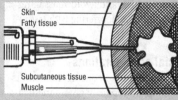

Pressure-jet injection

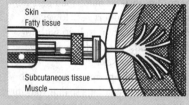

disposable oral syringe to measure the dose. *To ensure an accurate dose,* advise them to avoid using a teaspoon. Teach them how to use the oral syringe. Use written materials — such as a medication instruction sheet — to reinforce your teaching.

If appropriate, teach the child and his parents about subcutaneous injectors. (See *Using subcutaneous injectors.*)

Documentation
Record the medication, form, dosage, date, time, route, and site of administration. Also record the effect of the medication, the patient's tolerance of the procedure, complications, and nursing interventions. Note instructional activities related to medications.

DRUG IMPLANTATION

A newer method of advanced drug delivery involves implanting drugs beneath the skin — subdermally or subcutaneously — as well as targeting specific tissues with radiation implants.

With subdermal implants, flexible capsules are placed under the skin. The drug most commonly administered by this method is levonorgestrel, a synthetic hormone used for long-term contraception. Small Silastic capsules filled with the hormone are placed under the skin of the patient's upper arm, and the drug then diffuses through the capsule walls continuously.

With subcutaneous implants, drug pellets are injected into the skin's subcutaneous layer. The drug is then stored in one area of the body, called a depot. A newer treatment for prostate cancer cells calls for implants of goserelin acetate, a synthetic form of luteinizing hormone. By inhibiting pituitary gland secretion, goserelin implants reduce testosterone levels to those previously achieved only through castration. This reduction causes tumor regression and suppression of symptoms.

Radiation drug implants with a short half-life may be placed inside a body cavity, within a tumor or on its surface, or in the area from which a tumor has been removed. Implants that contain iodine 125 are used for lung and prostate tumors; gold 198, for oral and ocular tumors; and radium 226 and cesium 137, for tongue, lip, and skin therapy. These implants are usually inserted by a doctor with a nurse assisting. Some specially trained nurses may insert or inject intradermal implants. Radiation implants are usually put in place in an operating room or a radiation oncology suite.

Key nursing diagnoses and patient outcomes

Deficient knowledge related to lack of exposure to the procedure
The patient will:
▶ state or demonstrate an understanding of what has been taught
▶ demonstrate the ability to perform new health-related behaviors as they're taught.

Risk for injury related to improper technique
The patient will:
▶ identify factors that increase the risk of injury
▶ assist in identifying and applying safety measures to prevent injury.

Equipment
For subdermal implants
Sterile surgical drapes • sterile gloves • antiseptic solution • local anesthetic • set of implants • needles • 5-ml syringe • #11 scalpel • #10 trocar • forceps • sutures • sterile gauze • tape

For subcutaneous implants
Alcohol pad • drug implant in a preloaded syringe • local anesthetic (for some patients)

For radiation implants
RADIATION PRECAUTION sign for the patient's door • warning labels for the patient's wristband and personal belongings • film badge or pocket dosimeter • lead-lined container • long-handled forceps • masking tape • portable lead shield • optional: tracheostomy tray

Implementation
▶ Explain the procedure and its benefits and risks to the patient and show her a set of implants.

Inserting subdermal implants
▶ Assist the patient into a supine position on the examination table. During the procedure, stay and provide support as necessary.
▶ After anesthetizing the upper portion of the nondominant arm, the doctor will put on sterile gloves and use a trocar to insert each capsule through a 2-mm (⅛″) incision. After insertion, he'll remove the trocar and palpate the

area. He'll then close the incision and cover it with a dry compress and sterile gauze.

The steps below describe how levonorgestrel subdermal contraceptive implants are inserted:

▶ Have the patient lie supine on the examination table and flex the elbow of her nondominant arm so that her hand is opposite her head.

▶ Swab the insertion site with antiseptic solution. (The ideal insertion site is inside the upper arm about 3″ to 4″ [7.5 to 10 cm] above the elbow.)

▶ Cover the arm above and below the insertion site with sterile surgical drapes.

▶ The doctor puts on sterile gloves, fills a 5-ml syringe with a local anesthetic, inserts the needle under the skin, and injects a small amount of anesthetic into several areas, in a fanlike pattern.

▶ The doctor uses the scalpel to make a small, shallow incision (about 2 mm [⅛″]) through the skin.

▶ Next, he inserts the tip of the trocar through the incision at a shallow angle beneath the skin. He makes sure the trocar bevel is up *so that he can place the capsules in a superficial plane.* He advances the trocar slowly to the first mark near the hub of the trocar. The tip of the trocar should now be about 1½″ to 2″ (4 to 4.5 cm) from the incision site. The doctor then removes the obturator and loads the first capsule into the trocar.

▶ He gently advances the capsule with the obturator toward the tip of the trocar until he feels resistance. Next, he inserts each succeeding capsule beside the last one in a fanlike pattern. With the forefinger and middle finger of his free hand, he fixes the position of the previous capsule, advancing the trocar along the tips of his fingers. *This ensures a suitable distance of about 15 degrees between capsules and keeps the trocar from puncturing the previously inserted capsules.*

Inserting subcutaneous implants

▶ Help the patient into the supine position and drape him so that his abdomen is accessible. Remove the syringe from the package and make sure you can see the drug in the chamber. Put on gloves. Then, clean a small area on the patient's upper abdominal wall with the alcohol pad.

▶ As you stretch the skin at the injection site with one hand, grip the needle with the fingers of your other hand around the barrel of the syringe. Insert the needle into subcutaneous fat at a 45-degree angle. Don't attempt to aspirate. If blood appears in the syringe, withdraw the needle and inject a new preloaded syringe and needle at another site.

▶ Next, change the direction of the needle so that it's parallel to the abdominal wall. With the barrel hub touching the patient's skin, push the needle in. Then withdraw it about ½″ (1.3 cm) *to create a space for the drug.* Depress the plunger. Withdraw the needle and bandage the site with sterile gauze and tape.

▶ Inspect the tip of the needle. If you can see the metal tip of the plunger, the drug has been discharged.

▶ Remove and discard your gloves.

Inserting radiation implants

▶ To prepare for a radiation implant, place the lead-lined container and long-handled forceps in a corner of the patient's room. Also, place the lead shield in the back of the room so it can be worn when providing care. With masking tape, mark a safe line on the floor 6′ (1.8 m) from the bed *to warn visitors of the danger of radiation exposure.* Place a RADIATION PRECAUTION sign on the patient's door and warning labels on the patient's wristband and personal belongings.

▶ Place an emergency tracheotomy tray in the room if an implant will be inserted in the patient's mouth or neck.

▶ To insert the implant, the doctor puts on gloves, makes a small incision in the skin, and creates a pocket in the tissue. He inserts the implant and closes the incision. The doctor takes off the gloves and discards them. If the patient is being treated for tonsillar cancer, he'll undergo a bronchoscopy, during which radioactive pellets are implanted in tonsillar tissue.

▶ Your role in the implant procedure is to explain the treatment and its goals to the patient. Review radiation safety procedures and visitation policies. Talk with the patient about long-term physical and emotional aspects of the therapy and discuss home care.

Special considerations
Special care may be necessary, depending on the type of implant used.

Subdermal implants
▶ Tell the patient to resume normal activities but to protect the site during the first few days after implantation. Advise her not to bump the insertion site and to keep the area dry and covered with a gauze bandage for 3 days.

▶ Tell the patient to report signs of bleeding or infection at the insertion site.

▶ Tell the patient to notify the doctor immediately if one of the implanted

capsules falls out before the skin heals over the implants. If it's a contraceptive implant, it may no longer be effective. Advise the patient to use alternative means of contraception until she sees the doctor. If pregnancy is suspected, the implants must be removed immediately.

Subcutaneous implants
▶ Be aware that if an implant must be removed, a doctor will order an X-ray to locate it.

▶ Tell the patient to check the administration site for signs of infection or bleeding.

▶ Goserelin implants must be changed every 28 days. Female patients should be advised to use a nonhormonal form of contraception.

Radiation implants
▶ Know that if laboratory work is required during treatment, a technician wearing a film badge will obtain the specimen, affix a RADIATION PRECAUTION label to the specimen container, and alert laboratory personnel. If urine tests are needed, ask the radiation oncology department or laboratory technician how to transport the specimens safely.

▶ Minimize your own exposure to radiation. Wear a personal, nontransferable film badge or dosimeter at waist level during your entire shift. Turn in the film badge regularly. Pocket dosimeters measure immediate exposure.

▶ Use the principles of time, distance, and shielding. *Time:* Plan to give care in the shortest time possible. Less time equals less exposure. *Distance:* Work as far away from the radiation source as possible. Give care from the side opposite the implant or from a position that allows the greatest working distance possible. Prepare the patient's meal trays outside his room. *Shielding:* Wear a portable shield, if necessary.

▶ Make sure that the patient's room is monitored daily by the radiation oncology department and that disposable items are monitored and removed according to your facility's policy.

▶ Keep away staff members and visitors who are pregnant or trying to conceive or father a child. *The gonads and a developing embryo or fetus are highly susceptible to the damaging effects of ionizing radiation.*

▶ If you must take the patient out of his room, notify the appropriate department of the patient's status to allow time for the necessary preparations.

▶ Collect a dislodged implant with long-handled forceps and place it in a lead-lined container.

▶ A patient with a permanent implant may not be released until his radioactivity level is less than 5 millirems/hour at a distance of about 3′ (0.9 m).

▶ If a patient with an implant dies while on the unit, notify the radiation oncology staff *so that a temporary implant can be properly removed and stored.* If the implant was permanent, the staff will also determine which precautions should be followed after postmortem care measures.

Complications
Complications vary, depending on the type of implant used.

Subdermal implants
Possible adverse reactions to levonorgestrel include hyperpigmentation at the insertion site, menstrual irregularities, headache, nervousness, nausea, dizziness, adnexal enlargement, dermatitis, acne, appetite and weight changes, mastalgia, hirsutism, and alopecia. More serious reactions include breast abnormalities, mammographic changes, diabetes, elevated cholesterol or triglyceride levels, hypertension, seizures, depression, and gallbladder, heart, or kidney disease.

Subcutaneous implants
Goserelin implants may cause anemia, lethargy, pain, dizziness, insomnia, anxiety, depression, headache, chills, fever, edema, heart failure, arrhythmias, cerebrovascular accident, hypertension, peripheral vascular disease, nausea, vomiting, diarrhea, impotence, renal insufficiency, urinary obstruction, rash, sweating, hot flashes, gout, hyperglycemia, weight increase, and breast swelling and tenderness.

Radiation implants
Depending on the implant site and dosage, complications include implant dislodgment, tissue fibrosis, xerostomia, radiation pneumonitis, airway obstruction, muscle atrophy, sterility, vaginal dryness or stenosis, fistulas, altered bowel habits, diarrhea, hypothyroidism, infection, cystitis, myelosuppression, neurotoxicity, and secondary cancers.

Documentation
For subdermal and subcutaneous implants, document the name of the drug, insertion or administration site, date and time of insertion, and patient's response to the procedure. Note the date that implants should be removed and a new set inserted or the date of the next administration as appropriate.

For radiation implants, document radiation precautions taken during treatment, adverse reactions, patient and family teaching and their responses, patient's tolerance of isolation procedures and the family's compliance with procedures, and referrals to local cancer services.

DRUG THERAPY IN OLDER ADULTS

Four out of five persons over age 65 have one or more chronic disorders. This helps explain why elderly people consume more drugs than any other age-group. Although elderly people represent only 12% of the population, they take 30% to 40% of the prescription drugs dispensed. That is about 400 million prescriptions a year — twice the number of prescriptions filled for people under age 65.

Drug therapy for elderly patients presents a special set of problems rooted in age-related changes. Physiologically, aging alters body composition and triggers changes in the digestive system, liver, and kidneys. These changes affect drug metabolism, absorption, distribution, and excretion and, consequently, may lead to the need for altered drug dosages and administration techniques. They also potentiate adverse reactions to drugs and may interfere with therapeutic compliance. (See *How age affects drug action* and *Modifying I.M. injections,* page 236.)

Even when an elderly patient receives the optimum drug dosage, he's still at risk for an adverse drug reaction. Ongoing physiologic changes, poor compliance with the drug regimen, and greater drug consumption contribute to elderly patients experiencing twice as many adverse reactions as younger patients. In fact, about 40% of the people who experience adverse drug reactions are over age 60.

How age affects drug action

As the body ages, body structures and systems change. This affects how the body responds to medications. Some common changes that significantly affect medication administration follow.

Body composition
As a person grows older, his total body mass and lean body mass tend to decrease while body fat tends to increase. These factors affect the relationship between a drug's concentration and solubility in the body.

Digestive system
Decreases in gastric acid secretion and GI motility lead to the body's decreased ability to absorb many drugs well. This can cause problems with certain drugs — for example, digoxin, whose narrow therapeutic range is tied closely to absorption.

Hepatic system
Advancing age reduces blood supply, and certain liver enzymes become less active. As a result, the liver loses some of its ability to metabolize drugs. With reduced liver function comes more intense drug effects as higher levels of a drug remain in circulation. This increases the incidence of drug toxicity.

Renal system
Kidney function diminishes with age. This alone may impair drug elimination by 50% or more. In many cases, decreased kidney function leads to increased blood levels of certain drugs.

Many older patients who experience signs and symptoms of adverse drug reactions (such as confusion, weakness, and lethargy) blame them on the disease rather than on the drugs they're taking. If the adverse reaction is uniden-

Modifying I.M. injections

Before you give an I.M. injection to an elderly patient, remember the physical changes that accompany aging and choose your equipment, site, and technique accordingly.

Choosing a needle
Remember that an elderly patient usually has less subcutaneous tissue and less muscle mass than a younger patient—especially in the buttocks and deltoids. As a result, you may need to use a shorter needle than you would for a younger adult.

Selecting a site
Also, remember that an elderly patient typically has more fat around the hips, abdomen, and thigh areas. This makes the vastus lateralis muscle and ventrogluteal area (gluteus medius and minimus but not gluteus maximus muscles) the primary injection sites.

You should be able to palpate the muscle in these areas easily. However, if the patient is extremely thin, gently pinch the muscle *to elevate it and to avoid putting the needle completely through it (which will alter the absorption and distribution of the drug).*

Caution: Never give an I.M. injection in an immobile limb *because of poor drug absorption and the risk that a sterile abscess will form at the injection site.*

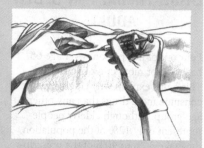

Checking technique
To avoid inserting the needle in a blood vessel, pull back on the plunger and look for blood before injecting the drug. Because of age-related vascular changes, elderly patients are also at greater risk for hematomas. *To check bleeding after an I.M. injection,* you may need to apply direct pressure over the puncture site for a longer time than usual.

Gently massage the injection site *to aid drug absorption and distribution.* However, avoid site massage with certain drugs given by the Z-track injection technique, such as iron dextran.

tified or misidentified, the patient will probably continue taking the drug. To compound the problem, if the patient has multiple physical dysfunctions or adverse drug reactions or both, he may consult several doctors or specialists who—unknown to one another—may prescribe more drugs. If the patient's drug history remains uninvestigated and the patient takes additional nonprescription drugs to relieve common complaints (such as indigestion, dizziness, and constipation), he may innocently fall into a pattern of inappropriate and excessive drug use. Known as polypharmacy, this pattern imperils the patient's safety and the drug regimen's effectiveness.

Although many drugs can cause adverse reactions, most serious reactions in elderly patients result from relatively few drugs—namely diuretics, anticoagulants, antihypertensives, digitalis glycosides, corticosteroids, sleeping aids, and nonprescription drugs.

Finally, the elderly patient may have difficulty complying with his drug regimen because of hearing and vision deficits, forgetfulness, the need for multiple drug therapy, poor understanding of dosage and directions, and various socioeconomic factors (such as poverty and social isolation). Ensuring successful compliance with drug therapy requires involving family members, the pharmacist, and other caregivers in supervision and teaching tailored to the patient's needs.

Key nursing diagnoses and patient outcomes

Noncompliance related to the medication regimen
The patient will:
► identify factors that influence noncompliance
► contract with the caregiver to adhere to the medication regimen
► demonstrate the ability to administer medications
► state the reason for adhering to the medication regimen.

Equipment

Patient's medication record • appropriate drugs • written dosage instructions • optional: compliance aids (such as pill containers, calendar or other large-print teaching aids, and premeasured injections)

Implementation

Noncompliance in elderly patients is so prevalent that most nurses rank handling it as a top priority when planning nursing care. Follow these procedures to assess the patient's ability or motivation to follow a drug regimen.

Assessing compliance ability

► Review the patient's complaint and obtain a comprehensive health and drug history. Question the patient about use of herbal preparations or other complementary therapies.
► Keeping in mind that discharge planning begins at admission, evaluate the patient's physical ability to take drugs. Can he read drug labels and directions? Does he identify drugs by sight or by touch? Can he open drug bottles easily? If he's disabled by Parkinson's disease or arthritis, for example, or if he lacks manual dexterity for any reason, advise him to ask his pharmacist for snap or screw caps (rather than childproof closures) for his drug containers.
► Evaluate the patient's cognitive skills. Can he remember to take prescribed drugs on time and regularly? Can he remember where he stored his drugs? If not, refer him to appropriate community resources for supervision.
► Assess the patient's lifestyle. Does he live with family or friends? If so, include them in your patient-teaching sessions, if possible. Does he live alone or with a debilitated spouse? If so, he'll need continuing support from a visiting nurse or other caregiver.
► Keep in mind that inadequate supervision may result in drug misuse. Make appropriate referrals and contact appropriate social agencies *to ensure compliance and safety and to provide financial assistance, if necessary.*
► Assess the patient's beliefs about drug use. For example, the patient may believe that chronic use of medication is a sign of illness or weakness and therefore may take his medications erratically.
► Ask the patient whether his prescribed medication regimen interferes with his daily routine.

Preventing reactions that impede compliance

▶ Discuss the patient's drug therapy with him. As he receives drugs, name them, explain their intended effect and describe possible adverse reactions to watch for and report. (See *Recognizing common adverse reactions in elderly patients.*)

▶ Tell the patient that you'll ask questions *to help identify (or reduce the risk of) harmful food or drug interactions (such as those caused by alcohol and caffeine) that may interfere with compliance.*

▶ Ask the patient about all drugs — prescription and nonprescription — he's currently taking and those he has taken in the past. If possible, ask to see samples. Have him name each drug and tell you why, when, and how often he takes it. Remember, the patient may have drugs prescribed by more than one doctor. Also ask whether he's taking any drugs originally prescribed for another person (a common occurrence).

▶ If your facility has a specially designed computer program, use it *to help prevent possible drug interactions.* Enter all the data you've collected on drug dosage, frequency, and administration route into a master file of drugs commonly used by elderly patients, such as anticoagulants (warfarin), benzodiazepines (diazepam), beta-adrenergic blockers (propranolol), calcium channel blockers (verapamil), digitalis glycosides (digoxin), and diuretics (furosemide). From this information the computer compiles a list of the patient's drugs, possible adverse reactions, potential interactions, and suggested interventions. Then review the findings with the patient. *If he knows what to expect, he'll be more likely to comply with treatment.* (If you don't have access to such technology, you can compile a similar list using a reputable drug reference.)

▶ Alternatively, encourage the patient to purchase drugs from only one pharmacy, preferably one that maintains a drug profile for each customer. Advise him to consult the pharmacist, who can anticipate drug interactions before they occur.

▶ Inform the patient about specific food-drug interactions. Based on the information in your drug history, provide a list of food items to avoid.

Boosting therapeutic compliance

▶ *To circumvent noncompliance caused by visual impairment,* provide dosage instructions in large print, if necessary.

▶ *To alter eating habits that lead to noncompliance,* emphasize which drugs the patient must take with food and which he must take on an empty stomach. Explain that taking some drugs on an empty stomach may cause nausea, whereas taking some drugs on a full stomach may interfere with absorption. Also find out whether the patient eats regularly or skips meals. If he skips meals, he may be skipping doses too. As needed, help him coordinate his drug administration schedule with his eating habits.

▶ *To correct problems related to drug form and administration,* help the patient find easier ways to take medicine. For example, if he can't swallow pills or capsules, switch to a liquid or powdered form of the drug, if possible. Or, suggest that he slide the tablet down with soft food such as applesauce. Keep in mind which tablets you can crush and which you can't. For example, enteric-coated tablets, timed-release capsules, and sublingual and buccal tablets shouldn't be crushed. *Doing so may affect absorption and effectiveness.*

Recognizing common adverse reactions in elderly patients

Common signs and symptoms of adverse reactions to medications include hives, impotence, incontinence, nausea, and rashes. Elderly patients are especially susceptible and may experience serious adverse reactions, such as orthostatic hypotension, dehydration, altered mental status, anorexia, blood disorders, and tardive dyskinesia.

Some adverse reactions, such as anxiety, confusion, and forgetfulness, may be dismissed as typical elderly behavior rather than recognized as drug effects.

Orthostatic hypotension

Marked by light-headedness or faintness and unsteady footing, orthostatic hypotension occurs as a common adverse effect of antidepressant, antihypertensive, antipsychotic, and sedative medications.

To prevent accidents such as falls, warn the patient not to sit up or get out of bed too rapidly. Instruct him to call for assistance in walking if he feels dizzy or faint.

Dehydration

If the patient is taking diuretics such as hydrochlorothiazide, be alert for dehydration and electrolyte imbalances. Monitor blood levels and provide potassium supplements as ordered.

Oral dryness results from many medications. If anticholinergic medications cause dryness, suggest sucking on sugarless candy for relief.

Altered mental status

Agitation or confusion may follow ingestion of alcohol or anticholinergic, antidiuretic, antihypertensive, antipsychotic, antianxiety, and antidepressant medications. Paradoxically, depression is a common adverse effect of antidepressant medications.

Anorexia

This is a warning sign of toxicity — especially from digoxin, bronchodilators, and antihistamines. That is why the doctor usually prescribes a very low initial dose.

Blood disorders

If the patient takes an anticoagulant such as warfarin, watch for signs of easy bruising or bleeding (such as excessive bleeding after toothbrushing). Easy bruising or bleeding may be a sign of other problems, such as blood dyscrasias and thrombocytopenia. Drugs that may cause these reactions include several antineoplastic agents (such as methotrexate), antibiotics (such as nitrofurantoin), and anticonvulsants (such as valproic acid and phenytoin). A patient who bruises easily should report this sign to his doctor immediately.

Tardive dyskinesia

Characterized by abnormal tongue movements, lip pursing, grimacing, blinking, and gyrating motions of the face and extremities, tardive dyskinesia may be triggered by psychotropic drugs, such as haloperidol and chlorpromazine.

Some crushed drugs may taste bitter and may stain or irritate oral mucosa.
► Suggest the use of compliance aids, such as pill containers and premeasured injections.
► If mobility or transportation deters compliance, help the patient locate a pharmacy that refills and delivers prescriptions. If appropriate, consider using a mail-order pharmacy.
► If forgetfulness interferes with compliance, devise a system for helping the patient remember to take his drugs properly. Suggest that the patient or a family member purchase or make a scheduling aid, such as a calendar, a

Using compliance aids

To help your patient comply with oral or injectable drug therapy safety, you or a family member may premeasure doses for him, using compliance aids such as those shown below or ones you create yourself. Most pharmacies or community service agencies can supply similar aids.

One-day pill pack

A plastic box with four lidded medication compartments marked "breakfast," "lunch," "dinner," and "bedtime" helps the patient see whether he has taken all of the medications prescribed for 1 day. The lids may be embossed with braille characters, if needed.

The patient, caregiver, or visiting nurse must remember to fill the device each day. Because it's small, the device doesn't hold many tablets or capsules.

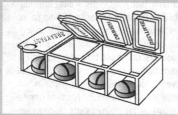

Seven-day pill reminder

The boxes shown here will help the patient remember whether he has taken all the tablets and capsules prescribed for each day of the week. (The days of the week appear in both braille characters and printed letters.)

Like the 1-day pill container, this device is inappropriate for large numbers of tablets or capsules that must be taken at different times each day.

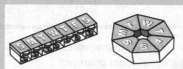

Homemade dosing aids

Show the patient and his caregivers how to make their own compliance aids by labeling clean, empty jars, extra prescription bottles (obtainable from pharmacists), or envelopes with the drug name, the time of day, and the day of the week to take the medication. Recommend that they use a separate container for each time and that they fill this container every morning with the correct doses of each medication.

Syringe-filling device

This device precisely measures insulin doses for a visually impaired diabetic patient. Designed for use with a disposable U-100 syringe and insulin bottle, the device is set by the caregiver to accommodate the syringe's width. She then positions the plunger at the point determined by the dose and tightens the stop. When the device is set, the patient can draw up the precise dose ordered for each injection.

As with any device, several drawbacks must be considered. This device can't be used if insulin needs to be mixed or if doses vary. The settings must be checked and adjusted whenever the syringe size or type changes. The screws must be checked regularly because they loosen with repeated use.

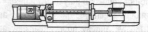

Syringe scale magnifier

This device helps a visually impaired diabetic patient read syringe markings, thereby enabling him to fill his own syringe. The plastic magnifier snaps onto the syringe barrel. This device may be impractical for a patient with arthritis who can't easily attach the magnifier to the syringe.

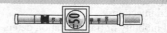

checklist, an alarm wristwatch, or a compartmented drug container. (See *Using compliance aids.*)

▶ Some patients may try to save money by not having prescriptions filled or refilled or by taking fewer doses than ordered to make the drug last longer. If financial considerations are preventing your patient's compliance, help him explore available resources. Suggest that he use the less expensive generic equivalents of name-brand drugs whenever possible. Also, explore ways that family members can help or refer the patient to the social services department and appropriate community agencies. Many states have programs to help low-income elderly patients buy needed medications.

Special considerations

▶ Advise the patient to contact you or his doctor before taking any nonprescription medications *to avoid adverse drug interactions.* If necessary, regularly monitor serum levels of such drugs as digoxin and potassium *to avoid toxicity.*

▶ When the doctor advises discontinuing a drug, instruct the patient to discard it — in the toilet, if possible. *This prevents others from using the drug and ensures that the patient won't continue taking it by mistake.*

▶ *To avoid improper storage and possible drug deterioration,* advise the patient to keep all prescribed drugs in their original containers. Tell him to keep in mind that some drugs deteriorate when exposed to light and that others decompose if they come in contact with other drugs, for example, in a pillbox. Before the patient stores drugs together, advise him to consult his pharmacist or doctor.

▶ Suggest that the patient store his medications in an area that is well-lit (but protected from direct sunlight), not too warm or humid (not the bathroom medicine cabinet), and some distance from his bedside (not on a bedside table). *If he keeps drugs at his bedside, he could accidentally overdose by taking them before he's fully awake and alert.*

Home care

If the patient is discharged from the facility with a new drug regimen, schedule him for follow-up care by a visiting nurse to assess his ability to follow the regimen and to monitor his response to therapy.

Documentation

Document all assessment findings and laboratory test results in the patient's chart. Record all instructions and teaching materials given to the patient, family members, or other caregivers. Keep a record of all drugs, dosages, adverse reactions, and interventions. Describe the patient's understanding of his drug regimen. Note all health and social service agency referrals.

DYING PATIENT CARE

A patient needs intensive physical and emotional support as he approaches death. Signs of impending death include reduced respiratory rate and depth, decreased or absent blood pressure, weak or erratic pulse rate, lowered skin temperature, decreased level of consciousness (LOC), diminished sensorium and neuromuscular control, diaphoresis, pallor, cyanosis, and mottling.

Emotional support for the dying patient and his family most commonly means simple reassurance and the nurse's physical presence to help ease fear and loneliness. More intense emotional support is important at much earlier stages, especially for patients with long-term progressive illnesses who can work through the stages of dying. (See *Five stages of dying*.)

Respect the patient's wishes about extraordinary means of supporting life. The patient may have signed a living will. This document, legally binding in most states, declares the patient's desire for a death unimpeded by the artificial support of defibrillators, ventilators, life-sustaining drugs, auxiliary hearts, and so on. If the patient has signed such a document, the nurse must respect his wishes and communicate the doctor's "no code" order to all staff members.

Key nursing diagnoses and patient outcomes

Death anxiety
The patient will:
▶ state a feeling of anxiety
▶ use support systems to assist with coping
▶ perform stress reduction techniques to avoid anxiety symptoms.

Powerlessness related to the disease outcome
The patient will:
▶ identify feelings of powerlessness associated with his disease
▶ describe modifications or adjustments to the environment that allow feelings of control
▶ participate in self-care activities (specify)
▶ state feelings of regained control.

Equipment

Bed linens • gowns • gloves • water-filled basin • soap • washcloth • towels • lotion • linen-saver pads • petroleum jelly • suction equipment as necessary • optional: indwelling urinary catheter

Implementation

▶ Assemble equipment at the patient's bedside as needed.

Meeting physical needs

▶ Take vital signs often and observe for pallor, diaphoresis, and decreased LOC.
▶ Reposition the patient in bed at least every 2 hours *because sensation, reflexes, and mobility diminish first in the legs and gradually in the arms.* Make sure the bed sheets cover him loosely *to reduce discomfort caused by pressure on arms and legs.*
▶ When the patient's vision and hearing start to fail, turn his head toward the light and speak to him from near the head of the bed. *Because hearing may be acute despite loss of consciousness,* avoid whispering or speaking inappropriately about the patient in his presence.
▶ Change the bed linens and the patient's gown as needed. Provide skin care during gown changes and adjust the room temperature for patient comfort, if necessary.
▶ Observe for incontinence or anuria, *which is a result of diminished neuromuscular control or decreased renal function.* If necessary, obtain an order to catheterize the patient or place linen-saver pads beneath the patient's buttocks. Put on gloves and provide perineal care with soap, a washcloth, and towels *to prevent irritation.*
▶ With suction equipment, suction the patient's mouth and upper airway *to re-*

Five stages of dying

According to Elisabeth Kübler-Ross, author of *On Death and Dying*, the dying patient may progress through five psychological stages in preparation for death. Although each patient experiences these stages differently, and not necessarily in this order, understanding the stages will help you meet the patient's needs.

Denial

When the patient first learns of his terminal illness, he'll refuse to accept the diagnosis. He may experience physical symptoms similar to a stress reaction—shock, fainting, pallor, sweating, tachycardia, nausea, and GI disorders. During this stage, be honest with the patient but not blunt or callous. Maintain communication with him so he can discuss his feelings when he accepts the reality of death. Don't force the patient to confront this reality.

Anger

When the patient stops denying his impending death, he may show deep resentment toward those who will live on after he dies—to you, to the facility staff, and to his own family. Although you may instinctively draw back from the patient or even resent this behavior, remember that he's dying and has a right to be angry. After you accept his anger, you can help him find different ways to express it and can help his family to understand it.

Bargaining

Although the patient acknowledges his impending death, he attempts to bargain with

God or fate for more time. He will probably strike this bargain secretly. If he does confide in you, don't urge him to keep his promises.

Depression

In this stage, the patient may first experience regrets about his past and then grieve about his current condition. He may withdraw from his friends, family, doctor, and from you. He may suffer from anorexia, increased fatigue, or self-neglect. You may find him sitting alone, in tears. Accept the patient's sorrow and if he talks to you, listen. Provide comfort by touch as appropriate. Resist the temptation to make optimistic remarks or cheerful small talk.

Acceptance

In this last stage, the patient accepts the inevitability and imminence of his death—without emotion. The patient may simply desire the quiet company of a family member or friend. If, for some reason, a family member or friend can't be present, stay with the patient to satisfy his final need. Remember, however, that many patients die before reaching this stage.

---

move secretions. Elevate the head of the bed *to decrease respiratory resistance.* As the patient's condition deteriorates, he may breathe mostly through his mouth.
▶ Offer fluids frequently and lubricate the patient's lips and mouth with petroleum jelly *to counteract dryness.*
▶ If the comatose patient's eyes are open, provide appropriate eye care *to*

prevent corneal ulceration. Such ulceration can cause blindness and prevent the use of these tissues for transplantation should the patient die.
▶ Provide ordered pain medication as needed. Keep in mind that, as circulation diminishes, medications given I.M. will be poorly absorbed. Medications

Understanding organ and tissue donation

A federal regulation enacted in 1998 requires facilities to report all deaths to the regional organ procurement organization. This regulation was enacted so that no potential donor is missed. The regulation ensures that the family of every potential donor will understand the option to donate. According to the American Medical Association, about 25 kinds of organs and tissues are being transplanted. Although the donor organ requirements vary, the typical donor must be between the ages of newborn and 60 years and free from transmissible disease. Tissue donations are less restrictive, and some tissue banks will accept skin from donors up to age 75.

Collection of most organs, such as the heart, liver, kidney, or pancreas, requires that the patient be pronounced brain dead and kept physically alive until the organs are harvested. Tissue such as eyes, skin, bone, and heart valves may be taken after death. Contact your regional organ procurement organization for specific organ donation criteria or to identify a potential donor. If you don't know the regional organ procurement organization in your area, call the United Network for Organ Sharing at (804) 330-8500.

should be given I.V., if possible, *for optimum results.*

Meeting emotional needs

▶ Fully explain all care and treatments to the patient even if he's unconscious *because he may still be able to hear.* Answer any questions as candidly as possible without sounding callous.
▶ Allow the patient to express his feelings, which may range from anger to loneliness. Take time to talk with the patient. Sit near the head of the bed and avoid looking rushed or unconcerned.
▶ Notify family members, if they're absent, when the patient wishes to see them. Let the patient and his family discuss death at their own pace.
▶ Offer to contact a member of the clergy or social services department, if appropriate.

Special considerations

▶ If the patient has signed a living will, the doctor will write a "no code" order on his progress notes and order sheets. Know your state's policy regarding the living will. If it's legal, transfer the "no code" order to the patient's chart or Kardex and, at the end of your shift, inform the incoming staff of this order.
▶ If family members remain with the patient, show them the location of bathrooms, lounges, and cafeterias. Explain the patient's needs, treatments, and plan of care to them. If appropriate, offer to teach them specific skills so they can take part in nursing care. Emphasize that their efforts are important and effective. As the patient's death approaches, give them emotional support.
▶ At an appropriate time, ask the family whether they have considered organ and tissue donation. Check the patient's records *to determine whether he completed an organ donor card.* (See *Understanding organ and tissue donation.*)

Documentation

Record changes in the patient's vital signs, intake and output, and LOC. Note the times of cardiac arrest and the end of respiration and notify the doctor when these occur.

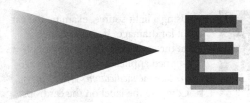

EARDROP INSTILLATION

Eardrops may be instilled to treat infection and inflammation, soften cerumen for later removal, produce local anesthesia, or facilitate removal of an insect trapped in the ear by immobilizing and smothering it.

Instillation of eardrops is usually contraindicated if the patient has a perforated eardrum, but it may be permitted with certain medications and adherence to sterile technique. Other conditions may also prohibit instillation of certain medications into the ear. For instance, instillation of drops containing hydrocortisone is contraindicated if the patient has herpes, another viral infection, or a fungal infection.

Key nursing diagnoses and patient outcomes

Deficient knowledge related to lack of exposure to eardrop instillation
The patient will:
▶ state or demonstrate an understanding of what has been taught
▶ demonstrate an ability to perform new health-related behaviors as they're taught.

Risk for injury related to improper technique
The patient will:

▶ identify factors that increase the risk of injury
▶ assist in identifying and applying safety measures to prevent injury.

Equipment

Prescribed eardrops • patient's medication record and chart • light source • facial tissue or cotton-tipped applicator • optional: cotton ball and bowl of warm water

Preparation of equipment

Verify the order on the patient's medication record by checking it against the doctor's order.

To avoid adverse effects (such as vertigo, nausea, and pain) resulting from instillation of eardrops that are too cold, warm the medication to body temperature in the bowl of warm water or carry it in your pocket for 30 minutes before administration. If necessary, test the temperature of the medication by placing a drop on your wrist. *(If the medication is too hot, it may burn the patient's eardrum.)*

Implementation

▶ Wash your hands.
▶ Confirm the patient's identity by asking his name and checking the name, room number, and bed number on his wristband.
▶ Provide privacy, if possible. Explain the procedure to the patient.

Positioning the patient for eardrop instillation

Before instilling eardrops, have the patient lie on his side. Then straighten the patient's ear canal to help the medication reach the eardrum. For an adult, gently pull the auricle up and back; for an infant or a young child, gently pull down and back.

Adult

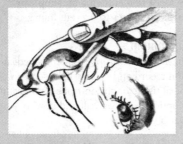

Child

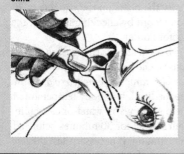

▶ Using a light source, examine the ear canal for drainage. If you find any, clean the canal with the tissue or cotton-tipped applicator *because drainage can reduce the medication's effectiveness.*

▶ Compare the label on the eardrops with the order on the patient's medication record. Check the label again while drawing the medication into the dropper. Check the label for the final time before returning the eardrops to the shelf or drawer.

▶ *To avoid damaging the ear canal with the dropper,* gently support the hand holding the dropper against the patient's head. Straighten the patient's ear canal once again and instill the ordered number of drops. *To avoid patient discomfort,* aim the dropper so that the drops fall against the sides of the ear canal, not on the eardrum. Hold the ear canal in position until you see the medication disappear down the canal. Then release the ear.

▶ Instruct the patient to remain on his side for 5 to 10 minutes *to let the medication run down into the ear canal.*

▶ If ordered, tuck the cotton ball loosely into the opening of the ear canal *to prevent the medication from leaking out.* Be careful not to insert it too deeply into the canal *because this would prevent drainage of secretions and increase pressure on the eardrum.*

▶ Clean and dry the outer ear.

▶ If ordered, repeat the procedure in the other ear after 5 to 10 minutes.

▶ Assist the patient into a comfortable position.

▶ Wash your hands.

Special considerations

▶ Remember that some conditions make the normally tender ear canal even more sensitive, so be especially gentle when performing this procedure. Wash your hands before and after car-

▶ Have the patient lie on the side opposite the affected ear.

▶ Straighten the patient's ear canal. For an adult, pull the auricle of the ear up and back. (See *Positioning the patient for eardrop instillation.*)

 Age alert For an infant or a child under age 3, gently pull the auricle down and back because the ear canal is straighter at this age.

ing for the patient's ear and between caring for each ear.

▶ *To prevent injury to the eardrum,* never insert a cotton-tipped applicator into the ear canal past the point where you can see the tip. After instilling eardrops to soften the cerumen, irrigate the ear as ordered *to facilitate its removal.*

▶ If the patient has vertigo, keep the side rails of his bed up and help him during the procedure as needed. Also, move slowly and unhurriedly *to avoid exacerbating his vertigo.*

▶ Teach the patient to instill the eardrops correctly so that he can continue treatment at home, if necessary. Review the procedure and let the patient try it while you observe.

Documentation

Record the medication used, the ear treated, and the date, time, and number of eardrops instilled. Also document any signs or symptoms that the patient experienced during the procedure, such as drainage, redness, vertigo, nausea, and pain.

EAR IRRIGATION

Irrigating the ear involves washing the external auditory canal with a stream of solution to clean the canal of discharges, soften and remove impacted cerumen, or dislodge a foreign body. Sometimes, irrigation aims to relieve localized inflammation and discomfort. The procedure must be performed carefully to avoid causing the patient discomfort or vertigo and to avoid increasing the risk of otitis externa. Because irrigation may contaminate the middle ear if the tympanic membrane is ruptured, an otoscopic examination always precedes ear irrigation.

This procedure is contraindicated when a vegetable (such as a pea) obstructs the auditory canal. This type of foreign body attracts and absorbs moisture. In contact with an irrigant or other solution, it swells, causing intense pain and complicating removal of the object by irrigation. Ear irrigation is also contraindicated if the patient has a cold, a fever, an ear infection, or an injured or ruptured tympanic membrane. The presence of a battery (or a battery part) in the ear also contraindicates irrigation because battery acid could leak, and irrigation would spread caustic material throughout the canal.

Key nursing diagnoses and patient outcomes

Deficient knowledge related to lack of exposure to ear irrigation
The patient will:

▶ state or demonstrate an understanding of what has been taught

▶ demonstrate an ability to perform new health related behaviors as they're taught.

Risk for injury related to improper technique
The patient will:

▶ identify factors that increase the risk of injury

▶ assist in identifying and applying safety measures to prevent injury.

Equipment

Ear irrigation syringe (rubber bulb) • otoscope with aural speculum • prescribed irrigant • large basin • linen-saver pad and bath towel • emesis basin • cotton-tipped applicators • 4″ × 4″ gauze pad • optional: adjustable light (such as a gooseneck lamp), container for irrigant, tubing, clamp, and syringe with ear tip, normal saline solution, gloves, and cotton

How to irrigate the ear canal

Follow these guidelines for irrigating the ear canal:
■ Gently pull the auricle up and back to straighten the ear canal. (For a child, pull the ear down and back.)
■ Have the patient hold an emesis basin beneath the ear to catch returning irrigant. Position the tip of the irrigating syringe at the meatus of the auditory canal (as shown below). Don't block the meatus because you'll impede backflow and raise pressure in the canal.

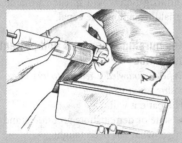

■ Tilt the patient's head toward the opposite ear and point the syringe tip upward and toward the posterior ear canal (as shown below). This angle prevents damage to the tympanic membrane and guards against pushing debris farther into the canal.

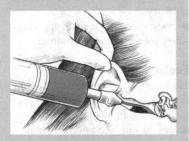

■ Direct a steady stream of irrigant against the upper wall of the ear canal, and inspect return fluid for cloudiness, cerumen, blood, or foreign matter.

Preparation of equipment

Select the appropriate syringe and obtain the prescribed irrigant. Put the container of irrigant into the large basin filled with hot water *to warm the solution to body temperature: 98.6° F (37° C).* Avoid extreme temperature changes *because they can affect inner ear fluids, causing nausea and dizziness.*

Test the temperature of the solution by sprinkling a few drops on your inner wrist. Inspect equipment (syringe or ear tips) for breaks or cracks; inspect all metal tips for roughness.

Implementation

▶ Explain the procedure to the patient, provide privacy, wash your hands, and put on gloves if you expect contact with drainage.
▶ If you haven't already done so, use the otoscope to inspect the auditory canal that will be irrigated.
▶ Help the patient to a sitting position. *To prevent the solution from running down his neck,* tilt his head slightly forward and toward the affected side. If he can't sit, have him lie on his back and tilt his head slightly forward and toward the affected ear.
▶ Make sure that you have adequate lighting.
▶ If the patient is sitting, place the linen-saver pad (covered with the bath towel) on his shoulder and upper arm, under the affected ear. If he's lying down, cover his pillow and the area under the affected ear.
▶ Have the patient hold the emesis basin close to his head under the affected ear.
▶ *To avoid getting foreign matter into the ear canal,* clean the auricle and the meatus of the auditory canal with a cotton-tipped applicator moistened

with normal saline solution or the prescribed irrigating solution.

▶ Draw the irrigant into the syringe and expel any air.

▶ Straighten the auditory canal; then insert the syringe tip and start the flow. (See *How to irrigate the ear canal.*)

▶ During irrigation, tell the patient to report pain or dizziness. If he reports either, stop the procedure, recheck the temperature of the irrigant, inspect the patient's ear with the otoscope, and resume irrigation as indicated.

▶ When the syringe is empty, remove it and inspect the return flow. Then, refill the syringe and continue the irrigation until the return flow is clear. Never use more than 500 ml of irrigant during this procedure.

▶ Remove the syringe and inspect the ear canal for cleanliness with the otoscope.

▶ Dry the patient's auricle and neck.

▶ Remove the bath towel and linen-saver pad. Help the seated patient lie on his affected side with the 4″ × 4″ gauze pad under his ear *to promote drainage of residual debris and solution.*

Special considerations

▶ Avoid dropping or squirting irrigant on the tympanic membrane. *This may startle the patient and cause discomfort.* If you're using an irrigating catheter instead of a syringe, adjust the flow of solution to a steady, comfortable rate with a flow clamp. Don't raise the container more than 6″ (15.2 cm) above the ear. *If the container is higher, the resulting pressure could damage the tympanic membrane.*

▶ If the doctor directs you to place a cotton pledget in the ear canal *to retain some of the solution,* pack the cotton

loosely. Instruct the patient not to remove it.

▶ If irrigation doesn't dislodge impacted cerumen, the doctor may order you to instill several drops of glycerin, carbamide peroxide (Debrox), or a similar preparation, two to three times daily for 2 to 3 days and then irrigate the ear again.

Complications

Possible complications include pain, vertigo, nausea, otitis externa, and otitis media (if the patient has a perforated or ruptured tympanic membrane). Forceful instillation of irrigant can rupture the tympanic membrane.

Documentation

Record the date and time of irrigation. Note which ear you irrigated. Also note the volume and the solution used, the appearance of the canal before and after irrigation, the appearance of the return flow, the patient's tolerance of the procedure, and any comments he made about his condition, especially related to his hearing acuity.

ELASTIC BANDAGE APPLICATION

Elastic bandages exert gentle, even pressure on a body part. By supporting blood vessels, these rolled bandages promote venous return and prevent pooling of blood in the legs. They're typically used in place of antiembolism stockings to prevent thrombophlebitis and pulmonary embolism in postoperative or bedridden patients who can't stimulate venous return by muscle activity.

Elastic bandages also minimize joint swelling after trauma to the musculoskeletal system. Used with a splint, they immobilize a fracture during healing. They can provide hemostatic pressure and anchor dressings over a fresh wound or after surgical procedures such as vein stripping.

Key nursing diagnoses and patient outcomes

Impaired physical mobility related to (specify)
The patient will:
▶ show no evidence of complications, such as venous stasis or thrombus formation
▶ carry out a mobility regimen
▶ achieve the highest level of mobility quickly to avoid complications.

Risk for peripheral neurovascular dysfunction related to immobility
The patient will:
▶ maintain circulation in the extremities
▶ demonstrate correct body positioning techniques
▶ have no symptoms of neurovascular compromise.

Equipment

Elastic bandage of appropriate width • tape, pins, or self-closures • gauze pads or absorbent cotton

Bandages usually come in 2″ to 6″ (5- to 15-cm) widths and 4′ and 6′ (1- and 2-m) lengths. The 3″ (7.6-cm) width is adaptable to most applications. An elastic bandage with self-closures is also available.

Preparation of equipment

Select a bandage that wraps the affected body part completely but isn't excessively long. In most cases, use a narrower bandage for wrapping the foot, lower leg, hand, or arm and a wider bandage for the thigh or trunk. The bandage should be clean and rolled before application.

Implementation

▶ Check the doctor's order and examine the area to be wrapped for lesions or skin breakdown. If these conditions are present, consult the doctor before applying the elastic bandage.
▶ Explain the procedure to the patient, provide privacy, and wash your hands thoroughly. Position him comfortably, with the body part to be bandaged in normal functioning position *to promote circulation and prevent deformity and discomfort.*
▶ Avoid applying a bandage to a dependent extremity. If you're wrapping an extremity, elevate it for 15 to 30 minutes before application *to facilitate venous return.*
▶ Apply the bandage so that two skin surfaces don't remain in contact when wrapped. Place gauze pads or absorbent cotton as needed between skin surfaces, such as between toes and fingers and under breasts and arms, *to prevent skin irritation.*
▶ Hold the bandage with the roll facing upward in one hand and the free end of the bandage in the other hand. Hold the bandage roll close to the part being bandaged *to ensure even tension and pressure.*
▶ Unroll the bandage as you wrap the body part in a spiral or spiral-reverse method. Never unroll the entire bandage before wrapping *because this could produce uneven pressure, which interferes with blood circulation and cell nourishment.*

Bandaging techniques

Circular
Each turn encircles the previous one, covering it completely. Use this technique to anchor a bandage.

Spiral
Each turn partially overlaps the previous one. Use this technique to wrap a long, straight body part or one of increasing circumference.

Spiral-reverse
Anchor the bandage and then reverse direction halfway through each spiral turn. Use this technique to accommodate the increasing circumference of a body part.

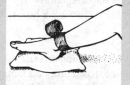

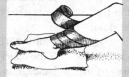

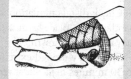

Figure eight
Anchor below the joint, and then use alternating ascending and descending turns to form a figure eight. Use this technique around joints.

Recurrent
This technique includes a combination of recurrent and circular turns. Hold the bandage as you make each recurrent turn and then use the circular turns as a final anchor. Use this technique for a stump, a hand, or the scalp.

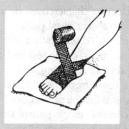

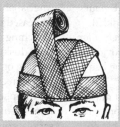

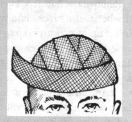

▶ Overlap each layer of bandage by one-half to two-thirds the width of the strip. (For specific instructions see *Bandaging techniques.*)

▶ Wrap firmly but not too tightly. As you wrap, ask the patient to tell you if the bandage feels comfortable. If he complains of tingling, itching, numbness, or pain, loosen the bandage.

▶ When wrapping an extremity, anchor the bandage initially by circling the body part twice. *To prevent the bandage from slipping out of place on the foot, wrap it in a figure eight around the foot, the ankle, and then the foot again before continuing. The same technique works on any joint, such as the knee, wrist, or elbow. Include the heel when wrapping the foot but never wrap the toes (or fingers) unless absolutely necessary *because the distal extremities are used to detect impaired circulation.*

▶ When you're finished wrapping, secure the end of the bandage with tape, pins, or self-closures, being careful not to scratch or pinch the patient. Avoid using metal clips *because they typically come loose when the patient moves and may get lost in the bed linens and injure him.*

▶ Check distal circulation after the bandage is in place *because the elastic may tighten as you wrap.*

▶ Elevate a wrapped extremity for 15 to 30 minutes *to facilitate venous return.*

▶ Check distal circulation once or twice every 8 hours *because an elastic bandage that is too tight may result in neurovascular damage.* Lift the distal end of the bandage and assess the skin underneath for color, temperature, and integrity.

▶ Remove the bandage every 8 hours or whenever it's loose and wrinkled. Roll it up as you unwrap *to ready it for reuse.* Observe the area and provide skin care before rewrapping the bandage.

▶ Change the bandage at least once daily. Bathe the skin, dry it thoroughly, and observe for irritation and breakdown before applying a fresh bandage.

Special considerations

▶ Wrap an elastic bandage from the distal area to the proximal area *to promote venous return.* Avoid leaving gaps in bandage layers or exposed skin surfaces *because this may result in uneven pressure on the body part.*

▶ Observe the patient for an allergic reaction *because some patients can't toler-*

ate the sizing in a new bandage. Laundering it reduces this risk.

▶ Launder the bandage daily or whenever it becomes limp *because laundering restores its elasticity.* Always keep two bandages handy *so one can be applied while the other bandage is being laundered.*

▶ When using an elastic bandage after a surgical procedure on an extremity (such as vein stripping) or with a splint to immobilize a fracture, remove it only as ordered rather than every 8 hours.

Home care

If the patient will be using an elastic bandage at home, teach him or a family member how to apply it correctly and how to assess for restricted circulation. Tell him to keep two bandages available *so he'll have one while the other is being laundered.*

Complications

Arterial obstruction characterized by a decreased or an absent distal pulse, blanching or bluish discoloration of skin, dusky nail beds, numbness and tingling or pain and cramping, and cold skin can result from elastic bandage application. Edema can occur from obstruction of venous return. Less serious complications include allergic reaction and skin irritation.

Documentation

Record the date and time of bandage application and removal; the application site, bandage size, skin condition before application, skin care provided after removal, and complications; the patient's tolerance of the treatment; and any patient teaching.

ELECTRICAL BONE GROWTH STIMULATION

By imitating the body's natural electrical forces, electrical bone growth stimulation initiates or accelerates the healing process in a fractured bone that fails to heal. About 1 in 20 fractures may fail to heal properly, possibly as a result of infection, insufficient reduction or fixation, pseudarthrosis, or severe tissue trauma around the fracture.

Recent discoveries about the stimulating effects of electrical currents on osteogenesis have led to using electrical bone stimulation to promote healing. The technique is also being investigated for treating spinal fusions.

Three basic electrical bone stimulation techniques are available: fully implantable direct current stimulation; semi-invasive percutaneous stimulation; and noninvasive electromagnetic coil stimulation. (See *Methods of electrical bone growth stimulation*.) Choice of technique depends on the fracture type and location, the doctor's preference, and the patient's ability and willingness to comply. The invasive device requires little or no patient involvement. With the other two methods, however, the patient must manage his own treatment schedule and maintain the equipment. Treatment time averages 3 to 6 months.

Key nursing diagnoses and patient outcomes

Deficient knowledge related to lack of exposure to electrical bone growth stimulation
The patient will:
▶ state or demonstrate an understanding of what has been taught
▶ demonstrate the ability to perform new health-related behaviors as they're taught.

Methods of electrical bone growth stimulation

Electrical bone growth stimulation may be invasive or noninvasive.

Invasive system
An invasive system involves placing a spiral cathode inside the bone at the fracture site. A wire leads from the cathode to a battery-powered generator, also implanted in local tissues. The patient's body completes the circuit.

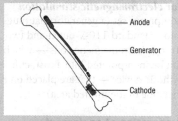

Noninvasive system
A noninvasive system may include a cuff-like transducer or fitted ring that wraps around the patient's limb at the level of the injury. Electric current penetrates the limb.

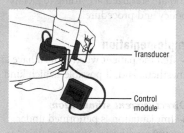

Risk for injury related to improper technique
The patient will:
▶ identify factors that increase the risk of injury
▶ assist in identifying and applying safety measures to prevent injury.

Equipment

For direct current stimulation

Equipment set (a small generator with leadwires that connect to a titanium cathode wire that is surgically implanted into the nonunited bone site)

For percutaneous stimulation

Equipment set (an external anode skin pad with a leadwire, lithium battery pack, and one to four Teflon-coated stainless steel cathode wires that are surgically implanted)

For electromagnetic stimulation

Equipment set (a generator that plugs into a standard 110-V outlet and two strong electromagnetic coils— which can be incorporated into a cast, cuff, or orthotic device—that are placed on either side of the injured area)

Preparation of equipment

All equipment comes in sets with instructions provided by the manufacturer. Follow the instructions carefully. Make sure that all parts are included and are sterilized according to facility policy and procedure.

Implementation

▶ Tell the patient whether he'll have an anesthetic and, if possible, which kind.

Direct current stimulation

▶ Implantation is performed under general anesthesia. Afterward, the doctor may apply a cast or external fixator to immobilize the limb. The patient is usually hospitalized for 2 to 3 days after implantation. Weight bearing may be ordered as tolerated.
▶ After the bone fragments join, the generator and leadwire can be removed

under local anesthesia. The titanium cathode remains implanted.

Percutaneous stimulation

▶ Remove excessive body hair from the injured site before applying the anode pad. Avoid stressing or pulling on the anode wire. Instruct the patient to change the anode pad every 48 hours. Tell him to report any local pain to his doctor and not to bear weight for the duration of treatment.

Electromagnetic stimulation

▶ Show the patient where to place the coils and tell him to apply them for 3 to 10 hours each day as ordered by his doctor. Many patients find it most convenient to perform the procedure at night.
▶ Urge the patient not to interrupt the treatments for more than 10 minutes at a time.
▶ Teach the patient how to use and care for the generator.
▶ Relay the doctor's instructions for weight bearing. Usually, the doctor will advise against bearing weight until evidence of healing appears on X-rays.

Special considerations

▶ A patient with a direct current electrical bone stimulation shouldn't undergo electrocauterization, diathermy, or magnetic resonance imaging (MRI). *Electrocautery may short the system; diathermy may potentiate the electrical current, possibly causing tissue damage; and MRI will interfere with or stop the current.*
▶ Percutaneous electrical bone stimulation is contraindicated in patients with any kind of inflammatory process. Ask the patient if he's sensitive to nickel

or chromium; *both are present in the electrical bone stimulation system.*

► Electromagnetic coils are contraindicated for a pregnant patient, a patient with a tumor, or a patient with an arm fracture and a pacemaker.

Home care

Teach the patient how to care for his cast or external fixation devices and for the electrical generator. Urge him to follow treatment instructions faithfully.

Complications

Complications associated with any surgical procedure, including increased risk of infection, may occur with direct current electrical bone stimulation equipment. Local irritation or skin ulceration may occur around cathode pin sites with percutaneous devices. No complications are associated with the use of electromagnetic coils.

Documentation

Record the type of electrical bone stimulation equipment provided, including date, time, and location, as appropriate. Note the patient's skin condition and tolerance of the procedure. Also record instructions given to the patient and family members as well as their ability to understand and act on those instructions.

ELECTROCARDIOGRAPHY

One of the most valuable and frequently used diagnostic tools, electrocardiography (ECG) measures the heart's electrical activity as waveforms. Impulses moving through the heart's conduction system create electric currents that can be monitored on the body's surface.

Electrodes attached to the skin can detect these electric currents and transmit them to an instrument that produces a record (the electrocardiogram) of cardiac activity.

ECG can be used to identify myocardial ischemia and infarction, rhythm and conduction disturbances, chamber enlargement, electrolyte imbalances, and drug toxicity.

The standard 12-lead ECG uses a series of electrodes placed on the extremities and the chest wall to assess the heart from 12 different views (leads). The 12 leads consist of three standard bipolar limb leads (designated I, II, III), three unipolar augmented leads (aV$_R$, aV$_L$, aV$_F$), and six unipolar precordial leads (V$_1$ to V$_6$). The limb leads and augmented leads show the heart from the frontal plane. The precordial leads show the heart from the horizontal plane.

The ECG device measures and averages the differences between the electrical potential of the electrode sites for each lead and graphs them over time. This creates the standard ECG complex, called P-QRS-T. The P wave represents atrial depolarization; the QRS complex, ventricular depolarization; and the T wave, ventricular repolarization. (See *Reviewing ECG waveforms and components,* page 256.)

Variations of standard ECG include exercise ECG (stress ECG) and ambulatory ECG (Holter monitoring). Exercise ECG monitors heart rate, blood pressure, and ECG waveforms as the patient walks on a treadmill or pedals a stationary bicycle. For ambulatory ECG, the patient wears a portable Holter monitor, which records heart activity continually over 24 hours.

Reviewing ECG waveforms and components

An electrocardiogram (ECG) waveform has three basic components: the P wave, QRS complex, and T wave. These elements can be further divided into the PR interval, J point, ST segment, U wave, and QT interval.

P wave and PR interval

The P wave represents atrial depolarization. The PR interval represents the time it takes an impulse to travel from the atria through the atrioventricular nodes and bundle of His. The PR interval measures from the beginning of the P wave to the beginning of the QRS complex.

QRS complex

The QRS complex represents ventricular depolarization (the time it takes for the impulse to travel through the bundle branches to the Purkinje fibers).

The Q wave appears as the first negative deflection in the QRS complex; the R wave, as the first positive deflection. The S wave appears as the second negative deflection or the first negative deflection after the R wave.

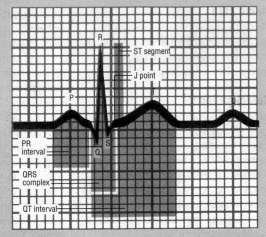

J point and ST segment

Marking the end of the QRS complex, the J point also indicates the beginning of the ST segment. The ST segment represents part of ventricular repolarization.

T wave and U wave

Usually following the same deflection pattern as the P wave, the T wave represents ventricular repolarization. The U wave follows the T wave, but isn't always seen.

QT interval

The QT interval represents ventricular depolarization and repolarization. It extends from the beginning of the QRS complex to the end of the T wave.

Today, ECG is typically accomplished using a multichannel method. All electrodes are attached to the patient at once, and the machine prints a simultaneous view of all leads.

Key nursing diagnoses and patient outcomes

Deficient knowledge related to lack of exposure to electrocardiography
The patient will:
▶ communicate a need to know the reasons for performing the procedure

▶ state an understanding of the procedure and the reasons for performing it.

Anxiety related to possible medical diagnosis
The patient will:
▶ state a feeling of anxiety
▶ use support systems to assist with coping
▶ cope with the threat of anxiety by being involved in decisions about care.

Equipment

ECG machine • recording paper • disposable pregelled electrodes • 4″ × 4″ gauze pads • optional: shaving supplies and marking pen

Preparation of equipment

Place the ECG machine close to the patient's bed and plug the power cord into the wall outlet. If the patient is already connected to a cardiac monitor, remove the electrodes to accommodate the precordial leads and minimize electrical interference on the ECG tracing. Keep the patient away from electrical fixtures and power cords.

Implementation

▶ As you set up the machine to record a 12-lead ECG, explain the procedure to the patient. Tell him that the test records the heart's electrical activity and that it may be repeated at certain intervals. Emphasize that no electrical current will enter his body. Also, tell him that the test typically takes about 5 minutes.
▶ Have the patient lie supine in the center of the bed with his arms at his sides. You may raise the head of the bed *to promote comfort*. Expose his arms and legs and cover him appropriately. His arms and legs should be relaxed *to*

minimize muscle trembling, which can cause electrical interference.
▶ If the bed is too narrow, place the patient's hands under his buttocks *to prevent muscle tension*. Also use this technique if the patient is shivering or trembling. Make sure his feet aren't touching the bed board.
▶ Select flat, fleshy areas to place the electrodes. Avoid muscular and bony areas. If the patient has an amputated limb, choose a site on the stump.
▶ If an area is excessively hairy, shave it. Clean excess oil or other substances from the skin *to enhance electrode contact*.
▶ Apply the electrode paste or gel or the disposable electrodes to the patient's wrists and to the medial aspects of his ankles. If you're using paste or gel, rub it into the skin. If you're using disposable electrodes, peel off the contact paper and apply them directly to the prepared site as recommended by the manufacturer's instructions. *To guarantee the best connection to the leadwire,* position disposable electrodes on the legs with the lead connection pointing superiorly.
▶ If you're using paste or gel, secure electrodes promptly after you apply the conductive medium. *This prevents drying of the medium, which could impair ECG quality.* Never use alcohol or acetone pads in place of the electrode paste or gel *because they impair electrode contact with the skin and diminish the transmission quality of electrical impulses.*
▶ Connect the limb leadwires to the electrodes. Make sure the metal parts of the electrodes are clean and bright. *Dirty or corroded electrodes prevent a good electrical connection.*
▶ You'll see that the tip of each leadwire is lettered and color-coded for easy

Positioning chest electrodes

To ensure accurate test results, position chest electrodes as follows:

V_1: Fourth intercostal space at right sternal border

V_2: Fourth intercostal space at left sternal border

V_3: Halfway between V_2 and V_4

V_4: Fifth intercostal space at midclavicular line

V_5: Fifth intercostal space at anterior axillary line (halfway between V_4 and V_6)

V_6: Fifth intercostal space at midaxillary line, level with V_4

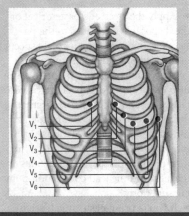

identification. The white or RA leadwire goes to the right arm; the green or RL leadwire, to the right leg; the red or LL leadwire, to the left leg; the black or LA leadwire, to the left arm; and the brown or V_1 to V_6 leadwires, to the chest.

▶ Now, expose the patient's chest. Put a small amount of electrode gel or paste or a disposable electrode at each electrode position. (See *Positioning chest electrodes.*)

▶ If your patient is a woman, place the chest electrodes below the breast tissue.

In a large-breasted woman, you may need to displace the breast tissue laterally.

▶ Check to see that the paper speed selector is set to the standard 25 mm/ second and that the machine is set to full voltage. The machine will record a normal standardization mark — a square that is the height of two large squares or 10 small squares on the recording paper. Then, if necessary, enter the appropriate patient identification data.

▶ If any part of the waveform extends beyond the paper when you record the ECG, adjust the normal standardization to half-standardization. Note this adjustment on the ECG strip *because this will need to be considered in interpreting the results.*

▶ Now you're ready to begin the recording. Ask the patient to relax and breathe normally. Tell him to lie still and not to talk when you record his ECG. Then press the AUTO button. Observe the tracing quality. The machine will record all 12 leads automatically, recording three consecutive leads simultaneously. Some machines have a display screen so you can preview waveforms before the machine records them on paper.

▶ When the machine finishes recording the 12-lead ECG, remove the electrodes and clean the patient's skin. After disconnecting the leadwires from the electrodes, dispose of or clean the electrodes as indicated.

Special considerations

▶ Small areas of hair on the patient's chest or extremities may be shaved, but this usually isn't necessary.

▶ If the patient's skin is exceptionally oily, scaly, or diaphoretic, rub the electrode site with a dry 4″ × 4″ gauze pad before applying the electrode *to help reduce interference in the tracing.* During the procedure, ask the patient to breathe normally. If his respirations distort the recording, ask him to hold his breath briefly *to reduce baseline wander in the tracing.*

▶ If the patient has a pacemaker, you can perform an ECG with or without a magnet, according to the doctor's orders. Note the presence of a pacemaker and the use of the magnet (to turn off the pacemaker) on the strip.

Documentation

Label the ECG recording with the patient's name, room number, and facility identification number. Document in your notes the test's date and time as well as significant responses by the patient. Record the date, time, and patient's name and room number on the ECG itself. Note any appropriate clinical information on the ECG.

ELECTROCARDIOGRAPHY, POSTERIOR CHEST LEAD

Because of the location of the heart's posterior surface, changes associated with myocardial damage aren't apparent on a standard 12-lead electrocardiogram (ECG). To help identify posterior involvement, some practitioners recommend adding posterior leads to the 12-lead ECG. Despite lung and muscle barriers, posterior leads may provide clues to posterior wall infarction so that appropriate treatment can begin.

Usually, the posterior lead ECG is performed with a standard ECG and only involves recording the additional posterior leads: V_7, V_8, and V_9.

Key nursing diagnoses and patient outcomes

Deficient knowledge related to lack of exposure to electrocardiography
The patient will:
▶ communicate a need to know the reasons for performing the procedure
▶ state an understanding of the procedure and the reasons for performing it.

Anxiety related to possible medical diagnosis
The patient will:
▶ state a feeling of anxiety
▶ use support systems to assist with coping
▶ cope with the threat of anxiety by being involved in decisions about care.

Equipment

Multichannel or single-channel ECG machine with recording paper • disposable pregelled electrodes • 4″ × 4″ gauze pads or moist cloth • optional: shaving supplies

Implementation

▶ Prepare the electrode sites according to the manufacturer's instructions. *To ensure good skin contact,* shave the site if the patient has considerable back hair.
▶ If you're using a multichannel ECG machine, begin by attaching a disposable electrode to the V_7 position on the left posterior axillary line, fifth intercostal space. Then attach the V_4 leadwire to the V_7 electrode.
▶ Next, attach a disposable electrode to the patient's back at the V_8 position on the left midscapular line, fifth intercostal space, and attach the V_5 leadwire to this electrode.
▶ Finally, attach a disposable electrode to the patient's back at the V_9 position, just left of the spinal column at the fifth

intercostal space (as shown below). Then attach the V_6 leadwire to the V_9 electrode.

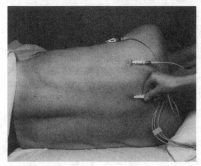

▶ If you're using a single-channel ECG machine, put electrode gel at locations for electrodes V_7, V_8, and V_9. Then connect the brown leadwire to the V_7 electrode.

▶ Turn on the machine and make sure that the paper speed is set for 25 mm/second. If necessary, standardize the machine. Press AUTO and the machine will record.

▶ If you're using a multichannel ECG machine, all leads will print out as a straight line except those labeled V_4, V_5, and V_6. Relabel those leads V_7, V_8, and V_9 respectively.

▶ If you're using a single-channel ECG machine, turn the selector knob to "V" to record the V_7 lead. Then stop the machine. Reposition the electrode to the V_8 position and record that lead. Repeat the procedure for the V_9 position.

▶ When the ECG is complete, remove the electrodes and clean the patient's skin with a gauze pad or a moist cloth. If you think you may need more than one posterior lead ECG, use a marking pen to mark the electrode sites on his skin *to permit accurate comparison for future tracings.*

Special considerations

▶ The number of leads may vary according to the cardiologist's preference. (If right posterior leads are requested, position the patient on his left side. These leads, known as V_{7R}, V_{8R}, and V_{9R}, are located at the same landmarks on the right side of the patient's back.)

▶ Some ECG machines won't operate unless you connect all leadwires. In that case, you may need to connect the limb leadwires and the leadwires for V_1, V_2, and V_3.

Documentation

Document the procedure in your nurse's notes. Make sure that the patient's name, age, and room number, the time and date, and the doctor's name are clearly written on the ECG along with the relabeled lead tracings. Document any patient teaching you may have performed as well as the patient's tolerance to the procedure.

ELECTROCARDIOGRAPHY, RIGHT CHEST LEAD

Unlike a standard 12-lead electrocardiogram (ECG), used primarily to evaluate left ventricular function, a right chest lead ECG reflects right ventricular function and provides clues to damage or dysfunction in this chamber. You might need to perform a right chest lead ECG for a patient with an inferior wall myocardial infarction (MI) and suspected right ventricular involvement. Between 25% and 50% of patients with this type of MI have right ventricular involvement. Many of these patients have high creatine kinase levels.

Early identification of a right ventricular MI is essential because its treatment differs from that for other MIs. For instance, in left ventricular MI, treatment involves withholding I.V. fluids or administering them judiciously to prevent heart failure. Conversely, in right ventricular MI, treatment usually requires administration of I.V. fluids to maintain adequate filling pressures on the right side of the heart. This helps the right ventricle eject an adequate volume of blood at an adequate pressure.

Key nursing diagnoses and patient outcomes

Deficient knowledge related to lack of exposure to electrocardiography
The patient will:
▶ communicate a need to know the reasons for the procedure
▶ state an understanding of the procedure and the reasons for performing it.

Anxiety related to possible medical diagnosis
The patient will:
▶ state a feeling of anxiety
▶ use support systems to assist with coping
▶ cope with the threat of anxiety by being involved in decisions about care.

Equipment

Multichannel ECG machine • paper • pregelled disposable electrodes • several 4″ × 4″ gauze pads

Implementation

▶ Take the equipment to the patient's bedside and explain the procedure to him. Inform him that the doctor has ordered a right chest lead ECG, a procedure that involves placing electrodes on his wrists, ankles, and chest. Reassure him that the test is painless and takes only a few minutes, during which he'll need to lie quietly on his back.
▶ Make sure that the paper speed is set at 25 mm/second and the amplitude at 1 mV/10 mm.
▶ Place the patient in a supine position or, if he has difficulty lying flat, in semi-Fowler's position. Provide privacy and expose his arms, chest, and legs. (Cover a female patient's chest with a drape until you apply the chest leads.)
▶ Examine the patient's wrists and ankles for the best areas to place the electrodes. Choose flat and fleshy (not bony or muscular), hairless areas such as the inner aspects of the wrists and ankles. Clean the sites with the gauze pads *to promote good skin contact.*
▶ Connect the leadwires to the electrodes. The leadwires are color-coded and lettered. Place the white or right arm (RA) wire on the right arm; the black or left arm (LA) wire on the left arm; the green or right leg (RL) wire on the right leg; and the red or left leg (LL) wire on the left leg.
▶ Then examine the patient's chest *to locate the correct sites for chest lead placement* (as shown below). If the patient is a woman, place the electrodes under the breast tissue.

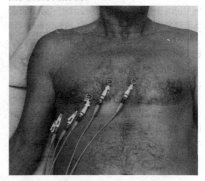

▶ Use your fingers to feel between the patient's ribs (the intercostal spaces). Start at the second intercostal space on the left (the notch felt at the top of the sternum, where the manubrium joins the body of the sternum). Count down two spaces to the fourth intercostal space. Then apply a disposable electrode to the site and attach leadwire V_{1R} to that electrode.

▶ Move your fingers across the sternum to the fourth intercostal space on the right side of the sternum. Apply a disposable electrode to that site and attach lead V_{2R}.

▶ Move your finger down to the fifth intercostal space and over to the midclavicular line. Place a disposable electrode here and attach lead V_{4R}.

▶ Visually draw a line between V_{2R} and V_{4R}. Apply a disposable electrode midway on this line and attach lead V_{3R}.

▶ Move your finger horizontally from V_{4R} to the right midaxillary line. Apply a disposable electrode to this site and attach lead V_{6R}.

▶ Move your fingers along the same horizontal line to the midpoint between V_{4R} and V_{6R}. This is the right anterior midaxillary line. Apply a disposable electrode to this site and attach lead V_{5R}.

▶ Turn on the ECG machine. Ask the patient to breathe normally but to refrain from talking during the recording *so that muscle movement won't distort the tracing.* Enter any appropriate patient information required by the machine you're using. If necessary, standardize the machine. This will cause a square tracing of 10 mm (two large squares) to appear on the ECG paper when the machine is set for 1 mV (1 mV = 10 mm).

▶ Press the AUTO key. The ECG machine will record all 12 leads automatically. Check your facility's policy for the number of readings to obtain. (Some facilities require at least two ECGs so that one copy can be sent out for interpretation while the other remains at the bedside.)

▶ When you're finished recording the ECG, turn off the machine. Clearly label the ECG with the patient's name, the date, and the time. Also label the tracing "Right chest ECG" to distinguish it from a standard 12-lead ECG. Remove the electrodes and help the patient get comfortable.

Special considerations

For best results, place the electrodes symmetrically on the limbs. If the patient's wrist or ankle is covered by a dressing, or if the patient is an amputee, choose an area that is available on both sides.

Documentation

Document the procedure in your nurse's notes, and document the patient's tolerance to the procedure. Place a copy of the tracing in the patient's chart.

ELECTROCARDIOGRAPHY, SIGNAL-AVERAGED

Signal-averaged electrocardiography (ECG) helps to identify patients at risk for sustained ventricular tachycardia. Because this cardiac arrhythmia can be a precursor of sudden death after a myocardial infarction (MI), the results of signal-averaged ECG can allow appropriate preventive measures.

Through a computer-based ECG, signal averaging detects low-amplitude signals or late electrical potentials, which reflect slow conduction or disorganized ventricular activity through abnormal or infarcted regions of the ventricles. The signal-averaged ECG is developed by recording the noise-free surface ECG in three specialized leads for several hundred beats.

Signal averaging enhances signals that would otherwise be missed because of increased amplitude and sensitivity to ventricular activity. For instance, on the standard 12-lead ECG, "noise" created by muscle tissue, electronic artifacts, and electrodes masks late potentials, which have a low amplitude.

This procedure identifies the risk of sustained ventricular tachycardia in patients with malignant ventricular tachycardia, a history of MI, unexplained syncope, nonischemic congestive cardiomyopathy, or nonsustained ventricular tachycardia.

Key nursing diagnoses and patient outcomes

Deficient knowledge related to lack of exposure to electrocardiography
The patient will:
▶ communicate a need to know the reasons for the procedure
▶ state an understanding of the procedure and the reasons for performing it.

Anxiety related to possible medical diagnosis
The patient will:
▶ state a feeling of anxiety
▶ use support systems to assist with coping
▶ cope with the threat of anxiety by being involved in decisions about care.

Equipment

Signal-averaged ECG machine • signal-averaged computer • record of patient's surface ECG for 200 to 300 QRS complexes • three bipolar electrodes or leads • shaving supplies

Implementation

▶ Inform the patient that this procedure will take 10 to 30 minutes and will help the doctor determine his risk for a certain type of arrhythmia. If appropriate, mention that it may be done along with other tests, such as echocardiography, Holter monitoring, and a stress test.
▶ Place the patient in the supine position and tell him to lie as still as possible. Tell him he shouldn't speak and should breathe normally during the procedure.
▶ If the patient has hair on his chest, shave the area, and dry it before placing the electrodes on it.
▶ Place the leads in the X, Y, and Z orthogonal positions. (See *Placing electrodes for signal-averaged ECG,* page 264.)
▶ The ECG machine gathers input from these leads and amplifies, filters, and samples the signals. The computer collects and stores data for analysis. The crucial values are those showing QRS complex duration, duration of the portion of the QRS complex with an amplitude under 40 V, and the root mean square voltage of the last 40 msec.

Special considerations

▶ *Because muscle movements may cause an abnormal result,* patients who are restless or in respiratory distress are poor candidates for signal-averaged ECG. Proper electrode placement and skin preparation are essential to this procedure.

Placing electrodes for signal-averaged ECG

To prepare your patient for signal-averaged electrocardiography (ECG), place the electrodes in the X, Y, and Z orthogonal positions. These positions bisect one another to provide a three-dimensional, composite view of ventricular activation.

Anterior chest

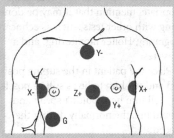

Posterior chest

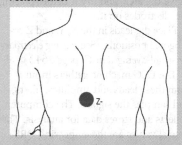

Key

X+   Fourth intercostal space, midaxillary line, left side

X-   Fourth intercostal space, midaxillary line, right side

Y+   Standard V_3 position (or proximal left leg)

Y-   Superior aspect of manubrium

Z+   Standard V_2 position

Z- V_2 position, posterior

G   Ground

▶ Results indicating low-amplitude signals include a QRS complex duration greater than 110 msec; a duration of more than 40 msec for the amplitude portion under 40 μV; and a root mean square voltage of less than 25 μV during the last 40 msec of the QRS complex. However, all three factors need not be present to consider the result normal or abnormal. The final interpretation hinges on individualized patient factors.

▶ Results of signal-averaged ECG help the doctor determine whether the patient is a candidate for invasive procedures, such as electrophysiologic testing or angiography.

▶ Keep in mind that the significance of signal-averaged ECG results in patients with bundle-branch heart block is unknown *because myocardial activation doesn't follow the usual sequence in these patients.*

Complications

Usually, there are no complications associated with this procedure.

Documentation

Document the time of the procedure, why the procedure was done, and how the patient tolerated it.

ELECTROLYTE TESTING WITH A VIA SYSTEM

The vascular intermittent access (VIA) system automatically measures electrolyte levels in patients who have an indwelling arterial or venous line. In just 1 minute, it obtains such critical indexes as potassium, calcium, sodium, and glucose levels; hematocrit; and arterial blood gas values. Then it reinfuses the blood sample into the patient.

By detecting changes in electrolyte levels almost as soon as they occur, the VIA system allows you to respond quickly to abnormalities. The arterial or venous line can be accessed as often as every 3 minutes. This avoids the need to collect blood manually for laboratory samples and eliminates the problems that an indwelling sensor sometimes causes. Easily transported with the patient from one area to another, the VIA system can be used in the operating room, intensive care unit, emergency department, and other special care units.

Abnormal levels measured by this system indicate electrolyte imbalances, which can disrupt various body systems and cause serious health problems.

Key nursing diagnoses and patient outcomes
Risk for fluid volume imbalance related to excessive loss
The patient will:
▶ maintain stable vital signs
▶ have normal electrolyte values.

Ineffective tissue perfusion (cardiopulmonary) related to decreased cellular exchange
The patient will:
▶ attain hemodynamic stability with a pulse not less than (specify) beats/minute and not greater than (specify) beats/minute and blood pressure not less than (specify) mm Hg and not greater than (specify) mm Hg
▶ exhibit no arrhythmias.

Equipment
VIA system with monitor and sensor array • isotonic I.V. solution (lactated Ringer's solution) • tubing and calibration additives • printer • tape • optional: armboard (see *Vascular intermittent access system,* page 266)

Implementation
▶ Set up the VIA system, following the manufacturer's directions. Place the sensor array at the distal end of the I.V. administration set by twisting the luer-lock connection.
▶ Turn on the monitor by pressing the ON/OFF key. Choose the appropriate mode by pressing the up or down arrow.
▶ Press the * key to advance the instructions. The monitor screen will display cues (or prompts) for continuing.
▶ Open the door on the monitor. Then pull the anti–free-flow lever down to open the pump mechanism.

Setting up the pump
▶ Holding the silicone portion of the tubing, place the tubing adapter into the top of the tubing retainer in the pump compartment.
▶ Hold the sensor disk so that the flat side faces the monitor. Pull down slightly and hook the disk under its retainer in the monitor.
▶ Holding the sensor disk in place, push the anti–free-flow lever up to close the pump. Now shut the monitor door.

Programming the sensor system
▶ Open the regulating clamp on the I.V. tubing all the way. Check the drip chamber *to make sure the solution isn't flowing.*
▶ Continue to advance the programming instructions by pressing the * key. When the previously infused volume appears on the screen, you may clear it

Vascular intermittent access system

Used to measure electrolyte levels automatically, the vascular intermittent access system includes a sensor set, an I.V. infusion set, I.V. solution with additives for sensor calibration, and a
monitor that processes signals from the sensors. A pumping mechanism infuses the solution
and withdraws blood samples.

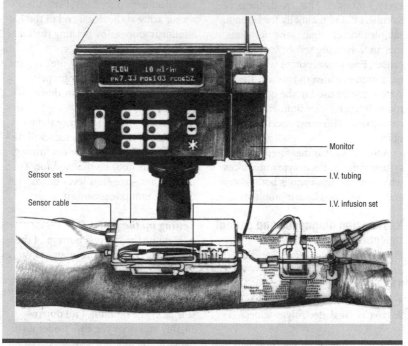

by pressing the CLEAR VOLUME INFUSED
key for 1 second.

▶ Select the intended infusion volume
(in 50-ml increments from 50 to 1,000)
by pressing the up and down arrows
until the desired total appears. Simultaneously press the SET VOL TO BE IN-
FUSED key. *To prevent the system from
running dry and to give yourself adequate
time to prepare a new I.V. solution,* enter a
volume that is 50 ml less than the volume in the I.V. bag. This accounts for
fluid in the tubing and fluid lost in

priming. After the selected volume infuses, an alarm will sound. The solution will continue to infuse at a rate of
10 ml/hour—the keep-vein-open rate.

Connecting the system to the patient

▶ Before connecting the system to the
patient, perform an initial two-point
calibration check of the sensor. Remember to perform this check each
time you use a new sensor. (See the operator's manual for complete instructions.) Use a four-way stopcock to con-

nect the end of the tubing from the sensor set to the patient's arterial line. Secure all luer-lock connections and be careful not to introduce air into the line.

▶ Press the * key again. This starts the infusion and maintains the flow rate at 10 ml/hour. The display screen will alternately present two messages: one identifying the flow rate and the other, the measurable values. The actual values will follow the equal signs when the blood is tested.

▶ Connect the monitor's sensor cable to the sensor set of the infusion tubing by lining up the cable with the sensor set and sliding it in place.

▶ Position the sensor upright and horizontal on the patient's arm as indicated by the label on the sensor cable and secure it with tape.

▶ Secure all the tubing and the cable lines to the patient's wrist so that they won't dislodge or pull out. As needed, use an armboard to stabilize the patient's wrist. Also, remind the patient to keep his wrist on top of the bed linens at all times.

Testing blood

▶ To start a sampling cycle and measure an electrolyte level, press the SAMPLE key. During the sampling cycle, the following steps occur automatically: The system calibrates its sensors, and the word *calibrating* and a countdown time appear on the screen (until the system segregates and analyzes a blood sample). After 8 seconds, the pumping system reverses its action and withdraws about 1.2 ml of blood, and the word *sampling* appears. As the patient's blood comes in contact with the sensors, the word *analyzing* appears on the screen. The word *purging* appears on

the screen when the system returns the blood and I.V. solution to the patient.

▶ Finally, blood chemistry values appear on the alternating screens. To hold the display for 30 seconds, press the DISPLAY FREEZE key. To resume the alternating display, press the same key again. Record the results promptly *because they appear for only 5 minutes, after which they automatically clear from the system*. If your monitor has an attached printer, you can print the results along with the date and time.

Special considerations

▶ Be aware that the VIA system doesn't require long-term compatibility between the sensors and the patient's blood. Except for the few seconds during which the measurement is being made, the sensors are exposed only to the I.V. solution, not the blood.

▶ Because the VIA system is closed, caregivers avoid handling blood and blood loss in the patient is prevented.

Documentation

Document the entire procedure, the results of the blood studies, any treatments given, and the patient's response.

ELECTRONIC VITAL SIGNS MONITOR USE

An electronic vital signs monitor allows you to track a patient's vital signs continually, without having to reapply a blood pressure cuff each time. What is more, the patient won't need an invasive arterial line to gather similar data.

Some automated vital signs monitors are lightweight and battery operated and can be attached to an I.V. pole for

> *Technology update*
>
> ## Blood pressure monitoring: A comfortable new approach
>
> A new blood pressure monitoring system provides a comfortable, noninvasive way to obtain continual blood pressure readings from the patient. Because the device is small and easily fits on the wrist, the patient experiences minimal sensation while wearing it. For this reason, the device is especially useful when monitoring obese patients and those with low cardiac output, hypothermia, or an abnormal heart rhythm.
>
> By measuring radial artery waveforms, the device can calculate the patient's systolic, diastolic, and mean pressures and display the initial measurement and waveform within 15 seconds. The device then provides continual updates, four to six times every minute. What is more, it can show trend lines and historical data on a graphics screen, and the data can be output to a standard serial port or the optional printer.

continual monitoring, even during patient transfers. Make sure you know the capacity of the monitor's battery and plug the machine in whenever possible to keep it charged.

Before using any monitor, check its accuracy. Determine the patient's pulse rate and blood pressure manually, using the same arm you'll use for the monitor cuff. Compare your results when you get initial readings from the monitor. If the results differ, call your supply department or the manufacturer's representative. (For a technology update on blood pressure monitors, see *Blood pressure monitoring: A comfortable new approach*.)

Key nursing diagnoses and patient outcomes

Ineffective tissue perfusion (cardiopulmonary) related to decreased cellular exchange The patient will:

▶ attain hemodynamic stability: pulse not less than (specify) beats/minute and not greater than (specify) beats/minute; blood pressure not less than (specify) mm Hg and not greater than (specify) mm Hg

▶ maintain adequate cardiac output.

Equipment

Automated vital signs monitor • properly grounded wall outlet

Implementation

▶ Explain the procedure to the patient. Describe the alarm system so he won't be frightened if it's triggered.

▶ Make sure the power switch is off, then plug the monitor into a properly grounded wall outlet. Next, secure the dual air hose to the front of the monitor.

▶ Connect the pressure cuff's tubing into the other ends of the dual air hose and tighten connections to prevent air leaks. Keep the air hose away from the patient to avoid accidental dislodgment.

▶ Squeeze all the air from the cuff and wrap it loosely around the patient's arm or leg, allowing two fingerbreadths between cuff and arm or leg. Never apply the cuff to a limb that has an I.V. line in place. Position the cuff's "artery" arrow over the palpated brachial artery. Then secure the cuff for a snug fit.

Selecting parameters

▶ When you turn on the monitor, it will default to a manual mode. (In this mode, you can obtain vital signs your-self before switching to the automatic mode.) Press the AUTO/MANUAL button to select the automatic mode. The mon-itor will give you the baseline data for the pulse rate and for the systolic and diastolic blood pressure.

▶ Compare your previous manual re-sults with these baseline data. If they match, you're ready to set the alarm pa-rameters. Press the SELECT button to blank all displays except systolic pres-sure.

▶ Use the HIGH and LOW limit buttons to set the specific parameters for sys-tolic pressure. (These limits range from a high of 240 to a low of 0.) You'll also do this three more times for mean arte-rial pressure, pulse rate, and baseline diastolic pressure. After you've set the parameters for diastolic pressure, press the SELECT button again to display all current data. Even if you forget to do this last step, the monitor will automat-ically display current data 10 seconds after you set the last parameter.

Collecting data
▶ You also need to program the moni-tor for the frequency that you want to obtain data. Press the SET button until you reach the desired time interval in minutes. If you've chosen the automatic mode, the monitor will display a de-fault cycle time of 3 minutes. You can override the default cycle time to set the interval, if you prefer.
▶ You can obtain a set of vital signs at any time by pressing the START button. Also, pressing the CANCEL button will stop the interval and deflate the cuff. You can retrieve stored data by pressing the PRIOR DATA button. The monitor will display the last data obtained along with the time elapsed since then.

Scrolling backward, you can retrieve data from the previous 99 minutes.

Special considerations
▶ If your patient is anxious or crying, delay blood pressure measurement, if possible, until the patient becomes calm *to avoid falsely elevated measure-ments.*
▶ Measure the blood pressure of pa-tients taking an antihypertensive while they're in a sitting position *to ensure ac-curate measurements.*
▶ For patients who have had a mastec-tomy, don't take blood pressure in the arm on the affected side *because doing so may decrease already compromised lym-phatic circulation, worsen edema, and damage the arm.* Likewise, don't take blood pressure on the same arm of an arteriovenous fistula or hemodialysis shunt *because blood flow through the vas-cular device may be compromised.*

Documentation
In the patient's chart, record blood pres-sure as systolic over diastolic pressures such as 120/78 mm Hg; if necessary, record systolic over the two diastolic pressures such as 120/78/20 mm Hg. If required by your facility, chart blood pressure on a graph, using dots or checkmarks. Also, document the ex-tremity used and the patient's position.

EMERGENCY DELIVERY

Emergency delivery, the unplanned birth of a neonate outside of a health care facility, may occur when labor pro-gresses quickly or when circumstances prevent the mother from entering a fa-cility. Whether assisting at an emer-gency delivery or instructing the person who is assisting your objectives include establishing a clean, safe, and private birth area; promoting a controlled delivery; and preventing injury, infection, and hemorrhage.

Key nursing diagnoses and patient outcomes

Risk for infection related to emergency delivery
The patient will:
▶ have no pathogens appear in culture
▶ show no evidence of infections such as foul-smelling lochia
▶ remain afebrile.

Risk for injury related to internal and external neonatal risk factors
The neonate will:
▶ have normal laboratory values
▶ be free from injury.

Hypothermia related to cold stress
The patient will:
▶ maintain a normal body temperature
▶ remain free from shivering
▶ have warm and dry skin
▶ maintain a normal cardiovascular status.

Equipment

Unopened newspaper or large cloth (such as a tablecloth, towel, or curtain) • bath towel, blanket, or coat • gloves • at least two small cloths • sharp object (such as scissors, new razor blade, knife, or nail file) • ligating material (such as string, yarn, ribbon, or new shoelaces) • blanket or towel (to cover the neonate) • boiling water

Preparation of equipment

Boil the ligating and cutting materials for at least 5 minutes, if possible.

Implementation

▶ Offer support and reassurance *to help relieve the patient's anxiety.* Encourage the patient to pant during contractions *to promote a controlled delivery.* As possible, provide privacy, wash your hands, and put on gloves.
▶ Position the patient comfortably on a bed, a couch, or the ground. Open the newspaper or the large, clean cloth and place it under the patient's buttocks *to provide a clean delivery area.* Elevate the buttocks slightly with the bath towel, blanket, or coat *to cushion and support the patient's buttocks.*
▶ Check for signs and symptoms of imminent delivery, such as bulging perineum, increase in bloody show, urgency to push, and crowning of the presenting part.
▶ As the fetal head reaches and begins to pass the perineum, instruct the patient to pant or blow through the contractions *because forceful bearing down could cause extensive maternal lacerations.* Place one hand gently on the perineum *to cover the fetal head, control birth speed, and prevent sudden expulsion.*
▶ Avoid forcibly restraining fetal descent *because undue pressure can cause cephalohematoma or scalp lacerations, head trauma, and vagal stimulation. Undue pressure can also occlude the umbilical cord, which may cause fetal bradycardia, circulatory depression, and hypoxia.*
▶ As the fetal head emerges, immediately break the amniotic sac if it's intact. Support the head as it emerges. Instruct the patient to continue blowing and panting.
▶ Locate the umbilical cord. Insert one or two fingers along the back of the emergent head *to be sure the cord isn't wrapped around the neck.* If the cord is wrapped loosely around the neck, slip

it over the head *to prevent prolonged cord compression, tearing of the cord, or interrupted delivery*. If it's wrapped tightly around the neck, ligate the cord in two places, using string, yarn, ribbon, or new shoelaces. Then carefully cut between the ligatures, using a clean, sharp object or, if possible, a sterile one.

▶ Carefully support the head with both hands as it rotates to one side (external rotation). Gently wipe mucus and amniotic fluid from the nose and mouth with a clean, small cloth *to prevent aspiration*.

▶ Instruct the patient to bear down with the next contraction *to aid delivery of the shoulders*. Position your hands on either side of the neonate's head and support the neck. Exert gentle downward pressure *to deliver the anterior shoulder*. Then exert gentle upward pressure *to deliver the posterior shoulder*.

▶ Remember that amniotic fluid and vernix are slippery, so take care to support the neonate's body securely after freeing the shoulders.

▶ Keep the neonate in a slightly head-down position *to encourage mucus to drain from the respiratory tract*. Wipe excess mucus from his face. If the neonate doesn't breathe spontaneously, gently pat the soles of his feet or stroke his back. *Never suspend a neonate by his feet.*

▶ Dry and cover the neonate quickly with the blanket or towel. Ensure that his head is well covered *to minimize exposure and prevent heat loss*.

▶ Cradle the neonate at the level of the maternal uterus until the umbilical cord stops pulsating. *This prevents the neonatal blood from flowing to or from the placenta and leading to hypovolemia or hypervolemia, respectively. Hypovolemia can lead to circulatory collapse and neona-*

tal death; hypervolemia can cause hyperbilirubinemia.

▶ Place the neonate on the mother's abdomen in a slightly head-down position.

▶ Ligate the umbilical cord at two points, 1″ to 2″ (2.5 to 5 cm) apart. Place the first ligature 4″ to 6″ (10 to 15 cm) from the neonate. *Ligation prevents autotransfusion, which may cause hemolysis and hyperbilirubinemia.*

▶ Cut the umbilical cord between the two ligatures, using sterile equipment, if available. *Using unsterile instruments may cause infection.*

▶ Watch for signs of placental separation, such as a slight gush of dark blood from the vagina, cord lengthening, and a firm uterine fundus rising within the abdominal area. Usually, the placenta separates from the uterus within 5 minutes after delivery (although it may take as long as 30 minutes). When you see these signs, encourage the patient to bear down *to expel the placenta*. As she does, apply gentle downward pressure on her abdomen *to aid placental delivery*. Never tug on the umbilical cord to initiate or aid placental delivery *because this may invert the uterus or sever the cord from the placenta*.

▶ Examine the expelled placenta for intactness. *Retained placental fragments may cause hemorrhage or lead to intrauterine infection.*

▶ Place the cord and the placenta inside the towel or blanket covering the neonate *to provide extra warmth and also to ensure that the cord and placenta will be transported to the hospital for closer examination*.

▶ Palpate the maternal uterus *to make sure it's firm*. Gently massage the atonic uterus *to encourage contraction and pre-*

vent hemorrhage. Encourage breast-feeding, if appropriate, *to stimulate uterine contraction.*

▶ Check the patient for excessive bleeding from perineal lacerations. Apply a perineal pad, if available, and instruct the patient to press her thighs together. Provide comfort and reassurance and offer fluids, if available. Have someone summon an emergency medical service or arrange transportation to the health care facility for the mother and neonate. Make sure that the mother and neonate are warm and dry while they await transport.

Special considerations

▶ Never introduce any object into the vagina to facilitate delivery. *Doing so increases the risk of intrauterine infection as well as injury to the cervix, uterus, fetus, cord, or placenta.*

▶ In a breech presentation, make every effort to transport the patient to a nearby health care facility. If the patient begins to deliver, carefully support the fetal buttocks with both hands. Gently lift the body to deliver the posterior shoulder. Then lower the neonate slightly to deliver the anterior shoulder. Flexion of the head usually follows. Never apply traction to the body *to avoid lodging the head in the cervix.* Allow the neonate to rotate and emerge spontaneously.

▶ If the umbilical cord emerges first, elevate the presenting part throughout delivery *to prevent occluding the cord and causing fetal hypoxia.* Because this obstetric emergency usually necessitates a cesarean section, arrange for immediate transport to a nearby health care facility.

▶ If the neonate fails to breathe spontaneously after birth, clear the airway and begin to breathe for him. Place your opened mouth over his nose and mouth. Using air collected in your cheeks, deliver two effective breaths (produce visible chest rise). Next, check the umbilical cord for pulsation. If the neonate's heart rate is less than 60 beats/minute, begin cardiopulmonary resuscitation (CPR). Compressions should be delivered on the lower third of the sternum. Place two thumbs on the sternum, superimposed or adjacent to each other depending on the infant's size, with fingers encircling the chest and supporting the back. Administer a breath of air; then use your thumbs gently but firmly to pump the heart. Pump three times for each ventilation. Continue performing CPR until the neonate breathes and his heart rate is 60 beats/minute or higher.

Documentation

Give the medical care team the following information, if possible: the time of delivery; the presentation and position of the fetus; any delivery complications, such as the cord wrapped around the neonate's neck; the color, character, and amount of amniotic fluid; and the mother's blood type and Rh factor, if known. Note the time of placental expulsion, the placental appearance and intactness, the amount of postpartum bleeding, the status of uterine firmness (tone) and contractions, and the mother's response.

Document the sex of the neonate, his estimated Apgar score, and any resuscitative measures used. Record whether the mother began breast-feeding the neonate. Also identify and quantify any fluids given to the mother.

ENDOTRACHEAL DRUG ADMINISTRATION

When an I.V. line isn't readily available, drugs can be administered into the respiratory system through an endotracheal (ET) tube. This route allows uninterrupted resuscitation efforts and avoids such complications as coronary artery laceration, cardiac tamponade, and pneumothorax, which can occur when emergency drugs are administered intracardially.

Drugs given endotracheally usually have a longer duration of action than drugs given I.V. because they're absorbed in the alveoli. For this reason, repeat doses and continuous infusions must be adjusted to prevent adverse effects. Drugs commonly given by this route include naloxone, atropine, diazepam, epinephrine, and lidocaine.

Endotracheal drugs are usually administered in an emergency situation by a doctor, an emergency medical technician, or a critical care nurse. Although guidelines may vary, depending on state, county, or city regulations, the basic administration method is the same. (See *Administering endotracheal drugs*.)

Endotracheal drugs may be given using the syringe method or the adapter method. Usually used for bronchoscopy suctioning, the swivel adapter can be placed on the end of the tube and, while ventilation continues through a bag-valve device, the drug can be delivered with a needle through the closed stopcock.

Administering endotracheal drugs

In an emergency, some drugs may be given through an endotracheal (ET) tube if I.V. access isn't available. They may be given using the syringe method or the adapter method.

Before injecting any drug, check for proper placement of the ET tube, using your stethoscope. Make sure that the patient is supine and that her head is level with or slightly higher than her trunk.

Syringe method

Remove the needle before injecting medication into the ET tube. Insert the tip of the syringe into the ET tube, and inject the drug deep into the tube (as shown below).

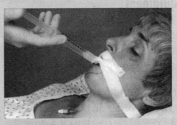

Adapter method

A device developed for ET drug administration provides a more closed system of drug delivery than the syringe method. A special adapter placed on the end of the ET tube (as shown below) allows needle insertion and drug delivery through the closed stopcock.

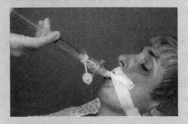

Key nursing diagnoses and patient outcomes

Deficient knowledge related to lack of exposure to endotracheal drug administration
The patient will:
▶ state or demonstrate an understanding of what has been taught
▶ demonstrate the ability to perform new health-related behaviors as they're taught.

Risk for injury related to improper technique
The patient will:
▶ identify factors that will increase injury
▶ help to identify and apply safety measures to prevent injury.

Equipment

ET tube or swivel adapter • gloves • stethoscope • handheld resuscitation bag • prescribed drug • syringe • sterile water or normal saline solution

Preparation of equipment

Verify the order on the patient's medication record by checking it against the doctor's order. Wash your hands. Check ET tube placement by using a handheld resuscitation bag and stethoscope.

Calculate the drug dose. Adult advanced cardiac life support guidelines recommend that drugs be administered at 2 to 2½ times the recommended I.V. dose. Next, draw the drug up into a syringe. Dilute it in 10 ml of sterile water or normal saline solution. *Dilution increases drug volume and contact with lung tissue.*

Implementation

▶ Put on gloves.
▶ Move the patient into the supine position and make sure his head is

level with or slightly higher than his trunk.
▶ Ventilate the patient three to five times with the resuscitation bag. Then remove the bag.
▶ Remove the needle from the syringe and insert the tip of the syringe into the ET tube or the swivel adapter. Inject the drug deep into the tube.
▶ After injecting the drug, reattach the resuscitation bag and ventilate the patient briskly. *This propels the drug into the lungs, oxygenates the patient, and clears the tube.*
▶ Discard the syringe in an appropriate sharps container.
▶ Remove and discard your gloves.

Special considerations

Be aware that the drug's onset of action may be quicker than it would be by I.V. administration. If the patient doesn't respond quickly, the doctor may order a repeat dose.

Complications

Potential complications of endotracheal drug administration result from the prescribed drug, not the administration route.

Documentation

Record the date and time of drug administration, drug administered, and the patient's response.

ENDOTRACHEAL INTUBATION

Endotracheal (ET) intubation involves the oral or nasal insertion of a flexible tube through the larynx into the trachea for the purposes of controlling the airway and mechanically ventilating the patient. Performed by a doctor, anesthetist, respiratory therapist, or nurse educated in the procedure, ET intubation usually occurs in emergencies, such as cardiopulmonary arrest or in diseases such as epiglottiditis. However, intubation may also occur under more controlled circumstances such as just before surgery. In such instances, ET intubation requires patient teaching and preparation.

Advantages of the procedure are that it establishes and maintains a patent airway, protects against aspiration by sealing off the trachea from the digestive tract, permits removal of tracheobronchial secretions in patients who can't cough effectively, and provides a route for mechanical ventilation. Disadvantages are that it bypasses normal respiratory defenses against infection, reduces cough effectiveness, and prevents verbal communication.

Oral ET intubation is contraindicated in patients with acute cervical spinal injury and degenerative spinal disorders, whereas nasal intubation is contraindicated in patients with apnea, bleeding disorders, chronic sinusitis, or nasal obstructions.

Key nursing diagnoses and patient outcomes

Risk for aspiration related to absence of protective mechanisms
The patient will:
▶ show no evidence of aspiration
▶ reveal no adventitious breath sounds on auscultation.

Ineffective airway clearance related to presence of secretions
The patient will:
▶ cough effectively

▶ expectorate sputum
▶ keep airway patent.

Equipment
Two ET tubes (one spare) in appropriate size • 10-ml syringe • stethoscope • gloves • lighted laryngoscope with a handle and blades of various sizes, curved and straight • sedative • local anesthetic spray • mucosal vasoconstricting agent (for nasal intubation) • overbed or other table • water-soluble lubricant • adhesive or other strong tape or Velcro tube holder • compound benzoin tincture • gloves • oral airway or bite block (for oral intubation) • suction equipment • handheld resuscitation bag with sterile swivel adapter • humidified oxygen source • optional: prepackaged intubation tray, sterile gauze pad, stylet, Magill forceps, sterile water, and sterile basin

Preparation of equipment
Quickly gather the individual supplies or use a prepackaged intubation tray, which will contain most of the necessary supplies. First, select an ET tube of the appropriate size—typically, 2.5 to 5.5 mm, uncuffed, for children and 6 to 10 mm, cuffed, for adults. The typical size of an oral tube is 7.5 mm for women and 9 mm for men. Select a slightly smaller tube for nasal intubation.

Check the light in the laryngoscope by snapping the appropriate-sized blade into place; if the bulb doesn't light, replace the batteries or the laryngoscope (whichever will be quicker).

Using sterile technique, open the package containing the ET tube and, if desired, open the other supplies on an overbed table. Pour the sterile water into the basin. Then, to ease insertion, lubricate 1″ (2.5 cm) of the distal end of the ET tube with the water-soluble lubricant using aseptic technique. Do this by squeezing the lubricant directly on the tube. Use only water-soluble lubricant *because it can be absorbed by mucous membranes.*

Next, attach the syringe to the port on the tube's exterior pilot cuff. Slowly inflate the cuff, observing for uniform inflation. Then use the syringe to deflate the cuff.

A stylet may be used on oral intubations *to stiffen the tube.* Lubricate the entire stylet. Insert the stylet into the tube so that its distal tip lies about ½″ (1.5 cm) inside the distal end of the tube. Make sure that the stylet doesn't protrude from the tube *to avoid vocal cord trauma.* Prepare the humidified oxygen source and the suction equipment for immediate use. If the patient is in bed, remove the headboard *to provide easier access.*

Implementation

▶ Administer a sedative as ordered *to induce amnesia or analgesia and help calm and relax the conscious patient.* Remove dentures and bridgework, if present.
▶ Administer oxygen until the tube is inserted *to prevent hypoxia.*
▶ Place the patient supine in the sniffing position so that his mouth, pharynx, and trachea are extended. For a blind intubation, place the patient's head and neck in a neutral position.
▶ Put on gloves.
▶ For oral intubation, spray a local anesthetic such as lidocaine deep into the posterior pharynx *to diminish the gag reflex and reduce patient discomfort.* For nasal intubation, spray a local anesthetic and a mucosal vasoconstrictor into the nasal passages *to anesthetize the nasal turbinates and reduce the chance of bleeding.*

▶ If necessary, suction the patient's pharynx just before tube insertion *to improve visualization of the patient's pharynx and vocal cords.*
▶ Time each intubation attempt, limiting attempts to less than 30 seconds *to prevent hypoxia.*

Intubation with direct visualization
▶ Stand at the head of the patient's bed. Using your right hand, hold the patient's mouth open by crossing your index finger over your thumb, placing your thumb on the patient's upper teeth and your index finger on his lower teeth. *This technique provides greater leverage.*
▶ Grasp the laryngoscope handle in your left hand and gently slide the blade into the right side of the patient's mouth. Center the blade and push the patient's tongue to the left. Hold the patient's lower lip away from his teeth *to prevent the lip from being traumatized.*
▶ Advance the blade *to expose the epiglottis.* When using a straight blade, insert the tip under the epiglottis; when using a curved blade, insert the tip between the base of the tongue and the epiglottis.
▶ Lift the laryngoscope handle upward and away from your body at a 45-degree angle *to reveal the vocal cords.* Avoid pivoting the laryngoscope against the patient's teeth to avoid damaging them.
▶ If desired, have an assistant apply pressure to the cricoid ring *to occlude the esophagus and minimize gastric regurgitation.*
▶ When performing an oral intubation, insert the ET tube into the right side of the patient's mouth. When performing a nasotracheal intubation, insert the ET tube through the nostril and into the pharynx. Then use Magill for-

ceps to guide the tube through the vocal cords.

▶ Guide the tube into the vertical openings of the larynx between the vocal cords, being careful not to mistake the horizontal opening of the esophagus for the larynx. If the vocal cords are closed because of a spasm, wait a few seconds for them to relax; then gently guide the tube past them *to avoid traumatic injury.*

▶ Advance the tube until the cuff disappears beyond the vocal cords. Avoid advancing the tube farther *to avoid occluding a major bronchus and precipitating lung collapse.*

▶ Holding the ET tube in place, quickly remove the stylet, if present.

Blind nasotracheal intubation

▶ Pass the ET tube along the floor of the nasal cavity. If necessary, use gentle force to pass the tube through the nasopharynx and into the pharynx.

▶ Listen and feel for air movement through the tube as it's advanced *to ensure that the tube is properly place in the airway.*

▶ Slip the tube between the vocal cords when the patient inhales *because the vocal cords separate on inhalation.*

▶ When the tube is past the vocal cords, the breath sounds should become louder. If, at any time during tube advancement, breath sounds disappear, withdraw the tube until they reappear.

After intubation

▶ Inflate the tube's cuff with 5 to 10 cc of air until you feel resistance. When the patient is mechanically ventilated, you'll use the minimal-leak technique or the minimal occlusive volume technique to establish correct inflation of the cuff. (For instructions, see "Tracheal cuff–pressure measurement," page 817.)

▶ Remove the laryngoscope. If the patient was intubated orally, insert an oral airway or a bite block *to prevent the patient from obstructing airflow or puncturing the tube with his teeth.*

▶ *To ensure correct tube placement,* observe for chest expansion and auscultate for bilateral breath sounds. If the patient is unconscious or uncooperative, use a handheld resuscitation bag while observing for upper chest movement and auscultating for breath sounds. Feel the tube's tip for warm exhalations and listen for air movement. Observe for condensation forming inside the tube.

▶ If you don't hear any breath sounds, auscultate over the stomach while ventilating with the resuscitation bag. Stomach distention, belching, or a gurgling sound indicates esophageal intubation. Immediately deflate the cuff and remove the tube. After reoxygenating the patient *to prevent hypoxia,* repeat insertion using a sterile tube *to prevent contamination of the trachea.*

▶ Auscultate bilaterally *to exclude the possibility of endobronchial intubation.* If you fail to hear breath sounds on both sides of the chest, you may have inserted the tube into one of the mainstem bronchi (usually the right one because of its wider angle at the bifurcation); such insertion occludes the other bronchus and lung and results in atelectasis on the obstructed side. Or the tube may be resting on the carina, resulting in dry secretions that obstruct both bronchi. (The patient's coughing and fighting the ventilator will alert you to the problem.) *To correct these situations,* deflate the cuff, withdraw the tube 1/8" (1 to 2 mm), auscultate for bilateral breath sounds, and reinflate the cuff.

▶ When you've confirmed correct tube placement, administer oxygen or initiate mechanical ventilation and suction, if indicated.

▶ *To secure tube position,* apply compound benzoin tincture to each cheek and let it dry. Tape the tube firmly with adhesive or other strong tape or use a Velcro tube holder. (See *Three methods to secure an ET tube.*)

▶ Inflate the cuff with the minimal-leak or minimal occlusive volume technique. For the minimal-leak technique, attach a 10-ml syringe to the port on the tube's exterior pilot cuff and place a stethoscope on the side of the patient's neck. Inject small amounts of air with each breath until you hear no leak. Then aspirate 0.1 cc of air from the cuff *to create a minimal air leak.* Record the amount of air needed to inflate the cuff. For the minimal occlusive volume technique, follow the first two steps of the minimal-leak technique but place the stethoscope over the trachea instead. Aspirate until you hear a small leak on inspiration and add just enough air to stop the leak. Record the amount of air needed to inflate the cuff *for subsequent monitoring of tracheal dilation or erosion.*

▶ Clearly note the centimeter marking on the tube where it exits the patient's mouth or nose. *By periodically monitoring this mark, you can detect tube displacement.*

▶ Make sure that a chest X-ray is taken *to verify tube position.*

▶ Place a swivel adapter between the tube and the humidified oxygen source *to allow for intermittent suctioning and to reduce tube tension.*

▶ Place the patient on his side with his head in a comfortable position *to avoid tube kinking and airway obstruction.*

▶ Auscultate both sides of the chest and watch chest movement as indicated by the patient's condition *to ensure correct tube placement and full lung ventilation.* Provide frequent oral care to the orally intubated patient and position the ET tube *to prevent formation of pressure ulcers* and avoid excessive pressure on the sides of the mouth. Provide frequent nasal and oral care to the nasally intubated patient *to prevent formation of pressure ulcers and drying of oral mucous membranes.*

▶ Suction secretions through the ET tube as the patient's condition indicates *to clear secretions and prevent mucus plugs from obstructing the tube.*

Special considerations

▶ Orotracheal intubation is preferred in emergencies *because insertion is easier and faster than it is with nasotracheal intubation.* However, maintaining exact tube placement is more difficult, and the tube must be well secured *to avoid kinking and prevent bronchial obstruction or accidental extubation.* Orotracheal intubation is also poorly tolerated by the conscious patient *because it stimulates salivation, coughing, and retching.*

▶ Nasotracheal intubation is preferred for elective insertion when the patient is capable of spontaneous ventilation for a short period. Blind intubation is typically used in conscious patients who risk imminent respiratory arrest or who have cervical spinal injury.

▶ Although nasotracheal intubation is more comfortable than oral intubation, it's also more difficult to perform. *Because the tube passes blindly through the nasal cavity,* the procedure causes greater tissue trauma, increases the risk of infection by nasal bacteria introduced into the trachea, and risks pressure necrosis of the nasal mucosa.

Three methods to secure an ET tube

Before taping an endotracheal (ET) tube in place, make sure the patient's face is clean, dry, and free of beard stubble. If possible, suction his mouth and dry the tube just before taping. Also, check the reference mark on the tube to ensure correct placement. After taping, always check for bilateral breath sounds to ensure that the tube hasn't been displaced by manipulation.

To tape the tube securely, use one of the following three methods.

Method 1

Cut two 2″ (5.1-cm) strips and two 15″ (38.1-cm) strips of 1″ cloth adhesive tape. Then cut a 13″ (33-cm) slit in one end of each 15″ strip (as shown below).

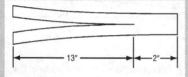

Apply compound benzoin tincture to the patient's cheeks. Place the 2″ strips on his cheeks, creating a new surface on which to anchor the tape securing the tube. *When frequent retaping is necessary, this helps preserve the patient's skin integrity.* If the patient's skin is excoriated or at risk, you can use a transparent semipermeable dressing to protect the skin.

Apply the benzoin tincture to the tape on the patient's face and to the part of the tube where you will be applying the tape. On the side of the mouth where the tube will be anchored, place the unslit end of the long tape on top of the tape on the patient's cheek.

Wrap the top half of the tape around the tube twice, pulling the tape tightly around the tube. Then, directing the tape over the patient's upper lip, place the end of the tape on his other cheek. Cut off any excess tape. Use the lower half of the tape to secure an oral airway, if necessary (as shown above right).

Or twist the lower half of the tape around the tube twice and attach it to the original

cheek (as shown in bottom illustration). *Taping in opposite directions places equal traction on the tube.*

If you've taped in an oral airway or are concerned about the tube's stability, apply the other 15″ strip of tape in the same manner, starting on the other side of the patient's

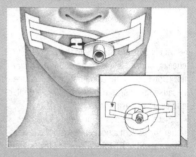

face. If the tape around the tube is too bulky, use only the upper part of the tape and cut off the lower part. If the patient has copious oral secretions, seal the tape by cutting a 1″ piece of paper tape, coating it with benzoin tincture, and placing the paper tape over the adhesive tape.

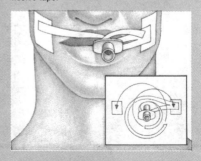

(continued)

Three methods to secure an ET tube *(continued)*

Method 2

Cut one piece of 1″ cloth adhesive tape long enough to wrap around the patient's head and overlap in front. Then cut an 8″ (20.3-cm) piece of tape and center it on the longer piece, sticky sides together. Next, cut a 5″ (12.7-cm) slit in each end of the longer tape (as shown below).

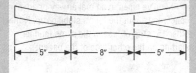

Apply benzoin tincture to the patient's cheeks, under his nose, and under his lower lip. (Don't spray benzoin directly on his face because the vapors can be irritating if inhaled and can also harm the eyes.)

Place the top half of one end of the tape under the patient's nose and wrap the lower half around the ET tube. Place the lower half of the other end of the tape along his lower lip and wrap the top half around the tube (as shown below).

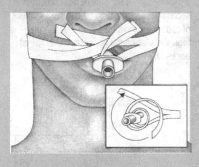

Method 3

Cut a tracheostomy tie in two pieces, one a few inches longer than the other, and cut two 6″ (15.2-cm) pieces of 1″ cloth adhesive tape. Then cut a 2″ slit in one end of both pieces of tape. Fold back the other end of the tape ½″ (1.3 cm) so that the sticky sides are together, and cut a small hole in it (as shown below).

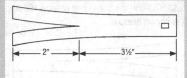

Apply benzoin tincture to the part of the ET tube that will be taped. Wrap the split ends of each piece of tape around the tube, one piece on each side. Overlap the tape to secure it.

Apply the free ends of the tape to both sides of the patient's face. Then insert tracheostomy ties through the holes in the tape and knot the ties (as shown below).

Bring the longer tie behind the patient's neck. *Knotting the ties on the side prevents the patient from lying on the knot and developing a pressure ulcer.*

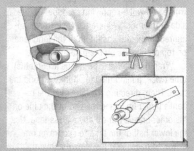

Retrograde intubation: An alternative form of airway maintenance

When a patient's airway can't be secured using conventional oral or nasal intubation, retrograde intubation should be considered. In this technique, a wire is inserted through the trachea and out the mouth and is then used to guide the insertion of an endotracheal (ET) tube (as shown below).

Only doctors, nurses, and paramedics who have been specially trained may perform retrograde intubation. However, the procedure has numerous advantages: It requires little or no head movement; it's less invasive than cricothyrotomy or tracheotomy and

doesn't leave a permanent scar; and it doesn't require direct visualization of the vocal cords.

Retrograde intubation is contraindicated in patients with complete airway obstruction, a thyroid tumor, an enlarged thyroid gland that overlies the cricothyroid ligament, or coagulopathy and in those whose mouths can't open wide enough to allow the guide wire to be retrieved. Possible complications include minor bleeding and hematoma formation at the puncture site, subcutaneous emphysema, hoarseness, and bleeding into the trachea.

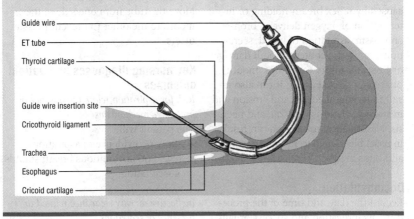

- Guide wire
- ET tube
- Thyroid cartilage
- Guide wire insertion site
- Cricothyroid ligament
- Trachea
- Esophagus
- Cricoid cartilage

However, exact tube placement is easier, and the risk of dislodgment is lower. The cuff on the ET tube maintains a closed system that permits positive-pressure ventilation and protects the airway from aspiration of secretions and gastric contents.

▶ Although low-pressure cuffs have significantly reduced the incidence of tracheal erosion and necrosis caused by cuff pressure on the tracheal wall, over-

inflation of a low-pressure cuff can negate the benefit. Use the minimal-leak technique to avoid these complications. Inflating the cuff a bit more to make a complete seal with the least amount of air is the next most desirable method.

▶ Always record the volume of air needed to inflate the cuff. A gradual increase in this volume indicates tracheal dilatation or erosion. A sudden increase in volume indicates rupture of the cuff and requires immediate reintubation if the patient is being ventilated or if he requires continuous cuff inflation to maintain a high concentration of delivered oxygen. When the cuff has been inflated, measure its pressure at least every 8 hours to avoid overinflation. Normal cuff pressure is about 18 mm Hg.

▶ When neither method of ET intubation is possible, consider the alternative of retrograde intubation. (See *Retrograde intubation: An alternative form of airway maintenance,* page 281.)

Complications
ET intubation can result in apnea caused by reflex breath-holding or interruption of oxygen delivery; bronchospasm; aspiration of blood, secretions, or gastric contents; tooth damage or loss; and injury to the lips, mouth, pharynx, or vocal cords. It can also result in laryngeal edema and erosion and in tracheal stenosis, erosion, and necrosis. Nasotracheal intubation can result in nasal bleeding, laceration, sinusitis, and otitis media.

Documentation
Record the date and time of the procedure; its indication and success or failure; tube type and size; cuff size, amount of inflation, and inflation technique; administration of medication; initiation of supplemental oxygen or ventilation therapy; results of chest auscultation and results of the chest X-ray; any complications and interventions; and the patient's reaction to the procedure.

ENDOTRACHEAL TUBE CARE

The intubated patient requires meticulous care to ensure airway patency and prevent complications until he can maintain independent ventilation. This care includes frequent assessment of airway status, maintenance of proper cuff pressure to prevent tissue ischemia and necrosis, repositioning of the tube to avoid traumatic manipulation, and constant monitoring for complications. Endotracheal (ET) tubes are repositioned for patient comfort or if a chest X-ray shows improper placement. Move the tube from one side of the mouth to the other to prevent pressure ulcers.

Key nursing diagnoses and patient outcomes
Risk for aspiration related to absence of protective mechanisms
The patient will:
▶ show no evidence of aspiration
▶ reveal no adventitious breath sounds on auscultation.

Ineffective airway clearance related to presence of secretions
The patient will:
▶ cough effectively
▶ expectorate sputum
▶ maintain a patent airway.

Equipment
For maintaining the airway
Stethoscope • suction equipment • gloves

For repositioning the tube
10-ml syringe • compound benzoin tincture • stethoscope • adhesive or hy-

poallergenic tape or Velcro tube holder
• suction equipment • sedative or 2%
lidocaine • gloves • handheld resuscitation bag with mask (in case of accidental extubation)

For removing the tube
10-ml syringe • suction equipment •
supplemental oxygen source with mask
• cool-mist, large-volume nebulizer •
handheld resuscitation bag with mask •
gloves • equipment for reintubation

Preparation of equipment
For repositioning the ET tube
Assemble all equipment at the patient's
bedside. Using sterile technique, set up
the suction equipment.

For removing the ET tube
Assemble all equipment at the patient's
bedside. Set up the suction and supplemental oxygen equipment. Have ready
all equipment for emergency reintubation.

Implementation
► Explain the procedure to the patient
even if he doesn't appear to be alert.
Provide privacy, wash your hands thoroughly, and put on gloves.

Maintaining airway patency
► Auscultate the patient's lungs at any
sign of respiratory distress. If you detect an obstructed airway, determine
the cause and treat it accordingly. If secretions are obstructing the lumen of
the tube, suction the secretions from
the tube. (See "Tracheal suction," page
819.)
► If the ET tube has slipped from the
trachea into the right or left mainstem
bronchus, breath sounds will be absent
over one lung. Obtain a chest X-ray as

ordered *to verify tube placement* and, if
necessary, reposition the tube.

Repositioning the ET tube
► Get help from a respiratory therapist
or another nurse *to prevent accidental
extubation during the procedure if the patient coughs.*
► Suction the patient's trachea through
the ET tube to remove any secretions,
*which can cause the patient to cough dur-
ing the procedure. Coughing increases the
risk of trauma and tube dislodgment.*
Then suction the patient's pharynx *to
remove any secretions that may have accumulated above the tube cuff. This helps to
prevent aspiration of secretions during cuff
deflation.*
► *To prevent traumatic manipulation of
the tube,* instruct the assisting nurse to
hold it as you carefully untape the tube
or unfasten the Velcro tube holder.
When freeing the tube, locate a landmark such as a number on the tube or
measure the distance from the patient's
mouth to the top of the tube *so that you
have a reference point when moving the
tube.*
► Next, deflate the cuff by attaching a
10-ml syringe to the pilot balloon port
and aspirating air until you meet resistance and the pilot balloon deflates.
Deflate the cuff before moving the tube
*because the cuff forms a seal within the
trachea and movement of an inflated cuff
can damage the tracheal wall and vocal
cords.*
► Reposition the tube as necessary,
noting new landmarks or measuring
the length. Then immediately reinflate
the cuff. To do this, instruct the patient
to inhale and slowly inflate the cuff using a 10-ml syringe attached to the pilot balloon port. As you do this, use
your stethoscope to auscultate the pa-

tient's neck *to determine the presence of an air leak.* When air leakage ceases, stop cuff inflation and, while still auscultating the patient's neck, aspirate a small amount of air until you detect a slight leak. *This creates a minimal air leak, which indicates that the cuff is inflated at the lowest pressure possible to create an adequate seal.* If the patient is being mechanically ventilated, aspirate to create a minimal air leak during the inspiratory phase of respiration *because the positive pressure of the ventilator during inspiration will create a larger leak around the cuff.* Note the number of cubic centimeters of air required to achieve a minimal air leak.

▶ Measure cuff pressure and compare the reading with previous pressure readings *to prevent overinflation.* Then use benzoin and tape to secure the tube in place, or refasten the Velcro tube holder.

▶ Make sure the patient is comfortable and the airway patent. Properly clean or dispose of equipment.

▶ When the cuff is inflated, measure its pressure at least every 8 hours *to avoid overinflation.* (See "Tracheal cuff–pressure measurement," page 817.)

Removing the ET tube

▶ When you're authorized to remove the tube, obtain another nurse's assistance *to prevent traumatic manipulation of the tube when it's untaped or unfastened.*

▶ Elevate the head of the patient's bed to approximately 90 degrees.

▶ Suction the patient's oropharynx and nasopharynx *to remove any accumulated secretions and to help prevent aspiration of secretions when the cuff is deflated.*

▶ Using a handheld resuscitation bag or the mechanical ventilator, give the patient several deep breaths through the ET tube *to hyperinflate his lungs and increase his oxygen reserve.*

▶ Attach a 10-ml syringe to the pilot balloon port and aspirate air until you meet resistance and the pilot balloon deflates. If you fail to detect an air leak around the deflated cuff, notify the doctor immediately and don't proceed with extubation. *Absence of an air leak may indicate marked tracheal edema, which can result in total airway obstruction if the ET tube is removed.*

▶ If you detect the proper air leak, untape or unfasten the ET tube while the assisting nurse stabilizes the tube.

▶ Insert a sterile suction catheter through the ET tube. Then apply suction and ask the patient to take a deep breath and to open his mouth fully and pretend to cry out. *This causes abduction of the vocal cords and reduces the risk of laryngeal trauma during withdrawal of the tube.*

▶ Simultaneously remove the ET tube and the suction catheter in one smooth, outward and downward motion, following the natural curve of the patient's mouth. *Suctioning during extubation removes secretions retained at the end of the tube and prevents aspiration.*

▶ Give the patient supplemental oxygen. For maximum humidity, use a cool-mist, large-volume nebulizer *to help decrease airway irritation, patient discomfort, and laryngeal edema.*

▶ Encourage the patient to cough and breathe deeply. Remind him that a sore throat and hoarseness are to be expected and will gradually subside.

▶ Make sure the patient is comfortable and the airway is patent. Clean or dispose of equipment.

▶ After extubation, auscultate the patient's lungs frequently and watch for signs of respiratory distress. Be especially alert for stridor or other evidence of upper airway obstruction. If ordered, draw an arterial sample for blood gas analysis.

Special considerations

▶ When repositioning an ET tube, be especially careful in patients with highly sensitive airways. Sedation or direct instillation of 2% lidocaine to numb the airway may be indicated in such patients. *Because the lidocaine is absorbed systemically, you must have a doctor's order to use it.*

▶ After extubation of a patient who has been intubated for an extended time, keep reintubation supplies readily available for at least 12 hours or until you're sure he can tolerate extubation.

▶ Never extubate a patient unless someone skilled at intubation is readily available.

▶ If you inadvertently cut the pilot balloon on the cuff, immediately call the person responsible for intubation in your facility, who will remove the damaged ET tube and replace it with one that is intact. Don't remove the tube *because a tube with an air leak is better than no airway.*

Complications

Traumatic injury to the larynx or trachea may result from tube manipulation, accidental extubation, or tube slippage into the right bronchus. Ventilatory failure and airway obstruction, due to laryngospasm or marked tracheal edema, are the gravest possible complications of extubation.

Documentation

After tube repositioning, record the date and time of the procedure, reason for repositioning (such as malposition shown by chest X-ray), new tube position, total amount of air in the cuff after the procedure, any complications and interventions, and the patient's tolerance of the procedure.

After extubation, record the date and time of extubation, presence or absence of stridor or other signs of upper airway edema, type of supplemental oxygen administered, any complications and required subsequent therapy, and the patient's tolerance of the procedure.

END-TIDAL CARBON DIOXIDE MONITORING

Monitoring of end-tidal carbon dioxide ($ETCO_2$) determines the carbon dioxide (CO_2) concentration in exhaled gas. In this technique, a photodetector measures the amount of infrared light absorbed by airway gas during inspiration and expiration. (Light absorption increases along with the CO_2 concentration.) A monitor converts these data to a CO_2 value and a corresponding waveform, or capnogram, if capnography is used. (See *How $ETCO_2$ monitoring works,* page 286.)

$ETCO_2$ monitoring provides information about the patient's pulmonary, cardiac, and metabolic status that aids patient management and helps prevent clinical compromise. This technique has become standard during anesthesia administration and mechanical ventilation.

The sensor, which contains an infrared light source and a photodetector, is positioned at one of two sites in the monitoring setup. With a mainstream monitor, it's positioned directly at the patient's airway with an airway adapter,

How ETCO$_2$ monitoring works

The optical portion of an end-tidal carbon dioxide (ETCO$_2$) monitor contains an infrared light source, a sample chamber, a special carbon dioxide (CO$_2$) filter, and a photodetector. The infrared light passes through the sample chamber and is absorbed in varying amounts, depending on the amount of CO$_2$ the patient has just exhaled. The photodetector measures CO$_2$ content and relays this information to the microprocessor in the monitor, which displays the CO$_2$ value and waveform.

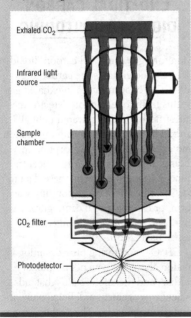

Exhaled CO$_2$

Infrared light source

Sample chamber

CO$_2$ filter

Photodetector

Some CO$_2$ detection devices provide semiquantitative indications of CO$_2$ concentrations, supplying an approximate range rather than a specific value for ETCO$_2$. Other devices simply indicate whether CO$_2$ is present during exhalation (See *Analyzing CO$_2$ levels.*)

ETCO$_2$ monitoring may be used to help wean a patient with a stable acid-base balance from mechanical ventilation. It also reduces the need for frequent arterial blood gas (ABG) measurements, especially when combined with pulse oximetry. Other uses for ETCO$_2$ monitoring include assessing resuscitation efforts and identifying the return of spontaneous circulation. Because no CO$_2$ is exhaled when breathing stops, this technique also detects apnea.

When used during ET intubation, ETCO$_2$ monitoring can avert neurologic injury and even death by confirming correct ET tube placement and detecting accidental esophageal intubation because CO$_2$ isn't normally produced by the stomach. Ongoing ETCO$_2$ monitoring throughout intubation can also prove valuable because an ET tube may become dislodged during manipulation or patient movement or transport.

Key nursing diagnoses and patient outcomes

Impaired gas exchange related to (specify)
The patient will:
▶ maintain adequate ventilation
▶ have ABG levels within acceptable limits (specify).

Dysfunctional ventilatory weaning response related to (specify)
The patient will:
▶ maintain a respiratory rate within plus or minus 5 breaths/minute of baseline during weaning

between the endotracheal (ET) tube and the breathing circuit tubing. With a sidestream monitor, the airway adapter is positioned at the airway (regardless of whether the patient is intubated) *to allow aspiration of gas from the patient's airway back to the sensor, which lies either within or close to the monitor.*

▶ stabilize mental and emotional states as ventilatory support is gradually withdrawn.

Equipment

Gloves • mainstream or sidestream CO_2 monitor • CO_2 sensor • airway adapter as recommended by the manufacturer (a neonatal adapter may have a much smaller dead space, making it appropriate for a smaller patient)

Preparation of equipment

If the monitor you're using isn't self-calibrating, calibrate it as the manufacturer directs. If you're using a sidestream CO_2 monitor, replace the water trap between patients, if directed. *The trap allows humidity from exhaled gases to be condensed into an attached container.* Newer sidestream models don't require water traps.

Implementation

▶ If the patient requires ET intubation, an $ETCO_2$ detector or monitor is usually applied immediately after the tube is inserted. If he doesn't require intubation or is already intubated and alert, explain the purpose and expected duration of monitoring. Tell an intubated patient that the monitor will painlessly measure the amount of CO_2 he exhales. Inform a nonintubated patient that the monitor will track his CO_2 concentration to make sure his breathing is effective.

▶ Wash your hands. After turning on the monitor and calibrating it (if necessary), position the airway adapter and sensor as the manufacturer directs. For an intubated patient, position the adapter directly on the ET tube. For a nonintubated patient, place the adapter at or near the patient's airway. (An oxygen-delivery cannula may have a sam-

Analyzing CO_2 levels

Depending on which end-tidal carbon dioxide ($ETCO_2$) detector you use, the meaning of color changes within the detector dome may differ from the analysis for the Easy Cap detector described below:

■ The rim of the Easy Cap is divided into four segments (clockwise from the top): CHECK, A, B, and C. The CHECK segment is solid purple, signifying the absence of carbon dioxide (CO_2).

■ The numbers in the other sections range from 0.03 to 5 and indicate the percentage of exhaled CO_2. The color should fluctuate during ventilation from purple (in section A) during inspiration to yellow (in section C) at the end of expiration. This indicates that the $ETCO_2$ levels are adequate: above 2%.

■ An end-expiratory color change from C to the B range may be the first sign of hemodynamic instability.

■ During cardiopulmonary resuscitation (CPR), an end-expiratory color change from the A or B range to the C range may mean the return of spontaneous ventilation.

■ During prolonged cardiac arrest, inadequate pulmonary perfusion leads to inadequate gas exchange. The patient exhales little or no CO_2, so the color stays in the purple range even with proper intubation. Ineffective CPR also leads to inadequate pulmonary perfusion.

Color indications on end-expiration

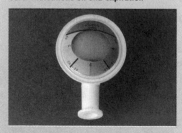

CO₂ waveform

The carbon dioxide (CO_2) waveform, or capnogram, produced in end-tidal carbon dioxide ($ETCO_2$) monitoring reflects the course of CO_2 elimination during exhalation. A normal capnogram (shown below) consists of several segments, which reflect the various stages of exhalation and inhalation.

Normally, any gas eliminated from the airway during early exhalation is dead-space gas, which hasn't undergone exchange at the alveolocapillary membrane. Measurements taken during this period contain no CO_2. As exhalation continues, CO_2 concentration rises sharply and rapidly. The sensor now detects gas that has undergone exchange, producing measurable quantities of CO_2.

The final stages of alveolar emptying occur during late exhalation. During the alveolar plateau phase, CO_2 concentration rises more gradually because alveolar emptying is more constant.

The point at which $ETCO_2$ value is derived is the end of exhalation, when CO_2 concentration peaks. Unless an alveolar plateau is present, this value doesn't accurately estimate alveolar CO_2. During inhalation, the CO_2 concentration declines sharply to zero.

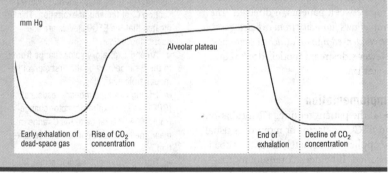

mm Hg

Alveolar plateau

Early exhalation of dead-space gas | Rise of CO_2 concentration | End of exhalation | Decline of CO_2 concentration

ple port through which gas can be aspirated for monitoring.)

▶ Turn on all alarms and adjust alarm settings as appropriate for your patient. Make sure the alarm volume is loud enough to hear.

Special considerations

▶ Wear gloves when handling the airway adapter *to prevent cross-contamination.* Make sure the adapter is changed with every breathing circuit and ET tube change.

▶ Place the adapter on the ET tube *to avoid contaminating exhaled gases with fresh gas flow from the ventilator.* If you're using a heat and moisture exchanger,

you may be able to position the airway adapter between the exchanger and breathing circuit.

▶ If your patient's $ETCO_2$ values differ from his partial pressure of arterial carbon dioxide, assess him for factors that can influence $ETCO_2$ — especially when the differential between arterial and $ETCO_2$ values (the arterial absolute difference of carbon dioxide [$a\text{-}ADCO_2$]) is above normal.

▶ The $a\text{-}ADCO_2$ value, if correctly interpreted, provides useful information about your patient's status. For example, an increased $a\text{-}ADCO_2$ may mean that your patient has worsening dead

Using a disposable $ETCO_2$ detector: Some do's and don'ts

When using a disposable end-tidal carbon dioxide ($ETCO_2$) detector, check the instructions and ensure ideal working conditions for the device. Here are some additional guidelines.

Avoiding high humidity, moisture, and heat

- Watch for changes indicating that the $ETCO_2$ detector's life span is decreasing — for example, sluggish color changes from breath to breath. A detector normally may be used for about 2 hours. However, using it with a ventilator that delivers high-humidity ventilation may shorten its life span to no more than 15 minutes.
- Don't use the detector with a heated humidifier or a nebulizer.
- Keep the detector protected from secretions, which would render the device useless. If secretions enter the dome, remove and discard the detector.
- Use a heat and moisture exchanger to protect the detector. In some detectors, this filter fits between the endotracheal (ET) tube and the detector.
- If you're using a heat and moisture exchanger, remember that it'll increase your patient's breathing effort. Be alert for in-creased resistance and breathing difficulties and remove the exchanger, if necessary.

Taking additional precautions

- Instilling epinephrine through the ET tube can damage the detector's indicator (the color may stay yellow). If this happens, discard the device.
- Take care when using an $ETCO_2$ detector on a child who weighs less than 30 lb (13.6 kg). A small patient who rebreathes air from the dead air space (about 38 cc) will inhale too much of his own carbon dioxide.
- Frequently spot-check the $ETCO_2$ detector you're using for effectiveness. If you must transport the patient to another area for testing or treatment, use another method to verify the tube's placement.
- Never reuse a disposable $ETCO_2$ detector; it's intended for one-time, one-patient use only.

space, especially if his tidal volume remains constant.

▶ Remember that $ETCO_2$ monitoring doesn't replace ABG measurements *because it doesn't assess oxygenation or blood pH.* Supplementing $ETCO_2$ monitoring with pulse oximetry may provide more complete information.

▶ If the CO_2 waveform is available, assess it for height, frequency, rhythm, baseline, and shape *to help evaluate gas exchange.* Make sure you know how to recognize a normal waveform and can identify any abnormal waveforms and their possible causes. If a printer is available, record and document any ab-normal waveforms in the patient's medical record. (See *CO_2 waveform.*)

▶ In a nonintubated patient, use $ETCO_2$ values to establish trends. Be aware that in a nonintubated patient, exhaled gas is more likely to mix with ambient air, and exhaled CO_2 may be diluted by fresh gas flow from the nasal cannula.

▶ $ETCO_2$ monitoring commonly is discontinued when the patient has been weaned effectively from mechanical ventilation or when he's no longer at risk for respiratory compromise. Carefully assess your patient's tolerance for weaning. After extubation, continuous

ETCO$_2$ monitoring may detect the need for reintubation.

▶ Disposable ETCO$_2$ detectors are available. When using a disposable ETCO$_2$ detector, always check its color under fluorescent or natural light *because the dome looks pink under incandescent light.* (See *Using a disposable ETCO$_2$ detector: Some do's and don'ts,* page 289.)

Complications

Inaccurate measurements — such as from poor sampling technique, calibration drift, contamination of optics with moisture or secretions, or equipment malfunction — can lead to misdiagnosis and improper treatment.

The effects of manual resuscitation or ingestion of alcohol or carbonated beverages can alter the detector's findings. Color changes detected after fewer than six ventilations can be misleading.

Documentation

Document the initial ETCO$_2$ value and all ventilator settings. Describe the waveform if one appears on the monitor. If the monitor has a printer, you may want to print out a sample waveform and include it in the patient's medical record.

Document ETCO$_2$ values at least as often as vital signs, whenever significant changes in waveform or patient status occur, and before and after weaning, respiratory, and other interventions. Periodically obtain samples for ABG analysis as the patient's condition dictates and document the corresponding ETCO$_2$ values.

ENEMA ADMINISTRATION

Enema administration involves instilling a solution into the rectum and colon. In a retention enema, the patient holds the solution within the rectum or colon for 30 minutes to 1 hour. In an irrigating enema, the patient expels the solution almost completely within 15 minutes. Both types of enema stimulate peristalsis by mechanically distending the colon and stimulating rectal wall nerves.

Enemas are used to clean the lower bowel in preparation for diagnostic or surgical procedures, to relieve distention and promote expulsion of flatus, to lubricate the rectum and colon, and to soften hardened stool for removal. They're contraindicated, however, after recent colon or rectal surgery or myocardial infarction and in a patient with an acute abdominal condition of unknown origin such as suspected appendicitis. Enemas should be administered cautiously to a patient with an arrhythmia.

Key nursing diagnoses and patient outcomes

Ineffective tissue perfusion (gastrointestinal) related to (specify)
The patient will:
▶ have intake equal to output
▶ have bowel function return to normal
▶ have no nausea, vomiting, or abdominal pain.

Constipation related to (specify)
The patient will:
▶ have bowel pattern return to normal
▶ state an understanding of factors causing constipation.

Understanding types of enemas

Enemas are used primarily for three purposes: cleansing, lubricating (or emollient), and carminative (to promote expulsion of flatus). This chart reveals the preparation steps and purposes of the common irrigating and retention enemas.

Solution	Preparation	Purpose
Irrigating enemas		
Tap water	Instill 1,000 ml of tap water.	Cleansing
Magnesium sulfate	Add 2 tbs of magnesium sulfate to 3 tbs of salt in 1,000 ml of tap water.	Carminative
Saline solution	If a commercially prepared solution isn't available, add 2 tsp of salt to 1,000 ml of tap water.	Cleansing
Soap and water	Add 1 packet of mild soap to 1,000 ml of tap water and remove all bubbles before administering solution.	Cleansing
Retention enemas		
Oil	Instill 150 ml of mineral, olive, or cottonseed oil.	Cleansing and emollient
1-2-3	Add 30 ml of 50% magnesium sulfate to 60 ml of glycerin. Add mixture to 90 ml of warm tap water.	Cleansing

Equipment

Prescribed solution • bath (utility) thermometer • enema administration bag with attached rectal tube and clamp • I.V. pole • gloves • linen-saver pads • bath blanket • two bedpans with covers, or bedside commode • water-soluble lubricant • toilet tissue • bulb syringe or funnel • plastic bag for equipment • water • gown • washcloth • soap and water • if observing enteric precautions: plastic trash bags and labels • optional (for patients who can't retain the solution): plastic rectal tube guard and indwelling urinary catheter or rectal catheter with 30-ml balloon and syringe

Prepackaged disposable enema sets are available, as are small-volume enema solutions in both irrigating and retention types and in pediatric sizes.

Preparation of equipment

Prepare the prescribed type and amount of solution as indicated. (See *Understanding types of enemas*.) The standard volume of an irrigating enema is 750 to 1,000 ml for an adult.

 Age alert Standard irrigating enema volumes for pediatric patients are 500 to 1,000 ml for a school-aged child; 250 to 500 ml for a toddler or preschooler; and 250 ml or less for an infant.

How to give an enema

Unless contraindicated, help the patient into the left-lateral Sims' position. After lubricating the end of the tube, separate the patient's buttocks and push the tube gently into the anus, aiming it toward the umbilicus. For an adult, insert the tube 2″ to 4″ (5 to 10 cm).

For a child, insert the tube only 2″ to 3″ (5 to 7.5 cm); for an infant, insert it only 1″ to 1½″ (2.5 to 4 cm).

Avoid forcing the tube to prevent rectal wall trauma. If it doesn't advance easily, allow a little solution to flow in to relax the inner sphincter enough to allow passage.

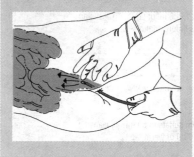

Because some ingredients may be mucosal irritants, make sure the proportions are correct and the agents are thoroughly mixed to avoid localized irritation. Warm the solution to reduce patient discomfort. Administer an adult's enema at 100° to 105° F (37.8° to 40.6° C). Check the temperature with a bath thermometer.

 Age alert Administer a child's enema at 100° F to avoid burning rectal tissues.

Clamp the tubing and fill the solution bag with the prescribed solution. Unclamp the tubing, flush the solution through the tubing, and then reclamp the tubing. *Flushing detects leaks and re-*

moves air that could cause discomfort if introduced into the colon.

Hang the solution container on the I.V. pole and take all supplies to the patient's room. If you're using an indwelling urinary catheter or rectal catheter, fill the syringe with 30 ml of water.

Implementation

▶ Check the doctor's order and assess the patient's condition.

▶ Provide privacy and explain the procedure. If you're administering an enema to a child, familiarize him with the equipment and allow a parent or another relative to remain with him during the procedure *to provide reassurance.* Instruct the patient to breathe through his mouth *to relax the anal sphincter, which will facilitate catheter insertion.*

▶ Ask the patient if he has had previous difficulty retaining an enema to determine whether you need to use a rectal tube guard or a catheter.

▶ Wash your hands and put on gloves.

▶ Assist the patient as necessary in putting on a hospital gown. *The gown makes enema administration easier, and the patient worries less about soiling it.*

▶ Assist the patient into the left-lateral Sims' position. *This will facilitate the solution's flow by gravity into the descending colon.* (See *How to give an enema.*) If contraindicated or if the patient reports discomfort, reposition him on his back or right side.

▶ Place linen-saver pads under the patient's buttocks *to prevent soiling the linens.* Replace the top bed linens with a bath blanket *to provide privacy and warmth.*

▶ Have a bedpan or commode nearby for the patient to use. If the patient may use the bathroom, make sure that it will be available when the patient needs it. Have toilet tissue within the patient's reach.

▶ Lubricate the distal tip of the rectal catheter with water-soluble lubricant *to facilitate rectal insertion and reduce irritation.*

▶ Separate the patient's buttocks and touch the anal sphincter with the rectal tube *to stimulate contraction.* Then, as the sphincter relaxes, tell the patient to breathe deeply through his mouth as you gently advance the tube.

▶ If the patient feels pain or the tube meets continued resistance, notify the doctor. *This may signal an unknown stricture or abscess.* If the patient has poor sphincter control, use a plastic rectal tube guard.

▶ You can also use an indwelling urinary catheter or rectal catheter as a rectal tube, if your facility's policy permits. Insert the lubricated catheter as you would a rectal tube. Then gently inflate the catheter's balloon with 20 to 30 ml of water. Gently pull the catheter back against the patient's internal anal sphincter *to seal off the rectum.* If leakage still occurs with the balloon in place, add more water to the balloon in small amounts. When using either catheter, avoid inflating the balloon above 45 ml *because overinflation can compromise blood flow to the rectal tissues and may cause necrosis from pressure on the rectal mucosa.*

▶ If you're using a rectal tube, hold it in place throughout the procedure because bowel contractions and the pressure of the tube against the anal sphincter can promote tube displacement.

▶ Hold the solution container slightly above bed level and release the tubing clamp. Then raise the container gradually to start the flow — usually at a rate of 75 to 100 ml/minute for an irrigating enema but at the slowest possible rate for a retention enema *to avoid stimulating peristalsis and to promote retention.* Adjust the flow rate of an irrigating enema by raising or lowering the solution container according to the patient's retention ability and comfort. However, make sure not to raise it higher than 18″ (45.7 cm) for an adult, 12″ (30.5 cm) for a child, and 6″ to 8″ (15 to 20.5 cm) for an infant *because excessive pressure can force colon bacteria into the small intestine or rupture the colon.*

▶ Assess the patient's tolerance frequently during instillation. If he complains of discomfort, cramps, or the need to defecate, stop the flow by pinching or clamping the tubing. Then hold the patient's buttocks together. Instruct him to gently massage his abdomen and to breathe slowly and deeply through his mouth *to help relax his abdominal muscles and promote retention.* Resume administration at a slower flow rate after a few minutes when discomfort passes but interrupt the flow any time the patient complains of discomfort.

▶ If the flow slows or stops, the catheter tip may be clogged with feces or pressed against the rectal wall. Gently turn the catheter slightly *to free it without stimulating defecation.* If the catheter tip remains clogged, withdraw the catheter, flush it with solution, and reinsert it.

▶ After administering most of the prescribed amount of solution, clamp the tubing. Stop the flow before the container empties completely *to avoid introducing air into the bowel.*

▶ To administer a commercially prepared, small-volume enema, first remove the cap from the rectal tube.

Insert the rectal tube into the rectum and squeeze the bottle *to deposit the contents in the rectum.* Remove the rectal tube, replace the used enema unit in its original container, and discard.

▶ For a flush enema, stop the flow by lowering the solution container below bed level and allowing gravity to siphon the enema from the colon. Continue to raise and lower the container until gas bubbles cease or the patient feels more comfortable and abdominal distention subsides. Don't allow the solution container to empty completely before lowering it *because this may introduce air into the bowel.*

▶ For an irrigating enema, instruct the patient to retain the solution for 15 minutes, if possible.

▶ For a retention enema, instruct the patient to avoid defecation for the prescribed time or as follows: 30 minutes or longer for oil retention and 15 to 30 minutes for anthelmintic and emollient enemas. If you're using an indwelling catheter, leave the catheter in place *to promote retention.*

▶ If the patient is apprehensive, position him on the bedpan and allow him to hold toilet tissue or a rolled washcloth against his anus. Place the call signal within his reach. If he'll be using the bathroom or the commode, instruct him to call for help before attempting to get out of bed *because the procedure may make the patient—particularly an elderly patient—feel weak or faint.* Also instruct him to call you if he feels weak at any time.

▶ When the solution has remained in the colon for the recommended time or for as long as the patient can tolerate it, assist the patient onto a bedpan or to the commode or bathroom as required.

▶ If an indwelling catheter is in place, deflate the balloon and remove the catheter, if applicable.

▶ Provide privacy while the patient expels the solution. Instruct the patient not to flush the toilet.

▶ While the patient uses the bathroom, remove and discard any soiled linen and linen-saver pads.

▶ Assist the patient with cleaning, if necessary, and help him to bed. Make sure he feels clean and comfortable and can easily reach the call signal. Place a clean linen-saver pad under him *to absorb rectal drainage* and tell him that he may need to expel additional stool or flatus later. Encourage him to rest *because the procedure may be tiring.*

▶ Cover the bedpan or commode and take it to the utility room for observation or observe the contents of the toilet as applicable. Carefully note fecal color, consistency, amount (such as minimal, moderate, or generous), and foreign matter, such as blood, rectal tissue, worms, pus, mucus, or other unusual matter.

▶ Send specimens to the laboratory if ordered.

▶ Rinse the bedpan or commode with cold water, and then wash it in hot soapy water. Return it to the patient's bedside.

▶ Properly dispose of the enema equipment. If additional enemas are scheduled, store clean, reusable equipment in a closed plastic bag in the patient's bathroom. Discard your gloves and wash your hands.

▶ Ventilate the room or use an air freshener, if necessary.

Special considerations

▶ *Because patients with salt-retention disorders, such as heart failure, may absorb sodium from the saline enema solution,* administer the solution to such patients cautiously and monitor electrolyte status.

▶ Schedule a retention enema before meals because a full stomach may stimulate peristalsis and make retention difficult. Follow an oil-retention enema with a soap and water enema 1 hour later *to help expel the softened feces completely.*

▶ Administer less solution when giving a hypertonic enema *because osmotic pull moves fluid into the colon from body tissues, increasing the volume of colon contents.* Alternative means of instilling the solution include using a bulb syringe or a funnel with the rectal tube.

▶ For the patient who can't tolerate a flat position (for example, a patient with shortness of breath), administer the enema with the head of the bed in the lowest position he can safely and comfortably maintain. For a bedridden patient who needs to expel the enema into a bedpan, raise the head of the bed to approximate a sitting or squatting position. Don't give an enema to a patient who is in a sitting position, unless absolutely necessary, *because the solution won't flow high enough into the colon and will only distend the rectum and trigger rapid expulsion.* If the patient has hemorrhoids, instruct him to bear down gently during tube insertion. This causes the anus to open and facilitates insertion.

▶ If the patient fails to expel the solution within 1 hour because of diminished neuromuscular response, you may need to remove the enema solution. First, review your facility's policy *because you may need a doctor's order.* Inform the doctor when a patient can't expel an enema spontaneously *because*

of possible bowel perforation or electrolyte imbalance. To siphon the enema solution from the patient's rectum, assist him to a side-lying position on the bed. Place a bedpan on a bedside chair so that it rests below mattress level. Disconnect the tubing from the solution container, place the distal end in the bedpan, and reinsert the rectal end into the patient's anus. If gravity fails to drain the solution into the bedpan, instill 30 to 50 ml of warm water (105° F [40.6° C] for an adult and 100° F [37.8° C] for a child or infant) through the tube. Then quickly direct the distal end of the tube into the bedpan. In both cases, measure the return *to make sure all of the solution has drained.*

▶ In patients with fluid and electrolyte disturbances, measure the amount of expelled solution *to assess for retention of enema fluid.*

▶ Double-bag all enema equipment and label it as isolation equipment if the patient is on enteric precautions.

▶ If the doctor orders enemas until returns are clear, give no more than three *to avoid excessive irritation of the rectal mucosa.* Notify the doctor if the returned fluid isn't clear after three administrations.

Home care

Describe the procedure to the patient and his family. Emphasize that administering an enema to a person in a sitting position or on the toilet could injure the rectal wall. Tell the patient how to prepare and care for the equipment.

Discuss relaxation techniques and review measures for preventing constipation, including regular exercise, dietary modifications, and adequate fluid intake.

Complications

Enemas may produce dizziness or faintness; excessive irritation of the colonic mucosa resulting from repeated administration or from sensitivity to the enema's ingredients; hyponatremia or hypokalemia from repeated administration of hypotonic solutions; and cardiac arrhythmias resulting from vasovagal reflex stimulation after insertion of the rectal catheter. Colonic water absorption may result from prolonged retention of hypotonic solutions, which may, in turn, cause hypervolemia or water intoxication.

Documentation

Record the date and time of enema administration; special equipment used; type and amount of solution; retention time; approximate amount returned; color, consistency, and amount of the return; abnormalities within the return; any complications that occurred; and the patient's tolerance of the treatment.

EPIDURAL ANALGESIC ADMINISTRATION

In epidural analgesic administration, the doctor injects or infuses medication into the epidural space, which lies just outside the subarachnoid space where cerebrospinal fluid (CSF) flows. The drug diffuses slowly into the subarachnoid space of the spinal canal and then into the CSF, which carries it directly into the spinal area, bypassing the blood-brain barrier. In some cases, the doctor injects medication directly into the subarachnoid space. (See *Understanding intrathecal injections.*)

Epidural analgesia helps manage acute and chronic pain, including moderate to severe postoperative pain. It's especially useful in patients with cancer or degenerative joint disease. This procedure works well because opioid receptors are located along the entire spinal cord. Narcotic drugs act directly on the receptors of the dorsal horn to produce localized analgesia without motor blockade. Narcotics, such as morphine, fentanyl, and hydromorphone are administered as an I.V. bolus dose or by continuous infusion, either alone or in combination with bupivacaine (a local anesthetic). Infusion through an epidural catheter is preferable because it allows a smaller drug dose to be given continuously.

The epidural catheter, which is inserted near the spinal cord, eliminates the risks of multiple I.M. injections, minimizes adverse cerebral and systemic effects, and eliminates the analgesic peaks and valleys that usually occur with intermittent I.M. injections. (See *Placement of a permanent epidural catheter,* page 298.)

Typically, epidural catheter insertion is performed by an anesthesiologist using aseptic technique. When the catheter has been inserted, the nurse is responsible for monitoring the infusion and assessing the patient.

Epidural analgesia is contraindicated in patients who have local or systemic infection, neurologic disease, coagulopathy, spinal arthritis or a spinal deformity, hypotension, marked hypertension, or an allergy to the prescribed medication and in those who are undergoing anticoagulant therapy.

Key nursing diagnoses and patient outcomes

Deficient knowledge related to lack of exposure to epidural analgesic administration

The patient will:
▶ state or demonstrate an understanding of what has been taught
▶ demonstrate the ability to perform behaviors that are taught.

Risk for injury related to improper technique
The patient will:
▶ identify factors that increase the risk of injury
▶ assist in identifying and applying safety measures to prevent injury.

Equipment

Volume infusion device and epidural infusion tubing (depending on your facility's policy) • patient's medication record and chart • prescribed epidural solutions • transparent dressing • epidural tray • labels for epidural infusion line • silk tape • optional: monitoring equipment for blood pressure and pulse and apnea monitor

For emergency use

oxygen • 0.4 mg of I.V. naloxone • 50 mg of I.V. ephedrine • intubation set • handheld resuscitation bag

Preparation of equipment

Prepare the infusion device according to the manufacturer's instructions and your facility's policy. Obtain an epidural tray. Make sure that the pharmacy has been notified ahead of time regarding the medication order *because epidural solutions require special preparation.* Check the medication concentration and infusion rate against the doctor's order.

Implementation

▶ Explain the procedure and its possible complications to the patient. Tell

Understanding intrathecal injections

An intrathecal injection allows the doctor to inject medication into the subarachnoid space of the spinal canal. Certain drugs— such as anti-infectives or antineoplastics used to treat meningeal leukemia— are administered by this route *because they can't readily penetrate the blood-brain barrier through the bloodstream.* Intrathecal injection may also be used to deliver anesthetics, such as lidocaine hydrochloride, to achieve regional anesthesia (as in spinal anesthesia and epidural block).

An invasive procedure performed by a doctor under sterile conditions with the nurse assisting, intrathecal injection requires informed patient consent. The injection site is usually between the third and fourth (or fourth and fifth) lumbar vertebrae, well below the spinal cord *to avoid the risk of paralysis.* This procedure may be preceded by aspiration of spinal fluid for laboratory analysis.

Contraindications to intrathecal injection include inflammation or infection at the puncture site, septicemia, and spinal deformities (especially when considered as an anesthesia route).

him that he'll feel some pain as the catheter is inserted. Answer any questions he has. Make sure that a consent form has been properly signed and witnessed.
▶ Position the patient on his side in the knee-chest position, or have him sit on the edge of the bed and lean over a bedside table.
▶ After the catheter is in place, prime the infusion device, confirm the appropriate medication and infusion rate, and then adjust the device for the correct rate.

Placement of a permanent epidural catheter

An epidural catheter is implanted beneath the patient's skin and inserted near the spinal cord at the first lumbar (L1) interspace. For temporary analgesic therapy (less than 1 week), the catheter may exit directly over the spine and be taped up the patient's back to the shoulder. For prolonged therapy, the catheter may be tunneled subcutaneously to an exit site on the patient's side or abdomen or over his shoulder.

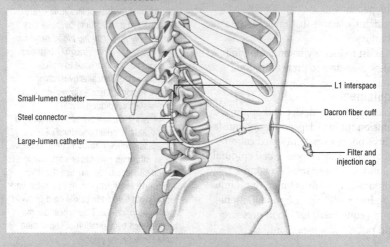

Small-lumen catheter

Steel connector

Large-lumen catheter

L1 interspace

Dacron fiber cuff

Filter and injection cap

▶ Help the anesthesiologist connect the infusion tubing to the epidural catheter. Then connect the tubing to the infusion pump.

▶ Bridge-tape all connection sites and apply an EPIDURAL INFUSION label to the catheter, infusion tubing, and infusion pump *to prevent accidental infusion of other drugs*. Then start the infusion.

▶ Tell the patient to immediately report any pain. Instruct him to use a pain scale from 0 to 10, with 0 denoting no pain and 10 denoting the worst pain imaginable. A response of 3 or less typically indicates tolerable pain. If the patient reports a higher pain score, the infusion rate may need to be increased. Call the doctor or change the rate within prescribed limits.

▶ If ordered, place the patient on an apnea monitor for the first 24 hours after beginning the infusion.

▶ Change the dressing over the catheter's exit site every 24 to 48 hours or as needed. The dressing is usually transparent *to allow inspection of drainage* and commonly appears moist or slightly blood-tinged.

▶ Change the infusion tubing every 48 hours or as specified by your facility's policy.

Removing an epidural catheter

▶ Typically, the anesthesiologist orders analgesics and removes the catheter. However, your facility's policy may allow a specially trained nurse to remove the catheter.

▶ If you feel resistance when removing the catheter, stop and call the doctor for further orders.

▶ Save the catheter. *The doctor will want to examine the catheter tip to rule out any damage during removal.*

Special considerations

▶ Assess the patient's respiratory rate and blood pressure every 2 hours for 8 hours and then every 4 hours for 8 hours during the first 24 hours after starting the infusion. Then assess the patient once per shift, depending on his condition or unless ordered otherwise. Notify the doctor if the patient's respiratory rate is less than 10 breaths/ minute or if his systolic blood pressure is less than 90 mm Hg.

▶ Assess the patient's sedation level, mental status, and pain-relief status every hour initially and then every 2 to 4 hours until adequate pain control is achieved. Notify the doctor if the patient appears drowsy; experiences nausea and vomiting, refractory itching, or inability to void, *which are adverse effects of certain narcotic analgesics;* or complains of unrelieved pain.

▶ Assess the patient's lower-extremity motor strength every 2 to 4 hours. If sensorimotor loss occurs, large motor nerve fibers have been affected and the dose may need to be decreased.

▶ Keep in mind that drugs given epidurally diffuse slowly and may cause adverse effects, including excessive sedation, up to 12 hours after the infusion has been discontinued.

▶ The patient should always have a peripheral I.V. line (either continuous infusion or saline lock) open *to allow immediate administration of emergency drugs.*

▶ If CSF leaks into the dura mater during removal of an epidural catheter, the patient usually experiences a headache. This postanalgesia headache worsens with postural changes, such as standing and sitting. The headache can be treated with a "blood patch," in which the patient's own blood (about 10 ml) is withdrawn from a peripheral vein and then injected into the epidural space. When the epidural needle is withdrawn, the patient is instructed to sit up. Because the blood clots seal off the leaking area, the blood patch should relieve the patient's headache immediately. The patient need not restrict his activity after this procedure.

Home care

Home use of epidural analgesia is possible only if the patient or a family member is willing and able to learn the care needed. The patient also must be willing and able to abstain from alcohol and street drugs *because these substances potentiate opioid action.*

Complications

The most common complication of epidural infusion is numbness and leg weakness, which may occur after the first 24 hours and are drug- and concentration-dependent. The doctor must titrate the dosage to identify the dose that provides adequate pain control without causing excessive numbness and weakness.

Other possible complications include respiratory depression, which usually occurs during the first 24 hours (treated with 0.2 to 0.4 mg of I.V. naloxone); pruritus (treated with 5 mg of I.V. nalbuphine or 25 mg of I.V. diphenhydramine); and nausea and vomiting (treated with 5 to 10 mg of

I.V. prochlorperazine or 10 mg of I.V. metoclopramide).

Documentation

Record the patient's response to treatment, catheter patency, condition of the dressing and insertion site, vital signs, and assessment results. Also document the labeling of the epidural catheter, changing of the infusion bags, ordered analgesics, if any, and patient's response.

ESOPHAGEAL TUBE CARE

Although the doctor inserts an esophageal tube, the nurse cares for the patient during and after intubation. Typically, the patient is in the intensive care unit for close observation and constant care. The environment may help to increase the patient's tolerance for the procedure and may help to control bleeding. Sedatives may be contraindicated, especially for a patient with portal systemic encephalopathy.

Most important, the patient who has an esophageal tube in place to control variceal bleeding (typically from portal hypertension) must be observed closely for esophageal rupture because varices weaken the esophagus. Additionally, possible traumatic injury from intubation or esophageal balloon inflation increases the chance of rupture. Emergency surgery is usually performed if a rupture occurs, but the operation has a low success rate.

Key nursing diagnoses and patient outcomes

Ineffective airway clearance related to the presence of secretions
The patient will:
▶ cough effectively

▶ expectorate sputum
▶ maintain a patent airway.

Risk for aspiration related to absence of protective mechanisms
The patient will:
▶ show no signs of aspiration
▶ reveal no adventitious breath sounds on auscultation.

Equipment

Manometer • two 2-L bottles of normal saline solution • irrigation set • water-soluble lubricant • several cotton-tipped applicators • mouth-care equipment • nasopharyngeal suction apparatus • several #12 French suction catheters • intake and output record sheets • gloves • goggles • sedatives • traction weights or football helmet • scissors

Implementation

▶ *To ease the patient's anxiety,* explain the care that you'll give.
▶ Provide privacy. Wash your hands and put on gloves and goggles.
▶ Monitor the patient's vital signs every 5 minutes to 1 hour as ordered. *A change in vital signs may signal complications or recurrent bleeding.*
▶ If the patient has a Sengstaken-Blakemore or Minnesota tube, check the pressure gauge on the manometer every 30 to 60 minutes *to detect any leaks in the esophageal balloon and to verify the set pressure.*
▶ Maintain drainage and suction on gastric and esophageal aspiration ports as ordered. This is important *because fluid accumulating in the stomach may cause the patient to regurgitate the tube, and fluid accumulating in the esophagus may lead to vomiting and aspiration.*
▶ Irrigate the gastric aspiration port as ordered, using the irrigation set and

normal saline solution. *Frequent irrigation keeps the tube from clogging. Obstruction in the tube can lead to regurgitation of the tube and vomiting.*

▶ *To prevent pressure ulcers,* clean the patient's nostrils and apply water-soluble lubricant frequently. Use warm water to loosen crusted nasal secretions before applying the lubricant with cotton-tipped applicators.

▶ Provide mouth care often *to rid the patient's mouth of foul-tasting matter and to relieve dryness from mouth breathing.*

▶ Use #12 French catheters to provide gentle oral suctioning, if necessary, *to help remove secretions.*

▶ Offer emotional support. Keep the patient as quiet as possible and administer sedatives, if ordered.

▶ A football helmet or traction weights may be used *to secure the tube.* If used, make sure that the traction weights hang from the foot of the bed at all times. Never rest them on the bed. Instruct housekeepers and other coworkers not to move the weights *because reduced traction may change the position of the tube.*

▶ Elevate the head of the bed about 25 degrees to ensure countertraction for the weights.

▶ Keep the patient on complete bed rest *because exertion, such as coughing or straining, increases intra-abdominal pressure, which may trigger further bleeding.*

▶ Keep the patient in semi-Fowler's position to reduce blood flow into the portal system and to prevent reflux into the esophagus.

▶ Monitor intake and output as ordered.

Special considerations

▶ Observe the patient carefully for esophageal rupture indicated by signs and symptoms of shock, increased res-

piratory difficulties, and increased bleeding. Tape scissors to the head of the bed *so you can cut the tube quickly to deflate the balloons if asphyxia develops.* When performing this emergency intervention, hold the tube firmly close to the nostril before cutting.

▶ If using traction, release the tension before deflating any balloons. If weights and pulleys supply traction, remove the weights. If a football helmet supplies traction, untape the esophageal tube from the face guard before deflating the balloons. *Deflating the balloon under tension triggers a rapid release of the entire tube from the nose, which may injure mucous membranes, initiate recurrent bleeding, and obstruct the airway.*

▶ If the doctor orders an X-ray study to check the tube's position or to view the chest, lift the patient in the direction of the pulley and then place the X-ray film behind his back. Never roll him from side to side *because pressure exerted on the tube in this way may shift the tube's position.* Similarly, lift the patient to make the bed or to assist him with the bedpan.

Complications

Esophageal rupture, the most life-threatening complication associated with esophageal balloon tamponade, can occur at any time but is most likely to occur during intubation or inflation of the esophageal balloon. Asphyxia may result if the balloon moves up the esophagus and blocks the airway. Aspiration of pooled esophageal secretions may also complicate this procedure.

Documentation

Read the manometer hourly and record the esophageal pressures. Note when the balloons are deflated and by whom.

Document vital signs, the condition of the patient's nostrils, routine care, and any drugs administered. Also note the color, consistency, and amount of gastric returns.

Record any signs and symptoms of complications and the nursing actions taken. Document gastric port and nasogastric tube irrigations. Maintain accurate intake and output records.

ESOPHAGEAL TUBE INSERTION AND REMOVAL

Used to control hemorrhage from esophageal or gastric varices, an esophageal tube is inserted nasally or orally and advanced into the esophagus or stomach. Ordinarily, a doctor inserts and removes the tube. In an emergency situation, a nurse may remove it.

Once the tube is in place, a gastric balloon secured at the end of the tube can be inflated and drawn tightly against the cardia of the stomach. The inflated balloon secures the tube and exerts pressure on the cardia. The pressure, in turn, controls the bleeding varices.

Most tubes also contain an esophageal balloon to control esophageal bleeding. (See *Types of esophageal tubes.*) Usually, gastric or esophageal balloons are deflated after 24 hours. If the balloon remains inflated longer than 24 hours, pressure necrosis may develop and cause further hemorrhage or perforation.

Other procedures to control bleeding include irrigation with tepid or iced saline solution and drug therapy with a vasopressor. Used with the esophageal tube, these procedures provide effective, temporary control of acute variceal hemorrhage.

Key nursing diagnoses and patient outcomes

Ineffective airway clearance related to presence of secretions
The patient will:
▶ cough effectively
▶ expectorate sputum
▶ maintain a patent airway.

Risk for aspiration related to absence of protective mechanisms
The patient will:
▶ show no signs of aspiration
▶ reveal no adventitious breath sounds on auscultation.

Equipment

Esophageal tube • nasogastric (NG) tube (if using a Sengstaken-Blakemore tube) • two suction sources • basin of ice • irrigation set • 2 L of normal saline solution • two 60-ml syringes • water-soluble lubricant • ½" or 1" adhesive tape • stethoscope • foam nose guard • four rubber-shod clamps (two clamps and two plastic plugs for a Minnesota tube) • anesthetic spray (as ordered) • traction equipment (football helmet or a basic frame with traction rope, pulleys, and a 1-lb [0.5-kg] weight) • mercury aneroid manometer • Y-connector tube (for Sengstaken-Blakemore or Linton tube) • basin of water • cup of water with straw • scissors • gloves • gown • waterproof marking pen • goggles • sphygmomanometer

Preparation of equipment

Keep the traction helmet at the bedside or attach traction equipment to the bed so that either is readily available after

ESOPHAGEAL TUBE INSERTION AND REMOVAL   303

Types of esophageal tubes

When working with patients who have an esophageal tube, remember the advantages of the most common types.

Sengstaken-Blakemore tube

This triple-lumen, double-balloon tube has a gastric aspiration port, which allows you to obtain drainage from below the gastric balloon and to instill medication.

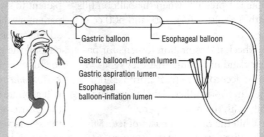

Linton tube

This triple-lumen, single-balloon tube has a port for gastric aspiration and one for esophageal aspiration, too. Additionally, the Linton tube reduces the risk of esophageal necrosis because it doesn't have an esophageal balloon.

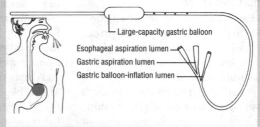

Minnesota esophagogastric tamponade tube

This esophageal tube has four lumens and two balloons. The device provides pressure-monitoring ports for both balloons without the need for Y-connectors. One port is used for gastric suction, the other for esophageal suction.

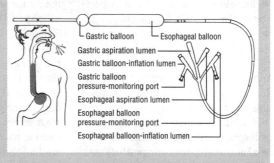

tube insertion. Place the suction machines nearby and plug them in. Open the irrigation set and fill the container with normal saline solution. Place all equipment within reach.

Test the balloons on the esophageal tube for air leaks by inflating them and submerging them in the basin of water. If no bubbles appear in the water, the balloons are intact. Remove them from the water and deflate them. Clamp the tube lumens, so that the balloons stay deflated during insertion.

To prepare the Minnesota tube, connect the mercury aneroid manometer to the gastric pressure monitoring port. Note the pressure when the balloon fills with 100, 200, 300, 400, and 500 cc of air.

Check the aspiration lumens for patency and make sure that they're labeled according to their purpose. If they aren't identified, label them carefully with the marking pen.

Chill the tube in a basin of ice. *This will stiffen it and facilitate insertion.*

Implementation

▶ Explain the procedure and its purpose to the patient and provide privacy.
▶ Wash your hands and put on gloves, gown, and goggles *to protect yourself from splashing blood.*
▶ Assist the patient into semi-Fowler's position and turn him slightly toward his left side. *This position promotes stomach emptying and helps prevent aspiration.*
▶ Explain that the doctor will inspect the patient's nostrils (for patency).
▶ *To determine the length of tubing needed,* hold the balloon at the patient's xiphoid process and then extend the tube to the patient's ear and forward to his nose. Using a waterproof pen, mark this point on the tubing.
▶ Inform the patient that the doctor will spray his throat (posterior pharynx) and nostril with an anesthetic *to minimize discomfort and gagging during intubation.*
▶ After lubricating the tip of the tube with water-soluble lubricant *to reduce friction and facilitate insertion,* the doctor will pass the tube through the more patent nostril. As he does, he'll direct the patient to tilt his chin toward his chest and to swallow when he senses the tip of the tube in the back of his throat. *Swallowing helps to advance the tube into the esophagus and prevents intubation of the trachea.* (If the doctor introduces the tube orally, he'll direct the patient to swallow immediately.) As the patient swallows, the doctor quickly advances the tube at least ½" (1.3 cm) beyond the previously marked point on the tube.
▶ *To confirm tube placement,* the doctor will aspirate stomach contents through the gastric port. He'll also auscultate the stomach with a stethoscope as he injects air. After partially inflating the gastric balloon with 50 to 100 cc of air, he'll order an X-ray of the abdomen *to confirm correct placement of the balloon.* Before fully inflating the balloon, he'll use the 60-ml syringe to irrigate the stomach with normal saline solution and empty the stomach as completely as possible. *This helps the patient avoid regurgitating gastric contents when the balloon inflates.*
▶ After confirming tube placement, the doctor will fully inflate the gastric balloon (250 to 500 cc of air for a Sengstaken-Blakemore tube; 700 to 800 cc of air for a Linton tube) and clamp the tube using rubber-shod clamps. If he's using a Minnesota tube, he'll connect the pressure-monitoring port for the gastric balloon lumen to the mercury manometer and then inflate the balloon in 100-cc increments until it fills with up to 500 cc of air. As he introduces the air, he'll monitor the intragastric balloon pressure *to make sure the balloon stays inflated.* Then he'll clamp the ports. For the Sengstaken-Blakemore or Minnesota tube, the doctor will gently pull on the tube until he feels resistance, *which indicates that the gastric balloon is inflated and exerting*

pressure on the cardia of the stomach.
When he senses that the balloon is engaged, he'll place the foam nose guard around the area where the tube emerges from the nostril.

▶ Be ready to tape the nose guard in place around the tube. *This helps to minimize pressure on the nostril from the traction and decreases the risk of necrosis.*

▶ With the nose guard secured, traction can be applied to the tube with a traction rope and a 1-lb (0.5-kg) weight, or the tube can be pulled gently and taped secure tightly to the face guard of a football helmet. (See *Securing an esophageal tube.*)

▶ With pulley-and-weight traction, lower the head of the bed to about 25 degrees *to produce countertraction.*

▶ Lavage the stomach through the gastric aspiration lumen with normal saline solution (iced or tepid) until the return fluid is clear. *The vasoconstriction thus achieved stops the hemorrhage; the lavage empties the stomach. Any blood detected later in the gastric aspirate indicates that bleeding remains uncontrolled.*

▶ Attach one of the suction sources to the gastric aspiration lumen. *This empties the stomach, helps prevent nausea and possible vomiting, and allows continuous observation of the gastric contents for blood.*

▶ If the doctor inserted a Sengstaken-Blakemore or a Minnesota tube, he'll inflate the esophageal balloon as he inflates the gastric balloon *to compress the esophageal varices and control bleeding.*

To do this with a Sengstaken-Blakemore tube, attach the Y-connector tube to the esophageal lumen. Then attach a sphygmomanometer inflation bulb to one end of the Y-connector and the manometer to the other end. Inflate the esophageal balloon until the pres-

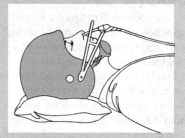
sure gauge ranges between 30 and 40 mm Hg and clamp the tube.

To do this with a Minnesota tube, attach the mercury manometer directly to the esophageal pressure-monitoring outlet. Then, using the 60-ml syringe and pushing the air slowly into the esophageal balloon port, inflate the balloon until the pressure gauge ranges from 35 to 45 mm Hg.

▶ Check the balloon pressure every 2 hours.

▶ Set up esophageal suction *to prevent accumulation of secretions that may cause vomiting and pulmonary aspiration.* This is important because swallowed secretions can't pass into the stomach if the patient has an inflated esophageal balloon in place. If the patient has a Linton or a Minnesota tube, attach the suction source to the esophageal aspiration port. If the patient has a Sengstaken-Blakemore tube, advance an NG tube through the other nostril into the esophagus to the point where the esophageal balloon begins and attach the suction source as ordered.

Removing the tube

▶ The doctor will deflate the esophageal balloon by aspirating the air with a syringe. (He may order the esophageal balloon to be deflated at 5-mm Hg increments every 30 minutes for several hours.) Then if bleeding doesn't recur, he'll remove the traction from the gastric tube and deflate the gastric balloon (also by aspiration). The gastric balloon is always deflated just before removing the tube *to prevent the balloon from riding up into the esophagus or pharynx and obstructing the airway or, possibly, causing asphyxia or rupture.*

▶ After disconnecting all suction tubes, the doctor will gently remove the esophageal tube. If he feels resistance, he'll aspirate the balloons again. (To remove a Minnesota tube, he'll grasp it near the patient's nostril and cut across all four lumens approximately 3″ [7.5 cm] below that point. *This ensures deflation of all balloons.*)

▶ After the tube has been removed, assist the patient with mouth care.

Special considerations

▶ If the patient appears cyanotic or if other signs of airway obstruction develop during tube placement, remove the tube immediately *because it may have entered the trachea instead of the esophagus.* After intubation, keep scissors taped to the head of the bed. If respira-

tory distress occurs, cut across all lumens while holding the tube at the nares and remove the tube quickly. Unless contraindicated, the patient can sip water through a straw during intubation *to facilitate tube advancement.*

▶ Keep in mind that the intraesophageal balloon pressure varies with respirations and esophageal contractions. Baseline pressure is the important pressure.

▶ The balloon on the Linton tube should stay inflated no longer than 24 hours *because necrosis of the cardia may result.* Usually, the doctor removes the tube only after a trial period (lasting at least 12 hours) with the esophageal balloon deflated or with the gastric balloon tension released from the cardia *to check for rebleeding.* In some facilities, the doctor may deflate the esophageal balloon for 5 to 10 minutes every hour *to temporarily relieve pressure on the esophageal mucosa.*

Complications

Erosion and perforation of the esophagus and gastric mucosa may result from the tension placed on these areas by the balloons during traction. Esophageal rupture may result if the gastric balloon accidentally inflates in the esophagus. Acute airway occlusion may result if the balloon dislodges and moves upward into the trachea. Other erosions, nasal tissue necrosis, and aspiration of oral secretions may also complicate the patient's condition.

Documentation

Record the date and time of insertion and removal, the type of tube used, and the name of the doctor who performed the procedure. Also document the intraesophageal balloon pressure (for

Sengstaken-Blakemore and Minnesota tubes), intragastric balloon pressure (for Minnesota tube), or amount of air injected (for Sengstaken-Blakemore and Linton tubes). Also record the amount of fluid used for gastric irrigation and the color, consistency, and amount of gastric returns, before and after lavage.

EXTERNAL FIXATION

In external fixation, a doctor inserts metal pins through skin and muscle layers into the broken bones and affixes them to an adjustable external frame that maintains their proper alignment. (See *Types of external fixation devices.*) This procedure is used most commonly to treat open, unstable fractures with extensive soft tissue damage, comminuted closed fractures, and septic, nonunion fractures and to facilitate surgical immobilization of a joint. Specialized types of external fixators may be used to lengthen leg bones or immobilize the cervical spine.

An advantage of external fixation over other immobilization techniques is that it stabilizes the fracture while allowing full visualization and access to open wounds. It also facilitates early ambulation, thus reducing the risk of complications from immobilization.

The Ilizarov fixator is a special type of external fixation device. This device is a combination of rings and tensioned transosseous wires used primarily in limb lengthening, bone transport, and limb salvage. Highly complex, it provides gradual distraction resulting in good-quality bone formation with a minimum of complications.

Types of external fixation devices

The doctor's selection of an external fixation device depends on the severity of the patient's fracture and on the type of bone alignment needed.

Universal day frame
This device is used to manage tibial fractures. The frame allows the doctor to readjust the position of bony fragments by angulation and rotation. The compression-distraction device allows compression and distraction of bony fragments.

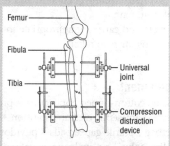

Portsmouth external fixation bar
This device is used to manage complicated tibial fractures. The locking nut adjustment on the mobile carriage only allows bone compression, so the doctor must accurately reduce bony fragments before applying the device.

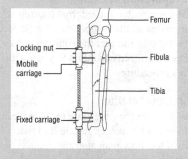

Key nursing diagnoses and patient outcomes

Impaired physical mobility related to neuromuscular impairment
The patient will:
▶ maintain muscle strength and joint range of motion
▶ show no evidence of complications, such as contractures, venous stasis, thrombus formation, or skin breakdown.

Acute pain related to musculoskeletal injury
The patient will:
▶ express a feeling of comfort and relief from pain
▶ state and carry out appropriate interventions for pain relief.

Equipment

Sterile cotton-tipped applicators • prescribed antiseptic cleaning solution • ice bag • sterile gauze pads • povidone-iodine solution • analgesic or narcotic •optional: antimicrobial ointment
   Equipment varies with the type of fixator and the type and location of the fracture. Typically, sets of pins, stabilizing rods, and clips are available from manufacturers. Don't reuse pins.

Preparation of equipment

Make sure that the external fixation set includes all the equipment it's supposed to include and that the equipment has been sterilized according to your facility's procedure.

Implementation

▶ Explain the procedure to the patient *to reduce his anxiety*. Assure him that he'll feel little pain after the fixation device is in place and that he'll be able to adjust to the apparatus.

▶ Tell the patient that he'll be able to move about with the apparatus in place, which may help him resume normal activities more quickly.
▶ After the fixation device is in place, perform neurovascular checks every 2 to 4 hours for 24 hours, then every 4 to 8 hours, as appropriate, *to assess for possible neurologic damage*. Assess color, motion, sensation, digital movement, edema, capillary refill, and pulses of the affected extremity. Compare with the unaffected side.
▶ Apply an ice bag to the surgical site as ordered *to reduce swelling, relieve pain, and lessen bleeding*.
▶ Administer analgesics or narcotics as ordered before exercising or mobilizing the affected extremity *to promote comfort*.
▶ Monitor the patient for pain not relieved by analgesics or narcotics and for burning, tingling, or numbness, *which may indicate nerve damage or circulatory impairment*.
▶ Elevate the affected extremity, if appropriate, *to minimize edema*.
▶ Perform pin-site care as ordered, *to prevent infection*. Pin-site care varies but you'll usually follow guidelines such as these: Use sterile technique; avoid digging at pin sites with the cotton-tipped applicator; if ordered, clean the pin site and surrounding skin with a cotton-tipped applicator dipped in ordered antiseptic solution; if ordered, apply an antimicrobial ointment to the pin site; apply a loose sterile dressing, or dress with sterile gauze pads soaked in povidone-iodine solution. Perform pin-site care as often as necessary, depending on the amount of drainage.
▶ Also check for redness, tenting of the skin, prolonged or purulent drainage from the pin site, swelling, elevated body or pin-site temperature, and any

bowing or bending of pins, which may stress the skin.

For the patient with an Ilizarov fixator

▶ When the device has been placed and preliminary calluses have begun to form at the insertion sites (in 5 to 7 days), gentle distraction is initiated by turning the appropriate screws one-quarter turn (1 mm) every 4 to 6 hours as ordered.

▶ Teach the patient that he must be consistent in turning the screws every 4 to 6 hours around the clock. Make sure he understands that he must be strongly committed to compliance with the protocol for the procedure to be successful. Because the treatment period may be prolonged (4 to 10 months), discuss with the patient and family members the psychological effects of long-term care.

▶ Don't administer nonsteroidal anti-inflammatory drugs (NSAIDs) to patients who are being treated with the Ilizarov fixator. *NSAIDs may decrease the necessary inflammation caused by the distraction, resulting in delayed bone formation.*

Special considerations

▶ Before discharge, teach the patient and family members how to provide pin-site care. This is a sterile procedure in the facility, but clean technique can be used at home. Teach them how to recognize signs of pin-site infection.

▶ Tell the patient to keep the affected limb elevated when sitting or lying down.

Complications

Complications of external fixation include loosening of pins and loss of fracture stabilization, infection of the pin tract or wound, skin breakdown, nerve damage, and muscle impingement.

Ilizarov fixator pin sites are more prone to infection *because of the extended treatment period and because of the pins' movement to accomplish distraction.* The pins are also more likely to break because of their small diameter. Also, the large number of pins used increases the patient's risk of neurovascular compromise.

Documentation

Assess and document the condition of the pin sites and skin. Also document the patient's reaction to the apparatus and to ambulation as well as his understanding of teaching instructions.

EXTERNAL RADIATION THERAPY

About 60% of all cancer patients are treated with some form of external radiation therapy. Also called radiotherapy, this treatment delivers X-rays or gamma rays directly to the cancer site.

Radiation doses are based on the type, stage, and location of the tumor as well as on the patient's size, condition, and overall treatment goals. Doses are given in increments, usually three to five times a week, until the total dose is reached.

The goals of radiation therapy include cure, in which the cancer is completely destroyed and not expected to recur; control, in which the cancer doesn't progress or regress but is expected to progress at some later time; or palliation, in which radiation is given to relieve signs or symptoms caused by the cancer (such as bone pain, bleeding, and headache).

External beam radiation therapy is delivered by machines that aim a concentrated beam of high-energy particles (photons and gamma rays) at the target site. Two types of machines are commonly used: units containing cobalt or cesium as radioactive sources for gamma rays and linear accelerators that use electricity to produce X-rays. Linear accelerators produce high energy with great penetrating ability. Some (known as orthovoltage machines) produce less powerful electron beams that may be used for superficial tumors.

Radiation therapy may be augmented by chemotherapy, brachytherapy (radiation implant therapy), or surgery as needed.

Key nursing diagnoses and patient outcomes

Disturbed body image related to presence of implants
The patient will:
▶ acknowledge change in body image
▶ participate in decision making about his radiation therapy
▶ express positive feelings about self.

Decisional conflict related to perceived threat to value system
The patient will:
▶ state feelings about the current situation
▶ identify desirable and undesirable consequences of available options
▶ accept assistance from family, friends, clergy, and other supportive persons.

Equipment
Radiation therapy machine

Implementation
▶ Explain the treatment to the patient and his family. Review the treatment goals and discuss the range of potential adverse effects as well as interventions to minimize them. Also discuss possible long-term complications and treatment issues. Educate the patient and his family about local cancer services.
▶ Make sure that the radiation oncology department has obtained informed consent.
▶ Review the patient's clinical record for recent laboratory and imaging results and alert the radiation oncology staff to any abnormalities or other pertinent results (such as myelosuppression, paraneoplastic syndromes, oncologic emergencies, and tumor progression).
▶ Transport the patient to the radiation oncology department.
▶ The patient begins by undergoing simulation (treatment planning), in which the target area is mapped out on his body using a machine similar to the radiation therapy machine. Then the target area is tattooed or marked in ink on his body *to ensure accurate treatments.*
▶ The doctor and radiation oncologist determine the duration and frequency of treatments, depending on the patient's body size, size of portal, extent and location of cancer, and treatment goals.
▶ The patient is positioned on the treatment table beneath the machine. Treatments last from a few seconds to a few minutes. Reassure the patient that he won't feel anything and won't be radioactive. After treatment is complete, the patient may return home or to his room.

Special considerations
▶ Explain to the patient that the full benefit of radiation treatments may not occur until several weeks or months af-

ter treatments begin. Instruct him to report long-term adverse effects.

▶ Instruct the patient about the importance of leaving the target area markings intact *to ensure treatment accuracy.*

▶ Emphasize the importance of keeping follow-up appointments with the doctor.

▶ Refer the patient to a support group such as a local chapter of the American Cancer Society.

Home care
Instruct the patient and his family on proper skin care and management of possible adverse effects.

Complications
Adverse effects arise gradually and diminish gradually after treatments. They may be acute, subacute (accumulating as treatment progresses), chronic (following treatment), or long-term (arising months to years after treatment). Adverse effects are localized to the area of treatment, and their severity depends on the total radiation dose, underlying organ sensitivity, and the patient's overall condition.

Common acute and subacute adverse effects can include altered skin integrity, altered GI and genitourinary function, altered fertility and sexual function, altered bone marrow production, fatigue, and alopecia.

Long-term complications or adverse effects may include radiation pneumonitis, neuropathy, skin and muscle atrophy, telangiectasia, fistulas, altered endocrine function, and secondary cancers. Other complications of treatment include headache, alopecia, xerostomia, dysphagia, stomatitis, altered skin integrity (wet or dry desquamation), nausea, vomiting, heartburn, diarrhea, cystitis, and fatigue.

Documentation
Record radiation precautions taken during treatment; interventions used and their effectiveness; grading of adverse effects; teaching given to the patient and his family and their responses to it; patient's tolerance of isolation procedures and the family's compliance with procedures; discharge plans and teaching; and referrals to local cancer services, if any.

EYE COMPRESS APPLICATION

Whether applied hot or cold, eye compresses are soothing and therapeutic. Hot compresses may be used to relieve discomfort. Because heat increases circulation (which enhances absorption and decreases inflammation), hot compresses may promote drainage of superficial infections. On the other hand, cold compresses can reduce swelling or bleeding and relieve itching. Because cold numbs sensory fibers, cold compresses may be ordered to ease periorbital discomfort between prescribed doses of pain medication. Typically, a hot or cold compress should be applied for 20-minute periods, four to six times per day. Ocular infection calls for the use of aseptic technique.

Key nursing diagnoses and patient outcomes
Deficient knowledge related to lack of exposure to eye compress application
The patient will:

▶ state or demonstrate an understanding of what has been taught

▶ demonstrate the ability to perform new health-related behaviors as they're taught.

Risk for injury related to improper technique

The patient will:

▶ identify factors that increase the risk of injury

▶ assist in identifying and applying safety measures to prevent injury.

Equipment

For hot compresses

Gloves • prescribed solution, usually sterile water or normal saline solution • sterile bowl • sterile 4″ × 4″ gauze pads • towel

For cold compresses

Small plastic bag (such as a sandwich bag) or glove • ice chips • ½″ hypoallergenic tape • towel • sterile 4″ × 4″ gauze pads • sterile water, normal saline solution, or prescribed ophthalmic irrigant • gloves

Preparation of equipment

For hot compresses

Place a capped bottle of sterile water or normal saline solution in a bowl of hot water or under a stream of hot tap water. Allow the solution to become warm, not hot (not higher than 120° F [48.9° C]). Pour the warm water or saline solution into a sterile bowl, filling the bowl about halfway. Place some sterile gauze pads in the bowl.

For cold compresses

Place ice chips in a plastic bag (or a glove, if necessary) to make an ice pack. Keep the ice pack small to avoid excessive pressure on the eye. Remove excess air from the bag or glove and knot the open end. Cut a piece of hypoallergenic tape to secure the ice pack. Place all equipment on the bedside stand near the patient.

Implementation

▶ Explain the procedure to the patient, make him comfortable, and provide privacy.

▶ When applying hot compresses, have the patient sit, if possible. When applying cold compresses, have the patient lie supine. Support his head with a pillow and turn his head slightly to the unaffected side. *This position will help hold the compress in place.*

▶ If the patient has an eye patch, remove it.

▶ Drape a towel around the patient's shoulders *to catch any spills.* Wash your hands and put on gloves.

Applying hot compresses

▶ Take two 4″ × 4″ gauze pads from the basin. Squeeze out the excess solution.

▶ Instruct the patient to close his eyes. Gently apply the pads — one on top of the other — to the affected eye. (If the patient complains that the compress feels too hot, remove it immediately.)

▶ Change the compress every few minutes as necessary, for the prescribed length of time. After removing each compress, check the patient's skin for signs that the compress solution is too hot.

Applying cold compresses

▶ Moisten the middle of one of the sterile 4″ × 4″ gauze pads with the sterile water, normal saline solution, or ophthalmic irrigating solution. *This helps to conduct the cold from the ice pack.* Keep the edges dry *so that they can absorb excess moisture.*

▶ Tell the patient to close his eyes, then place the moist gauze pad over the affected eye.

Applying an eye patch

With a doctor's order, you may apply an eye patch for various reasons: to protect the eye after injury or surgery, to prevent accidental damage to an anesthetized eye, to promote healing, to absorb secretions, to protect the eye from drying when the patient is comatose or unable to close the eye as in Bell's palsy, or to prevent the patient from touching or rubbing his eye.

A thicker patch, called a pressure patch, may be used to help corneal abrasions heal, compress postoperative edema, or control hemorrhage from traumatic injury. Application requires an ophthalmologist's prescription and supervision.

To apply a patch, choose a gauze pad of appropriate size for the patient's face, place it gently over the closed eye (as shown), and secure it with two or three strips of tape. Extend the tape from midforehead across the eye to below the earlobe.

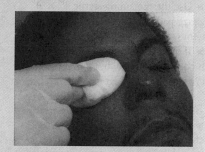

A pressure patch, which is markedly thicker than a single-thickness gauze patch, exerts extra tension against the closed eye. After placing the initial gauze pad, build it up with additional gauze pieces. Tape it firmly so that the patch exerts even pressure against the closed eye (as shown).

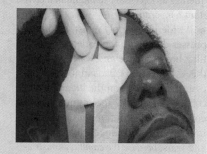

For increased protection of an injured eye, place a plastic or metal shield (as shown) on top of the gauze pads and apply tape over the shield.

Occasionally, you may use a head dressing to secure a pressure patch. The dressing applies additional pressure or, in burn patients, holds the patch in place without tape.

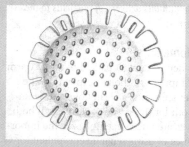

▶ Place the ice pack on top of the gauze pad and tape it in place. If the patient complains of pain, remove the ice pack. Some patients may have an adverse reaction to cold.

▶ After 15 to 20 minutes, remove the tape, ice pack, and gauze pad and discard them.

Concluding the procedure

▶ Use the remaining sterile 4″ × 4″ gauze pads to clean and dry the patient's face.

▶ If ordered, apply ophthalmic ointment or an eye patch. (See *Applying an eye patch,* page 313.)

Special considerations

▶ When applying hot compresses, change the prescribed solution as frequently as necessary *to maintain a constant temperature.*

▶ If ordered to apply moist, cold compresses directly to the patient's eyelid, fill a bowl with ice and water and soak the 4″ × 4″ gauze pads in it. Place a compress directly on the lid and change compresses every 2 to 3 minutes. Cold compresses are contraindicated in treating eye inflammation, such as keratitis and iritis, *because the capillary constriction inhibits delivery of nutrients to the cornea.*

Home care

When teaching a patient to apply warm compresses at home, explain that he can substitute a clean bowl and washcloth for the sterile equipment. If both eyes are infected, emphasize the importance of using separate equipment for each eye. Inform the patient that this will keep him from passing infection back and forth between the eyes. Also

direct him to wash his hands thoroughly before and after treating each eye.

Documentation

Record the time and duration of the procedure. Describe the eye's appearance before and after treatment. Note any ointments (and amounts) or dressings applied to the eye. Also note the patient's tolerance of the procedure.

EYE IRRIGATION

Used mainly to flush secretions, chemicals, and foreign objects from the eye, eye irrigation also provides a way to administer medications for corneal and conjunctival disorders. In an emergency, tap water may serve as an irrigant.

The amount of solution needed to irrigate an eye depends on the contaminant. Secretions require a moderate volume; major chemical burns require a copious amount. Usually, an I.V. bottle or bag of normal saline solution (with I.V. tubing attached) supplies enough solution for continuous irrigation of a chemical burn. (See *Three devices for eye irrigation.*)

Key nursing diagnoses and patient outcomes

Risk for infection related to (specify)
The patient will:
▶ be free from elevated body temperature
▶ identify signs of infection, such as redness, swelling, or drainage.

Risk for injury related to (specify)
The patient will:
▶ be free from injury
▶ take appropriate safety precautions.

Three devices for eye irrigation

Depending on the type and extent of injury, the patient's eye may need to be irrigated using different devices.

Squeeze bottle

For moderate-volume irrigation — to remove eye secretions, for example — apply sterile ophthalmic irrigant to the eye directly from the squeeze bottle container. Direct the stream at the inner canthus and position the patient so that the stream washes across the cornea and exits at the outer canthus.

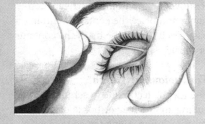

I.V. tube

For copious irrigation — to treat chemical burns, for example — set up an I.V. bag and tubing without a needle. Use the procedure described for moderate irrigation to flush the eye for at least 15 minutes. Alkali burns may require irrigation for several hours.

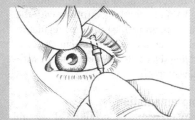

Morgan lens

Connected to irrigation tubing, a Morgan lens permits continuous lavage and also delivers medication to the eye. Use an adapter to connect the lens to the I.V. tubing and the solution container. Begin the irrigation at the prescribed flow rate. To insert the device, ask the patient to look down as you insert the lens under the upper eyelid. Then have her look up as you retract and release the lower eyelid over the lens.

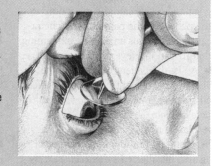

Equipment

Gloves • goggles • towels • eyelid retractor • sterile gauze pads • I.V. pole • optional: litmus paper and proparacaine hydrochloride topical anesthetic

For moderate-volume irrigation

Prescribed sterile ophthalmic irrigant

For copious irrigation

One or more 1 L bottles or bags of normal saline solution • standard I.V. infusion set without needle

Commercially prepared bottles of sterile ophthalmic irrigant are available. All solutions should be at body temperature: 98.6° F (37° C).

Preparation of equipment

Read the label on the sterile ophthalmic irrigant. Double-check its sterility, strength, and expiration date.

For moderate-volume irrigation

Remove the cap from the irrigant container and place the container within easy reach. (Keep the tip of the container sterile.)

For copious irrigation

Use aseptic technique to set up the I.V. tubing and the bag or bottle of normal saline solution. Hang the container on an I.V. pole, fill the I.V. tubing with the solution, and adjust the drip regulator valve *to ensure an adequate but not forceful flow.* Place all other equipment within easy reach.

Implementation

▶ Wash your hands, put on gloves and goggles, and explain the procedure to the patient. If the patient has a chemical burn, ease his anxiety by explaining that irrigation prevents further damage.
▶ Assist the patient in lying supine. Turn his head slightly toward the affected side *to prevent solution flowing over his nose and into the other eye.*
▶ Place a towel under the patient's head and let him hold another towel against his affected side *to catch excess solution.*
▶ Using the thumb and index finger of your nondominant hand, separate the patient's eyelids.
▶ If ordered, instill ophthalmic anesthetic eyedrops *as a comfort measure.* Use them only once *because repeated use retards healing.*
▶ To irrigate the conjunctival cul-de-sac, continue holding the eyelids apart with your thumb and index finger.

▶ To irrigate the upper eyelid (the superior fornix), use an eyelid retractor. Steady the hand holding the retractor by resting it on the patient's forehead. *The retractor prevents the eyelid from closing involuntarily when solution touches the cornea and conjunctiva.*

For moderate irrigation

▶ Holding the bottle of sterile ophthalmic irrigant about 1″ (2.5 cm) from the eye, direct a constant, gentle stream at the inner canthus *so that the solution flows across the cornea to the outer canthus.*
▶ Evert the lower eyelid and then the upper eyelid *to inspect for retained foreign particles.*
▶ Remove any foreign particles by gently touching the conjunctiva with a wet sterile gauze pad. Don't touch the cornea.
▶ Resume irrigating the eye until it's clean of all visible foreign particles.

For copious irrigation

▶ Hold the control valve on the I.V. tubing about 1″ above the eye and direct a constant, gentle stream of normal saline solution at the inner canthus *so that the solution flows across the cornea to the outer canthus.*
▶ Ask the patient to rotate his eye periodically while you continue the irrigation. *This action may dislodge foreign particles.*
▶ Evert the lower eyelid and then the upper eyelid *to inspect for retained foreign particles.* (This inspection is especially important when the patient has caustic lime in his eye.)

For aftercare

▶ After eye irrigation, gently dry the eyelid with a sterile gauze pad, wiping from the inner to the outer canthus. Use a new sterile gauze pad for each wipe. *This reduces the patient's need to rub his eye.*

▶ Remove and discard your gloves and goggles.

▶ When indicated, arrange for follow-up care.

▶ Wash your hands *to avoid burning from residual chemical contaminants.*

Special considerations

▶ When irrigating both eyes, have the patient tilt his head toward the side being irrigated *to avoid cross-contamination.*

▶ For chemical burns, irrigate each eye for at least 15 minutes with normal saline solution *to dilute and wash the harsh chemical.* If the patient can't identify the specific chemical, use litmus paper *to determine whether the chemical is acidic or alkaline, or to be sure that the eye has been irrigated adequately.* (After irrigating for a chemical burn, note the time, date, and chemical for your own reference *in case you develop contact dermatitis.*)

▶ If an ophthalmic anesthetic agent was used, instruct the patient to avoid touching the eye. *Touching the eye before the anesthetic has worn off may cause damage to the cornea or conjunctiva.*

Documentation

Note the duration of irrigation, the type and amount of solution, and characteristics of the drainage. Record your assessment of the patient's eye before and after irrigation. Also note his response to the procedure.

EYE MEDICATION ADMINISTRATION

Eye medications — drops, ointments, and disks — serve diagnostic and therapeutic purposes. During an eye examination, eyedrops can be used to anesthetize the eye, dilate the pupil to facilitate examination, and stain the cornea to identify corneal abrasions, scars, and other anomalies. Eye medications can also be used to lubricate the eye, treat certain eye conditions (such as glaucoma and infections), protect the vision of neonates, and lubricate the eye socket for insertion of a prosthetic eye.

Understanding the ocular effects of medications is important because certain drugs may cause eye disorders or have serious ocular effects. For example, anticholinergics, which are commonly used during eye examinations, can precipitate acute glaucoma in patients with a predisposition to the disorder.

Key nursing diagnoses and patient outcomes

Deficient knowledge related to lack of exposure to eye medication administration
The patient will:

▶ state or demonstrate an understanding of what has been taught

▶ demonstrate the ability to perform new health-related behaviors as they're taught.

Risk for injury related to improper technique
The patient will:

▶ identify factors that increase the risk of injury

▶ assist in identifying and applying safety measures to prevent injury.

Equipment

Prescribed eye medication • patient's medication record and chart • gloves • warm water or normal saline solution • sterile gauze pads • facial tissues • optional: ocular dressing

Preparation of equipment

Make sure the medication is labeled for ophthalmic use. Then check the expiration date. Remember to date the container the first time you use the medication. After it's opened, an eye medication may be used for a maximum of 2 weeks *to avoid contamination.*

Inspect ocular solutions for cloudiness, discoloration, and precipitation but remember that some eye medications are suspensions and normally appear cloudy. Don't use any solution that appears abnormal. If the tip of an eye ointment tube has crusted, turn the tip on a sterile gauze pad to remove the crust.

Implementation

▶ Verify the order on the patient's medication record by checking it against the doctor's order on his chart.
▶ Wash your hands.
▶ Check the medication label against the patient's medication record.

 Nursing alert **Make sure you know which eye to treat because different medications or doses may be ordered for each eye.**
▶ Confirm the patient's identity by asking his name and checking the name, room number, and bed number on his wristband.
▶ Explain the procedure to the patient and provide privacy. Put on gloves.
▶ If the patient is wearing an eye dressing, remove it by gently pulling it down and away from his forehead. Take care not to contaminate your hands.
▶ Remove any discharge by cleaning around the eye with sterile gauze pads moistened with warm water or normal saline solution. With the patient's eye closed, clean from the inner to the outer canthus, using a fresh sterile gauze pad for each stroke.
▶ To remove crusted secretions around the eye, moisten a gauze pad with warm water or normal saline solution. Ask the patient to close the eye, and then place the gauze pad over it for 1 or 2 minutes. Remove the pad and then reapply moist sterile gauze pads as necessary, until the secretions are soft enough to be removed without traumatizing the mucosa.
▶ Have the patient sit or lie in the supine position. Instruct him to tilt his head back and toward the side of the affected eye *so that excess medication can flow away from the tear duct, minimizing systemic absorption through the nasal mucosa.*

Instilling eyedrops

▶ Remove the dropper cap from the medication container, if necessary, and draw the medication into it. Be careful to avoid contaminating the dropper tip or bottle top.
▶ Before instilling the eyedrops, instruct the patient to look up and away. *This moves the cornea away from the lower lid and minimizes the risk of touching the cornea with the dropper if the patient blinks.*
▶ You can steady the hand holding the dropper by resting it against the patient's forehead. Then, with your other hand, gently pull down the lower lid of the affected eye and instill the drops in

the conjunctival sac. Try to avoid placing the drops directly on the eyeball *to prevent the patient from experiencing discomfort.* (See *Instilling eye medications.*)

Applying eye ointment
▶ Squeeze a small ribbon of medication on the edge of the conjunctival sac from the inner to the outer canthus. Cut off the ribbon by turning the tube. You can steady the hand holding the medication tube by bracing it against the patient's forehead or cheek.

Using a medication disk
▶ A medication disk can release medication in the eye for up to 1 week before needing to be replaced. Pilocarpine, for example, can be administered this way to treat glaucoma. (For specific instructions, see *How to insert and remove an eye medication disk,* pages 320 and 321.)

After instilling eyedrops or eye ointment
▶ Instruct the patient to close his eyes gently, without squeezing the lids shut. If you instilled drops, tell the patient to blink. If you applied ointment, tell him to roll his eyes behind closed lids *to help distribute the medication over the surface of the eyeball.*
▶ Use a clean tissue to remove any excess solution or ointment leaking from the eye. Remember to use a fresh tissue for each eye *to prevent cross-contamination.*
▶ Apply a new eye dressing, if necessary.
▶ Return the medication to the storage area. Store it according to the label's instructions.
▶ Wash your hands.

Instilling eye medications

To instill eyedrops, pull the lower lid down to expose the conjunctival sac. Have the patient look up and away and then squeeze the prescribed number of drops into the sac. Release the patient's eyelid and have him blink to distribute the medication.

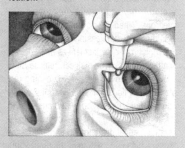

To apply an ointment, gently lay a thin strip of the medication along the conjunctival sac from the inner canthus to the outer canthus. Avoid touching the tip of the tube to the patient's eye. Then release the eyelid and have the patient roll his eye behind closed lids to distribute the medication.

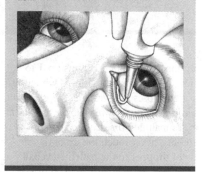

Special considerations
▶ When administering an eye medication that may be absorbed systemically (such as atropine), gently press your

How to insert and remove an eye medication disk

Small and flexible, an oval eye medication disk consists of three layers: two soft outer layers and a middle layer that contains the medication. Floating between the eyelids and the sclera, the disk stays in the eye while the patient sleeps and even during swimming and athletic activities. The disk frees the patient from having to remember to instill his eyedrops. When the disk is in place, ocular fluid moistens it, releasing the medication. Eye moisture or contact lenses don't adversely affect the disk. The disk can release medication for up to 1 week before needing replacement. Pilocarpine, for example, can be administered this way to treat glaucoma.

Contraindications include conjunctivitis, keratitis, retinal detachment, and any condition in which constriction of the pupil should be avoided.

To insert an eye medication disk
Arrange to insert the disk before the patient goes to bed. *This minimizes the blurring that usually occurs immediately after disk insertion.*
- Wash your hands and put on gloves.

- Press your fingertip against the oval disk so that it lies lengthwise across your fingertip. It should stick to your finger. Lift the disk out of its packet.
- Gently pull the patient's lower eyelid away from the eye and place the disk in the conjunctival sac. It should lie horizontally, not vertically. The disk will adhere to the eye naturally.

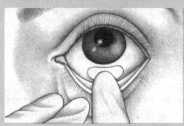

- Pull the lower eyelid out, up, and over the disk. Tell the patient to blink several times. If the disk is still visible, pull the lower lid out and over the disk again. Tell the patient that when the disk is in place, he can adjust its position by gently pressing his finger against his closed lid. Caution him against rubbing his eye or moving the disk across the cornea.

thumb on the inner canthus for 1 to 2 minutes after instilling drops while the patient closes his eyes. *This helps prevent medication from flowing into the tear duct.*
▶ To maintain the drug container's sterility, never touch the tip of the bottle or dropper to the patient's eyeball, lids, or lashes. Discard any solution remaining in the dropper before returning the dropper to the bottle. If the dropper or bottle tip has become contaminated, discard it and obtain another sterile dropper. *To prevent cross-contamination, never use a container of eye medication for more than one patient.*
▶ Teach the patient to instill eye medications *so that he can continue treatment at home, if necessary.* Review the procedure and ask for a return demonstration.

Complications
Instillation of some eye medications may cause transient burning, itching, and redness. Rarely, systemic effects may also occur.

■ If the disk falls out, wash your hands, rinse the disk in cool water, and reinsert it. If the disk appears bent, replace it.

■ If both of the patient's eyes are being treated with medication disks, replace both disks at the same time so that both eyes receive medication at the same rate.

■ If the disk repeatedly slips out of position, reinsert it under the upper eyelid. To do this, gently lift and evert the upper eyelid and insert the disk in the conjunctival sac. Then gently pull the lid back into position and tell the patient to blink several times. Again, the patient may press gently on the closed eyelid to reposition the disk. The more the patient uses the disk, the easier it should be for him to retain it. If he can't retain it, notify the doctor.

■ If the patient will continue therapy with an eye medication disk after discharge, teach him how to insert and remove it himself. To check his mastery of these skills, have him demonstrate insertion and removal for you.

■ Also, teach the patient about possible adverse reactions. Foreign-body sensation in the eye, mild tearing or redness, increased mucous discharge, eyelid redness, and itchiness can occur with the use of disks. Blurred vision, stinging, swelling, and headaches can occur with pilocarpine, specifically. Mild symptoms are common but should subside within the first 6 weeks of use. Tell the patient to report persistent or severe symptoms to his doctor.

To remove an eye medication disk

■ You can remove an eye medication disk with one or two fingers. To use one finger, put on gloves and evert the lower eyelid to expose the disk. Then use the forefinger of your other hand to slide the disk onto the lid and out of the patient's eye. To use two fingers, evert the lower lid with one hand to expose the disk. Then pinch the disk with the thumb and forefinger of your other hand and remove it from the eye.

■ If the disk is located in the upper eyelid, apply long circular strokes to the patient's closed eyelid with your finger until you can see the disk in the corner of the patient's eye. When the disk is visible, you can place your finger directly on the disk and move it to the lower sclera. Then remove it as you would a disk located in the lower lid.

Documentation

Record the medication instilled or applied, eye or eyes treated, and date, time, and dose. Note any adverse effects and the patient's response.

EYE PROPHYLAXIS (CREDÉ'S TREATMENT)

Named for its developer, Credé's treatment prevents damage and blindness from conjunctivitis due to *Neisseria gonorrhoeae,* which is transmitted to the neonate during birth if the mother has gonorrhea. It's also used to treat chlamydial conjunctivitis transmitted during birth.

Required by law in all states in the United States, Credé's treatment consists of instilling 1% tetracycline ointment or 0.5% erythromycin ophthalmic ointment. Erythromycin is the drug of choice. The nurse instills the ointment in the conjunctival sac (from the eye's inner canthus to its outer can-

How to instill medication for Credé's treatment

Using your nondominant hand, gently raise the neonate's upper eyelid with your index finger and pull down the lower eyelid with your thumb. Using your dominant hand, apply the ordered ophthalmic antibiotic ointment in a line along the lower conjunctival sac (as shown). Repeat the procedure for the other eye.

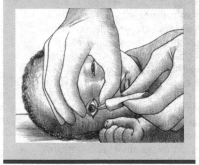

thus). The ointment should be administered as soon after birth as possible.

Key nursing diagnoses and patient outcomes

Risk for injury related to improper technique

The patient will:
▶ identify factors that increase the risk of injury
▶ assist in identifying and applying safety measures to prevent injury.

Equipment

Ophthalmic antibiotic ointment as ordered • gloves

Preparation of equipment

Remove the cap from the ointment container. A single-dose ointment tube should be used *to prevent contamination and spread of infection.*

Implementation

▶ If the parents are present for the procedure, explain that state law mandates Credé's treatment. Forewarn them that the neonate may have blurry vision from the ointment. Reassure them that these are temporary effects.

▶ Put on gloves. *To ensure comfort and effectiveness,* shield the neonate's eyes from direct light, tilt his head slightly to the side of the intended treatment, and instill the medication. (See *How to instill medication for Credé's treatment.*)

▶ Close and manipulate the eyelids to spread the medication over the eye.

Special considerations

▶ Treatment should be administered immediately upon admission if the neonate is born outside the facility.

Complications

Chemical conjunctivitis may cause redness, swelling, and drainage.

Documentation

If you perform Credé's treatment in the delivery room, record the treatment on the delivery room form. If you perform it in the nursery, document it in your notes.

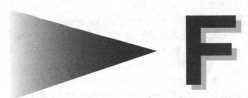

FALL PREVENTION AND MANAGEMENT

Falls are a major cause of injury and death among elderly people. In fact, the older the person, the more likely he's to die of a fall or its complications. In people age 75 or older, falls account for three times as many accidental deaths as motor vehicle accidents.

Factors that contribute to falls among elderly patients include lengthy convalescent periods, a greater risk of incomplete recovery, medications, and increasing physical disability. For example, once impaired, equilibrium takes longer to be restored in elderly people than in younger adults. Naturally, loss of balance increases the risk of falling. In addition to causing physical harm, injuries from falls can trigger psychological problems, leading to a loss of self-confidence and hastening dependence and a move to a long-term care facility or nursing home.

Falls may be caused by environmental factors, such as poor lighting, slippery throw rugs, and highly waxed floors. However, they commonly result from physiologic factors, such as temporary muscle paralysis, vertigo, orthostatic hypotension, central nervous system lesions, dementia, failing eyesight, and decreased strength or coordination.

Who is at risk for a fall?

Preventing falls begins with identifying the patients at greatest risk. Consider a patient with one or more of the following characteristics to be at risk:
- age 65 or older
- poor general health with a chronic disease
- a history of falls
- altered mental status
- decreased mobility
- improperly fitted shoes or slippers
- inappropriate use of restraints
- urinary frequency or diarrhea
- sensory deficits — particularly visual deficits
- use of certain drugs, such as diuretics, strong analgesics, antipsychotics, and hypnotics.

In a health care facility, an accidental fall can change a short stay for a minor problem into a prolonged stay for serious — and possibly life-threatening — problems. The risk of falling is highest during the 1st week of a stay in a health care facility or nursing home. The adage "an ounce of prevention is worth a pound of cure" is worth remembering when working with elderly patients (See *Who is at risk for a fall?*)

Key nursing diagnoses and patient outcomes

Risk for injury related to sensory or motor difficulties
The patient will:
▶ identify factors that increase the risk of injury
▶ assist in identifying and applying safety measures to prevent injury
▶ optimize activities of daily living with sensorimotor limitations.

Equipment

Stethoscope • sphygmomanometer • analgesics • cold and warm compresses • pillows • blankets • emergency resuscitation equipment (crash cart), if needed • electrocardiograph (ECG) monitor, if needed

Preparation of equipment

If you're helping a fallen patient, send an assistant to collect the assessment or resuscitation equipment you need.

Implementation

▶ Whether your plan of care focuses on preventing a fall or managing one in an elderly patient, you'll need to proceed with patience and caution.

Preventing falls

▶ Assess your patient's risk of falling at least once each shift (or at least every 3 months if the patient is in a long-term care facility.) Note any changes in his condition—such as decreased mental status—that increase his chances of falling. If you decide that he's at risk, take steps to reduce the danger. (See *Risk assessment for falls.*)
▶ Correct potential dangers in the patient's room. Position the call light so that he can reach it. Provide adequate nighttime lighting.

▶ Place the patient's personal belongings and aids (such as a purse, a wallet, books, tissues, a urinal, a commode, and a cane or walker) within easy reach.
▶ Instruct him to rise slowly from a supine position *to avoid possible dizziness and loss of balance.*
▶ Lower the bed to its lowest position *so the patient can easily reach the floor when he gets out of bed. This also reduces the distance to the floor in case he falls.* Lock the bed's wheels and place the bed against the wall, if possible. If side rails are to be raised, observe the patient frequently.
▶ Advise the patient to wear nonskid footwear.
▶ Respond promptly to the patient's call light *to help limit the number of times he gets out of bed without help.*
▶ Check the patient at least every 2 hours. Check a high-risk patient every 30 minutes.
▶ Alert other caregivers to the patient's risk of falling and to the interventions you've implemented.
▶ Consider other precautions, such as placing two high-risk patients in the same room and having someone with them at all times.
▶ Encourage the patient to perform active range-of-motion (ROM) exercises *to improve flexibility and coordination.*

Managing falls

▶ If you're with a patient as he falls, try to break his fall with your body.
▶ As you gently guide him to the floor, support his body, particularly his head and trunk. If possible, help him to a supine position.
▶ While guiding the patient, concentrate on maintaining proper body alignment yourself to keep the center of gravity within your support base.

Risk assessment for falls

This standardized assessment tool can help you evaluate your patient's risk for falls and plan preventive measures, if needed. A score above 4 indicates the need for intervention.

Parameters	4	3	2	1	Patient score
Age		Over age 80	70 to 79		2
Mental status	Intermittent confusion or disorientation		Confused or disoriented at times		4
Elimination	Independent and incontinent	Needs assistance		Indwelling catheter or ostomy	3
History of falling	History of multiple falls (3 or more)		Has fallen 1 or 2 times		2
Activity level	Confined to bed or chair	Out of bed with assistance		Bathroom privileges	3
Gait and balance	Unsteady, poor balance standing or walking	Orthostatic hypotension	Spastic or jerky gait		4
Medications (current or in the past 7 days)	3 or more medications	2 medications	1 medication		4
				Total Risk Score	22

Medications		Patient scores
__ Anesthetic	✓ Cathartic	11 to 24 = extremely high risk
✓ Antidiabetic	✓ Diuretic	5 to 10 = high risk
__ Antihistamine	__ Narcotic	0 to 4 = low risk
✓ Antihypertensive	__ Psychotropic	If score is greater than 4, patient is at
__ Anticonvulsant	__ Sedative	high risk for falling, and fall-prevention
__ Benzodiazepine	__ Hypnotic	protocol must be implemented.
	__ Other (specify)	

Courtesy of Abington Memorial Hospital Department of Nursing, Abington, Pa.

Spread your feet to widen your support base. Remember, the wider the base, the better your balance will be. Bend your knees—rather than your back—*to support the patient and to avoid injuring yourself.*

▶ Remain calm and stay with the patient *to prevent any further injury.*

▶ Ask another nurse to collect any tools you may need, such as a stethoscope, a sphygmomanometer and, if necessary, an ECG monitor.

▶ Assess the patient's airway, breathing, and circulation *to be sure the fall wasn't caused by respiratory or cardiac arrest.* If you don't detect respirations or a pulse, call a code and begin emergency resuscitation measures. Also note his level of consciousness (LOC) and assess pupil size, equality, and reaction to light.

▶ *To determine the extent of the patient's injuries,* look for lacerations, abrasions, and obvious deformities. Note any deviations from the patient's baseline condition. Notify the doctor.

▶ If you weren't present during the fall, ask the patient or a witness what happened. Ask if the patient experienced pain or a change in LOC.

▶ Don't move the patient until you evaluate his status fully. Provide reassurance as needed and observe for such signs and symptoms as confusion, tremor, weakness, pain, and dizziness.

▶ Assess the patient's limb strength and motion. Don't perform any ROM exercises if you suspect a fracture or if the patient complains of any odd sensations or limited movement. If you suspect any disorder, don't move the patient until a doctor examines him. Spinal cord injuries from patient falls are rare, *but if injury has occurred, any movement may cause irreversible spinal damage.*

▶ While the patient lies on the floor until the doctor arrives, offer pillows and blankets *for comfort.* If you suspect a spinal cord injury, however, don't place a pillow under his head.

▶ If you don't detect any problems, return the patient to his bed with the help of another staff member. Never try to lift a patient alone *because you may injure yourself or the patient.*

▶ Take steps to control bleeding (if indicated) and to obtain an X-ray if you suspect a fracture. Provide first aid for minor injuries as needed. Then monitor the patient's status for the next 24 hours.

▶ Even if the patient shows no signs of distress or has sustained only minor injuries, monitor his vital signs every 15 minutes for 1 hour, then every 30 minutes for 1 hour, then every hour for 2 hours or until his condition stabilizes. Notify the doctor if you note any change from the baseline.

▶ Perform necessary measures to relieve the patient's pain and discomfort. Give analgesics as ordered. Apply cold compresses for the first 24 hours and warm compresses thereafter.

▶ Reassess the patient's environment and his risk of falling. Talk to him about the fall. Discuss why it occurred and how he thinks it could have been prevented. Review the events that preceded the fall. Did the patient change position abruptly? Does he wear corrective lenses, and was he wearing them when he fell? Review medications that may have contributed to the fall, such as tranquilizers and narcotics. (See *Medications associated with falls.*) In addition, assess gait disturbances or improper use of canes, crutches, or a walker.

Special considerations

▶ After a fall, review the patient's medical history *to determine whether he's at risk for other complications.* For example, if he hit his head, check his history to see whether he takes anticoagulants. If he does, he's at greater risk for intracranial bleeding, and you'll need to monitor him accordingly.

▶ Consider beginning a fall prevention program in your facility if you don't already have one.

▶ Devise an alternative to restraints for a high-risk patient. For example, investigate using a device such as a pressure-pad alarm. The pressure sensor pad lies under the bed linens. The reduced pressure that results as the patient gets out of bed triggers an alarm at the nurses' station. One such system consists of a lightweight plastic sensor sheet and a control unit. The system adapts to both bed and chair, and setting it up according to the manufacturer's directions prevents false alarms. An alternative alarm device can be worn by the patient just above the knee. The alarm sounds when the patient moves his leg to a vertical position.

▶ *To promote patient safety,* consider drawing a red arrow next to the patient's room number on the call-light console and making a red dot on the AT RISK card on the patient's door. Also add an appropriate notation to the Kardex and chart.

▶ Provide emotional support, whether you're managing a fall or preventing one. Let the elderly patient know that you recognize his limitations and acknowledge his fears. Point out measures that you'll take to provide a safe environment.

▶ Teach the patient how to fall safely. Show him how to protect his hands

Medications associated with falls

This chart highlights some classes of drugs that are commonly prescribed for older patients and the possible adverse effects of each that may increase a patient's risk of falling.

Drug Class	Adverse effects
Diuretics	Hypovolemia Orthostatic hypotension Electrolyte imbalance Urinary incontinence
Antihypertensives	Hypotension
Tricyclic antidepressants	Orthostatic hypotension
Antipsychotics	Orthostatic hypotension Muscle rigidity Sedation
Benzodiazepines and antihistamines	Excessive sedation Confusion Paradoxical agitation Loss of balance
Narcotics	Hypotension Sedation Motor incoordination Agitation
Hypnotics	Excessive sedation Ataxia Poor balance Confusion Paradoxical agitation
Antidiabetics	Acute hypoglycemia
Alcohol	Intoxication Motor incoordination Agitation Sedation Confusion

Promoting safety in the home

Before your patient leaves the health care facility, provide him with the following tips for ensuring a safe home environment:

■ Secure all carpets and floor coverings around the edges and tack down worn spots. Never use lightweight, loose mats or rugs on bare floors.

■ Make sure potential hazards such as stairs are well lit. White paint on either side of a staircase can enhance visibility.

■ Install strong banisters along all indoor and outdoor steps.

■ Use a bedside lamp or low-wattage night-light in the bedroom to avoid having to grope around in the dark when getting out of bed.

■ Fit secure handrails in convenient places in the shower, bathtub, and toilet. Use nonskid mats both inside and alongside every tub or shower.

■ Minimize clutter. Store children's toys, especially those on wheels, when not in use.

■ Walk carefully if a pet, such as a dog or a cat, is present.

■ Secure wires from electrical appliances to walls or moldings.

■ Store frequently used clothing and other items in places where they can be reached without standing on a stool or chair.

■ Reduce the risk of accidental slips and falls by selecting properly fitted shoes with nonskid soles, avoiding long robes, and wearing glasses, if needed.

■ Sit on the edge of a bed or chair for a few minutes before rising.

■ Use a walking stick, cane, or walker whenever an unsteady feeling arises.

and face. If he uses a walker or a wheelchair, demonstrate how to cope with and recover from a fall. Instruct him to survey the room for a low, sturdy, supportive piece of furniture (such as a coffee table). Then review the proper procedure for lifting himself off the floor and either standing up with the walker or getting into the wheelchair.

Home care

Before discharge, teach the patient and his family how to prevent accidental falls at home by correcting common household hazards. Encourage them to take steps to ensure safety. (See *Promoting safety in the home*.)

As needed, refer the patient to the local visiting nurse association so that nursing services can continue after discharge and during convalescence.

Documentation

After a fall, complete a detailed incident report in case the patient takes legal action. Primarily for your facility's insurance carrier, this report isn't considered part of the patient's record. A copy, however, will go to the facility's administrator, who will evaluate care given in the unit and propose new safety policies as appropriate.

The incident report should note where and when the fall occurred, how the patient was found, and in what position. Include the events preceding the fall, the names of witnesses, the patient's reaction to the fall, and a detailed description of his condition based on assessment findings. Note any interventions taken and the names of other staff members who helped care for him after the fall. Record the doctor's name and the date and time that he was notified. Include a copy of the doctor's report.

Also, note whether the patient was sent for diagnostic tests or transferred to another unit.

Include all of the information about the fall in the patient's record. Also, document his vital signs. If you're monitoring the patient for a severe complication, record this as well.

FECAL IMPACTION REMOVAL (DIGITAL)

Fecal impaction — a large, hard, dry mass of stool in the folds of the rectum and, at times, in the sigmoid colon — results from prolonged retention and accumulation of stool. Common causes include poor bowel habits, inactivity, dehydration, improper diet (especially inadequate fluid intake), the use of constipation-inducing drugs, and incomplete bowel cleaning after a barium enema or barium swallow. Digital removal of fecal impaction is used when oil retention and cleansing enemas, suppositories, and laxatives fail to clear the impaction. It typically requires a doctor's order.

This procedure is contraindicated during pregnancy; after rectal, genitourinary, abdominal, perineal, or gynecologic reconstructive surgery; in patients with myocardial infarction, coronary insufficiency, pulmonary embolus, heart failure, heart block, or Stokes-Adams syndrome (without pacemaker treatment); and in patients with GI or vaginal bleeding, hemorrhoids, rectal polyps, or blood dyscrasias.

Key nursing diagnoses and patient outcomes

Constipation related to (specify)

The patient will:
▶ experience return of normal elimination
▶ experience bowel movements every (specify) days without laxatives, enemas, or suppositories
▶ state an understanding of the causes of constipation
▶ describe changes in personal habits to maintain normal elimination patterns.

Deficient knowledge related to lack of exposure to digital removal of fecal impaction
The patient will:
▶ state an understanding of the procedure.

Equipment

Gloves (two pairs) • linen-saver pad • bedpan • plastic disposal bag • soap • water-filled basin • towel • water-soluble lubricant • washcloth • bath blanket

Implementation

▶ Explain the procedure to the patient and provide privacy.
▶ Position the patient on his left side and flex his knees *to allow easier access to the sigmoid colon and rectum.*
▶ Drape the patient with a bath blanket and place a linen-saver pad beneath the buttocks *to prevent soiling the bed linens.*
▶ Put on gloves and moisten an index finger with water-soluble lubricant *to reduce friction during insertion, thereby avoiding injury to sensitive tissue.*
▶ Instruct the patient to breathe deeply to promote relaxation. Then gently insert your lubricated index finger beyond the anal sphincter until you touch the impaction. Rotate your finger gently around the stool *to dislodge and break it into small fragments.* Then work the

fragments downward to the end of the rectum and remove each one separately.

▶ Before removing your finger, gently stimulate the anal sphincter with a circular motion two or three times *to increase peristalsis and encourage evacuation.*

▶ Remove your finger and change your gloves. Then clean the anal area with soap and water and lightly pat it dry with a towel.

▶ Offer the patient the bedpan or commode *because digital manipulation stimulates the urge to defecate.*

▶ Place disposable items in the plastic bag and discard the bag properly. If necessary, clean the bedpan and return it to the bedside stand.

▶ Wash your hands.

Special considerations

If the patient experiences pain, nausea, rectal bleeding, changes in pulse rate or skin color, diaphoresis, or syncope, stop the procedure immediately and notify the doctor.

Complications

Digital removal of fecal impaction can stimulate the vagus nerve and may decrease heart rate and cause syncope.

Documentation

Record the time and date of the procedure, the patient's response, and stool color, consistency, and odor.

FECAL OCCULT BLOOD TEST

Fecal occult blood tests are valuable for determining the presence of occult blood (hidden GI bleeding) and for distinguishing between true melena and melena-like stools. Certain medications, such as iron supplements and bismuth compounds, can darken stools so that they resemble melena.

Two common occult blood screening tests are Hematest (an orthotolidin reagent tablet) and the Hemoccult slide (filter paper impregnated with guaiac). Both tests produce a blue reaction in a fecal smear if occult blood loss exceeds 5 ml in 24 hours. A newer test, ColoCARE, requires no fecal smear.

Occult blood tests are particularly important for early detection of colorectal cancer because 80% of patients with this disorder test positive. However, a single positive test result doesn't necessarily confirm GI bleeding or indicate colorectal cancer. To confirm a positive result, the test must be repeated at least three times while the patient follows a meatless, high-residue diet. Even then, a confirmed positive test doesn't necessarily indicate colorectal cancer. It does indicate the need for further diagnostic studies because GI bleeding can result from many causes other than cancer, such as ulcers and diverticula. These tests are easily performed on collected specimens or smears from a digital rectal examination.

Key nursing diagnoses and patient outcomes

Deficient knowledge related to lack of exposure to fecal occult blood tests
The patient will:
▶ state the need for performing fecal occult blood tests.

Anxiety related to results of fecal occult blood tests
The patient will:

▶ verbalize feelings about potential outcome of procedure
▶ use available support systems, such as family and significant others.

Equipment
Test kit • gloves • glass or porcelain plate • tongue blade or other wooden applicator

Implementation
▶ Put on gloves and collect a stool specimen.

Hematest reagent tablet test
▶ Use a wooden applicator to smear a bit of the stool specimen on the filter paper supplied with the test kit. Or, after performing a digital rectal examination, wipe the finger you used for the examination on a square of the filter paper.
▶ Place the filter paper with the stool smear on a glass plate.
▶ Remove a reagent tablet from the bottle and immediately replace the cap tightly. Then place the tablet in the center of the stool smear on the filter paper.
▶ Add one drop of water to the tablet and allow it to soak in for 5 to 10 seconds. Add a second drop, letting it run from the tablet onto the specimen and filter paper. If necessary, tap the plate gently to dislodge any water from the top of the tablet.
▶ After 2 minutes, the filter paper will turn blue if the test is positive. Don't read the color that appears on the tablet itself or that develops on the filter paper after the 2-minute period.
▶ Note the results and discard the filter paper.
▶ Remove and discard your gloves and wash your hands thoroughly.

Hemoccult slide test
▶ Open the flap on the slide packet and use a wooden applicator to apply a thin smear of the stool specimen to the guaiac-impregnated filter paper exposed in box A. Or, after performing a digital rectal examination, wipe the finger you used for the examination on a square of the filter paper.
▶ Apply a second smear from another part of the specimen to the filter paper exposed in box B *because some parts of the specimen may not contain blood.*
▶ Allow the specimens to dry for 3 to 5 minutes.
▶ Open the flap on the reverse side of the slide package and place 2 drops of Hemoccult developing solution on the paper over each smear. A blue reaction will appear in 30 to 60 seconds if the test is positive.
▶ Record the results and discard the slide package.
▶ Remove and discard your gloves and wash your hands thoroughly.

Special considerations
▶ Make sure stool specimens aren't contaminated with urine, soap solution, or toilet tissue and test them as soon as possible after collection.
▶ Test samples from several portions of the same specimen *because occult blood from the upper GI tract isn't always evenly dispersed throughout the formed stool; likewise, blood from colorectal bleeding may occur mostly on the outer stool surface.*
▶ Check the condition of the reagent tablets and note their expiration date. Use only fresh tablets and discard outdated ones. Protect Hematest tablets from moisture, heat, and light.
▶ If repeat testing is necessary after a positive screening test, explain the test

Home tests for fecal occult blood

Most fecal occult blood tests require the patient to collect a specimen of his stool and smear some of it on a slide. In contrast, some new tests don't require the patient to handle stool, making the procedure safer and simpler. One example is a test called ColoCARE.

If the patient will be performing the ColoCARE test at home, tell him to avoid red meat and vitamin C supplements for 2 days before the test. He should check with his doctor about discontinuing any medications before the test. Some drugs that may interfere with test results are aspirin, indomethacin, corticosteroids, phenylbutazone, reserpine, dietary supplements, anticancer drugs, and anticoagulants.

Tell the patient to flush the toilet twice just before performing the test to remove any toilet-cleaning chemicals from the tank. Tell him to defecate into the toilet but to throw no toilet paper into the bowl. Within 5 minutes, he should remove the test pad from its pouch and float it printed side up on the surface of the water. Tell him to watch the pad for 15 to 30 seconds for any evidence of blue or green color changes and have him record the result on the reply card.

Emphasize that he should perform this test with three consecutive bowel movements and then send the completed card to his doctor. However, he should call his doctor immediately if he notes a positive color change in the first test.

collection period *because these substances may alter test results.*

▶ As ordered, have the patient discontinue the use of iron preparations, bromides, iodides, rauwolfia derivatives, indomethacin, colchicine, salicylates, potassium, phenylbutazone, oxyphenbutazone, bismuth compounds, steroids, and ascorbic acid for 48 to 72 hours before the test and during it *to ensure accurate test results and avoid possible bleeding, which some of these compounds may cause.*

Home care

If the patient will be using the Hemoccult slide packet at home, advise him to complete the label on the slide packet before specimen collection. If he'll be using a ColoCARE test packet, inform him that this test is a preliminary screen for occult blood in his stool. Tell him that he won't have to obtain a stool specimen to perform the test but that he should follow your instructions carefully. (See *Home tests for fecal occult blood.*)

Documentation

Record the time and date of the test, the result, and any unusual characteristics of the stool tested. Report positive results to the doctor.

FEEDING

Confusion, arm or hand immobility, injury, weakness, or restrictions on activities or positions may prevent a patient from feeding himself. Feeding the patient then becomes a key nursing responsibility. Injured or debilitated patients may experience depression and subsequent anorexia. Meeting such pa-

to the patient. Instruct him to maintain a high-fiber diet and to refrain from eating red meat, poultry, fish, turnips, and horseradish for 48 to 72 hours before the test as well as throughout the tients' nutritional needs requires determining food preferences, conducting the feeding in a friendly, unhurried manner, encouraging self-feeding to promote independence and dignity, and documenting intake and output. (See *Recording fluid intake and output.*)

Key nursing diagnoses and patient outcomes

Imbalanced nutrition: Less than body requirements related to (specify)
The patient will:
▶ consume at least (specify) calories daily
▶ gain (specify) lb (kg) weekly or maintain normal body weight.

Feeding self-care deficit related to (specify)
The patient will:
▶ express feelings about feeding limitations
▶ maintain a weight of (specify)
▶ demonstrate the correct use of assistive feeding devices.

Equipment
Meal tray • overbed table • linen-saver pad or towels • clean linens • alcohol • flexible straw • basin of water • soap • washcloth • hand towel • spoon or feeding syringe • assistive feeding devices, if necessary

Implementation
▶ *Because many adults consider being fed demeaning,* allow the patient some control over mealtime, such as letting him set the pace of the meal or decide the order in which he eats various foods.
▶ Raise the head of the bed, if allowed. *Fowler's or semi-Fowler's position makes swallowing easier and reduces the risk of aspiration and choking.*

Better charting

Recording fluid intake and output

Accurate intake and output records help evaluate a patient's fluid and electrolyte balance, suggest various diagnoses, and influence the choice of fluid therapy. These records are mandatory for patients with burns, renal failure, electrolyte imbalance, recent surgical procedures, heart failure, or severe vomiting and diarrhea, and for patients receiving diuretics or corticosteroids. Intake and output records are also significant in monitoring patients with nasogastric (NG) tubes or drainage collection devices and those receiving I.V. therapy.

Fluid intake comprises all fluid entering the patient's body, including beverages, fluids contained in solid foods taken by mouth, and foods that are liquid at room temperature, such as flavored gelatin, custard, ice cream, and some beverages. Additional intake includes GI instillations, bladder irrigations, and I.V. fluids.

Fluid output consists of all fluid that leaves the patient's body, including urine, loose stools, vomitus, aspirated fluid loss, and drainage from surgical drains, NG tubes, and chest tubes.

When recording fluid intake and output, enlist the patient's help, if possible. Record amount in cubic centimeters (cc) or milliliters (ml). Measure; don't estimate. For a small child, weigh diapers, if appropriate. Monitor intake and output during each shift and notify the doctor if amounts differ significantly over a 24-hour period. Document your findings in the appropriate location; describe any fluid restrictions and the patient's compliance.

▶ Before the meal tray arrives, give the patient soap, a basin of water or a wet washcloth, and a hand towel *to clean his*

Using assistive feeding devices

Various feeding devices can help the patient who has limited arm mobility, grasp, range of motion, or coordination. Before introducing your patient to an assistive feeding device, assess his ability to master it. Don't introduce a device he can't manage. If his condition is progressively disabling, encourage him to use the device only until his mastery of it falters.

Introduce the assistive device before mealtime, with the patient seated in a natural position. Explain its purpose, show the patient how to use it, and encourage him to practice. After meals, wash the device thoroughly and store it in the patient's bedside stand. Document the patient's progress and share it with staff and family members to help reinforce the patient's independence. Specific devices include the following:

Plate guard

A plate guard blocks food from spilling off the plate. Attach the guard to the side of the plate opposite the hand the patient uses to feed himself. Guiding the patient's hand, show him how to push food against the guard to secure it on the utensil. Then have him try again with food of a different consistency. When the patient tires, feed him the rest of the meal. At subsequent meals, encourage the patient to feed himself for progressively longer periods until he can feed himself an entire meal.

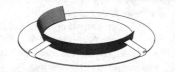

Swivel spoon

A swivel spoon helps the patient with limited range of motion (ROM) in his forearm and will fit in universal cuffs.

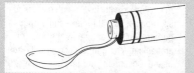

Universal cuffs

Universal cuffs are flexible bands that help the patient with flail hands or diminished grasp. Each cuff contains a slot that holds a fork or spoon. Attach the cuff to the hand the patient uses to feed himself. Then place the fork or spoon in the cuff slot. Bend the utensil to facilitate feeding.

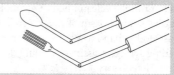

Long-handled utensils

Long-handled utensils have jointed stems to help the patient with limited ROM in his elbow and shoulder.

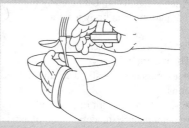

Utensils with built-up handles

Utensils with built-up handles can help the patient with diminished grasp. They can be purchased or can be improvised by wrapping tape around the handles.

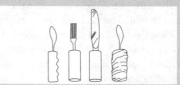

hands. If necessary, you may wash his hands for him.

▶ Wipe the overbed table with soap and water or alcohol, especially if a urinal or bedpan was on it.

▶ When the meal tray arrives, compare the name on the tray with the name on the patient's wristband. Check the tray to make sure it contains foods appropriate for the patient's condition.

▶ Encourage the patient to feed himself, if he can. If he's restricted to the prone or the supine position but can use his arms and hands, encourage him to try foods he can pick up such as sandwiches. If he can assume Fowler's or semi-Fowler's position but has limited use of his arms or hands, teach him how to use assistive feeding devices. (See *Using assistive feeding devices.*)

▶ If necessary, tuck a napkin or towel under his chin *to protect his gown from spills.* Use a linen-saver pad or towel *to protect bed linens.*

▶ Position a chair next to the patient's bed *so you can sit comfortably if you need to feed him yourself.*

▶ Set up the patient's tray, remove the plate from the tray warmer, and discard all plastic wrappings. Then cut the food into bite-sized pieces.

▶ To help the blind or visually impaired patient feed himself, tell him that placement of various foods on his plate corresponds to the hours on a clock face. Maintain consistent placement for subsequent meals.

▶ Ask the patient which food he prefers to eat first *to promote his sense of control over the meal.* Some patients prefer to eat one food at a time, while others prefer to alternate foods.

▶ If the patient has difficulty swallowing, offer liquids carefully with a spoon or feeding syringe to help prevent aspi-

ration. Pureed or soft foods, such as custard or flavored gelatin, may be easier to swallow than liquids. If the patient doesn't have difficulty swallowing, use a flexible straw *to reduce the risk of spills.*

▶ Ask the patient to indicate when he's ready for another mouthful. Pause between courses and whenever the patient wants to rest. During the meal, wipe the patient's mouth and chin as needed.

▶ When the patient finishes eating, remove the tray. If necessary, clean up spills and change the bed linens. Provide mouth care.

Special considerations

▶ Don't feed the patient too quickly *because this can upset him and impair digestion.*

▶ If the patient is restricted to the supine position, provide foods that he can chew easily. Feed him liquids carefully and only after he has swallowed his food *to reduce the risk of aspiration.*

▶ If the patient won't eat, try to find out why. For example, confirm his food preferences. Also, make sure that the patient isn't in pain at mealtimes or that he hasn't received any treatments immediately before a meal that could upset or nauseate him. Find out if any medications cause anorexia, nausea, or sedation. Of course, clear the bedside of emesis basins, urinals, bedpans, and similar distractions at mealtimes.

▶ Establish a pattern for feeding the patient and share this information with the rest of the staff *so the patient doesn't need to repeatedly instruct staff members about the best way to feed him.*

▶ If the patient and his family are willing, suggest that family members assist with feeding. This will make the patient feel more comfortable at mealtimes and may ease discharge planning.

Complications

Choking and aspiration of food can occur if the patient is fed too quickly or is given excessively large mouthfuls.

Documentation

Describe the feeding technique used in the nursing plan of care to ensure continuity of care. In your notes, record the amount of food and fluid consumed; also note the fluids consumed on the intake and output record, if required. Note which foods the patient consistently fails to eat, then try to find the reason. Record the patient's level of independence. For the blind patient, record the pattern of feeding on the nursing plan of care.

FEEDING TUBE INSERTION AND REMOVAL

Inserting a feeding tube nasally or orally into the stomach or duodenum allows a patient who can't or won't eat to receive nourishment. The feeding tube also permits administration of supplemental feedings to a patient who has very high nutritional requirements, such as an unconscious patient or one with extensive burns. Typically, a feeding tube is inserted by a nurse as ordered. The preferred feeding tube route is nasal, but the oral route may be used for patients with such conditions as a deviated septum or a head or nose injury.

The doctor may order duodenal feeding when the patient can't tolerate gastric feeding or when he expects gastric feeding to produce aspiration. Absence of bowel sounds or possible intestinal obstruction contraindicates using a feeding tube.

Feeding tubes differ somewhat from standard nasogastric tubes. Made of silicone, rubber, or polyurethane, feeding tubes have small diameters and great flexibility. This reduces oropharyngeal irritation, necrosis from pressure on the tracheoesophageal wall, distal esophageal irritation, and discomfort from swallowing. To facilitate passage, some feeding tubes are weighted with tungsten, and some need a guide wire to keep them from curling in the back of the throat.

These small-bore tubes usually have radiopaque markings and a water-activated coating, which provides a lubricated surface.

Key nursing diagnoses and patient outcomes

Imbalanced nutrition: Less than body requirements related to (specify)
The patient will:
▶ avoid aspiration
▶ avoid episodes of diarrhea
▶ gain (specify) lb (kg) weekly
▶ communicate an understanding of special dietary needs.

Deficient knowledge related to lack of exposure to the procedure
The patient will:
▶ communicate a need to know the reasons for performing the procedure
▶ state an understanding of the reasons for performing the procedure.

Anxiety related to lack of exposure to the procedure
The patient will:
▶ communicate feelings of anxiety about the procedure

▶ use available support systems, such as family and significant others.

Equipment
For insertion
Feeding tube (#6 to #18 French, with or without guide) • linen-saver pad • gloves • hypoallergenic tape • water-soluble lubricant • cotton-tipped applicators • skin preparation (such as compound benzoin tincture) • facial tissues • penlight • small cup of water with straw, or ice chips • emesis basin • 60-ml syringe • stethoscope • water

During use
Mouthwash or normal saline solution • toothbrush

For removal
Linen-saver pad • tube clamp • bulb syringe

Preparation of equipment
Have the proper size tube available. Usually, the doctor orders the smallest-bore tube that will allow free passage of the liquid feeding formula. Read the instructions on the tubing package carefully *because tube characteristics vary according to manufacturer.* (For example, some tubes have marks at the appropriate lengths for gastric, duodenal, and jejunal insertion.)

Examine the tube *to make sure it's free from defects,* such as cracks or rough or sharp edges. Next, run water through the tube. *This checks for patency, activates the coating, and facilitates removal of the guide.*

Implementation
▶ Explain the procedure to the patient and show him the tube *so that he knows what to expect and can cooperate more fully.*
▶ Provide privacy. Wash your hands and put on gloves.
▶ Assist the patient into semi-Fowler's or high Fowler's position.
▶ Place a linen-saver pad across the patient's chest *to protect him from spills.*
▶ *To determine the tube length needed to reach the stomach,* first extend the distal end of the tube from the tip of the patient's nose to his earlobe. Coil this portion of the tube around your fingers *so the end will remain curved until you insert it.* Then extend the uncoiled portion from the earlobe to the xiphoid process. Use a small piece of hypoallergenic tape to mark the total length of the two portions.

Inserting the tube nasally
▶ Using a penlight, assess nasal patency. Inspect nasal passages for a deviated septum, polyps, or other obstructions. Occlude one nostril, then the other, *to determine which has the better airflow.* Assess the patient's history of nasal injury or surgery.
▶ Lubricate the curved tip of the tube (and the feeding tube guide, if appropriate) with a small amount of water-soluble lubricant *to ease insertion and prevent tissue injury.*
▶ Ask the patient to hold the emesis basin and facial tissues in case he needs them.
▶ To advance the tube, insert the curved, lubricated tip into the more patent nostril and direct it along the nasal passage toward the ear on the same side. When it passes the nasopharyngeal junction, turn the tube 180 degrees *to aim it downward into the esophagus.* Tell the patient to lower his chin to his chest *to close the trachea.* Then give

him a small cup of water with a straw, or ice chips. Direct him to sip the water or suck on the ice and swallow frequently. *This will ease the tube's passage.* Advance the tube as he swallows.

Inserting the tube orally

▶ Have the patient lower his chin *to close his trachea* and ask him to open his mouth.

▶ Place the tip of the tube at the back of the patient's tongue, give water, and instruct the patient to swallow as above. Remind him to avoid clamping his teeth down on the tube. Advance the tube as he swallows.

Positioning the tube

▶ Keep passing the tube until the tape marking the appropriate length reaches the patient's nostril or lips.

▶ *To check tube placement,* attach the syringe filled with 10 cc of air to the end of the tube. Gently inject the air into the tube as you auscultate the patient's abdomen with the stethoscope about 3″ (7.5 cm) below the sternum. Listen for a whooshing sound, *which signals that the tube has reached its target in the stomach.* If the tube remains coiled in the esophagus, you'll feel resistance when you inject the air, or the patient may belch.

▶ If you hear a whooshing sound, gently try to aspirate gastric secretions. Successful aspiration confirms correct tube placement. If no gastric secretions return, the tube may be in the esophagus. You'll need to advance the tube or reinsert it before proceeding.

▶ After confirming proper tube placement, remove the tape marking the tube length.

▶ Tape the tube to the patient's nose and remove the guide wire. *Note:* In

some cases, X-rays may be ordered to verify tube placement.

▶ *To advance the tube to the duodenum,* especially a tungsten-weighted tube, position the patient on his right side. *This lets gravity assist tube passage through the pylorus.* Move the tube forward 2″ to 3″ (5 to 7.5 cm) hourly until X-ray studies confirm duodenal placement. (An X-ray must confirm placement before feeding begins *because duodenal feeding can cause nausea and vomiting if accidentally delivered to the stomach.*)

▶ Apply a skin preparation to the patient's cheek before securing the tube with tape. *This helps the tube adhere to the skin and also prevents irritation.*

▶ Tape the tube securely to the patient's cheek *to avoid excessive pressure on his nostrils.*

Removing the tube

▶ Protect the patient's chest with a linen-saver pad.

▶ Flush the tube with air, clamp or pinch it *to prevent fluid aspiration during withdrawal,* and withdraw it gently but quickly.

▶ Promptly cover and discard the used tube.

Special considerations

▶ Flush the feeding tube every 8 hours with up to 60 ml of normal saline solution or water *to maintain patency.* Retape the tube at least daily and as needed. Alternate taping the tube toward the inner and outer side of the nose *to avoid constant pressure on the same nasal area.* Inspect the skin for redness and breakdown.

▶ Provide nasal hygiene daily using the cotton-tipped applicators and water-soluble lubricant *to remove crusted secre-*

tions. Also help the patient brush his teeth, gums, and tongue with mouthwash or saline solution at least twice daily.

▶ If the patient can't swallow the feeding tube, use a guide *to aid insertion.*

▶ Precise feeding-tube placement is especially important *because small-bore feeding tubes may slide into the trachea without causing immediate signs of respiratory distress, such as coughing, choking, gasping, or cyanosis.* However, the patient will usually cough if the tube enters the larynx. To be sure that the tube clears the larynx, ask the patient to speak. If he can't, the tube is in the larynx. Withdraw the tube at once and reinsert.

▶ When aspirating gastric contents to check tube placement, pull gently on the syringe plunger *to prevent trauma to the stomach lining or bowel.* If you meet resistance during aspiration, stop the procedure *because resistance may result simply from the tube lying against the stomach wall.* If the tube coils above the stomach, you won't be able to aspirate stomach contents. To rectify this, change the patient's position or withdraw the tube a few inches, readvance it, and try to aspirate again. If the tube was inserted with a guide wire, don't use the guide wire to reposition the tube. The doctor may do so, using fluoroscopic guidance.

Home care

If your patient will use a feeding tube at home, make appropriate home care nursing referrals and teach the patient and caregivers how to use and care for a feeding tube. Teach them how to obtain equipment, insert and remove the tube, prepare and store feeding formu-

la, and solve problems with tube position and patency.

Complications

Prolonged intubation may lead to skin erosion at the nostril, sinusitis, esophagitis, esophagotracheal fistula, gastric ulceration, and pulmonary and oral infection.

Documentation

For tube insertion, record the date, time, tube type and size, insertion site, area of placement, and confirmation of proper placement. Also record the name of the person performing the procedure. For tube removal, record the date and time and the patient's tolerance of the procedure.

FETAL HEART RATE ASSESSMENT

A major clue to fetal well-being during gestation and labor, fetal heart rate (FHR) may be assessed by auscultating with a fetoscope or a Doppler ultrasound stethoscope placed on the maternal abdomen. This ultrasound device emits low-energy, high-frequency sound waves that rebound from the fetal heart to a transducer, which transmits the impulses to a monitor strip for recording.

Because FHR normally ranges from 120 to 160 beats/minute, auscultation yields only an average rate at best. However, because auscultation can detect gross (but often late) fetal distress signs (such as tachycardia and bradycardia), the technique remains useful in an uncomplicated, low-risk pregnancy. In a high-risk pregnancy, external (indi-

Instruments for hearing fetal heart tones

The fetoscope and the Doppler stethoscope are basic instruments for auscultating fetal heart tones and assessing fetal heart rate.

Fetoscope

This instrument can detect fetal heartbeats as early as the 20th gestational week. As an assessment tool during labor, the fetoscope is helpful for hearing fetal heart tones when contractions are mild and infrequent.

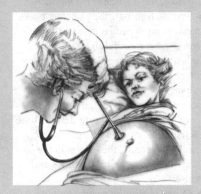

Doppler stethoscope

This instrument can detect fetal heartbeats as early as the 10th gestational week. Useful throughout labor, the Doppler stethoscope has greater sensitivity than the fetoscope.

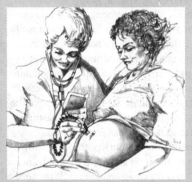

Portable Doppler stethoscope

With a clear sound that the mother and the examiner can easily hear, this device provides a digital display of the fetal heart rate. Features include a "freeze" button to hold the reading until it's recorded, an optional 10-second manual count mode, and an automatic shutoff to save power.

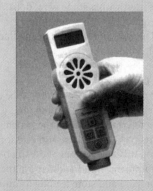

rect) or internal (direct) electronic fetal monitoring provides more accurate information on fetal status.

Key nursing diagnoses and patient outcomes

Deficient knowledge related to lack of exposure to the procedure
The patient will:
▶ verbalize an understanding of the procedure
▶ recognize that increased knowledge will help her cope better with the procedure.

Equipment

Fetoscope or Doppler stethoscope • water-soluble lubricant (for ultrasound instrument) • watch with second hand (see *Instruments for hearing fetal heart tones*)

Implementation

▶ Explain the procedure to the patient, wash your hands, and provide privacy. Reassure the patient that you may reposition the listening instrument frequently *to hear the loudest fetal heart tones.*
▶ Assist the patient to a supine position and drape her in a way that minimizes exposure. If you're using a Doppler stethoscope, apply the water-soluble lubricant to the patient's abdomen or Doppler stethoscope. *The gel or paste creates an airtight seal between the skin and the instrument and promotes optimal ultrasound wave conduction and reception.*

Calculating FHR during gestation

▶ To assess FHR in a fetus age 20 weeks or older, place the earpieces in your ears and position the bell of the fetoscope or Doppler stethoscope on the abdominal midline above the pubic

hairline. After 20 weeks, when you can palpate the fetal position, use Leopold's maneuvers *to locate the back of the fetal thorax.* Then position the listening instrument over the fetal back. (See *Performing Leopold's maneuvers,* page 342.)

Note: Because the presentation and position of the fetus may change, most clinicians don't perform Leopold's maneuvers until 32 to 34 weeks' gestation.
▶ Using a Doppler stethoscope, place the earpieces in your ears and press the bell gently on the patient's abdomen. Start listening at the midline, midway between the umbilicus and the symphysis pubis. Or, using a fetoscope, place the earpieces in your ears with the fetoscope positioned centrally on your forehead. Gently press the bell about $\frac{1}{2}''$ (1.5 cm) into the patient's abdomen. Remove your hands from the fetoscope *to avoid extraneous noise.*
▶ Move the bell of either instrument slightly from side to side as necessary, *to locate the loudest heart tones.* After locating these tones, palpate the maternal pulse.
▶ While monitoring the maternal pulse rate *(to avoid confusing maternal heart tones with fetal heart tones),* count the fetal heartbeats for at least 15 seconds. If the maternal radial pulse and FHR are the same, try to locate the fetal thorax by using Leopold's maneuvers; then reassess FHR. Usually, the fetal heart beats faster than the maternal heart does. Record FHR.

Counting FHR during labor

▶ Allow the mother and her support person to listen to the fetal heart, if they wish. *This helps to make the fetus a greater reality for them.* Record their participation.
▶ Place the fetoscope or Doppler stethoscope on the abdomen — midway

Performing Leopold's maneuvers

You can determine fetal position, presentation, and attitude by performing Leopold's maneuvers. Ask the patient to empty her bladder, assist her to a supine position, and place a small rolled towel under her right hip *to prevent supine hypotension syndrome*. Expose her abdomen and then perform the four maneuvers in order.

First maneuver

Face the patient and warm your hands. Place them on her abdomen to determine fetal position in the uterine fundus. Curl your fingers around the fundus. With the fetus in vertex position, the buttocks feel irregularly shaped and firm. With the fetus in breech position, the head feels hard, round, and movable.

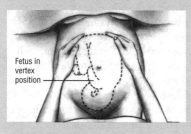

Fetus in
vertex
position

Second maneuver

Move your hands down the sides of the abdomen and apply gentle pressure. If the fetus lies in vertex position, you'll feel a smooth, hard surface on one side — the fetal back. Opposite, you'll feel lumps and knobs — the knees, hands, feet, and elbows. If the fetus lies in breech position, you may not feel the back at all.

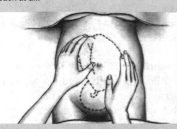

Third maneuver

Spread apart the thumb and fingers of one hand. Place them just above the patient's symphysis pubis. Bring your fingers together. If the fetus lies in vertex position (and hasn't descended), you'll feel the head. If the fetus lies in vertex position (and has descended), you'll feel a less distinct mass. Apply gentle pressure to the fundus with your other hand to help facilitate the maneuver.

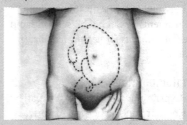

Fourth maneuver

Use this maneuver in late pregnancy. The purpose of the fourth maneuver is to determine flexion or extension of the fetal head and neck. Place your hands on both sides of the lower abdomen. Apply gentle pressure with your fingers as you slide your hands downward, toward the symphysis pubis. If the head presents, one hand's descent will be stopped by the cephalic prominence. The other hand will be unobstructed.

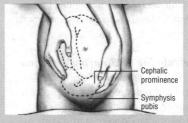

Cephalic
prominence

Symphysis
pubis

between the umbilicus and symphysis pubis *for cephalic presentation,* or at the umbilicus or above *for breech presentation.* Locate the loudest heartbeats and simultaneously palpate the maternal pulse *to ensure that you're monitoring fetal rather than maternal pulse.*

▶ Monitor maternal pulse rate and count fetal heartbeats for 60 seconds during the relaxation period between contractions *to determine baseline FHR.* In a low-risk labor, assess FHR every 60 minutes during the latent phase, every 30 minutes during the active phase, and every 15 minutes during the second stage of labor. In a high-risk labor, assess FHR every 30 minutes during the latent phase, every 15 minutes during the active phase, and every 5 minutes during the second stage of labor.

▶ Auscultate FHR during a contraction and for 30 seconds afterward *to identify the response to the contraction.*

▶ Notify the doctor or nurse-midwife immediately if you observe marked changes in FHR from baseline values (especially during or immediately after a contraction when signs of fetal distress typically occur). If fetal distress develops, begin indirect or direct electronic fetal monitoring.

▶ Repeat the procedure as ordered.

▶ Also auscultate before administration of medications, before ambulation, and before artificial rupture of membranes.

▶ Auscultate after rupture of membranes, after any changes in the characteristics of the contractions, after ambulation, after vaginal examinations, and after administration of medications.

Special considerations

▶ If you're auscultating FHR with a Doppler stethoscope, be aware that obesity and hydramnios can interfere with sound-wave transmission, making accurate results more difficult to obtain. If the doctor orders continuous FHR monitoring, apply the ultrasound transducer to the patient's abdomen. The monitor will provide a printed record of FHR.

▶ The tocotransducer may also be applied to monitor the contractile pattern at this time.

Documentation

Record both FHR and maternal pulse rate on the flowchart. Also record each auscultation and note the patient's tolerance to activity or treatment.

FETAL MONITORING, EXTERNAL

An indirect, noninvasive procedure, external fetal monitoring uses two devices strapped to the mother's abdomen to evaluate fetal well-being during labor. One device, an ultrasound transducer, transmits high-frequency sound waves through soft body tissues to the fetal heart. The waves rebound from the heart and the transducer relays them to a monitor. The other, a pressure-sensitive tocotransducer, responds to the pressure exerted by uterine contractions and simultaneously records their duration and frequency. (See *Applying external fetal monitoring devices,* page 344.) The monitoring apparatus traces fetal heart rate (FHR) and uterine contraction data onto the same printout paper.

Indications for external fetal monitoring include high-risk pregnancy, oxytocin-induced labor, and antepartum nonstress and contraction stress tests. Many labor and delivery units use external fetal monitoring for all pa-

Applying external fetal monitoring devices

To ensure clear tracings that define fetal status and labor progress, precisely position external monitoring devices, such as an ultrasound transducer and a tocotransducer.

Fetal heart monitor
Palpate the uterus to locate the fetus's back. If possible, place the ultrasound transducer over this site where the fetal heartbeat sounds the loudest. Then tighten the belt. Use the fetal heart tracing on the monitor strip to confirm the transducer's position.

Labor monitor
A tocotransducer records uterine motion during contractions. Place the tocotransducer over the uterine fundus where it contracts, either midline or slightly to one side. Place your hand on the fundus, and palpate a contraction to verify proper placement. Secure the tocotransducer's belt; then adjust the pen set so that the baseline values read between 5 and 15 mm Hg on the monitor strip.

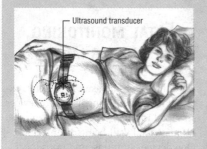
Ultrasound transducer

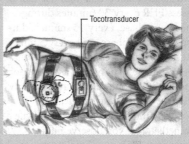
Tocotransducer

tients. The procedure has no contraindications, but it may be difficult to perform on patients with hydramnios, on obese patients, or on hyperactive or premature fetuses.

Key nursing diagnoses and patient outcomes
Anxiety related to the procedure
The patient will:
▶ communicate feelings of anxiety
▶ use available emotional support
▶ show decreased signs of anxiety.

Deficient knowledge related to lack of exposure to the procedure
The patient will:
▶ state an understanding of the procedure

▶ recognize that increased knowledge will help her cope with the procedure.

Equipment
Electronic fetal monitor • ultrasound transducer • tocotransducer • conduction gel • transducer straps • damp cloth • printout paper

Monitoring devices, such as phonotransducers and abdominal electrocardiogram transducers, are commercially available. However, facilities use these devices less frequently than they use the ultrasound transducer.

Preparation of equipment
Because fetal monitor features and complexity vary, review the operator's manual before proceeding. If the monitor has

two paper speeds, select the higher speed (typically 3 cm/minute) *to ensure an easy-to-read tracing.* At slower speeds (for example, 1 cm/minute), the printed tracings are difficult to decipher and interpret accurately.

Then plug the tocotransducer cable into the uterine activity jack and the ultrasound transducer cable into the phono-ultrasound jack. Attach the straps to the tocotransducer and the ultrasound transducer.

Label the printout paper with the patient's identification number or birth date and name, the date, maternal vital signs and position, the paper speed, and the number of the strip paper *to maintain accurate, consecutive monitoring records.*

If your facility has central monitoring capabilities, enter the patient data into the central computer *to ensure accurate labeling of monitor strips.*

Implementation

▶ Explain the procedure to the patient and provide emotional support. Inform her that the monitor may make noise if the pen set tracer moves above or below the printed paper. Reassure her that this doesn't indicate fetal distress. As appropriate, explain other aspects of the monitor *to help reduce maternal anxiety about fetal well-being.*

▶ Make sure the patient has signed a consent form, if required.

▶ Wash your hands and provide privacy.

Beginning the procedure

▶ Assist the patient to the semi-Fowler or left-lateral position with her abdomen exposed. Don't let her lie supine *because pressure from the gravid uterus on the maternal inferior vena cava may cause mater-*

nal hypotension and decreased uterine perfusion and may induce fetal hypoxia.

▶ Palpate the patient's abdomen to locate the fundus — the area of greatest muscle density in the uterus. Then, using transducer straps, secure the tocotransducer over the fundus.

▶ Adjust the pen set tracer controls so that the baseline values read between 5 and 15 mm Hg on the monitor strip. *This prevents triggering the alarm that indicates the tracer has dropped below the paper's margins.* The proper setting varies among tocotransducers.

▶ Apply conduction gel to the ultrasound transducer crystals *to promote an airtight seal and optimal sound-wave transmission.*

▶ Use Leopold's maneuvers to palpate the fetal back, through which fetal heart tones resound most audibly.

▶ Start the monitor. Then apply the ultrasound transducer directly over the site having the strongest heart tones.

▶ Activate the control that begins the printout. On the printout paper, note any coughing, position changes, drug administration, vaginal examinations, and blood pressure readings that may affect interpretation of the tracings.

▶ Explain to the patient and her support person how to time and anticipate contractions with the monitor. Inform them that the distance from one dark vertical line to the next on the printout grid represents 1 minute. The support person can use this information to prepare the patient for the onset of a contraction and to guide and slow her breathing as the contraction subsides.

Monitoring the patient

▶ Observe the tracings *to identify the frequency and duration of uterine contrac-*

tions but palpate the uterus *to determine intensity of contractions.*

▶ Mentally note the baseline FHR— the rate between contractions— *to compare with suspicious-looking deviations.* FHR normally ranges from 120 to 160 beats/minute.

▶ Assess periodic accelerations or decelerations from the baseline FHR. Compare the FHR patterns with those of the uterine contractions. Note the time relationship between the onset of an FHR deceleration and the onset of a uterine contraction, the time relationship of the lowest level of an FHR deceleration to the peak of a uterine contraction, and the range of FHR deceleration. *These data help distinguish fetal distress from benign head compression.*

▶ Move the tocotransducer and the ultrasound transducer *to accommodate changes in maternal or fetal position.* Readjust both transducers every hour and assess the patient's skin for reddened areas caused by the strap pressure. Document skin condition.

▶ Clean the ultrasound transducer periodically with a damp cloth *to remove dried conduction gel, which can interfere with ultrasound transmission.* Apply fresh gel as necessary. After using the ultrasound transducer, replace the cover over it.

Special considerations

▶ If the monitor fails to record uterine activity, palpate for contractions. Check for equipment problems as the manufacturer directs and readjust the tocotransducer.

▶ If the patient reports discomfort in the position that provides the clearest signal, try to obtain a satisfactory 5- or 10-minute tracing with the patient in this position before assisting her to a more comfortable position. As the patient progresses through labor and abdominal pressure increases, the pen set tracer may exceed the alarm boundaries.

Documentation

Make sure you number each monitor strip in sequence and label each printout sheet with the patient's identification number or birth date and name, the date, the time, and the paper speed. Record the time of any vaginal examinations, membrane rupture, drug administration, and maternal or fetal movements. Also, record maternal vital signs and the intensity of uterine contractions. Document each time that you moved or readjusted the tocotransducer and ultrasound transducer and summarize this information in your notes.

FETAL MONITORING, INTERNAL

Also called direct fetal monitoring, this sterile, invasive procedure uses a spiral electrode and an intrauterine catheter to evaluate fetal status during labor. By providing an electrocardiogram (ECG) of the fetal heart rate (FHR), internal electronic fetal monitoring assesses fetal response to uterine contractions more accurately than external fetal monitoring. Internal FHR monitoring allows evaluation of short- and long-term FHR variability. The intrauterine catheter measures uterine pressure during contraction and relaxation.

Internal fetal monitoring is indicated whenever direct, beat-to-beat FHR monitoring is required. Specific indications include maternal diabetes or hypertension, fetal postmaturity, suspected intrauterine growth retardation, and meconium-stained fluid. However, internal monitoring is performed only if the amniotic sac has ruptured, the cervix is dilated at least 2 cm, and the presenting part of the fetus is at least at the −1 station.

Contraindications for internal fetal monitoring include maternal blood dyscrasias, suspected fetal immune deficiency, placenta previa, face presentation or uncertainty about the presenting part, maternal HIV-positive status, and cervical or vaginal herpetic lesions.

A spiral electrode is the most commonly used device for internal fetal monitoring. Shaped like a corkscrew, the electrode is attached to the presenting fetal part (usually the scalp). It detects the fetal heartbeat and then transmits it to the monitor, which converts the signals to a fetal ECG waveform.

A pressure-sensitive intrauterine catheter, although not as widely used as the tocotransducer, is the most accurate method of determining the true intensity of contractions. It's especially helpful in dysfunctional labor and in preventing or rapidly determining the need for a cesarean birth. However, the risk of infection or uterine perforation associated with this device is high.

Key nursing diagnoses and patient outcomes

Anxiety related to the invasive procedure and potential outcomes
The patient will:
▶ state feelings of anxiety
▶ use available emotional support
▶ show fewer signs of anxiety
▶ identify positive aspects of her efforts to cope during childbirth.

Deficient knowledge related to lack of exposure to the invasive procedure
The patient will:
▶ state an understanding of the invasive procedure
▶ demonstrate the ability to perform skills needed for coping with labor.

Equipment

Electronic fetal monitor • spiral electrode and a drive tube • disposable leg plate pad or reusable leg plate with Velcro belt • conduction gel • antiseptic solution • sterile drape • hypoallergenic tape • sterile gloves (two pairs) • intrauterine catheter connection cable and pressure-sensitive catheter • printout paper • operator's manual.

Preparation of equipment

Review the operator's manual before using the equipment. If the monitor has two paper speeds, set the speed at 3 cm/minute *to ensure a readable tracing*. A tracing at 1 cm/minute is more condensed and harder to interpret accurately.

Connect the intrauterine cable to the uterine activity outlet on the monitor. Wash your hands and open the sterile equipment, maintaining aseptic technique.

Implementation

▶ Describe the procedure to the patient and her partner, if present, and explain how the equipment works. Tell the patient that a doctor or specially trained nurse will perform a vaginal examination to identify the position of the fetus.
▶ Make sure that the patient is fully informed about the procedure and obtain a signed consent form.

Applying an internal electronic fetal monitor

During internal electronic fetal monitoring, a spiral electrode monitors the fetal heart rate (FHR) and an internal catheter monitors uterine contractions.

Monitoring FHR

The spiral electrode is inserted after a vaginal examination determines the position of the fetus. As shown at right, the electrode is attached to the presenting fetal part, usually the scalp or buttocks.

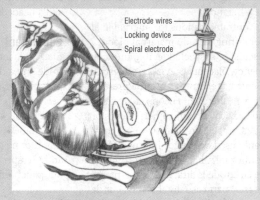

Electrode wires
Locking device
Spiral electrode

Monitoring uterine contractions

The intrauterine catheter is inserted up to a premarked level on the tubing and then connected to a monitor that interprets uterine contraction pressures.

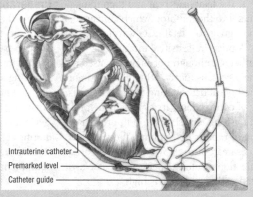

Intrauterine catheter
Premarked level
Catheter guide

▶ Label the printout paper with the patient's identification number or name and birth date, the date, the paper speed, and the number on the monitor strip.

Monitoring contractions

▶ Assist the patient into the lithotomy position for a vaginal examination. The doctor puts on sterile gloves.

▶ Attach the connection cable to the appropriate outlet on the monitor marked UA (uterine activity). Connect the cable to the intrauterine catheter. Next, zero the catheter with a gauge provided on the distal end of the catheter. *This will help determine the resting tone of the uterus, which is usually 5 to 15 mm Hg.*

Reading a fetal monitor strip

Presented in two parallel recordings, the fetal monitor strip records the fetal heart rate (FHR) in beats per minute in the top recording and uterine activity (UA) in millimeters of mercury (mm Hg) in the bottom recording. You can obtain information on fetal status and labor progress by reading the strips horizontally and vertically.

Reading the FHR or the UA strip horizontally, you see that each small block represents 10 seconds. Six consecutive small blocks, separated by a dark vertical line, rep-

resent 1 minute. Reading the FHR strip vertically, you see that each block represents an amplitude of 10 beats/minute. Reading the UA strip vertically, you see that each block represents 5 mm Hg of pressure.

Assess the baseline FHR — the "resting" heart rate — between uterine contractions when fetal movement diminishes. This baseline FHR (normal range: 120 to 160 beats/minute) pattern serves as a reference for subsequent FHR tracings produced during contractions.

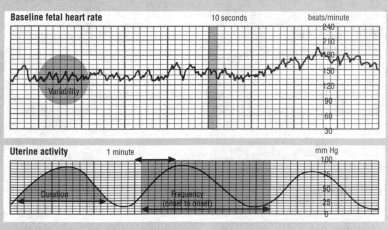

Cover the patient's perineum with a sterile drape, if facility policy so dictates. Then clean the perineum with antiseptic solution, according to facility policy. Using aseptic technique, the doctor inserts the catheter into the uterine cavity while performing a vaginal examination. The catheter is advanced to the black line on the catheter and secured with hypoallergenic tape along the inner thigh.

Observe the monitoring strip *to verify proper placement of the catheter guide*

and to ensure a clear tracing. Periodically evaluate the monitoring strip to determine the exact amount of pressure exerted with each contraction. Note all such data on the monitoring strip and on the patient's medical record.

The intrauterine catheter is usually removed during the second stage of labor or at the doctor's discretion. Dispose of the catheter and clean and store the cable according to facility policy. (See *Applying an internal electronic fetal monitor.*)

(*Text continues on page 352.*)

Identifying baseline FHR irregularities

Irregularity	Possible causes

Baseline tachycardia
beats/minute

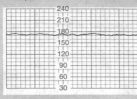

- Early fetal hypoxia
- Maternal fever
- Parasympathetic agents, such as atropine and scopolamine
- Beta-adrenergics, such as ritodrine and terbutaline
- Amnionitis (inflammation of inner layer of fetal membrane, or amnion)
- Maternal hyperthyroidism
- Fetal anemia
- Fetal heart failure
- Fetal arrhythmias

Baseline bradycardia
beats/minute

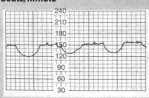

- Late fetal hypoxia
- Beta-adrenergic blocking agents, such as propranolol and anesthetics
- Maternal hypotension
- Prolonged umbilical cord compression
- Fetal congenital heart block

Early decelerations
beats/minute

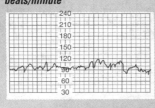

- Fetal head compression

mm Hg

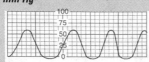

Clinical significance	Nursing interventions
Persistent tachycardia without periodic changes doesn't usually adversely affect fetal well-being, especially when associated with maternal fever. However, tachycardia is an ominous sign when associated with late decelerations, severe variable decelerations, or lack of variability.	■ Intervene to alleviate the cause of fetal distress and provide supplemental oxygen as ordered. Also administer I.V. fluids as prescribed. ■ Discontinue oxytocin infusion to reduce uterine activity. ■ Turn the patient onto her left side and elevate her legs. ■ Continue to observe the fetal heart rate (FHR). ■ Document interventions and outcomes. ■ Notify the doctor; further medical intervention may be necessary.
Bradycardia with good variability and no periodic changes doesn't signal fetal distress if FHR remains higher than 80 beats/minute. However, bradycardia caused by hypoxia and acidosis is an ominous sign when associated with loss of variability and late decelerations.	■ Intervene to correct the cause of fetal distress. Administer supplemental oxygen as ordered. Start an I.V. line and administer fluids as prescribed. ■ Discontinue oxytocin infusion to reduce uterine activity. ■ Turn the patient onto her left side, and elevate her legs. ■ Continue observing the FHR. ■ Document interventions and outcomes. ■ Notify the doctor; further medical intervention may be necessary.
Early decelerations are benign, indicating fetal head compression at dilation of 4 to 7 cm.	■ Reassure the patient that the fetus isn't at risk. ■ Observe the FHR. ■ Document the frequency of decelerations.

(continued)

Identifying baseline FHR irregularities *(continued)*

Irregularity	Possible causes

Late decelerations
beats/minute

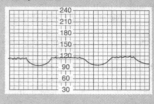

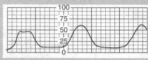
mm Hg

■ Uteroplacental circulatory insufficiency (placental hypo-perfusion) caused by decreased intervillous blood flow during contractions or a structural placental defect such as abruptio placentae
■ Uterine hyperactivity caused by excessive oxytocin infusion
■ Maternal hypotension
■ Maternal supine hypotension

Variable decelerations
beats/minute

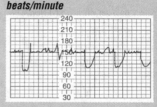

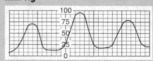
mm Hg

■ Umbilical cord compression causing decreased fetal oxygen perfusion

Monitoring FHR

► Apply conduction gel to the leg plate. Then secure the leg plate to the patient's inner thigh with Velcro straps or 2″ tape. Connect the leg plate cable to the ECG outlet on the monitor.

► Inform the patient that she'll undergo a vaginal examination to identify the fetal presenting part (which is usually the scalp or buttocks), to determine the level of fetal descent, and to apply the electrode. Explain that this examination is done to ensure that the electrode isn't

Clinical significance	Nursing interventions
Late decelerations indicate uteroplacental circulatory insufficiency and may lead to fetal hypoxia and acidosis if the underlying cause isn't corrected.	■ Turn the patient onto her left side to increase placental perfusion and decrease contraction frequency. ■ Increase the I.V. fluid rate to boost intravascular volume and placental perfusion as prescribed. ■ Administer oxygen by mask to increase fetal oxygenation as ordered. ■ Assess for signs of the underlying cause, such as hypotension or uterine tachysystole. ■ Take other appropriate measures such as discontinuing oxytocin as prescribed. ■ Document interventions and outcomes. ■ Notify the doctor; further medical intervention may be necessary.
Variable decelerations are the most common deceleration pattern in labor because fetal movement during contractions compresses the umbilical cord.	■ Help the patient change position to relieve pressure on the cord. No other intervention is necessary unless you detect fetal distress. ■ Assure the patient that the fetus tolerates cord compression well. Explain that cord compression affects the fetus the same way that holding her breath affects her. ■ Assess the deceleration pattern for reassuring signs: a baseline FHR that isn't increasing, short-term variability that isn't decreasing, abruptly beginning and ending decelerations, and decelerations lasting less than 50 seconds. If assessment doesn't reveal reassuring signs, notify the doctor. ■ Start I.V. fluids and administer oxygen by mask at 10 L/minute as prescribed. ■ Document interventions and outcomes. ■ Discontinue oxytocin infusion to decrease uterine activity.

attached to the suture lines, fontanels, face, or genitalia of the fetus. The spiral electrode will be placed in a drive tube and advanced through the vagina to the fetal presenting part. *To secure the electrode,* mild pressure will be applied and the drive tube will be turned clockwise 360 degrees.

▶ After the electrode is in place and the drive tube has been removed, connect the color-coded electrode wires to the corresponding color-coded leg plate posts.

▶ Turn on the recorder and note the time on the printout paper.

▶ Help the patient to a comfortable position and evaluate the strip *to verify proper placement and a clear FHR tracing.*

Monitoring the patient

▶ Begin by noting the frequency, duration, and intensity of uterine contractions. Normal intrauterine pressure ranges from 8 to 12 mm Hg. (See *Reading a fetal monitor strip,* page 349.)

▶ Next, check the baseline FHR. Assess periodic accelerations or decelerations from the baseline FHR.

▶ Compare the FHR pattern with the uterine contraction pattern. Note the interval between the onset of an FHR deceleration and the onset of a uterine contraction; the interval between the lowest level of an FHR deceleration and the peak of a uterine contraction; and the range of FHR deceleration.

▶ Check for FHR variability, which is a measure of fetal oxygen reserve and neurologic integrity and stability.

Special considerations

▶ Interpret FHR and uterine contractions at regular intervals. Guidelines of the Association of Women's Health, Obstetric, and Neonatal Nurses specify that high-risk patients need continuous FHR monitoring, whereas low-risk patients should have FHR auscultated every 30 minutes after a contraction during the first stage and every 15 minutes after a contraction during the second stage.

▶ First determine the baseline FHR within 10 beats/minute; then assess the degree of baseline variability. Note the presence or absence of short-term or long-term variability. Identify periodic FHR changes such as decelerations

(early late, variable, or mixed) and nonperiodic changes such as a sinusoidal pattern.

▶ Keep in mind that acute fetal distress can result from any change in the baseline FHR that causes fetal compromise. If necessary, take steps to counteract FHR changes. (See *Identifying baseline FHR irregularities,* pages 350 to 353.)

▶ If vaginal delivery isn't imminent (within 30 minutes) and fetal distress patterns don't improve, a cesarean birth will be necessary.

Complications

Maternal complications of internal uterine monitoring may include uterine perforation and intrauterine infection. Fetal complications caused by scalp electrode application may include abscess, hematoma, and infection.

Documentation

Document all activity related to monitoring. (A fetal monitoring strip becomes part of the patient's permanent record, so it's considered a legal document.) Record the type of monitoring your patient received as well as all interventions. Identify the monitoring strip with the patient's name, her doctor's name, your name, and the date and time. Also document the paper speed and electrode placement.

Record the patient's vital signs at regular intervals. Note her pushing efforts and record any change in her position. Document any I.V. line insertion and any changes in the I.V. solution or infusion rate. Note the use of oxytocin, regional anesthetics, or other medications.

After a vaginal examination, document cervical dilation and effacement as well as fetal station, presentation, and position. Also document membrane rupture, including the time it occurred and whether it was spontaneous or artificial. Note the amount, color, and odor of the fluid.

FOOT CARE

Daily bathing of feet and regular trimming of toenails promotes cleanliness, prevents infection, stimulates peripheral circulation, and controls odor by removing debris from between toes and under toenails. It's particularly important for the bedridden patient and those especially susceptible to foot infection. Increased susceptibility may be caused by peripheral vascular disease, diabetes mellitus, poor nutritional status, arthritis, or any condition that impairs peripheral circulation. In such a patient, proper foot care should include meticulous cleanliness and regular observation for signs of skin breakdown. (For additional instructions, see *Foot care for diabetic patients,* page 356.)

Toenail trimming is contraindicated in patients with a toe infection, diabetes mellitus, neurologic disorders, renal failure, or peripheral vascular disease, unless performed by a doctor or podiatrist. Some facilities prohibit nurses from trimming toenails. Check facility policy before performing the procedure.

Key nursing diagnoses and patient outcomes

Impaired skin integrity related to (specify)
The patient will:
▶ experience no skin breakdown
▶ maintain muscle strength.

Risk for infection related to (specify)
The patient will:
▶ have a normal body temperature
▶ have a normal white blood cell and differential counts
▶ remain free from all signs and symptoms of infection
▶ state infection risk factors
▶ communicate an understanding of signs and symptoms of infection.

Deficient knowledge related to lack of exposure to the procedure for foot care
The patient will:
▶ state an understanding of the procedure for foot care
▶ return demonstrate the correct procedure for foot care
▶ identify risk factors associated with foot care and health-seeking behaviors.

Equipment

Bath blanket • large basin • soap • water • towel • linen-saver pad • pillow • washcloth • toenail clippers • orangewood stick • emery board • cotton-tipped applicator • cotton • lotion • water-absorbent powder • bath thermometer • gloves (if the patient has open lesions)

Preparation of equipment

Fill the basin halfway with warm water. Test water temperature with a bath thermometer *because patients with diminished peripheral sensation could burn their feet in excessively hot water (over 105° F [40.6° C]) without feeling any warning pain.* If a bath thermometer isn't available, test the water by inserting your elbow. The water temperature should feel comfortably warm.

Foot care for diabetic patients

Because diabetes mellitus can reduce blood supply to the feet, normally minor foot injuries can lead to dangerous infection. When caring for a diabetic patient, keep the following foot care guidelines in mind:

■ Exercising the feet daily can help improve circulation. While the patient is sitting on the edge of the bed, ask him to point his toes upward, then downward, 10 times. Then have him make a circle with each foot 10 times.

■ A diabetic's shoes must fit properly. Instruct the patient to break in new shoes gradually by increasing wearing time by 30 minutes each day. Also tell the patient to check old shoes frequently in case they develop rough spots in the lining.

■ Tell the patient to wear clean socks daily and to avoid socks with holes, darned spots, or rough, irritating seams.

■ Advise the patient to see a doctor if he has corns or calluses.

■ Tell the patient to wear warm socks or slippers and use extra blankets to avoid cold feet. The patient shouldn't use heating pads and hot water bottles because these may cause burns.

■ Teach the patient to regularly inspect the skin on the feet for cuts, cracks, blisters, or red, swollen areas. Even slight cuts on the feet should receive a doctor's attention. As a first-aid measure, tell him to wash the cut thoroughly and apply a mild antiseptic. Urge the patient to avoid harsh antiseptics, such as iodine, because they can damage tissue.

■ Advise the diabetic patient to avoid tight-fitting garments or activities that can decrease circulation. He should especially avoid wearing elastic garters, sitting with knees crossed, picking at sores or rough spots on the feet, walking barefoot, or applying adhesive tape to the skin on the feet.

Implementation

▶ Assemble equipment at the patient's bedside. Wash your hands and put on gloves, if necessary.

▶ Tell the patient that you'll wash his feet and provide foot and toenail care.

▶ Cover the patient with a bath blanket. Fanfold the top linen to the foot of the bed.

▶ Place a linen-saver pad and a towel under the patient's feet *to keep the bottom linen dry.* Then position the basin on the pad.

▶ Insert a pillow beneath the patient's knee *to provide support* and cushion the rim of the basin with the edge of the towel *to prevent pressure on patient's leg.*

▶ Immerse one foot in the basin. Wash it with soap and then allow it to soak for about 10 minutes. Soaking softens

the skin and toenails, loosens debris under toenails, and comforts and refreshes the patient.

▶ After soaking the foot, rinse it with a washcloth, remove it from the basin and place it on the towel.

▶ Dry the foot thoroughly, especially between the toes, *to avoid skin breakdown.* Blot gently to dry *because harsh rubbing may damage the skin.*

▶ Empty the basin, refill it with warm water, and clean and soak the other foot.

▶ While the second foot is soaking, give the first one a pedicure. Using the cotton-tipped applicator, carefully clean the toenails. Using an orangewood stick, gently remove any dirt beneath the toenails; avoid injuring subungual skin.

▶ Consult a podiatrist if nails need trimming, if your facility's policy prevents you from trimming them.

▶ Rinse the foot that has been soaking, dry it thoroughly, and give it a pedicure.

▶ Apply lotion *to moisten dry skin,* or lightly dust water-absorbent powder between the toes *to absorb moisture.*

▶ Remove and clean all equipment and dispose of gloves.

Special considerations

▶ While providing foot care, observe the color, shape, and texture of the toenails. If you see redness, drying, cracking, blisters, discoloration, or other signs of traumatic injury, especially in a patient with impaired peripheral circulation, notify the doctor. *Because such patients are vulnerable to infection and gangrene,* they need prompt treatment.

▶ If a patient's toenail grows inward at the corners, tuck a wisp of cotton under it *to relieve pressure on the toe.*

▶ When giving the bedridden patient foot care, perform range-of-motion exercises unless contraindicated *to stimulate circulation and prevent foot contractures or muscle atrophy.* Tuck folded 2″ × 2″ gauze pads between overlapping toes *to protect the skin from the toenails.* Apply heel protectors *to prevent skin breakdown.*

Documentation

Record the date and time of bathing and toenail trimming in your notes. Record and report any abnormal findings and any nursing actions you take.

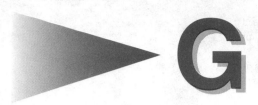

Gastric lavage

After poisoning or a drug overdose, especially in patients who have central nervous system depression or an inadequate gag reflex, gastric lavage flushes the stomach and removes ingested substances through a gastric lavage tube. The procedure is also used to empty the stomach in preparation for endoscopic examination. For patients with gastric or esophageal bleeding, lavage with tepid or iced water or normal saline solution may be used to stop bleeding. However, some controversy exists over the effectiveness of iced lavage for this purpose. (See *Is iced lavage effective?*)

Gastric lavage can be continuous or intermittent. Typically, this procedure is done in the emergency department or intensive care unit by a doctor, gastroenterologist, or nurse; a wide-bore lavage tube is almost always inserted by a gastroenterologist.

Gastric lavage is contraindicated after ingestion of a corrosive substance (such as lye, petroleum distillates, ammonia, alkalis, or mineral acids) because the lavage tube may perforate the already compromised esophagus.

Correct lavage tube placement is essential for patient safety because accidental misplacement (in the lungs, for example) followed by lavage can be fa-

tal. Other complications of gastric lavage include bradyarrhythmias and aspiration of gastric fluids.

Key nursing diagnoses and patient outcomes

Risk for poisoning related to (specify)
The patient will:
▶ be free from effects of poisoning
▶ communicate an understanding of self-protection
▶ state a method for safekeeping of dangerous or potentially dangerous products.

Anxiety related to lack of exposure to gastric lavage
The patient will:
▶ state an understanding of the need for the procedure
▶ use available support systems
▶ exhibit few if any signs of anxiety.

Equipment

Lavage setup (two graduated containers for drainage, three pieces of large-lumen rubber tubing, Y-connector, and a clamp or hemostat) • 2 to 3 L of normal saline solution, tap water, or appropriate antidote as ordered • I.V. pole • basin of ice, if ordered • Ewald tube or any large-lumen gastric tube, typically #36 to #40 French (see *Using wide-bore gastric tubes,* page 360) • water-soluble lubricant or anesthetic ointment • stethoscope • ½″ hypoallergenic tape • 50-ml bulb or catheter-tip syringe • gloves • face shield • linen-saver pad or towel • Yankauer or tonsil-tip suction device • suction apparatus • labeled specimen container • laboratory request form • norepinephrine • optional: patient restraints and charcoal tablets

A prepackaged, syringe-type irrigation kit may be used for intermittent lavage. For poisoning or a drug overdose, however, the continuous lavage setup may be more appropriate to use because it's a faster and more effective means of diluting and removing the harmful substance.

Preparation of equipment

Set up the lavage equipment. (See *Preparing for gastric lavage,* page 361.) If iced lavage is ordered, chill the desired irrigant (water or normal saline solution) in a basin of ice. Lubricate the end of the lavage tube with the water-soluble lubricant or anesthetic ointment.

Implementation

▶ Explain the procedure to the patient, provide privacy, and wash your hands.
▶ Put on gloves and a face shield.
▶ Drape the towel or linen-saver pad over the patient's chest *to protect him from spills.*
▶ The doctor inserts the lavage tube nasally and advances it slowly and gently *because forceful insertion may injure tissues and cause epistaxis.* He checks the tube's placement by injecting about 30 cc of air into the tube with the bulb syringe and then auscultating the patient's abdomen with a stethoscope. If the tube is in place, he'll hear the sound of air entering the stomach.

Is iced lavage effective?

Some experts question the effectiveness of using an iced irrigant for gastric lavage to treat GI bleeding. Here is why.

Iced irrigating solutions stimulate the vagus nerve, which triggers increased hydrochloric acid secretion. In turn, this stimulates gastric motility, which can irritate the bleeding site.

Some doctors prefer using unchilled normal saline solution (which may prevent rapid electrolyte loss) or even water if the patient must avoid sodium. They point out that no research exists to support the use of iced irrigant to stop acute GI bleeding.

▶ *Because the patient may vomit when the lavage tube reaches the posterior pharynx during insertion,* be prepared to suction the airway immediately with either a Yankauer or a tonsil-tip suction device.
▶ When the lavage tube passes the posterior pharynx, help the patient into Trendelenburg's position and turn him toward his left side in a three-quarter prone posture. *This position minimizes passage of gastric contents into the duodenum and may prevent the patient from aspirating vomitus.*
▶ After securing the lavage tube nasally or orally with tape and making sure the irrigant inflow tube on the lavage setup is clamped, connect the unattached end of this tube to the lavage tube. Allow the stomach contents to empty into the drainage container before instilling any irrigant. *This confirms proper tube placement and decreases the risk of overfilling the stomach with irrigant and inducing vomiting.* If you're using a syringe irrigation set, aspirate stomach contents with

Using wide-bore gastric tubes

If you need to deliver a large volume of fluid rapidly through a gastric tube (when irrigating the stomach of a patient with profuse gastric bleeding or poisoning, for example), a wide-bore gastric tube usually serves best. Typically inserted orally, these tubes remain in place only long enough to complete the lavage and evacuate stomach contents.

Ewald tube

In an emergency, using this single-lumen tube with several openings at the distal end allows you to aspirate large amounts of gastric contents quickly.

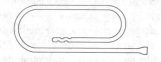

Levacuator tube

This tube has two lumens. Use the larger lumen for evacuating gastric contents; the smaller, for instilling an irrigant.

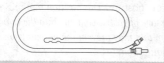

Edlich tube

This single-lumen tube has four openings near the closed distal tip. A funnel or syringe may be connected at the proximal end. Like the Ewald tube, the Edlich tube allows you to withdraw large quantities of gastric contents quickly.

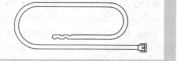

a 50-ml bulb or catheter-tip syringe before instilling the irrigant.

▶ When you confirm proper tube placement, begin gastric lavage by instilling about 250 ml of irrigant *to assess the patient's tolerance and prevent vomiting.* If you're using a syringe, instill about 50 ml of solution at a time until you've instilled between 250 and 500 ml.

▶ Clamp the inflow tube and unclamp the outflow tube *to allow the irrigant to flow out.* If you're using the syringe irrigation kit, aspirate the irrigant with the syringe and empty it into a calibrated container. Measure the outflow amount to make sure that it equals at least the amount of irrigant you instilled. *This prevents accidental stomach distention and vomiting.* If the drainage amount falls significantly short of the instilled amount, reposition the tube until sufficient solution flows out. Gently massage the abdomen over the stomach *to promote outflow.*

▶ Repeat the inflow-outflow cycle until returned fluids appear clear. *This signals that the stomach no longer holds harmful substances or that bleeding has stopped.*

▶ Assess the patient's vital signs, urine output, and level of consciousness (LOC) every 15 minutes. Notify the doctor of any changes.

▶ If ordered, remove the lavage tube.

Special considerations

▶ *To control GI bleeding,* the doctor may order continuous irrigation of the stomach with an irrigant and a vasoconstrictor, such as norepinephrine. After the stomach absorbs norepinephrine, the portal system delivers the drug directly to the liver, where it's metabolized. *This prevents the drug from circulating systemically and initiating a hypertensive response.* Or the doctor may direct you to clamp the outflow tube for a prescribed period after instilling the irrigant and the vasoconstrictive medication and before withdrawing it. *This allows the mucosa time to absorb the drug.*

▶ Never leave a patient alone during gastric lavage. Observe continuously for any changes in LOC and monitor vital signs frequently *because the natural vagal response to intubation can depress the patient's heart rate.*

▶ If you need to restrain the patient, secure restraints on the same side of the bed or stretcher *so you can free them quickly without moving to the other side of the bed.*

▶ Remember also to keep tracheal suctioning equipment nearby and watch closely for airway obstruction caused by vomiting or excess oral secretions. Throughout gastric lavage, you may need to suction the oral cavity frequently *to ensure an open airway and prevent aspiration.* For the same reasons, and if he doesn't exhibit an adequate gag reflex, the patient may require an endotracheal tube before the procedure.

▶ When aspirating the stomach for ingested poisons or drugs, save the contents in a labeled container to send to the laboratory for analysis, along with a laboratory request form. If ordered, after lavage to remove poisons or drugs, mix charcoal tablets with the irrigant (water or normal saline solution) and administer the mixture through the NG tube. The charcoal will absorb any remaining toxic substances. The tube may be clamped temporarily, allowed to drain via gravity, attached to intermittent suction, or removed.

▶ When performing gastric lavage to stop bleeding, keep precise intake and output records *to determine the amount*

Preparing for gastric lavage

Prepare the lavage setup as follows:
■ Connect one of the three pieces of large-lumen tubing to the irrigant container.
■ Insert the stem of the Y-connector in the other end of the tubing.
■ Connect the remaining two pieces of tubing to the free ends of the Y-connector.
■ Place the unattached end of one of the tubes into one of the drainage containers. (Later, you'll connect the other piece of tubing to the patient's gastric tube.)
■ Clamp the tube leading to the irrigant.
■ Suspend the entire setup from the I.V. pole, hanging the irrigant container at the highest level.

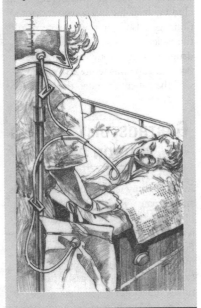

of bleeding. When large volumes of fluid are instilled and withdrawn, serum electrolyte and arterial blood gas levels may be measured during or at the end of lavage.

Complications

Vomiting and subsequent aspiration, the most common complication of gastric lavage, occur more commonly in a groggy patient. Bradyarrhythmias also may occur. After iced lavage especially, the patient's body temperature may drop, thereby triggering cardiac arrhythmias.

Documentation

Record the date and time of lavage, size and type of NG tube used, volume and type of irrigant, and amount of drained gastric contents. Document this information on the intake and output record sheet and include your observations, including the color and consistency of drainage. Also keep precise records of the patient's vital signs and LOC, any drugs instilled through the tube, the time the tube was removed, and how well the patient tolerated the procedure.

GASTROSTOMY FEEDING BUTTON CARE

A gastrostomy feeding button serves as an alternative feeding device for an ambulatory patient who is receiving long-term enteral feedings. Approved by the Food and Drug Administration for 6-month implantation, feeding buttons can be used to replace gastrostomy tubes, if necessary.

The feeding button has a mushroom dome at one end and two wing tabs and a flexible safety plug at the other. When inserted into an established stoma, the button lies almost flush with the skin, with only the top of the safety plug visible.

The button can usually be inserted into a stoma in less than 15 minutes. In addition to its cosmetic appeal, the device is easily maintained, reduces skin irritation and breakdown, and is less likely to become dislodged or to migrate than an ordinary feeding tube. A one-way, antireflux valve mounted just inside the mushroom dome prevents accidental leakage of gastric contents. The device usually requires replacement after 3 to 4 months, typically because the antireflux valve wears out.

Key nursing diagnoses and patient outcomes

Imbalanced nutrition: Less than body requirements related to (specify)
The patient will:
▶ consume at least (specify) calories
▶ gain (specify) lb (kg) weekly or maintain normal body weight.

Impaired skin integrity related to the feeding button
The patient will:
▶ experience no skin breakdown at the feeding button site
▶ communicate an understanding of skin care of the feeding button site.

Deficient knowledge related to a lack of exposure to feeding button care
The patient will:
▶ state an understanding of care of the feeding button
▶ demonstrate the correct procedure for inserting the feeding button
▶ identify available resources that can provide assistance.

Equipment

Gastrostomy feeding button of the correct size (all three sizes, if the correct one isn't known) • obturator • water-soluble lubricant • gloves • feeding accessories, including adapter, feeding catheter, food syringe or bag, and formula • catheter clamp • cleaning equipment, including water, a syringe, cotton-tipped applicator, pipe cleaner, and mild soap or povidone-iodine solution • optional: I.V. pole and pump to provide continuous infusion over several hours

Implementation

▶ Explain the insertion, reinsertion, and feeding procedure to the patient. Tell him the doctor will perform the initial insertion.
▶ Wash your hands and put on gloves. (See *How to reinsert a gastrostomy feeding button,* page 364.)
▶ Attach the adapter and feeding catheter to the syringe or feeding bag. Clamp the catheter and fill the syringe or bag and catheter with formula. Refill the syringe before it's empty. *These steps prevent air from entering the stomach and distending the abdomen.*
▶ Open the safety plug and attach the adapter and feeding catheter to the button. Elevate the syringe or feeding bag above stomach level and gravity-feed the formula for 15 to 30 minutes, varying the height as needed *to alter the flow rate.* Use a pump for continuous infusion or for feedings lasting several hours.
▶ After the feeding, flush the button with 10 ml of water and clean the inside of the feeding catheter with a cotton-tipped applicator and water *to preserve patency and to dislodge formula or food particles.* Then lower the syringe or bag below stomach level *to allow burping.* Remove the adapter and feeding catheter. The antireflux valve should prevent gastric reflux. Then

snap the safety plug into place *to keep the lumen clean and prevent leakage if the antireflux valve fails.* If the patient feels nauseated or vomits after the feeding, vent the button with the adapter and feeding catheter *to control emesis.*
▶ Wash the catheter and syringe or feeding bag in warm soapy water and rinse thoroughly. Clean the catheter and adapter with a pipe cleaner. Rinse well before using for the next feeding. Soak the equipment once per week according to the manufacturer's recommendations.

Special considerations

▶ If the button pops out while feeding, reinsert it, estimate the formula already delivered, and resume feeding.
▶ Once daily, clean the peristomal skin with mild soap and water or povidone-iodine and let the skin air-dry for 20 minutes *to avoid skin irritation.* Also, clean the site whenever spillage from the feeding bag occurs.

Home care

Before discharge, make sure the patient can insert and care for the gastrostomy feeding button. If necessary, teach him or a family member how to reinsert the button by first practicing on a model. Offer written instructions and answer his questions on obtaining replacement supplies.

Documentation

Record the feeding time and duration, amount and type of feeding formula used, and the patient's tolerance of the procedure. Maintain intake and output records as necessary. Note the appearance of the stoma and surrounding skin.

How to reinsert a gastrostomy feeding button

If your patient's gastrostomy feeding button pops out (with coughing, for instance), you or he will need to reinsert the device. Here are some steps to follow.

Prepare the equipment

Collect the feeding button, an obturator, and water-soluble lubricant. If the button will be reinserted, wash it with soap and water and rinse it thoroughly.

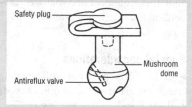

Safety plug

Mushroom dome

Antireflux valve

Insert the button

■ Check the depth of the patient's stoma to make sure you have a feeding button of the correct size. Then clean around the stoma.
■ Lubricate the obturator with a water-soluble lubricant and distend the button several times to ensure the patency of the antireflux valve within the button.
■ Lubricate the mushroom dome and the stoma. Gently push the button through the stoma into the stomach.

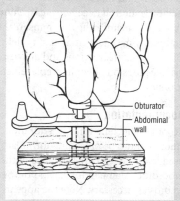

Obturator

Abdominal wall

■ Remove the obturator by gently rotating it as you withdraw it, *to keep the antireflux valve from adhering to it.* If the valve sticks nonetheless, gently push the obturator back into the button until the valve closes.
■ After removing the obturator, make sure the valve is closed. Then close the flexible safety plug, which should be relatively flush with the skin surface.

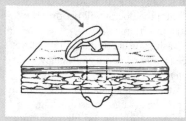

■ If you need to administer a feeding right away, open the safety plug and attach the feeding adapter and feeding tube. Deliver the feeding as ordered.

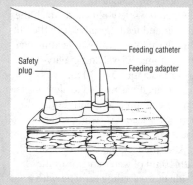

Feeding catheter

Safety plug

Feeding adapter

GAVAGE FEEDING

Gavage feeding involves passing nutrients directly to the neonate's stomach by a tube advanced nasally or orally. If a neonate can't suck (because of prematurity, illness, or congenital deformity) or is at risk for aspiration (because of gastroesophageal reflux, ineffective gag reflex, or easy tiring), gavage feeding may supply nutrients until he can take food by mouth.

Unless the neonate has problems with the feeding tube, the nurse usually inserts it orally before each feeding and withdraws it after the feeding. This intermittent method stimulates the sucking reflex. If the neonate can't tolerate this, the nurse advances the tube nasally and leaves it in place for 24 to 72 hours. Gavage feeding is contraindicated for neonates without bowel sounds or with suspected intestinal obstruction, severe respiratory distress, or massive gastroesophageal reflux.

Key nursing diagnoses and patient outcomes

Ineffective infant feeding pattern related to (specify)
The infant will:
▶ not lose more than 10% of birth weight within the first week of life
▶ gain 4 to 7 oz (113.5 to 198.5 g) per week after the first week of life
▶ not experience dehydration
▶ receive adequate nutrition until able to suckle efficiently.

Ineffective family coping: Compromised related to compromised neonatal health
The family will:
▶ communicate feelings regarding the neonate's condition
▶ become involved in planning and providing the neonate's care
▶ express a feeling of having greater control over the situation.

Equipment

Feeding tube (#3½ to #6 French for nasogastric [NG] feeding of premature neonate; #8 French for others) • feeding reservoir or large (20- to 50-ml) syringe • prescribed formula or breast milk • sterile water • tape measure • tape • stethoscope • gloves • optional: bowl and pacifier

A commercial feeding reservoir is available.

Preparation of equipment

Allow the formula or breast milk to warm to room temperature, if necessary. Wash your hands and open the sterile water if it comes in a small-sized disposable container. Remove the syringe or reservoir and the feeding tube from the packaging.

Implementation

▶ Identify the neonate and verify the doctor's orders.
▶ Using a tape measure or the feeding tube, determine how far you should insert the tubing to ensure placement in the stomach. You'll usually measure from the tip of the nose to the tip of the earlobe to the xiphoid process. Mark the tube at the appropriate distance with a piece of tape. Measure from the bottom.
▶ Place the neonate in a supine position. Elevate the head of his mattress one notch. Otherwise, place him supine or tilted slightly to his right with head and chest slightly elevated.
▶ Put on gloves. Stabilize the neonate's head with one hand and lubricate the

feeding tube with sterile water with the other hand.

▶ Insert the tube smoothly and quickly up to the premeasured tape mark. For oral insertion, pass the tube toward the back of the throat. For nasal insertion, pass the tube toward the occiput in a horizontal plane.

▶ Synchronize tube insertion with throat movement if the neonate swallows *to facilitate tube passage into the stomach.* During insertion, watch for choking and cyanosis, signs that a tube has entered the trachea. If these occur, remove the tube and reinsert it. Also watch for bradycardia and apnea resulting from vagal stimulation.

▶ If the tube will remain in place, tape it flat to the neonate's cheek. *To prevent possible nasal skin breakdown,* don't tape the tube to the bridge of his nose.

▶ Make sure the tube is in the stomach (and not the lungs) by aspirating residual stomach contents with the syringe. Check the content's pH *because gastric contents are highly acidic. This helps confirm tube placement.* Note the volume obtained and then reinject it *to avoid altering the neonate's buffer system and electrolyte balance.* Or, as ordered, reduce the feeding volume by the residual amount, or prolong the interval between feedings.

▶ Alternatively, or additionally, check placement of the feeding tube in the stomach by injecting 0.5 to 1 cc of air into the tube while listening with the stethoscope for air sounds in the stomach and on each side of the anterior chest.

▶ If you suspect that the tube is displaced, advance it several centimeters further and test again. *Don't begin feeding until you're certain the tube is in the stomach.*

▶ When the tube is in place, fill the feeding reservoir or syringe with formula or breast milk. Connect the feeding reservoir or syringe to the top of the tube and start the feeding.

▶ If the neonate is on your lap, hold the container about 4″ (10 cm) above his abdomen. If he's lying down, hold it between 6″ and 8″ (15 and 20.5 cm) above his head. When using a commercial feeding reservoir, look for air bubbles in the container, which is an indicator of formula passage.

▶ Regulate the flow by raising and lowering the container so that the feeding takes 15 to 20 minutes, which is the average time for a bottle-feeding. *To prevent stomach distention, reflux, and vomiting,* don't let the feeding proceed too rapidly.

▶ When the feeding is finished, pinch off the tubing before air enters the neonate's stomach. *This helps prevent distention, fluid leakage into the pharynx during tube removal, and consequent aspiration.*

▶ Withdraw the tube smoothly and quickly. If the tube will remain in place, flush it with several milliliters of sterile water, if ordered.

▶ Burp the neonate *to decrease abdominal distention.* Hold him upright or in a sitting position. Use one hand to support his head and chest and your other hand to gently rub or pat his back until he expels the air.

▶ Place him on his stomach (only if he's being monitored with a cardiac-respiratory monitor) or right side for 1 hour after feeding *to facilitate gastric emptying and to prevent aspiration if he regurgitates.*

▶ Don't perform postural drainage and percussion until 1 hour or more after feeding.

Special considerations
▶ Use the NG approach for the neonate who must keep the feeding tube in place *because this approach holds the tube more securely than the orogastric approach.* Alternate the nostril used at each insertion *to prevent skin and mucosal irritation.*

Note: When possible, the oral route should be used for gavage feedings rather than the nasal route *because the neonate is an obligatory nose breather.*

▶ Observe the premature neonate for indications that he's ready to begin bottle- or breast-feeding, such as strong sucking reflex, coordinated sucking and swallowing, alertness before feeding, and sleep after feeding.

▶ Provide the neonate with a pacifier during feeding *to soothe him, help prevent gagging, and promote an association between sucking and the full feeling that follows feeding.*

Complications
Gagging with regurgitation causes loss of nutrients. An indwelling NG tube can irritate mucous membranes and cause nasal airway obstruction, epistaxis, and stomach perforation. A feeding tube may kink, coil, or knot and become obstructed, preventing feeding.

Documentation
Record the amount of residual fluid and the amount currently taken. Note the type and amount of any vomitus as well as any adverse reactions to tube insertion or feeding.

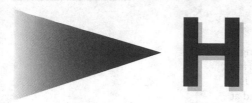

HALO-VEST TRACTION

Halo-vest traction immobilizes the head and neck after traumatic injury to the cervical vertebrae — the most common of all spinal injuries. This procedure, which can prevent further injury to the spinal cord, is performed by an orthopedic surgeon, with nursing assistance, in the emergency department, a specially equipped room, or in the operating room after surgical reduction of vertebral injuries. The halo-vest traction device consists of a metal ring that fits over the patient's head and metal bars that connect the ring to a plastic vest that distributes the weight of the entire apparatus around the chest. (See *Comparing halo-vest traction devices.*)

When in place, halo-vest traction allows the patient greater mobility than traction with skull tongs. It also carries less risk of infection because it doesn't require skin incisions and drill holes to position skull pins.

Key nursing diagnoses and patient outcomes

Ineffective individual coping related to personal vulnerability
The patient will:
▶ become actively involved in planning own care

▶ identify effective and ineffective coping techniques.

Deficient knowledge related to lack of exposure to procedure
The patient will:
▶ communicate a need to know
▶ state or demonstrate an understanding of what has been taught.

Equipment

Halo-vest traction unit • halo ring • cervical collar or sandbags (if needed) • plastic vest • board or padded headrest • tape measure • halo ring conversion chart • scissors and razor • 4″ × 4″ gauze pads • povidone-iodine solution • sterile gloves • Allen wrench • four positioning pins • multiple-dose vial of 1% lidocaine (with or without epinephrine) • alcohol pads • 3-ml syringe • 25G needles • five sterile skull pins (one more than needed) • torque screwdriver • sheepskin liners • cotton-tipped applicators • ordered cleaning solution • medicated powder or cornstarch • sterile water or normal saline solution • optional: hair dryer and pain medication (such as an analgesic)

Most facilities supply packaged halo-vest traction units that include software (such as jacket and sheepskin liners), hardware (such as halo, head pins, upright bars, and screws), and tools (such

Comparing halo-vest traction devices

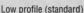

Type	Description	Advantages
Low profile (standard) 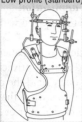	■ Traction and compression are produced by threaded support rods on either side of the halo ring. ■ Flexion and extension are obtained by moving the swivel arm to an anterior or posterior position, depending on the location of the skull pins.	■ Immobilizes cervical spine fractures while allowing patient mobility ■ Facilitates surgery of the cervical spine and permits flexion and extension ■ Allows airway intubation without losing skeletal traction ■ Facilitates necessary alignment by an adjustment at the junction of the threaded support rods and horizontal frame
Mark II (type of low profile) 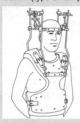	■ Traction and compression are produced by threaded support rods on either side of the halo ring. ■ Flexion and extension are obtained by swivel clamps, which allow the bars to intersect and hold at any angle.	■ Enables doctors to assemble the metal framework more quickly ■ Allows unobstructed access for anteroposterior and lateral X-rays of the cervical spine ■ Allows the patient to wear his usual clothing because uprights are shaped closer to the body
Mark III (update of Mark II) 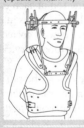	■ Traction and compression are produced by threaded support rods on either side of the halo ring. ■ Flexion and extension are accommodated by a serrated split articulation coupling attached to the halo ring, which can be adjusted in 4-degree increments.	■ Simplifies application while promoting patient comfort ■ Eliminates shoulder pressure and discomfort by using a flexible padded strap instead of the vest's solid plastic shoulder ■ Accommodates the tall patient with modified hardware and shorter uprights and allows unobstructed access for medial and lateral X-rays
Trippi-Wells tongs 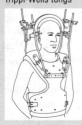	■ Traction is produced by four pins that compress the skull. ■ Flexion and extension are obtained by adjusting the midline vertical plate.	■ Applies tensile force to the neck or spine while allowing patient mobility ■ Makes it possible to change from mobile to stationary traction without interrupting traction ■ Adjusts to three planes for mobile and stationary traction ■ Allows unobstructed access for medial and lateral X-rays

as torque screwdriver, two conventional wrenches, Allen wrench, and screws and bolts). These units don't include sterile gloves, povidone-iodine solution, sterile drapes, cervical collars, or equipment for local anesthetic injection.

Preparation of equipment

Obtain a halo-vest traction unit with halo rings and plastic vests in several sizes. Check the expiration date of the prepackaged tray and check the outside covering for damage *to ensure the sterility of the contents.* Then assemble the equipment at the patient's bedside.

Implementation

▶ Check the support that was applied to the patient's neck on the way to the hospital. If necessary, apply the cervical collar immediately or immobilize the head and neck with sandbags. Keep the cervical collar or sandbags in place until the halo is applied. This support will then be carefully removed *to facilitate application of the vest. Because the patient is likely to be frightened,* try to reassure him.

▶ Remove the headboard and any furniture at the head of the bed *to provide ample working space.* Then carefully place the patient's head on a board or on a padded headrest that extends beyond the edge of the bed.

⚠ **Nursing alert** **Never put the patient's head on a pillow before applying the halo to avoid further injury to the spinal cord.**

▶ Elevate the bed to a working level that gives the doctor easy access to the front and back of the halo unit.

▶ Stand at the head of the bed and see if the patient's chin lines up with his midsternum, indicating proper alignment. If ordered, support the patient's head in your hands and gently rotate the neck into alignment without flexing or extending it.

Assisting with halo application

▶ Ask another nurse to help you with the procedure.

▶ Explain the procedure to the patient, wash your hands, and provide privacy.

▶ Have the assisting nurse hold the patient's head and neck stable while the doctor removes the cervical collar or sandbags. Maintain this support until the halo is secure while you assist with pin insertion.

▶ The doctor measures the patient's head with a tape measure and refers to the halo ring conversion chart to determine the correct ring size. (The ring should clear the head by ⅝" [1.6 cm] and fit ½" [1.3 cm] above the bridge of the nose.)

▶ The doctor selects four pin sites: ½" above the lateral one-third of each eyebrow and ½" above the top of each ear in the occipital area. He also takes into account the degree and type of correction needed to provide proper cervical alignment.

▶ Trim and shave the hair at the pin sites with scissors or a razor *to facilitate subsequent care and help prevent infection.* Put on gloves. Then use 4" × 4" gauze pads soaked in povidone-iodine solution to clean the sites.

▶ Open the halo-vest unit using sterile technique *to avoid contamination.* The doctor puts on the sterile gloves and removes the halo and the Allen wrench. He then places the halo over the patient's head and inserts the four positioning pins *to hold the halo in place temporarily.*

▶ Help the doctor prepare the anesthetic. First, clean the injection port of the multiple-dose vial of lidocaine with the alcohol pad. Then invert the vial so the doctor can insert a 25G needle attached to the 3-ml syringe and withdraw the anesthetic.

▶ The doctor injects the anesthetic at the four pin sites. He may change needles on the syringe after each injection.

▶ The doctor removes four of the five skull pins from the sterile setup and firmly screws in each pin at a 90-degree angle to the skull. When the pins are in place, he removes the positioning pins. He then tightens the skull pins with the torque screwdriver.

Applying the vest

▶ After the doctor measures the patient's chest and abdomen, he selects a vest of appropriate size.

▶ Place the sheepskin liners inside the front and back of the vest *to make it more comfortable and help prevent pressure ulcers.*

▶ Help the doctor carefully raise the patient while the other nurse supports the head and neck. Slide the back of the vest under the patient and gently lay him down. The doctor then fastens the front of the vest on the patient's chest using Velcro straps.

▶ The doctor attaches the metal bars to the halo and vest and tightens each bolt in turn *to avoid tightening any single bolt completely, causing maladjusted tension.* When halo-vest traction is in place, X-rays should be taken immediately *to check the depth of the skull pins and verify proper alignment.*

Caring for the patient

▶ Take routine and neurologic vital signs at least every 2 hours for 24 hours

(preferably every hour for 48 hours) and then every 4 hours until stable.

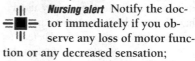 **Nursing alert** Notify the doctor immediately if you observe any loss of motor function or any decreased sensation; *these findings could indicate spinal cord trauma.*

▶ Put on gloves. Gently clean the pin sites every 4 hours with cotton-tipped applicators dipped in cleaning solution. Rinse the sites with sterile water or normal saline solution *to remove any excess cleaning solution.* Then clean the pin sites with povidone-iodine solution or other ordered solution. *Meticulous pin-site care prevents infection and removes debris that might block drainage and lead to abscess formation.* Watch for signs of infection — a loose pin, swelling or redness, purulent drainage, pain at the site — and notify the doctor if these signs develop.

▶ The doctor retightens the skull pins with the torque screwdriver 24 and 48 hours after the halo is applied. If the patient complains of a headache after the pins are tightened, obtain an order for an analgesic. If pain occurs with jaw movement, notify the doctor *because this may indicate that pins have slipped onto the thin temporal plate.*

▶ Examine the halo-vest unit every shift *to make sure that everything is secure and that the patient's head is centered within the halo.* If the vest fits correctly, you should be able to insert one or two fingers under the jacket at the shoulder and chest when the patient is lying in a supine position.

▶ Wash the patient's chest and back daily. First, place the patient on his back. Loosen the bottom Velcro straps *so you can get to the chest and back.* Then, reaching under the vest, wash and dry the skin. Check for tender, reddened areas or pressure spots that may develop into ulcers. If necessary, use a hair dryer to dry damp sheepskin *because moisture predisposes the skin to pressure ulcer formation.* Lightly dust the skin with medicated powder or cornstarch *to prevent itching.* If itching persists, check to see if the patient is allergic to sheepskin and if any drug he's taking might cause a skin rash. If your facility's policy allows, change the vest lining as necessary.

▶ Turn the patient on his side (less than 45 degrees) to wash his back. Then close the vest.

▶ Be careful not to put any stress on the apparatus, *which could knock it out of alignment and lead to subluxation of the cervical spine.*

Special considerations

 Nursing alert Keep two conventional wrenches available at all times. In case of cardiac arrest, use them to remove the distal anterior bolts. Pull the two upright bars outward. Unfasten the Velcro straps and remove the front of the vest. Use the sturdy back of the vest as a board for cardiopulmonary resuscitation (CPR). *To prevent subluxating the cervical injury,* start CPR with the jaw thrust maneuver, which avoids hyperextension of the neck. Pull the patient's mandible forward while maintaining proper head and neck alignment. *This pulls the tongue forward to open the airway.*

▶ Never lift the patient up by the vertical bars. *This could strain or tear the skin at the pin sites or misalign the traction.*

▶ *To prevent falls,* walk with the ambulatory patient. Remember, he'll have trouble seeing objects at or near his

feet, and the weight of the halo-vest unit (about 10 lb [4.5 kg]) may throw him off balance. If the patient is in a wheelchair, lower the leg rests *to prevent the chair from tipping backward.*

▶ *Because the vest limits chest expansion,* routinely assess pulmonary function, especially in a patient with pulmonary disease.

Home care

Teach the patient to turn slowly — in small increments — *to avoid losing his balance.* Remind him to avoid bending forward *because the extra weight of the halo apparatus could cause him to fall.* Teach him to bend at the knees rather than the waist.

Have a physical therapist teach the patient how to use assistive devices to extend his reach and to help him put on socks and shoes. Suggest that he wear shirts that button in front and that are larger than usual to accommodate the halo-vest.

Most important, teach the patient about pin-site care, shampooing, and hair care.

Complications

Manipulating the patient's neck during application of halo-vest traction may cause subluxation of the spinal cord, or it could push a bone fragment into the spinal cord, possibly compressing the cord and causing paralysis below the break.

Inaccurate positioning of the skull pins can lead to a puncture of the dura mater, causing a loss of cerebrospinal fluid and a serious central nervous system infection. Nonsterile technique during application of the halo or inadequate pin-site care can also lead to infection at the pin sites. Pressure ulcers can develop if the vest fits poorly or chafes the skin.

Documentation

Record the date and time that the halovest traction was applied. Also note the length of the procedure and the patient's response. After application, record routine and neurologic vital signs. Document pin-site care and note any signs of infection.

HANDHELD OROPHARYNGEAL INHALERS

Handheld oropharyngeal inhalers include the metered-dose inhaler (or nebulizer), the turbo-inhaler, and the nasal inhaler. These devices deliver topical medications to the respiratory tract, producing local and systemic effects. The mucosal lining of the respiratory tract absorbs the inhalant almost immediately. Examples of common inhalants are bronchodilators, which are used to improve airway patency and facilitate mucous drainage; mucolytics, which attain a high local concentration to liquefy tenacious bronchial secretions; and corticosteroids, which are used to decrease inflammation.

The use of these inhalers may be contraindicated in patients who can't form an airtight seal around the device and in patients who lack the coordination or clear vision necessary to assemble a turbo-inhaler. Specific inhalant drugs may also be contraindicated. For example, bronchodilators are contraindicated if the patient has tachycardia or a history of cardiac arrhythmias associated with tachycardia.

Key nursing diagnoses and patient outcomes

Deficient knowledge related to a lack of exposure to the use of handheld oropharyngeal inhalers
The patient will:
▶ communicate a need to know more about using an inhaler
▶ set realistic learning goals
▶ state or demonstrate an understanding of what has been taught.

Ineffective breathing pattern related to (specify)
The patient will:
▶ maintain a respiratory rate within 5 breaths/minute of baseline
▶ have normal arterial blood gas levels
▶ demonstrate correct use of the inhaler
▶ report the ability to breathe comfortably.

Equipment

Patient's medication record and chart • metered-dose inhaler, turbo-inhaler, or nasal inhaler • prescribed medication • normal saline solution (or another appropriate solution) for gargling • optional: emesis basin (see *Types of handheld inhalers,* page 374)

Implementation

▶ Verify the order on the patient's medication record by checking it against the doctor's order.
▶ Wash your hands.
▶ Check the label on the inhaler against the order on the medication record. Verify the expiration date.
▶ Confirm the patient's identity by asking his name and by checking his name, room number, and bed number on his wristband.
▶ Explain the procedure to the patient.

Types of handheld inhalers

Handheld inhalers use air under pressure to produce a mist containing tiny droplets of medication. Drugs delivered in this form (such as mucolytics and bronchodilators) can travel deep into the lungs.

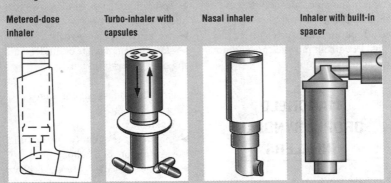

Metered-dose inhaler **Turbo-inhaler with capsules** **Nasal inhaler** **Inhaler with built-in spacer**

Using a metered-dose inhaler

▶ Shake the inhaler bottle *to mix the medication and aerosol propellant.*

▶ Remove the mouthpiece and cap. *Note:* Some metered-dose inhalers have a spacer built into the inhaler. Pull the spacer away from the section holding the medication canister until it clicks into place.

▶ Insert the metal stem on the bottle into the small hole on the flattened portion of the mouthpiece. Then turn the bottle upside down.

▶ Have the patient exhale; then place the mouthpiece in his mouth and close his lips around it.

▶ As you firmly push the bottle down against the mouthpiece, ask the patient to inhale slowly and to continue inhaling until his lungs feel full. *This action draws the medication into his lungs.* Compress the bottle against the mouthpiece only once.

▶ Remove the mouthpiece from the patient's mouth and tell him to hold his breath for several seconds *to allow the medication to reach the alveoli.* Then instruct him to exhale slowly through pursed lips *to keep the distal bronchioles open, allowing increased absorption and diffusion of the drug and better gas exchange.*

▶ Have the patient gargle with normal saline solution *to remove medication from the mouth and back of the throat.* (The lungs retain only about 10% of the inhalant; most of the remainder is exhaled but substantial amounts may remain in the oropharynx.)

▶ Rinse the mouthpiece thoroughly with warm water *to prevent accumulation of residue.*

Using a turbo-inhaler

▶ Hold the mouthpiece in one hand, and with the other hand, slide the sleeve away from the mouthpiece as far as possible.

▶ Unscrew the tip of the mouthpiece by turning it counterclockwise.

▶ Firmly press the colored portion of the medication capsule into the propeller stem of the mouthpiece.

▶ Screw the inhaler together again securely.

▶ Holding the inhaler with the mouthpiece at the bottom, slide the sleeve all the way down and then up again *to puncture the capsule and release the medication*. Do this only once.

▶ Have the patient exhale and tilt his head back. Tell him to place the mouthpiece in his mouth, close his lips around it, and inhale once — quickly and deeply — through the mouthpiece.

▶ Tell the patient to hold his breath for several *seconds to allow the medication to reach the alveoli*. (Instruct him not to exhale through the mouthpiece.)

▶ Remove the inhaler from the patient's mouth and tell him to exhale as much air as possible.

▶ Repeat the procedure until all the medication in the device is inhaled.

▶ Have the patient gargle with normal saline solution *to remove medication from the mouth and back of the throat*. Make sure you provide an emesis basin if the patient needs one.

▶ Discard the empty medication capsule, put the inhaler in its can, and secure the lid. Rinse the inhaler with warm water at least once per week.

Using a nasal inhaler

▶ Have the patient blow his nose *to clear his nostrils*.

▶ Shake the medication cartridge and then insert it in the adapter. (Before inserting a refill cartridge, remove the protective cap from the stem.)

▶ Remove the protective cap from the adapter tip.

▶ Hold the inhaler with your index finger on top of the cartridge and your thumb under the nasal adapter. The adapter tip should be pointing toward the patient.

▶ Have the patient tilt his head back. Tell him to place the adapter tip into one nostril while occluding the other nostril with his finger.

▶ Instruct the patient to inhale gently as he presses the adapter and the cartridge together firmly to release a measured dose of medication. Make sure you follow the manufacturer's instructions. *With some medications, such as dexamethasone sodium phosphate (Turbinaire), inhaling during administration isn't desirable.*

▶ Tell the patient to remove the inhaler from his nostril and exhale through his mouth.

▶ Shake the inhaler and have the patient repeat the procedure in the other nostril.

▶ Have the patient gargle with normal saline solution *to remove medication from his mouth and throat*.

▶ Remove the medication cartridge from the nasal inhaler and wash the nasal adapter in lukewarm water. Let the adapter dry thoroughly before reinserting the cartridge.

Special considerations

▶ When using a turbo-inhaler or nasal inhaler, make sure the pressurized cartridge isn't punctured or incinerated. Store the medication cartridge below 120° F (48.9° C).

▶ If you're using a turbo-inhaler, keep the medication capsules wrapped until needed *to keep them from deteriorating.*

▶ Spacer inhalers may be recommended to provide greater therapeutic benefit for children and for patients who have difficulty with coordination. A spacer attachment is an extension to the inhaler's mouthpiece that provides more dead-air space for mixing the medication. Some inhalers have built-in spacers.

▶ Teach the patient how to use the inhaler *so that he can continue treatments himself after discharge, if necessary.* Explain that overdosage — which is common — can cause the medication to lose its effectiveness. Tell him to record the date and time of each inhalation as well as his response *to prevent overdosage and to help the doctor determine the drug's effectiveness.* Also, note whether the patient uses an unusual amount of medication — for example, more than one cartridge for a metered-dose nebulizer every 3 weeks. Inform the patient of possible adverse reactions.

▶ If more than one inhalation is ordered, advise the patient to wait at least 2 minutes before repeating the procedure.

▶ If the patient is also using a steroid inhaler, instruct him to use the bronchodilator first and then wait 5 minutes before using the steroid. *This allows the bronchodilator to open the air passages for maximum effectiveness.*

Documentation
Record the inhalant administered as well as the dose and time. Note any significant change in the patient's heart rate and any other adverse reactions.

HAND WASHING

The hands are the conduits for almost every transfer of potential pathogens from one patient to another, from a contaminated object to the patient, or from a staff member to the patient. Thus, hand washing is the single most important procedure for preventing infection. To protect patients from nosocomial infections, hand washing must be performed routinely and thoroughly. In effect, clean and healthy hands with intact skin, short fingernails, and no rings minimize the risk of contamination. Artificial nails may serve as a reservoir for microorganisms, and microorganisms are more difficult to remove from rough or chapped hands.

Key nursing diagnoses and patient outcomes
Risk for infection related to improper technique
The patient will:
▶ remain free from all signs and symptoms of infection
▶ identify signs and symptoms of infection
▶ state factors that put him at risk for infection.

Equipment
Soap or detergent (from a dispenser) • warm running water • paper towels • optional: antiseptic cleaning agent, fingernail brush, disposable sponge brush or plastic cuticle stick

Implementation
▶ Remove rings as your facility's policy dictates *because they harbor dirt and skin microorganisms.* Remove your watch or wear it well above the wrist. *Note:*

Artificial fingernails and nail polish must be kept in good repair to minimize their potential to harbor microorganisms; refer to your facility's policy pertaining to nail polish and artificial nails.

▶ Wet your hands and wrists with warm water and apply soap from a dispenser. Don't use bar soap *because it allows cross-contamination.* Hold your hands below elbow level *to prevent water from running up your arms and back down, thus contaminating clean areas.* (See *Proper hand-washing technique.*)

▶ Work up a generous lather by rubbing your hands together vigorously for about 10 seconds. *Soap and warm water reduce surface tension and this, aided by friction, loosens surface microorganisms, which wash away in the lather.*

▶ Pay special attention to the area under fingernails and around cuticles and to the thumbs, knuckles, and sides of the fingers and hands *because microorganisms thrive in these protected or overlooked areas.* If you don't remove your wedding band, move it up and down your finger *to clean beneath it.*

▶ Avoid splashing water on yourself or the floor *because microorganisms spread more easily on wet surfaces and because slippery floors are dangerous.*

▶ Avoid touching the sink or faucets *because they're considered contaminated.*

▶ Rinse hands and wrists well *because running water flushes suds, soil, soap or detergent, and microorganisms away.*

▶ Pat hands and wrists dry with a paper towel. Avoid rubbing, *which can cause abrasion and chapping.*

▶ If the sink isn't equipped with knee or foot controls, turn off faucets by gripping them with a dry paper towel *to avoid recontaminating your hands.*

Proper hand-washing technique

To minimize the spread of infection, follow these basic hand-washing instructions. With your hands angled downward under the faucet, adjust the water temperature until it's comfortably warm.

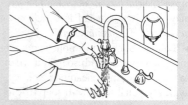

Work up a generous lather by scrubbing vigorously for 10 seconds. Make sure you clean beneath your fingernails, around your knuckles, and along the sides of your fingers and hands.

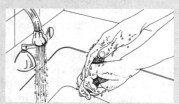

Rinse your hands completely to wash away suds and microorganisms. Pat dry with a paper towel. To prevent recontaminating your hands on the faucet handles, cover each one with a dry paper towel when turning off the water.

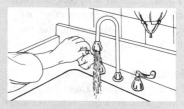

Special considerations

▶ Before participating in any sterile procedure or whenever your hands are grossly contaminated, wash your forearms also, and clean under the fingernails and in and around the cuticles with a fingernail brush, disposable sponge brush, or plastic cuticle stick. Use these softer implements *because brushes, metal files, or other hard objects may injure your skin and, if reused, may be a source of contamination.*

▶ Follow your facility's policy concerning when to wash with soap and when to use an antiseptic cleaning agent. Typically, you'll wash with soap before coming on duty; before and after direct or indirect patient contact; before and after performing any bodily functions, such as blowing your nose or using the bathroom; before preparing or serving food; before preparing or administering medications; after removing gloves or other personal protective equipment; and after completing your shift.

▶ Use an antiseptic cleaning agent before performing invasive procedures, wound care, and dressing changes and after contamination. Antiseptics are also recommended for hand washing in isolation rooms and neonate and special care nurseries as well as before caring for any highly susceptible patient.

▶ Wash your hands before and after performing patient care or procedures or having contact with contaminated objects, even though you may have worn gloves. Always wash your hands after removing gloves.

Home care

If you're providing care in the patient's home, bring your own supply of soap and disposable paper towels. If there is no running water, disinfect your hands with an antiseptic cleaning agent.

Complications

Because frequent hand washing strips the skin of natural oils, this simple procedure can result in dryness, cracking, and irritation. However, these effects are probably more common after repeated use of antiseptic cleaning agents, especially in people with sensitive skin. *To help minimize irritation,* rinse your hands thoroughly, making sure they're free from any residue.

To prevent your hands from becoming dry or chapped, apply an emollient hand cream after each washing or switch to a different cleaning agent. Make sure that the hand cream or lotion you use won't cause the material in your gloves to deteriorate. If you develop dermatitis, your employee health care provider may need to evaluate you *to determine whether you should continue to work until the condition resolves.*

HEAT APPLICATION

Heat applied directly to the patient's body raises tissue temperature and enhances the inflammatory process by causing vasodilation and increasing local circulation. This promotes leukocytosis, suppuration, drainage, and healing. Heat also increases tissue metabolism, reduces pain caused by muscle spasm, and decreases congestion in deep visceral organs.

Direct heat may be dry or moist. Dry heat can be delivered at a higher temperature and for a longer time. Devices for applying dry heat include the hot-water bottle, electric heating pad, K pad, and chemical hot pack.

Moist heat softens crusts and exudates, penetrates deeper than dry heat, is less drying to the skin, produces less perspiration, and usually is more comfortable for the patient. Devices for applying moist heat include warm compresses for small body areas and warm packs for large areas.

Direct heat treatment can't be used on a patient at risk for hemorrhage. It's also contraindicated if the patient has a sprained limb in the acute stage (because vasodilation would increase pain and swelling) or if he has a condition associated with acute inflammation such as appendicitis. Direct heat should be applied cautiously to pediatric and elderly patients and to patients with impaired renal, cardiac, or respiratory function; arteriosclerosis or atherosclerosis; or impaired sensation. It should be applied with extreme caution to heat-sensitive areas, such as scar tissue and stomas.

Key nursing diagnoses and patient outcomes

Risk for injury related to heat application
The patient will:
▶ experience no injury from heat application
▶ identify the factors that increase potential for injury
▶ verbalize an understanding of the safety measures necessary for preventing injury during heat application.

Acute pain related to (specify)
The patient will:
▶ express relief from pain after the application of heat
▶ identify specific characteristics of pain
▶ use available resources to understand pain phenomenon.

Equipment

Patient thermometer • towel • adhesive tape or roller gauze • absorbent, protective cloth covering • gloves, if the patient has an open lesion

For a hot-water bottle
Hot tap water • pitcher • bath thermometer • absorbent, protective cloth covering

For an electric heating pad
Absorbent, protective cloth covering

For a K pad
Distilled water • temperature-adjustment key • absorbent, protective cloth covering

For a chemical hot pack (disposable)
Absorbent, protective cloth covering

For a warm compress or pack (sterile or nonsterile)
Basin of hot tap water or container of sterile water, normal saline, or other solution as ordered • bath thermometer • hot-water bottle, K pad, or chemical hot pack • linen-saver pad • optional: forceps

The following items may be sterile or nonsterile as needed: compress material (such as flannel and 4" × 4" gauze pads) or pack material (such as absorbent towels and large absorbent pads) • cotton-tipped applicators • forceps • bowl or basin • bath thermometer • waterproof covering • towel • dressing

Preparation of equipment
Hot-water bottle
Fill the bottle with hot tap water *to detect leaks and warm the bottle;* then empty it. Run hot tap water into a pitcher

and measure the water temperature with the bath thermometer. Adjust the temperature as ordered, usually 115° to 125° F (46.1° to 51.7° C) for adults.

 Age alert **Adjust the water temperature to 105° to 115° F (40.6° to 46.1° C) for elderly patients or children younger than age 2.**

Next, pour hot water into the bottle, filling it one-half to two-thirds full. *Partially filling the bottle keeps it lightweight and flexible to mold to the treatment area.* Squeeze the bottle until the water reaches the neck *to expel any air that would make the bottle inflexible and reduce heat conduction.* Fasten the top and cover the bag with an absorbent cloth. Secure the cover with tape or roller gauze.

Electric heating pad

Check the cord for frayed or damaged insulation. Then plug in the pad and adjust the control switch to the desired setting. Wrap the pad in a protective cloth covering and secure the cover with tape or roller gauze.

K pad

Check the cord for frayed or damaged insulation and fill the control unit two-thirds full with distilled water, according to the manufacturer's directions. Don't use tap water *because it leaves mineral deposits in the unit.* Check for leaks and then tilt the unit in several directions *to clear the pad's tubing of air.* Tighten the cap and then loosen it a quarter turn *to allow heat expansion within the unit.* After making sure the hoses between the control unit and the pad are free of tangles, place the unit on the bedside table, slightly above the patient *so that gravity can assist water*

flow. If the central supply department hasn't preset the temperature, use the temperature-adjustment key provided to set the temperature on the control unit. The usual temperature is 105° F. Place the pad in a protective cloth covering and secure the cover with tape or roller gauze. Plug in the unit, turn it on, and allow the pad to warm for 2 minutes.

Chemical hot pack

Select a pack of the correct size. Follow the manufacturer's directions (strike, squeeze, or knead) *to activate the heat-producing chemicals.* Place the pack in a protective cloth covering, and secure the cover with tape or roller gauze.

Sterile warm compress or pack

Warm the container of sterile water or solution by setting it in a sink or basin of hot water. Measure its temperature with a sterile bath thermometer. If a sterile thermometer is unavailable, pour some heated sterile solution into a clean container, check the temperature with a regular bath thermometer, and then discard the tested solution. Adjust the temperature by adding hot or cold water to the sink or basin until the solution reaches 131° F (55° C) for adults.

Pour the heated solution into a sterile bowl or basin. Then using sterile technique, soak the compress or pack in the heated solution. If necessary, prepare a hot-water bottle, K pad, or chemical hot pack to keep the compress or pack warm.

Nonsterile warm compress or pack

Fill a bowl or basin with hot tap water or other solution, and measure the temperature of the fluid with a bath thermometer. Adjust the temperature as ordered, usually to 131° F (55° C) for adults.

Soak the compress or pack in the hot liquid. If necessary, prepare a hot-water bottle, K pad, or chemical hot pack *to keep the compress or pack warm.*

Implementation
▶ Check the doctor's order and assess the patient's condition.
▶ Explain the procedure to the patient and tell him not to lean or lie directly on the heating device *because this reduces air space and increases the risk of burns.* Warn him against adjusting the temperature of the heating device or adding hot water to a hot-water bottle. Advise him to report pain immediately and remove the device if necessary.
▶ Provide privacy and make sure the room is warm and free from drafts.
▶ Wash your hands.
▶ Take the patient's temperature, pulse, and respiration *to serve as a baseline.* If heat treatment is being applied to raise the patient's body temperature, monitor temperature, pulse, and respirations throughout the application.
▶ Expose only the treatment area *because vasodilation will make the patient feel chilly.*

Applying a hot-water bottle, an electric heating pad, a K pad, or a chemical hot pack
▶ Before applying the heating device, press it against your inner forearm *to test its temperature and heat distribution.* If it heats unevenly, obtain a new device.
▶ Apply the device to the treatment area and, if necessary, secure it with tape or roller gauze. Begin timing the application.

▶ Assess the patient's skin condition frequently and remove the device if you observe increased swelling or excessive redness, blistering, maceration, or pallor or if the patient reports discomfort. Refill the hot-water bottle as necessary *to maintain the correct temperature.*
▶ Remove the device after 20 to 30 minutes, or as ordered.
▶ Dry the patient's skin with a towel and redress the site, if necessary. Take the patient's temperature, pulse, and respiration *for comparison with the baseline.* Position him comfortably in bed.
▶ If the treatment is to be repeated, store the equipment in the patient's room, out of his reach; otherwise, return it to its proper place.

Applying a warm compress or pack
▶ Place a linen-saver pad under the site.
▶ Remove the warm compress or pack from the bowl or basin. (Use sterile forceps throughout the procedure if needed.)
▶ Wring excess solution from the compress or pack. *Excess moisture increases the risk of burns.*
▶ Apply the compress gently to the affected site. After a few seconds, lift the compress and check the skin for excessive redness, maceration, or blistering. When you're sure the compress isn't causing a burn, mold it firmly to the skin *to keep air out, which reduces the temperature and effectiveness of the compress.* Work quickly *so the compress retains its heat.*
▶ Apply a waterproof covering (sterile, if necessary) to the compress. Secure it with tape or roller gauze *to prevent it from slipping.*
▶ Place a hot-water bottle, K pad, or chemical hot pack over the compress

Using moist heat to relieve muscle spasm

Tell patients to choose moist heat rather than dry heat when attempting to ease muscle tension or spasm. Moist heat is less drying to the skin, less apt to cause burns, less likely to cause excessive fluid and salt loss through sweating, and more likely to penetrate deeper tissues. Instruct the patient to apply heat for 20 to 30 minutes, as follows:

■ Place a moist towel over the painful area.

■ Cover the towel with a hot-water bottle properly filled and at the correct temperature.

■ Remove the hot-water bottle and wet pack after 20 to 30 minutes. Don't continue application for longer than 30 minutes because therapeutic value decreases after that time.

and waterproof covering *to maintain the correct temperature.* Begin timing the application.

▶ Check the patient's skin every 5 minutes for tissue tolerance. Remove the device if the skin shows excessive redness, maceration, or blistering or if the patient experiences pain or discomfort. Change the compress as needed *to maintain the correct temperature.*

▶ After 15 to 20 minutes or as ordered, remove the compress. Discard the compress into a waterproof trash bag.

▶ Dry the patient's skin with a towel (sterile, if necessary). Note the condition of the skin and redress the area, if necessary. Take the patient's temperature, pulse, and respiration *for comparison with baseline.* Make sure the patient is comfortable.

Special considerations

▶ If the patient is unconscious, anesthetized, irrational, neurologically impaired, or insensitive to heat, stay with him throughout the treatment.

▶ When direct heat is ordered to decrease congestion within internal organs, the application must cover a large enough area *to increase blood volume at the skin's surface.* For relief of pelvic organ congestion, for example, apply heat over the patient's lower abdomen, hips, and thighs. To achieve local relief, you may concentrate heat only over the specified area. (See *Using moist heat to relieve muscle spasm.*)

▶ As an alternative method of applying sterile moist compresses, use a bedside sterilizer to sterilize the compresses. Saturate the compress with tap water or another solution and wring it dry. Then place it in the bedside sterilizer at 275° F (135° C) for 15 minutes. Remove the compress with sterile forceps or sterile gloves, and wring out the excess solution. Then place the compress in a sterile bowl and measure its temperature with a sterile thermometer.

Complications

Because tissue damage may result from direct heat application, monitor the temperature of the compress carefully. Assess frequently the condition of the patient's skin under the heat application device.

Documentation

Record the time and date of heat application including type, temperature or heat setting, duration, and site of application; the patient's temperature, pulse, respirations, and skin condition before, during, and after treatment; signs of complications; and the patient's tolerance of the treatment.

HEMODIALYSIS

Hemodialysis is performed to remove toxic wastes from the blood of patients in renal failure. This potentially life-saving procedure removes blood from the body, circulates it through a purifying dialyzer and then returns the blood to the body. Various access sites can be used for this procedure. (See *Hemodialysis access sites,* page 384.) The most common access device for long-term treatment is an arteriovenous (AV) fistula.

The underlying mechanism in hemodialysis is differential diffusion across a semipermeable membrane, which extracts by-products of protein metabolism, such as urea and uric acid, as well as creatinine and excess body water. This process restores or maintains the balance of the body's buffer system and electrolyte level. Hemodialysis thus promotes a rapid return to normal serum values and helps prevent complications associated with uremia. (See *How hemodialysis works,* pages 385 and 386.)

Hemodialysis provides temporary support for patients with acute reversible renal failure. It's also used for regular long-term treatment of patients with chronic end-stage renal disease. A less common indication for hemodialysis is acute poisoning, such as a barbiturate or analgesic overdose. The patient's condition (such as rate of creatinine accumulation and weight gain) determines the number and duration of hemodialysis treatments.

Specially prepared personnel usually perform this procedure in a hemodialysis unit. However, if the patient is acutely ill and unstable, hemodialysis can be done at bedside in the intensive care unit. Special hemodialysis units are available for use at home.

Key nursing diagnoses and patient outcomes

Ineffective individual therapeutic regimen management related to hemodialysis
The patient will:
▶ express personal beliefs about illness and its management
▶ identify necessary dietary modifications
▶ develop a plan for integrating the components of the therapeutic regimen into a pattern of daily living.

Ineffective individual coping related to hemodialysis
The patient will:
▶ identify personal coping mechanisms
▶ become actively involved in planning own care
▶ use available support systems, such as family and significant others, to develop and maintain effective coping skills.

Risk for infection related to hemodialysis
The patient will:
▶ remain free from elevated temperature
▶ remain free from other signs and symptoms of infection.

Equipment
For preparing the hemodialysis machine
Hemodialysis machine with appropriate dialyzer • I.V. solution, administration sets, lines, and related equipment • dialysate • optional: heparin, 3-ml syringe with needle, medication label, and hemostat

(Text continues on page 386.)

Hemodialysis access sites

Hemodialysis requires vascular access. The site and type of access may vary, depending on the expected duration of dialysis, the surgeon's preference, and the patient's condition.

Subclavian vein catheterization

Using the Seldinger technique, the doctor or surgeon inserts an introducer needle into the subclavian vein. He then inserts a guide wire through the introducer needle and removes the needle. Using the guide wire, he then threads a 5″ to 12″ (12.5- to 30.5-cm) plastic or Teflon catheter (with a Y hub) into the patient's vein.

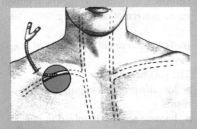

Femoral vein catheterization

Using the Seldinger technique, the doctor or surgeon inserts an introducer needle into the left or right femoral vein. He then inserts a guide wire through the introducer needle and removes the needle.

Using the guide wire, he then threads a 5″ to 12″ plastic or Teflon catheter with a Y hub or two catheters, one for inflow and another placed about ½″ (1.3 cm) distal to the first for outflow.

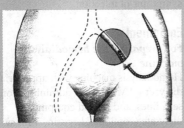

Arteriovenous fistula

To create a fistula, the surgeon makes an incision into the patient's wrist or lower forearm, then a small incision in the side of an artery and another in the side of a vein. He sutures the edges of the incisions together to make a common opening 3 to 7 mm long.

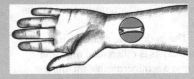

Arteriovenous shunt

To create a shunt, the surgeon makes an incision in the patient's wrist, lower forearm, or (rarely) an ankle. He then inserts a 6″ to 10″ (15- to 25-cm) transparent Silastic cannula into an artery and another into a vein. Finally, he tunnels the cannulas out through stab wounds and joins them with a piece of Teflon tubing.

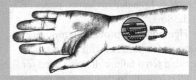

Arteriovenous graft

To create a graft, the surgeon makes an incision in the patient's forearm, upper arm, or thigh. He then tunnels a natural or synthetic graft under the skin and sutures the distal end to an artery and the proximal end to a vein.

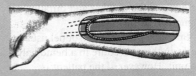

How hemodialysis works

In hemodialysis, blood flows from the patient to an external dialyzer (or artificial kidney) through an arterial access site. Inside the dialyzer, blood and dialysate flow countercurrently divided by a semipermeable membrane. The composition of the dialysate resembles normal extracellular fluid. The blood contains an excess of specific solutes (such as metabolic waste products and some electrolytes), and the dialysate contains electrolytes that may be at abnormal levels in the patient's bloodstream. The dialysate's electrolyte composition can be modified to raise or lower electrolyte levels, depending on need.

Excretory function and electrolyte homeostasis are achieved by *diffusion*, the movement of a molecule across the dialyzer's semipermeable membrane, from an area of higher solute concentration to an area of lower concentration. Water (solvent) crosses the membrane from the blood into the dialysate by *ultrafiltration*. This process removes excess water, waste products, and other metabolites through *osmotic pressure* and *hydrostatic pressure*. Osmotic pressure is the movement of water across the semipermeable membrane from an area of lesser solute concentration to one of greater solute concentration. Hydrostatic pressure forces water from the blood compartment into the dialysate compartment. Cleaned of impurities and excess water, the blood returns to the body through a venous site.

Types of dialyzers

There are three types of dialyzers: the hollow-fiber, the flat-plate or parallel flow-plate, and the coil.

The *hollow-fiber dialyzer*, the most common type, contains fine capillaries, with a semipermeable membrane enclosed in a plastic cylinder. Blood flows through these capillaries as the system pumps dialysate in the opposite direction on the outside of the capillaries.

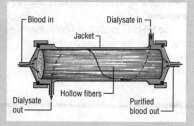

The *flat-plate* or *parallel flow-plate dialyzer* has two or more layers of semipermeable membrane, bound by a semirigid or rigid structure. Blood ports are located at both ends, between the membranes. Blood flows between the membranes, and dialysate flows in the opposite direction along the outside of the membranes.

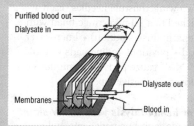

The *coil dialyzer* (no longer widely used) consists of one or more semipermeable

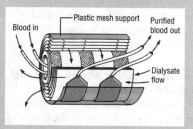

(continued)

How hemodialysis works *(continued)*

membrane tubes supported by mesh and wrapped concentrically around a central core. Blood passes through the coils as dialysate circulates at high speed around the coils and meshwork.

The flat-plate and hollow-fiber dialyzers may be used several times on each patient. Heparin is used to prevent clot formation during hemodialysis.

Three system types can be used to deliver dialysate. The *batch system* uses a reservoir for recirculating dialysate. The *regenerative system* uses sorbents to purify and regenerate recirculating dialysate. The *proportioning system* (the most common) mixes concentrate with water to form dialysate, which then circulates through the dialyzer and goes down a drain after a single pass, followed by fresh dialysate.

For hemodialysis with a double-lumen catheter

Povidone-iodine pads • two sterile 4″ × 4″ gauze pads • two 3-ml and two 5-ml syringes • tape • heparin bolus syringe • gloves

For hemodialysis with an AV fistula

Two winged fistula needles (each attached to a 10-ml syringe filled with heparin flush solution) • linen-saver pad • povidone-iodine pads • sterile 4″ × 4″ gauze pads • tourniquet • gloves • adhesive tape

For hemodialysis with an AV shunt

Povidone-iodine pads • alcohol pads • sterile gloves • two sterile shunt adapters • sterile Teflon connector • two bulldog clamps • two 10-ml syringes • normal saline solution • four short strips of adhesive tape • optional: sterile shunt spreader

For discontinuing hemodialysis with a double-lumen catheter

Sterile 4″ × 4″ gauze pads • povidone-iodine pad • precut gauze dressing • clean and sterile gloves • normal saline solution • alcohol pads • heparin flush

solution • luer-lock injection caps • optional: transparent occlusive dressing, skin barrier preparation, tape, and materials for culturing drainage

For discontinuing hemodialysis with an AV fistula

Gloves • sterile 4″ × 4″ gauze pads • two adhesive bandages • two hemostats • optional: sterile absorbable gelatin sponges (Gelfoam)

For discontinuing hemodialysis with an AV shunt

Sterile gloves • two bulldog clamps • two hemostats • povidone-iodine solution • sterile 4″ × 4″ gauze pads • alcohol pads • elastic gauze bandages • plasticized or hypoallergenic tape

Preparation of equipment

Prepare the hemodialysis equipment following the manufacturer's instructions and your facility's protocol. Maintain strict sterile technique *to prevent introducing pathogens into the patient's bloodstream during dialysis.* Make sure you test the dialyzer and dialysis machine for residual disinfectant after rinsing, and test all the alarms.

Implementation

▶ Weigh the patient. *To determine ultrafiltration requirements,* compare his present weight to his weight after the last dialysis and his target weight. Record his baseline vital signs, taking his blood pressure while he's sitting and standing. Auscultate his heart for rate, rhythm, and abnormalities. Observe respiratory rate, rhythm, and quality. Assess for edema. Check his mental status and the condition and patency of the access site. Also check for problems since the last dialysis and evaluate previous laboratory data.

▶ Help the patient into a comfortable position (such as supine or sitting in recliner chair with feet elevated). Make sure the access site is well supported and resting on a clean drape.

▶ If the patient is undergoing hemodialysis for the first time, explain the procedure in detail.

▶ Use standard precautions in all cases *to prevent transmission of infection.* Wash your hands before beginning.

Beginning hemodialysis with a double-lumen catheter

▶ Prepare venous access. If extension tubing isn't already clamped, clamp it *to prevent air from entering the catheter.* Then clean each catheter extension tube, clamp, and luer-lock injection cap with povidone-iodine pads *to remove contaminants.* Next, place a sterile 4″ × 4″ gauze pad under the extension tubing and place two 5-ml syringes and two sterile gauze pads on the drape.

▶ Prepare the anticoagulant regimen as ordered.

▶ Identify arterial and venous blood lines and place them near the drape.

▶ *To remove clots and ensure catheter patency,* remove catheter caps, attach syringes to each catheter port, open one clamp, and aspirate 1.5 to 3 ml of blood. Close the clamp and repeat the procedure with the other port. Flush each port with 5 ml of heparin flush solution.

▶ Attach blood lines to patient access. First, remove the syringe from the arterial port, and attach the line to the arterial port. Then administer the heparin according to protocol. *This prevents clotting in the extracorporeal circuit.*

▶ Grasp the venous blood line and attach it to the venous port. Open the clamps on the extension tubing, and secure the tubing to the patient's extremity with tape *to reduce tension on the tube and minimize trauma to the insertion site.*

▶ Begin hemodialysis according to your unit's protocol.

Beginning hemodialysis with an AV fistula

▶ Flush the fistula needles, using attached syringes containing heparin flush solution, and set them aside.

▶ Place a linen-saver pad under the patient's arm.

▶ Using aseptic technique, clean a 3″ × 10″ (7.6 × 25 cm) area of skin over the fistula with povidone-iodine pads. Discard each pad after one wipe. (If the patient is sensitive to iodine, use chlorhexidine gluconate [Hibiclens] or alcohol instead.)

▶ Apply a tourniquet above the fistula *to distend the veins and facilitate venipuncture.* Make sure you avoid occluding the fistula.

▶ Put on gloves. Perform the venipuncture with a fistula needle. Remove the needle guard and squeeze the wing tips firmly together. Insert the arterial needle at least 1″ (2.5 cm) above the anastomosis, being careful not to puncture the fistula.

▶ Release the tourniquet and flush the needle with heparin flush solution *to prevent clotting*. Clamp the arterial needle tubing with a hemostat and secure the wing tips of the needle to the skin with adhesive tape *to prevent it from dislodging within the vein*.

▶ Perform another venipuncture with the venous needle a few inches above the arterial needle. Flush the needle with heparin flush solution. Clamp the venous needle tubing, and secure the wing tips of the venous needle as you did the arterial needle.

▶ Remove the syringe from the end of the arterial tubing, uncap the arterial line from the hemodialysis machine, and connect the two lines. Tape the connection securely *to prevent it from separating during the procedure*. Repeat these two steps for the venous line.

▶ Release the hemostat and start hemodialysis.

Beginning hemodialysis with an AV shunt

▶ Remove the bulldog clamps and place them within easy reach of the sterile field. Remove the shunt dressing and clean the shunt, using sterile technique, as you would for daily care. (See "Arteriovenous shunt care," page 38.) Clean the bulldog clamps with an alcohol pad.

▶ Assemble the shunt adapters according to the manufacturer's directions.

▶ Clean the arterial and venous shunt connection with povidone-iodine pads *to remove contaminants*. Use a separate pad for each tube and wipe in one direction only, from the insertion site to the connection sites. Allow the tubing to air-dry.

▶ Put on sterile gloves.

▶ Clamp the arterial side of the shunt with a bulldog clamp *to prevent blood from flowing through it*. Clamp the venous side *to prevent leakage when the shunt is opened*.

▶ Open the shunt by separating its sides with your fingers or with a sterile shunt spreader, if available. Both sides of the shunt should be exposed. Always inspect the Teflon connector on one side of the shunt *to see if it's damaged or bent*. If necessary, replace it before proceeding. Note which side contains the connector *so you can use the new one to close the shunt after treatment*.

▶ *To adapt the shunt to the lines of the machine*, attach a shunt adapter and 10-ml syringe filled with about 8 ml of normal saline solution to the side of the shunt containing the Teflon connector. Attach the new Teflon connector to the other side of the shunt with the second adapter. Attach the second 10-ml syringe filled with about 8 ml of normal saline solution to the same side.

▶ Flush the shunt's arterial tubing by releasing its clamp and gently aspirating it with the normal saline solution–filled syringe. Then flush the tubing slowly, observing it for signs of fibrin buildup. Repeat the procedure on the venous side of the shunt.

▶ Secure the shunt to the adapter connection with adhesive tape *to prevent separation during treatment*.

▶ Connect the arterial and venous lines to the adapters and secure the connections with tape. Tape each line to the patient's arm *to prevent unnecessary strain on the shunt during treatment*.

▶ Begin hemodialysis according to your unit's protocol.

Discontinuing hemodialysis with a double-lumen catheter

▶ Wash your hands.

▶ Clamp the extension tubing *to prevent air from entering the catheter.* Clean all connection points on the catheter and blood lines as well as the clamps *to reduce the risk of systemic or local infections.*

▶ Place a clean drape under the catheter and place two sterile 4″ × 4″ gauze pads on the drape beneath the catheter lines. Soak the pads with povidone-iodine solution. Then prepare the catheter flush solution with normal saline or heparin flush solution, as ordered.

▶ Put on clean gloves. Grasp each blood line with a gauze pad and disconnect each line from the catheter.

▶ Flush each port with normal saline solution *to clean the extension tubing and catheter of blood.* Administer additional heparin flush solution as ordered *to ensure catheter patency.* Then attach luerlock injection caps *to prevent entry of air or loss of blood.*

▶ Clamp the extension tubing.

▶ When hemodialysis is complete, redress the catheter insertion site; also redress it if it's occluded, soiled, or wet. Place the patient in a supine position with his face turned away from the insertion site *so that he doesn't contaminate the site by breathing on it.*

▶ Wash your hands and remove the outer occlusive dressing. Then put on sterile gloves, remove the old inner dressing, and discard the gloves and the inner dressing.

▶ Set up a sterile field and observe the site for drainage. Obtain a drainage sample for culture if necessary. Notify the doctor if the suture appears to be missing.

▶ Put on sterile gloves and clean the insertion site with an alcohol pad *to remove skin oils.* Then clean the site with a povidone-iodine pad and allow it to air-dry.

▶ Put a precut gauze dressing over the insertion site and under the catheter, and place another gauze dressing over the catheter.

▶ Apply a skin barrier preparation to the skin surrounding the gauze dressing. Then cover the gauze and catheter with a transparent occlusive dressing.

▶ Apply a 4″ to 5″ piece of 2″ tape over the cut edge of the dressing *to reinforce the lower edge.*

Discontinuing hemodialysis with an AV fistula

▶ Wash your hands. Turn the blood pump on the hemodialysis machine to 50 to 100 ml/minute.

▶ Put on gloves and remove the tape from the connection site of the arterial lines. Clamp the needle tubing with the hemostat and disconnect the lines. The blood in the machine's arterial line will continue to flow toward the dialyzer, followed by a column of air. Just before the blood reaches the point where the normal saline solution enters the line, clamp the blood line with another hemostat.

▶ Unclamp the normal saline solution *to allow a small amount to flow through the line.* Unclamp the hemostat on the machine line. *This allows all blood to flow into the dialyzer where it passes through the filter and back to the patient through the venous line.*

▶ After blood is retransfused, clamp the venous needle tubing and the machine's venous line with hemostats. Turn off the blood pump.

▶ Remove the tape from the connection site of the venous lines and disconnect the lines.

▶ Remove the venipuncture needle, and apply pressure to the site with a folded 4″ × 4″ gauze pad until all bleeding stops, usually within 10 minutes. Apply an adhesive bandage. Repeat the procedure on the arterial line.

▶ When hemodialysis is complete, assess the patient's weight, vital signs (including standing blood pressure), and mental status. Then compare your findings with your predialysis assessment data. Document your findings.

▶ Disinfect and rinse the delivery system according to the manufacturer's instructions.

Discontinuing hemodialysis with an AV shunt

▶ Wash your hands. Turn the blood pump on the hemodialysis machine to 50 to 100 ml/minute.

▶ Put on the sterile gloves and remove the tape from the connection site of the arterial lines. Clamp the arterial cannula with a bulldog clamp, and then disconnect the lines. The blood in the machine's arterial line will continue to flow toward the dialyzer, followed by a column of air. Just before the blood reaches the point where the normal saline solution enters the line, clamp the blood line with a hemostat.

▶ Unclamp the normal saline solution *to allow a small amount to flow through the line.* Reclamp the normal saline solution line and unclamp the hemostat on the machine line. *This allows all blood to flow into the dialyzer where it's circulated through the filter and back to the patient through the venous line.*

▶ Just before the last volume of blood enters the patient, clamp the venous cannula with a bulldog clamp and the machine's venous line with a hemostat.

▶ Remove the tape from the connection site of the venous lines. Turn off the blood pump and disconnect the lines.

▶ Reconnect the shunt cannula. Remove the older of the two Teflon connectors and discard it. Connect the shunt, taking care to position the Teflon connector equally between the two cannulas. Remove the bulldog clamps.

▶ Secure the shunt connection with plasticized or hypoallergenic tape *to prevent accidental disconnection.*

▶ Clean the shunt and its site with the povidone-iodine pads. When the cleaning procedure is finished, remove the povidone-iodine with alcohol pads.

▶ Make sure blood flows through the shunt adequately.

▶ Apply a dressing to the shunt site and wrap it securely (but not too tightly) with elastic gauze bandages. Attach the bulldog clamps to the outside dressing.

▶ When hemodialysis is complete, assess the patient's weight, vital signs, and mental status. Then compare your findings with your predialysis assessment data. Document your findings.

▶ Disinfect and rinse the delivery system according to the manufacturer's instructions.

Special considerations

▶ Obtain blood samples from the patient as ordered. Samples are usually drawn before beginning hemodialysis.

▶ *To avoid pyrogenic reactions and bacteremia with septicemia resulting from contamination,* use strict aseptic technique during preparation of the machine. Discard equipment that has fallen on the floor or that has been disconnected and exposed to the air.

► Immediately report any machine malfunction or equipment defect.

► Avoid unnecessary handling of shunt tubing. However, make sure you inspect the shunt carefully for patency by observing its color. Also look for clots and serum and cell separation, and check the temperature of the Silastic tubing. Assess the shunt insertion site for signs of infection, such as purulent drainage, inflammation, and tenderness, *which may indicate the body's rejection of the shunt.* Also check to see if the shunt insertion tips are exposed.

► Make sure you complete each step in this procedure correctly. Overlooking a single step or performing it incorrectly can cause unnecessary blood loss or inefficient treatment from poor clearances or inadequate fluid removal. For example, never allow a saline solution bag to run dry while priming and soaking the dialyzer. This can cause air to enter the patient portion of the dialysate system. Ultimately, failure to perform hemodialysis accurately can lead to patient injury and even death.

► If bleeding continues after you remove an AV fistula needle, apply pressure with a sterile, absorbable gelatin sponge. If bleeding persists, apply a similar sponge soaked in topical thrombin solution.

► Throughout hemodialysis, carefully monitor the patient's vital signs. Read blood pressure at least hourly or as often as every 15 minutes, if necessary. Monitor the patient's weight before and after the procedure *to ensure adequate ultrafiltration during treatment.* (Many dialysis units are now equipped with bed scales.)

► Perform periodic tests for clotting time on the patient's blood samples and samples from the dialyzer. If the patient receives meals during treatment, make sure they're light.

► Continue necessary drug administration during dialysis unless the drug would be removed in the dialysate; if so, administer the drug after dialysis.

Home care

Before the patient leaves the facility, teach him how to care for his vascular access site. Instruct him to keep the incision clean and dry *to prevent infection,* and to clean it daily until it heals completely and the sutures are removed (usually 10 to 14 days after surgery). He should notify the doctor of pain, swelling, redness, or drainage in the accessed arm. Teach him how to use a stethoscope to auscultate for bruits and how to palpate a thrill.

Explain that after the access site heals, he may use the arm freely. In fact, exercise is beneficial *because it helps stimulate vein enlargement.* Remind him not to allow any treatments or procedures on the accessed arm, including blood pressure monitoring or needle punctures. Also tell him to avoid putting excessive pressure on the arm. He shouldn't sleep on it, wear constricting clothing over it, or lift heavy objects or strain with it. He also should avoid getting wet for several hours after dialysis.

Teach the patient exercises for the affected arm *to promote vascular dilation and enhance blood flow.* He may start by squeezing a small rubber ball or other soft object for 15 minutes, when advised by the doctor.

If the patient will be performing hemodialysis at home, thoroughly review all aspects of the procedure with the patient and his family. Give them the phone number of the dialysis center. Emphasize that training for home hemodialysis is a complex process requiring 2 to 3 months *to ensure that the patient or family member performs it safely and competently.* Keep in mind that this procedure is stressful.

Complications

Bacterial endotoxins in the dialysate may cause fever. Rapid fluid removal and electrolyte changes during hemodialysis can cause early dialysis disequilibrium syndrome. Signs and symptoms include headache, nausea, vomiting, restlessness, hypertension, muscle cramps, backache, and seizures.

Excessive removal of fluid during ultrafiltration can cause hypovolemia and hypotension. Diffusion of the sugar and sodium content of the dialysate solution into the blood can cause hyperglycemia and hypernatremia. These conditions, in turn, can cause hyperosmolarity.

Cardiac arrhythmias can occur during hemodialysis as a result of electrolyte and pH changes in the blood. They can also develop in patients taking antiarrhythmic drugs because the dialysate removes these drugs during treatment. Angina may develop in patients with anemia or preexisting arteriosclerotic cardiovascular disease because of the physiologic stress on the blood during purification and ultrafiltration. Reduced oxygen levels due to extracorporeal blood flow or membrane sensitivity may require increasing oxygen administration during hemodialysis.

Some complications of hemodialysis can be fatal. For example, an air embolism can result if the dialyzer retains air, if tubing connections become loose, or if the saline solution container empties. Symptoms include chest pain, dyspnea, coughing, and cyanosis.

Hemolysis can result from obstructed flow of the dialysate concentrate or from incorrect setting of the conductivity alarm limits. Symptoms include chest pain, dyspnea, cherry red blood, arrhythmias, acute decrease in hematocrit, and hyperkalemia.

Hyperthermia, another potentially fatal complication, can result if the dialysate becomes overheated. Exsanguination can result from separations of the blood lines or from rupture of the blood lines or dialyzer membrane.

Documentation

Record the time treatment began and any problems with it. Note the patient's vital signs and weight before and during treatment. Note the time blood samples were taken for testing, the test results, and treatment for complications. Record the time the treatment was completed and the patient's response to it.

Hip spica cast care

After orthopedic surgery to correct a fracture or deformity, a patient may need a hip spica cast to immobilize both legs. Occasionally, the doctor may apply a hip spica cast to treat an orthopedic deformity that doesn't require surgery.

Caring for a patient in a hip spica cast poses several challenges, including protecting the cast from urine and feces, keeping the cast dry, ensuring proper blood supply to the legs, and teaching the patient and his parents how to care for the cast at home.

Infants usually adapt more easily to the cast than older children but both need encouragement, support, and diversionary activity during their prolonged immobilization.

Key nursing diagnoses and patient outcomes

Impaired physical mobility related to fracture or deformity
The patient will:
▶ show no evidence of complications, such as venous stasis or skin breakdown
▶ carry out mobility regimen
▶ achieve the highest level of mobility.

Ineffective tissue perfusion (peripheral) related to fracture
The patient will:
▶ have strong peripheral pulses
▶ have normal skin color and temperature
▶ have no numbness, tingling, or pain in body parts distal to the cast.

Equipment
Waterproof adhesive tape • moleskin or plastic petals • cast cutter or saw • scissors • nonabrasive cleaner • hair dryer • damp sponge or cloth • optional: disposable diaper or perineal pad

Implementation
▶ Before the doctor applies the cast, describe the procedure to the patient and his parents. For patients ages 3 to 12, illustrate your explanation. Draw a picture, present a diagram, or use a doll with a cast or an elastic gauze dressing

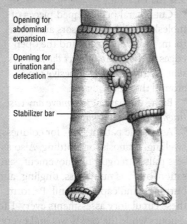

Understanding the hip spica cast

As you talk with parents about their child's hip spica cast, describe how it will extend from the child's lower rib margin (or sometimes from the nipple line) down to the tips of the toes on the affected side and to the knee on the opposite unaffected side. Also mention that it expands at the waist to allow the child to eat comfortably. A stabilizer bar positioned between the legs keeps the hips in slight abduction and separates the legs.

Opening for abdominal expansion

Opening for urination and defecation

Stabilizer bar

wrapped around its trunk and limbs. (See *Understanding the hip spica cast.*)
▶ After the doctor constructs the cast, keep all but the perineal area uncovered. Provide privacy by draping a small cover over this opening. Turn the patient every 1 to 2 hours *to speed drying time.* Make sure you turn the patient to his unaffected side *to prevent adding pressure to the affected side.* If the patient is an infant, you can turn him by yourself. If the patient is an older child or an adolescent, seek assistance before attempting to turn him. When turning

the patient, don't use the stabilizer bar between his legs for leverage. *Excessive pressure on this bar may disrupt the cast.* Handle a damp cast only with your palms *to avoid misshaping the cast material.*

▶ After the cast dries, inspect the inside edges of the cast for stray pieces of casting material *that can irritate the skin.* (A traditional hip spica cast requires 24 to 48 hours to dry. However, a hip spica cast made from newer, quick-drying substances takes only 8 to 10 hours to dry. If made of fiberglass, it will dry in less than 1 hour.)

▶ Cut several petal-shaped pieces of moleskin using the scissors and place them, overlapping, around the open edges of the cast *to protect the patient's skin.* Use waterproof adhesive tape around the perineal area.

▶ Bathe the patient *to remove any cast fragments from his skin.*

▶ Assess the patient's legs for coldness, swelling, cyanosis, or mottling. Also assess pulse strength, toe movement, sensation (such as numbness, tingling, and burning), and capillary refill. Perform these circulatory assessments every 1 to 2 hours while the cast is wet and every 2 to 4 hours after the cast dries.

▶ If the cast is applied after surgery, remember that the most accurate way to assess for bleeding is to monitor vital signs. A visible blood spot on the cast can be misleading: One drop of blood can produce a circle 3″ (7.6 cm) in diameter.

▶ Check the patient's exposed skin for redness or irritation, and observe the patient for pain or discomfort caused by hot spots (pressure-sensitive areas under the cast). Also be alert for a foul odor. *These signs and symptoms suggest a pressure ulcer or infection.*

▶ *To relieve itching,* set a handheld hair dryer on "cool" and blow air under the cast. Warn the patient and his parents not to insert any object (such as a ruler, coat hanger, or knitting needle) into the cast to relieve itching by scratching *because these objects could disrupt the suture line, break adjacent skin, and introduce infection.* Also, be vigilant in ensuring that small objects or food particles don't become lodged under the cast and cause skin breakdown and infection.

▶ Encourage the patient's family to visit and participate in his care and recreation. *This increases the patient's sense of security and enhances the parents' sense of participation and control.*

Special considerations

▶ If the patient is incontinent (or not toilet-trained), *protect the cast from soiling.* Tuck a folded disposable diaper or perineal pad around the perineal edges of the cast. Then apply a second diaper to the patient, over the top of the cast, to hold the first diaper in place. Also, tuck plastic petals into the cast *to channel urine and feces into a bedpan.* If the cast still becomes soiled, wipe it with a nonabrasive cleaner and a damp sponge or cloth. Then air-dry it with a hair dryer set on "cool."

▶ Keep a cast cutter or saw available at all times *to remove the cast quickly in case of an emergency.*

▶ During mealtimes, position older children on their abdomens *to promote safer eating and swallowing.*

▶ Before removing the cast, reassure the parents and the patient that the noisy sawing process is painless. If necessary, explain how the saw works.

Home care

Before discharge, teach the parents how to care for the cast and give them an opportunity to demonstrate their understanding. Include instructions for checking circulatory status, recognizing signs of circulatory impairment, and notifying the doctor. Also demonstrate how to turn the child, apply moleskin, clean the cast, and ensure adequate nourishment.

Teach the parents to treat dry, scaly skin around the cast by washing the child's skin frequently. After the cast is removed, they may apply baby oil or other lotion to soothe the skin. Urge them to schedule and keep all follow-up medical appointments.

Teach the parents how to use a car restraint device, such as the E-Z-ON Vest, because the child won't be able to use a conventional car seat.

Complications

Complications associated with a hip spica cast come from immobility. They include constipation, urinary stasis, kidney stones, skin breakdown, respiratory compromise, and contractures. Frequent turnings, range-of-motion exercises, and adequate hydration and nutrition can minimize complications.

Documentation

Record the date and time of cast care. Describe circulatory status in the patient's legs and record measurements of any bleeding or drainage. Note the condition of the cast and the patient's skin. Describe all skin care given.

Record findings of bowel and bladder assessments. Note patient and family tolerance of the cast. Document patient- and family-teaching topics discussed as well.

HOUR OF SLEEP CARE

Hour of sleep (h.s.) care meets the patient's physical and psychological needs in preparation for sleep. It includes providing for the patient's hygiene, making the bed clean and comfortable, and ensuring safety. For example, raising the bed's side rails can prevent the drowsy or sedated patient from falling out. This type of care also provides an opportunity to answer the patient's questions about the next day's tests and procedures and to discuss his worries and concerns.

Effective h.s. care prepares the patient for a good night's sleep. Ineffective care may contribute to sleeplessness, which can intensify patient anxiety and interfere with treatment and recuperation.

Key nursing diagnoses and patient outcomes

Anxiety related to (specify)
The patient will:
▶ express feelings of anxiety
▶ use support systems to assist with coping
▶ perform stress-reduction techniques to avoid symptoms of anxiety.

Risk for injury
The patient will:
▶ remain free from injury
▶ identify factors that increase risk of injury
▶ assist in identifying and applying safety measures to prevent injury.

Equipment

Bedpan, urinal, or commode• basin• soap• towel• washcloth• toothbrush and toothpaste• denture cup and commercial denture cleaner, if necessary • lotion • linens, if necessary • gown, if necessary • blanket • facial tissues • soft restraints, if necessary

Preparation of equipment

Assemble the equipment at the patient's bedside. For the ambulatory patient who is capable of self-care, assemble soap, a washcloth, a towel, and oral hygiene items at the sink.

Implementation

▶ Tell the patient you'll help him prepare for sleep and provide privacy.
▶ Offer the patient on bed rest a bedpan, urinal, or commode. Otherwise, assist the ambulatory patient to the bathroom.
▶ Fill the basin with warm water and bring it to the patient's bedside. Immerse the lotion in the basin *to warm it for back massage.* Then wash the patient's face and hands and dry them well. Encourage the patient to do this himself, if possible, *to promote independence.*
▶ Provide toothpaste or a properly labeled denture cup and commercial denture cleaner. Assist the patient with oral hygiene as necessary. (See "Mouth care," page 524.) If the patient prefers to wear dentures until bedtime, leave denture-care items within easy reach.
▶ After providing mouth care, turn the patient on his side or stomach. Wash, rinse, and dry the patient's back and buttocks. Massage well with lotion *to help relax the patient.* (See "Back care," page 47, for complete information on massage.)
▶ While providing back care, observe the skin for redness, cracking, or other signs of breakdown. If the patient's gown is soiled or damp, provide a clean

one and help him put it on, if necessary.
▶ Check dressings, binders, antiembolism stockings, or other aids, changing or readjusting them as needed.
▶ Refill the water container, and place it and a box of facial tissues within the patient's easy reach *to prevent falls if patient needs to reach for these items.*
▶ Straighten or change bed linens, as necessary, and fluff the patient's pillow. Cover him with a blanket or place one within his easy reach *to prevent chills during the night.* Position him comfortably. If he appears distressed, restless, or in pain, give ordered drugs as needed.
▶ After making the patient comfortable, evaluate his mental and physical condition. Place the bed in a low position and raise the side rails. Place the call button within the patient's easy reach, and instruct him to call you whenever necessary. Tidy the patient's environment: Move all breakables from the overbed table out of his reach and remove any equipment and supplies that could cause falls should the patient get up during the night. Finally, turn off the overhead light and put on the night-light.

Special considerations

▶ Ask the patient about his sleep routine at home and, whenever possible, let him follow it.
▶ Also try to observe certain rituals, such as a bedtime snack, *which can aid sleep.* A back massage, a tub bath, or a shower also help relax the patient and promote a restful night. If the patient normally bathes or showers before bedtime, let him do so if his condition and doctor's orders permit it.

Documentation

Record the time and type of h.s. care in your notes. Include application of soft restraints or any other special procedures.

HUMIDIFIER THERAPY

Humidifiers, which deliver a maximum amount of water vapor without producing particulate water, are used to prevent drying and irritation of the upper airway in conditions such as croup, in which the upper airway is inflamed, or when secretions are particularly thick and tenacious.

Some humidifiers heat the water vapor, which raises the moisture-carrying capacity of gas and thus increases the amount of humidity delivered to the patient. Room humidifiers add humidity to an entire room, while humidifiers added to gas lines humidify only the air being delivered to the patient. (See *Comparing humidifiers,* page 398.)

Key nursing diagnoses and patient outcomes

Risk for infection related to humidification equipment
The patient will:
▶ be free from signs and symptoms of infection
▶ state an understanding of the potential risk of infection with home use of humidification equipment
▶ demonstrate the correct procedure for preventing bacterial buildup in the equipment during home use.

Ineffective airway clearance related to (specify)
The patient will:
▶ maintain a patent airway

▶ drink 3 to 4 qt (3 to 4 L) of fluid daily (if not contraindicated)
▶ demonstrate correct procedures for performing breathing exercises
▶ perform activities of daily living to level of ability.

Equipment

Humidifier • sterile distilled water, or tap water if the unit has demineralizing capability • container for waste water • bleach • white vinegar

Preparation of equipment

For a bedside humidifier
Open the reservoir and add sterile distilled water to the fill line; then close the reservoir. Keep all room windows and doors tightly closed *to maintain adequate humidification.* Plug the unit into the electrical outlet.

For a heated vaporizer
Remove the top and fill the reservoir to the fill line with tap water. Replace the top securely. Place the vaporizer about 4′ (1 m) from the patient, directing the steam toward but not directly onto the patient. Place the unit in a spot where it can't be overturned *to avoid hot water burns.* This is especially important if children will be in the room.

Plug the unit into an electrical outlet. Steam should soon rise from the unit into the air. Close all windows and doors to maintain adequate humidification.

For a diffusion head humidifier
Unscrew the humidifier reservoir, and add sterile distilled water to the appropriate level. (If using a disposable unit, screw the cap with the extension onto the top of the unit.) Then screw the reservoir back onto the humidifier and

Comparing humidifiers

Type	Description and uses	Advantages	Disadvantages
Bedside 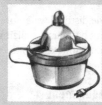	■ Spinning disk splashes water against baffle, creating small drops and increasing evaporation; motor disperses mist to directly humidify room air	■ May be used with all oxygen masks and nasal cannulas ■ Easy to operate ■ Inexpensive	■ Produces humidity inefficiently ■ Can't be used for patients with bypassed upper airway ■ May harbor bacteria and molds
Heated vaporizer 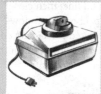	■ Provides direct humidification to room air by heating the water in the reservoir	■ May be used with all oxygen masks and nasal cannulas ■ Easy to operate ■ Inexpensive	■ Can't guarantee the amount of humidity delivered ■ Risk of burn injury if the machine is knocked over
Diffusion head 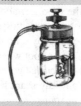	■ In-line humidifier most commonly used with low-flow oxygen delivery systems; gas flows through porous diffuser in reservoir to increase gas-liquid interface; provides humidification to patients using a nasal cannula or oxygen mask (except the Venturi mask)	■ Easy to use ■ Inexpensive	■ Provides only 20% to 30% humidity at body temperature ■ Can't be used for a patient with bypassed upper airway
Cascade bubble diffusion 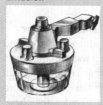	■ Forces gas through a plastic grid in reservoir of warmed water to create fine bubbles; commonly used in patients receiving mechanical ventilation or continuous positive airway pressure therapy	■ Delivers 100% humidity at body temperature ■ The most effective of all evaporative humidifiers	■ If correct water level isn't maintained, mucosa can become irritated

attach the flowmeter to the oxygen source.

Screw the humidifier onto the flowmeter until the seal is tight. Then set the flowmeter at a rate of 2 L/minute and check for gentle bubbling. Next, check the positive-pressure release valve by occluding the end valve on the humidifier. The pressure should back up into the humidifier, signaled by a high-pitched whistle. If this doesn't occur, tighten all connections and try again.

For a cascade bubble diffusion humidifier

Unscrew the cascade reservoir and add sterile distilled water to the fill line. Screw the top back onto the reservoir. Plug in the heater unit, and set the temperature between 95° F (35° C) and 100.4° F (38° C).

Implementation

▶ Check to make sure that the humidifier or vaporizer has been prepared properly.

For a bedside humidifier

▶ Direct the humidifier unit's nozzle away from the patient's face (but toward the patient) for effective treatment. Check for a fine mist emission from the nozzle, which indicates proper operation.

▶ Check the unit every 4 hours for proper operation and the water level every 8 hours. When refilling, unplug the unit, discard any old water, wipe with a disinfectant, rinse the reservoir container, and refill with sterile distilled water as necessary.

▶ Keep the unit cleaned and refilled with sterile water *to reduce the risk of bacterial growth.* Replace the unit every

7 days and send used units for proper decontamination.

For a heated vaporizer

▶ Check the unit every 4 hours for proper functioning.

▶ If steam production seems insufficient, unplug the unit, discard the water, and refill with half distilled water and half tap water or clean the unit well.

▶ Check the water level in the unit every 8 hours. To refill, unplug the unit, discard any old water, wipe with a disinfectant, rinse the reservoir container, and refill with tap water as necessary.

For a diffusion head humidifier

▶ Attach the oxygen delivery device to the humidifier and then to the patient. Then adjust the flowmeter to the appropriate oxygen flow rate.

▶ Check the reservoir every 4 hours. If the water level drops too low, empty the remaining water, rinse the jar, and refill it with sterile water. (As the reservoir water level decreases, the evaporation of water in the gas decreases, reducing humidification of the delivered gas.)

▶ Change the humidification system regularly *to prevent bacterial growth and invasion.*

▶ Periodically assess the patient's sputum; sputum that is too thick can hinder mobilization and expectoration. If this occurs, the patient requires a device that can provide higher humidity.

For a cascade bubble diffusion humidifier

▶ Assess the temperature of the inspired gas near the patient's airway every 2 hours when used in critical care and every 4 hours when used in general patient care. If the cascade becomes too hot, drain the water and replace it. *Overheated water vapor can cause respiratory tract burns.*

▶ Check the reservoir's water level every 2 to 4 hours, and fill as necessary. *If the water level falls below the minimum water level mark, humidity will decrease to that of room air.*

▶ Be alert for condensation buildup in the tubing, which can result from the very high humidification produced by the cascade.

▶ Check the tubing frequently and empty the condensate as necessary *so it can't drain into the patient's respiratory tract, encourage growth of microorganisms, or obstruct dependent sections of tubing.* To do so, disconnect the tubing, drain the condensate into a container, and dispose of it properly. Never drain the condensate into the humidification system.

▶ Change the cascade regularly according to your facility's policy.

Special considerations

▶ Because it creates a humidity level comparable to that of ambient air, the diffusion head humidifier is only used for oxygen flow rates greater than 4 L/ minute.

▶ Because the bedside humidifier doesn't deliver a precise amount of humidification, assess the patient regularly *to determine the effectiveness of therapy.* Ask him if he has noticed any improvement and evaluate his sputum.

▶ Like the bedside humidifier, the heated vaporizer doesn't deliver a precise amount of humidification, so assess the patient regularly by asking if he's feeling better and by examining his sputum.

▶ Keep in mind that a humidifier, if not kept clean, can cause or aggravate respiratory problems, especially for people allergic to molds. Refer to your facility's policy for changing and disposing of humidification equipment.

Home care

Make sure the patient and his family understand the reason for using a humidifier and know how to use the equipment. Give them specific written guidelines concerning all aspects of home care.

Instruct the patient using a bedside humidifier at home to fill it with plain tap water and to periodically use sterile distilled water *to prevent mineral buildup.* Also tell him to run white vinegar through the unit *to help clean it, prevent bacterial buildup, and dissolve deposits.*

Tell the patient using a heated vaporizer unit to rinse it with bleach and water every 5 days. Also tell him to run white vinegar through it *to help clean it, prevent bacterial buildup, and dissolve any deposits.*

Complications

Cascade humidifiers can cause aspiration of tubal condensation and, if the air is heated, can cause pulmonary burns. Humidifiers, if contaminated, can cause infection.

Documentation

Record the date and time humidification began and was discontinued; the type of humidifier; the flow rate (of a gas system); thermometer readings (if heated); any complications and the nursing action taken; and the patient's reaction to humidification.

HYDROTHERAPY

Treating diseases or injuries by immersing part or all of the patient's body in water is known as hydrotherapy. Commonly used to debride serious burns and to hasten healing, hydrotherapy also promotes circulation and comfort in patients with peripheral vascular disease and musculoskeletal disorders such as arthritis. Although hydrotherapy usually involves immersing the patient in a tub of water ("tubbing"), showers or other water-spray techniques may replace tubbing in some health care facilities and burn centers. (See *Positioning the patient for hydrotherapy.*)

The nurse or physical therapist usually assists the patient into the tub or shower area if he's ambulatory. If he isn't ambulatory, he can enter the water using a stretcher or hoist device.

Hydrotherapy is contraindicated in the presence of sudden changes: fever, electrolyte or fluid imbalance, or unstable vital signs. Always follow the standard precautions guidelines.

Key nursing diagnoses and patient outcomes

Deficient knowledge related to lack of exposure to hydrotherapy
The patient will:
▶ communicate a need to know more about hydrotherapy
▶ state or demonstrate an understanding of what has been taught.

Risk for injury related to hydrotherapy
The patient will:
▶ experience no injury from the procedure

Positioning the patient for hydrotherapy

To perform hydrotherapy, you'll immerse the patient in a tub or Hubbard tank as shown. Alternatively, you may spray the patient's wounds with water as he lies on a special shower table. Either way, hydrotherapy is traumatic and painful for the burn patient. Provide continual support and encouragement as you proceed.

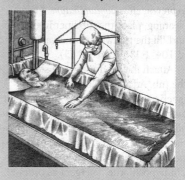

▶ identify factors that increase the potential of injury
▶ state an understanding of the safety measures necessary for preventing injury.

Equipment

Water tank or tub or shower table • plastic tub liner • chemical additives as ordered • plinth (padded table for patient to sit or lie on while performing exercises) • stretcher • headrest • hydraulic hoist • gown • surgical cap • mask • gloves (for removing dressings) • shoulder-length gloves (for tubbing) • apron • debridement instruments • razor, shaving cream, mild soap, shampoo and washcloth (for general cleaning) • fluffed gauze pads • cotton-tipped applicators • sterile sheets • warm, sterile bath blankets • optional: analgesic

Barriers, sheets, and bath blankets may be sterile or clean, depending on the patient's condition and your facility's infection-control policies.

Preparation of equipment

Thoroughly clean and disinfect the tub or shower, its equipment, and the tub or shower room before each treatment *to prevent cross-contamination.* After cleaning, place the tub liner in the tub and fill the tub with warm water (98° to 104° F [36.6° to 40° C]).

Attach the headrest to the sides of the tub. Add prescribed chemicals (such as sodium chloride) to the water *to maintain the normal isotonic level (usually 0.9%) and to prevent dialysis and tissue irritation.* Also add potassium chloride *to prevent potassium loss* and calcium hypochlorite detergent as ordered. Warm the bath blankets and ensure that the room is warm enough *to avoid chilling the patient.*

Implementation

▶ If this is the patient's first treatment, explain the procedure to him *to allay his fears and promote cooperation.* As necessary (before debridement, for example), administer an analgesic about 20 minutes before the procedure.
▶ Check the patient's vital signs.
▶ If the patient is receiving an I.V. infusion, make sure that he has enough I.V. solution to last through the procedure.
▶ Transfer the patient to a stretcher and transport him to the therapy room. If he's ambulatory, he may walk unassisted, provided that the therapy room is nearby.

▶ Wash your hands and put on your gown, gloves, mask, and surgical cap.
▶ Remove the outer dressings and dispose of them properly before immersing the patient. Leave the inner gauze layer on the wound unless it can be easily removed.
▶ If the patient is ambulatory, position him on the plinth for transfer to the tub, or assist him into the tub and situate him on the already lowered plinth.
▶ If the patient isn't ambulatory, attach the stretcher to the overhead hydraulic hoist. Ensure that the hoist hooks are fastened securely. Use the hoist to transfer the patient to and from the tub.
▶ Lower the patient into the tub. Position him so that the headrest supports his head. Allow him to soak for 3 to 5 minutes.
▶ Remove your gloves, wash your hands, and put on the shoulder-length tubbing gloves and apron.
▶ Remove remaining gauze dressings, if any, from the patient's wounds.
▶ If ordered, place the tub's agitator into the water and turn it on. *The motor may burn out if it's turned on out of the water.* Some tubs have aerators to agitate the water.
▶ Clean all unburned areas first (encourage the patient to do this if he can). Wash unburned skin, and clip or shave hair near the wound. Shave facial hair, shampoo the scalp, and give mouth care, as appropriate. Provide perineal care, and clean inside the patient's nose and the folds of the ears and eyes with cotton-tipped applicators.
▶ Gently scrub burned areas with fluffed gauze pads *to remove topical agents, exudates, necrotic tissue, and other debris.* Debride the wound after turning off the agitator.

▶ Exercise the patient's extremities with active or passive range of motion, depending on his condition and exercise tolerance. Alternatively, you may have the physical therapist exercise the patient.

▶ After you've completed the treatment, use the hoist to raise the patient above the water.

▶ With the patient still suspended over the water, spray-rinse his body *to remove debris from shaving, cleaning, and debridement.*

▶ Transfer the patient to a stretcher covered with a clean sheet and bath blanket, and cover him with a warm sterile sheet (a blanket may be added for warmth). Pat unburned areas dry *to prevent chilling.*

▶ Remove the wet or damp sheets and cover the patient with dry sheets. Remove your gown, gloves, and mask before transporting the patient to the dressing area for further debridement, if needed, and new sterile dressings.

▶ Have the tub drained, cleaned, and disinfected according to facility policy.

Special considerations

▶ Remain with the patient at all times *to prevent accidents in the tub.* Limit hydrotherapy to 20 or 30 minutes. Watch the patient closely for adverse reactions.

▶ Patients with an endotracheal tube may receive hydrotherapy. Spray their wounds while they're suspended over the tub on a plinth. Immerse patients with long-standing tracheostomies only with a doctor's order.

▶ If necessary, weigh the patient during hydrotherapy *to assess nutritional status and fluid shift.* Use a hoist that has a table scale.

▶ Whirlpool treatments should be discontinued when the wounds are assessed as clean *because the whirlpool's agitating water may result in trauma to the regenerating tissue.*

Complications

Incomplete disinfection of tub, drains, and faucets or cross-contamination from members of the tubbing team may cause infection. The patient may chill easily from decreased resistance to temperature changes. A fluid or electrolyte imbalance (or both) may result from a chemical imbalance between the patient and the tub solution.

Documentation

Record the date, time, and patient's reaction. Note the patient's condition (including vital signs and wound appearance). Document any wound infection or bleeding. Note treatments given, such as debridement, and dressing changes. Record any special treatments in the nursing plan of care.

HYPERTHERMIA-HYPOTHERMIA THERAPY

A blanket-sized aquathermia K pad, the hyperthermia-hypothermia blanket raises, lowers, or maintains body temperature through conductive heat or cold transfer between the blanket and the patient. It can be operated manually or automatically.

In manual operation, the nurse or doctor sets the temperature on the unit. The blanket reaches and maintains this temperature regardless of the patient's temperature. The temperature control must be adjusted manually to reach a different setting. The nurse monitors the patient's body temperature with a conventional thermometer.

In automatic operation, the unit directly and continually monitors the patient's temperature by means of a thermistor probe (rectal, skin, or esophageal) and alternates heating and cooling cycles as necessary to achieve and maintain the desired body temperature. The thermistor probe also may be used in conjunction with manual operation but isn't essential. The unit is equipped with an alarm to warn of abnormal temperature fluctuations and a circuit breaker that protects against current overload.

The blanket is most commonly used to reduce high fever when more conservative measures — such as baths, ice packs, and antipyretics — are unsuccessful. Other uses include maintaining normal temperature during surgery or shock; inducing hypothermia during surgery to decrease metabolic activity and thereby reduce oxygen requirements; reducing intracranial pressure; controlling bleeding and intractable pain in patients with amputations, burns, or cancer; and providing warmth in cases of severe hypothermia.

Key nursing diagnoses and patient outcomes

Hypothermia related to (specify)
The patient will:
▶ maintain a normal body temperature
▶ not shiver
▶ express feelings of comfort
▶ exhibit warm, dry skin
▶ maintain a heart rate and blood pressure within normal limits
▶ show no complications associated with hypothermia and rapid warming, such as soft-tissue injury, fracture, dehydration, and hypovolemia shock.

Hyperthermia related to (specify)
The patient will:
▶ maintain a normal body temperature
▶ experience no seizure activity
▶ state increased comfort.

Deficient knowledge related to lack of exposure to hyperthermia-hypothermia blanket
The patient will:
▶ communicate feelings of anxiety
▶ state an understanding of the blanket's use.

Equipment

Hyperthermia-hypothermia control unit • operation manual • fluid for the control unit (distilled water or distilled water and 20% ethyl alcohol) • thermistor probe (such as rectal, skin, or esophageal) • patient thermometer • one or two hyperthermia-hypothermia blankets • one or two disposable blanket covers (or one or two sheets or bath blankets) • lanolin or a mixture of lanolin and cold cream • adhesive tape • towel • sphygmomanometer • gloves and gown, if necessary • optional: protective wraps for the patient's hands and feet

Disposable hyperthermia-hypothermia blankets are available for single-patient use.

Preparation of equipment

First, read the operation manual. Inspect the control unit and each blanket for leaks and the plugs and connecting wires for broken prongs, kinks, and fraying. If you detect or suspect malfunction, don't use the equipment.

Review the doctor's order, and prepare one or two blankets by covering them with disposable covers (or use a sheet or bath blanket when positioning the blanket on the patient). *The cover absorbs perspiration and condensation, which could cause tissue breakdown if left on the skin.* Connect the blanket to the control unit, and set the controls for manual or automatic operation and for the desired blanket or body temperature. Make sure the machine is properly grounded before plugging it in.

Turn on the machine and add liquid to the unit reservoir, if necessary, as fluid fills the blanket. Allow the blanket to preheat or precool *so that the patient receives immediate thermal benefit.*

Implementation

▶ Assess the patient's condition and explain the procedure to him. Provide privacy and make sure the room is warm and free from drafts. Check facility policy and, if necessary, make sure the patient or a responsible family member has signed a consent form.
▶ Wash your hands thoroughly. If the patient isn't already wearing a patient gown, ask him to put one on. Use a gown with cloth ties rather than metal snaps or pins *to prevent heat or cold injury.*
▶ Take the patient's temperature, pulse, respirations, and blood pressure *to serve as a baseline* and assess his level of consciousness, pupil reaction, limb strength, and skin condition.
▶ Keeping the bottom sheet in place and the patient recumbent, roll the patient to one side and slide the blanket halfway underneath him so that its top edge aligns with his neck. Then roll the patient back, and pull and flatten the blanket across the bed. Place a pillow under the patient's head. Make sure that his head doesn't lie directly on the blanket *because the blanket's rigid surface may be uncomfortable and the heat or cold*

may lead to tissue breakdown. If necessary, use a sheet or bath blanket as insulation between the patient and the blanket.
▶ Apply lanolin or a mixture of lanolin and cold cream to the patient's skin where it touches the blanket *to help protect the skin from heat or cold sensation.*
▶ In automatic operation, insert the thermistor probe in the patient's rectum and tape it in place to prevent accidental dislodgment. If rectal insertion is contraindicated, tuck a skin probe deep into the axilla and secure it with tape. If the patient is comatose or anesthetized, insert an esophageal probe. Plug the other end of the probe into the correct jack on the unit's control panel.
▶ Place a sheet or, if ordered, the second hyperthermia-hypothermia blanket over the patient. *This increases the thermal benefit by trapping cooled or heated air.*
▶ Wrap the patient's hands and feet if he wishes *to minimize chilling and promote comfort.* Monitor vital signs and perform a neurologic assessment every 5 minutes until the desired body temperature is reached and then every 15 minutes until temperature is stable or as ordered.
▶ Check fluid intake and output hourly or as ordered. Observe the patient regularly for color changes in skin, lips, and nail beds and for edema, induration, inflammation, pain, and sensory impairment. If they occur, discontinue the procedure and notify the doctor.
▶ Reposition the patient every 30 minutes to 1 hour, unless contraindicated, *to prevent skin breakdown.* Keep the patient's skin, bedclothes, and blanket cover free from perspiration and con-

Using a warming system

Shivering, which is the compensatory response to falling body temperature, may use more oxygen than the body can supply—especially in a surgical patient. In the past, you would cover the patient with blankets to warm his body. Now, health care facilities may supply a warming system, such as the Bair Hugger patient-warming system (shown below).

This new system helps to gradually increase body temperature. Like a large hair dryer, the warming unit draws air through a filter, warms the air to the desired temperature, and circulates it through a hose connected to a warming blanket that is placed over the patient.

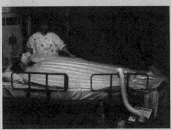

When using the warming system, follow these guidelines:

■ Use a bath blanket in a single layer over the warming blanket to minimize heat loss.

■ Place the warming blanket directly over the patient with the paper side facing down and the clear tubular side facing up.

■ Make sure the connection hose is at the foot of the bed.

■ Take the patient's temperature during the first 15 to 30 minutes and at least every 30 minutes while the warming blanket is in use.

■ Obtain guidelines from the patient's doctor for discontinuing use of the warming blanket.

densation and reapply cream to exposed body parts as needed.

▶ After turning off the machine, follow the manufacturer's directions. *Some units must remain plugged in for at least 30 minutes to allow the condenser fan to remove water vapor from the mechanism.* Continue to monitor the patient's temperature until it stabilizes *because body temperature can fall as much as 5° F (2.8° C) after this procedure.*

▶ Remove all equipment from the bed. Dry the patient and make him comfortable. Supply a fresh patient gown, if necessary. Cover him lightly.

▶ Continue to perform neurologic checks and monitor vital signs, fluid intake and output, and general condition every 30 minutes for 2 hours and then hourly or as ordered.

▶ Return the equipment to the central supply department for cleaning, servicing, and storage.

Special considerations

▶ If the patient shivers excessively during hypothermia treatment, discontinue the procedure and notify the doctor immediately. *By increasing metabolism, shivering elevates body temperature.*

▶ Avoid lowering the temperature more than 1 degree every 15 minutes *to prevent premature ventricular contractions.*

▶ Don't use pins to secure catheters, tubes, or blanket covers *because an accidental puncture can result in fluid leakage and burns.*

▶ With hyperthermia or hypothermia therapy, the patient may experience a secondary defense reaction (such as vasoconstriction or vasodilation, respectively) that causes body temperature to rebound and thus defeat the treatment's purpose.

▶ If the patient requires isolation, place the blanket, blanket cover, and probe in a plastic bag clearly marked with the type of isolation *so that the central supply department can give it special handling.* If the blanket is disposable, discard it, using appropriate precautions.

▶ To avoid bacterial growth in the reservoir or blankets, always use sterile distilled water and change it monthly. Check to see if facility policy calls for adding a bacteriostatic agent to the water. Avoid using deionized water *because it may corrode the system.*

▶ To gradually increase body temperature, especially in postoperative patients, the doctor may order a disposable warming system. (See *Using a warming system.*)

Complications

Use of a hyperthermia-hypothermia blanket can cause shivering, marked changes in vital signs, increased intracranial pressure, respiratory distress or arrest, cardiac arrest, oliguria, and anuria.

Documentation

Record the patient's pulse, respirations, blood pressure, neurologic signs, fluid intake and output, skin condition, and position change. Record the patient's temperature and that of the blanket every 30 minutes while the blanket is in use. Also document the type of hyperthermia-hypothermia unit used; control settings (manual or automatic and temperature settings); date, time, duration, and patient's tolerance of treatment; and signs of complications.

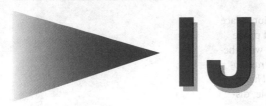

I.M. INJECTION

Intramuscular (I.M.) injections deposit medication deep into muscle tissue. This route of administration provides rapid systemic action and absorption of relatively large doses (up to 5 ml in appropriate sites). I.M. injections are recommended for patients who can't take medication orally, when I.V. administration is inappropriate, and for drugs that are altered by digestive juices. Because muscle tissue has few sensory nerves, I.M. injection allows less painful administration of irritating drugs.

The site for an I.M. injection must be chosen carefully, taking into account the patient's general physical status and the purpose of the injection. I.M. injections shouldn't be administered at inflamed, edematous, or irritated sites or at sites that contain moles, birthmarks, scar tissue, or other lesions. I.M. injections may also be contraindicated in patients with impaired coagulation mechanisms, occlusive peripheral vascular disease, edema, and shock; after thrombolytic therapy; and during an acute myocardial infarction because these conditions impair peripheral absorption. I.M. injections require sterile technique to maintain the integrity of muscle tissue.

Oral or I.V. routes are preferred for administration of drugs that are poorly absorbed by muscle tissue, such as phenytoin, digoxin, chlordiazepoxide, and diazepam.

Key nursing diagnoses and patient outcomes

Deficient knowledge related to a lack of exposure to I.M. injections
The patient will:
▶ state or demonstrate understanding of what has been taught
▶ demonstrate an ability to perform new health-related behaviors as they're taught.

Risk for injury related to improper technique
The patient will:
▶ identify factors that increase risk of injury
▶ assist in identifying and applying safety measures to prevent injury.

Equipment

Patient's medication record and chart • prescribed medication • diluent or filter needle, if needed • 3- or 5-ml syringe • 20G to 25G 1″ to 3″ needle • gloves • alcohol pads • optional: gauze pad, 1″ tape, and ice

The prescribed medication must be sterile. The needle may be packaged separately or already attached to the syringe. Needles used for I.M. injections are longer than subcutaneous needles because they must reach deep into the muscle. Needle length also depends on the injection site, patient's size, and amount of subcutaneous fat covering the muscle. The needle gauge for I.M. injections should be larger to accommodate viscous solutions and suspensions.

Preparation of equipment

Verify the order on the patient's medication record by checking it against the doctor's order. Also note whether the patient has any allergies, especially before the first dose.

Check the prescribed medication for color and clarity. Also note the expiration date. Never use medication that is cloudy or discolored or contains a precipitate unless the manufacturer's instructions allow it. Remember that for some drugs (such as suspensions), the presence of drug particles is normal. Observe for abnormal changes. If in doubt, check with the pharmacist.

Choose equipment appropriate to the prescribed medication and injection site, and make sure it works properly. The needle should be straight, smooth, and free from burrs.

For single-dose ampules

Wrap an alcohol pad around the ampule's neck and snap off the top, directing the force away from your body. Attach a filter needle to the needle and withdraw the medication, keeping the needle's bevel tip below the level of the solution. Tap the syringe *to clear air from it.* Cover the needle with the needle sheath.

Before discarding the ampule, check the medication label against the patient's medication record. Discard the filter needle and the ampule. Attach the appropriate needle to the syringe.

For single-dose or multidose vials

Reconstitute powdered drugs according to instructions. Make sure all crystals have dissolved in the solution. Warm the vial by rolling it between your palms *to help the drug dissolve faster.*

Wipe the stopper of the medication vial with an alcohol pad and draw up the prescribed amount of medication. Read the medication label as you select the medication, as you draw it up, and after you've drawn it up *to verify the correct dosage.*

Don't use an air bubble in the syringe. *A holdover from the days of reusable syringes, air bubbles can affect the medication dosage by 5% to 100%.* Modern disposable syringes are calibrated to administer the correct dose without an air bubble.

Gather all necessary equipment and proceed to the patient's room.

Implementation

▶ Confirm the patient's identity by asking his name and checking his wristband for name, room number, and bed number.

▶ Provide privacy, explain the procedure to the patient, and wash your hands.

▶ Select an appropriate injection site. The gluteal muscles (gluteus medius and minimus and the upper outer corner of the gluteus maximus) are used most commonly for healthy adults, although the deltoid muscle may be used for a small-volume injection (2 ml or less). Remember to rotate injection sites for patients who require repeated injections.

Age alert For infants and children, the vastus lateralis muscle of the thigh is used most often because *it's usually the best developed and contains no large nerves or blood vessels, minimizing the risk of serious injury.* **The rectus femoris muscle may also be used in infants but is usually contraindicated in adults.**

▶ Position and drape the patient appropriately, making sure the site is well exposed and that lighting is adequate.

▶ Loosen the protective needle sheath but don't remove it.

▶ After selecting the injection site, gently tap it *to stimulate the nerve endings and minimize pain when the needle is inserted.* (See *Locating I.M. injection sites.*) Clean the skin at the site with an alcohol pad. Move the pad outward in a circular motion to a circumference of about 2″ (5 cm) from the injection site and allow the skin to dry. Keep the alcohol pad for later use.

▶ Put on gloves. With the thumb and index finger of your nondominant hand, gently stretch the skin of the injection site taut.

▶ While you hold the syringe in your dominant hand, remove the needle sheath by slipping it between the free fingers of your nondominant hand and then drawing back the syringe.

▶ Position the syringe at a 90-degree angle to the skin surface with the needle a couple of inches from the skin. Tell the patient that he'll feel a prick as you insert the needle. Then quickly and firmly thrust the needle through the skin and subcutaneous tissue, deep into the muscle.

▶ Support the syringe with your nondominant hand, if desired. Pull back slightly on the plunger with your dominant hand to aspirate for blood. If no blood appears, slowly inject the medication into the muscle. *A slow, steady injection rate allows the muscle to distend gradually and accept the medication under minimal pressure.* You should feel little or no resistance against the force of the injection.

▶ If blood appears in the syringe on aspiration, the needle is in a blood vessel. If this occurs, stop the injection, withdraw the needle, prepare another injection with new equipment, and inject another site. Don't inject the bloody solution.

▶ After the injection, gently but quickly remove the needle at a 90-degree angle.

▶ Using a gloved hand, cover the injection site immediately with the used alcohol pad, apply gentle pressure and, unless contraindicated, massage the relaxed muscle to help distribute the drug.

▶ Remove the alcohol pad and inspect the injection site for signs of active bleeding or bruising. If bleeding continues, apply pressure to the site; if bruising occurs, you may apply ice.

▶ Watch for adverse reactions at the site for 10 to 30 minutes after the injection.

Age alert **An elderly patient will probably bleed or ooze from the site after the injection because of decreased tissue elasticity. Applying a small pressure bandage may be helpful.**

▶ Discard all equipment according to standard precautions and your facility's policy. Don't recap needles; dispose of them in an appropriate sharps container *to avoid needle-stick injuries.*

Special considerations

▶ To slow their absorption, some drugs for I.M. administration are dissolved in

Locating I.M. injection sites

Deltoid
Find the lower edge of the acromial process and the point on the lateral arm in line with the axilla. Insert the needle 1″ to 2″ (2.5 to 5 cm) below the acromial process, usually two or three fingerbreadths, at a 90-degree angle or angled slightly toward the process. Typical injection: 0.5 ml (range: 0.5 to 2.0 ml).

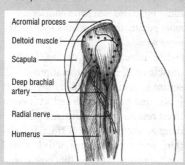

Ventrogluteal
Locate the greater trochanter of the femur with the heel of your hand. Then spread your index and middle fingers from the anterior superior iliac spine to as far along the iliac crest as you can reach. Insert the needle between the two fingers at a 90-degree angle to the muscle. (Remove your fingers before inserting the needle.) Typical injection: 1 to 4 ml (range: 1 to 5 ml).

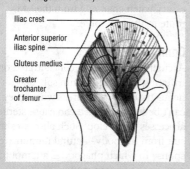

Dorsogluteal
Inject above and outside a line drawn from the posterior superior iliac spine to the greater trochanter of the femur. Or, divide the buttock into quadrants and inject in the upper outer quadrant, about 2″ to 3″ (5 to 7.5 cm) below the iliac crest. Insert the needle at a 90-degree angle. Typical injection: 1 to 4 ml (range: 1 to 5 ml).

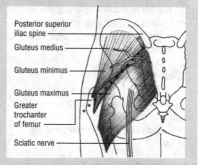

Vastus lateralis
Use the lateral muscle of the quadriceps group, from a handbreadth below the greater trochanter to a handbreadth above the knee. Insert the needle into the middle third of the muscle parallel to the surface on which the patient is lying. You may have to bunch the muscle before insertion. Typical injection: 1 to 4 ml (range: 1 to 5 ml; 1 to 3 ml for infants).

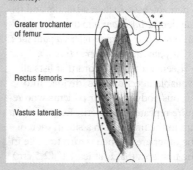

Documenting administration of narcotics

Regulations require narcotics to be counted after each nursing shift to ensure an accurate drug count. Before administering a narcotic, verify the amount of drug in the container, and sign out the medication on the appropriate form.

Another regulation requires that a second nurse document your activity and observe you if part of a narcotic dose must be wasted.

What to report

If you discover a discrepancy in the narcotic count, follow your facility's policy for reporting this. You'll need to file an incident report as well. An investigation will follow.

---

oil or other special solutions. Mix these preparations well before drawing them into the syringe.

 Age alert **The gluteal muscles can be used as the injection site only after a toddler has been walking for about 1 year.**

▶ Never inject into sensitive muscles, especially those that twitch or tremble when you assess site landmarks and tissue depth. *Injections into these trigger areas may cause sharp or referred pain such as the pain caused by nerve trauma.*

▶ Keep a rotation record that lists all available injection sites, divided into various body areas, for patients who require repeated injections. Rotate from a site in the first area to a site in each of the other areas. Then return to a site in the first area that is at least 1″ (2.5 cm)

away from the previous injection site in that area.

▶ If the patient has experienced pain or emotional trauma from repeated injections, consider numbing the area before cleaning it by holding ice on it for several seconds. If you must inject more than 5 ml of solution, divide the solution and inject it at two separate sites.

▶ Always encourage the patient to relax the muscle you'll be injecting *because injections into tense muscles are more painful than usual and may bleed more readily.*

▶ I.M. injections can damage local muscle cells, causing elevations in serum enzyme levels (creatine kinase [CK]) that can be confused with elevations resulting from cardiac muscle damage such as in myocardial infarction. *To distinguish between skeletal and cardiac muscle damage,* diagnostic tests for suspected myocardial infarction must identify the isoenzyme of CK specific to cardiac muscle (CK-MB) and include tests to determine lactate dehydrogenase and aspartate aminotransferase levels. If it's important to measure these enzyme levels, suggest that the doctor switch to I.V. administration and adjust dosages accordingly.

▶ Dosage adjustments are usually necessary when changing from the I.M. route to the oral route.

Complications

Accidental injection of concentrated or irritating medications into subcutaneous tissue or other areas where they can't be fully absorbed can cause sterile abscesses to develop. Such abscesses result from the body's natural immune response in which phagocytes attempt to remove the foreign matter.

Failure to rotate sites in patients who require repeated injections can lead to deposits of unabsorbed medications. Such deposits can reduce the desired pharmacologic effect and may lead to abscess formation or tissue fibrosis.

 Age alert Because elderly patients have decreased muscle mass, I.M. medications can be absorbed more quickly than expected.

Documentation

Chart the drug administered, dose, date, time, route of administration, and injection site. Also note the patient's tolerance of the injection and the injection's effects, including any adverse effects. (See *Documenting administration of narcotics.*)

INCENTIVE SPIROMETRY

Incentive spirometry involves using a breathing device to help the patient achieve maximal ventilation. The device measures respiratory flow or respiratory volume and induces the patient to take a deep breath and hold it for several seconds. This deep breath increases lung volume, boosts alveolar inflation, and promotes venous return. This exercise also establishes alveolar hyperinflation for a longer time than is possible with a normal deep breath, thus preventing and reversing the alveolar collapse that causes atelectasis and pneumonitis.

Devices used for incentive spirometry provide a visual incentive to breathe deeply. Some are activated when the patient inhales a certain volume of air; the device then estimates the amount of air inhaled. Others contain plastic floats, which rise according to the amount of air the patient pulls through the device when he inhales.

Patients at low risk for developing atelectasis may use a flow incentive spirometer. Patients at high risk may need a volume incentive spirometer, which measures lung inflation more precisely.

Incentive spirometry benefits the patient on prolonged bed rest, especially the postoperative patient who may regain his normal respiratory pattern slowly due to such predisposing factors as abdominal or thoracic surgery, advanced age, inactivity, obesity, smoking, and decreased ability to cough effectively and expel lung secretions.

Key nursing diagnoses and patient outcomes

Ineffective breathing pattern related to decreased energy
The patient will:
▶ achieve maximum lung expansion with adequate ventilation
▶ report feeling comfortable with breathing.

Impaired gas exchange related to altered oxygen supply
The patient will:
▶ cough effectively
▶ expectorate sputum.

Equipment

Flow or volume incentive spirometer, as indicated, with sterile disposable tube and mouthpiece (the tube and mouthpiece are sterile on first use and clean on subsequent uses) • stethoscope • watch • pencil and paper

Better charting

Documenting flow and volume levels

If you've used a flow incentive spirometer, compute the volume by multiplying the setting by the duration that the patient kept the ball (or balls) suspended. For example, if the patient suspended the ball for 3 seconds at a setting of 500 cc during each of 10 breaths, multiply 500 cc by 3 seconds and then record this total (1,500 cc) and the number of breaths as follows: 1,500 cc × 10 breaths.

If you've used a volume incentive spirometer, take the volume reading directly from the spirometer. For example, record 1,000 cc × 5 breaths.

Preparation of equipment

Assemble the ordered equipment at the patient's bedside. Read the manufacturer's instructions for spirometer setup and operation.

Remove the sterile flow tube and mouthpiece from the package and attach them to the device. Set the flow rate or volume goal as determined by the doctor or respiratory therapist and based on the patient's preoperative performance. Turn on the machine if necessary.

Implementation

▶ Assess the patient's condition.
▶ Explain the procedure to the patient, making sure that he understands the importance of performing incentive spirometry regularly *to maintain alveolar inflation*. Wash your hands.
▶ Help the patient into a comfortable sitting or semi-Fowler's position *to promote optimal lung expansion*. If you're using a flow incentive spirometer and

the patient is unable to assume or maintain this position, he can perform the procedure in any position as long as the device remains upright. *Tilting a flow incentive spirometer decreases the required patient effort and reduces the exercise's effectiveness.*
▶ Auscultate the patient's lungs *to provide a baseline for comparison with posttreatment auscultation.*
▶ Instruct the patient to insert the mouthpiece and close his lips tightly around it *because a weak seal may alter flow or volume readings.*
▶ Instruct the patient to exhale normally and then inhale as slowly and as deeply as possible. If he has difficulty with this step, tell him to suck as he would through a straw but more slowly. Ask the patient to retain the entire volume of air he inhaled for 3 seconds or, if you're using a device with a light indicator, until the light turns off. This deep breath creates sustained transpulmonary pressure near the end of inspiration and is sometimes called a sustained maximal inspiration.
▶ Tell the patient to remove the mouthpiece and exhale normally. Allow him to relax and take several normal breaths before attempting another breath with the spirometer. Repeat this sequence 5 to 10 times during every waking hour. Note tidal volumes.
▶ Evaluate the patient's ability to cough effectively and encourage him to cough after each effort *because deep lung inflation may loosen secretions and facilitate their removal.* Observe any expectorated secretions.
▶ Auscultate the patient's lungs, and compare findings with the first auscultation.
▶ Instruct the patient to remove the mouthpiece. Wash the device in warm

water and shake it dry. Avoid immersing the spirometer itself *because this enhances bacterial growth and impairs the internal filter's effectiveness in preventing inhalation of extraneous material.*

▶ Place the mouthpiece in a plastic storage bag between exercises and label it and the spirometer, if applicable, with the patient's name *to avoid inadvertent use by another patient.*

Special considerations

▶ If the patient is scheduled for surgery, make a preoperative assessment of his respiratory pattern and capability *to ensure the development of appropriate postoperative goals.* Teach the patient how to use the spirometer before surgery *so that he can concentrate on your instructions and practice the exercise.* A preoperative evaluation will also help in establishing a postoperative therapeutic goal.

▶ Avoid exercising at mealtime *to prevent nausea.* Provide paper and *pencil so the patient can note exercise times.* Exercise frequency varies with condition and ability.

▶ Immediately after surgery, monitor the exercise frequently *to ensure compliance and assess achievement.*

Documentation

Record any preoperative teaching you provided. Document preoperative flow or volume levels, the date and time of the procedure, the type of spirometer, the flow or volume levels achieved, and the number of breaths taken. (See *Documenting flow and volume levels.*) Also note the patient's condition before and after the procedure, his tolerance of the procedure, and the results of both auscultations.

INCONTINENCE DEVICE APPLICATION AND REMOVAL

Many patients don't require an indwelling urinary catheter to manage their incontinence. For male patients, a male incontinence device reduces the risk of urinary tract infection from catheterization, promotes bladder retraining when possible, helps prevent skin breakdown, and improves the patient's self-image. The device consists of a condom catheter secured to the shaft of the penis and connected to a leg bag or drainage bag. It has no contraindications but can cause skin irritation and edema.

Key nursing diagnoses and patient outcomes

Impaired urinary elimination related to use of an incontinence device
The patient will:
▶ maintain fluid balance (intake will equal output)
▶ experience few, if any, complications
▶ describe feelings and concerns about use of an incontinence device.

Risk for infection related to use of an incontinence device
The patient will:
▶ have no pathogens in cultures
▶ remain afebrile
▶ show no evidence of urinary tract infection, such as cloudy, malodorous, or sediment-containing urine.

Equipment

Condom catheter • drainage bag • extension tubing • hypoallergenic tape or incontinence sheath holder • commercial adhesive strip or skin-bond cement

How to apply a condom catheter

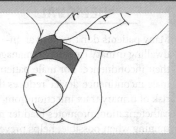

Apply an adhesive strip to the shaft of the penis about 1″ (2.5 cm) from the scrotal area.

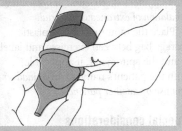

Roll the condom catheter onto the penis past the adhesive strip, leaving about ½″ (1 cm) clearance at the end. Press the sheath gently against the strip until it adheres.

• elastic adhesive or Velcro, if needed • gloves • razor, if needed • basin • soap • washcloth • towel

Preparation of equipment

Fill the basin with lukewarm water. Then bring the basin and the remaining equipment to the patient's bedside.

Implementation

▶ Explain the procedure to the patient, wash your hands thoroughly, put on gloves, and provide privacy.

Applying the device

▶ If the patient is circumcised, wash the penis with soap, water, and a washcloth, rinse well, and pat dry with a towel. If the patient is uncircumcised, gently retract the foreskin and clean beneath it. Rinse well but don't dry *because moisture provides lubrication and prevents friction during foreskin replacement*. Replace the foreskin to avoid penile constriction. Then, if necessary, shave the base and shaft of the penis to *prevent the adhesive strip or skin-bond cement from pulling pubic hair.*

▶ If you're using a precut commercial adhesive strip, insert the glans penis through its opening, and position the strip 1″ (2.5 cm) from the scrotal area. If you're using uncut adhesive, cut a strip to fit around the shaft of the penis. Remove the protective covering from one side of the adhesive strip and press this side firmly to the penis *to enhance adhesion*. Then remove the covering from the other side of the strip. If a commercial adhesive strip isn't available, apply skin-bond cement and let it dry for a few minutes.

▶ Position the rolled condom catheter at the tip of the penis, leaving 1″ between the condom and the tip of the penis, with the drainage opening at the urinary meatus.

▶ Unroll the catheter upward, past the adhesive strip on the shaft of the penis. Gently press the sheath against the strip until it adheres. (See *How to apply a condom catheter.*)

▶ After the condom catheter is in place, secure it with hypoallergenic tape or an incontinence sheath holder.

▶ Using extension tubing, connect the condom catheter to the leg bag or drainage bag. Remove and discard your gloves.

Removing the device

▶ Put on gloves and simultaneously roll the condom catheter and adhesive strip off the penis and discard them. If you've used skin-bond cement rather than an adhesive strip, remove it with solvent. Also remove and discard the hypoallergenic tape or incontinence sheath holder.

▶ Clean the penis with lukewarm water, rinse thoroughly, and dry. Check for swelling or signs of skin breakdown.

▶ Remove the leg bag by closing the drain clamp, unlatching the leg straps, and disconnecting the extension tubing at the top of the bag. Discard your gloves.

Special considerations

▶ If hypoallergenic tape or an incontinence sheath holder isn't available, secure the condom with a strip of elastic adhesive or Velcro. Apply the strip snugly — but not too tightly — to *prevent circulatory constriction*.

▶ Inspect the condom catheter for twists and the extension tubing for kinks *to prevent obstruction of urine flow, which could cause the condom to balloon, eventually dislodging it.*

Documentation

Record the date and time of application and removal of the incontinence device. Also note skin condition and the patient's response to the device, including voiding pattern, to assist with bladder retraining.

INCONTINENCE MANAGEMENT

In elderly patients, incontinence commonly follows any loss or impairment of urinary or anal sphincter control. The incontinence may be transient or permanent. In all, about 10 million adults experience some form of urinary incontinence; this includes about 50% of the 1.5 million people in extended care facilities. Fecal incontinence affects up to 10% of the patients in such facilities.

Contrary to popular opinion, urinary incontinence is neither a disease nor a part of normal aging. Incontinence may be caused by confusion, dehydration, fecal impaction, or restricted mobility. It's also a sign of various disorders, such as prostatic hyperplasia, bladder calculus, bladder cancer, urinary tract infection (UTI), cerebrovascular accident (CVA), diabetic neuropathy, Guillain-Barré syndrome, multiple sclerosis, prostatic cancer, prostatitis, spinal cord injury, and urethral stricture. It may also result from urethral sphincter damage after prostatectomy. In addition, certain drugs, including diuretics, hypnotics, sedatives, anticholinergics, antihypertensives, and alpha antagonists, may trigger urinary incontinence.

Urinary incontinence is classified as acute or chronic. Acute urinary incontinence results from disorders that are potentially reversible, such as delirium, dehydration, urine retention, restricted mobility, fecal impaction, infection or inflammation, drug reactions, and polyuria. Chronic urinary incontinence occurs as four distinct types: stress, overflow, urge, and functional incontinence.

Artificial urinary sphincter implant

An artificial urinary sphincter implant can help restore continence to a patient with a neurogenic bladder. Criteria for inserting an implant include:

■ incontinence associated with a weak urinary sphincter

■ incoordination between the detrusor muscle and the urinary sphincter (if drug therapy fails)

■ inadequate bladder storage (if intermittent catheterization and drug therapy are unsuccessful).

Configuration and placement

An implant consists of a control pump, an occlusive cuff, and a pressure-regulating balloon. The cuff is placed around the bladder neck, and the balloon is placed under the rectus muscle in the abdomen. The balloon holds fluid that inflates the cuff. In men, the surgeon places the control pump in the scrotum; in women, the surgeon places the pump in the labium.

Using the implant

To void, the patient squeezes the bulb to deflate the cuff, which opens the urethra by returning fluid to the balloon. After voiding, the cuff reinflates automatically, sealing the urethra until the patient needs to void again.

Complications and care

If complications develop, the implant may need to be repaired or removed. Possible complications include cuff leakage (uncommon), trapped blood or other fluid contaminants (which can cause control pump problems), skin erosion around the bulb or erosion in the bladder neck or the urethra, infection, inadequate occlusion pressures, and kinked tubing. If the bladder holds residual urine, intermittent self-catheterization may be needed.

Care includes avoiding strenuous activity for about 6 months after surgery and having regular checkups.

Implant position in a man

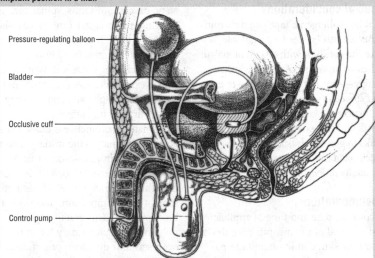

Pressure-regulating balloon

Bladder

Occlusive cuff

Control pump

In *stress incontinence,* leakage results from a sudden physical strain, such as a sneeze, cough, or quick movement. In *overflow incontinence,* urine retention causes dribbling because the distended bladder can't contract strongly enough to force a urine stream. In *urge incontinence,* the patient can't control the impulse to urinate. Finally, in *functional (total) incontinence,* urine leakage occurs despite the fact that the bladder and urethra are functioning normally. This condition is usually related to cognitive or environmental factors, such as mental impairment or lack of appropriate or timely care.

Fecal incontinence, the involuntary passage of feces, may occur gradually (as in dementia) or suddenly (as in spinal cord injury). It usually results from fecal stasis and impaction secondary to reduced activity, inappropriate diet, or untreated painful anal conditions. It can also result from chronic laxative use; reduced fluid intake; neurologic deficit; pelvic, prostatic, or rectal surgery; and the use of certain medications, including antihistamines, psychotropics, and iron preparations. Not usually a sign of serious illness, fecal incontinence can seriously impair an elderly patient's physical and psychological well-being.

Patients with urinary or fecal incontinence should be carefully assessed for underlying disorders. Most can be treated; some can even be cured. Treatment aims to control the condition through bladder or bowel retraining or other behavior management techniques, diet modification, drug therapy, and possibly surgery. Corrective surgery for urinary incontinence includes transurethral resection of the prostate in men, repair of the anterior vaginal wall or retropelvic suspension of the bladder in women, urethral sling, and bladder augmentation. (See *Artificial urinary sphincter implant,* page 418, and *Correcting urinary incontinence with bladder retraining,* page 420.)

Key nursing diagnoses and patient outcomes

Functional urinary incontinence related to (specify)
The patient will:
▶ void in an appropriate situation using a suitable receptacle
▶ void at specific times
▶ have no wet episodes
▶ demonstrate skill in managing incontinence
▶ discuss the impact of incontinence on self and significant other
▶ identify resources to assist with care after discharge.

Bowel incontinence related to (specify)
The patient will:
▶ establish and maintain a regular pattern of bowel care
▶ state an understanding of the bowel care routine
▶ demonstrate skill in carrying out the bowel care routine.

Social isolation related to incontinence
The patient will:
▶ express feelings associated with social isolation
▶ participate in developing a plan for increasing social activity
▶ report improved social relationships and diminished negative feelings
▶ achieve expected state of wellness.

Equipment
Bladder retraining record sheet • gloves • stethoscope (to assess bowel sounds)

Correcting urinary incontinence with bladder retraining

The incontinent patient typically feels frustrated, embarrassed, and hopeless. Fortunately, his problem can usually be corrected by bladder retraining—a program that aims to establish a regular voiding pattern. Follow these guidelines.

Assess elimination patterns

First, assess the patient's intake and voiding patterns and reason for each accidental voiding (such as a coughing spell). Use an incontinence monitoring record for 3 to 7 days. Evaluate the record and note if there is a pattern of incontinence.

Establish a voiding schedule

Encourage the patient to void regularly, for example, every 2 hours. After he can stay dry for 2 hours, increase the interval by 30 minutes every day until he achieves a 3- to 4-hour voiding schedule. Teach the patient to practice relaxation techniques such as deep breathing, which help decrease the sense of urgency.

Record results and remain positive

Use the incontinence monitoring record to evaluate the effectiveness of the voiding schedule. Revise the schedule as necessary. Remember, both your own and your patient's positive attitudes are crucial to his successful bladder retraining.

Take steps for success

Here are some additional tips to boost the patient's success:
- Situate the patient's bed near a bathroom or portable toilet. Leave a light on at night. If the patient needs assistance getting out of bed or a chair, promptly answer the call for help.
- Teach the patient measures to prevent urinary tract infections, such as adequate fluid intake (at least 2 qt [2 L]/day unless contraindicated), drinking cranberry juice to help acidify urine, wearing cotton underpants, and bathing with nonirritating soaps.
- Encourage the patient to empty his bladder completely before and after meals and at bedtime.
- Advise him to urinate whenever the urge arises and never to ignore it.
- Instruct the patient to take prescribed diuretics upon rising in the morning.
- Advise him to limit the use of sleeping aids, sedatives, and alcohol; *they decrease the urge to urinate and can increase incontinence, especially at night.*
- If the patient is overweight, encourage weight loss.
- Suggest exercises to strengthen pelvic muscles.
- Instruct the patient to increase dietary fiber *to decrease constipation and incontinence.*
- Monitor the patient for signs of anxiety and depression.
- Reassure the patient that periodic incontinent episodes don't mean that the program has failed. Encourage persistence, tolerance, and a positive attitude.

• lubricant • moisture barrier cream • incontinence pads • bedpan • specimen container • label • laboratory request form • optional: stool collection kit and urinary catheter

Implementation

Whether the patient reports urinary or fecal incontinence or both, you'll need to perform initial and continuing assessments to plan effective interventions.

For urinary incontinence

▶ Ask the patient when he first noticed urine leakage and whether it began suddenly or gradually. Have him describe his typical urinary pattern: Does he usually experience incontinence during the day or at night? Ask him to rate his urinary control: Does he have moderate control, or is he completely incontinent? If he sometimes urinates with control, ask him to identify when and how much he usually urinates.

▶ Evaluate related problems, such as urinary hesitancy, frequency, urgency, nocturia, and decreased force or interrupted urine stream. Ask the patient to describe any previous treatment he has had for incontinence or measures he has performed by himself. Also ask about medications, including nonprescription drugs.

▶ Assess the patient's environment. Is a toilet or commode readily available, and how long does the patient take to reach it? When the patient is in the bathroom, assess his manual dexterity; for example, how easily does he manipulate his clothes?

▶ Evaluate the patient's mental status and cognitive function.

▶ Quantify the patient's normal daily fluid intake.

▶ Review the patient's medication and diet history for drugs and foods that affect digestion and elimination.

▶ Review or obtain the patient's medical history, noting especially the number and route of births (in women) and any incidence of UTI, prostate disorders, spinal injury or tumor, CVA, and bladder, prostate, or pelvic surgery. Also assess for such disorders as delirium, dehydration, urine retention, restricted mobility, fecal impaction, infection, inflammation, and polyuria.

▶ Inspect the urethral meatus for obvious inflammation or anatomic defects. Have the female patient bear down while you note any urine leakage. Gently palpate the abdomen for bladder distention, which signals urine retention. If possible, have the patient examined by a urologist.

▶ Obtain specimens for appropriate laboratory tests as ordered. Label each specimen container, and send it to the laboratory with a request form.

▶ Begin incontinence management by implementing an appropriate bladder retraining program.

▶ *To ensure healthful hydration and to prevent UTI,* make sure that the patient maintains an adequate daily intake of fluids (six to eight 8-oz glasses). Restrict fluid intake after 6 p.m.

▶ *To manage stress incontinence,* begin an exercise program to help strengthen the pelvic floor muscles. (See *Strengthening pelvic floor muscles,* page 422.)

▶ *To manage functional incontinence,* frequently assess the patient's mental and functional status. Regularly remind him to void. Respond to his calls promptly and help him get to the bathroom quickly. Provide positive reinforcement.

For fecal incontinence

▶ Ask the patient with fecal incontinence to identify its onset, duration, severity, and pattern (for instance, determine whether it occurs at night or with diarrhea). Focus the history on GI, neurologic, and psychological disorders.

▶ Note the frequency, consistency, and volume of stool passed in the past 24 hours. Obtain a stool specimen if ordered. Protect the patient's bed with an incontinence pad.

Strengthening pelvic floor muscles

Stress incontinence, the most common kind of urinary incontinence in women, usually results from weakening of the urethral sphincter. In men, it may sometimes occur after a radical prostatectomy.

You can help a patient prevent or minimize stress incontinence by teaching her pelvic floor (Kegel) exercises to strengthen the pubococcygeal muscles. Here is how.

Learning Kegel exercises

First, explain how to locate the muscles of the pelvic floor. Instruct the patient to tense the muscles around the anus, as if to retain stool.

Next, teach her to tighten the muscles of the pelvic floor to stop the flow of urine while urinating and then to release the muscles to restart the flow. When learned, these exercises can be done anywhere at any time.

Establishing a regimen

Explain to the patient that contraction and relaxation exercises are essential to muscle retraining. Suggest that she start out by contracting the pelvic floor muscles for 10 seconds, relax for 10 seconds, and then repeat the procedure as often as needed.

Typically, the patient starts with 15 contractions in the morning and afternoon and 20 at night. Or, she may exercise for 10 minutes three times per day, working up to 25 contractions at a time as strength improves.

Advise the patient not to use stomach, leg, or buttock muscles. Also discourage leg crossing or breath holding during these exercises.

▶ Assess for chronic constipation, GI and neurologic disorders, and laxative abuse. Inspect the abdomen for distention, and auscultate for bowel sounds. If not contraindicated, put on gloves, apply lubricant, and check for fecal impaction (a factor in overflow incontinence). Remove gloves when finished. Checking for fecal impaction may stimulate a bowel movement, so keep a bedpan readily available.

▶ Assess the patient's medication regimen. Check for drugs that affect bowel activity, such as aspirin, some anticholinergic antiparkinsonians, aluminum hydroxide, calcium carbonate antacids, diuretics, iron preparations, opiates, tranquilizers, tricyclic antidepressants, and phenothiazines.

▶ For the neurologically capable patient with chronic incontinence, provide bowel retraining.

▶ Advise the patient to consume a fiber-rich diet that includes lots of raw, leafy vegetables (such as carrots and lettuce), unpeeled fruits (such as apples), and whole grains (such as wheat or rye breads and cereals). If the patient has a lactase deficiency, suggest that he take calcium supplements to replace calcium lost by eliminating dairy products from the diet.

▶ Encourage adequate fluid intake.

▶ Teach the elderly patient to gradually eliminate laxative use. Point out that using laxatives to promote regular bowel movement may have the opposite effect, producing either constipation or incontinence over time. Suggest natural laxatives, such as prunes and prune juice, instead.

▶ Promote regular exercise by explaining how it helps to regulate bowel motility. Even a nonambulatory patient can perform some exercises while sitting or lying in bed.

Special considerations

▶ To rid the bladder of residual urine, teach the patient to perform Valsalva's or Credé's maneuver or institute clean intermittent catheterization. Use an indwelling urinary catheter only as a last resort *because of the risk of UTI.*

▶ For fecal incontinence, maintain effective hygienic care *to increase the patient's comfort and prevent skin breakdown and infection.* Clean the perineal area frequently and apply a moisture barrier cream. Control foul odors as well.

▶ Schedule extra time to provide encouragement and support for the patient, who may feel shame, embarrassment, and powerlessness from loss of control.

Complications

Skin breakdown and infection may result from incontinence. Psychological problems resulting from incontinence include social isolation, loss of independence, lowered self-esteem, and depression.

Documentation

Record all bladder and bowel retraining efforts, noting scheduled bathroom times, food and fluid intake, and elimination amounts, as appropriate. Document the duration of continent periods. Note any complications, including emotional problems and signs of skin breakdown and infection as well as the treatments given for them.

INDWELLING URINARY CATHETER CARE AND REMOVAL

Intended to prevent infection and other complications by keeping the catheter insertion site clean, routine catheter care typically is performed daily after the patient's morning bath and immediately after perineal care. (Bedtime catheter care may have to be performed before perineal care.)

Because some studies suggest that catheter care increases the risk of infection and other complications rather than lowers it, many health care facilities don't recommend daily catheter care. Thus, individual facility policy dictates whether a patient receives such care. Regardless of the catheter care policy, the equipment and the patient's genitalia require inspection twice daily.

An indwelling urinary catheter should be removed when bladder decompression is no longer necessary, when the patient can resume voiding, or when the catheter is obstructed. Depending on the length of the catheterization, the doctor may order bladder retraining before catheter removal.

Key nursing diagnoses and patient outcomes

Impaired urinary elimination related to presence of an indwelling urinary catheter The patient will:

▶ maintain fluid balance (intake will equal output)

▶ have few if any complications

▶ describe feelings and concerns regarding the indwelling urinary catheter.

Risk for infection related to presence of an indwelling urinary catheter
The patient will:
▶ have no pathogens appear in cultures
▶ remain afebrile
▶ show no evidence of urinary tract infection, such as cloudy or malodorous urine or urine with sediment.

Equipment

For catheter care
Soap and water • sterile gloves • eight sterile 4″ × 4″ gauze pads • basin • washcloth • leg bag • collection bag • adhesive tape or leg band • waste receptacle • optional: safety pin, rubber band, gooseneck lamp or flashlight, adhesive remover, and specimen container

For perineal cleaning
Washcloth • additional basin • soap and water

For catheter removal
Gloves • alcohol pad • 10-ml syringe with a luer-lock • bedpan • linen-saver pad • optional: clamp for bladder retraining

Preparation of equipment
Wash your hands and bring all equipment to the patient's bedside. Open the gauze pads, place several in the first basin, and pour some povidone-iodine or other cleaning agent over them.

Some facilities specify that, after wiping the urinary meatus with cleaning solution, you should wipe it off with wet, sterile gauze pads *to prevent possible irritation from the cleaning solution.* If this is your facility's policy, pour water into the second basin, and moisten three more gauze pads.

Implementation
▶ Explain the procedure and its purpose to the patient.
▶ Provide privacy.

Catheter care
▶ Make sure that the lighting is adequate *so that you can see the perineum and catheter tubing clearly.* Place a gooseneck lamp or flashlight at the bedside if needed.
▶ Inspect the catheter for any problems and check the urine drainage for mucus, blood clots, sediment, and turbidity. Then pinch the catheter between two fingers *to determine if the lumen contains any material.* If you notice any of these conditions (or if your facility's policy requires it), obtain a urine specimen (collect at least 3 ml of urine, but don't fill the specimen cup more than halfway) and notify the doctor.
▶ Inspect the outside of the catheter where it enters the urinary meatus for encrusted material and suppurative drainage. Also inspect the tissue around the meatus for irritation or swelling.
▶ Remove the leg band, or if adhesive tape was used to secure the catheter, remove the adhesive tape. Inspect the area for signs and symptoms of adhesive burns—redness, tenderness, or blisters.
▶ Put on the gloves. Clean the outside of the catheter and the tissue around the meatus using soap and water. *To avoid contaminating the urinary tract,* always clean by wiping away from—never toward—the urinary meatus. Use a dry gauze pad to remove encrusted material.

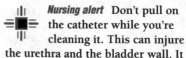 **Nursing alert** Don't pull on the catheter while you're cleaning it. This can injure the urethra and the bladder wall. It

can also expose a section of the catheter that was inside the urethra, so that when you release the catheter, the newly contaminated section will reenter the urethra, introducing potentially infectious organisms.

▶ Remove your gloves, reapply the leg band, and reattach the catheter to the leg band. If a leg band isn't available, tear a piece of adhesive tape from the roll.

▶ *To prevent skin hypersensitivity or irritation*, retape the catheter on the opposite side.

၊|၊ ***Nursing alert*** **Provide enough**
≡■≡ **slack before securing the**
‖၊ **catheter to prevent tension on the tubing, which could injure the urethral lumen or bladder wall.**

▶ Most drainage bags have a plastic clamp on the tubing to attach them to the sheet. If this isn't available, wrap a rubber band around the drainage tubing, insert the safety pin through a loop of the rubber band, and pin the tubing to the sheet below bladder level. Then attach the collection bag, below bladder level, to the bed frame.

▶ If necessary, clean residue from the previous tape site with adhesive remover. Dispose of all used supplies in a waste receptacle.

Catheter removal

▶ Wash your hands. Assemble the equipment at the patient's bedside. Explain the procedure and tell him that he may feel slight discomfort. Tell him that you'll check him periodically during the first 6 to 24 hours after catheter removal *to make sure he resumes voiding.*

▶ Put on gloves. Place a linen-saver pad under the patient's buttocks. Attach the syringe to the luer-lock mechanism on the catheter.

▶ Pull back on the plunger of the syringe. *This deflates the balloon by aspirating the injected fluid.* The amount of fluid injected is usually indicated on the tip of the catheter's balloon lumen and on the Kardex and the patient's chart.

▶ *Because urine may leak as the catheter is removed*, offer the patient a bedpan. Grasp the catheter and pinch it firmly with your thumb and index finger *to prevent urine from flowing back into the urethra.* Gently pull the catheter from the urethra. If you meet resistance, don't apply force, instead notify the doctor. Remove the bedpan.

▶ Measure and record the amount of urine in the collection bag before discarding it. Remove and discard gloves, and wash your hands. For the first 24 hours after catheter removal, note the time and amount of each voiding.

Special considerations

▶ Your facility may require the use of specific cleaning agents for catheter care, so check the policy manual before beginning this procedure.

▶ Avoid raising the drainage bag above bladder level. *This prevents reflux of urine, which may contain bacteria. To avoid damaging the urethral lumen or bladder wall,* always disconnect the drainage bag and tubing from the bed linen and bed frame before helping the patient out of bed.

▶ When possible, attach a leg bag *to allow the patient greater mobility*. If the patient will be discharged with an indwelling catheter, teach him how to use a leg bag. (See *Teaching about leg bags,* page 426.)

▶ Encourage patients with unrestricted fluid intake to increase intake to at least 3 qt (3 L)/day. *This helps flush the urinary system and reduces sediment forma-*

Teaching about leg bags

A urine drainage bag attached to the leg provides the catheterized patient with greater mobility. Because the bag is hidden under clothing, it may also help him feel more comfortable about catheterization. Leg bags are usually worn during the day and are replaced with a standard collection device at night.

If your patient will be discharged with an indwelling catheter, teach him how to attach and remove a leg bag. To demonstrate, you'll need a bag with a short drainage tube, two straps, an alcohol pad, adhesive tape, and a screw clamp or hemostat.

Attaching the leg bag
- Provide privacy and explain the procedure. Describe the advantages of a leg bag but caution the patient that a leg bag is smaller than a standard collection device and may have to be emptied more frequently.
- Remove the protective covering from the tip of the drainage tube. Then show the patient how to clean the tip with an alcohol pad, wiping away from the opening to avoid contaminating the tube. Show him how to attach the tube to the catheter.
- Place the drainage bag on the patient's calf or thigh. Have him fasten the straps securely (as shown), and show him how to tape the catheter to his leg. Emphasize that he must leave slack in the catheter to minimize pressure on the bladder, urethra, and related structures. *Excessive pressure or tension can lead to tissue breakdown.*
- Also tell him not to fasten the straps too tightly *to avoid interfering with his circulation.*

Avoiding complications
- Although most leg bags have a valve in the drainage tube that prevents urine reflux into the bladder, urge the patient to keep the drainage bag lower than his bladder at all

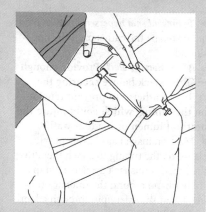

times *because urine in the bag is a perfect growth medium for bacteria.* Also, caution him not to go to bed or take long naps while wearing the drainage bag.
- *To prevent a full leg bag from damaging the bladder wall and urethra,* encourage the patient to empty the bag when it's only half full. He should also inspect the catheter and drainage tube periodically for compression or kinking, *which could obstruct urine flow and result in bladder distention.*
- Tell the patient to wash the leg bag with soap and water or a bacteriostatic solution before each use *to prevent infection.*

tion. *To prevent urinary sediment and calculi from obstructing the drainage tube,* some patients are placed on an acid-ash diet to acidify the urine. Cranberry juice, for example, may help to promote urinary acidity.

▶ After catheter removal, assess the patient for incontinence (or dribbling), urgency, persistent dysuria or bladder spasms, fever, chills, or palpable bladder distention. Report these to the doctor.

▶ When changing catheters after long-term use (usually 30 days), you may need a larger size catheter because the meatus enlarges, causing urine to leak around the catheter.

Home care

Instruct patients discharged with indwelling catheters to wash the urinary meatus and perineal area with soap and water twice daily and the anal area after each bowel movement.

Complications

Sediment buildup can occur anywhere in a catheterization system, especially in bedridden and dehydrated patients. *To prevent this,* keep the patient well hydrated if he isn't on fluid restriction. Change the indwelling catheter as ordered or when malfunction, obstruction, or contamination occurs.

Acute renal failure may result from a catheter obstructed by sediment. Be alert for sharply reduced urine flow from the catheter. Assess for bladder discomfort or distention.

Urinary tract infection can result from catheter insertion or from intraluminal or extraluminal migration of bacteria up the catheter. Signs and symptoms may include cloudy urine, foul-smelling urine, hematuria, fever, malaise, tenderness over the bladder, and flank pain.

Major complications in removing an indwelling catheter are failure of the balloon to deflate and rupture of the balloon. If the balloon ruptures, cystoscopy is usually performed to ensure removal of any balloon fragments.

Documentation

Record the care you performed, any modifications, patient complaints, and the condition of the perineum and urinary meatus. Note the character of the urine in the drainage bag, any sediment buildup, and whether a specimen was sent for laboratory analysis. Also record fluid intake and output. An hourly record is usually necessary for critically ill patients and those with renal insufficiency who are hemodynamically unstable.

For bladder retraining, record the date and time the catheter was clamped, the time it was released, and the volume and appearance of the urine. For catheter removal, record the date and time and the patient's tolerance of the procedure. Record when and how much he voided after catheter removal and any associated problems.

INDWELLING URINARY CATHETER INSERTION

Also known as a Foley or retention catheter, an indwelling urinary catheter remains in the bladder to provide continuous urine drainage. A balloon inflated at the catheter's distal end prevents it from slipping out of the bladder after insertion.

Indwelling catheters are used most commonly to relieve bladder distention caused by urine retention and to allow continuous urine drainage when the urinary meatus is swollen from childbirth, surgery, or local trauma. Other indications for an indwelling catheter include urinary tract obstruction (caused by a tumor or enlarged prostate), urine retention or infection from neurogenic bladder paralysis caused by spinal cord injury or disease, and any illness in which the patient's urine output must be monitored closely.

An indwelling catheter is inserted using sterile technique and only when absolutely necessary. Insertion should be performed with extreme care to prevent injury and infection.

Key nursing diagnoses and patient outcomes

Impaired urinary elimination related to presence of an indwelling urinary catheter
The patient will:
▶ maintain fluid balance (intake will equal output)
▶ have few if any complications
▶ describe feelings and concerns regarding the indwelling urinary catheter.

Risk for infection related to presence of an indwelling urinary catheter
The patient will:
▶ have no pathogens appear in cultures
▶ remain afebrile
▶ show no evidence of urinary tract infection, such as cloudy or malodorous urine or urine with sediment.

Equipment

Sterile indwelling catheter (latex or silicone #10 to #22 French [average adult sizes are #16 to #18 French]) • syringe filled with 5 to 8 ml of sterile water (normal saline solution is sometimes used) • washcloth • towel • soap and water • two linen-saver pads • sterile gloves • sterile drape • sterile fenestrated drape • sterile cotton-tipped applicators (or cotton balls and plastic forceps) • povidone-iodine or other antiseptic cleaning agent • urine receptacle • sterile water-soluble lubricant • sterile drainage collection bag • intake and output sheet • adhesive tape • optional:

urine specimen container and laboratory request form, leg band with Velcro closure, gooseneck lamp or flashlight, pillows or rolled blankets or towels

Prepackaged sterile disposable kits that usually contain all the necessary equipment are available. The syringes in these kits are prefilled with 10 ml of normal saline solution.

Preparation of equipment

Check the order on the patient's chart *to determine if a catheter size or type has been specified.* Then wash your hands, select the appropriate equipment and assemble it at the patient's bedside.

Implementation

▶ Explain the procedure to the patient and provide privacy. Check his chart and ask when he voided last. Percuss and palpate the bladder *to establish baseline data.* Ask if he feels the urge to void.
▶ Have a coworker hold a flashlight or place a gooseneck lamp next to the patient's bed *so that you can see the urinary meatus clearly in poor lighting.*
▶ Place the female patient in the supine position, with her knees flexed and separated and her feet flat on the bed, about 2' (0.6 m) apart. If she finds this position uncomfortable, have her flex one knee and keep the other leg flat on the bed.

 Age alert **The elderly patient may need pillows or rolled blankets or towels** *to provide support with positioning.*

▶ You may need an assistant to help the patient stay in position or to direct the light. Place the male patient in the supine position with his legs extended and flat on the bed. Ask the patient to hold the position *to give you a clear view*

of the urinary meatus and to prevent contamination of the sterile field.

▶ Use the washcloth to clean the patient's genital area and perineum thoroughly with soap and water. Dry the
area with the towel. Then wash your
hands.

▶ Place the linen-saver pads on the
bed between the patient's legs and under the hips. To create the sterile field,
open the prepackaged kit or equipment
tray and place it between the female patient's legs or next to the male patient's
hip. If the sterile gloves are the first
item on the top of the tray, put them
on. Place the sterile drape under the
patient's hips. Drape the patient's lower
abdomen with the sterile fenestrated
drape so only the genital area remains
exposed. Take care not to contaminate
your gloves.

▶ Open the rest of the kit or tray. Put
on the sterile gloves if you haven't already done so.

▶ Make sure the patient isn't allergic
to iodine solution; if he is allergic, another antiseptic cleaning agent must be
used.

▶ Tear open the packet of povidone-
iodine or other antiseptic cleaning
agent and use it to saturate the sterile
cotton balls or applicators. Be careful
not to spill the solution on the equipment.

▶ Open the packet of water-soluble lubricant and apply it to the catheter tip;
attach the drainage collection bag to the
other end of the catheter. (If you're using a commercial kit, the drainage bag
may be attached.) Make sure all tubing
ends remain sterile and make sure the
clamp at the emptying port of the
drainage bag is closed to prevent urine
leakage from the bag. Some drainage systems have an air-lock chamber to pre-

vent bacteria from traveling to the bladder
from urine in the drainage bag.

Note: Some urologists and nurses use
a syringe prefilled with water-soluble
lubricant and instill the lubricant directly into the male urethra, instead of
on the catheter tip. This method helps
prevent trauma to the urethral lining as
well as possible urinary tract infection.
Check your facility's policy.

▶ Before inserting the catheter, inflate
the balloon with sterile water or normal
saline solution to inspect it for leaks. To
do this, attach the prefilled syringe to
the luer-lock, then push the plunger
and check for seepage as the balloon
expands. Aspirate the solution to deflate
the balloon. Also inspect the catheter for
resiliency. Rough, cracked catheters can
injure the urethral mucosa during insertion, which can predispose the patient to
infection.

▶ For the female patient, separate the
labia majora and labia minora as widely
as possible with the thumb, middle,
and index fingers of your nondominant
hand so you have a full view of the urinary meatus. Keep the labia well separated throughout the procedure (as
shown below), so they don't obscure the
urinary meatus or contaminate the area
after it's cleaned.

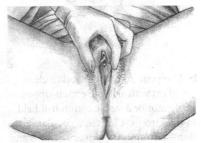

▶ With your dominant hand, use a
sterile, cotton-tipped applicator (or
pick up a sterile cotton ball with the

plastic forceps) and wipe one side of the urinary meatus with a single downward motion (as shown below).

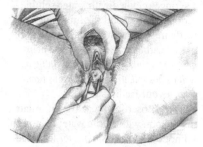

▶ Wipe the other side with another sterile applicator or cotton ball in the same way. Then wipe directly over the meatus with still another sterile applicator or cotton ball. Take care not to contaminate your sterile glove.
▶ For the male patient, hold the penis with your nondominant hand. If he's uncircumcised, retract the foreskin. Then gently lift and stretch the penis to a 60- to 90-degree angle. Hold the penis this way throughout the procedure *to straighten the urethra and maintain a sterile field* (as shown below).

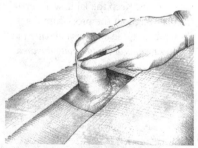

▶ Use your dominant hand to clean the glans with a sterile cotton-tipped applicator or a sterile cotton ball held in the forceps. Clean in a circular motion, starting at the urinary meatus and working outward.
▶ Repeat the procedure, using another sterile applicator or cotton ball and tak-ing care not to contaminate your sterile glove.
▶ Pick up the catheter with your dominant hand and prepare to insert the lubricated tip into the urinary meatus. *To facilitate insertion by relaxing the sphincter,* ask the patient to cough as you insert the catheter. Tell him to breathe deeply and slowly *to further relax the sphincter and spasms.* Hold the catheter close to its tip *to ease insertion and control its direction.*

Nursing alert Never force a catheter during insertion. Maneuver the catheter gently, angling it slightly toward the symphysis pubis as the patient bears down or coughs. If you still meet resistance, stop and notify the doctor. Sphincter spasms, strictures, misplacement in the vagina (in females), or an enlarged prostate (in males) may cause resistance.

▶ For the female patient, advance the catheter 2″ to 3″ (5 to 7.6 cm)—while continuing to hold the labia apart—until urine begins to flow (as shown below).

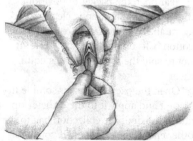

If the catheter is inadvertently inserted into the vagina, leave it there as a landmark. Then begin the procedure over again using new supplies.
▶ For the male patient, advance the catheter to the bifurcation 5″ to 7½″ (13 to 19 cm) and check for urine flow

(as shown below). If the foreskin was retracted, replace it *to prevent compromised circulation and painful swelling.*

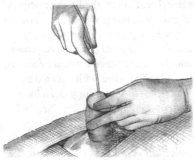

▶ When urine stops flowing, attach the saline-filled syringe to the luer-lock.
▶ Push the plunger and inflate the balloon (as shown below) *to keep the catheter in place in the bladder.*

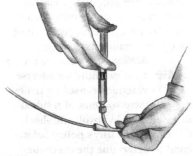

Nursing alert **Never inflate a balloon without first establishing urine flow,** *which assures you that the catheter is in the bladder.*

▶ Hang the collection bag below bladder level *to prevent urine reflux into the bladder, which can cause infection, and to facilitate gravity drainage of the bladder.* Make sure the tubing doesn't get tangled in the bed's side rails.
▶ Tape the catheter to the female patient's thigh *to prevent possible tension on the urogenital trigone* (as shown at top of next column).

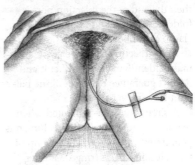

▶ Tape the catheter to the male patient's anterior thigh *to prevent pressure on the urethra at the penoscrotal junction, which can lead to formation of urethrocutaneous fistulas. Taping this way also prevents traction on the bladder and alteration in the normal direction of urine flow in males.*
▶ As an alternative, secure the catheter to the patient's thigh using a leg band with a Velcro closure (as shown below). *This decreases skin irritation, especially in patients with long-term indwelling catheters.*

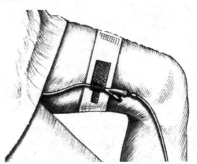

▶ Dispose of all used supplies properly.

Special considerations

▶ Several types of catheters are available with balloons of various sizes. Each type has its own method of inflation and closure. For example, in one type of catheter, sterile solution or air is injected through the inflation lumen, then the end of the injection port is folded over itself and fastened with a clamp or rubber band.

Note: Injecting a catheter with air makes identifying leaks difficult and doesn't guarantee deflation of the balloon for removal.

► A similar catheter is inflated when a seal in the end of the inflation lumen is penetrated with a needle or the tip of the solution-filled syringe. Another type of balloon catheter self-inflates when a prepositioned clamp is loosened. The balloon size determines the amount of solution needed for inflation, and the exact amount is usually printed on the distal extension of the catheter used for inflating the balloon.

► If necessary, ask the female patient to lie on her side with her knees drawn up to her chest during the catheterization procedure (as shown below).

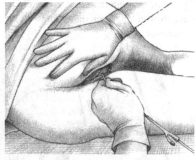

This position may be especially helpful for elderly or disabled patients such as those with severe contractures.

► If the doctor orders a urine specimen for laboratory analysis, obtain it from the urine receptacle with a specimen collection container at the time of catheterization and send it to the laboratory with the appropriate laboratory request form. Connect the drainage bag when urine stops flowing.

► Inspect the catheter and tubing periodically while they're in place *to detect compression or kinking that could obstruct urine flow.* Explain the basic principles of gravity drainage *so that the patient realizes the importance of keeping the drainage tubing and collection bag lower than his bladder at all times.* If necessary, provide the patient with detailed instructions for performing clean intermittent self-catheterization. (See "Self-catheterization," page 720.)

► For monitoring purposes, empty the collection bag at least every 8 hours. Excessive fluid volume may require more frequent emptying *to prevent traction on the catheter,* which would cause the patient discomfort, and *to prevent injury to the urethra and bladder wall.* Some facilities encourage changing catheters at regular intervals, such as every 30 days, if the patient will have long-term continuous drainage.

Nursing alert Observe the patient carefully for adverse reactions caused by removing excessive volumes of residual urine such as hypovolemic shock. Check your facility's policy beforehand to determine the maximum amount of urine that may be drained at one time (some facilities limit the amount to 700 to 1,000 ml). Whether to limit the amount of urine drained is currently controversial. Clamp the catheter at the first sign of an adverse reaction and notify the doctor.

Home care

If the patient will be discharged with a long-term indwelling catheter, teach him and his family all aspects of daily catheter maintenance, including care of the skin and urinary meatus, signs and symptoms of urinary tract infection or obstruction, how to irrigate the catheter (if appropriate), and the importance of adequate fluid intake to maintain patency. Explain that a home care nurse should visit every 4 to 6 weeks, or more often if needed, to change the catheter.

Complications

Urinary tract infection can result from the introduction of bacteria into the bladder. Improper insertion can cause traumatic injury to the urethral and bladder mucosa. Bladder atony or spasms can result from rapid decompression of a severely distended bladder.

Documentation

Record the date, time, and size and type of indwelling catheter used. Also describe the amount, color, and other characteristics of urine emptied from the bladder. Your hospital may require only the intake and output sheet for fluid-balance data. If large volumes of urine have been emptied, describe the patient's tolerance for the procedure. Note whether a urine specimen was sent for laboratory analysis.

INTERMITTENT INFUSION DEVICE INSERTION

Also called a saline lock, an intermittent infusion device consists of a cannula with an injection cap attached. Filled with saline solution to prevent blood clot formation, the device maintains venous access in patients who are receiving I.V. medication regularly or intermittently but who don't require

continuous infusion. An intermittent infusion device is superior to an I.V. line that is maintained at a moderately slow infusion rate because it minimizes the risk of fluid overload and electrolyte imbalance. It also cuts costs, reduces the risk of contamination by eliminating I.V. solution containers and administration sets, increases patient comfort and mobility, reduces patient anxiety and, if inserted in a large vein, allows collection of multiple blood samples without repeated venipuncture.

Key nursing diagnoses and patient outcomes

Risk for infection related to the intermittent infusion device
The patient will:
▶ maintain a normal body temperature
▶ show no signs of infection at the I.V. puncture site
▶ remain free from all signs and symptoms of infection.

Deficient knowledge related to lack of exposure to the intermittent infusion device
The patient will:
▶ communicate a need to know
▶ state an understanding of what has been taught
▶ ask questions related to therapy with an intermittent infusion device.

Equipment

Intermittent infusion device • needleless system device • normal saline solution • tourniquet • gloves • alcohol pads or other approved antimicrobial solution, such as tincture of iodine 2% or 10% povidone-iodine solution • venipuncture equipment, transparent semipermeable dressing, and tape

Converting an I.V. line to an intermittent infusion device

Many types of adapter caps, such as the ones shown below, allow you to convert an existing I.V. line to an intermittent infusion device. To make the conversion, follow these steps:

■ Prime the adapter cap with normal saline solution, as appropriate.

■ Clamp the I.V. tubing and remove the administration set from the cannula hub.

■ Insert the male adapter cap.

■ Inject the remaining normal saline solution to fill the line and prevent clot formation.

Long male adapter
This long adapter cap slides into place.

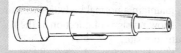

Short male adapter
This short luer-lock adapter cap twists into place.

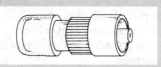

Prefilled saline cartridges are available in both doses for use in a syringe cartridge holder.

Implementation

▶ Wash your hands thoroughly to prevent contamination of the venipuncture site.

▶ Explain the procedure to the patient and describe the purpose of the intermittent infusion device.

▶ Remove the set from its packaging, wipe the port with an alcohol pad and inject normal saline solution to fill the tubing and needleless system. This removes air from the system, preventing formation of an air embolus.

▶ Select a venipuncture site. Put on gloves. Apply a tourniquet 2″ (5 cm) proximal to the chosen area.

▶ Clean the venipuncture site with alcohol or other approved antimicrobial solution according to your facility's policy, wiping outward from the site in a circular motion.

▶ Perform the venipuncture, and ensure correct needle placement in the vein. Then release the tourniquet. (See "Venipuncture" on page 920 for complete instructions.)

▶ Tape the set in place. Loop the tubing, if applicable, so that the injection port is free and easily accessible.

▶ Apply a transparent semipermeable dressing. On a dressing label, write the time, date, and your initials, and place the label on the dressing.

▶ Remove and discard gloves.

▶ Inject normal saline solution every 8 to 24 hours or according to your facility's policy to maintain the patency of the intermittent infusion device.

Special considerations

▶ When accessing an intermittent infusion device, make sure you stabilize the device to prevent dislodging it from the vein.

▶ Change the intermittent infusion device every 48 to 72 hours, according to your facility's policy, using a new venipuncture site. Some facilities use a transparent semipermeable dressing. This allows more patient freedom and better observation of the injection site.

▶ If the doctor orders an I.V. infusion discontinued and an intermittent infusion device inserted in its place, convert the existing line by disconnecting the I.V. tubing and inserting a male adapter cap into the device. (See *Converting an I.V. line to an intermittent infusion device.*)

▶ Most health organizations require the use of luer-locking systems on all infusion cannulas and lines.

Home care

If you're caring for a patient who will be going home with a peripheral line, teach him how to care for the I.V. site and identify complications. If he must observe movement restrictions, make sure he understands which movements to avoid.

Because the patient may have special drug delivery equipment that differs from the type used in the facility, make sure you demonstrate the equipment and have the patient give a return demonstration.

Teach the patient to examine the site and to notify the nurse if the dressing becomes moist, if blood appears in the tubing, or if redness, swelling, or discomfort develops.

Also tell the patient to report any problems with the I.V. line, for instance, if the solution stops infusing or if an alarm goes off on the infusion pump controller. Explain that the I.V. site will be changed at established intervals by a home care nurse.

Teach the patient or caregiver how and when to flush the device. Finally, teach the patient to document daily whether the I.V. site is free from pain, swelling, and redness.

Complications

Use of an intermittent infusion device has the same potential complications as the use of a peripheral I.V. line. (See "Peripheral I.V. line insertion," page 625.)

Documentation

Record the date and time of insertion; type and gauge of the needle and length of the cannula; anatomic location of the insertion site; patient's tolerance of the procedure; and date and time of each saline flush.

INTERMITTENT INFUSION DEVICE USE

An intermittent infusion injection device, or saline lock, eliminates the need for multiple venipunctures or for maintaining venous access with a continuous I.V. infusion. This device allows intermittent administration by infusion or by the I.V. bolus or I.V. push injection method.

Dilute saline solution is typically injected as the final step in this procedure *to prevent clotting in the device.*

Key nursing diagnoses and patient outcomes

Risk for infection related to the intermittent infusion device
The patient will:
▶ maintain a normal body temperature
▶ show no signs of infection at the I.V. puncture site
▶ remain free from all signs and symptoms of infection.

Deficient knowledge related to a lack of exposure to the intermittent infusion device

The patient will:
▶ communicate a need to know
▶ state an understanding of what has been taught
▶ ask questions related to therapy with an intermittent infusion device.

Equipment

Patient's medication record and chart • gloves • alcohol pads • three 3-ml syringes with needleless adapter • normal saline solution • extra intermittent infusion device • prescribed medication in an I.V. container with administration set and needle (for infusion) or in a syringe with needle (for I.V. bolus or push) • tourniquet • optional: T-connector and sterile bacteriostatic water

Preparation of equipment

Verify the order on the patient's medication record by checking it against the doctor's order. Wash your hands; then wipe the tops of the normal saline solution and medication containers with alcohol pads.

Fill two of the 3-ml syringes (bearing 22G needles) with normal saline solution. If you'll be infusing medication, insert the administration set spike into the I.V. container, attach the needleless adapter, and prime the line. If you'll be giving an I.V. injection, fill a syringe with the prescribed medication.

Implementation

▶ Confirm the patient's identity by asking his name and checking the name, room number, and bed number on his wristband. Explain the procedure.
▶ Put on gloves. Wipe the injection port of the intermittent infusion device with an alcohol pad and insert the needleless adapter of a saline-filled syringe.

▶ Aspirate the syringe and observe for blood *to verify the patency of the device.* If none appears, apply a tourniquet slightly above the site, keep it in place for about 1 minute and then aspirate again. If blood still doesn't appear, remove the tourniquet and inject the normal saline solution slowly.

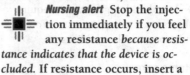 **Nursing alert** Stop the injection immediately if you feel any resistance *because resistance indicates that the device is occluded.* If resistance occurs, insert a new saline lock.

▶ If you feel no resistance, watch for signs of infiltration (such as puffiness and pain at the site) as you slowly inject the saline solution. If these signs occur, insert a new intermittent infusion device.
▶ If blood is aspirated, slowly inject the saline solution and observe for signs of infiltration.
▶ Withdraw the saline syringe and needleless adapter.

Administering I.V. bolus or push injections

▶ Insert the needleless adapter and syringe with the medication for the I.V. bolus or push injection into the injection port of the device.
▶ Inject the medication at the required rate. Then remove the needleless adapter and syringe from the injection port.
▶ Insert the needleless adapter of the remaining saline-filled syringe into the injection port and slowly inject the saline solution *to flush all medication through the device.*
▶ Remove the needleless adapter and syringe; then insert and inject the saline flush solution *to prevent clotting in the device.*

Administering an infusion

▶ Insert and secure the needleless adapter attached to the administration set.

▶ Open the infusion line and adjust the flow rate as necessary.

▶ Infuse medication for the prescribed length of time; then flush the device with normal saline solution, as you would after a bolus or push injection, according to your facility's policy.

▶ To administer fluids and drugs simultaneously or to administer a medication incompatible with the primary I.V. solution, you may want to use a T-connector or needleless adapter. (See *Using a needleless system for intermittent infusions.*)

Special considerations

▶ If you're giving a bolus injection of a drug that is incompatible with saline solution, such as diazepam (Valium), flush the device with bacteriostatic water.

▶ Intermittent infusion devices should be changed regularly (usually every 48 to 72 hours), according to standard precautions and your facility's policy.

▶ If you can't rotate injection sites because the patient has fragile veins, document this fact.

Complications

Infiltration and a specific reaction to the infused medication are the most common complications.

Documentation

Record the type and amount of drug administered and times of administration. Include all I.V. solutions used to dilute the medication and flush the line on the intake record. Also document the use of saline solution.

Using a needleless system for intermittent infusions

You can use a needleless I.V. system, such as InterLink (shown here), to administer intermittent infusion medication when you need to convert an I.V. line to a saline lock. To make the conversion:

■ clamp the I.V. tubing and remove the administration set from the catheter or needle hub

■ connect the adapter

■ inject the remaining saline solution to prevent clot formation.

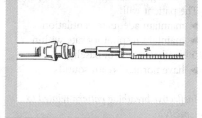

INTERMITTENT POSITIVE-PRESSURE BREATHING

Intermittent positive-pressure breathing (IPPB) delivers room air or oxygen into the lungs at a pressure higher than atmospheric pressure. This delivery ceases when pressure in the mouth or in the breathing circuit tube increases to a predetermined airway pressure.

IPPB was formerly the mainstay of pulmonary therapy, with its proponents claiming that the device delivered aerosolized medications deeper into the lungs, decreased the work of breathing, and assisted in the mobilization of secretions. Studies now show that IPPB has no clinical benefit over handheld nebulizers. However, IPPB may be useful in helping asthmatics with hypercapnia and impending respiratory failure avoid intubation and mechanical ventilation. Although IPPB easily inflates healthy alveoli, it may have little effect on alveoli with thickened or obstructed walls — the walls most difficult to inflate.

Typically, personnel from the respiratory therapy department deliver these treatments.

Key nursing diagnoses and patient outcomes

Impaired gas exchange related to (specify)
The patient will:
▶ maintain adequate ventilation
▶ maintain respiratory rate within 5 breaths/minute of baseline
▶ have normal breath sounds.

Ineffective breathing pattern related to (specify)
The patient will:
▶ demonstrate diaphragmatic pursed-lip breathing
▶ achieve maximum lung expansion with adequate ventilation
▶ demonstrate skill in conserving energy while carrying out activities of daily living.

Anxiety related to difficulty breathing
The patient will:
▶ state feelings of anxiety
▶ use support systems to assist with coping
▶ perform relaxation techniques every 4 hours.

Equipment

IPPB machine • breathing circuit tubing • other necessary tubing (usually one or two sections) • mouthpiece or mask • noseclips, if necessary • source of pressurized gas at 50 psi, if necessary • oxygen, if desired • prescribed medication, such as isoetharine hydrochloride (Bronkosol) and normal saline solution • 3-ml syringe with needle • sphygmomanometer • stethoscope • facial tissues and waste bag or specimen cup • warm, soapy water • optional: glutaraldehyde solution and suction equipment

Preparation of equipment

Follow the manufacturer's instructions to set up the equipment properly.

Implementation

▶ Explain the procedure to the patient *to ensure his cooperation.* Tell him to sit erect in a chair, if possible, *to allow for optimal lung expansion.* Otherwise, place him in semi-Fowler's position. Wash your hands.
▶ Take baseline blood pressure and heart rate, especially if a bronchodilator will be administered, and listen to breath sounds for posttreatment comparisons.
▶ Instruct the patient to breathe deeply and slowly through his mouth as if sucking on a straw. Encourage the patient to let the machine do the work.
▶ During treatment, instruct the patient to hold his breath for a few seconds after full inspiration *to allow for greater distribution of gas and medication.* Then instruct him to exhale normally.
▶ During treatment, take the patient's blood pressure and heart rate. *IPPB treatment increases intrathoracic pressure and may temporarily decrease cardiac output and venous return, resulting in tachycardia, hypotension, or headache. Monitoring also detects reactions to the bronchodilator.* If you find a sudden change in blood pressure or an increase

in heart rate of 20 beats/minute or more, stop the treatment and notify the doctor.

▶ If the patient is tolerating the treatment, continue until the medication in the nebulizer is exhausted, usually about 10 minutes.

▶ After treatment or as needed, have the patient expectorate into tissues and discard into waste bag or expectorate in a specimen cup, or suction him as necessary. Listen to his breath sounds, and compare them to the pretreatment assessment.

▶ Shake excess moisture from the nebulizer and the mouthpiece or mask. After 24 hours of use, either discard the equipment or clean it with warm, soapy water. After washing, rinse with warm water and immerse in glutaraldehyde solution for 10 minutes. Then remove the equipment, rinse in warm water, and air dry. When it's dry, store it in a clean plastic bag.

Special considerations

▶ If possible, avoid administering IPPB treatment immediately before or after a meal *because the treatment may induce nausea and because a full stomach reduces lung expansion.*

▶ Never give IPPB treatment without medication in the nebulizer *because this could dry the patient's airways and make secretions more difficult to mobilize.* If the purpose of treatment is to mobilize secretions, use a specimen cup to measure the secretions obtained.

▶ If the patient wears dentures, leave them in place *to ensure a proper seal* but remove them if they slide out of position. If the patient has an artificial airway, use a special adapter, such as mechanical ventilation tubing, to give IPPB treatments. When using a mask to

administer treatments, allow the patient frequent rest periods and observe for gastric distention *because this is more likely to occur with a mask.*

▶ If the patient's blood pressure is stable during the initial treatment, you may not need to check it during subsequent treatments unless he has a history of cardiovascular disease, hypotension, or sensitivity to any drug delivered in the treatment.

▶ If the patient will be using IPPB at home, provide appropriate patient teaching.

Complications

Gastric insufflation may result from swallowed air and occurs more commonly with a mask than with a mouthpiece. Dizziness can result from hyperventilation. The work of breathing can be increased, especially if the patient is uncomfortable with or frightened by the machine. Decreased blood pressure can result from decreased venous return, especially in the patient with hypovolemia or cardiovascular disease. Increased intracranial pressure can result from impeded venous return from the brain. Spontaneous pneumothorax may result from increased intrathoracic pressure; this complication is rare but is most likely to occur in patients with emphysematous blebs.

Documentation

Record the date, time, and duration of treatment; medication administered; pressure used; vital signs; breath sounds before and after treatment; amount of sputum produced; any complications and nursing actions taken; and the patient's tolerance of the procedure.

INTERNAL FIXATION

In internal fixation, also known as surgical reduction or open reduction — internal fixation, the doctor implants fixation devices to stabilize the fracture. Internal fixation devices include nails, screws, pins, wires, and rods, all of which may be used in combination with metal plates. These devices remain in the body indefinitely unless the patient experiences adverse reactions after the healing process is complete. (See *Reviewing internal fixation devices*.)

Internal fixation is typically used to treat fractures of the face and jaw, spine, arm or leg bones, and fractures involving a joint (most commonly, the hip). Internal fixation permits earlier mobilization and can shorten hospitalization, particularly in elderly patients with hip fractures.

Key nursing diagnoses and patient outcomes

Pain related to fracture
The patient will:
▶ identify specific characteristics of pain
▶ use available resources (such as pamphlets or a pain specialist) to understand the pain phenomenon
▶ express relief from pain.

Ineffective tissue perfusion (peripheral) related to fracture
The patient will:
▶ have strong peripheral pulses
▶ have normal skin color and temperature
▶ have no numbness, tingling, or pain in body parts distal to the fracture.

Impaired physical mobility related to fracture

The patient will:
▶ state relief from pain
▶ show no evidence of such complications as contractures, venous stasis, thrombus formation, or skin breakdown
▶ displays increased mobility and attains the highest degree of mobility within the confines of the disease.

Equipment

Ice bag • pain medication (analgesic or narcotic) • incentive spirometer • elastic stockings

Patients with leg fractures may also need: overhead frame with trapeze • pressure-relief mattress • crutches or walker • pillow (hip fractures may require abductor pillows).

Preparation of equipment

Equipment is collected and prepared in the operating room.

Implementation

▶ Explain the procedure to the patient *to allay his fears.* Tell him what to expect during postoperative assessment and monitoring, teach him how to use an incentive spirometer, and prepare him for proposed exercise and progressive ambulation regimens if necessary. Instruct him to tell the doctor if he feels pain.
▶ After the procedure, monitor the patient's vital signs every 2 to 4 hours for 24 hours, then every 4 to 8 hours, according to your facility's protocol. *Changes in vital signs may indicate hemorrhage or infection.*
▶ Monitor fluid intake and output every 4 to 8 hours.
▶ Perform neurovascular checks every 2 to 4 hours for 24 hours, then every 4 to 8 hours as appropriate. Assess color, motion, sensation, digital movement,

Reviewing internal fixation devices

Choice of a specific internal fixation device depends on the location, type, and configuration of the fracture.

In trochanteric or subtrochanteric fractures, the surgeon may use a hip pin or nail, with or without a screw plate. A pin or plate with extra nails stabilizes the fracture by impacting the bone ends at the fracture site.

In an uncomplicated fracture of the femoral shaft, the surgeon may use an intramedullary rod. This device permits early ambulation with partial weight bearing.

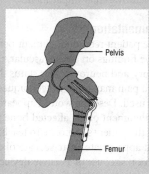

Pelvis

Femur

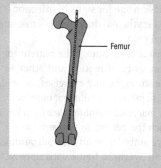

Femur

Another choice for fixation of a long-bone fracture is a screw plate, shown here on the tibia.

In an arm fracture, the surgeon may fix the involved bones with a plate, rod, or nail. Most radial and ulnar fractures may be fixed with plates, whereas humeral fractures are commonly fixed with rods.

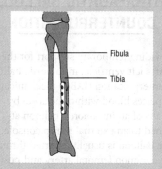

Fibula

Tibia

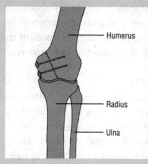

Humerus

Radius

Ulna

edema, capillary refill, and pulses of the affected area. Compare findings with the unaffected side.

▶ Apply an ice bag to the operative site, as ordered, *to reduce swelling, relieve pain, and lessen bleeding.*

▶ *To promote comfort,* administer analgesics or narcotics, as ordered, before exercising or mobilizing the affected area. If the patient is using patient-controlled analgesia, instruct him to administer a dose before exercising or mobilizing.

▶ Monitor the patient for pain unrelieved by analgesics or narcotics and for burning, tingling, or numbness, *which may indicate infection or impaired circulation.*

▶ Elevate the affected limb on a pillow, if appropriate, *to minimize edema.*

▶ Check surgical dressings for excessive drainage or bleeding. Also check the incision site for signs of infection, such as erythema, drainage, edema, and unusual pain.

▶ Assist and encourage the patient to perform range-of-motion and other muscle strengthening exercises, as ordered, *to promote circulation, improve muscle tone, and maintain joint function.*

▶ Teach the patient to perform progressive ambulation and mobilization using an overhead frame with trapeze, or crutches or a walker, as appropriate.

Special considerations

To avoid the complications of immobility after surgery, have the patient use an incentive spirometer. Apply elastic stockings and sequential compression device, as appropriate. The patient may also require a pressure-relief mattress.

Home care

Before discharge, teach the patient and family members how to care for the incision site and recognize signs and symptoms of wound infection. Also teach them about administering pain medication, practicing an exercise regimen (if any), and using assistive ambulation devices (such as crutches or a walker), if appropriate.

Complications

Wound infection and, more critically, infection involving metal fixation devices may require reopening the incision, draining the suture line and, possibly, removing the fixation device. Any such infection would require wound dressings and antibiotic therapy. Other complications may include malunion, nonunion, fat or pulmonary embolism, and neurovascular impairment.

Documentation

In the patient record, document perioperative findings on cardiovascular, respiratory, and neurovascular status. Note which pain management techniques were used. Describe wound appearance and alignment of the affected bone. Note the patient's response to teaching about appropriate exercise, care of the infection site, use of assistive devices (if appropriate), and symptoms that should be reported to the doctor.

INTRA-AORTIC BALLOON COUNTERPULSATION

Providing temporary support for the heart's left ventricle, intra-aortic balloon counterpulsation (IABC) mechanically displaces blood within the aorta by means of an intra-aortic balloon attached to an external pump console. The balloon is usually inserted through the common femoral artery and positioned with its tip just distal to the left subclavian artery. It monitors myocardial perfusion and the effects of drugs on myocardial function and perfusion. When used correctly, IABC improves two key aspects of myocardial physiology: It increases the supply of oxygen-rich blood to the myocardium, and it decreases myocardial oxygen demand.

IABC is recommended for patients with a wide range of low-cardiac-output disorders or cardiac instability, including refractory anginas, ventricular arrhythmias associated with ischemia, and pump failure caused by cardiogenic shock, intraoperative myocardial infarction (MI), or low cardiac output after bypass surgery. IABC is also indicated for patients with low cardiac output secondary to acute mechanical defects after MI (such as ventricular septal defect, papillary muscle rupture, or left ventricular aneurysm).

Perioperatively, the technique is used to support and stabilize patients with a suspected high-grade lesion who are undergoing such procedures as angioplasty, thrombolytic therapy, cardiac surgery, and cardiac catheterization.

IABC is contraindicated in patients with severe aortic regurgitation, aortic aneurysm, or severe peripheral vascular disease.

Key nursing diagnoses and patient outcomes

Decreased cardiac output related to (specify)
The patient will:
▶ maintain hemodynamic stability as evidenced by normal pulse rate and blood pressure
▶ experience no dizziness, syncope, or arrhythmias
▶ experience a decrease in cardiac workload.

Anxiety related to invasive monitoring and treatment
The patient will:
▶ express feelings of anxiety

▶ use support systems to assist with coping
▶ cope with the threat of anxiety by being involved in decisions about care.

Equipment

IABC console and balloon catheters • insertion kit • Dacron graft (for surgically inserted balloon) • electrocardiogram (ECG) monitor and electrodes • sedative • pain medication • pulmonary artery (PA) catheter setup • temporary pacemaker setup • 18G angiography needle • sterile drape • sterile gloves • gown • mask • sutures • povidone-iodine solution • suction setup • oxygen setup and ventilator, if necessary • defibrillator and emergency medications • fluoroscope • indwelling urinary catheter • urinometer • arterial blood gas (ABG) kits and tubes for laboratory studies • povidone-iodine swabs • dressing materials • 4″ × 4″ gauze pads • shaving supplies • optional: I.V. heparin

Preparation of equipment

Depending on your facility's policy, you or a perfusionist must balance the pressure transducer in the external pump console and calibrate the oscilloscope monitor to ensure accuracy.

Implementation

▶ Explain to the patient that the doctor will place a special balloon catheter in his aorta *to help his heart pump more easily.* Briefly explain the insertion procedure, and mention that the catheter will be connected to a large console next to his bed. Tell him that the balloon will temporarily reduce his heart's workload *to promote rapid healing of the ventricular muscle.* Let him know that it will be removed after his heart can resume an

How the intra-aortic balloon pump works

Made of polyurethane, the intra-aortic balloon is attached to an external pump console by means of a large-lumen catheter. The illustrations here show the direction of blood flow when the pump inflates and deflates the balloon.

Balloon inflation
The balloon inflates as the aortic valve closes and diastole begins. Diastole increases perfusion to the coronary arteries.

Balloon deflation
The balloon deflates before ventricular ejection, when the aortic valve opens. This permits ejection of blood from the left ventricle against a lowered resistance. As a result, aortic end-diastolic pressure and afterload decrease and cardiac output rises.

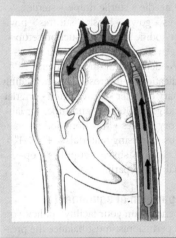

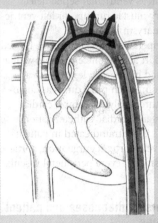

adequate workload. (See *How the intra-aortic balloon pump works.*)

Preparing for intra-aortic balloon insertion

▶ Make sure the patient or a family member understands and signs a consent form. Verify that the form is attached to his chart.

▶ Obtain the patient's baseline vital signs, including pulmonary artery pressure (PAP). (A PA line should already be in place.) Attach the patient to an ECG machine for continuous monitoring. Apply chest electrodes in a stan-

dard lead II position — or in whatever position produces the largest R wave — *because the R wave triggers balloon inflation and deflation.* Obtain a baseline ECG.

▶ Attach another set of ECG electrodes to the patient unless the ECG pattern is being transmitted from the patient's bedside monitor to the balloon pump monitor through a phone cable. Administer oxygen as ordered and as necessary.

▶ Make sure the patient has an arterial line, a PA line, and a peripheral I.V. line in place. *The arterial line is used for with-*

drawing blood samples, monitoring blood pressure, and assessing the timing and effectiveness of therapy. The PA line allows measurement of PAP, aspiration of blood samples, and cardiac output studies. Increased PAP indicates increased myocardial workload and ineffective balloon pumping. Cardiac output studies are usually performed with and without the balloon *to check the patient's progress.* The central lumen of the intra-aortic balloon, which is used to monitor central aortic pressure, produces an augmented pressure waveform that allows you to check for proper timing of the inflation-deflation cycle and demonstrates the effects of counterpulsation, elevated diastolic pressure, and reduced end-diastolic and systolic pressures. (See *Interpreting intra-aortic balloon waveforms,* pages 446 and 447.)

▶ Insert an indwelling urinary catheter with a urinometer *so you can measure the patient's urine output and assess his fluid balance and renal function. To reduce the risk of infection,* shave or clip hair bilaterally from the lower abdomen to the lower thigh, including the pubic area.

▶ Observe and record the patient's peripheral leg pulse and document sensation, movement, color, and temperature of the legs.

▶ Administer a sedative as ordered. Shave the insertion site if needed.

▶ Have the defibrillator, suction setup, temporary pacemaker setup, and emergency medications readily available in case the patient develops complications during insertion, such as an arrhythmia.

▶ Before the doctor inserts the balloon, he puts on sterile gloves, gown, and mask. He cleans the site with povidone-iodine solution, and drapes the area using a sterile drape.

Inserting the intra-aortic balloon percutaneously

▶ The doctor may insert the balloon percutaneously through the femoral artery into the descending thoracic aorta, using a modified Seldinger technique. First, he accesses the vessel with an 18G angiography needle and removes the inner stylet.

▶ Then he passes the guide wire through the needle and removes the needle.

▶ Next, the doctor passes an introducer (dilator and sheath assembly) over the guide wire into the vessel until about 1″ (2.5 cm) remains above the insertion site. He then removes the inner dilator, leaving the introducer sheath and guide wire in place.

▶ After passing the balloon over the guide wire into the introducer sheath, the doctor advances the catheter into position, ⅜″ to ¾″ (1 to 2 cm) distal to the left subclavian artery under fluoroscopic guidance.

▶ The doctor attaches the balloon to the control system to initiate counterpulsation. The balloon catheter then unfurls.

Inserting the intra-aortic balloon surgically

▶ If the doctor chooses not to insert the catheter percutaneously, he usually inserts it by femoral arteriotomy. (See *Surgical insertion sites for the intra-aortic balloon,* page 448.)

▶ After making an incision and isolating the femoral artery, the doctor attaches a Dacron graft to a small opening in the arterial wall.

▶ He then passes the catheter through this graft. Using fluoroscopic guidance as necessary, he advances the catheter up the descending thoracic aorta and

Interpreting intra-aortic balloon waveforms

During intra-aortic balloon counterpulsation, you can use electrocardiogram and arterial pressure waveforms to determine whether the balloon pump is functioning properly.

Normal inflation-deflation timing

Balloon inflation occurs after aortic valve closure; deflation, during isovolumetric contraction, just before the aortic valve opens. In a properly timed waveform, like the one shown at right, the inflation point lies at or slightly above the dicrotic notch. Both inflation and deflation cause a sharp V. Peak diastolic pressure exceeds peak systolic pressure; peak systolic pressure exceeds assisted peak systolic pressure.

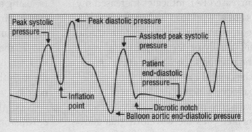

Early inflation

With early inflation, the inflation point lies before the dicrotic notch. Early inflation dangerously increases myocardial stress and decreases cardiac output.

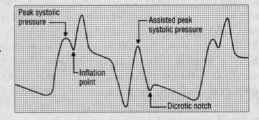

Early deflation

With early deflation, a U shape appears and peak systolic pressure is less than or equal to assisted peak systolic pressure. This won't decrease afterload or myocardial oxygen consumption.

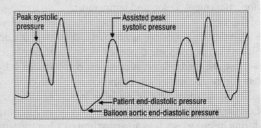

places the catheter tip between the left subclavian artery and the renal arteries.
▶ The doctor sews the Dacron graft around the catheter at the insertion point and connects the other end of the catheter to the pump console.

▶ If the balloon can't be inserted through the femoral artery, the doctor inserts it in an antegrade direction through the anterior wall of the ascending aorta. He positions it ⅜" to ¾" (1 to 2 cm) beyond the left subclavian artery

Interpreting intra-aortic balloon waveforms *(continued)*

Late inflation

With late inflation, the dicrotic notch precedes the inflation point, and the notch and the inflation point create a W shape. This can lead to a reduction in peak diastolic pressure, coronary and systemic perfusion augmentation time, and augmented coronary perfusion pressure.

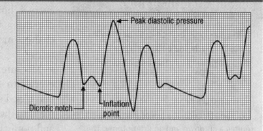

Late deflation

With late deflation, peak systolic pressure exceeds assisted peak systolic pressure. This threatens the patient by increasing afterload, myocardial oxygen consumption, cardiac workload, and preload. It occurs when the balloon has been inflated for too long.

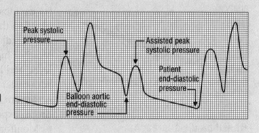

and brings the catheter out through the chest wall.

Monitoring the patient after balloon insertion

Nursing alert If the control system malfunctions or becomes inoperable, don't let the balloon catheter remain dormant for more than 30 minutes. Get another control system and attach it to the balloon; then resume pumping. In the meantime, inflate the balloon manually, using a 60-ml syringe and room air a minimum of once every 5 minutes, *to prevent thrombus formation in the catheter.*

▶ The doctor will clean the insertion site with povidone-iodine swabs and apply a sterile dressing.

▶ Obtain a chest X-ray *to verify correct balloon placement.*

▶ Assess and record pedal and posterior tibial pulses as well as color, sensation, and temperature in the affected limb every 15 minutes for 1 hour, then hourly. Notify the doctor immediately if you detect circulatory changes *because the balloon may need to be removed.*

▶ Observe and record the patient's baseline arm pulses, arm sensation and movement, and arm color and temperature every 15 minutes for 1 hour after balloon insertion, then every 2 hours while the balloon is in place. *Loss of left arm pulses may indicate upward balloon displacement.* Notify the doctor of any changes.

▶ Monitor the patient's urine output every hour. Note baseline blood urea

Surgical insertion sites for the intra-aortic balloon

If an intra-aortic balloon can't be inserted percutaneously, the doctor will insert it surgically, using a femoral or transthoracic approach.

Femoral approach

Insertion through the femoral artery requires a cutdown and an arteriotomy. The doctor passes the balloon through a Dacron graft that has been sewn to the artery.

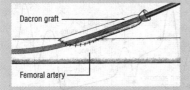

Dacron graft

Femoral artery

Transthoracic approach

If femoral insertion is unsuccessful, the doctor may use a transthoracic approach. He inserts the balloon in an antegrade direction through the subclavian artery and then positions it in the descending thoracic aorta.

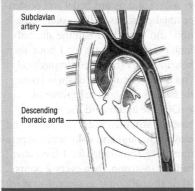

Subclavian artery

Descending thoracic aorta

nitrogen (BUN) and serum creatinine levels, and monitor these levels daily. *Changes in urine output, BUN, and serum creatinine levels may signal reduced renal*

perfusion from downward balloon displacement.

▶ Auscultate and record bowel sounds every 4 hours. Check for abdominal distention and tenderness as well as changes in the patient's elimination patterns.

▶ Measure the patient's temperature every 1 to 4 hours. If it's elevated, obtain blood samples for a culture, send them to the laboratory immediately, and notify the doctor. Culture any drainage at the insertion site.

▶ Monitor the patient's hematologic status. Observe for bleeding gums, blood in the urine or stools, petechiae, and bleeding at the insertion site. Monitor his platelet count, hemoglobin level, and hematocrit daily. Expect to administer blood products *to maintain hematocrit at 30%.* If the platelet count drops, expect to administer platelets.

▶ Monitor partial thromboplastin time (PTT) every 6 hours while the heparin dose is adjusted *to maintain PTT at $1\frac{1}{2}$ to 2 times the normal value,* then every 12 to 24 hours while the balloon remains in place.

▶ Measure PAP and pulmonary artery wedge pressure (PAWP) every 1 to 2 hours as ordered. A rising PAWP reflects preload, signaling increased ventricular pressure and workload; notify the doctor if this occurs. Some patients require I.V. nitroprusside during IABC *to reduce preload and afterload.*

▶ Obtain samples for ABG analysis as ordered.

▶ Monitor serum electrolyte levels— especially sodium and potassium—*to assess the patient's fluid and electrolyte balance and help prevent arrhythmias.*

▶ Watch for signs and symptoms of a dissecting aortic aneurysm, such as a blood pressure differential between the left and right arms, elevated blood pressure, syncope, pallor, diaphoresis, dyspnea, a throbbing abdominal mass, a reduced red blood cell count with an elevated white blood cell count, and pain in the chest, abdomen, or back. Notify the doctor immediately if you detect any of these complications.

Weaning the patient from IABC

▶ Assess the cardiac index, systemic blood pressure, and PAWP *to help the doctor evaluate the patient's readiness for weaning* — usually about 24 hours after balloon insertion. The patient's hemodynamic status should be stable on minimal doses of inotropic agents, such as dopamine (Intropin) or dobutamine (Dobutrex).

▶ To begin weaning, gradually decrease the frequency of balloon augmentation to 1:2 and 1:4, as ordered. Although your facility has its own weaning protocol, be aware that assist frequency is usually maintained for an hour or longer. If the patient's hemodynamic indices remain stable during this time, weaning may continue.

▶ Avoid leaving the patient on a low augmentation setting for more than 2 hours *to prevent embolus formation.*

▶ Assess the patient's tolerance of weaning. Signs and symptoms of poor tolerance include confusion and disorientation, urine output below 30 ml/hour, cold and clammy skin, chest pain, arrhythmias, ischemic ECG changes, and elevated PAP. If the patient develops any of these problems, notify the doctor at once.

Removing the intra-aortic balloon

▶ The balloon is removed when the patient's hemodynamic status remains stable after the frequency of balloon augmentation is decreased. The control system is turned off and the connective tubing is disconnected from the catheter *to ensure balloon deflation.*

▶ The doctor withdraws the balloon until the proximal end of the catheter contacts the distal end of the introducer sheath.

▶ The doctor then applies pressure below the puncture site and removes the balloon and introducer sheath as a unit, allowing a few seconds of free bleeding *to prevent thrombus formation.*

▶ *To promote distal bleedback,* the doctor applies pressure above the puncture site.

▶ Apply direct pressure to the site for 30 minutes or until bleeding stops. (In some facilities, this is the doctor's responsibility.)

▶ If the balloon was inserted surgically, the doctor will close the Dacron graft and suture the insertion site. The cardiologist usually removes a percutaneous catheter.

▶ After balloon removal, provide wound care according to your facility's policy. Record the patient's pedal and posterior tibial pulses, and the color, temperature, and sensation of the affected limb. Enforce bed rest as appropriate (usually for 24 hours).

Special considerations

▶ Before using the IABC control system, make sure you know what the alarms and messages mean and how to respond to them.

 Nursing alert You must respond immediately to alarms and messages.

▶ Change the dressing at the balloon insertion site every 24 hours or as needed, using strict sterile technique. Don't let povidone-iodine solution come in contact with the catheter.

▶ Make sure the head of the bed is elevated no more than 30 degrees.

▶ Watch for pump interruptions, which may result from loose ECG electrodes or leadwires, static or 60-cycle interference, catheter kinking, or improper body alignment.

▶ Make sure PTT is within normal limits before the balloon is removed *to prevent hemorrhage at insertion site.*

Complications

IABC may cause numerous complications. The most common, arterial embolism, stems from clot formation on the balloon surface. Other potential complications include extension or rupture of an aortic aneurysm, femoral or iliac artery perforation, femoral artery occlusion, and sepsis. Bleeding at the insertion site may become aggravated by pump-induced thrombocytopenia caused by platelet aggregation around the balloon.

Documentation

Document all aspects of patient assessment and management, including the patient's response to therapy. If you're responsible for the IABC device, document all routine checks, problems, and troubleshooting measures. If a technician is responsible for the IABC device, record only when and why the technician was notified and the result of his actions on the patient, if any. Also document any teaching of the patient, family, or close friends as well as their responses.

INTRACRANIAL PRESSURE MONITORING

Intracranial pressure (ICP) monitoring measures pressure exerted by the brain, blood, and cerebrospinal fluid (CSF)

against the inside of the skull. Indications for monitoring ICP include head trauma with bleeding or edema, overproduction or insufficient absorption of CSF, cerebral hemorrhage, and space-occupying brain lesions. ICP monitoring can detect elevated ICP early, before clinical danger signs develop. Prompt intervention can then help avert or diminish neurologic damage caused by cerebral hypoxia and shifts of brain mass.

The four basic ICP monitoring systems are intraventricular catheter, subarachnoid bolt, epidural sensor, and intraparenchymal pressure monitoring. (See *Understanding ICP monitoring systems.*)

Regardless of which system is used, the procedure is typically performed by a neurosurgeon in the operating room, emergency department, or intensive care unit.

Insertion of an ICP monitoring device requires sterile technique to reduce the risk of central nervous system (CNS) infection. Setting up equipment for the monitoring systems also requires strict asepsis.

Key nursing diagnoses and patient outcomes

Decreased adaptive capacity: Intracranial related to (specify)
The patient will:
▶ experience a decrease in intracranial pressure
▶ show signs of improving level of consciousness (LOC).

Risk for infection related to invasive monitoring procedure
The patient will:
▶ maintain a normal body temperature

Understanding ICP monitoring systems

Intracranial pressure (ICP) can be monitored using one of four systems.

Intraventricular catheter monitoring

In intraventricular catheter monitoring, which monitors ICP directly, the doctor inserts a small polyethylene or silicone rubber catheter into the lateral ventricle through a burr hole.

Although this method measures ICP most accurately, it carries the greatest risk of infection. This is the only type of ICP monitoring that allows evaluation of brain compliance and drainage of significant amounts of cerebrospinal fluid (CSF).

Contraindications usually include stenotic cerebral ventricles, cerebral aneurysms in the path of catheter placement, and suspected vascular lesions.

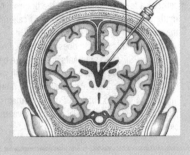

Ventricular catheter

Subarachnoid bolt monitoring

Subarachnoid bolt monitoring involves insertion of a special bolt into the subarachnoid space through a twist-drill burr hole that is positioned in the front of the skull behind the hairline.

Placing the bolt is easier than placing an intraventricular catheter, especially if a computed tomography scan reveals that the cerebrum has shifted or the ventricles have collapsed. This type of ICP monitoring also carries less risk of infection and parenchymal damage because the bolt doesn't penetrate the cerebrum.

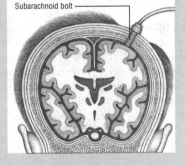

Subarachnoid bolt

Epidural or subdural sensor monitoring

ICP can also be monitored from the epidural or subdural space. For epidural monitoring, a fiber-optic sensor is inserted into the epidural space through a burr hole. This system's main drawback is its questionable accuracy because ICP isn't being measured directly from a CSF-filled space.

For subdural monitoring, a fiber-optic transducer-tipped catheter is tunneled through a burr hole, and its tip is placed on brain tissue under the dura mater. The main drawback to this method is its inability to drain CSF.

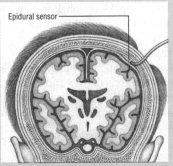

Epidural sensor

(continued)

Understanding ICP monitoring systems *(continued)*

Intraparenchymal monitoring

In intraparenchymal monitoring, the doctor inserts a catheter through a small subarachnoid bolt and, after puncturing the dura, advances the catheter a few centimeters into the brain's white matter. There is no need to balance or calibrate the equipment after insertion.

Although this method doesn't provide direct access to CSF, measurements are accurate because brain tissue pressures correlate well with ventricular pressures. Intraparenchymal monitoring may be used to obtain ICP measurements in patients with compressed or dislocated ventricles.

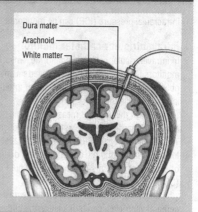

Dura mater
Arachnoid
White matter

▶ show no signs or symptoms of infection from the invasive procedure.

Equipment

Monitoring unit and transducers as ordered • 16 to 20 sterile 4″ × 4″ gauze pads • linen-saver pads • shave preparation tray or hair scissors • sterile drapes • povidone-iodine solution • sterile gown • surgical mask • sterile gloves • head dressing supplies (including two rolls of 4″ elastic gauze dressing, one roll of 4″ roller gauze, and adhesive tape) • optional: suction apparatus, I.V. pole, and yardstick

Preparation of equipment

Monitoring units and setup protocols are varied and complex and differ among health care facilities. Check your facility's guidelines for your particular unit.

Various types of preassembled ICP monitoring units are also available, each with its own setup protocols. These units are designed to reduce the risk of infection by eliminating the need for multiple stopcocks, manometers, and transducer dome assemblies. Some facilities use units that have miniaturized transducers rather than transducer domes.

Implementation

▶ Explain the procedure to the patient or his family. Make sure the patient or a responsible family member has signed a consent form.
▶ Determine whether the patient is allergic to iodine preparations.
▶ Provide privacy if the procedure is being done in an open emergency department or intensive care unit. Wash your hands.
▶ Obtain baseline routine and neurologic vital signs *to aid in prompt detection of decompensation during the procedure.*
▶ Place the patient in the supine position and elevate the head of the bed 30 degrees (or as ordered). Document the number of bed crank rotations, or hang

a yardstick on an I.V. pole and mark the exact elevation.

▶ Place linen-saver pads under the patient's head. Shave or clip his hair at the insertion site, as indicated by the doctor, *to decrease the risk of infection.* Carefully fold and remove the linen-saver pads *to avoid spilling loose hair onto the bed.* Drape the patient with sterile drapes. Then scrub the insertion site for 2 minutes with povidone-iodine solution.

▶ The doctor puts on the sterile gown, mask, and sterile gloves. He then opens the interior wrap of the sterile supply tray and proceeds with insertion of the catheter or bolt.

▶ *To facilitate placement of the device,* hold the patient's head in your hands or attach a long strip of 4″ roller gauze to one side rail, and bring it across the patient's forehead to the opposite rail. Reassure the conscious patient *to help ease his anxiety.* Talk to him frequently *to assess his LOC and detect signs of deterioration.* Watch for cardiac arrhythmias and abnormal respiratory patterns.

▶ After insertion, put on sterile gloves and apply povidone-iodine solution and a sterile dressing to the site. If not done by the doctor, connect the catheter to the appropriate monitoring device, depending on the system used. (See *Setting up a ventriculostomy ICP monitoring system,* pages 454 and 455.)

▶ If the doctor has set up a ventriculostomy drainage system, attach the drip chamber to the headboard or bedside I.V. pole as ordered.

> **Nursing alert** Positioning the drip chamber too high may raise ICP; positioning it too low may cause excessive CSF drainage.

▶ Inspect the insertion site at least every 24 hours (or according to facility policy) for redness, swelling, and drainage. Clean the site, reapply povidone-iodine solution, and apply a fresh sterile dressing.

▶ Assess the patient's clinical status and take routine and neurologic vital signs every hourly or as ordered. Make sure you've obtained orders for waveforms and pressure parameters from the doctor.

▶ Calculate cerebral perfusion pressure (CPP) hourly; use the equation: CPP = MAP − ICP (MAP refers to mean arterial pressure).

▶ Observe digital ICP readings and waves. Remember, the pattern of readings is more significant than any single reading. (See *Interpreting ICP waveforms,* pages 456 and 457.) If you observe continually elevated ICP readings, note how long they're sustained. If they last several minutes, notify the doctor immediately. Finally, record and describe any CSF drainage.

Special considerations

> **Age alert** In infants, ICP monitoring can be performed without penetrating the scalp. In this external method, a photoelectric transducer with a pressure-sensitive membrane is taped to the anterior fontanel. The transducer responds to pressure at the site and transmits readings to a bedside monitor and recording system. The external method is restricted to infants because pressure readings can be obtained only at fontanels, the incompletely ossified areas of the skull.

▶ Osmotic diuretic agents, such as mannitol, reduce cerebral edema by shrinking intracranial contents. Given

Setting up a ventriculostomy ICP monitoring system

To set up a ventriculostomy intracranial pressure (ICP) monitoring system, follow these steps, using strict aseptic technique:

■ Begin by opening a sterile towel. On the sterile field, place a 20-ml luer-lock syringe, an 18G needle, a 250-ml bag filled with normal saline solution (with outer wrapper removed), and a disposable transducer.
■ Put on sterile gloves and gown and fill the 20-ml syringe with normal saline solution from the I.V. bag.
■ Remove the injection cap from the patient line and attach the syringe. Turn the system stopcock off to the short end of the patient line and flush through to the drip chamber (as shown below). Allow a few drops to flow through the flow chamber (the manometer), the tubing, and the one-way valve into the drainage bag. (Fill the tubing and the manometer slowly to minimize air bubbles. If air bubbles surface, make sure to force them from the system.)

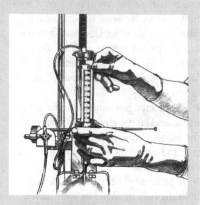

■ Next, connect the transducer to the monitor.
■ Put on a new pair of sterile gloves.
■ Keeping one hand sterile, turn the patient stopcock off to the patient.
■ Align the zero point with the center line of the patient's head, level with the middle of the ear (as shown below).

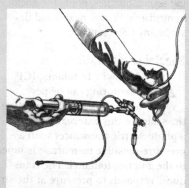

■ Attach the manometer to the I.V. pole at the head of the bed.
■ Slide the drip chamber onto the manometer and align the chamber to the zero point (as shown at top of next column).

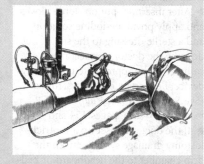

■ Lower the flow chamber to zero and turn the stopcock off to the dead-end cap. With a clean hand, balance the system according to monitor guidelines.

Setting up a ventriculostomy ICP monitoring system *(continued)*

■ Turn the system stopcock off to drainage and raise the flow chamber to the ordered height (as shown at right).
■ Return the stopcock to the ordered position and observe the monitor for the return of ICP patterns.

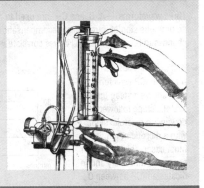

by I.V. drip or bolus, mannitol draws water from tissues into plasma; it doesn't cross the blood-brain barrier. Monitor serum electrolyte levels and osmolality readings closely because the patient may become dehydrated very quickly. Be aware that a rebound increase in ICP may occur. (See *Nursing management of increased ICP*, page 458.) To avoid rebound increased ICP, 50 ml of albumin may be given with the mannitol bolus. Note, however, that you'll see a residual rise in ICP before it decreases. If your patient has heart failure or severe renal dysfunction, monitor for problems in adapting to the increased intravascular volumes.

▶ Fluid restriction, usually 1,200 to 1,500 ml/day, prevents cerebral edema from developing or worsening.

▶ Although their use is controversial, steroids may be used to lower elevated ICP by reducing sodium and water concentration in the brain. They're usually given with antacids and famotidine or ranitidine *because they may produce peptic ulcers.* Observe for possible GI bleeding. Also monitor blood glucose

levels *because steroids may cause hyperglycemia.*

▶ A barbiturate-induced coma depresses the reticular activating system and reduces the brain's metabolic demand. Reduced demand for oxygen and energy reduces cerebral blood flow, thereby lowering ICP.

▶ Hyperventilation with oxygen from a handheld resuscitation bag or ventilator helps rid the patient of excess carbon dioxide, thereby constricting cerebral vessels and reducing cerebral blood volume and ICP. However, only normal brain tissues respond because blood vessels in damaged areas have reduced vasoconstrictive ability.

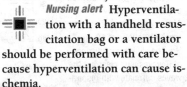 *Nursing alert* **Hyperventilation with a handheld resuscitation bag or a ventilator should be performed with care because hyperventilation can cause ischemia.**

▶ Before tracheal suctioning, hyperventilate the patient with 100% oxygen as ordered. Apply suction for a maximum of 15 seconds. Avoid inducing

Interpreting ICP waveforms

Three waveforms—A, B, and C—are used to monitor intracranial pressure (ICP). A waves are an ominous sign of intracranial decompensation and poor compliance. B waves correlate with changes in respiration, and C waves correlate with changes in arterial pressure.

Normal waveform

A normal ICP waveform typically shows a steep upward systolic slope followed by a downward diastolic slope with a dicrotic notch. In most cases, this waveform occurs continuously and indicates an ICP between 0 and 15 mm Hg—normal pressure.

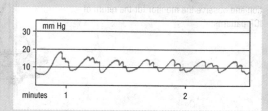

A waves

The most clinically significant ICP waveforms are A waves, which may reach elevations of 50 to 100 mm Hg, persist for 5 to 20 minutes, then drop sharply—signaling exhaustion of the brain's compliance mechanisms. A waves may come and go, spiking from temporary rises in thoracic pressure or from any condition that increases ICP beyond the brain's compliance limits. Activities, such as sustained coughing or straining during defecation, can cause temporary elevations in thoracic pressure.

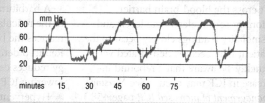

B waves

B waves, which appear sharp and rhythmic with a sawtooth pattern, occur every 1½ to 2 minutes and may reach elevations of 50 mm Hg. The clinical significance of B waves isn't clear but the waves correlate with respiratory changes and may occur more frequently with decreasing compensation. Because B waves sometimes precede A waves, notify the doctor if B waves occur frequently.

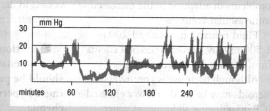

Interpreting ICP waveforms *(continued)*

C waves

Like B waves, C waves are rapid and rhythmic but they aren't as sharp. Clinically insignificant, they may fluctuate with respirations or systemic blood pressure changes.

Waveform showing equipment problem

A waveform such as the one shown at right signals a problem with the transducer or monitor. Check for line obstruction and determine whether the transducer needs rebalancing.

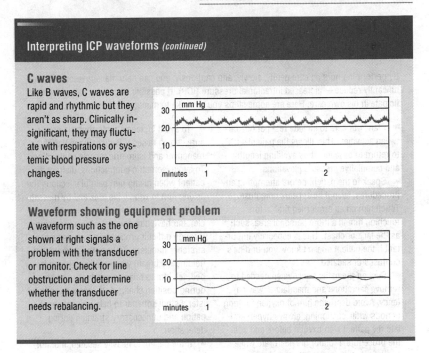

hypoxia *because this condition greatly increases cerebral blood flow.*

▶ Because fever raises brain metabolism, which increases cerebral blood flow, fever reduction (achieved by administering acetaminophen, sponge baths, or a hypothermia blanket) also helps to reduce ICP. However, rebound increases in ICP and brain edema may occur if rapid rewarming takes place after hypothermia or if cooling measures induce shivering.

▶ Withdrawal of CSF through the drainage system reduces CSF volume and thus reduces ICP. Although less commonly used, surgical removal of a skull-bone flap provides room for the swollen brain to expand. If this procedure is performed, keep the site clean and dry *to prevent infection* and maintain sterile technique when changing the dressing.

Complications

CNS infection, the most common hazard of ICP monitoring, can result from contamination of the equipment setup or of the insertion site.

Nursing alert **Excessive loss of CSF can result from faulty stopcock placement or a drip chamber that is positioned too low. Such loss can rapidly decompress the cranial contents and damage bridging cortical veins, leading to hematoma formation. Decompression can also lead to rupture of existing hematomas or aneurysms, causing hemorrhage.**

Watch for signs of impending or overt decompensation: pupillary dilation (unilateral or bilateral); decreased pupillary response to light; decreasing LOC; rising systolic blood pressure and widening pulse pressure; bradycardia;

Nursing management of increased ICP

By performing nursing care gently, slowly, and cautiously, you can help manage—or even significantly reduce—increased intracranial pressure (ICP). If possible, urge your patient to participate in his own care. Here are some steps you can take to manage increased ICP:

- Plan your care to include rest periods between activities. This allows the patient's ICP to return to baseline, thus avoiding lengthy and cumulative pressure elevations.
- Speak to the patient before attempting any procedures, even if he appears comatose. Touch him on an arm or leg first before touching him in a more personal area, such as the face or chest. This is especially important if the patient doesn't know you or if he's confused or sedated.
- Suction the patient only when needed to remove secretions and maintain airway patency. Avoid depriving him of oxygen for long periods while suctioning; always hyperventilate the patient with oxygen before and after the procedure. Monitor his heart rate while suctioning. If multiple catheter passes are needed to clear secretions, hyperventilate the patient between them to bring ICP as close to baseline as possible.
- To promote venous drainage, keep the patient's head in the midline position, even when he's positioned on his side. Avoid flexing the neck or hip more than 90 degrees, and keep the head of the bed elevated 30 to 45 degrees.

- To avoid increasing intrathoracic pressure, which raises ICP, discourage Valsalva's maneuver and isometric muscle contractions. To avoid isometric contractions, distract the patient when giving him painful injections (by asking him to wiggle his toes and by massaging the area before injection to relax the muscle) and have him concentrate on breathing through difficult procedures such as bed-to-stretcher transfers. To keep the patient from holding his breath when moving around in bed, tell him to relax as much as possible during position changes. If necessary, administer a stool softener to help prevent constipation and unnecessary straining during defecation.
- If the patient is heavily sedated, monitor his respiratory rate and blood gas levels. Depressed respirations will compromise ventilations and oxygen exchange. Maintaining adequate respiratory rate and volume will help reduce ICP.
- If you're in a specialty unit, you may be able to routinely hyperventilate the patient to counter sustained ICP elevations. This procedure is one of the best ways to reduce high ICP at bedside for short periods. Consult your facility's protocol.

slowed, irregular respirations; and, in late decompensation, decerebrate posturing.

Documentation

Record the time and date of the insertion procedure and the patient's response. Note the insertion site and the type of monitoring system used. Record ICP digital readings and waveforms and CCP hourly in your notes, in a flow-

chart, or directly on readout strips, depending on your facility's policy. Document any factors that may affect ICP (for example, drug administration, stressful procedures, or sleep).

Record routine and neurologic vital signs hourly and describe the patient's clinical status. Note the amount, character, and frequency of any CSF drainage (for example, "between 6 p.m. and 7 p.m., 15 ml of blood-tinged

CSF"). Also record the ICP reading in response to drainage.

INTRADERMAL INJECTION

Because little systemic absorption of intradermally injected agents takes place, this type of injection is used primarily to produce a local effect, such as in allergy or tuberculin testing. Intradermal injections are administered in small volumes (usually 0.5 ml or less) into the outer layers of the skin.

The ventral forearm is the most commonly used site for intradermal injection because of its easy accessibility and lack of hair. In extensive allergy testing, the outer aspect of the upper arms may be used as well as the area of the back located between the scapulae. (See *Intradermal injection sites*.)

Key nursing diagnoses and patient outcomes

Deficient knowledge related to lack of exposure to intradermal injections
The patient will:
▶ state or demonstrate an understanding of what has been taught
▶ demonstrate an ability to perform new health-related behaviors as they're taught.

Risk for injury related to intradermal injections
The patient will:
▶ identify factors that increase the potential for injury
▶ assist in identifying and applying safety measures to prevent injury.

Equipment
Patient's medication record and chart • tuberculin syringe with a 26G or 27G

Intradermal injection sites

The most common intradermal injection site is the ventral forearm. Other sites (indicated by dotted areas) include the upper chest, upper arm, and shoulder blades. Skin in these areas is usually lightly pigmented, thinly keratinized, and relatively hairless, facilitating detection of adverse reactions.

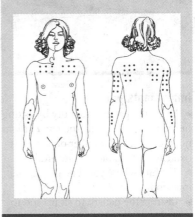

½″ to ⅜″ needle • prescribed medication • gloves • alcohol pads

Preparation of equipment
Verify the order on the patient's medication record by checking it against the doctor's orders. Inspect the medication to make sure it isn't abnormally discolored or cloudy and doesn't contain precipitates. Wash your hands.

Choose equipment appropriate to the prescribed medication and injection site and make sure it works properly. Check the medication label against the patient's medication record. Read the label again as you draw up the medication for injection.

Giving an intradermal injection

Secure the forearm. Insert the needle at a 10- to 15-degree angle so that it just punctures the skin's surface. The antigen should raise a small wheal as it's injected.

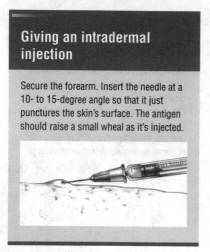

Implementation

▶ Verify the patient's identity by asking his name and checking the name, room number, and bed number on his wristband against his medical record.

▶ Tell him where you'll be giving the injection.

▶ Instruct the patient to sit up and to extend his arm and support it on a flat surface, with the ventral forearm exposed.

▶ Put on gloves.

▶ With an alcohol pad, clean the surface of the ventral forearm about two or three fingerbreadths distal to the antecubital space. Make sure the test site you have chosen is free from hair or blemishes. Allow the skin to dry completely before administering the injection.

▶ While holding the patient's forearm in your hand, stretch the skin taut with your thumb.

▶ With your free hand, hold the needle at a 10- to 15-degree angle to the patient's arm, with its bevel up.

▶ Insert the needle about ¹⁄₈″ (0.3 cm) below the epidermis at sites 2″ (5 cm)

apart. Stop when the needle's bevel tip is under the skin and inject the antigen slowly. You should feel some resistance as you do this, and a wheal should form as you inject the antigen. (See *Giving an intradermal injection.*)

If no wheal forms, you have injected the antigen too deeply; withdraw the needle, and administer another test dose at least 2″ from the first site.

▶ Withdraw the needle at the same angle at which it was inserted. Don't rub the site. *This could irritate the underlying tissue, which may affect test results.*

▶ Circle each test site with a marking pen and label each site according to the recall antigen given. Instruct the patient to refrain from washing off the circles until the test is completed.

▶ Dispose of needles and syringes according to your facility's policy.

▶ Remove and discard your gloves and wash your hands.

▶ Assess the patient's response to the skin testing in 24 to 48 hours.

Special considerations

In patients who are hypersensitive to the test antigens, a severe anaphylactic response can result. This requires immediate epinephrine injection and other emergency resuscitation procedures. Be especially alert after giving a test dose of penicillin or tetanus antitoxin.

Documentation

On the patient's medication record, document the type and amount of medication given, the time it was given, and the injection site. Note skin reactions and other adverse reactions.

INTRAOSSEOUS INFUSION

When rapid venous infusion is difficult or impossible, intraosseous infusion allows delivery of fluids, medications, or whole blood into the bone marrow. Performed on infants and children, this technique is used in such emergencies as cardiopulmonary arrest, circulatory collapse, hypokalemia from traumatic injury or dehydration, status epilepticus, status asthmaticus, burns, near-drowning, and overwhelming sepsis.

Any drug that can be given I.V. can be given by intraosseous infusion with comparable absorption and effectiveness. Intraosseous infusion has been used as an acceptable alternative for infants and children.

Intraosseous infusion is commonly undertaken at the anterior surface of the tibia. Alternative sites include the iliac crest, spinous process and, rarely, the upper anterior portion of the sternum. Only personnel trained in this procedure should perform it. Usually, a nurse assists. (See *Understanding intraosseous infusion.*)

This procedure is contraindicated in patients with osteogenesis imperfecta, osteopetrosis, and ipsilateral fracture because of the potential for subcutaneous extravasation. Infusion through an area with cellulitis or an infected burn increases the risk of infection.

Key nursing diagnoses and patient outcomes

Deficient knowledge related to lack of exposure to intraosseous infusion
The patient will:
▶ state or demonstrate an understanding of what has been taught

Understanding intraosseous infusion

During intraosseous infusion, the bone marrow serves as a noncollapsible vein; thus, fluid infused into the marrow cavity rapidly enters the circulation by way of an extensive network of venous sinusoids. Here, the needle is shown positioned in the patient's tibia.

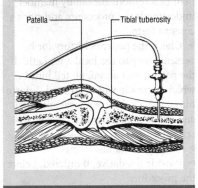

▶ demonstrate an ability to perform new health-related behaviors as they are taught.

Risk for injury related to intraosseous infusion
The patient will:
▶ identify factors that increase the potential for injury
▶ assist in identifying and applying safety measures to prevent injury.

Equipment

Bone marrow biopsy needle or specially designed intraosseous infusion needle (cannula and obturator) • povidone-iodine pads • sterile gauze pads • sterile gloves • sterile drape • heparin flush solution • I.V. fluids and tubing • 1%

lidocaine • 3- or 5-ml syringe • tape • optional: sedative, if ordered

Preparation of equipment
Prepare I.V. fluids and tubing as ordered.

Implementation
▶ If the patient is conscious, explain the procedure *to allay his fears and promote his cooperation.* Ensure that the patient or a responsible family member understands the procedure and signs a consent form.
▶ Check the patient's history for hypersensitivity to the local anesthetic. If the patient isn't an infant, tell him which bone site will be infused. Inform him that he'll receive a local anesthetic and will feel pressure from needle insertion.
▶ Wash your hands.
▶ Provide a sedative, if ordered, before the procedure.
▶ Position the patient based on the selected puncture site.
▶ Using sterile technique, the doctor cleans the puncture site with a povidone-iodine pad and allows it to dry. He then covers the area with a sterile drape.
▶ Using sterile technique, hand the doctor the 3- or 5-ml syringe with 1% lidocaine *so that he can anesthetize the infusion site.*
▶ The doctor inserts the infusion needle through the skin and into the bone at an angle of 10 to 15 degrees from vertical. He advances it with a forward and backward rotary motion through the periosteum until it penetrates the marrow cavity. The needle should "give" suddenly as it enters the marrow and stand erect when released.
▶ Then the doctor removes the obturator from the needle and attaches a 5-ml

syringe. He aspirates some bone marrow *to confirm needle placement.*
▶ The doctor replaces this syringe with a syringe containing 5 ml of heparin flush solution and flushes the cannula *to confirm needle placement and clear the cannula of clots and bone particles.*
▶ Next, the doctor removes the syringe of flush solution and attaches I.V. tubing to the cannula *to allow infusion of medications and I.V. fluids.*
▶ Put on sterile gloves.
▶ Clean the infusion site with povidone-iodine pads and then secure the site with tape and a sterile gauze dressing.
▶ Monitor vital signs and check the infusion site for bleeding and extravasation.

Special considerations
▶ Intraosseous infusion should be discontinued as soon as conventional vascular access is established (within 2 to 4 hours, if possible). *Prolonged infusion significantly increases the risk of infection.*
▶ After the needle has been removed, place a sterile dressing over the injection site, and apply firm pressure to the site for 5 minutes.
▶ Intraosseous flow rates are determined by needle size and flow through the bone marrow. Fluids should flow freely if needle placement is correct. Normal saline solution has been given intraosseously at a rate of 600 ml/minute and up to 2,500 ml/hour when delivered under pressure of 300 mm Hg through a 13G needle.

Complications
Common complications include extravasation of fluid into subcutaneous tissue, resulting from incorrect needle placement; subperiosteal effusion, resulting from failure of fluid to enter the

marrow space; and clotting in the needle, resulting from delayed infusion or failure to flush the needle after placement. Other complications include subcutaneous abscess, osteomyelitis, and epiphyseal injury.

Documentation
Record the time, date, location, and patient's tolerance of the procedure. Document the amount of fluid infused on the input and output record.

INTRAPLEURAL DRUG ADMINISTRATION

An intrapleural drug is injected through the chest wall into the pleural space or instilled through a chest tube placed intrapleurally for drainage. Doctors use intrapleural administration to promote analgesia, treat spontaneous pneumothorax, resolve pleural effusions, and administer chemotherapy.

Intrapleurally administered drugs diffuse across the parietal pleura and innermost intercostal muscles to affect the intercostal nerves. During intrapleural injection of a drug, the needle passes through the intercostal muscles and parietal pleura on its way to the pleural space.

The internal intercostal muscle is a key landmark for needle placement. It resists the advancing needle, becoming the posterior intercostal membrane in the posterior chest region.

Drugs commonly given by intrapleural injection include tetracycline, streptokinase, anesthetics, and chemotherapeutic agents (to treat malignant pleural effusion or lung adenocarcinoma).

Contraindications for this route include pleural fibrosis or adhesions, which interfere with diffusion of the drug to the intended site; pleural inflammation; sepsis; and infection at the puncture site. Patients with bullous emphysema and those receiving respiratory therapy using positive end-expiratory pressure also shouldn't have intrapleural injections because the injections may exacerbate an already compromised pulmonary condition.

Key nursing diagnoses and patient outcomes
Deficient knowledge related to lack of exposure to intrapleural drug instillation
The patient will:
▶ state or demonstrate an understanding of what has been taught
▶ demonstrate an ability to perform new health-related behaviors as they're taught.

Risk for injury related to intrapleural drug instillation
The patient will:
▶ identify factors that increase the potential for injury
▶ assist in identifying and applying safety measures to prevent injury.

Equipment
An intrapleural drug is given through a #16 to #20 or #28 to #40 chest tube if the patient has empyema, pleural effusion, or pneumothorax. Otherwise, it's given through a 16G to 18G blunt-tipped intrapleural (epidural) needle and catheter. Accessory equipment depends on the type of access device the doctor uses. All equipment must be sterile.

Giving intrapleural drugs

In intrapleural administration, the doctor injects a drug into the pleural space using a catheter.

Help the patient lie on one side with the affected side up. The doctor inserts a needle into the fourth to eighth intercostal space, 3″ to 4″ (7.5 to 10 cm) from the posterior midline. He then advances the needle medially over the superior edge of the patient's rib through the intercostal muscles until it tangentially penetrates the parietal pleura, as shown. The catheter is advanced into the pleural space through the needle, which is then removed.

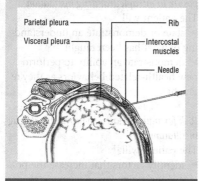

Parietal pleura — Rib
Visceral pleura — Intercostal muscles
— Needle

For intrapleural catheter insertion

Gloves • gauze • antiseptic solution such as povidone-iodine • drape • local anesthetic such as 1% lidocaine • 3- or 5-ml syringe with 22G 1″ and 25G ⅝″ needles • 18G needle or scalpel • saline-lubricated glass syringe • dressings • sutures • tape

For chest tube insertion

Towels • gloves • gauze • antiseptic solution such as povidone-iodine • 3- or 5-ml syringe • local anesthetic such as 1% lidocaine • 18G needle or scalpel • chest tube with or without trocar (#16 to #20 catheter for air or serous fluid, #28 to #40 catheter for blood, pus, or thick fluid) • two rubber-tipped clamps • sutures • drain dressings • tape • thoracic drainage system and tubing

For drug administration

Gloves • sterile gauze pads • antiseptic solution such as povidone-iodine • prescribed medication • appropriate-sized needles and syringes • 1% lidocaine, if necessary • dressings • tape

Implementation

▶ Explain the procedure to the patient *to allay his fears.* Encourage him to follow instructions.

Inserting an intrapleural catheter

▶ The doctor inserts the intrapleural catheter at the patient's bedside with the nurse assisting.
▶ Position the patient on his side with the affected side up. The doctor will insert the catheter into the fourth to eighth intercostal space, 3″ to 4″ (7.5 to 10 cm) from the posterior midline. (See *Giving intrapleural drugs.*)
▶ The doctor puts on sterile gloves, cleans around the puncture site with antiseptic-soaked gauze, and covers the area with a sterile drape. Next, he fills the 3- or 5-ml syringe with local anesthetic and injects it into the skin and deep tissues.
▶ The doctor punctures the skin with the 18G needle or scalpel, which helps the blunt-tipped intrapleural needle penetrate the skin over the superior edge of the lower rib in the chosen interspace. Keeping the bevel tilted upward, he directs the needle medially at a 30- to 40-degree angle to the skin. When the needle tip punctures the posterior intercostal membrane, he re-

moves the stylet and attaches a saline-lubricated glass syringe containing 2 to 4 cc of air to the needle hub.

▶ During puncture, tell the patient to hold his breath (or momentarily disconnect him from mechanical ventilation) until the needle is removed. *This helps prevent the needle from injuring lung tissue.*

▶ The doctor advances the needle slowly. When the needle punctures the parietal pleura, negative intrapleural pressure moves the plunger outward. He then removes the syringe from the needle and threads the intrapleural catheter through the needle until he has advanced it about 2″ (5 cm) into the pleural space. Without removing the catheter, he carefully withdraws the needle.

▶ Tell the patient that he can breathe again (or reconnect mechanical ventilation).

▶ After inserting the catheter, the doctor coils it to prevent kinking and then sutures it securely to the patient's skin. He confirms placement by aspirating the catheter. Resistance indicates correct placement in the pleural space; aspirated blood means that the catheter probably is misplaced in a blood vessel, and aspirated air means that it's probably in a lung. He'll then order a chest X-ray *to detect pneumothorax.*

▶ Apply a sterile dressing over the insertion site *to prevent catheter dislodgment.* Take the patient's vital signs every 15 minutes for the 1st hour after the procedure and then as needed.

Inserting a chest tube

▶ The doctor inserts the chest tube with the nurse assisting. (For more information see "Chest tube insertion," page 158.)

▶ First, position the patient with the affected side up, and drape him with sterile towels.

▶ The doctor puts on gloves and cleans the appropriate site with antiseptic-soaked gauze. If the patient has a pneumothorax, the doctor uses the second intercostal space as the access site *because air rises to the top of the pleural space.* If the patient has a hemothorax or pleural effusion, the doctor uses the sixth to eighth intercostal space *because fluid settles to the bottom of the pleural space.*

▶ The doctor fills the 3- or 5-ml syringe with a local anesthetic and injects it into the site. He makes a small incision with the 18G needle or scalpel, inserts the appropriate-sized chest tube, and immediately connects it to the thoracic drainage system or clamps it close to the patient's chest. He then sutures the tube to the patient's skin.

▶ Tape the chest tube to the patient's chest distal to the insertion site *to help prevent accidental dislodgment.* Also tape the junction of the chest tube and drainage tube *to prevent their separation.* Apply sterile drain dressings and tape them to the site.

▶ After insertion, the doctor checks tube placement with an X-ray. Check the patient's vital signs every 15 minutes for 1 hour and then as needed. Auscultate his lungs at least every 4 hours to assess air exchange in the affected lung. Diminished or absent breath sounds mean that the lung hasn't reexpanded.

Administering medication

▶ The doctor injects medication through the intrapleural catheter or chest tube with the nurse assisting.

▶ If the patient will receive chemotherapy, expect to give an antiemetic at least 30 minutes beforehand.

▶ Position the patient with the affected side up. Help the doctor move the dressing away from the intrapleural catheter or chest tube and clamp the drainage tube, if present.

▶ The doctor disinfects the access port of the catheter or chest tube with antiseptic-soaked gauze. Draw up the appropriate medication dose and hand it to the doctor with the vial for verification.

▶ The doctor injects the medication. If it's an anesthetic, he gives a bolus or loading dose initially and then a continuous infusion. For tetracycline, he mixes it with an anesthetic, such as lidocaine, *to alleviate pain during injection.*

▶ Reapply the dressings around the catheter. Monitor the patient closely during and after drug administration *to gauge the effectiveness of drug therapy and to check for complications and adverse effects.*

Special considerations

▶ Make sure the patient has signed a consent form.

▶ Before catheter insertion, ask the patient to urinate *to reduce the risk of bladder perforation and promote comfort.* If the patient is receiving a continuous infusion, label the solution bag clearly. Cover all injection ports *so that other drugs aren't injected into the pleural space accidentally.*

▶ If the chest tube dislodges, cover the site at once with a sterile gauze pad and tape it in place. Stay with the patient, monitor his vital signs, and observe carefully for signs and symptoms of tension pneumothorax: hypotension, distended neck veins, absent breath sounds, tracheal shift, hypoxemia, dyspnea, tachypnea, diaphoresis, chest pain, and weak, rapid pulse. Have another nurse call the doctor and gather the equipment for reinsertion.

▶ Keep rubber-tipped clamps at the bedside. If a commercial chest tube system cracks or a tube disconnects, use the clamps to clamp the chest tube close to the insertion site temporarily. Make sure to observe the patient closely for signs of tension pneumothorax *because no air can escape from the pleural space while the tube is clamped.*

▶ You can wrap a piece of petroleum gauze around the chest tube at the insertion site to make an airtight seal; then apply the sterile dressing. After the chest tube is removed, use petroleum gauze to dress the wound; then cover it with a new piece of sterile gauze.

▶ After the catheter is removed, inspect the skin at the entry site for signs of infection and then cover the wound with a sterile dressing.

Complications

Pneumothorax or tension pneumothorax may occur if the doctor accidentally injects air into the pleural cavity. These complications are more likely to occur in a patient who is on mechanical ventilation.

Accidental catheter placement in the lung can lead to respiratory distress; catheter placement within a vessel can increase the medication's effects. With catheter fracture, lung puncture may occur. Laceration of intercostal vessels can cause bleeding.

Local anesthetic toxicity can lead to tinnitus, metallic taste, light-headedness, somnolence, visual and auditory disturbances, restlessness, delirium, slurred speech, nystagmus, muscle tremor, seizures, arrhythmias, and cardiovascular collapse. A local anesthetic containing epinephrine can cause tachycardia and hypertension.

Intrapleural chemotherapeutic drugs can irritate the pleura chemically and cause such systemic effects as neutropenia and thrombocytopenia. Administering intrapleural tetracycline without an anesthetic can cause pain.

The insertion site can become infected. However, meticulous skin preparation, strict sterile technique, and sterile dressings usually prevent infection.

Documentation
Document the drug administered, drug dosage, patient's response to the treatment, and condition of the catheter insertion site.

IONTOPHORESIS

Iontophoresis is a technique for delivering dermal analgesia quickly (in 10 to 20 minutes) with minimal discomfort and without distorting the tissue. The Numby 900 inotophoretic drug-delivery system is a handheld device with two electrodes that uses a mild electric current to deliver charged ions of lidocaine 2% and epinephrine 1:100,000 solution into the skin. The device is powered by a 9-volt battery. Because iontophoresis acts quickly, it's an excellent choice for numbing an I.V. injection site, especially in children.

Key nursing diagnoses and patient outcomes
Deficient knowledge related to lack of exposure to iontophoresis
The patient will:

▶ state an understanding of iontophoresis
▶ verbalize decreased anxiety related to gained knowledge.

Equipment
Dose-control device with battery • drug-delivery electrode kit • lidocaine 2% with epinephrine 1:100,000 solution • alcohol pads • syringe with needle • gloves • tongue blade

Implementation
▶ Ask the patient—or if the patient is a child, ask the parents—if the patient has any allergies or a sensitivity to any medications. Avoid using iontophoresis in patients with implanted devices such as a pacemaker.
▶ Explain the procedure to the patient and tell him that he may feel tingling or warmth under the electrode pads while they're on the skin.
▶ Assess the patient for appropriate electrode placement. You'll place a medication-delivery electrode over the intended I.V. insertion site. The second electrode, which drives drug ions into the skin, must be applied over a muscle 4″ to 6″ (10 to 15 cm) away.
▶ Put on gloves. Examine the patient's skin and select intact electrode placement sites, avoiding areas with pimples, unhealed wounds, or ingrown hairs. With alcohol pads, briskly rub an area slightly larger than the electrode at each site.
▶ Remove the paper flap from the back of the drug-delivery electrode.
▶ Draw up the lidocaine with epinephrine in a syringe. Remove the needle from the syringe and saturate the medication pad with the amount of lidocaine and epinephrine solution indicated on the electrode pad (see photo be-

low). The amount of lidocaine and epinephrine solution required to saturate the pad varies with pad size: for a standard-sized pad, use about 1 ml; for a large pad, use about 2.5 ml.

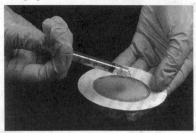

▶ Remove the remaining backing from the drug-delivery pad and apply the pad to the selected site. Remove the backing from the grounding electrode and apply it to the second prepared site.

▶ Connect the lead clips: red (positive charge) to the drug-delivery electrode and black (negative charge) to the grounding electrode.

▶ Turn on the device. (See photo below.)

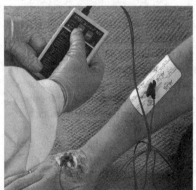

As indicated by the green light, the device will automatically operate at the lowest current, 2 milliamperes (mA), unless you increase the level to 3 mA or 4 mA by pressing the ON button. If your patient has discomfort at a higher

setting, reduce the current by pushing the ON button until the appropriate light indicates the desired level. The device will stop automatically after delivering 40 mA-minutes. The device is calibrated to deliver a dose of 40 mA-minutes. If the setting remains at 4 mA, treatment is completed in 10 minutes. However, if you decrease the setting because the patient has discomfort, the device will automatically adjust to a longer treatment time to deliver the entire dose.

▶ After the dose has been delivered remove the electrodes. Assess the skin at the drug-delivery site for numbness by touching it with a blunt object such as a tongue blade.

▶ Promptly prepare the site and perform the venipuncture because the numbness may only last a few minutes.

▶ Discard gloves and wash your hands.

Special considerations

▶ *To avoid interfering with energy emission,* don't tape or compress the electrodes.

▶ If you need to stop the treatment for any reason, press the OFF button and hold it. The lights will indicate decreasing current levels, then the device will beep and turn off. Don't disconnect the lead clips or the electrodes until all signals have stopped *because the device is still transmitting energy until it turns off.*

Complications

Allergic reaction may occur in patients sensitive to lidocaine or epinephrine.

Documentation

Document the treatment, the sites used, and whether analgesia was achieved. Also document an allergic response, if any.

ISOLATION EQUIPMENT USE

Isolation procedures may be implemented to prevent the spread of infection from patient to patient, from the patient to health care workers, or from health care workers to the patient. They may also be used to reduce the risk of infection in immunocompromised patients. Central to the success of these procedures is the selection of the proper equipment and the adequate training of those who use it.

Key nursing diagnoses and patient outcomes

Risk for infection related to hospital admission
The patient will:
▶ remain free from all signs and symptoms of infection
▶ have no pathogens appear in cultures
▶ state factors that put him at risk for infection
▶ identify signs and symptoms of infection.

Social isolation
The patient will:
▶ express feelings associated with social isolation
▶ participate in developing a plan for increasing social activity
▶ achieve the expected state of wellness
▶ develop use of support systems to overcome a sense of isolation.

Equipment

Materials required for isolation typically include barrier clothing, an isolation cart or anteroom for storing equipment,

and a door card announcing that isolation precautions are in effect.

Barrier clothing
Gowns • gloves • goggles • masks
Each staff member must be trained on the proper use of these items.

Isolation supplies
Specially marked laundry bags (and water-soluble laundry bags, if used) • plastic trash bags
An isolation cart may be used when the patient's room has no anteroom. It should include a work area (such as a pull-out shelf), drawers or a cabinet area for holding isolation supplies and, possibly, a pole on which to hang coats or jackets.

Preparation of equipment

Remove the cover from the isolation cart if necessary, and set up the work area. Check the cart or anteroom *to ensure that correct and sufficient supplies are in place for the designated isolation category.*

Implementation

▶ Remove your watch (or push it well up your arm) and your rings according to facility policy. *These actions help to prevent the spread of microorganisms hidden under your watch or rings.*
▶ Wash your hands with an antiseptic cleaning agent *to prevent the growth of microorganisms under gloves.*

Putting on isolation garb
▶ Put the gown on and wrap it around the back of your uniform. Tie the strings or fasten the snaps or pressure-sensitive tabs at the neck. Make sure your uniform is completely covered and secure the gown at the waist.

Putting on a face mask

To avoid spreading airborne particles, wear a sterile or nonsterile face mask as indicated. Position the mask to cover your nose and mouth and secure it high enough to ensure stability. Tie the top strings at the back of your head above the ears. Then tie the bottom strings at the base of your neck.

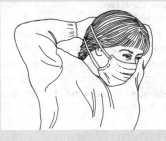

Adjust the metal nose strip if the mask has one.

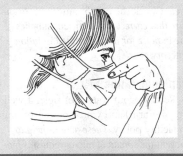

▶ Place the mask snugly over your nose and mouth. Secure ear loops around your ears or tie the strings behind your head high enough so the mask won't slip off. If the mask has a metal strip, squeeze it to fit your nose firmly but comfortably. (See *Putting on a face mask.*) If you wear eyeglasses, tuck the mask under their lower edge.

▶ Put on the gloves. Pull the gloves over the cuffs to cover the edges of the gown's sleeves.

Removing isolation garb

▶ Remember that the outside surfaces of your barrier clothes are contaminated.

▶ Wearing gloves, untie the gown's waist strings.

▶ With your gloved left hand, remove the right glove by pulling on the cuff, turning the glove inside out as you pull. Don't touch any skin with the outside of either glove. (See *Removing contaminated gloves.*) Remove the left glove by wedging one or two fingers of your right hand inside the glove and pulling it off, turning it inside out as you remove it. Discard the gloves in a trash container that contains a plastic trash bag.

▶ Untie your mask, holding it only by the strings. Discard the mask in the trash container. If the patient has a disease spread by airborne pathogens, you may prefer to remove the mask last.

▶ Untie the neck straps of your gown. Grasp the outside of the gown at the back of the shoulders and pull the gown down over your arms, turning it inside out as you remove it *to ensure containment of the pathogens.*

▶ Holding the gown well away from your uniform, fold it inside out. Discard it in the specially marked laundry bags or trash container as necessary.

▶ If the sink is inside the patient's room, wash your hands and forearms with soap or antiseptic before leaving the room. Turn off the faucet using a paper towel and discard the towel in the room. Grasp the door handle with a clean paper towel to open it and discard the towel in a trash container in-

Removing contaminated gloves

Proper removal techniques are essential for preventing the spread of pathogens from gloves to your skin surface. Follow these steps carefully.

1. Using your left hand, pinch the right glove near the top. Avoid allowing the glove's outer surface to buckle inward against your wrist.

2. Pull downward, allowing the glove to turn inside out as it comes off. Keep the right glove in your left hand after removing it.

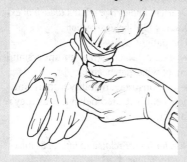

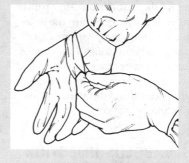

3. Now insert the first two fingers of your ungloved right hand under the edge of the left glove. Avoid touching the glove's outer surface or folding it against your left wrist.

4. Pull downward so that the glove turns inside out as it comes off. Continue pulling until the left glove completely encloses the right one and its uncontaminated inner surface is facing out.

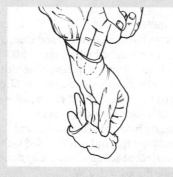

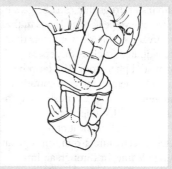

side the room. Close the door from the outside with your bare hand.

▶ If the sink is in an anteroom, wash your hands and forearms with soap or antiseptic after leaving the room.

Special considerations

▶ Use gowns, gloves, goggles, and masks only once, and discard them in the appropriate container before leaving a contaminated area. If your mask is reusable, retain it for further use unless it's damaged or damp. Be aware that isolation garb loses its effectiveness when wet because moisture permits organisms to seep through the material. Change masks and gowns as soon as moisture is noticeable or according to the manufacturer's recommendations or your facility's policy.

▶ At the end of your shift, restock used items for the next person. After patient transfer or discharge, return the isolation cart to the appropriate area for cleaning and restocking of supplies. An isolation room or other room prepared for isolation purposes must be thoroughly cleaned and disinfected before use by another patient.

I.V. BOLUS INJECTION

The I.V. bolus injection method allows rapid drug administration. It can be used in an emergency to provide an immediate drug effect. It can also be used to administer drugs that can't be given I.M., to achieve peak drug levels in the bloodstream, and to deliver drugs that can't be diluted, such as diazepam, digoxin, and phenytoin. The term bolus usually refers to the concentration or amount of a drug. I.V. push is a technique for rapid I.V. injection.

Bolus doses of medication may be injected directly into a vein, through an existing I.V. line, or through an implanted vascular access port (VAP). The medication administered by these methods usually takes effect rapidly, so the patient must be monitored for an adverse reaction, such as cardiac arrhythmia and anaphylaxis. I.V. bolus injections are contraindicated when rapid drug administration could cause life-threatening complications. For certain drugs, the safe rate of injection is specified by the manufacturer.

Some facilities permit only specially trained nurses (such as emergency department, critical care, and chemotherapy nurses) to give bolus injections.

Key nursing diagnoses and patient outcomes

Deficient knowledge related to lack of exposure to I.V. bolus injection
The patient will:
▶ state or demonstrate an understanding of what has been taught
▶ demonstrate an ability to perform new health-related behaviors as they're taught.

Risk for injury related to improper injection technique
The patient will:
▶ identify factors that increase risk of injury
▶ assist in identifying and applying safety measures to prevent injury.

Equipment

Patient's medication record and chart • gloves • prescribed medication • 20G needle and syringe • diluent, if needed • tourniquet • povidone-iodine or alcohol pad • sterile 2″ × 2″ gauze pad • adhesive bandage • tape • optional: winged-tip needle with catheter and second syringe (and needle) filled with normal saline solution and a noncoring needle if used with a VAP

Winged-tip needles are commonly used for this purpose because they can be quickly and easily inserted. They're ideal for repeated drug administration, such as in weekly or monthly chemotherapy. Another useful dosage form is the ready injectable. (See *Using a ready injectable.*)

Preparation of equipment

Verify the order on the patient's medication record by checking it against the doctor's order. Know the actions, adverse effects, and administration rate of the medication to be injected. Draw up the prescribed medication in the syringe and dilute it if necessary.

Implementation

▶ Confirm the patient's identity, wash your hands, put on gloves, and explain the procedure.

Giving direct injections

▶ Select the largest vein suitable for an injection. *The larger the vein, the more diluted the drug will become, minimizing vascular irritation.*

▶ Apply a tourniquet above the injection site *to distend the vein.*

▶ Clean the injection site with an alcohol or a povidone-iodine pad, working outward from the puncture site in a circular motion *to prevent recontamination with skin bacteria.*

▶ If you're using the drug syringe's needle, insert it into the vein at a 30-degree angle with the bevel up. The bevel should reach ¼″ (0.6 cm) into the vein. If you're using a winged-tip needle, insert the needle (bevel up), tape the butterfly wings in place when you see blood return in the tubing, and attach the syringe containing the medication.

▶ Pull back on the syringe plunger and check for blood backflow, *which indicates that the needle is in the vein.*

▶ Remove the tourniquet and inject the medication at the appropriate rate.

▶ Pull back slightly on the syringe plunger and check for blood backflow again. *If blood appears, this indicates that*

Using a ready injectable

A commercially premeasured medication packaged with a syringe and needle, the ready injectable allows for rapid drug administration in an emergency. Usually, preparing a ready injectable takes only 15 to 20 seconds. Other advantages include the reduced risk of breaking sterile technique during administration and the easy identification of medication and dose.

When using a commercially prefilled syringe, make sure you give the precise dose prescribed. For example, if a 50 mg/ml cartridge is supplied but the patient's prescribed dose is 25 mg, you must administer only 0.5 ml — half of the volume contained in the cartridge. Be alert for potential medication errors whenever dispensing medications in premeasured dosage forms.

---

the needle remained in place and all the injected medication entered the vein.

▶ Flush the line with the normal saline solution from the second syringe *to ensure delivery of all the medication.*

▶ Withdraw the needle and apply pressure to the injection site with a sterile gauze pad for at least 3 minutes *to prevent hematoma formation.*

▶ Apply the adhesive bandage to the site after bleeding has stopped.

Giving injections through an existing I.V. line

▶ Check the compatibility of the medication with the I.V. solution.

▶ Close the flow clamp, wipe the injection port with an alcohol pad, and inject the medication as you would a direct injection. (Some I.V. lines have a secondary injection port or a T-connector; others have a needleless adapter or latex cap at the end of the I.V. tubing where the needle is attached.)

▶ Open the flow clamp and readjust the flow rate.

▶ If the drug isn't compatible with the I.V. solution, flush the line with normal saline solution before and after the injection. (For additional information, see "Intermittent infusion device use," page 435.)

Giving a bolus injection through a VAP

▶ Wash your hands, put on gloves, and clean the injection site with an alcohol or a povidone-iodine pad, starting at the center of the port and working outward in a circular motion over a 4″ to 5″ (10- to 12.7-cm) diameter. Do this three times.

▶ Palpate the area over the port *to locate the port septum.*

▶ Anchor the port between the thumb and first two fingers of your nondominant hand. Then using your dominant hand, insert a noncoring needle into the appropriate area of the device and deliver the injection.

Special considerations

▶ *Because drugs administered by I.V. bolus or push injections are delivered directly into the circulatory system and can produce an immediate effect,* an acute allergic reaction or anaphylaxis can develop rapidly. If signs of anaphylaxis (such as dyspnea, cyanosis, seizures, and increasing respiratory distress) occur, notify the doctor immediately and begin emergency procedures, as necessary. Also watch for signs of extravasation (such as redness and swelling). If extravasation occurs, stop the injection, estimate the amount of infiltration, and notify the doctor.

▶ If you're giving diazepam or chlordiazepoxide hydrochloride through a winged-tip needle or an I.V. line, flush with bacteriostatic water instead of normal saline solution *to prevent drug precipitation resulting from incompatibility.*

Complications

Excessively rapid administration may cause adverse effects, depending on the medication administered.

Documentation

Record the amount and type of drug administered, time of injection, appearance of the site, duration of administration, and patient's tolerance of the procedure. Also note the drug's effect and any adverse reactions.

I.V. CONTROLLERS AND PUMPS

Various types of controllers and pumps electronically regulate the flow of I.V. solutions or drugs with great accuracy. Controllers regulate gravity flow by counting drops and achieve the desired infusion rate by compressing the I.V. tubing. Because controllers count drops, which aren't always of equal size, they fail to achieve the accuracy of volumetric pumps, which measure flow rate in milliliters per hour.

Volumetric pumps, used for high-pressure infusion of drugs or for highly accurate delivery of fluids or drugs, have mechanisms to propel the solution at the desired rate under pressure. (Pressure is exerted only when gravity flow rates are insufficient to maintain preset infusion rates.) The peristaltic pump applies pressure to the I.V. tubing to force the solution through it. (Not all peristaltic pumps are volumetric; some count drops.) The piston-cylinder pump pushes the solution through special disposable cassettes. Most of these pumps operate at high pressures (up to 45 psi), delivering from 1 to 999 ml/hour with about 98% accuracy. (Some pumps operate at 10 to 25 psi.) The portable syringe pump, another type of volumetric pump, delivers very small amounts of fluid over a long period. It's used for administering fluids to infants and for delivering intra-arterial drugs. Other specialized devices include the controlled-release infusion system, secondary syringe converter, and patient-controlled analgesia device.

Controllers and pumps have various detectors and alarms that automatically signal or respond to the completion of an infusion, air in the line, low battery power, and occlusion or inability to deliver at the set rate. Depending on the problem, these devices may sound or flash an alarm, shut off, or switch to a keep-vein-open rate.

Key nursing diagnoses and patient outcomes
Risk for injury related to I.V. therapy
The patient will:
▶ remain free from injury
▶ show signs of fluid and electrolyte balance
▶ show no signs of fluid volume excess or depletion from use of controllers or pumps
▶ communicate the importance of not altering rates on controllers and pumps.

Deficient knowledge related to lack of exposure to I.V. control equipment

The patient will:
▶ communicate a need to know about the use of I.V. control equipment
▶ communicate an understanding of the I.V. control equipment.

Equipment
Controller or peristaltic pump • I.V. pole • I.V. solution • sterile administration set • sterile peristaltic tubing or cassette, if needed (tubing and cassettes vary among manufacturers) • alcohol pads • adhesive tape (see *Controllers and infusion pumps,* page 476)

Preparation of equipment
To set up a controller
Attach the controller to the I.V. pole. Clean the port on the I.V. solution container with an alcohol pad, insert the administration set spike, and fill the drip chamber no more than halfway *to avoid miscounting the drops.* Rotate the chamber so that the fluid touches all sides *to remove any vapor that could interfere with correct drop counting.* Now prime the tubing and close the clamp. Position the drop sensor above the fluid level in the drip chamber and below the drop port to ensure correct drop counting. Insert the peristaltic tubing into the controller, close the door, and open the flow clamp completely.

To set up a volumetric pump
Attach the pump to the I.V. pole. Swab the port on the I.V. container with alcohol, insert the administration set spike, and fill the drip chamber completely *to prevent air bubbles from entering the tubing.* Next, prime the tubing and close the clamp. Follow the manufacturer's instructions for placement of tubing.

Controllers and infusion pumps

Controllers and infusion pumps, such as the two shown below, electronically regulate the flow of I.V. solutions and drugs. You'll use them when a precise flow rate is needed, for instance, when administering total parenteral nutrition solutions and chemotherapeutic or cardiovascular agents.

Controller

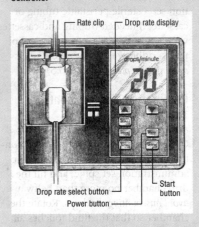

Infusion pump

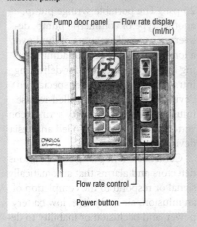

Implementation

▶ Position the controller or pump on the same side of the bed as the I.V. or anticipated venipuncture site *to avoid crisscrossing I.V. lines over the patient.* If necessary, perform the venipuncture.

▶ Plug in the machine and attach its tubing to the needle or catheter hub. If you're using a controller, position the drip chamber 30″ (76.2 cm) above the infusion site *to ensure accurate gravity flow.*

▶ Depending on the machine, turn it on and press the START button. Set the appropriate dials on the front panel to the desired infusion rate and volume. Always set the volume dial at 50 ml less than the prescribed volume or 50 ml less than the volume in the container *so*

that you can hang a new container before the old one empties.

▶ Check the patency of the I.V. line and watch for infiltration. If you're using a controller, monitor the accuracy of the infusion rate.

▶ Tape all connections and recheck the controller's drip rate *because taping may alter it.*

▶ Turn on the alarm switches. Explain the alarm system to the patient *to prevent anxiety when a change in the infusion activates the alarm.*

Special considerations

▶ Monitor the pump or controller and the patient frequently to ensure the device's correct operation and flow rate and to detect infiltration and such complications as infection and air embolism.

▶ If electrical power fails, the pumps automatically switch to battery power.

▶ Check the manufacturer's recommendations before administering opaque fluids, such as blood, *because some pumps fail to detect opaque fluids and others may cause hemolysis of infused blood.*

▶ Move the tubing in controllers every few hours *to prevent permanent compression or tubing damage.* Change the tubing and cassette every 48 hours or according to your facility's policy.

▶ Remove I.V. solutions from the refrigerator 1 hour before infusing them to help release small gas bubbles from the solutions. *Small bubbles in the solution can join to form larger bubbles, which can activate the pump's air-in-line alarm.*

Home care

Make sure the patient and his family understand the purpose of using the pump or controller. If necessary, demonstrate how the device works. Also demonstrate how to maintain the system (including tubing, solution, and site assessment and care) until you're confident that the patient and family can proceed safely. As time permits, have the patient repeat the demonstration. Discuss which complications to watch for, such as infiltration, and review measures to take if complications occur. Schedule a teaching session with the patient or family *so you can answer questions they may have about the procedure before the patient's discharge.* (See *Home I.V. therapy.*)

Complications

Complications associated with I.V. controllers and pumps are the same as

Technology update

Home I.V. therapy

Home I.V. therapy has become easier with the Baxter's Intermate system, which uses pressure instead of gravity or an infusion pump to dispense medication. To use the system, the patient simply has the pharmacy fill the Intermate with medication; then, the patient attaches the Intermate to the I.V. access device. (The Intermate doesn't need to be hung on an I.V. pole or attached to an infusion pump.) The medication is dispensed according to the size of the system: small (which can deliver 105 ml at rates of 50 or 200 ml/hour), large (which can deliver 275 ml at rates of 50, 100, or 250 ml/hour), or extra large (which can deliver 550 ml at a rate of 250 ml/hour).

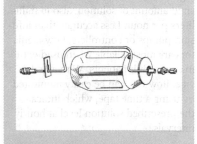

those associated with peripheral lines. (See "Peripheral I.V. line insertion," page 625.) Keep in mind that infiltration can develop rapidly with infusion by a volumetric pump because the increased subcutaneous pressure won't slow the infusion rate until significant edema occurs.

Documentation

In addition to routine documentation of the I.V. infusion, record the use of a controller or pump on the I.V. record and in your notes.

I.V. FLOW RATE CALCULATION AND MANUAL CONTROL

Calculated from a doctor's orders, flow rate is usually expressed as the total volume of I.V. solution infused over a prescribed interval or as the total volume given in milliliters per hour. Many devices can regulate the flow of I.V. solution, including clamps, controllers, the flow regulator (or rate minder), and the volumetric pump. (See *Using I.V. clamps*.)

When regulated by a clamp or controller, flow rate is usually measured in drops per minute; by a volumetric pump, in milliliters per hour. The flow regulator can be set to deliver the desired amount of solution, also in milliliters per hour. Less accurate than infusion pumps or controllers, flow regulators are most reliable when used with inactive adult patients. With any device, flow rate can be easily monitored by using a time tape, which indicates the prescribed solution level at hourly intervals.

Key nursing diagnoses and patient outcomes

Deficient fluid volume related to (specify)
The patient will:
▶ maintain normal vital signs
▶ maintain normal skin turgor and moist mucous membranes
▶ maintain an adequate urine output
▶ maintain a normal electrolyte level.

Equipment

I.V. administration set with clamp • 1″ paper or adhesive tape (or premarked time tape) • infusion pump and controller (if infusing medication) • watch

Using I.V. clamps

With a roller clamp or screw clamp, you can increase or decrease the flow through the I.V. line by turning a wheel or screw.

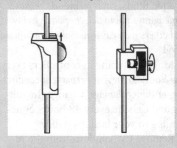

With a slide clamp, you can open or close the line by moving the clamp horizontally. However, you can't make fine adjustments to flow rate.

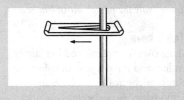

with second hand • drip rate chart, as necessary • pen

Standard macrodrip sets deliver from 10 to 20 drops/ml, depending on the manufacturer; microdrip sets, 60 drops/ml; and blood transfusion sets, 10 drops/ml. A commercially available adapter can convert a macrodrip set to a microdrip system.

Implementation

▶ Flow rate requires close monitoring and correction *because such factors as venous spasm, venous pressure changes, patient movement or manipulation of the clamp, and bent or kinked tubing can cause the rate to vary markedly.*

Calculating flow rates

When calculating the flow rate of I.V. solutions, remember that the number of drops required to deliver 1 ml varies with the type and manufacturer of the administration set used. The illustration on the left shows a standard (macrodrip) set, which delivers from 10 to 20 drops/ml. The illustration in the center shows a pediatric (microdrip) set, which delivers about 60 drops/ml. The illustration on the right shows a blood transfusion set, which delivers about 10 drops/ml.

To calculate the flow rate, you must know the calibration of the drip rate for each manufacturer's product. Use this formula to calculate specific drip rates:

$$\frac{\text{volume of infusion (in ml)}}{\text{time of infusion (in minutes)}} \times \text{drip factor (in drops/ml)} = \text{drops/minute}$$

Macrodrip set   **Microdrip set**   **Blood transfusion set**

 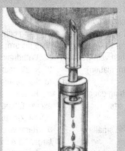 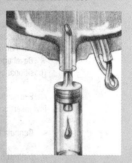

Calculating and setting the drip rate

▶ Follow the steps in *Calculating flow rates* to determine the proper drip rate or use your unit's drip rate chart.

▶ After calculating the desired drip rate, remove your watch and hold it next to the drip chamber *so that you can observe the watch and drops simultaneously.*

▶ Release the clamp to the approximate drip rate. Then count drops for 1 minute *to account for flow irregularities.*

▶ Adjust the clamp, as necessary, and count drops for 1 minute. Continue to adjust the clamp and count drops until the correct rate is achieved.

Making a time tape

▶ Calculate the number of milliliters to be infused per hour. Place a piece of tape vertically on the container alongside the volume-increment markers.

▶ Starting at the current solution level, move down the number of milliliters to be infused in 1 hour and use the pen to mark the appropriate time and a horizontal line on the tape at this level. Then continue to mark 1-hour intervals until you reach the bottom of the container.

▶ Check the flow rate every 15 minutes until stable, then every hour or according to facility policy; adjust as needed.

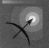

Troubleshooting

Managing I.V. flow rate deviations

Problem	Cause	Intervention
Flow rate too slow	■ Venous spasm after insertion	■ Apply warm soaks over site.
	■ Venous obstruction from bending arm	■ Secure with an arm board if necessary.
	■ Pressure change (decreasing fluid in bottle causes solution to run slower because of decreasing pressure)	■ Readjust flow rate.
	■ Elevated blood pressure	■ Readjust flow rate. Use infusion pump or controller to ensure correct flow rate.
	■ Cold solution	■ Allow solution to warm to room temperature before hanging.
	■ Change in solution viscosity from medication added	■ Readjust flow rate.
	■ I.V. container too low or patient's arm or leg too high	■ Hang container higher or remind patient to keep his arm below heart level.
	■ Bevel against vein wall (positional cannulation)	■ Withdraw needle slightly, or place a folded 2″ × 2″ gauze pad over or under catheter hub to change angle.
	■ Excess tubing dangling below insertion site	■ Replace tubing with shorter piece, or tape excess tubing to I.V. pole, below flow clamp. (Make sure tubing isn't kinked.)
	■ Cannula too small	■ Remove cannula in use and insert a larger-bore cannula, or use an infusion pump.
	■ Infiltration or clotted cannula	■ Remove cannula in use and insert a new cannula.
	■ Kinked tubing	■ Check tubing over its entire length and unkink it.
	■ Clogged filter	■ Remove filter and replace with a new one.
	■ Tubing memory (tubing compressed at area clamped)	■ Massage or milk tubing by pinching and wrapping it around a pencil four or five times. Quickly pull pencil out of coiled tubing.
Flow rate too fast	■ Patient or visitor manipulating clamp	■ Instruct patient not to touch clamp. Place tape over it. Restrain patient, or administer I.V. solution with infusion pump or controller if necessary.
	■ Tubing disconnected from catheter	■ Wipe distal end of tubing with alcohol, reinsert firmly into catheter hub, and tape at connection site. Consider using tubing with luer-lock connections.
	■ Change in patient position	■ Administer I.V. solution with infusion pump or controller to ensure correct flow rate.
	■ Bevel against vein wall (position cannulation)	■ Manipulate cannula and place a 2″ × 2″ gauze pad under or over catheter hub to change angle. Reset flow clamp at desired rate. If necessary, remove cannula and reinsert.
	■ Flow clamp drifting because of patient movement	■ Place tape below clamp.

▶ With each check, inspect the I.V. site for complications and assess the patient's response to therapy.

Special considerations
▶ If the infusion rate slows significantly, a slight rate increase may be necessary. If the rate must be increased by more than 30%, consult the doctor. When infusing drugs, use an I.V. pump or controller, if possible, to avoid flow rate inaccuracies. Always use a pump or controller when infusing solutions by way of a central line.
▶ Large-volume solution containers have about 10% more fluid than the amount indicated on the bag to allow for tubing purges. Thus, a 1,000-ml bag or bottle contains an additional 100 ml; similarly, a 500-ml container holds an extra 50 ml; and a 250-ml container, 25 ml.

Complications
An excessively slow flow rate may cause insufficient intake of fluids, drugs, and nutrients; an excessively rapid rate of fluid or drug infusion may cause circulatory overload — possibly leading to heart failure and pulmonary edema — as well as adverse drug effects. (See *Managing I.V. flow rate deviations.*)

Documentation
Record the original flow rate when setting up a peripheral line. If you adjust the rate, record the change, date and time, and your initials.

I.V. THERAPY, PEDIATRIC

In children, I.V. therapy may be prescribed to administer medications or to correct a fluid deficit, improve serum electrolyte balance, or provide nourishment. Primary nursing concerns related to pediatric I.V. therapy include correlating the I.V. site and equipment with the reason for therapy and the patient's age, size, and activity level. For example, a scalp vein is a typical I.V. site for infants, whereas a peripheral hand, wrist, or foot vein may suit older children.

During I.V. therapy, the nurse must continually assess the patient and the infusion to prevent fluid overload and other complications.

Key nursing diagnoses and patient outcomes
Risk for infection related to I.V. therapy
The patient will:
▶ have normal vital signs, temperature, and laboratory values
▶ have no pathogens appear in cultures
▶ show no signs or symptoms of infection at the I.V. insertion site.

Risk for fluid volume imbalance related to the need for I.V. therapy
The patient will:
▶ exhibit no signs of dehydration
▶ maintain a urine output of at least (specify) ml/hour
▶ have normal electrolyte values
▶ maintain fluid balance (intake will equal output).

Equipment
Prescribed I.V. fluid • volume-control set with microdrip tubing • infusion pump • I.V. pole • normal saline solution or sterile dextrose 5% in water (D_5W) for injection • povidone-iodine solution • alcohol pads • 3-ml syringe • child-sized butterfly needle or I.V. catheter • tourniquet • ½″or 1″ tape • gloves • transparent semipermeable

Easing the pain of venipuncture

For some patients, receiving a needle stick—especially during venipuncture—can be a traumatic experience. You can lessen your patient's anxiety, reduce his pain, and improve compliance during the procedure by applying a transdermal anesthesia cream before the use of this cream. Here are a few guidelines for the use of this cream:

■ Transdermal anesthesia cream (commonly known by the brand name EMLA Cream) is supplied in a eutectic mixture of lidocaine 2.5% and prilocaine 2.5%. A eutectic mixture has a melting point below room temperature, allowing it to penetrate intact skin as far as the fat layer. The onset, depth, and duration of the anesthesia depend on how long the cream is allowed to stay on the skin. The minimum duration of application is 60 minutes; the maximum is 180 minutes.

■ Apply the cream in a thick layer to clean, dry, intact skin at the intended venipuncture site. Then cover it with a transparent occlu-sive dressing, being careful not to spread the cream.

■ Note the time of application on the dressing with a marking pen. When you're ready to perform the venipuncture, carefully remove the dressing. Wipe off the cream, clean the site with an antiseptic solution, and perform the venipuncture as usual.

■ EMLA Cream is also indicated for pain relief for various other procedures, including lumbar puncture, port access, bone marrow aspiration, insertion of a peripherally inserted central venous catheter, withdrawal of blood samples for arterial blood gas analysis and other laboratory tests, I.M. injection, and superficial skin surgery. It can be used on adults and on children who are at least 1 month old. Local reactions may include erythema and edema. Avoid administering EMLA Cream to individuals with a known sensitivity to lidocaine or prilocaine.

dressing • optional: arm board and insulated foam or medicine cup

Whenever possible, use a catheter instead of a needle. *A flexible catheter is less likely to perforate the vein wall. To promote compliance and reduce the discomfort associated with catheter insertion,* consider using a transdermal anesthetic cream. (See *Easing the pain of venipuncture.*)

Preparation of equipment

Gather the I.V. equipment and take it to the patient's bedside. Check the expiration date on the I.V. fluid and inspect the I.V. container (an I.V. bag for leakage and a bottle for cracks). Examine the I.V. tubing for defects or cracks. Make sure that the packaging sur-rounding the I.V. catheter or needle remains intact.

Open the wrappings on the I.V. solution and the volume-control tubing set. Close all clamps on the tubing set; then insert the tip of the tubing set into the entry port of the I.V. bag or bottle. (If you're using an I.V. bag, make sure you hold the bag upright when attaching the tubing. *This will keep the sterile air inside the bag from escaping and making the fluid level difficult to read.*)

Hang the bottle or bag from the I.V. pole. Open the clamp between the bag and the volume-control set and allow 30 to 50 ml of solution to flow into the calibrated chamber. Close the clamp.

Squeeze the drip chamber located below the calibrated chamber or volume-control set *to create a vacuum.* Release the drip chamber and allow it to fill halfway with solution. Then release the clamp below the drip chamber *so that fluid flows into the remaining tubing, removing any air.* After the tubing fills, close the clamp.

If you're using an infusion pump, attach the I.V. tubing to the infusion cassette and insert the cassette into the infusion pump. Prime the cassette tubing according to the manufacturer's instructions. If you're using an air eliminator I.V. filter, attach the filter to the end of the cassette tubing. *To prevent any air bubbles from entering the patient's circulatory system,* place the filter as close to the patient as possible. *To minimize the risk of infection,* maintain sterility at the tip of the I.V. tubing until you connect it to the I.V. needle.

Cut as many strips of ½″ or 1″ tape as you'll need to secure the I.V. line. Prepare a syringe with 3 ml of flush solution — either the normal saline solution or D_5W.

Implementation

▶ Match the name on the patient's wristband with the name on the doctor's order (or on the medication card). Ask the patient (or his parents) whether he's allergic to povidone-iodine solution or to any type of tape.

▶ Explain the reason for the I.V. therapy. Reassure the parents and enlist their assistance in explaining the procedure to the patient in terms he can understand.

▶ Make sure you have a staff member available to assist you. Inform the parents that the staff member will help the patient remain still, if necessary, during the procedure.

▶ Wash your hands and put on gloves.

Common pediatric I.V. sites

The most common sites for I.V. therapy in infants and children are shown below. Peripheral hand, wrist, or foot veins are typically used with older children, whereas scalp veins are used with an infant.

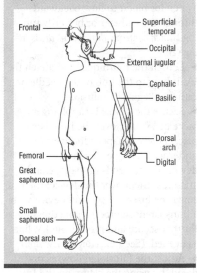

▶ Select the insertion site for the butterfly needle or catheter. (See *Common pediatric I.V. sites.*) Aim for the most distal site possible and avoid placing the I.V. line in the patient's dominant arm or in areas of flexion if possible. Avoid previously used or sclerotic veins.

▶ To locate an appropriate scalp vein, carefully palpate the site for arterial pulsations. If you feel these pulsations, select another site. Before inserting the I.V. line, prepare the selected site as ordered.

▶ To find an appropriate peripheral site, apply a tourniquet to the patient's arm or leg and palpate a suitable vein.

▶ If you're inserting a butterfly needle, flush the tubing connected to the butterfly with D_5W or normal saline solution.

▶ Clean the insertion site. Unless contraindicated, use a povidone-iodine pad. Wipe with a circular motion from the insertion site's center to the outer rim. Let the solution dry.

▶ Insert the I.V. needle into the vein. Watch for blood to flow backward through the catheter or butterfly tubing, *which confirms that the needle is in the vein.*

▶ Loosen the tourniquet and attach the I.V. tubing to the hub of the needle or catheter. Begin the infusion.

▶ Secure the device by applying a piece of ½″ tape over the hub. Next, place a piece of tape, adhesive side up, underneath and perpendicular to the device. Lift the ends of the tape and crisscross them over the device; then cover the insertion site and device with a transparent semipermeable dressing. Further secure and protect the I.V. line as needed. (See *Protecting an I.V. site.*)

▶ Adjust the infusional flow, as ordered, by using the clamp on the I.V. volume-control tubing or by setting the infusion rate on the infusion pump.

▶ Add solution hourly (or as needed) from the I.V. bag to the volume-control set.

▶ Assess the I.V. site frequently for signs of infiltration and check the I.V. bottle or bag for the amount of solution infused.

▶ Change the I.V. dressing every 24 hours or as needed *to prevent infection.* Also change the I.V. tubing every 48 to 72 hours and the I.V. solution bottle or bag every 24 hours. Label the I.V. bottle or bag, tubing, and volume control set with the time and date of change.

▶ Change the I.V. insertion site every 72 hours, if possible, *to minimize the risk of infection.* If you inserted the I.V.

line without proper skin preparation (during an emergency, for example), change the site sooner.

Special considerations

▶ When selecting an I.V. site, try not to use a site that impairs the child's ability to seek comfort. For example, if an infant typically sucks his right thumb, avoid placing the I.V. needle or catheter in his right arm.

▶ Forewarn parents if you'll start the I.V. infusion in a scalp vein. Also tell them that you may have to shave hair from a small section of the infant's head.

▶ Ask an older child to participate in selecting the I.V. site, if possible, *to give him a sense of control.* If the child is mobile, aim for an I.V. site on the upper extremity *so that he can still get out of bed.* Avoid starting the I.V. infusion in the same arm as the patient's identification band, unless you first remove the band and replace it on the other arm, *to prevent potential circulatory impairment.*

▶ Evaluate the need for restraints after inserting the I.V. line. Apply them only if I.V. needle displacement seems imminent. If you must use restraints, assess the patient's skin integrity and provide hourly skin care *to prevent skin breakdown.* Remove the restraints at frequent intervals *to let the patient move freely.* Encourage the parents to hold and comfort the patient when he's unrestrained.

▶ *For precise regulation of the I.V. infusion,* use a volumetric infusion pump. These pumps infuse fluids at a predetermined rate regardless of temperature fluctuations, vessel variations, or fluid volume changes. Before using an infusion pump, review the operator's manual.

Protecting an I.V. site

Protecting a child's I.V. site can be a challenge. An active child can easily dislodge an I.V. line, which will necessitate your reinserting it, thus causing him further discomfort; or he may injure himself.

To prevent a child from dislodging an I.V. line, you'll first need to secure the needle or catheter carefully. Tape the I.V. site as you would for an adult, so that the skin over the tip of the venipuncture device is easily visible. However, avoid overtaping the site; doing so makes it harder to inspect the site and the surrounding tissue.

If the child is old enough to understand, warn him not to play with or jostle the equipment and teach him how to walk with an I.V. pole to minimize tension on the line. If necessary, you can restrain the extremity.

You should also create a protective barrier between the I.V. site and the environment using one of the following methods.

Paper cup

Consider using a small paper cup to protect a scalp site. First, cut off the cup's bottom. (Make sure there are no sharp edges that could damage the child's skin.)

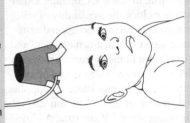

Next, cut a small slot through the top rim to accommodate the I.V. tubing. Place the cup upside down over the insertion site, so the I.V. tubing extends through the slot. Secure the cup with strips of tape (as shown). The opening you cut in the cup allows you to examine the site.

Stockinette

Place the child's arm on an arm board and secure the arm board to the child's arm with tape. Cut a piece of 4" (10.2-cm) stockinette the same length as the patient's arm. Slip the stockinette over the patient's arm, as shown.

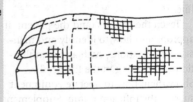

Note: You may also protect a scalp site by placing a stockinette on the patient's head, leaving a hole to allow access to the site.

I.V. shield

Peel off the strips covering the adhesive backing on the bottom of the shield. Position the shield over the site so that the I.V. tubing runs through one of the shield's two slots. Then firmly press the shield's adhesive backing against the patient's skin. The shield's clear plastic composition allows you to see the I.V. site clearly.

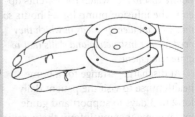

If the shield is too large to fit securely over the site, just cut off the shield's narrow end below the two air holes. Now you can easily shape the device to the patient's arm.

▶ After inserting the I.V. needle or catheter, reward preschool and school-age patients. Popular rewards are colorful stickers to wear on clothes or on the I.V. dressing.

Home care

Children who require long-term I.V. medications or nourishment may continue receiving I.V. therapy at home. Assess for conditions that promote successful home I.V. therapy—first and foremost, a patient and a parent (or other caregiver) who can and want to participate in home I.V. therapy. Other factors include the availability of relief caregivers to provide occasional assistance (especially in an emergency) and a conducive home environment with electricity, running water, a telephone, refrigeration, storage space for supplies, and an area set up for solution and tubing changes and I.V. site care. Additionally, a hospital should be accessible should the patient need emergency assistance or routine reinsertion of an I.V. line.

Teach the parents (and the patient, if appropriate) how to identify and manage complications, such as site infiltration and clotting in the I.V. needle. Show them how to operate equipment such as the infusion pump. Supplement verbal instructions with written patient-teaching materials for later reference. Before discharge, watch the parents operate the infusion pump for 24 hours *so that you can identify areas in which they need further instruction and skills that require refinement.*

At discharge, arrange for a home health nurse to visit the patient daily for 2 to 3 days to support and guide initial home therapy. Inform the parents that after her daily visits, the home health nurse will probably visit every 2 to 3 days to assess the I.V. site, provide care, and answer questions.

Complications

Infection, fluid overload, electrolyte imbalance, infiltration, and circulatory impairment are complications of I.V. therapy.

Documentation

Record the date and time of the I.V. infusion, the insertion site, and the type and size of I.V. needle or catheter. Note the patient's tolerance of the procedure. Describe patient- and parent-teaching activities. Document the condition of the I.V. site according to facility policy. If infiltration affects the I.V. site, document the condition of the site at every shift change until the condition resolves.

I.V. THERAPY PREPARATION

Selection and preparation of appropriate equipment are essential for accurate delivery of an I.V. solution. Selection of an I.V. administration set depends on the rate and type of infusion desired and the type of I.V. solution container used. Two types of drip sets are available: the macrodrip and the microdrip. The macrodrip set can deliver a solution in large quantities at rapid rates because it delivers a larger amount with each drop than the microdrip set. The microdrip set, used for pediatric patients and certain adult patients who require small or closely regulated amounts of I.V. solution, delivers a smaller quantity with each drop.

Administration tubing with a secondary injection port permits separate or simultaneous infusion of two solutions; tubing with a piggyback port and a backcheck valve permits intermittent infusion of a secondary solution and, on its completion, a return to infusion of the primary solution. Vented I.V. tubing is selected for solutions in nonvented bottles; nonvented tubing is selected for solutions in bags or vented bottles. Assembly of I.V. equipment requires aseptic technique to prevent contamination, which can cause local or systemic infection.

Key nursing diagnoses and patient outcomes

Risk for infection related to I.V. therapy
The patient will:
▶ maintain a normal body temperature
▶ show no signs of infection at the I.V. site
▶ take precautions to keep the I.V. site dry.

Deficient knowledge related to lack of exposure to I.V. therapy
The patient will:
▶ state an understanding of the need for I.V. therapy
▶ state an understanding of the precautions and care associated with the I.V. site.

Equipment

I.V. solution • alcohol pad • I.V. administration set • in-line filter, if needed • I.V. pole • medication and label, if necessary

Preparation of equipment

Verify the type, volume, and expiration date of the I.V. solution. Discard outdated solution. If the solution is contained in a glass bottle, inspect the bottle for chips and cracks; if it's in a plastic bag, squeeze the bag to detect leaks. Examine the I.V. solution for particles, abnormal discoloration, and cloudiness. If present, discard the solution and notify the pharmacy or dispensing department. If ordered, add medication to the solution and place a completed medication-added label on the container. Remove the administration set from its box and check for cracks, holes, and missing clamps.

Implementation

▶ Wash your hands thoroughly *to prevent introducing contaminants during preparation.*
▶ Slide the flow clamp of the administration set tubing down to the drip chamber or injection port and close the clamp.

Preparing a bag

▶ Place the bag on a flat, stable surface or hang it on an I.V. pole.
▶ Remove the protective cap or tear the tab from the tubing insertion port.
▶ Remove the protective cap from the administration set spike.
▶ Holding the port firmly with one hand, insert the spike with your other hand.
▶ Hang the bag on the I.V. pole, if you haven't already, and squeeze the drip chamber until it's half full.

Preparing a nonvented bottle

▶ Remove the bottle's metal cap and inner disk, if present.
▶ Place the bottle on a stable surface and wipe the rubber stopper with an alcohol pad.
▶ Remove the protective cap from the administration set spike and push the

When to use an in-line filter

An in-line filter removes pathogens and particles from I.V. solutions, helping to reduce the risk of infusion phlebitis. However, because in-line filters are expensive and their installation cumbersome and time-consuming, they aren't used routinely. Many facilities require that a filter be used only when administering an admixture. If you're unsure of whether to use a filter, check your facility's policy or follow this list of do's and don'ts.

Do's

Use an in-line filter:

■ when administering solutions to an immunodeficient patient.

■ when administering total parenteral nutrition.

■ when using additives comprising many separate particles, such as antibiotics requiring reconstitution, or when administering several additives.

■ when using rubber injection ports or plastic diaphragms repeatedly.

■ when phlebitis is likely to occur.

Change the in-line filter according to the manufacturer's recommendations (typically every 24 to 36 hours). If you don't, bacteria trapped in the filter releases endotoxin, a pyrogen small enough to pass through the filter into the bloodstream.

Use an add-on filter of larger pore size (1.2 microns) when infusing lipid emulsions and albumin mixed with nutritional solutions and amphotericin B.

Don'ts

Don't use an in-line filter:

■ when administering solutions with large particles that will clog a filter and stop I.V. flow, such as blood and its components, suspensions, lipid emulsions, and high-molecular-volume plasma expanders.

■ when administering a drug dose of 5 mg or less (because the filter may absorb it).

---

spike through the center of the bottle's rubber stopper. Avoid twisting or angling the spike *to prevent pieces of the stopper from breaking off and falling into the solution.*

▶ Invert the bottle. If its vacuum is intact, you'll hear a hissing sound and see air bubbles rise (this may not occur if you've already added medication). If the vacuum isn't intact, discard the bottle and begin again.

▶ Hang the bottle on the I.V. pole and squeeze the drip chamber until it's half full.

Preparing a vented bottle

▶ Remove the bottle's metal cap and latex diaphragm to release the vacuum. If the vacuum isn't intact (except after medication has been added), discard the bottle and begin again.

▶ Place the bottle on a stable surface and wipe the rubber stopper with an alcohol pad.

▶ Remove the protective cap from the administration set spike and push the spike through the insertion port next to the air vent tube opening.

▶ Hang the bottle on the I.V. pole, and squeeze the drip chamber until it's half full.

Priming the I.V. tubing

▶ If necessary, attach an in-line filter to the opposite end of the I.V. tubing, and follow the manufacturer's instructions

Teaching your patient about I.V. therapy

Many patients are apprehensive about peripheral I.V. therapy. So before you begin therapy, tell your patient what to expect before, during, and after the procedure. Thorough patient teaching can reduce anxiety, making therapy easier. Follow these guidelines.

Before insertion

■ Describe the procedure. Tell him that "intravenous" means inside the vein and that a plastic catheter or needle will be placed in his vein. Explain that fluids containing certain nutrients or medications will flow from a bag or bottle through a length of tubing and then through the plastic catheter or needle into his vein.

■ Tell him about how long the catheter or needle will stay in place. Explain that the doctor will decide how much and what type of fluid the patient needs.

■ If the patient will receive a local anesthetic at the insertion site, ask him if he's allergic to lidocaine. If in doubt, use another anesthetic. Tell him that this injection will numb the site to reduce the pain of I.V. device insertion.

■ If no anesthetic will be used, tell the patient that he may feel transient pain at the insertion site but that the discomfort will stop when the catheter or needle is in place.

■ Tell him that I.V. fluid may feel cold at first but that this sensation should last only a few minutes.

During therapy

■ Instruct the patient to report any discomfort after the catheter or needle has been inserted and the fluid has begun to flow.

■ Explain any restrictions as ordered. As appropriate, tell the patient that he may be able to walk and, depending on the insertion site and the device, to shower or take a tub bath during therapy.

■ Teach him how to care for the I.V. line. Tell him not to pull at the insertion site or tubing, not to remove the container from the I.V. pole, and not to kink the tubing or lie on it. Instruct him to call a nurse if the flow rate suddenly slows or speeds up.

At removal

■ Explain that removing a peripheral I.V. line is a simple procedure. Tell the patient that pressure will be applied to the site until the bleeding stops. Reassure him that when the device is out and the bleeding stops, he'll be able to use the affected arm or leg as before therapy.

---

for filling and priming it. Purge the tubing before attaching the filter *to avoid forcing air into the filter and, possibly, clogging some filter channels.* Most filters are positioned with the distal end of the tubing facing upward *so that the solution will completely wet the filter membrane and all air bubbles will be eliminated from the line.* (See *When to use an in-line filter.*)

▶ If you aren't using a filter, aim the distal end of the tubing over a wastebasket or sink and slowly open the flow clamp. (Most distal tube coverings allow the solution to flow without having to remove the protective cover.)

▶ Leave the clamp open until the I.V. solution flows through the entire length of tubing *to release trapped air bubbles and force out all the air.*

▶ Invert all Y-ports and backcheck valves and tap them, if necessary, *to fill them with solution.*

▶ After priming the tubing, close the clamp. Then loop the tubing over the I.V. pole.

Better charting

Documenting insertion of a venipuncture device

After you establish an I.V. route, remember to document the date, time, and venipuncture site together with the equipment used, such as the type and gauge of catheter or needle. Record how the patient tolerated the procedure and any patient teaching that you performed with the patient and his family, such as explaining the purpose of I.V. therapy, describing the procedure itself, and discussing any possible complications.

You'll need to update your records each time you change the insertion site and change the venipuncture device or the I.V. tubing. Also document any reason for changing the I.V. site, such as extravasation, phlebitis, occlusion, patient removal, or routine change according to facility policy.

1/6/01	0200	A #20 FR. angiocath inserted
		in the anterior portion of the
		right hand. Good blood return
		noted. I.V. of 1,000 ml
		D5¹/₂ NSS with 20 mEq KCL
		running at 125 ml/hr. On
		infusion pump. I.V. tolerated
		well. Taught pt. about the
		need for I.V. therapy, its
		complications, and how to
		ambulate with I.V. Pt. stated
		that he understood.—
		————Pat Natting, RN

▶ Label the container with the patient's name and room number, date and time, container number, ordered rate and duration of infusion, and your initials.

Special considerations

▶ Before initiation of I.V. therapy, the patient should be told what to expect. (See *Teaching your patient about I.V. therapy*, page 489.)

▶ Always use sterile technique when preparing I.V. solutions. If you contaminate the administration set or container, replace it with a new one *to prevent introducing contaminants into the system.*

▶ If necessary, you can use vented tubing with a vented bottle. To do this, don't remove the latex diaphragm. Instead, insert the spike into the larger indentation in the diaphragm.

▶ Change I.V. tubing every 48 or 72 hours according to your facility's policy or more frequently if you suspect cont-

amination. Change the filter according to the manufacturer's recommendations or sooner if it becomes clogged.

Documentation

Document the type of solution used and any additives to the solution. (See *Documenting insertion of a venipuncture device.*)

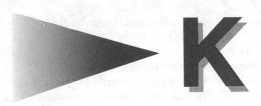

KNEE EXTENSION THERAPY

Stretching therapy uses various techniques to lengthen pathologically shortened soft tissues (such as ligaments, tendons, joint capsules, and other related structures), thereby restoring functional range of motion (ROM) to limbs stiffened by immobility and possibly contractures or adhesions. One kind of stretching therapy involves the use of dynamic splinting to apply a low-load, prolonged-duration stretching force to the joint.

A knee extension system helps the patient regain ROM by applying dynamic stress continuously while he's sleeping or resting. The system provides support to the upper and lower leg by means of struts fitted with tension rods that apply gentle but firm force to coax muscles and connective tissues to stretch. During stretching, new tissue is synthesized to a permanently elongated state. When dynamic splinting is applied early in the patient's treatment program, rehabilitation time usually is greatly reduced.

These extension systems are indicated for the treatment of joint stiffness and limited ROM resulting from fractures, dislocations, ligament and tendon repairs, joint arthroplasty, burns,

total knee replacement, hemophilia, spinal cord injuries, rheumatoid arthritis, tendon release, cerebral palsy, multiple sclerosis, and other traumatic and nontraumatic disorders.

Units can be used for both extension and flexion of the elbow, wrist, ankle, finger, and toe as well as the knee. Units are available in pediatric and adult sizes.

General protocol

A knee extension system consists of two stainless-steel struts (medial and lateral), each provided with a tension adjuster; four Velcro cuffs (two each for the upper and lower legs); cuff padding; and two anterior counterforce (over-the-knee) straps. The system is custom fitted, and tension is adjusted to the patient's tolerance. The system should be worn at the optimal tolerable tension for the longest time (usually 8 to 10 continuous hours) and preferably at night.

On the 1st day, the patient should wear the system for up to 4 continuous hours with the tension screws set on both struts at the first setting (or 1). If the patient reports more than 1 hour of stiffness or discomfort after wearing the system, tension on each strut is reduced (by increments of 0.5 or more) if necessary until he can tolerate wearing the device for 4 continuous hours during the day.

When the patient has learned to tolerate wearing the system for 4 continuous hours (usually by days 2 to 4), he begins wearing the system overnight. Initially, he wears it for 8 to 20 hours with the tension set at 1. Tension is then increased in increments of 0.5, as tolerated, to produce no more than 1 hour of beyond-normal discomfort or stiffness after wearing the system. Higher tension settings don't usually achieve better results. In most cases, knee system tension can be set to between 5 and 8 after several weeks of use.

The patient should be inactive and relaxed while wearing the system. The extremity should be supported but not in a hanging position. Place the patient on one side with a pillow between his legs, or elevate the affected leg. Don't let the leg dangle. If the patient can't tolerate the splint overnight, he can wear it during the day.

Patients who have neurologic involvement may begin treatment with the tension set higher than 1 initially; the tension is then lowered if spasticity or agitation increases. Alternatively, the system may be applied on a 2-hours-on, 4-hours-off routine.

Key nursing diagnoses and patient outcomes

Deficient knowledge related to a lack of exposure to knee extension therapy
The patient will:
▶ communicate a need to know about the procedure
▶ state an understanding of what is taught.

Impaired physical mobility related to (specify)
The patient will:
▶ state relief from pain
▶ show no evidence of complications, such as contractures, venous stasis, thrombus formation, or skin breakdown
▶ attain the highest level of mobility possible within the confines of the disease
▶ maintain muscle strength and joint ROM.

Equipment
Knee extension system and tension adjustment tool (as shown below) • optional: pillow, adhesive tape, and marking pen

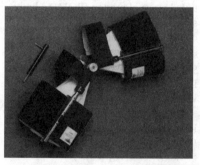

Implementation
▶ Explain the procedure to the patient.
▶ Hold the system so that the adjustment scale is visible on one of the struts.
▶ To read the tension, turn the system right side up. The tension spacer will be visible in the window next to the tension scale. The flat top of the tension spacer inside the strut lines up with a number on the scale.
▶ If the top of the tension spacer isn't lined up with the "0" on the tension scale with each strut, adjust the tension

screw in the top of each spacer with the tension adjustment tool until they're lined up.

Adjusting strut length

▶ To shorten or lengthen the distal strut, first remove the ⅛″ screw or screws located near the cam, using the tension adjustment tool.

▶ Slide the smaller tube in or out of the larger tube *to obtain the correct strut length*. Line up the screw holes and re-place and gently tighten the screw or screws. Repeat as necessary for all struts.

▶ Open the front-of-thigh, shin, and over-the-knee straps. As you open each cuff, pull it out of the D-wire attached to the strut and fold the strap's Velcro closure onto itself.

▶ Next, loosen the back-of-thigh and calf cuffs. *This widens the splint to accommodate the patient's calf and thigh dimensions.*

▶ Place the system under the patient's leg.

▶ Position the distal struts, which are the larger tubes with the tension adjusters, beneath the calf. Pull the proximal and distal struts up with both hands until the struts are even with the midlines of the sides of the thigh and calf.

▶ Next, align the cams across the knee axis, making sure they're in a straight line.

▶ With the cams aligned, close the over-the-knee straps. Make sure that you can slide one finger under the upper and lower edges of each strap.

▶ Next, close the front-of-thigh cuffs and shin cuffs. Then adjust and close the back-of-thigh cuffs and calf cuffs. If necessary, adjust strut length so that

cuffs are positioned on the bulk of the muscle mass at mid-thigh and mid-calf.

Setting splint tension

▶ Insert the tension adjustment tool into the open end of the lower strut.

▶ Increase the tension by turning the tool clockwise; reduce the tension by turning it counterclockwise.

▶ Make sure that cams are aligned across the knee axis, struts are placed on the medial and lateral axes of the leg, and cuffs are evenly contoured across the leg (as shown below).

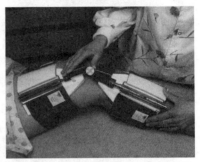

▶ Tape or mark the backs of both cuffs *to keep the patient from changing the fitting.*

▶ Mark a reference line with a pen on the over-the-knee straps and the front-of-thigh and shin cuffs *so that the patient knows where to close them.* Make sure the patient practices applying and removing the splint.

Special considerations

The knee extension system is contraindicated if passive ROM treatments are inappropriate, as in unhealed or unstable fractures. It should be used cautiously in patients with thrombophlebitis, osteoporosis, spasticity, edema, gross ligament instability, and circulatory impairment.

Complications

Pain and stiffness usually can be minimized by reducing the tension on the struts.

Documentation

In the patient record, record the time and date of the procedure, the tension ordered by the doctor, the length of time that the patient can tolerate the amount of tension, any increase or decrease in the tension, and the reason for the change in tension.

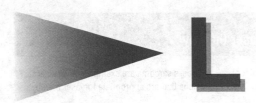

LASER THERAPY

Using the highly focused and intense energy of a laser beam, the surgeon can treat various skin lesions. Laser surgery has several advantages. As a surgical instrument, the laser offers precise control. It spares normal tissue, speeds healing, and deters infection by sterilizing the operative site. In addition, by sealing tiny blood vessels as it vaporizes tissue, the laser beam leaves a nearly bloodless operative field. In addition, the procedure can be performed on an outpatient basis.

The lasers used most commonly to treat skin lesions are vascular, pigment, and carbon dioxide (CO_2) lasers. (See *Understanding types of laser therapy*, page 496.)

In general, laser surgery is safe, although bleeding and scarring can result. One pronounced hazard — to the patient and treatment staff alike — is eye damage or other injury caused by unintended laser beam reflection. For this reason, everyone in the surgical suite, including the patient, must wear special goggles to filter laser light. Also, the surgeon must use special nonreflective instruments. Access to the room must be strictly controlled, and all windows must be covered.

Key nursing diagnoses and patient outcomes

Deficient knowledge related to a lack of exposure to laser therapy
The patient will:
▶ state or demonstrate an understanding of what has been taught
▶ demonstrate an ability to perform new health-related behaviors as they're taught.

Risk for injury related to improper technique
The patient will:
▶ identify factors that increase risk of injury
▶ assist in identifying and applying safety measures to prevent injury.

Equipment

Laser • filtration face masks • protective eyewear • laser vacuum • extra vacuum filters • prescribed cleaning solution • surgical drape • sterile gauze • nonadherent dressings • surgical tape • cotton-tipped applicators • nonreflective surgical instruments • gowns • sterile gloves

Preparation of equipment

Before the procedure begins, prepare the tray. It should include a local anesthetic, as ordered, and dry and wet gauze. The gauze will be used *to control bleeding, protect healthy tissue, and*

Understanding types of laser therapy

Laser therapy has become an essential tool for treating many types of skin lesions. The number of lasers used in dermatology is growing, and each type is used for specific conditions. The term *laser* is an acronym for Light Amplification by the Stimulated Emission of Radiation. When directed toward the skin, most of this light energy is absorbed by chromophores, which are substances that absorb specific wavelengths of light. This is the basis of selective photothermolysis, which has revolutionized cutaneous laser surgery. Melanin is the target chromophore in pigmented lesions, and oxyhemoglobin in microvessels is the target chromophore in vascular lesions.

It's important to be familiar with the various types of lasers and the indications for each.

Lasers for vascular lesions
The laser most commonly used for vascular lesions is the flashlamp-pumped dye laser (FLPDL). Other types include copper vapor, argon, KTP, krypton, neodymium: yttrium-aluminum-garnet (Nd:YAG), and frequency-doubled Q-switched Nd:YAG lasers. The type of laser used depends on the type of vascular lesion. Port-wine stains, hemangiomas, venous lake, rosacea, telangiectasia, and Kaposi's sarcoma are examples of vascular lesions that are appropriate for laser therapy.

Lasers for pigmented lesions
Lasers that are effective in treating tattoos and dermal and epidermal pigmented lesions include Q-switched ruby, Q-switched Nd:YAG, Q-switched alexandrite, FLPDL, copper vapor, krypton, and KTP. Among the pigmented lesions appropriate for laser treatment are nevi of Ota, melasma, solar lentigo, café-au-lait spots, Becker's nevi, and epidermal nevi.

Carbon-dioxide laser
Although it's one of the oldest lasers, the carbon-dioxide laser is used less commonly since the advent of lasers that work on the principle of selective photothermolysis. This laser causes thermal injury, resulting in ablation in the defocused mode and cut tissue in the focused mode. It's used to treat actinic cheilitis, rhinophyma, warts, keloids, and other lesions.

Lasers for hair removal
Lasers used to eliminate unwanted hair include ruby, diode, alexondrite, and Nd:YAG. Laser treatment is only effective in removing dark-colored hair; it isn't effective for removing blonde, red, white, or gray hair.

abrade and remove any eschar, which would otherwise inhibit laser absorption. Prepare surgical instruments as needed.

Implementation
▶ Put on gown, filtration face mask, and protective eyewear.
▶ Tell the patient how the laser works and review its benefits. Point out the equipment and outline the procedure *to help allay the patient's concerns.*

▶ Just before the surgeon begins, position the patient comfortably, drape him, and place protective gauze, if needed, around the operative site. Confirm that everyone in the room — including the patient — has protective eyewear on *to filter the laser light.*
▶ Lock the door to the surgical suite *to keep unprotected persons from inadvertently entering the room.*
▶ After the surgeon administers the anesthetic and it takes effect, activate

the laser vacuum. The CO_2 laser has a vacuum hose attached to a separate apparatus. Use this apparatus *to clear the surgical site.* The vacuum has a filter that traps and collects most of the vaporized tissue. Change the filter whenever suction decreases and follow facility guidelines for filter disposal.

▶ When the surgeon finishes the procedure, apply direct pressure with a sterile gauze pad to any bleeding wound for 20 minutes. (Wear sterile gloves.) If the wound continues to bleed, notify the doctor.

▶ Once the bleeding is controlled, use aseptic technique to clean the area with a cotton-tipped applicator dipped in the prescribed cleaning solution. Then size and cut a nonadherent dressing. Secure the dressing with surgical tape.

▶ Vascular and pigment lasers won't result in a wound; only superficial skin changes will occur.

Special considerations
▶ The surgeon uses the laser beam much as he would a scalpel to excise the lesion. Explain that the laser causes a burnlike wound that can be deep. Inform the patient that the wound will appear charred. Also, tell the patient that some of the eschar will be removed during the initial postoperative cleaning and that more will gradually dislodge at home.

▶ Warn the patient to expect a burning odor and smoke during the procedure. A machine called a smoke evacuator, which sounds like a vacuum cleaner, will clear it away. Advise the patient that he may sense heat from the laser. Urge him to tell the doctor immediately if pain develops.

▶ The nurse must have thorough knowledge of how each laser operates and of laser safety considerations for both the patient and the health care providers.

Home care
Teach the patient how to dress his wound or care for his skin daily as ordered by the surgeon. Tell him that he can take showers but shouldn't immerse the wound site in water *to promote wound healing and prevent infection.*

If the wound bleeds at home, demonstrate how to apply direct pressure on the site with clean gauze or a washcloth for 20 minutes. If pressure doesn't control the bleeding, tell the patient to call his doctor.

If the patient's foot or leg was operated on, urge him to keep the extremity elevated and to use it as little as possible *because pressure can inhibit healing.*

Warn the patient to protect the treated area from exposure to the sun *to avoid changes in pigmentation.* Tell him to call the doctor if a fever of 100° F (37.8° C) or higher persists longer than 1 day.

Complications
Bleeding, scarring, and infection are rare complications of laser surgery.

Documentation
Most patients who have laser surgery for skin lesions are treated as outpatients. Note the patient's skin condition before and after the procedure. Also document any bleeding, record the type of dressing applied, and list the patient's complaints of pain. Note whether the patient comprehends home care instructions.

LATEX ALLERGY PROTOCOL

Latex—a natural product of the rubber tree—is used in many products in the health care field as well as other areas. With the increased use of latex in barrier protection and medical equipment, more and more nurses and patients are becoming hypersensitive to it. Certain groups of people are at an increased risk for developing latex allergy. These groups include people who have had or will undergo multiple surgical procedures (especially those with a history of spina bifida), health care workers (especially those in the emergency department and operating room), workers who manufacture latex and latex-containing products, and people with a genetic predisposition to latex allergy.

People who are allergic to certain "cross-reactive" foods, including apricots, cherries, grapes, kiwis, passion fruit, bananas, avocados, chestnuts, tomatoes, and peaches, may also be allergic to latex. Exposure to latex elicits an allergic response similar to the one elicited by the foods.

For people with latex allergy, latex becomes a hazard when the protein in latex comes in direct contact with mucous membranes or is inhaled, which happens when powdered latex surgical gloves are used. People with asthma are at greater risk for developing worsening symptoms from airborne latex.

The diagnosis of latex allergy is based on the patient's history and physical examination. Laboratory testing should be performed to confirm or eliminate the diagnosis. Skin testing can be done but the Alastat test, Hycor assay, and Pharmacia Cap test are the only Food and Drug Administration-approved blood tests available. Some laboratories may also choose to perform an enzyme-linked immunosorbent assay.

Latex allergy can produce a myriad of symptoms, including generalized itching (on the hands and arms, for example); itchy, watery, or burning eyes; sneezing and coughing (hay fever–type symptoms); rash; hives; bronchial asthma, scratchy throat, or difficulty breathing; edema of the face, hands, or neck; and anaphylaxis.

To help identify people at risk for latex allergy, ask latex allergy–specific questions during the health history. (See *Latex allergy screening.*) If the patient's history reveals a latex sensitivity, the doctor assigns him to one of three categories based on the extent of his sensitization. Group 1 includes patients who have a history of anaphylaxis or a systemic reaction when exposed to a natural latex product. Group 2 patients have a clear history of an allergic reaction of a nonsystemic type. Group 3 patients don't have a previous history of latex hypersensitivity but are designated as "high risk" because of an associated medical condition, occupation, or "cross-over" allergy.

If you determine that your patient has a sensitivity to latex, make sure that he doesn't come in contact with latex *because such contact could result in a life-threatening hypersensitivity reaction.* Creating a latex-free environment is the only way to safeguard your patient. Many facilities now designate "latex-free" equipment, which is usually kept on a cart that can be moved into the patient's room.

Key nursing diagnoses and patient outcomes

Latex allergy response
The patient will:
▶ remain free from latex complications
▶ show no signs or symptoms of latex allergy, such as generalized itching; itchy, watery, or burning eyes; sneezing and coughing; rash; hives; or difficulty breathing.

Deficient knowledge related to a lack of exposure to latex allergy protocol
The patient will:
▶ state an understanding of latex allergy
▶ communicate a need to know about latex allergy
▶ express knowledge of cross-reactive foods
▶ express knowledge of signs and symptoms of latex allergy, such as generalized itching; itchy, watery, or burning eyes; sneezing and coughing; rash; hives; or difficulty breathing.

Equipment

Latex allergy patient identification wristband • latex-free equipment, including room contents • anaphylaxis kit • optional: LATEX ALLERGY sign

Preparation of equipment

After you've determined that the patient has a latex allergy or is sensitive to latex, arrange for him to be placed in a private room. If that isn't possible, make the room latex-free, even if the roommate hasn't been designated as hypersensitive to latex. *This prevents the spread of airborne particles from latex products used on the other patient.*

Latex allergy screening

To determine if your patient has a latex sensitivity or allergy, ask the following screening questions:
■ What is your occupation?
■ Have you experienced an allergic reaction, local sensitivity, or itching following exposure to any latex products, such as balloons or condoms?
■ Do you have shortness of breath or wheezing after blowing up balloons or after a dental visit?
■ Do you have itching in or around your mouth after eating a banana?
   If your patient answers "yes" to any of these questions, proceed with the following questions:
■ Do you have a history of allergies, dermatitis, or asthma? If so, what type of reaction do you have?
■ Do you have any congenital abnormalities? If yes, explain.
■ Do you have any food allergies? If so, what specific allergies do you have? Describe your reaction.
■ If you experience shortness of breath or wheezing when blowing up latex balloons, describe your reaction.
■ Have you had any previous surgical procedures? Did you experience associated complications? If so, describe them.
■ Have you had previous dental procedures? Did complications result? If so, describe them.
■ Are you exposed to latex in your occupation? Do you experience a reaction to latex products at work? If so, describe your reaction.

Implementation

For all patients in groups 1 and 2
▶ Assess for possible latex allergy in all patients being admitted to the delivery

Anesthesia induction and latex allergy

Latex allergy can cause signs and symptoms in both conscious and anesthetized patients.

Causes of intraoperative reaction	Signs and symptoms in conscious patient	Signs and symptoms in anesthetized patient
■ Latex contact with mucous membrane ■ Latex contact with intraperitoneal serosal lining ■ Inhalation of airborne latex particles during anesthesia ■ Injection of antibiotics and anesthetic agents through latex ports	■ Abnormal cramping ■ Anxiety ■ Bronchoconstriction ■ Diarrhea ■ Feeling of faintness ■ Generalized pruritus ■ Itchy eyes ■ Nausea ■ Shortness of breath ■ Swelling of soft tissue (such as the hands, face, and tongue) ■ Vomiting	■ Bronchospasm ■ Cardiopulmonary arrest ■ Facial edema ■ Flushing ■ Hypotension ■ Laryngeal edema ■ Tachycardia ■ Urticaria ■ Wheezing

room or short procedure unit or having a surgical procedure.

▶ If the patient has a confirmed latex allergy, bring a cart with latex-free supplies into his room.

▶ Document in the patient's chart (according to facility policy) that the patient has a latex allergy. If policy requires that the patient wear a latex allergy identification bracelet, place it on the patient.

▶ If the patient will be receiving anesthesia, make sure that "LATEX ALLERGY" is clearly visible on the front of his chart. (See Anesthesia induction and latex allergy.) Notify the circulating nurse in the surgical unit, the postanesthesia care unit nurses, and any other team members that the patient has a latex allergy.

▶ If the patient must be transported to another area of the hospital, make certain that the latex-free cart accompanies him and that all health care workers who come in contact with him are wearing nonlatex gloves. The patient should wear a mask with cloth ties when leaving his room to protect him from inhaling airborne latex particles.

▶ If the patient will have an I.V. line, make sure that I.V. access is accomplished using all latex-free products. Post a LATEX ALLERGY sign on the I.V. tubing to prevent access of the line using latex products.

▶ Flush I.V. tubing with 50 ml of I.V. solution because of latex ports in the I.V. tubing.

▶ Place a warning label on I.V. bags that says "Do not use latex injection ports."

▶ Use a nonlatex tourniquet. If none are available, use a latex tourniquet over clothing.

▶ Use latex-free oxygen administration equipment. Remove the elastic and tie equipment on with gauze.

Managing a latex allergy reaction

If you determine that your patient is having an allergic reaction to a latex product, act immediately. Make sure that you perform emergency interventions using latex-free equipment. If the latex product that caused the reaction is known, remove it and perform the following measures:

■ If the allergic reaction develops during medication administration or a procedure, stop the medication or procedure immediately.

■ Assess airway, breathing, and circulation.

■ Administer 100% oxygen with continuous pulse oximetry.

■ Start I.V. volume expanders with lactated Ringer's solution or normal saline solution.

■ Administer epinephrine according to the patient's symptoms, as follows:

– cutaneous manifestations of anaphylaxis (urticaria and angioedema): 0.3 to 0.5 ml of 1:1,000 aqueous epinephrine subcutaneously; may be repeated every 15 to 20 minutes as needed for a maximum of 3 doses

– pulmonary manifestations of anaphylaxis (primarily laryngeal and pharyngeal edema) without airway obstruction or apnea: 0.3 to 0.5 ml of 1:1,000 aqueous epinephrine subcutaneously; may be repeated every 15 to 20 minutes as needed to a maximum of three doses.

– patients with circulatory shock: 1 to 2 ml of aqueous epinephrine in 1:10,000 dilution (0.1 to 0.2 mg) I.V. over 2 to 3 minutes. In refractory cases, an epinephrine infusion through a

1:1,000,000 dilution can be administered using 1 ml of epinephrine 1:1,000 in 100 ml of dextrose 5% in water and adjusting the infusion rate from 6 to 30 ml/hour for a dosage range of 1 to 5 mcg/minute. This infusion rate should be titrated to the patient's blood pressure response or the development of arrhythmias.

■ Administer famotidine 20 mg I.V. push for 2 to 5 minutes and then switch to oral administration as ordered.

■ If bronchospasm is evident, treat it with nebulized albuterol (0.25 to 0.5 ml diluted in 2.5 ml normal saline solution), as ordered.

■ Secondary treatment for latex allergy reaction is aimed at treating the swelling and tissue reaction to the latex as well as breaking the chain of events associated with the allergic reaction. It includes:

– diphenhydramine 1 mg/kg I.V. (to a maximum dose of 50 mg)

– methylprednisolone 2 mg/kg I.V. (to maximum dose of 125 mg)

– famotidine 20 mg every 12 hours I.V. push over 2 over 5 minutes (to a maximum dose of 40 mg).

■ Document the event and the exact cause (if known). If latex particles have entered the I.V. line, insert a new I.V. line with a new catheter, new tubing, and new infusion attachments as soon as possible.

Adapted with permission from North Penn Hospital, Lansdale, Pa.

▶ Wrap your stethoscope with a nonlatex product *to protect the patient from latex contact.*

▶ Wrap Tegaderm over the patient's finger before using pulse oximetry.

▶ Use latex-free syringes when administering medication through a syringe.

▶ Make sure an anaphylaxis kit is readily available. If the patient has an allergic reaction to latex, you must act immediately. (See *Managing a latex allergy reaction.*)

Special considerations

▶ Remember that signs and symptoms of latex allergy usually occur within 30 minutes of anesthesia induction. However, the time of onset can range from 10 minutes to 5 hours.

▶ Don't forget that, as a health care worker, you're in a position to develop a latex hypersensitivity. If you suspect that you're sensitive to latex, contact the employee health services department concerning facility protocol for latex-sensitive employees. Use latex-free products whenever possible *to help reduce your exposure to latex.*

▶ Don't assume that if something doesn't look like rubber it isn't latex. Latex can be found in a wide variety of equipment, including electrocardiograph leads, oral and nasal airway tubing, tourniquets, nerve stimulation pads, temperature strips, and blood pressure cuffs.

LIPID EMULSION ADMINISTRATION

Typically given as separate solutions in conjunction with parenteral nutrition, lipid emulsions are a source of calories and essential fatty acids. A deficiency in essential fatty acids can hinder wound healing, adversely affect the production of red blood cells, and impair prostaglandin synthesis.

Lipid emulsions may also be given alone. They can be administered through either a peripheral or a central venous line.

Lipid emulsions are contraindicated in patients who have a condition that disrupts normal fat metabolism, such as pathologic hyperlipidemia, lipid nephrosis, or acute pancreatitis. They must be used cautiously in patients who have liver disease, pulmonary disease, anemia, or coagulation disorders and in those who are at risk for developing a fat embolism.

Key nursing diagnoses and patient outcomes

Imbalanced nutrition: Less than body requirements related to (specify)
The patient will:
▶ show no further evidence of weight loss
▶ gain _____ pounds weekly
▶ tolerate lipid emulsion infusion without adverse effects.

Deficient knowledge related to a lack of exposure to the administration of lipid emulsions
The patient will:
▶ express an interest in learning the treatment regimen
▶ communicate an understanding of special dietary needs.

Equipment

Lipid emulsion • I.V. administration set with vented spike (a separate adapter may be used if an administration set with vented spike isn't available) • access pin with reflux valve • tape • time tape • alcohol pads

If administering the lipid emulsion as part of a 3-in-1 solution, also obtain a filter that is 1.2 microns or greater because lipids will clog a smaller filter.

Preparation of equipment

Inspect the lipid emulsion for opacity and consistency of color and texture. If the emulsion looks frothy or oily or contains particles or if you think its stability or sterility is questionable, return the bottle to the pharmacy. To prevent aggregation of fat globules, don't shake the lipid container excessively. Protect the emulsion from freezing and never add anything to it. Make sure you have the correct lipid emulsion and verify the doctor's order and the patient's name.

Implementation
▶ Explain the procedure to the patient *to promote his cooperation.*

Connecting the tubing
▶ First, connect the I.V. tubing to the access pin. Access pins with reflux valves take the place of needles when connecting piggyback tubing to primary tubing.
▶ Close the flow clamp on the I.V. tubing. If the tubing doesn't contain luerlock connections, tape all connections securely *to prevent accidental separation, which can lead to air embolism, exsanguination, and sepsis.*
▶ Using sterile technique, remove the protective cap from the lipid emulsion bottle and wipe the rubber stopper with an alcohol pad.
▶ Hold the bottle upright and, using strict sterile technique, insert the vented spike through the inner circle of the rubber stopper.
▶ Invert the bottle and squeeze the drip chamber until it fills to the level indicated in the tubing package instructions.
▶ Open the flow clamp and prime the tubing. Gently tap the tubing *to dislodge air bubbles trapped in the Y-ports.* If necessary, attach a time tape to the lipid emulsion container *to allow accurate measurement of fluid intake.*
▶ Label the tubing, noting the date and time the tubing was hung.

Starting the infusion
▶ If this is the patient's first lipid infusion, administer a test dose at the rate of 1 ml/minute for 30 minutes.
▶ Monitor the patient's vital signs and watch for signs and symptoms of an adverse reaction, such as fever; flushing, sweating, or chills; a pressure sensation over the eyes; nausea; vomiting; headache; chest and back pain; tachycardia; dyspnea; and cyanosis. An allergic reaction is usually due either to the source of lipids or to eggs, which occur in the emulsion as egg phospholipids, which is an emulsifying agent.
▶ If the patient has no adverse reactions to the test dose, begin the infusion at the prescribed rate. Use an infusion pump if you'll be infusing the lipids at less than 20 ml/hour. The maximum infusion rate is 125 ml/hour for a 10% lipid emulsion and 60 ml/hour for a 20% lipid emulsion.

Special considerations
▶ Always maintain strict sterile technique while preparing and handling equipment.
▶ Observe the patient's reaction to the lipid emulsion. Most patients report a feeling of satiety; some complain of an unpleasant metallic taste.
▶ Change the I.V. tubing and the lipid emulsion container every 24 hours.
▶ Monitor the patient for hair and skin changes. Also, closely monitor his lipid tolerance rate. Cloudy plasma in a centrifuged sample of citrated blood indicates that the lipids haven't been cleared from the patient's bloodstream.
▶ A lipid emulsion may clear from the blood at an accelerated rate in patients with full-thickness burns, multiple traumatic injuries, or a metabolic imbalance. This is because catecholamines,

adrenocortical hormones, thyroxine, and growth hormone enhance lipolysis and embolization of fatty acids.

▶ Obtain weekly laboratory tests as ordered. The usual tests include liver function studies, prothrombin time, platelet count, and serum triglyceride levels. Whenever possible, draw blood for triglyceride levels at least 6 hours after the completion of the lipid emulsion infusion *to avoid falsely elevated results.*

▶ A lipid emulsion is an excellent medium for bacterial growth. Therefore, never rehang a partially empty bottle of emulsion.

Complications

Immediate or early adverse reactions to lipid emulsion therapy, which occur in fewer than 1% of patients, include fever, dyspnea, cyanosis, nausea, vomiting, headache, flushing, diaphoresis, lethargy, syncope, chest and back pain, slight pressure over the eyes, irritation at the infusion site, hyperlipidemia, hypercoagulability, and thrombocytopenia.

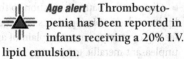 **Age alert** Thrombocytopenia has been reported in infants receiving a 20% I.V. lipid emulsion.

Delayed but uncommon complications associated with prolonged administration of lipid emulsion include hepatomegaly, splenomegaly, jaundice secondary to central lobular cholestasis, and blood dyscrasias (such as thrombocytopenia, leukopenia, and transient increases in liver function studies). Dry or scaly skin, thinning hair, abnormal liver function studies, and thrombocytopenia may indicate a deficiency of essential fatty acids. For unknown reasons, some patients develop brown pigmentation in the reticuloendothelial system.

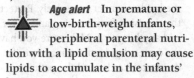 **Age alert** In premature or low-birth-weight infants, peripheral parenteral nutrition with a lipid emulsion may cause lipids to accumulate in the infants' lungs.

Report any adverse reactions to the patient's doctor so that he can change the parenteral nutrition regimen as needed.

Documentation

Record the times of all dressing changes and solution changes, the condition of the catheter insertion site, your observations of the patient's condition, and any complications and resulting treatments.

LUMBAR PUNCTURE

Lumbar puncture involves the insertion of a sterile needle into the subarachnoid space of the spinal canal, usually between the third and fourth lumbar vertebrae. This procedure is used to detect increased intracranial pressure (ICP) or the presence of blood in cerebrospinal fluid (CSF), to obtain CSF specimens for laboratory analysis, and to inject dyes or gases for contrast in radiologic studies. It's also used to administer drugs or anesthetics and to relieve ICP by removing CSF.

Performed by a doctor with a nurse assisting, lumbar puncture requires sterile technique and careful patient positioning. This procedure is contraindicated in patients with lumbar deformity or infection at the puncture site. It should be performed cautiously in patients with increased ICP because the rapid reduction in pressure that follows withdrawal of CSF can cause tonsillar herniation and medullary compression.

Key nursing diagnoses and patient outcomes

Anxiety related to a lack of exposure to lumbar puncture
The patient will:
▶ express feelings of anxiety
▶ perform stress-reduction techniques
▶ use support systems to assist with coping
▶ demonstrate abated physical symptoms of anxiety.

Acute pain related to adverse effects of the procedure
The patient will:
▶ maintain a flat position for 8 to 12 hours after the procedure
▶ identify pain characteristics if present
▶ express a feeling of comfort and relief from pain.

Equipment

Overbed table • one or two pairs of sterile gloves for the doctor • sterile gloves for the nurse • povidone-iodine solution • sterile gauze pads • alcohol sponges • sterile fenestrated drape • 3-ml syringe for local anesthetic • 25G 3/4″ sterile needle for injecting anesthetic • local anesthetic (usually 1% lidocaine) • 18G or 20G 1/2″ spinal needle with stylet (22G needle for children) • three-way stopcock • manometer • small adhesive bandage • three sterile collection tubes with stoppers • laboratory request forms • labels • light source such as a gooseneck lamp • optional: patient-care reminder

Disposable lumbar puncture trays contain most of the needed sterile equipment.

Preparation of equipment

Gather the equipment and take it to the patient's bedside.

Implementation

▶ Explain the procedure to the patient *to ease his anxiety and ensure his cooperation.* Make sure a consent form has been signed.
▶ Inform the patient that he may experience headache after lumbar puncture but reassure him that his cooperation during the procedure minimizes such an effect.
▶ Immediately before the procedure, provide privacy and instruct the patient to void.
▶ Wash your hands thoroughly.
▶ Open the equipment tray on an overbed table, being careful not to contaminate the sterile field when you open the wrapper.
▶ Provide adequate lighting at the puncture site using a gooseneck lamp and adjust the height of the patient's bed *to allow the doctor to perform the procedure comfortably.*
▶ Position the patient and reemphasize the importance of remaining as still as possible *to minimize discomfort and trauma.* (See *Positioning for lumbar puncture,* page 506.)
▶ The doctor cleans the puncture site with sterile gauze pads soaked in povidone-iodine solution, wiping in a circular motion away from the puncture site; he uses three different pads *to prevent contamination of spinal tissues by the body's normal skin flora.* Next, he drapes the area with the fenestrated drape *to provide a sterile field.* (If the

Positioning for lumbar puncture

Have the patient lie on his side at the edge of the bed, with his chin tucked to his chest and his knees drawn up to his abdomen. Make sure the patient's spine is curved and his back is at the edge of the bed (as shown below). This position widens the spaces between the vertebrae, easing insertion of the needle.

To help the patient maintain this position, place one of your hands behind his neck and the other hand behind his knees and pull gently. Hold the patient firmly in this position throughout the procedure to prevent accidental needle displacement.

Patient positioning

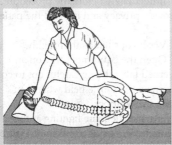

Typically, the doctor inserts the needle between the third and fourth lumbar vertebrae (as shown below).

Needle insertion

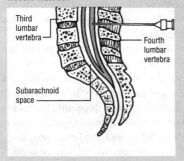

Third lumbar vertebra

Fourth lumbar vertebra

Subarachnoid space

doctor uses povidone-iodine pads instead of sterile gauze pads, he may remove his sterile gloves and put on another pair *to avoid introducing povidone-iodine into the subarachnoid space with the lumbar puncture needle.*)

▶ If no ampule of anesthetic is included on the equipment tray, clean the injection port of a multidose vial of anesthetic with an alcohol pad. Then invert the vial 45 degrees so that the doctor can insert a 25G needle and syringe and withdraw the anesthetic for injection.

▶ Before the doctor injects the anesthetic, tell the patient he'll experience a transient burning sensation and local pain. Ask him to report any other persistent pain or sensations *because they may indicate irritation or puncture of a nerve root, requiring repositioning of the needle.*

▶ When the doctor inserts the sterile spinal needle into the subarachnoid space between the third and fourth lumbar vertebrae, instruct the patient to remain still and breathe normally. If necessary, hold the patient firmly in position *to prevent sudden movement that may displace the needle.*

▶ If the lumbar puncture is being performed to administer contrast media for radiologic studies or spinal anesthetic, the doctor injects the dye or anesthetic at this time.

▶ When the needle is in place, the doctor attaches a manometer with a three-way stopcock to the needle hub to read CSF pressure. If ordered, help the patient extend his legs *to provide a more accurate pressure reading.*

▶ The doctor then detaches the manometer and allows CSF to drain from the needle hub into the collection tubes. When he has collected 2 to 3 ml in each tube, mark the tubes in sequence, insert a stopper to secure them, and label them.

▶ If the doctor suspects an obstruction in the spinal subarachnoid space, he may check for Queckenstedt's sign. After he takes an initial CSF pressure reading, compress the patient's jugular vein for 10 seconds as ordered. *This increases ICP and — if no subarachnoid block exists — causes CSF pressure to rise as well.* The doctor then takes pressure readings every 10 seconds until the pressure stabilizes.

▶ Put on sterile gloves.

▶ After the doctor collects the specimens and removes the spinal needle, clean the puncture site with povidone-iodine and apply a small adhesive bandage.

▶ Remove and discard gloves.

▶ Send the CSF specimens to the laboratory immediately, with completed laboratory request forms.

Special considerations

▶ During lumbar puncture, watch closely for signs of adverse reaction: elevated pulse rate, pallor, and clammy skin. Alert the doctor immediately to any significant changes.

▶ The patient may be ordered to lie flat for 8 to 12 hours after the procedure. If necessary, place a patient-care reminder on his bed to this effect.

▶ Collected CSF specimens must be sent to the laboratory immediately; they can't be refrigerated for later transport.

Complications

Headache is the most common adverse effect of lumbar puncture. Others include a reaction to the anesthetic, meningitis, epidural or subdural abscess, bleeding into the spinal canal,

CSF leakage through the dural defect remaining after needle withdrawal, local pain caused by nerve root irritation, edema or hematoma at the puncture site, transient difficulty voiding, and fever. The most serious complications of lumbar puncture, although rare, are tonsillar herniation and medullary compression.

Documentation

Record the initiation and completion times of the procedure, the patient's response, administration of drugs, number of specimen tubes collected, time of transport to the laboratory, and color, consistency, and any other characteristics of the collected specimens.

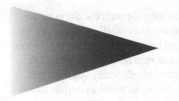

MANUAL VENTILATION

A handheld resuscitation bag is an inflatable device that can be attached to a face mask or directly to an endotracheal (ET) or tracheostomy tube to allow manual delivery of oxygen or room air to the lungs of a patient who can't breathe by himself. Usually used in an emergency, manual ventilation also can be performed while the patient is disconnected temporarily from a mechanical ventilator, such as during a tubing change, during transport, or before suctioning. In such instances, the use of the handheld resuscitation bag maintains ventilation. Oxygen administration with a resuscitation bag can help improve a compromised cardiorespiratory system.

Key nursing diagnoses and patient outcomes

Ineffective breathing pattern related to decreased energy
The patient will:
▶ achieve maximum lung expansion with adequate ventilation
▶ report feeling comfortable with breathing.

Impaired gas exchange related to altered oxygen supply
The patient will:

▶ cough effectively
▶ expectorate sputum.

Equipment
Handheld resuscitation bag • mask • oxygen source (wall unit or tank) • oxygen tubing • nipple adapter attached to oxygen flowmeter • optional: suction equipment, oxygen accumulator and positive end-expiratory pressure (PEEP) valve (see *Using a PEEP valve*).

Preparation of equipment
Unless the patient is intubated or has a tracheostomy, select a mask that fits snugly over the mouth and nose. Attach the mask to the resuscitation bag.

If oxygen is readily available, connect the handheld resuscitation bag to the oxygen. Attach one end of the tubing to the bottom of the bag and the other end to the nipple adapter on the flowmeter of the oxygen source.

Turn on the oxygen and adjust the flow rate according to the patient's condition. For example, if the patient has a low partial pressure of arterial oxygen, he'll need a higher fraction of inspired oxygen (FIO_2). To increase the concentration of inspired oxygen, you can add an oxygen accumulator (also called an oxygen reservoir). This device, which attaches to an adapter on the bottom of the bag, permits an FIO₂ of up to 100%. Then, if time allows, set up suction equipment.

Implementation

▶ Before using the handheld resuscitation bag, check the patient's upper airway for foreign objects. If any are present, remove them *because this alone may restore spontaneous respirations in some instances. Also, foreign matter or secretions can obstruct the airway and impede resuscitation efforts.* Suction the patient *to remove any secretions that may obstruct the airway.* If necessary, insert an oropharyngeal or nasopharyngeal airway *to maintain airway patency.* If the patient has a tracheostomy or ET tube in place, suction the tube.

▶ If appropriate, remove the bed's headboard and stand at the head of the bed *to help keep the patient's neck extended and to free space at the side of the bed for other activities such as cardiopulmonary resuscitation.*

▶ Tilt the patient's head backward, if not contraindicated, and pull his jaw forward *to move the tongue away from the base of the pharynx and prevent obstruction of the airway.* (See *How to apply a handheld resuscitation bag and mask,* page 510.)

▶ Keeping your nondominant hand on the patient's mask, exert downward pressure to seal the mask against his face. For an adult patient, use your dominant hand to compress the bag every 5 seconds to deliver approximately 1 L of air.

 Age alert For infants and children, use a pediatric handheld resuscitation bag. For a child, deliver 15 breaths/minute, or one compression of the

Using a PEEP valve

Add positive end-expiratory pressure (PEEP) to manual ventilation by attaching a PEEP valve to the resuscitation bag. This may improve oxygenation if the patient hasn't responded to increased fraction of inspired oxygen levels. Always use a PEEP valve to manually ventilate a patient who has been receiving PEEP on the ventilator.

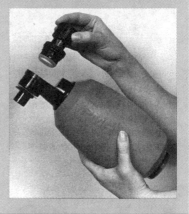

bag every 4 seconds; for an infant, 20 breaths/minute, or one compression every 3 seconds. Infants and children should receive 250 to 500 cc of air with each bag compression.

▶ Deliver breaths with the patient's own inspiratory effort, if any is present. Don't attempt to deliver a breath as the patient exhales.

▶ Observe the patient's chest *to ensure that it rises and falls with each compression.* If ventilation fails to occur, check the fit of the mask and the patency of the patient's airway; if necessary, reposition his head and ensure patency with an oral airway.

How to apply a handheld resuscitation bag and mask

Place the mask over the patient's face so that the apex of the triangle covers the bridge of his nose and the base lies between his lower lip and chin.

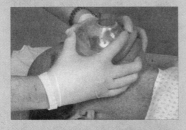

Make sure that the patient's mouth remains open underneath the mask. Attach the bag to the mask and to the tubing leading to the oxygen source.

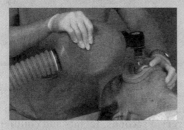

Or, if the patient has a tracheostomy tube or an endotracheal tube in place, remove the mask from the bag and attach the handheld resuscitation bag directly to the tube.

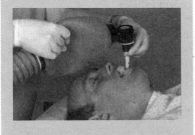

Special considerations

► Avoid neck hyperextension if the patient has a possible cervical injury; instead, use the jaw-thrust technique to open the airway. If you need both hands to keep the patient's mask in place and maintain hyperextension, use the lower part of your arm to compress the bag against your side.

► Observe for vomiting through the clear part of the mask. If vomiting occurs, stop the procedure immediately, lift the mask, wipe and suction the vomitus, and resume resuscitation.

► Underventilation commonly occurs because the handheld resuscitation bag is difficult to keep positioned tightly on the patient's face while ensuring an open airway. In addition, the volume of air delivered to the patient varies with the type of bag used and the hand size of the person compressing the bag. An adult with a small- or medium-sized hand may not consistently deliver 1 L of air. For these reasons, have someone assist with the procedure, if possible.

Complications

Aspiration of vomitus can result in pneumonia, and gastric distention may result from air forced into the patient's stomach.

Documentation

In an emergency, record the date and time of the procedure, manual ventilation efforts, any complications and the nursing action taken, and the patient's response to treatment according to your facility's protocol for respiratory arrest.

In a nonemergency situation, record the date and time of the procedure, reason and length of time the patient was disconnected from mechanical ventilation and received manual ventilation, any complications and the nursing action taken, and the patient's tolerance of the procedure.

MECHANICAL DEBRIDEMENT

Debridement involves removing necrotic tissue by mechanical, chemical, or surgical means to allow underlying healthy tissue to regenerate. Mechanical debridement procedures include irrigation, hydrotherapy, and excision of dead tissue with forceps and scissors. The procedure may be done at the bedside or in a specially prepared room.

Depending on the type of burn, a combination of debridement techniques may be used. Other debridement techniques include chemical debridement (with wound-cleaning beads or topical agents that absorb exudate and debris) or surgical excision and skin grafting (usually reserved for deep burns or ulcers). Typically, the patient receives a local or general anesthetic.

Burn wound debridement removes eschar (hardened, dead tissue). This prevents or controls infection, promotes healing, and prepares the wound surface to receive a graft. Ideally, the wound should be debrided daily during the dressing change. Frequent, regular debridement guards against possible hemorrhage resulting from more extensive and forceful debridement. It also reduces the need to conduct extensive debridement under anesthesia.

Closed blisters over partial-thickness burns shouldn't be debrided. (For additional information, see "Hydrotherapy," page 401.)

Key nursing diagnoses and patient outcomes

Disturbed body image related to appearance of wounds
The patient will:
▶ communicate feelings about changed body image
▶ express positive feelings about self
▶ demonstrate the ability to practice two new coping behaviors.

Acute pain related to physical, biological, or chemical agents
The patient will:
▶ identify pain characteristics
▶ articulate factors that intensify pain and modify behavior accordingly
▶ express feelings of comfort and relief from pain
▶ state and carry out appropriate interventions for pain relief.

Equipment
Ordered pain medication • two pairs of sterile gloves • two gowns or aprons • mask • cap • sterile scissors • sterile forceps • 4″ × 4″ sterile gauze pads • sterile solutions and medications as ordered • hemostatic agent as ordered

Be sure to have the following equipment immediately available to control hemorrhage: needle holder, gut suture with needle, and silver nitrate sticks.

Implementation
▶ Explain the procedure to the patient *to allay his fears and promote cooperation.* Teach him distraction and relaxation techniques, if possible, *to minimize his discomfort.*
▶ Provide privacy. Administer an analgesic 20 minutes before debridement begins, or give an I.V. analgesic immediately before the procedure.

▶ Keep the patient warm. Expose only the area to be debrided *to prevent chilling and fluid and electrolyte loss.*

▶ Wash your hands and put on a cap, mask, gown or apron, and sterile gloves.

▶ Remove the burn dressings and clean the wound. (For detailed directions, see "Burn care," page 84.)

▶ Remove your gown or apron and dirty gloves and change to another gown or apron and sterile gloves.

▶ Lift loosened edges of eschar with forceps. Use the blunt edge of scissors or forceps to probe the eschar. Cut the dead tissue from the wound with the scissors. Leave a ¼" (0.6-cm) edge on remaining eschar *to avoid cutting into viable tissue.*

▶ Because debridement removes only dead tissue, bleeding should be minimal. If bleeding occurs, apply gentle pressure on the wound with sterile 4" × 4" gauze pads. Then apply the hemostatic agent. If bleeding persists, notify the doctor and maintain pressure on the wound until he arrives. Excessive bleeding or spurting vessels may require ligation.

▶ Perform additional procedures, such as application of topical medications and dressing replacements as ordered.

Special considerations

▶ Work quickly, with an assistant, if possible, to complete this painful procedure as soon as possible. Limit the procedure time to 20 minutes, if possible.

▶ Acknowledge the patient's discomfort and provide emotional support.

▶ Debride no more than a 4" (10.2 cm) square area at one time.

Complications

Because burns damage or destroy the protective skin barrier, infection may develop despite the use of aseptic technique and equipment. In addition, some blood loss may occur if debridement exposes an eroded blood vessel or if you inadvertently cut a vessel. Fluid and electrolyte imbalances may result from exudate lost during the procedure.

Documentation

Record the date and time of wound debridement, the area debrided, and solutions and medications used. Describe wound condition, noting signs of infection or skin breakdown. Record the patient's tolerance of and reaction to the procedure. Note indications for additional therapy.

MECHANICAL VENTILATION

A mechanical ventilator moves air in and out of a patient's lungs. Although the equipment serves to ventilate a patient, it doesn't ensure adequate gas exchange. Mechanical ventilators may use either positive or negative pressure to ventilate patients.

Positive-pressure ventilators exert a positive pressure on the airway, which causes inspiration while increasing tidal volume (V_T). The inspiratory cycles of these ventilators may vary in volume, pressure, or time. For example, a volume-cycled ventilator — the type used most commonly — delivers a preset volume of air each time, regardless of the amount of lung resistance. A pressure-cycled ventilator generates flow until the machine reaches a preset pressure regardless of the volume delivered or the time required to achieve the pressure. A time-cycled ventilator generates flow for a preset amount of time. A high-frequency ventilator uses high respiratory rates and low V_T to maintain alveolar ventilation.

Negative-pressure ventilators act by creating negative pressure, which pulls the thorax outward and allows air to flow into the lungs. Examples of such ventilators are the iron lung, the cuirass (chest shell), and the body wrap. Negative-pressure ventilators are used mainly to treat neuromuscular disorders, such as Guillain-Barré syndrome, myasthenia gravis, and poliomyelitis.

Other indications for ventilator use include central nervous system disorders, such as cerebral hemorrhage and spinal cord transsection; adult respiratory distress syndrome; pulmonary edema; chronic obstructive pulmonary disease; flail chest; and acute hypoventilation.

Key nursing diagnoses and patient outcomes

Ineffective breathing pattern related to decreased energy
The patient will:
▶ achieve maximum lung expansion with adequate ventilation
▶ report feeling comfortable with breathing.

Impaired gas exchange related to altered oxygen demand
The patient will:
▶ cough effectively
▶ expectorate sputum.

Equipment

Oxygen source • air source that can supply 50 psi • mechanical ventilator • humidifier • ventilator circuit tubing, connectors, and adapters • condensation collection trap • in-line thermometer • gloves • handheld resuscitation bag with reservoir • suction equipment • sterile distilled water • equipment for arterial blood gas (ABG) analysis • optional: oximeter and soft restraints

Preparation of equipment

In most facilities, respiratory therapists assume responsibility for setting up the ventilator. If necessary, check the manufacturer's instructions for setting it up. In most cases, you'll need to add sterile distilled water to the humidifier and connect the ventilator to the appropriate gas source.

Implementation

▶ Verify the doctor's order for ventilator support. If the patient isn't already intubated, prepare him for intubation. (See "Endotracheal intubation," page 274.)
▶ When possible, explain the procedure to the patient and his family *to help reduce anxiety and fear.* Assure the patient and his family that staff members are nearby to provide care.
▶ Perform a complete physical assessment and draw blood for ABG analysis *to establish a baseline.*
▶ Suction the patient, if necessary.
▶ Plug the ventilator into the electrical outlet and turn it on. Adjust the settings on the ventilator as ordered. (See *Mechanical ventilation glossary,* page 514.) Make sure that the ventilator's alarms are set as ordered and that the humidifier is filled with sterile distilled water.

Mechanical ventilation glossary

Although a respiratory therapist usually monitors ventilator settings based on the doctor's order, you should understand all of the following terms.

Assist-control mode: The assist-control mode allows the ventilator to deliver a preset rate; however, the patient can initiate additional breaths, which trigger the ventilator to deliver the preset tidal volume at positive pressure.

Continuous positive airway pressure (CPAP): The continuous positive airway pressure setting prompts the ventilator to deliver positive pressure to the airway throughout the respiratory cycle. It works only on patients who can breathe spontaneously.

Control mode: The control mode allows the ventilator to deliver a preset tidal volume at a fixed rate regardless of whether or not the patient is breathing spontaneously.

Fraction of inspired oxygen (FIO_2): The fraction of inspired oxygen is the amount of oxygen delivered to the patient by the ventilator. The dial on the ventilator that sets this percentage is labeled by the term oxygen concentration or oxygen percentage.

I:E ratio: The I:E ratio compares the duration of inspiration with the duration of expiration. The I:E ratio of normal, spontaneous breathing is 1:2, meaning that expiration is twice as long as inspiration.

Inspiratory flow rate (IFR): The inspiratory flow rate denotes the tidal volume delivered within a certain time. Its value can range from 20 to 120 L/minute.

Minute ventilation or minute volume (V_E): The minute ventilation or minute volume measurement results from the multiplication of respiratory rate and tidal volume.

Peak inspiratory pressure (PIP): Measured by the pressure manometer on the ventilator, the peak inspiratory pressure reflects the amount of pressure required to deliver a preset tidal volume.

Positive end-expiratory pressure (PEEP): In the positive end-expiratory pressure mode, the ventilator is triggered to apply positive pressure at the end of each expiration to increase the area for oxygen exchange by helping to inflate and keep open collapsed alveoli.

Pressure support ventilation (PSV): The pressure support ventilation mode allows the ventilator to apply a preset amount of positive pressure when the patient inspires spontaneously. PSV increases tidal volume while decreasing the patient's breathing workload.

Respiratory rate: The respiratory rate is the number of breaths per minute delivered by the ventilator— also called frequency.

Sensitivity setting: The sensitivity setting determines the amount of effort the patient must exert to trigger the inspiratory cycle.

Sigh volume: The sigh volume is a ventilator-delivered breath that is 1½ times as large as the patient's tidal volume.

Synchronized intermittent mandatory ventilation (SIMV): The synchronized intermittent mandatory ventilation allows the ventilator to deliver a preset number of breaths at a specific tidal volume. The patient may supplement these mechanical ventilations with his own breaths, in which case the tidal volume and rate are determined by his own inspiratory ability.

Tidal volume (V_T): Tidal volume refers to the volume of air delivered to the patient with each cycle, usually 12 to 15 cc/kg.

► Put on gloves, if you haven't already. Connect the endotracheal tube to the ventilator. Observe for chest expansion, and auscultate for bilateral breath sounds *to verify that the patient is being ventilated.*

► Monitor the patient's ABG values after the initial ventilator setup (usually 20 to 30 minutes), after any changes in ventilator settings, and as the patient's clinical condition indicates *to determine whether the patient is being adequately ventilated and to avoid oxygen toxicity.* Be prepared to adjust ventilator settings based on ABG analysis.

► Check the ventilator tubing frequently for condensation, which can cause resistance to airflow and may also be aspirated by the patient. As needed, drain the condensate into a collection trap or briefly disconnect the patient from the ventilator (ventilating him with a handheld resuscitation bag, if necessary), and empty the water into a receptacle. Don't drain the condensate into the humidifier *because the condensate may be contaminated with the patient's secretions.*

► Check the in-line thermometer *to make sure that the temperature of the air delivered to the patient is close to body temperature.*

► When monitoring the patient's vital signs, count spontaneous breaths as well as ventilator-delivered breaths.

► Change, clean, or dispose of the ventilator tubing and equipment according to your facility's policy *to reduce the risk of bacterial contamination.* Typically, ventilator tubing should be changed every 48 to 72 hours and sometimes more often.

► When ordered, begin to wean the patient from the ventilator. (See *Weaning a patient from the ventilator,* page 516.)

Special considerations

► Provide emotional support to the patient during all phases of mechanical ventilation *to reduce his anxiety and promote successful treatment.* Even if the patient is unresponsive, continue to explain all procedures and treatments to him.

► Make sure that the ventilator alarms are on at all times. *These alarms alert the nursing staff to potentially hazardous conditions and changes in patient status.* If an alarm sounds and the problem can't be identified easily, disconnect the patient from the ventilator and use a handheld resuscitation bag to ventilate him. (See *Responding to ventilator alarms,* page 517.)

► Unless contraindicated, turn the patient from side to side every 1 to 2 hours *to facilitate lung expansion and removal of secretions.* Perform active or passive range-of-motion exercises for all extremities *to reduce the hazards of immobility.* If the patient's condition permits, position him upright at regular intervals *to increase lung expansion.* When moving the patient or the ventilator tubing, be careful to prevent condensation in the tubing from flowing into the lungs *because aspiration of this contaminated moisture can cause infection.* Provide care for the patient's artificial airway as needed.

► Assess the patient's peripheral circulation and monitor his urine output for signs of decreased cardiac output. Watch for signs and symptoms of fluid volume excess or dehydration.

► Place the call light within the patient's reach and establish a method of communication such as a communication board *because intubation and mechanical ventilation impair the patient's ability to speak.* An artificial airway may

(Text continues on page 518.)

Weaning a patient from the ventilator

Successful weaning depends on the patient's ability to breathe on his own. This means he must have a spontaneous respiratory effort that can keep him ventilated, a stable cardiovascular system, and sufficient respiratory muscle strength and level of consciousness to sustain spontaneous breathing. He also should meet some or all of the following criteria.

Criteria

■ Partial pressure of arterial oxygen of 60 mm Hg (50 mm Hg or the ability to maintain baseline levels if he has chronic lung disease) or a fraction of inspired oxygen (FIO_2) of 0.4 or less

■ Partial pressure of arterial carbon dioxide ($PaCO_2$) of less than 40 mm Hg (or normal for the patient) or an FIO_2 of 0.4 or less if $PaCO_2$ is 60 mm Hg or more

■ Vital capacity of more than 10 ml/kg of body weight

■ Maximum inspiratory pressure of more than 20 cm H_2O

■ Minute ventilation less than10 L/minute with a respiratory frequency of less than 30 breaths/minute

■ Forced expiratory volume in the first second of more than 10 ml/kg of body weight

■ Ability to double his spontaneous resting minute ventilation

■ Adequate natural airway or a functioning tracheostomy

■ Ability to cough and mobilize secretions

■ Successful withdrawal of any neuromuscular blocker such as pancuronium bromide

■ Clear or clearing chest X-ray

■ Absence of infection, acid-base or electrolyte imbalance, hyperglycemia, arrhythmia, renal failure, anemia, fever, or excessive fatigue

Short-term ventilation

If the patient has received mechanical ventilation for a short time, weaning may be accomplished by progressively decreasing the frequency and tidal volume of the ventilated breaths. Then the patient's endotracheal tube can be converted to a T tube to assess whether his spontaneous respirations are adequate before extubation. If the patient has been mechanically ventilated with 5 cm H_2O or less of positive end-expiratory pressure, the adequacy of his spontaneous breathing can be assessed by using a trial of continuous positive airway pressure on the ventilator.

Long-term ventilation

If the patient has received mechanical ventilation for a long time, weaning is usually accomplished by switching the ventilator to pressure support ventilation (PSV) with or without intermittent mandatory ventilation (IMV). That way, each of the patient's spontaneous breaths is augmented by the ventilator. As the patient's own respirations improve, IMV and PSV can be decreased.

If the patient doesn't progress satisfactorily using one of these methods, an alternative method of weaning is to disconnect him from the ventilator and place him on a T tube or tracheostomy collar for the ordered amount of time before reconnecting him to the ventilator. The patient then alternates between being on and off the ventilator, increasing the time off the ventilator with each trial.

Eventually, the patient will be able to breathe on his own all day. However, even then, he should be reconnected to the ventilator for a few nights so that he can obtain adequate rest and conserve the energy required to breathe on his own the next day.

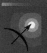

Responding to ventilator alarms

Signal	Possible cause	Interventions
Low-pressure alarm	■ Tube disconnected from ventilator	■ Reconnect the tube to the ventilator.
	■ Endotracheal (ET) tube displaced above vocal cords or tracheostomy tube extubated	■ Check tube placement and reposition, if needed. If extubation or displacement has occurred, ventilate the patient manually and call the doctor immediately.
	■ Leaking tidal volume from low cuff pressure (from an underinflated or ruptured cuff or a leak in the cuff or one-way valve)	■ Listen for a whooshing sound around the tube, indicating an air leak. If you hear one, check cuff pressure. If you can't maintain pressure, call the doctor; he may need to insert a new tube.
	■ Ventilator malfunction	■ Disconnect the patient from the ventilator and ventilate him manually, if necessary. Obtain another ventilator.
	■ Leak in ventilator circuitry (from loose connection or hole in tubing, loss of temperature-sensitive device, or cracked humidification jar)	■ Make sure all connections are intact. Check for holes or leaks in the tubing and replace, if necessary. Check the humidification jar and replace, if cracked.
High-pressure alarm	■ Increased airway pressure or decreased lung compliance caused by worsening disease	■ Auscultate the lungs for evidence of increasing lung consolidation, barotrauma, or wheezing. Call the doctor, if indicated.
	■ Patient biting on oral ET tube	■ Insert a bite block if needed.
	■ Secretions in airway	■ Look for secretions in the airway. To remove them, suction the patient or have him cough.
	■ Condensate in large-bore tubing	■ Check tubing for condensate and remove any fluid.
	■ Intubation of right mainstem bronchus	■ Check tube position. If it has slipped, call the doctor; he may need to reposition it.
	■ Patient coughing, gagging, or attempting to talk	■ If the patient fights the ventilator, the doctor may order a sedative or neuromuscular blocking agent.
	■ Chest wall resistance	■ Reposition the patient to see if doing so improves chest expansion. If repositioning doesn't help, administer the prescribed analgesic.
	■ Failure of high-pressure relief valve	■ Have the faulty equipment replaced.
	■ Bronchospasm	■ Assess the patient for the cause. Report to the doctor and treat as ordered.

help the patient to speak *by allowing air to pass through his vocal cords.*

▶ Administer a sedative or neuromuscular blocking agent as ordered *to relax the patient or eliminate spontaneous breathing efforts that can interfere with the ventilator's action.* Remember that the patient receiving a neuromuscular blocking drug requires close observation *because of his inability to breathe or communicate.*

▶ If the patient is receiving a neuromuscular blocking agent, make sure that he also receives a sedative. *Neuromuscular blocking agents cause paralysis without altering the patient's level of consciousness.* Reassure the patient and his family that the paralysis is temporary. Also, make sure that emergency equipment is readily available in case the ventilator malfunctions or the patient is extubated accidentally. Continue to explain all procedures to the patient and take additional steps to ensure his safety, such as raising the side rails of his bed while turning him and covering and lubricating his eyes.

▶ Ensure that the patient gets adequate rest and sleep *because fatigue can delay weaning from the ventilator.* Provide subdued lighting, safely muffle equipment noises, and restrict staff access to the area *to promote quiet during rest periods.*

▶ When weaning the patient, continue to observe for signs of hypoxia. Schedule weaning to fit comfortably and realistically with the patient's daily regimen. Avoid scheduling sessions after meals, baths, or lengthy therapeutic or diagnostic procedures. Have the patient help you set up the schedule *to give him some sense of control over a frightening procedure.* As the patient's tolerance for weaning increases, help him sit up out of bed *to improve his breathing and sense*

of well-being. Suggest diversionary activities *to take his mind off breathing.*

Home care

If the patient will be discharged on a ventilator, evaluate the family's or the caregiver's ability and motivation to provide such care. Well before discharge, develop a teaching plan that will address the patient's needs. For example, teaching should include information about ventilator care and settings, artificial airway care, suctioning, respiratory therapy, communication, nutrition, therapeutic exercise, the signs and symptoms of infection, and ways to troubleshoot minor equipment malfunctions.

Also, evaluate the patient's need for adaptive equipment, such as a hospital bed, wheelchair or walker with a ventilator tray, patient lift, and bedside commode. Determine whether the patient needs to travel; if so, select appropriate portable and backup equipment.

Before discharge, have the patient's caregiver demonstrate his ability to use the equipment. At discharge, contact a durable medical equipment vendor and a home health nurse to follow up with the patient. Also, refer the patient to community resources, if available.

Complications

Mechanical ventilation can cause tension pneumothorax, decreased cardiac output, oxygen toxicity, fluid volume excess caused by humidification, infection, and such GI complications as distention or bleeding from stress ulcers.

Documentation

Document the date and time of initiation of mechanical ventilation. Name the type of ventilator used for the patient, and note its settings. Describe the patient's subjective and objective response to mechanical ventilation, including vital signs, breath sounds, use of accessory muscles, intake and output, and weight. List any complications and nursing actions taken. Record all pertinent laboratory data, including ABG analysis results and oxygen saturation levels.

During weaning, record the date and time of each session, the weaning method, and baseline and subsequent vital signs, oxygen saturation levels, and ABG values. Again, describe the patient's subjective and objective responses, including level of consciousness, respiratory effort, arrhythmia, skin color, and need for suctioning.

List all complications and nursing actions taken. If the patient was receiving pressure support ventilation (PSV) or using a T-piece or tracheostomy collar, note the duration of spontaneous breathing and the patient's ability to maintain the weaning schedule. If using intermittent mandatory ventilation, with or without PSV, record the control breath rate, the time of each breath reduction, and the rate of spontaneous respirations.

MIST TENT THERAPY

Also known as a croupette for infants or a cool-humidity tent for children, a mist tent houses a nebulizer that transforms distilled water into mist. Mist tent therapy benefits the patient by providing a cool, moist environment. This atmosphere eases breathing and helps to decrease respiratory tract edema, liquefy secretions, and reduce fever.

Oxygen may also be administered along with the mist.

Mist tents are commonly used to treat croup and such infections or inflammations as bronchiolitis and pneumonia.

Key nursing diagnoses and patient outcomes

Impaired gas exchange related to altered oxygen supply
The patient will:
▶ maintain respiratory rate within 5 breaths/minute of baseline
▶ express feelings of comfort while maintaining air exchange
▶ have normal breath sounds
▶ return to baseline arterial blood gas levels: (specify) pH; (specify) partial pressure of arterial oxygen; and (specify) partial pressure of arterial carbon dioxide.

Ineffective breathing pattern related to (specify)
The patient will:
▶ achieve maximum lung expansion with adequate ventilation.

Equipment
Mist tent frame and plastic tenting • bed sheets • plastic sheet or linen-saver pad • two bath blankets • nebulizer with water reservoir and filter • oxygen flowmeter and oxygen analyzer, if ordered • sterile distilled water • optional: stockinette cap or booties and infant seat

Preparation of equipment
Review facility policy to determine who sets up a mist tent. In some facilities the nurse sets up the tent; in others a respiratory therapist may do so. In setting up the tent, first wash your hands

and then place the tent frame and the plastic tenting at the head of the crib or bed. Then cover the mattress with a bed sheet, cover the bed sheet with a plastic sheet or linen-saver pad (tucked under the mattress), and cover these layers with a bath blanket.

Next, fill the reservoir of the nebulizer with sterile distilled water and make sure that the inlet for air contains a clean filter. If the patient will have oxygen in the tent, make sure that the oxygen flowmeter connects to the tent. Then turn the flowmeter to the desired setting. Be sure to analyze the percentage of oxygen being delivered. Wait 2 minutes after the mist begins filling the tent before placing the patient in it.

Implementation

▶ Carefully explain the mist tent's purpose to the patient and his parents *to alleviate anxiety and promote cooperation.* Use terms that both generations can understand. When talking with the parents, you might compare the mist tent with a vaporizer. When talking with the patient, however, you might compare the tent with a teepee or a spaceship cabin.

▶ Elevate the head of the bed to a position that enhances patient comfort. If the patient is an infant, consider placing him in an infant seat. *The more upright position will help him to mobilize secretions.* If the patient will be in the room alone, position him on his side *to prevent him from aspirating mucus from liquefied secretions and productive coughing.*

▶ Use a stockinette cap, booties, and the other bath blanket as needed *to keep the patient from becoming chilled as the mist condenses inside the tent.*

▶ Change the patient's bed sheets and clothing as they dampen and check his temperature frequently *to detect impending hypothermia.*

▶ Monitor the patient frequently for a change in condition, keeping in mind that the mist may make observation difficult.

▶ Encourage parents to stay with the patient. If he grows irritable and uncooperative while in the tent, the parent may enter the tent to comfort him *because excessive irritability causes labored breathing and increases oxygen consumption.*

▶ If secretions coat the inside of the tent, wipe the tent down with a hospital-approved cleaner such as soap and water. Also, clean the reservoir with sterile water *to prevent bacterial growth.*

Nursing alert Because the tent alone won't stop an infant or a small child from falling out of bed, raise the side rails all the way. Check on the patient frequently; if possible, place him near the nurses' station.

Special considerations

▶ Allow the patient to have toys in the mist tent *to provide distraction.* To amuse infants, string plastic toys across the top bar of the tent. However, discourage playing with cloth or stuffed toys in the tent *because these objects absorb moisture and supply a medium for bacterial growth.*

▶ *To prevent a fire,* forbid toys or games that may spark or trigger an electric shock such as battery-operated toys. Also, remove the electric call light and give older children a hand bell instead. If the patient is receiving oxygen, check the percentage of oxygen delivered at least every 4 hours.

▶ For bathing, remove the patient from the tent *to prevent hypothermia.*

Home care

If the mist tent will be used at home, show the parents how to set up, use, and clean the tent properly.

Documentation

Record the date and time the patient was placed in the tent. Describe the patient's respiratory status, including breath sounds, sputum production, and perfusion. Document his vital signs. Also, note the date and time that the patient was removed from the tent. Record the percentage of oxygen being delivered, the date and time of all analyses, and the oxygen saturation.

MIXED VENOUS OXYGEN SATURATION MONITORING

Mixed venous oxygen saturation (SvO_2) monitoring uses a fiber-optic thermodilution pulmonary artery (PA) catheter to continuously monitor oxygen delivery to tissues and oxygen consumption by tissues. It allows rapid detection of impaired oxygen delivery, as from decreased cardiac output, hemoglobin level, or arterial oxygen saturation. It also helps evaluate a patient's response to drug therapy, endotracheal tube suctioning, ventilator setting changes, positive end-expiratory pressure, and fraction of inspired oxygen. SvO_2 usually ranges from 60% to 80%; the normal value is 75%.

Key nursing diagnoses and patient outcomes

Impaired gas exchange related to altered oxygen supply

The patient will:

▶ maintain respiratory rate within 5 breaths/minute of baseline
▶ express feelings of comfort while maintaining air exchange
▶ have normal breath sounds
▶ return to baseline arterial blood gas levels: (specify) pH; (specify) partial pressure of arterial oxygen; and (specify) partial pressure of arterial carbon dioxide.

Ineffective tissue perfusion (cardiopulmonary) related to decreased cellular exchange

The patient will:

▶ attain hemodynamic stability as evidenced by pulse not less than (specify) beats/minute and not greater than (specify) beats/minute; blood pressure not less than (specify) mm Hg and not greater than (specify) mm Hg; and respiration within 5 breaths/minute of baseline
▶ have warm and dry skin
▶ not experience arrhythmia
▶ maintain adequate cardiac output
▶ have an SvO_2 value between 60% and 80%.

Equipment

Fiber-optic PA catheter • co-oximeter • optical module and cable • gloves

Preparation of equipment

Review the manufacturer's instructions for assembly and use of the fiber-optic PA catheter. Connect the optical module and cable to the monitor. Next, peel back the wrapping covering the catheter just enough to uncover the fiber-optic connector. Attach the fiber-optic connector to the optical module while allowing the rest of the catheter to remain in its sterile wrapping. Calibrate the fiber-optic catheter by following the manufacturer's instructions.

To prepare for the rest of the procedure, follow the instructions for pulmonary catheter insertion as described in "PAP and PAWP monitoring," page 608. (See also *SvO₂ monitoring equipment*.)

Implementation

▶ Wash your hands and put on gloves.
▶ Explain the procedure to the patient *to allay his fears and promote cooperation.*
▶ Assist with the insertion of the fiber-optic catheter just as you would for a PA catheter.
▶ After the catheter is inserted, confirm that the light intensity tracing on the graphic printout is within normal range *to ensure correct positioning and function of the catheter.*
▶ Observe the digital readout and record the SvO₂ on graph paper. Repeat readings at least once each hour *to monitor and document trends.*
▶ Set the machine alarms 10% above and 10% below the patient's current SvO₂ reading.

Recalibrating the monitor

▶ Draw a mixed venous blood sample from the distal port of the PA catheter. Send it to the laboratory for analysis *to compare the laboratory's SvO₂ reading with that of the fiber-optic catheter.*
▶ If the catheter values and the laboratory values differ by more than 4%, follow the manufacturer's instructions to enter the SvO₂ value obtained by the laboratory into the co-oximeter.
▶ Recalibrate the monitor every 24 hours or whenever the catheter has been disconnected from the optical module.

Special considerations

▶ If the patient's SvO₂ drops below 60% or varies by more than 10% for 3 minutes or longer, reassess the patient. If the SvO₂ doesn't return to the baseline value after nursing interventions, notify the doctor. A decreasing SvO₂ or a value less than 60% indicates impaired oxygen delivery, as occurs in hemorrhage, hypoxia, shock, arrhythmia, or suctioning. SvO₂ may also decrease as a result of increased oxygen demand from hyperthermia, shivering, or seizures, for example.
▶ If the intensity of the tracing is low, ensure that all connections between the catheter and co-oximeter are secure and that the catheter is patent and not kinked.
▶ If the tracing is damped or erratic, try to aspirate blood from the catheter *to check for patency.* If you can't aspirate blood, notify the doctor *so that he can replace the catheter.* Also, check the PA waveform *to determine whether the catheter has wedged.* If the catheter has wedged, try to flush the line. Also, turn the patient from side to side and instruct him to cough. If the catheter remains wedged, notify the doctor immediately.
▶ If the tracing shows a high intensity, the catheter may be pressing against a vessel wall. Flush the line. If the tracing doesn't return to normal, notify the doctor *so he can reposition the catheter.*

Complications

Thrombosis can result from local irritation by the catheter; however, a heparin flush helps prevent this complication. Thromboembolism also can occur if a thrombus breaks off and lodges in the circulatory system. Monitor the patient for signs and symptoms of infection,

Svo₂ monitoring equipment

The mixed venous oxygen saturation (Svo_2) monitoring system consists of a flow-directed pulmonary artery (PA) catheter with fiber-optic filaments, an optical module, and a co-oximeter. The co-oximeter displays a continuous digital Svo_2 value; the strip recorder prints a permanent record.

Catheter insertion follows the same technique as with any thermodilution flow-directed PA catheter. The distal lumen connects to an external PA pressure monitoring system; the proximal or central venous pressure lumen connects to another monitoring system or to a continuous-flow administration unit; and the optical module connects to the co-oximeter unit.

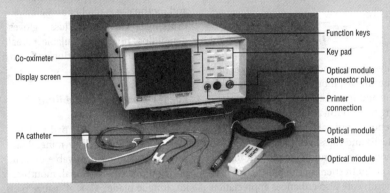

Co-oximeter

Display screen

PA catheter

Function keys

Key pad

Optical module connector plug

Printer connection

Optical module cable

Optical module

Normal Svo₂ waveform

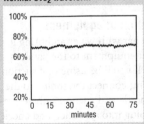

Svo₂ with patient activities

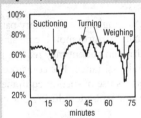

Svo₂ with PEEP and Fio₂ changes

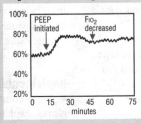

such as redness or drainage, at the catheter site.

Documentation

Record the Svo_2 value on a flowchart and attach a tracing as ordered. Note any significant changes in the patient's status and the results of any interventions. For comparison, note the Svo_2 as measured by the fiber-optic catheter whenever a blood sample is obtained for laboratory analysis of Svo_2.

MOUTH CARE

Given in the morning, at bedtime, or after meals, mouth care entails brushing and flossing the teeth and inspecting the mouth. It removes soft plaque deposits and calculus from the teeth, cleans and massages the gums, reduces mouth odor, and helps prevent infection. By freshening the patient's mouth, mouth care also enhances appreciation of food, thereby aiding appetite and nutrition.

Although the ambulatory patient can usually perform mouth care alone, the bedridden patient may require partial or full assistance. The comatose patient requires use of suction equipment to prevent aspiration during oral care.

Key nursing diagnoses and patient outcomes

Impaired oral mucous membrane related to (specify)
The patient will:
▶ state feelings of increased comfort
▶ maintain pink and moist oral mucous membranes
▶ explain oral hygiene routine.

Bathing and hygiene self-care deficit related to (specify)
The patient will:
▶ communicate feelings about limitations
▶ have self-care needs met
▶ achieve the highest possible level of functioning.

Equipment

Towel or facial tissues • emesis basin • trash bag • mouthwash • toothbrush and toothpaste • pitcher and glass • drinking straw • dental floss • gloves • dental floss holder, if available • small mirror, if necessary • optional: oral irrigating device

For the comatose or debilitated patients

(As needed) Linen-saver pad • bite-block • petroleum jelly • mineral oil • sponge-tipped mouth swab • oral suction equipment • optional: mouth-care kit, tongue blade, 4″ × 4″ gauze pads, and adhesive tape

Preparation of equipment

Fill a pitcher with water and bring it and other equipment to the patient's bedside. If you'll be using oral suction equipment, connect the tubing to the suction bottle and suction catheter, insert the plug into an outlet, and check for correct operation. If necessary, devise a bite-block to protect yourself from being bitten during the procedure. Wrap a gauze pad over the end of a tongue blade, fold the edge in, and secure it with adhesive tape.

Implementation

▶ Wash your hands thoroughly, put on gloves, explain the procedure to the patient, and provide privacy.

Supervising mouth care

► For the bedridden patient capable of self-care, encourage him to perform his own mouth care.

► If allowed, place the patient in Fowler's position. Place the overbed table in front of the patient and arrange the equipment on it. Open the table and set up the built-in mirror, if available, or position a small mirror on the table.

► Drape a towel over the patient's chest *to protect his gown.* Tell him to floss his teeth while looking into the mirror.

► Observe the patient *to make sure he's flossing correctly,* and correct him, if necessary. Tell him to wrap the floss around the second or third fingers of both hands. Starting with his back teeth and without injuring the gums, he should insert the floss as far as possible into the space between each pair of teeth. Then he should clean the surfaces of adjacent teeth by pulling the floss up and down against the side of each tooth. After the patient flosses a pair of teeth, remind him to use a clean 1″ (2.5 cm) section of floss for the next pair.

► After the patient flosses, mix mouthwash and water in a glass, place a straw in the glass, and position the emesis basin nearby. Then instruct the patient to brush his teeth and gums while looking into the mirror. Encourage him to rinse frequently during brushing and provide facial tissues for him to wipe his mouth.

Performing mouth care

► For the comatose patient or the conscious patient incapable of self-care, you'll perform mouth care. If the patient wears dentures, clean them thoroughly. (See *Dealing with dentures,* page

526.) Some patients may benefit from using an oral irrigating device such as a Water Pik. (See *Using an oral irrigating device,* page 527.)

► Raise the bed to a comfortable working height *to prevent back strain.* Then lower the head of the bed and position the patient on his side, with his face extended over the edge of the pillow *to facilitate drainage and prevent fluid aspiration.*

► Arrange the equipment on the overbed table or bedside stand, including the oral suction equipment, if necessary. Turn on the machine. If a suction machine isn't available, wipe the inside of the patient's mouth frequently with a moist, sponge-tipped swab.

► Place a linen-saver pad under the patient's chin and an emesis basin near his cheek *to absorb or catch drainage.*

► Lubricate the patient's lips with petroleum jelly *to prevent dryness and cracking.* Reapply lubricant as needed during oral care.

► If necessary, insert the bite-block *to hold the patient's mouth open during oral care.*

► Using a dental floss holder, hold the floss against each tooth and direct it as close to the gum as possible without injuring the sensitive tissues around the tooth.

► After flossing the patient's teeth, mix mouthwash and water in a glass and place the straw in it.

► Wet the toothbrush with water. If necessary, use hot water *to soften the bristles.* Apply toothpaste.

► Brush the patient's lower teeth from the gum line up; the upper teeth, from the gum line down. Place the brush at a 45-degree angle to the gum line and press the bristles gently into the gingival sulcus. Using short, gentle strokes

(Text continues on page 528.)

Dealing with dentures

Prostheses made of acrylic resins, vinyl composites, or both, dentures replace some or all of the patient's natural teeth. Dentures require proper care to remove soft plaque deposits and calculus and to reduce mouth odor. Such care involves removing and rinsing dentures after meals, daily brushing and removal of tenacious deposits, and soaking in a commercial denture cleaner. Dentures must be removed from the comatose or presurgical patient to prevent possible airway obstruction.

Equipment and preparation
Emesis basin • labeled denture cup • toothbrush or denture brush • gloves • toothpaste • commercial denture cleaner • paper towel • sponge-tipped mouth swab • mouthwash • gauze • optional: adhesive denture liner

Start by assembling the equipment at the patient's bedside. Wash your hands and put on gloves.

Removing dentures
■ To remove a full upper denture, grasp the front and palatal surfaces of the denture with your thumb and forefinger. Position the index finger of your opposite hand over the upper border of the denture and press to break the seal between denture and palate. Grasp the denture with gauze *because saliva can make it slippery.*
■ To remove a full lower denture, grasp the front and lingual surfaces of the denture with your thumb and index finger and gently lift up.
■ To remove partial dentures, first ask the patient or caregiver how the prosthesis is retained and how to remove it. If the partial denture is held in place with clips or snaps, then exert equal pressure on the border of each side of the denture. Avoid lifting the clasps, which easily bend or break.

Oral and denture care
■ After removing dentures, place them in a properly labeled denture cup. Add warm water and a commercial denture cleaner to remove stains and hardened deposits. Follow package directions. Avoid soaking dentures in mouthwash containing alcohol *because it may damage a soft liner.*
■ Instruct the patient to rinse with mouthwash to remove food particles and reduce mouth odor. Then stroke the palate, buccal surfaces, gums, and tongue with a soft toothbrush or sponge-tipped mouth swab to clean the mucosa and stimulate circulation. Inspect for irritated areas or sores *because they may indicate a poorly fitting denture.*
■ Carry the denture cup, emesis basin, toothbrush, and toothpaste to the sink. After lining the basin with a paper towel, fill it with water to cushion the dentures in case you drop them. Hold the dentures over the basin, wet them with warm water, and apply toothpaste to a denture brush or long-bristled toothbrush. Clean the dentures using only moderate pressure to prevent scratches and warm water to prevent distortion.
■ Clean the denture cup, and place the dentures in it. Rinse the brush, and clean and dry the emesis basin. Return all equipment to the patient's bedside stand.

Wearing dentures
■ If the patient desires, apply an adhesive liner to the dentures. Moisten them with water, if necessary, *to reduce friction and ease insertion.*
■ Encourage the patient to wear his dentures to enhance his appearance, facilitate eating and speaking, and prevent changes in the gum line that may affect denture fit.

Using an oral irrigating device

An oral irrigating device, such as the Water Pik, directs a pulsating jet of water around the teeth to massage gums and remove debris and food particles. It's especially useful for cleaning areas missed by brushing, such as around bridgework, crowns, and dental wires. Because this device enhances oral hygiene, it benefits patients undergoing head and neck irradiation, which can damage teeth and cause severe caries. The device also maintains oral hygiene in a patient with a fractured jaw or with mouth injuries that limit standard mouth care.

Equipment and preparation
Oral irrigating device • towel • emesis basin • pharyngeal suction apparatus • salt solution or mouthwash, if ordered • soap

To use the device, first assemble the equipment. Wash your hands and put on gloves.

Implementation
■ Turn the patient to his side to prevent aspiration of water. Then place a towel under his chin and an emesis basin next to his cheek to absorb or catch drainage.
■ Insert the oral irrigating device's plug into a nearby electrical outlet. Remove the device's cover, turn it upside down, and fill it with lukewarm water or with a mouthwash or salt solution as ordered. When using a salt solution, dissolve the salt beforehand in a separate container. Then pour the solution into the cover.
■ Secure the cover to the base of the device. Remove the water hose handle from the base and snap the jet tip into place. If necessary, wet the grooved end of the tip to ease insertion. Adjust the pressure dial to the setting most comfortable for the patient. If his gums are tender and prone to bleed, choose a low setting.

■ Adjust the knurled knob on the handle to direct the water jet, place the jet tip in the patient's mouth, and turn on the device. Instruct the alert patient to keep his lips partially closed to avoid spraying water.
■ Direct the water at a right angle to the gum line of each tooth and between teeth. Avoid directing water under the patient's tongue *because this may injure sensitive tissue.*

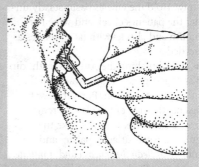

■ After irrigating each tooth, pause briefly and instruct the patient to expectorate the water or solution into the emesis basin. If he's unable to do so, suction it from the sides of the mouth with the pharyngeal suction apparatus. After irrigating all teeth, turn off the device and remove the jet tip from the patient's mouth.
■ Empty the remaining water or solution from the cover, remove the jet tip from the handle, and return the handle to the base. Clean the jet tip with soap and water, rinse the cover, and dry them both and return them to storage.

to prevent gum damage, brush the buccal surfaces (toward the cheek) and the lingual surfaces (toward the tongue) of the bottom teeth. Use just the tip of the brush for the lingual surfaces of the front teeth. Then, using the same technique, brush the buccal and lingual surfaces of the top teeth. Next, brush the biting surfaces of the bottom and top teeth, using a back and forth motion. If possible, ask the patient to rinse frequently during brushing by taking the mouthwash solution through the straw. Hold the emesis basin steady under the patient's cheek and wipe his mouth and cheeks with facial tissues as needed.

▶ After brushing the patient's teeth, dip a sponge-tipped mouth swab into the mouthwash solution. Press the swab against the side of the glass to remove excess moisture. Gently stroke the gums, buccal surfaces, palate, and tongue *to clean the mucosa and stimulate circulation.* Replace the swab as necessary for thorough cleaning. Avoid inserting the swab too deeply *to prevent gagging and vomiting.*

After mouth care

▶ Assess the patient's mouth for cleanliness and tooth and tissue condition.
▶ Then rinse the toothbrush and clean the emesis basin and glass. Empty and clean the suction bottle, if used. Remove your gloves.
▶ Place a clean suction catheter on the tubing. Return reusable equipment to the appropriate storage location and properly discard disposable equipment in the trash bag.

Special considerations

▶ Use sponge-tipped mouth swabs to clean the teeth of a patient with sensi-

tive gums. These swabs produce less friction than a toothbrush but don't clean as well.

▶ Remember that mucous membranes dry quickly in the patient breathing through his mouth or receiving oxygen therapy. Moisten his mouth and lips regularly with mineral oil, moistened sponge-tipped swabs, or water. If you use water as the lubricant, place a short straw in a glass of water and stop the open end with your finger. Remove the straw from the water and, with your finger in place, position it in the patient's mouth. Release your finger slightly to let the water flow out gradually. If the patient is comatose, suction excess water to prevent aspiration.

Documentation

Record the date and time of mouth care in your notes. Also note any unusual conditions, such as bleeding, edema, mouth odor, excessive secretions, or plaque on the tongue.

MUCUS CLEARANCE

Patients with chronic respiratory disorders, such as cystic fibrosis, bronchitis, and bronchiectasis, require therapy to mobilize and remove mucus secretions from the lungs. A handheld mucus clearance device, also known as "the flutter," can help such patients cough up secretions more easily. This device is basically a ball valve that vibrates as the patient exhales vigorously through it. The vibrations propagate throughout the airways during expiration, thereby loosening the mucus. As the patient repeats this process, the mucus progressively moves up the airways until it can be coughed out easily. The frequency and duration with which this device can be used should be determined by a licensed practitioner.

Key nursing diagnoses and patient outcomes

Ineffective breathing pattern related to the patient's physical condition
The patient will:
▶ maintain respiratory rate within 5 breaths/minute of baseline
▶ express feeling of comfort while maintaining air exchange
▶ have normal breath sounds.

Impaired gas exchange related to altered oxygen supply
The patient will:
▶ cough effectively
▶ have normal breath sounds
▶ expectorate sputum.

Equipment

Mucus clearance device • emesis basin • tissues

Implementation

▶ Begin by explaining the procedure to the patient. Tell him that this device will help move the mucus through his airways so that he can eventually expectorate it.
▶ Then have the patient sit with his back straight and his head tilted backward slightly so that his throat and trachea are wide open. *This position allows exhaled air to flow smoothly from the lungs and out through the device.*
▶ If the patient prefers, he may place his elbows on a table at a height that prevents him from slouching, *which would interfere with smooth breathing.*
▶ Tell the patient to hold the device so that the stem is parallel to the floor. *This places the interior cone of the device*

at a 30-degree tilt, which allows the ball inside the device to bounce and roll freely in the cone.
▶ Next, have the patient draw a deep breath and hold it for 2 to 3 seconds. This inhalation step is very important; *the inspired air is evenly distributed throughout the lungs, especially in the small airways, where infection and airway damage can occur.*
▶ After 2 to 3 seconds, instruct the patient to place the device in his mouth and then exhale at a steady rate for as long as he can. *Explain that if he breathes out too quickly and forcefully, the ball won't vibrate or flutter properly, thereby defeating the purpose of the device.*
▶ Tell the patient to keep his cheeks as flat and hard as possible while exhaling *to direct the air out through the device most effectively.* Suggest that he hold his cheeks lightly with his other hand *to help learn the technique.*
▶ After the patient has completely exhaled, he can remove the device from his mouth, take in another full breath, and cough. The entire procedure can be repeated several times as recommended by a licensed practitioner.
▶ Tell the patient to expectorate the mucus into an emesis basin or tissue.

Special considerations

▶ Alternatively, after completely exhaling, the patient can leave the device in his mouth, draw another big breath through his nose, hold it for 2 to 3 seconds, and repeat the exhalation maneuver. He can breathe through the device up to five times before taking the final breath and coughing.
▶ *To help the patient achieve the best fluttering effect,* you may need to place one hand on his back and the other on his chest as he exhales through the device.

If he's achieving the maximum effect, you'll feel the vibrations in his lungs as he exhales. If results are unsatisfactory at first, tell the patient to adjust the angle at which he's holding the device until optimal fluttering occurs.

▶ If the patient's final cough doesn't seem to work, he can try repeated, controlled, short, rapid exhalations ("huffing") as though he were trying to cough a bread crumb out of his throat, *to aid mucus removal.*

▶ Make sure that the patient cleans the device after each use *to remove mucus from the internal components.* Instruct him to clean it more thoroughly every 2 days. All parts should be washed in a solution of mild soap or detergent. Tell him not to use bleach or other chlorine-containing products. After thorough cleaning, all parts should be rinsed under a stream of hot tap water, wiped with a clean towel, and reassembled and stored in a clean, dry place.

▶ Auscultate for the patient's breath sounds to determine the effectiveness of his coughing.

Documentation

Record your patient teaching as well as the patient's tolerance of the procedure. Record the amount, color, and odor of any secretions that the patient is able to expectorate. Document the patient's breath sounds before and after he has used the device and coughed. Also, record the amount of times that the patient repeated the procedure and the success of his coughing efforts.

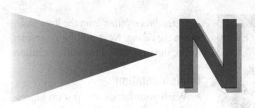

NASAL IRRIGATION

Irrigation of the nasal passages soothes irritated mucous membranes and washes away crusted mucus, secretions, and foreign matter. Left unattended, these deposits may impede sinus drainage and nasal airflow and cause headaches, infections, and unpleasant odors. Irrigation may be done with a bulb syringe or an electronic oral irrigating device.

Nasal irrigation benefits patients with acute or chronic nasal conditions, including sinusitis, rhinitis, Wegener's granulomatosis, and Sjögren's syndrome. In addition, the procedure may help people who regularly inhale toxins or allergens — paint fumes, sawdust, pesticides, or coal dust, for example. Nasal irrigation is routinely recommended after some nasal surgeries to enhance healing by removal of postoperative eschar and to aid remucosolization of the sinus cavities and ostia.

Contraindications for nasal irrigation may include advanced destruction of the sinuses, frequent nosebleeds, and foreign bodies in the nasal passages (which could be driven farther into the passages by the irrigant). However, some patients with these conditions may benefit from irrigation.

Key nursing diagnoses and patient outcomes

Risk for infection related to (specify)
The patient will:
▶ maintain a normal body temperature
▶ show no signs or symptoms of infection
▶ express an understanding of the signs and symptoms of infection and report them to the health care provider.

Deficient knowledge related to lack of exposure to nasal irrigation
The patient will:
▶ express a desire to become informed about the procedure
▶ correctly demonstrate the procedure if it will be performed independently at home.

Equipment
Bulb syringe or an oral irrigating device (such as a Water Pik) • rigid or flexible disposable irrigation tips (for one-patient use) • hypertonic saline solution • plastic sheet • apron or towels • facial tissues • bath basin • gloves

Preparation of equipment
Warm the saline solution to about 105° F (40.5° C). If you'll be irrigating with a bulb syringe, draw some irrigant into the bulb and then expel it. *This will rinse any residual solution from the previous irrigation and warm the bulb.*

Positioning the patient for nasal irrigation

Whether you're teaching a patient to perform nasal irrigation with a bulb syringe or an oral irrigating device, the irrigation will progress more easily once the patient learns how to hold her head for optimal safety, comfort, and effectiveness.

Help the patient sit upright with her head bent forward over the basin or sink and well-flexed on her chest. Her nose and ear should be on the same vertical plane.

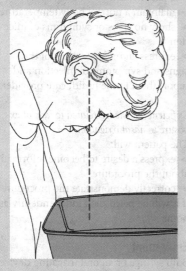

Explain that she's less likely to breathe in the irrigant when holding her head in this position. Also, this position should keep the irrigant from entering the eustachian tubes, which will now lie above the level of the irrigation stream.

If you're using an oral irrigating device, plug the instrument into an electrical outlet in an area near the patient. Then, run about 1 cup (240 ml) of saline solution through the tubing *to rinse residual solution from the lines and warm the tubing.* Next, fill the reservoir of the device with warm saline solution.

Implementation

▶ Wash your hands and put on gloves.
▶ Explain the procedure to the patient and place an apron or towel on his upper body to protect his clothing from getting wet. Place a plastic sheet on the bed, if indicated.
▶ Have the patient sit comfortably near the equipment in a position that allows the bulb or catheter tip to enter his nose and the returning irrigant to flow into the bath basin or sink. (See *Positioning the patient for nasal irrigation.*)
▶ Remind the patient to keep his mouth open and to breathe rhythmically during irrigation. *This causes the soft palate to seal the throat, allowing the irrigant to stream out the opposite nostril and carry discharge with it.*
▶ Instruct the patient not to speak or swallow during the irrigation *to avoid forcing infectious material into the sinuses or eustachian tubes.*
▶ *To avoid injuring the nasal mucosa,* remove the irrigating tip from the patient's nostril if he reports the need to sneeze or cough.

Using a bulb syringe
▶ Fill the bulb syringe with saline solution and insert the tip ½″ (1.3 cm) into the patient's nostril.
▶ Squeeze the bulb until a gentle stream of warm irrigant washes through the nose. Avoid forceful squeezing, *which may drive debris from the nasal passages into the sinuses or eustachian tubes and introduce infection.* Alternate the nostrils until the return irrigant runs clear.

Using an oral irrigating device

▶ Insert the irrigation tip into the nostril about ½" to 1" (1.3 to 2.5 cm) and turn on the irrigating device. Begin with a low pressure setting (increasing the pressure as needed) *to obtain a gentle stream of irrigant.* Again, be careful not to drive material from the nose into the sinuses or eustachian tubes. Irrigate both nostrils.

▶ Inspect returning irrigant. Changes in color, viscosity, or volume may signal an infection and should be reported to the doctor. Also, report blood or necrotic material.

Concluding the procedure

▶ After irrigation, have the patient wait a few minutes before blowing excess fluid from both nostrils at once. *Gentle blowing through both nostrils prevents fluid or pressure buildup in the sinuses. This action also helps to loosen and expel crusted secretions and mucus.*

▶ Clean the bulb syringe or irrigating device with soap and water and then disinfect as recommended. Rinse and dry the device. Remove your gloves.

Special considerations

▶ Expect fluid to drain from the patient's nose for a brief time after the irrigation and before he blows his nose.

▶ Insert the irrigation tip far enough to ensure that the irrigant cleans the nasal membranes before draining out. A typical amount of irrigant is 500 to 1,000 ml.

Home care

To continue nasal irrigations at home, teach the patient how to prepare saline solution. Tell him to fill a clean 1-L plastic bottle with bottled or distilled water (4 cups + 1 oz = 1 L), add 1 tsp of salt, and shake the solution until the salt dissolves. Teach him how to disinfect used irrigating devices.

Documentation

Write down the time and duration of the procedure and the amount of irrigant used. Describe the appearance of the returned solution. Record your assessment of the patient's comfort level and breathing ease before and after the procedure. Document patient-teaching content.

NASAL PACKING

In the highly vascular nasal mucosa, even seemingly minor injuries can cause major bleeding and blood loss. When routine therapeutic measures, such as direct pressure, cautery, and vasoconstrictive drugs, fail to control epistaxis (nosebleed), the patient's nose may have to be packed to stop anterior bleeding (which runs out of the nose) or posterior bleeding (which runs down the throat). If blood drains into the nasopharyngeal area or lacrimal ducts, the patient may also appear to bleed from the mouth and eyes.

Most nasal bleeding originates at a plexus of arterioles and venules in the anteroinferior septum. Only about 1 in 10 nosebleeds occurs in the posterior nose, which usually bleeds more heavily than the anterior location.

A nurse typically assists a doctor with anterior or posterior nasal packing. (See *Types of nasal packing,* page 534.) Or, she may assist with nasal balloon catheterization, which applies pressure to a posterior bleeding site. (See *Nasal balloon catheters,* page 535.)

(Text continues on page 536.)

Types of nasal packing

Anterior nasal packing

The doctor may treat an anterior nosebleed by packing the anterior nasal cavity with a 3' to 4' (0.9- to 1.2-m) strip of antibiotic-impregnated petroleum gauze (as shown below) or with a nasal tampon.

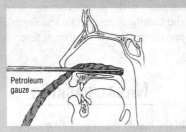

A nasal tampon is made of tightly compressed absorbent material with or without a central breathing tube. The doctor inserts a lubricated tampon along the floor of the nose and, with the patient's head tilted backward, instills 5 to 10 ml of antibiotic or normal saline solution. This causes the tampon to expand, stopping the bleeding. The tampon should be moistened periodically, and the central breathing tube should be suctioned regularly.

In a child or a patient with blood dyscrasias, the doctor may fashion an absorbable pack by moistening a gauzelike, regenerated cellulose material with a vasoconstrictor. Applied to a visible bleeding point, this substance will swell to form a clot. The packing is absorbable and doesn't need removal.

Posterior nasal packing

Posterior packing consists of a gauze roll shaped and secured by three sutures (one suture at each end and one in the middle) or a balloon-type catheter. To insert the packing, the doctor advances one or two soft catheters into the patient's nostrils (as shown at top of next column). When the catheter tips

appear in the nasopharynx, the doctor grasps them with a Kelly clamp or bayonet forceps and pulls them forward through the mouth. He secures the two end sutures to the catheter tip and draws the catheter back through the nostrils.

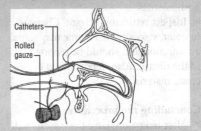

This step brings the packing into place with the end sutures hanging from the patient's nostril. (The middle suture emerges from the patient's mouth to free the packing, when needed.)

The doctor may weight the nose sutures with a clamp. Then he will pull the packing securely into place behind the soft palate and against the posterior end of the septum (nasal choana).

After he examines the patient's throat (to ensure that the uvula hasn't been forced under the packing), he inserts anterior packing and secures the whole apparatus by tying the posterior pack strings around rolled gauze or a dental roll at the nostrils (as shown below).

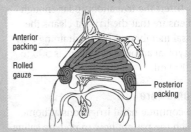

Nasal balloon catheters

To control epistaxis, the doctor may use a balloon catheter instead of nasal packing. Self-retaining and disposable, the catheter may have a single or double balloon to apply pressure to bleeding nasal tissues. If bleeding is still uncontrolled, the doctor may choose to use arterial ligation, cryotherapy, or arterial embolization.

Once inserted and inflated, the single-balloon catheter (shown below) compresses the blood vessels while a soft, collapsible external bulb prevents the catheter from dislodging posteriorly.

Single-balloon catheter

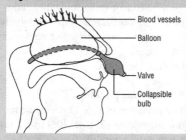

The double-balloon catheter (shown below) is used for simultaneous anterior and posterior nasal packing. The posterior balloon compresses the posterior vessels serving the nose, including the bleeding vessels; the anterior balloon compresses bleeding intranasal vessels. This catheter contains a central airway for breathing comfort.

Double-balloon catheter

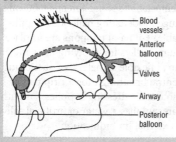

Assisting with insertion

To assist with inserting a single- or double-balloon catheter, prepare the patient as you would for nasal packing. Discuss the procedure thoroughly *to alleviate the patient's anxiety and promote his cooperation.*

Explain that the catheter tip will be lubricated with an antibiotic or a water-soluble lubricant *to ease passage and to prevent infection.*

Providing routine care

The tip of the single-balloon catheter will be inserted in one of the nostrils until it reaches the posterior pharynx. Then the balloon will be inflated with normal saline solution, pulled gently into the posterior nasopharynx, and secured at the nostrils with the collapsible bulb. With a double-balloon catheter, the posterior balloon is inflated with normal saline solution; then the anterior balloon is inflated.

To check catheter placement, mark the catheter at the nasal vestibule; then inspect for that mark and observe the oropharynx for the posteriorly placed balloon. Assess the nostrils for irritation or erosion. Remove secretions by gently suctioning the airway of a double-balloon catheter or by dabbing away crusted external secretions if the patient has a catheter with no airway.

Recognizing complications

The patient may report difficulty breathing, swallowing, or eating, and the nasal mucosa may sustain damage from pressure. Balloon deflation may dislodge clots and nasal debris into the oropharynx, which could prompt coughing, gagging, or vomiting.

Whichever procedure the patient undergoes, the nurse should provide ongoing encouragement and support to reduce his discomfort and anxiety. The nurse should also perform ongoing assessment to determine the procedure's success and to detect possible complications.

Key nursing diagnoses and patient outcomes

Anxiety related to lack of exposure to nasal packing procedure
The patient will:
▶ communicate feelings of anxiety
▶ discuss healthy coping strategies
▶ use available support systems to aid coping
▶ perform stress-reduction techniques to prevent anxiety symptoms.

Risk for aspiration related to nasal packing
The patient will:
▶ show no signs of aspiration
▶ maintain a patent airway
▶ exhibit normal skin color.

Equipment
For anterior and posterior packing
Gowns • goggles • masks • sterile gloves • emesis basin • facial tissues • patient drape (towels, incontinence pads, or gown) • nasal speculum and tongue depressors (may be in preassembled head and neck examination kit) • directed illumination source (such as headlamp or strong flashlight) or fiber-optic nasal endoscope, light cables, and light source • suction apparatus with sterile suction-connecting tubing and sterile nasal aspirator tip • sterile bowl and sterile normal saline solution for flushing out suction apparatus • sterile tray or sterile towels • sterile cotton-tipped applicators • local anesthetic spray (topical 4% lidocaine) or vial of local anesthetic solution (such as 2% lidocaine or 1% to 2% lidocaine with epinephrine 1:100,000) • sedative or analgesic • sterile cotton balls or cotton pledgets • 10-ml syringe with 22G 1½" needle • silver nitrate sticks • electrocautery device with grounding plate and small tip • topical vasoconstrictor (such as 0.5% phenylephrine) • absorbable hemostatic (such as Gelfoam, Avitene, Surgicel, or thrombin) • sterile normal saline solution (1-g container and 60-ml syringe with luer-lock tip, or 5-ml bullets for moistening nasal tampons) • hypoallergenic tape • antibiotic ointment • petroleum jelly • equipment for measuring vital signs • equipment for drawing blood

For anterior packing
Two packages of 1½" (3.8-cm) petroleum strip gauze (3' to 4' [0.9 to 1.2 m]) • two nasal tampons

For posterior packing
Two #14 or #16 French catheters with 30-cc balloon or two single- or double-chamber nasal balloon catheters • bayonet forceps • marking pen

For assessment and bedside use
Tongue depressors • flashlight • long hemostat or sponge forceps • 60-ml syringe for deflating balloons (if applicable) • if nasal tampons are in place: saline bullets for applying moisture and small flexible catheters for suctioning central breathing tube • drip pad or moustache dressing supplies • mouth care supplies • water or artificial saliva • external humidification

Preparation of equipment

Wash your hands. Assemble all equipment at the patient's bedside. Make sure the headlamp works. Plug in the suction apparatus and connect the tubing from the collection bottle to the suction source. Test the suction equipment to make sure it works properly. At the bedside, create a sterile field. (Use the sterile towels or the sterile tray.) Using aseptic technique, place all sterile equipment on the sterile field.

If the doctor will inject a local anesthetic rather than spray it into the nose, place the 22G 1½″ needle attached to the 10-ml syringe on the sterile field. When the doctor readies the syringe, clean the stopper on the anesthetic vial and hold the vial so he can withdraw the anesthetic. *This practice allows the doctor to avoid touching his sterile gloves to the nonsterile vial.*

Open the packages containing the sterile suction-connecting tubing and aspirating tip and place them on the sterile field. Fill the sterile bowl with sterile normal saline solution *so that the suction tubing can be flushed as necessary.* Thoroughly lubricate the anterior or posterior packing with antibiotic ointment.

If the patient needs a nasal balloon catheter, test the balloon for leaks by inflating the catheter with normal saline solution. Remove the solution before insertion.

Implementation

▶ Ensure that all people caring for the patient wear gowns, gloves, masks, and goggles during insertion of packing *to prevent possible contamination from splattered blood.*

▶ Check the patient's vital signs and observe for hypotension with postural

changes. *Hypotension suggests significant blood loss.* Also, monitor airway patency *because the patient will be at risk for aspirating or vomiting swallowed blood.*

▶ Explain the procedure to the patient and offer reassurance *to reduce his anxiety and promote cooperation.*

▶ If ordered, administer a sedative or analgesic *to reduce the patient's anxiety and pain and decrease sympathetic stimulation, which can exacerbate a nosebleed.*

▶ Help the patient sit with his head tilted forward *to minimize blood drainage into the throat and prevent aspiration.*

▶ Turn on the suction apparatus and attach the connecting tubing *so the doctor can aspirate the nasal cavity to remove clots before locating the bleeding source.*

▶ To inspect the nasal cavity, the doctor will use a nasal speculum and an external light source, or a fiber-optic nasal endoscope. To remove collected blood and help visualize the bleeding vessel, he will use suction or cotton-tipped applicators. The nose may be treated early with a topical vasoconstrictor such as phenylephrine *to slow bleeding and aid visualization.*

For anterior nasal packing

▶ Help the doctor apply a topical vasoconstrictor to control bleeding or to use chemical cautery with silver nitrate sticks.

▶ *To enhance the vasoconstrictor's action,* apply manual pressure to the nose for about 10 minutes.

▶ If bleeding persists, you may help insert an absorbable hemostatic nasal pack directly on the bleeding site. The pack swells to form an artificial clot.

▶ If these methods fail, prepare to assist with electrocautery or insertion of petroleum strip gauze. (Even if only one side is bleeding, both sides may require packing to control bleeding.)

▶ While the anterior pack is in place, use the cotton-tipped applicators to apply petroleum jelly to the patient's lips and nostrils *to prevent drying and cracking.*

For posterior nasal packing

▶ Wash your hands and put on sterile gloves.

▶ If the doctor identifies the bleeding source in the posterior nasal cavity, lubricate the soft catheters *to ease insertion.*

▶ Instruct the patient to open his mouth and to breathe normally through his mouth during catheter insertion *to minimize gagging as the catheters pass through the nostrils.*

▶ Help the doctor insert the packing as directed.

▶ Help the patient assume a comfortable position with his head elevated 45 to 90 degrees. Assess him for airway obstruction or any respiratory changes.

▶ Monitor the patient's vital signs regularly *to detect changes that may indicate hypovolemia or hypoxemia.*

Special considerations

▶ Patients with posterior packing usually are hospitalized for monitoring. If mucosal oozing persists, apply a moustache dressing by securing a folded gauze pad over the nasal vestibules with tape or a commercial nasal dressing holder. Change the pad when soiled.

▶ Test the patient's call bell to make sure he can summon help, if needed. Also, keep emergency equipment (flashlight, tongue depressor, syringe, and hemostat) at the patient's bedside *to speed packing removal if it becomes displaced and occludes the airway.*

▶ Once the packing is in place, compile assessment data carefully to help detect the underlying cause of nosebleeds. Mechanical factors include a deviated septum, injury, and a foreign body. Environmental factors include drying and erosion of the nasal mucosa. Other possible causes are upper respiratory tract infection, anticoagulant or salicylate therapy, blood dyscrasias, cardiovascular or hepatic disorders, tumors of the nasal cavity or paranasal sinuses, chronic nephritis, and familial hemorrhagic telangiectasia.

▶ If significant blood loss occurs or if the underlying cause remains unknown, expect the doctor to order a complete blood count and coagulation profile as soon as possible. Blood transfusion may be necessary. After the procedure, the doctor may order arterial blood gas analysis *to detect any pulmonary complications* and arterial oxygen saturation monitoring *to assess for hypoxemia.* If necessary, prepare to administer supplemental humidified oxygen with a face mask and to give antibiotics and decongestants as ordered.

▶ Because a patient with nasal packing must breathe through his mouth, provide thorough mouth care often. Artificial saliva, room humidification, and ample fluid intake also relieve dryness caused by mouth breathing.

▶ Until the pack is removed, the patient should be on modified bed rest. As ordered, administer moderate doses of nonaspirin analgesics, decongestants, and sedatives along with prophylactic antibiotics *to prevent sinusitis or related infections.*

▶ Nasal packing is usually removed in 2 to 5 days. After an anterior pack is removed, instruct the patient to avoid rubbing or picking his nose, inserting any object into his nose, and blowing his nose forcefully for 48 hours or as ordered.

Home care

Tell the patient to expect reduced smell and taste ability. Make sure he has a working smoke detector at home. Advise him to eat soft foods *because his eating and swallowing abilities will be impaired.* Instruct him to drink fluids often or to use artificial saliva *to cope with dry mouth.* Teach him measures to prevent nosebleeds and instruct him to seek medical help if these measures fail to stop bleeding. (See *Preventing recurrent nosebleeds.*)

Complications

The pressure of a posterior pack on the soft palate may lead to hypoxemia. Patients with posterior packing are at special risk for aspiration of blood. Patients with underlying pulmonary conditions, such as chronic obstructive pulmonary disease and asthma, are at special risk for exacerbation of the condition or for hypoxemia while nasal packing is in place. Hypoxemia can be detected with pulse oximetry; signs and symptoms include tachycardia, confusion, cyanosis, and restlessness.

Airway obstruction may occur if a posterior or anterior nasal pack slips backward. The patient may complain of difficulty swallowing, pain, or discomfort. In patients with posterior packs, otitis media may develop. Other possible complications include sinusitis, hematotympanum, and pressure necrosis of nasal structures, especially the septum.

Sedation may cause hypotension in a patient with significant blood loss and may also increase the patient's risk of aspiration and hypoxemia.

Preventing recurrent nosebleeds

Review the following self-care guidelines with your patient to reduce his risk of developing recurrent nosebleeds:

■ *Because nosebleeds can result from dry mucous membranes,* suggest that the patient use a cool mist vaporizer or humidifier as needed, especially in dry environments.

■ Teach the patient how to minimize pressure on nasal passages. Advise him, for instance, to avoid constipation and consequent straining during defecation. Recommend a fiber-rich diet and adequate fluid intake and warn him to avoid extreme physical exertion for 24 hours after the nosebleed stops. Also, caution him to avoid aspirin (which has anticoagulant properties), alcoholic beverages, and tobacco for at least 5 days.

■ If the patient gets a nosebleed despite these precautions, tell him to keep his head higher than his heart and, using his thumb and forefinger, to press the soft portion of the nostrils together and against the facial bones. (Recommend against direct pressure if he has a facial injury or nasal fracture.) Tell him to maintain pressure for up to 10 minutes and then to reassess bleeding. If it's uncontrolled, he should reapply pressure for another 10 minutes with ice between the thumb and forefinger.

■ After a nosebleed or after nasal packing is removed, caution the patient to avoid rubbing or picking his nose, putting a handkerchief or tissue in his nose, or blowing his nose forcefully for at least 48 hours. After this time, he may blow his nose gently and use salt-water nasal spray to clear nasal clots.

Documentation

Record the type of pack used *to ensure its removal at the appropriate time.* On the intake and output record, document the estimated blood loss and all fluid administered. Also, note the patient's vital signs, his response to sedation or position changes, the results of any laboratory tests, and any drugs administered, including topical agents. Record any complications. Document discharge instructions and clinical follow-up plans.

NASOENTERIC-DECOMPRESSION TUBE CARE

The patient with a nasoenteric-decompression tube needs special care and continuous monitoring to ensure tube patency, to maintain suction and bowel decompression, and to detect such complications as fluid-electrolyte imbalances related to aspiration of intestinal contents. Precise intake and output records are an integral part of the patient's care. Frequent mouth and nose care is also essential to provide comfort and to prevent skin breakdown. Lastly, a patient with a nasoenteric-decompression tube will need encouragement and support during insertion and removal of the tube and while the tube is in place.

Key nursing diagnoses and patient outcomes

Risk for deficient fluid volume related to enteric decompression
The patient will:
▶ maintain normal vital signs, skin color, and turgor

▶ maintain urine output of at least (specify) ml/hr
▶ have an output equal to or greater than input
▶ maintain normal electrolyte levels.

Risk for impaired skin integrity related to presence of nasoenteric tube
The patient will:
▶ show no signs of skin breakdown in nares
▶ maintain adequate circulation to nares
▶ report signs of discomfort at nares.

Anxiety related to presence of nasoenteric decompression tube
The patient will:
▶ verbalize feelings of anxiety
▶ decrease anxiety by asking questions related to the plan of care
▶ use available support systems to aid coping
▶ perform stress-reducing techniques to prevent symptoms of anxiety.

Equipment

Suction apparatus with intermittent suction capability (stationary or portable unit) • container of water • intake and output record sheets • mouthwash and water mixture • sponge tipped swabs • water-soluble lubricant or petroleum jelly • cotton-tipped applicators • safety pin • tape or rubber band • disposable irrigation set • irrigant • labels for tube lumens • optional: throat comfort measures, such as gargle, viscous lidocaine, throat lozenges, ice collar, sour hard candy, or gum

Preparation of equipment

Assemble the suction apparatus and set up the suction unit. If indicated, test the unit by turning it on and placing the end of the suction tubing in a container of water. If the tubing draws in water, the unit works.

Implementation

▶ Explain to the patient and his family the purpose of the procedure. Answer questions clearly and thoroughly *to ease anxiety and enhance cooperation.*

▶ After tube insertion, have the patient lie quietly on his right side for about 2 hours *to promote the tube's passage.* After the tube advances past the pylorus, the tube can be advanced 2″ (5 cm) per hour as ordered.

▶ After the tube advances to the desired position, coil the excess external tubing and secure it to the patient's gown or bed linens with a safety pin attached to tape or a rubber band looped around it. *This prevents kinks in the tubing, which would interrupt suction.* When in the desired location, the tube may be taped to the patient's face.

▶ Maintain slack in the tubing *so the patient can move comfortably and safely in bed.* Show him how far he can move without dislodging the tube.

▶ After securing the tube, connect it to the tubing on the suction machine *to begin decompression.*

▶ Check the suction machine at least every 2 hours *to confirm proper functioning and to ensure tube patency and bowel decompression.* Excessive negative pressure may draw the mucosa into the tube openings, impair the suction's effectiveness, and injure the mucosa. By using intermittent suction, you may avoid these problems. *To check functioning in an intermittent suction unit,* look for drainage in the connecting tube and dripping into the collecting container. Empty the container every 8 hours and measure the contents.

▶ After decompression and before extubation, as ordered, provide a clear-to-full liquid diet *to assess bowel function.*

▶ Record intake and output accurately to monitor fluid balance. If you irrigate the tube, its length may prohibit aspiration of the irrigant, so record the amount of instilled irrigant as "intake." Typically, normal saline solution supersedes water as the preferred irrigant *because water, which is hypotonic, may increase electrolyte loss through osmotic action, especially if you irrigate the tube often.*

▶ Observe the patient for signs and symptoms of disorders related to suctioning and intubation. Signs and symptoms of dehydration, a fluid-volume deficit, or a fluid-electrolyte imbalance include dry skin and mucous membranes, decreased urine output, lethargy, exhaustion, and fever.

▶ Watch for signs and symptoms of pneumonia related to the patient's inability to clear his pharynx or cough effectively with a tube in place. Be alert for fever, chest pain, tachypnea or labored breathing, and diminished breath sounds over the affected area.

▶ Observe drainage characteristics: color, amount, consistency, odor, and any unusual changes.

▶ Provide mouth care frequently (at least every 4 hours) *to increase the patient's comfort and promote a healthy oral cavity. If the tube remains in place for several days, mouth-breathing will leave the lips, tongue, and other tissues dry and cracked.*

▶ Encourage the patient to brush his teeth or rinse his mouth with the mouthwash and water mixture.

▶ Lubricate the patient's lips with either wet sponge tipped swabs or petroleum jelly applied with a cotton-tipped applicator.

Clearing a nasoenteric-decompression tube obstruction

If your patient's nasoenteric-decompression tube appears to be obstructed, notify the doctor right away. He may order measures such as those below to restore patency quickly and efficiently.

■ First, disconnect the tube from the suction source and irrigate with normal saline solution. Use gravity flow to help clear the obstruction unless ordered otherwise.

■ If irrigation doesn't reestablish patency, the tube may be obstructed by its position against the gastric mucosa. To rectify this, tug slightly on the tube to move it away from the mucosa.

■ If gentle tugging doesn't restore patency, the tube may be kinked and may need additional manipulation. Before proceeding, though, take the following precautions:

– Never reposition or irrigate a nasoenteric-decompression tube (without a doctor's order) in a patient who has had GI surgery.

– Avoid manipulating a tube in a patient who had the tube inserted during surgery. To do so may disturb new sutures.

– Don't try to reposition a tube in a patient who was difficult to intubate (because of an esophageal stricture, for example).

▶ At least every 4 hours, gently clean and lubricate the patient's external nostrils with either petroleum jelly or water-soluble lubricant on a cotton-tipped applicator *to prevent skin breakdown.*

▶ Watch for peristalsis to resume, signaled by bowel sounds, passage of flatus, decreased abdominal distention and possibly, a spontaneous bowel movement. *These signs may require tube removal.*

Special considerations

▶ For a Miller-Abbott tube, clamp the lumen leading to the mercury balloon and label it DO NOT TOUCH. Label the other lumen SUCTION. *Marking the tube may prevent accidentally instilling irrigant into the wrong lumen.*

▶ If the suction machine works improperly, replace it immediately. If the machine works properly but no drainage accumulates in the collection container, suspect an obstruction in the tube.

▶ As ordered, irrigate the tube with the irrigation set to clear the obstruction. (See *Clearing a nasoenteric-decompression tube obstruction.*)

▶ If your patient is ambulatory and his tube connects to a portable suction unit, he may move short distances while connected to the unit. Or, if feasible and ordered, the tube can be disconnected and clamped briefly while he moves around.

▶ If the tubing irritates the patient's throat or makes him hoarse, offer relief with mouthwash, gargles, viscous lidocaine, throat lozenges, an ice collar, sour hard candy, or gum as appropriate.

▶ If the tip of the balloon falls below the ileocecal valve (confirmed by X-ray), the tube can't be removed nasally. It has to be advanced and removed through the anus.

▶ If the balloon at the end of the tube protrudes from the anus, notify the doctor. Most likely, the tube can be disconnected from suction, the proximal end severed, and the remaining tube removed gradually through the anus either manually or by peristalsis.

Complications

In addition to fluid-volume deficit, electrolyte imbalance, and pneumonia, potential complications include mercury poisoning (from a ruptured mercury-filled balloon) and intussusception of the bowel (from the weight of the mercury in the balloon).

Documentation

Record the frequency and type of mouth and nose care provided. Describe the therapeutic effect, if any. Document in your notes the amount, color, consistency, and odor of the drainage obtained each time you empty the collection container.

Record the amount of drainage on the intake and output sheet. Always document the amount of any irrigant or other fluid introduced through the tube or taken orally by the patient.

If the suction machine malfunctions, note the length of time it wasn't functioning and the nursing action taken. Document the amount and character of any vomitus. Also, note the patient's tolerance of the tube's insertion and removal.

NASOENTERIC-DECOMPRESSION TUBE INSERTION AND REMOVAL

The nasoenteric-decompression tube is inserted nasally and advanced beyond the stomach into the intestinal tract. It's used to aspirate intestinal contents for analysis and to treat intestinal obstruction. The tube may also help to prevent abdominal distention after GI surgery. A doctor usually inserts or removes a nasoenteric-decompression tube; sometimes, however, a nurse removes it.

A balloon or rubber bag at one end of the tube holds mercury (or air or water) to stimulate peristalsis and facilitate the tube's passage through the pylorus and into the intestinal tract. (See *Common types of nasoenteric-decompression tubes,* page 544.)

Key nursing diagnoses and patient outcomes

Risk for deficient fluid volume related to enteric decompression
The patient will:
▶ maintain normal vital signs, skin color, and turgor
▶ maintain urine output of at least (specify) ml/hr
▶ have an output equal to or greater than input
▶ maintain normal electrolyte levels.

Risk for impaired skin integrity related to presence of nasoenteric tube
The patient will:
▶ show no signs of skin breakdown in nares
▶ maintain adequate circulation to nares
▶ report signs of discomfort at nares.

Anxiety related to presence of nasoenteric decompression tube
The patient will:
▶ verbalize feelings of anxiety
▶ decrease anxiety by asking questions about the plan of care
▶ use available support systems to assist with coping
▶ perform stress-reducing techniques to prevent symptoms of anxiety.

Common types of nasoenteric-decompression tubes

The type of nasoenteric-decompression tube chosen for your patient will depend on the size of the patient and his nostrils, the estimated duration of intubation, and the reason for the procedure. For example, to remove viscous material from the patient's intestinal tract, the doctor may select a tube with a wide bore and a single lumen.

Whichever tube you use, you'll need to provide good mouth care and check the patient's nostrils often for signs of irritation. If you see any signs of irritation, retape the tube so that it doesn't cause tension and then lubricate the nostril. Or check with the doctor to see if the tube can be inserted through the other nostril.

Most tubes are impregnated with a radiopaque mark so that placement can easily be confirmed by X-ray or other imaging technique. The following are among the most commonly use types of nasoenteric-decompression tubes.

Cantor tube

The Cantor tube is a 10' (3-m) long, single-lumen tube with a balloon that can hold mercury at its distal tip. The tube may be used to relieve bowel obstructions and to aspirate intestinal contents.

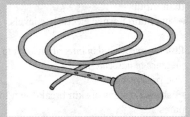

Miller-Abbott tube

The Miller-Abbott tube is a 10' long tube with two lumens: one for inflating the distal balloon with air and one for instilling mercury or water. Also used for bowel obstruction, the tube allows aspiration of intestinal contents.

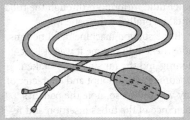

Harris tube

Measuring only 6' (1.8 m) long, the Harris tube is a single-lumen tube that also ends with a balloon that holds mercury. Used primarily for treating a bowel obstruction, the tube allows lavage of the intestinal tract — usually with a Y-tube attached.

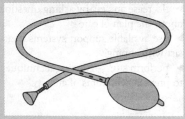

Dennis tube

The Dennis tube is a 10' long, three-lumen sump tube and is used to decompress the intestinal tract before or after GI surgery. Each lumen is marked to denote its use: irrigation, drainage, and balloon inflation.

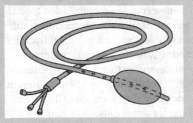

Equipment

Sterile 10-ml syringe • 21G needle • nasoenteric-decompression tube • container of water • 5 to 10 ml of mercury or water, as ordered • suction-decompression equipment • gloves • towel or linen-saver pad • water-soluble lubricant • 4″ × 4″ gauze pad • ½″ hypoallergenic tape • bulb syringe or 60-ml catheter-tip syringe • rubber band • safety pin • clamp • specimen container • basin of ice or warm water • penlight • waterproof marking pen • glass of water with straw • optional: ice chips and local anesthetic

Preparation of equipment

Stiffen a flaccid tube by chilling it in a basin of ice to facilitate insertion. To make a stiff tube flexible, dip it into warm water.

Check the tube's balloon for leaks. If you're using a Cantor or Harris tube, inject 10 cc of air into the balloon with a 10-ml syringe and 21G needle. If you're using a Miller-Abbott or Dennis tube, attach a 10-ml syringe to the distal balloon port. Immerse the balloon in a container of water and watch for air bubbles. *Bubble-free water means that the balloon is free of leaks.* Then remove the balloon from the water. Mercury, air, or water is added to the balloon either before or after insertion of the tube, depending on the type of tube used. Follow the manufacturer's recommendations.

Set up suction-decompression equipment, if ordered, and make sure it works properly.

Implementation

▶ Explain the procedure to the patient, forewarning him that he may experience some discomfort. Provide privacy and adequate lighting. Wash your hands and put on gloves.

▶ Position the patient as the doctor specifies, usually in semi-Fowler's or high Fowler's position. You may also need to help the patient hold his neck in a hyperextended position.

▶ Protect the patient's chest with a linen-saver pad or towel.

▶ Agree with the patient on a signal that can be used to stop the insertion briefly, if necessary.

Assisting with insertion

▶ The doctor assesses the patency of the patient's nostrils. *To evaluate which nostril has better airflow in a conscious patient,* he holds one nostril closed and then the other as the patient breathes. In an unconscious patient, he examines each nostril with a penlight *to check for polyps, a deviated septum, or other obstruction.*

▶ *To decide how far the tube must be inserted to reach the stomach,* the doctor places the tube's distal end at the tip of the patient's nose and then extends the tube to the earlobe and down to the xiphoid process. He either marks the tube with a waterproof marking pen or holds it at this point.

▶ The doctor applies water-soluble lubricant to the first few inches of the tube *to reduce friction and tissue trauma and to facilitate insertion.*

▶ If the balloon already contains mercury or water, the doctor holds it so the fluid runs to the bottom. Then he pinches the balloon closed *to retain the fluid as the insertion begins.*

▶ Tell the patient to breathe through his mouth or to pant as the balloon enters his nostril. After the balloon begins its descent, the doctor releases his grip on it, allowing the weight of the fluid to pull the tube into the nasopharynx. When the tube reaches the nasopharynx, the doctor instructs the patient to lower his chin and to swallow. In some cases, the patient may sip water through a straw *to facilitate swallowing as the tube advances*, but not after the tube reaches the trachea. *This prevents injury from aspiration.* The doctor continues to advance the tube slowly *to prevent it from curling or kinking in the stomach.*

▶ *To confirm the tube's passage into the stomach,* the doctor aspirates stomach contents with a bulb syringe.

▶ When the doctor confirms proper placement of a Miller-Abbott tube, he injects the appropriate amount of mercury (commonly between 2 and 5 ml) into the balloon lumen.

▶ *To keep the tube out of the patient's eyes and to help avoid undue skin irritation,* fold a 4″ × 4″ gauze pad in half and tape it to the patient's forehead with the fold directed toward the patient's nose. The doctor can slide the tube through this sling, leaving enough slack for the tube to advance.

▶ Position the patient as directed *to help advance the tube.* He'll typically lie on his right side until the tube clears the pylorus (about 2 hours). The doctor will confirm passage by X-ray.

▶ After the tube clears the pylorus, the doctor may direct you to advance it 2″ to 3″ (5 to 7.5 cm) every hour and to reposition the patient until the premeasured mark reaches the patient's nostril. Gravity and peristalsis will help advance the tube. (Notify the doctor if you can't advance the tube.)

▶ Keep the remaining premeasured length of tube well lubricated *to ease passage and prevent irritation.*

▶ Don't tape the tube while it advances to the premeasured mark unless the doctor asks you to do so.

▶ After the tube progresses the necessary distance, the doctor will order an X-ray *to confirm tube positioning.* When the tube is in place, secure the external tubing with tape *to help prevent further progression.*

▶ Loop a rubber band around the tube and pin the rubber band to the patient's gown with a safety pin.

▶ If ordered, attach the tube to intermittent suction.

Removing the tube

▶ Assist the patient into semi-Fowler's or high Fowler's position. Drape a linen-saver pad or towel across the patient's chest.

▶ Wash your hands and put on gloves.

▶ Clamp the tube and disconnect it from the suction. *This prevents the patient from aspirating any gastric contents that leak from the tube during withdrawal.*

▶ If your patient has a double-lumen Miller-Abbott tube or a triple-lumen Dennis tube, attach a 10-ml syringe to the balloon port and withdraw the mercury. Place the mercury in a specimen container and follow your facility's protocol for safe disposal. (If you're working with a single-lumen Cantor or Harris tube, you'll withdraw the mercury after you remove the tube.)

▶ Slowly withdraw between 6″ and 8″ (15 and 20.5 cm) of the tube. Wait 10 minutes and withdraw another 6″ to 8″. Wait another 10 minutes. Continue this procedure until the tube reaches the patient's esophagus (with about 18″ [45.5 cm] of the tube remaining inside the patient). At this point, you can gently withdraw the tube completely with the mercury in the balloon.

Special considerations

▶ For a double- or triple-lumen tube, note which lumen accommodates balloon inflation and which accommodates drainage.

▶ An alternative method for removing a single-lumen tube is to withdraw it gently into the pharynx. Ask the patient to open his mouth. Then grasp the tube and mercury balloon and gently pull them outside of the patient's mouth. Remove mercury from the bag with a needle and syringe. Then pull the tube and empty balloon through the patient's nose. Never forcibly remove a tube if you meet resistance. Notify the doctor instead.

▶ Apply a local anesthetic, if ordered, to the nostril or the back of the throat *to dull sensations and the gag reflex for intubation.* Letting the patient gargle with a liquid anesthetic or hold ice chips in his mouth for a few minutes serves the same purpose.

▶ Mercury can be disposed of only by a licensed hazardous-waste disposal company. Put the container of mercury into a plastic bag, and send it to the appropriate department for disposal, according to your facility's policy.

Complications

Nasoenteric-decompression tubes may cause reflux esophagitis, nasal or oral inflammation, and nasal, laryngeal, or esophageal ulceration.

Documentation

Record the date and time the nasoenteric-decompression tube was inserted and by whom. Note the patient's tolerance of the procedure; the type of tube used; the suction type and amount; and the color, amount, and consistency of drainage. Also, note the date, time, and name of the person removing the tube and the patient's tolerance of the removal procedure.

NASOGASTRIC TUBE CARE

Providing effective nasogastric (NG) tube care requires meticulous monitoring of the patient and the equipment. Monitoring the patient involves checking drainage from the NG tube and assessing GI function. Monitoring the equipment involves verifying correct tube placement and irrigating the tube to ensure patency and to prevent mucosal damage.

Specific care measures vary only slightly for the most commonly used NG tubes: the single-lumen Levin tube and the double-lumen Salem sump tube.

Key nursing diagnoses and patient outcomes

Risk for deficient fluid volume related to presence of an NG tube
The patient will:

▶ maintain normal vital signs, skin color, and turgor

▶ maintain urine output of at least (specify) ml/hr

▶ have an output equal to or greater than input

▶ maintain normal electrolyte levels.

Risk for impaired skin integrity related to presence of an NG tube
The patient will:

▶ show no signs of skin breakdown in nares

▶ maintain adequate circulation to nares

▶ report signs of discomfort at nares.

Common gastric suction devices

Various suction devices are available for applying negative pressure to nasogastric (NG) and other drainage tubes. Two common types are shown here.

Portable suction machine

In the portable suction machine, a vacuum created intermittently by an electric pump draws gastric contents up the NG tube and into the collecting bottle.

Stationary suction machine

A stationary wall-unit apparatus can provide intermittent or continuous suction. On-off switches and variable power settings let you set and adjust the suction force on either machine.

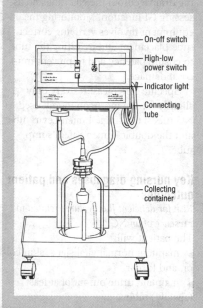

On-off switch
High-low power switch
Indicator light
Connecting tube
Collecting container

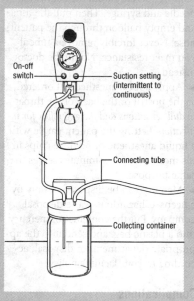

On-off switch
Suction setting (intermittent to continuous)
Connecting tube
Collecting container

Anxiety related to presence of an NG tube
The patient will:
▶ verbalize feelings of anxiety
▶ decrease anxiety by asking questions about the plan of care
▶ use available support systems to aid coping
▶ perform stress-reducing techniques to prevent symptoms of anxiety.

Equipment

Irrigant (usually normal saline solution) • irrigant container • 60-ml catheter-tip syringe • bulb syringe • suction equipment • sponge-tipped swabs or toothbrush and toothpaste • petroleum jelly • ½" or 1" hypoallergenic tape • water-soluble lubricant • gloves • stethoscope • linen-saver pad • optional: emesis basin

Preparation of equipment

Make sure the suction equipment works properly. (See *Common gastric suction devices*.) When using a Salem sump tube with suction, connect the larger, primary lumen (for drainage and suction) to the suction equipment and select the appropriate setting as ordered (usually low constant suction). If the doctor doesn't specify the setting, follow the manufacturer's directions. A Levin tube usually calls for intermittent low suction.

Implementation

▶ Explain the procedure and provide privacy.
▶ Wash your hands and put on gloves.

Irrigating an NG tube

▶ Review the irrigation schedule (usually every 4 hours), if the doctor orders this procedure.
▶ Inject 10 cc of air and auscultate the epigastric area with a stethoscope and aspirate stomach contents *to check correct positioning in the stomach and to prevent the patient from aspirating the irrigant.*
▶ Measure the amount of irrigant in the bulb syringe or in the 60-ml catheter-tip syringe (usually 10 to 20 ml) *to maintain an accurate intake and output record.*
▶ When using suction with a Salem sump tube or a Levin tube, unclamp and disconnect the tube from the suction equipment while holding it over a linen-saver pad or an emesis basin *to collect any drainage.*
▶ Slowly instill the irrigant into the NG tube. (When irrigating the Salem sump tube, you may instill small amounts of solution into the vent lumen without interrupting suction;

however, you should instill greater amounts into the larger, primary lumen.)
▶ Gently aspirate the solution with the bulb syringe or 60-ml catheter-tip syringe or connect the tube to the suction equipment as ordered. *Gentle aspiration prevents excessive pressure on a suture line and on delicate gastric mucosa.* Report any bleeding.
▶ Reconnect the tube to suction after completing irrigation.

Instilling a solution through an NG tube

▶ If the doctor orders instillation, inject the solution, and don't aspirate it. Note the amount of instilled solution as "intake" on the intake and output record.
▶ Reattach the tube to suction as ordered.
▶ After attaching the Salem sump tube's primary lumen to suction, instill 10 to 20 cc of air into the vent lumen *to verify patency.* Listen for a soft hiss in the vent. If you don't hear this sound, suspect a clogged tube; recheck patency by instilling 10 ml of normal saline solution and 10 to 20 cc of air in the vent.

Monitoring patient comfort and condition

▶ Provide mouth care once a shift or as needed. Depending on the patient's condition, use sponge-tipped swabs to clean his teeth or assist him to brush them with toothbrush and toothpaste. Coat the patient's lips with petroleum jelly *to prevent dryness from mouth breathing.*
▶ Change the tape securing the tube as needed or at least daily. Clean the skin,

apply fresh tape, and dab water-soluble lubricant on the nostrils as needed.

▶ Regularly check the tape that secures the tube *because sweat and nasal secretions may loosen the tape.*

▶ Assess bowel sounds regularly (every 4 to 8 hours) *to verify GI function.*

▶ Measure the drainage amount and update the intake and output record every 8 hours. Be alert for electrolyte imbalances with excessive gastric output.

▶ Inspect gastric drainage and note its color, consistency, odor, and amount. Normal gastric secretions have no color or appear yellow-green from bile and have a mucoid consistency. Immediately report any drainage with a coffee-bean color; *this may indicate bleeding.* If you suspect that the drainage contains blood, use a screening test (such as Hematest) for occult blood according to your facility's policy.

Special considerations

▶ Irrigate the NG tube with 30 ml of irrigant before and after instilling medication. Wait for about 30 minutes, or as ordered, after instillation, before reconnecting the suction equipment *to allow sufficient time for the medication to be absorbed.*

▶ When no drainage appears, check the suction equipment for proper function. Then, holding the NG tube over a linen-saver pad or an emesis basin, separate the tube and the suction source. Check the suction equipment by placing the suction tubing in an irrigant container. If the apparatus draws the water, check the NG tube for proper function. Note the amount of water drawn into the suction container on the intake and output record.

▶ A dysfunctional NG tube may be clogged or incorrectly positioned. At-

tempt to irrigate the tube, reposition the patient, or rotate and reposition the tube. However, if the tube was inserted during surgery, avoid this maneuver *to ensure that the movement doesn't interfere with gastric or esophageal sutures.* Notify the doctor.

▶ If you can ambulate the patient and interrupt suction, disconnect the NG tube from the suction equipment. Clamp the tube *to prevent stomach contents from draining out of the tube.*

▶ If the patient has a Salem sump tube, watch for gastric reflux in the vent lumen when pressure in the stomach exceeds atmospheric pressure. This problem may result from a clogged primary lumen or from a suction system that is set up improperly. Assess the suction equipment for proper functioning. Then irrigate the NG tube and instill 30 cc of air into the vent tube *to maintain patency.* Don't attempt to stop reflux by clamping the vent tube. Unless contraindicated, elevate the patient's torso more than 30 degrees, and keep the vent tube above his midline *to prevent a siphoning effect.*

Complications

Epigastric pain and vomiting may result from a clogged or improperly placed tube. Any NG tube — the Levin tube in particular — may move and aggravate esophagitis, ulcers, or esophageal varices, causing hemorrhage. Perforation may result from aggressive intubation. Dehydration and electrolyte imbalances may result from removing body fluids and electrolytes by suctioning. Pain, swelling, and salivary dysfunction may signal parotitis, which occurs in dehydrated, debilitated patients. Intubation can cause nasal skin breakdown and discomfort and increased mucous secretions. Aspiration pneumonia may result from gastric reflux. Vigorous suction may damage the gastric mucosa and cause significant bleeding, possibly interfering with endoscopic assessment and diagnosis.

Documentation

Regularly record tube placement confirmation (usually every 4 to 8 hours). Keep a precise record of fluid intake and output, including the instilled irrigant in fluid input. Track the irrigation schedule and note the actual time of each irrigation. Describe drainage color, consistency, odor, and amount. Also, note tape change times and condition of the nares.

NASOGASTRIC TUBE INSERTION AND REMOVAL

Usually inserted to decompress the stomach, a nasogastric (NG) tube can prevent vomiting after major surgery. An NG tube is typically in place for 48 to 72 hours after surgery, by which time peristalsis usually resumes. It may remain in place for shorter or longer periods, however, depending on its use.

The NG tube has other diagnostic and therapeutic applications, especially in assessing and treating upper GI bleeding, collecting gastric contents for analysis, performing gastric lavage, aspirating gastric secretions, and administering medications and nutrients.

Inserting an NG tube requires close observation of the patient and verification of proper placement. Removing the tube requires careful handling to prevent injury or aspiration. The tube must be inserted with extra care in pregnant patients and in those with an increased risk of complications. For example, the doctor will order an NG tube for a patient with aortic aneurysm, myocardial infarction, gastric hemorrhage, or esophageal varices only if he believes that the benefits outweigh the risks of intubation.

Most NG tubes have a radiopaque marker or strip at the distal end so that the tube's position can be verified by X-ray studies. If the position can't be confirmed, the doctor may order fluoroscopy to verify placement.

The most common NG tubes are the Levin tube, which has one lumen, and the Salem sump tube, which has two lumens, one for suction and drainage and a smaller one for ventilation. Air flows through the vent lumen continuously. This protects the delicate gastric mucosa by preventing a vacuum from forming should the tube adhere to the stomach lining. The Moss tube, which has a triple lumen, is usually inserted during surgery. (See *Types of NG tubes,* page 552.)

Key nursing diagnoses and patient outcomes

Risk for deficient fluid volume related to presence of an NG tube
The patient will:
▶ maintain normal vital signs, skin color, and turgor
▶ maintain urine output of at least (specify) ml/hr
▶ have an output equal to or greater than input
▶ maintain normal electrolyte levels.

Risk for impaired skin integrity related to presence of an NG tube
The patient will:
▶ show no signs of skin breakdown in nares

Types of NG tubes

The doctor will choose the type and diameter of nasogastric (NG) tube that best suits the patient's needs, including lavage, aspiration, enteral therapy, or stomach decompression. Choices may include the Levin and Salem sump tubes.

Levin tube

The Levin tube is a rubber or plastic tube with a single lumen, a length of 42″ to 50″ (106.5 to 127 cm), and holes at the tip and along the side.

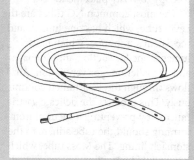

Salem sump tube

The Salem sump tube is a double-lumen tube made of clear plastic and has a blue sump port (pigtail) that allows atmospheric air to enter the patient's stomach. Thus, the tube floats freely and doesn't adhere to or damage gastric mucosa. The larger port of this 48″ (121.9-cm) tube serves as the main suction conduit. The tube has openings at 45, 55, 65, and 75 cm as well as a radiopaque line to verify placement.

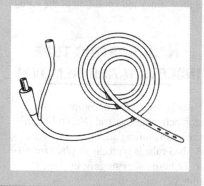

▶ maintain adequate circulation to nares
▶ report signs of discomfort at nares.

Equipment

For inserting an NG tube

Tube (usually #12, #14, #16, or #18 French for a normal adult) • towel or linen-saver pad • facial tissues • emesis basin • penlight • 1″ or 2″ hypoallergenic tape • gloves • water-soluble lubricant • cup or glass of water with straw (if appropriate) • stethoscope • tongue blade • catheter-tip or bulb syringe or irrigation set • safety pin • or-

dered suction equipment • optional: metal clamp, ice, alcohol pad, warm water, large basin or plastic container, and rubber band

For removing an NG tube

Stethoscope • gloves • catheter-tip syringe • normal saline solution • towel or linen-saver pad • adhesive remover • optional: clamp

Preparation of equipment

Inspect the NG tube for defects, such as rough edges or partially closed lumens. Then check the tube's patency by flushing it with water. To ease insertion, increase a stiff tube's flexibility by coiling it around your gloved fingers for a few seconds or by dipping it into warm water. Stiffen a limp rubber tube by briefly chilling it in ice.

Implementation

▶ Whether you're inserting or removing an NG tube, provide privacy, wash your hands, and put on gloves before inserting the tube. Check the doctor's order to determine the type of tube that should be inserted.

Inserting an NG tube

▶ Explain the procedure to the *patient to ease anxiety and promote cooperation.* Inform her that she may experience some nasal discomfort, that she may gag, and that her eyes may water. Emphasize that swallowing will ease the tube's advancement.
▶ Agree on a signal that the patient can use if she wants you to stop briefly during the procedure.
▶ Gather and prepare all necessary equipment.
▶ Help the patient into high Fowler's position unless contraindicated.
▶ Stand at the patient's right side if you're right-handed or at her left side if you're left-handed *to ease insertion.*
▶ Drape the towel or linen-saver pad over the patient's chest *to protect her gown and bed linens from spills.*
▶ Have the patient gently blow her nose to clear her nostrils.
▶ Place the facial tissues and emesis basin well within the patient's reach.
▶ Help the patient face forward with her neck in a neutral position.
▶ *To determine how long the NG tube must be to reach the stomach,* hold the end of the tube at the tip of the patient's nose. Extend the tube to the patient's earlobe and then down to the xiphoid process (as shown below).

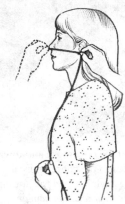

▶ Mark this distance on the tubing with the tape. (Average measurements for an adult range from 22″ to 26″ [56 to 66 cm].) It may be necessary to add 2″ (5 cm) to this measurement in tall individuals *to ensure entry into the stomach.*
▶ *To determine which nostril will allow easier access,* use a penlight and inspect for a deviated septum or other abnormalities. Ask the patient if she ever had nasal surgery or a nasal injury. Assess airflow in both nostrils by occluding one nostril at a time while the patient breathes through her nose. Choose the nostril with the better airflow.
▶ Lubricate the first 3″ (7.6 cm) of the tube with a water-soluble gel *to minimize injury to the nasal passages. Using a water-soluble lubricant prevents lipoid pneumonia,* which may result from aspiration of an oil-based lubricant or from accidental slippage of the tube into the trachea.
▶ Instruct the patient to hold her head straight and upright.
▶ Grasp the tube with the end pointing downward, curve it, if necessary,

and carefully insert it into the more patent nostril (as shown below).

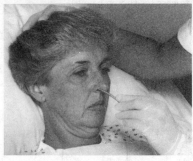

▶ Aim the tube downward and toward the ear closer to the chosen nostril. Advance it slowly *to avoid pressure on the turbinates and resultant pain and bleeding.*
▶ When the tube reaches the naso-pharynx, you'll feel resistance. Instruct the patient to lower her head slightly *to close the trachea and open the esophagus.* Then rotate the tube 180 degrees toward the opposite nostril *to redirect it so that the tube won't enter the patient's mouth.*
▶ Unless contraindicated, offer the patient a cup or glass of water with a straw. Direct her to sip and swallow as you slowly advance the tube (as shown below).

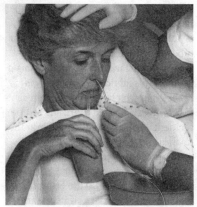

This helps the tube pass to the esophagus. (If you aren't using water, ask the patient to swallow.)

Ensuring proper tube placement
▶ Use a tongue blade and penlight to examine the patient's mouth and throat for signs of a coiled section of tubing (especially in an unconscious patient). *Coiling indicates an obstruction.*
▶ Keep an emesis basin and facial tissues readily available for the patient.
▶ As you carefully advance the tube and the patient swallows, watch for respiratory distress signs, *which may mean the tube is in the bronchus and must be removed immediately.*
▶ Stop advancing the tube when the tape mark reaches the patient's nostril.
▶ Attach a catheter-tip or bulb syringe to the tube and try to aspirate stomach contents (as shown below). If you don't

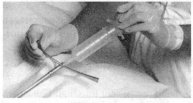

obtain stomach contents, position the patient on her left side to move the contents into the stomach's greater curvature, and aspirate again.

Note: When confirming tube placement, never place the tube's end in a container of water. *If the tube should be mispositioned in the trachea, the patient may aspirate water.* Also, water without bubbles doesn't confirm proper placement. *Instead, the tube may be coiled in the trachea or the esophagus.*
▶ If you still can't aspirate stomach contents, advance the tube 1″ to 2″ (2.5 to 5 cm). Then inject 10 cc of air into the tube. At the same time, auscultate

for air sounds with your stethoscope placed over the epigastric region. You should hear a whooshing sound if the tube is patent and properly positioned in the stomach.

▶ If these tests don't confirm proper tube placement, you'll need X-ray verification.

▶ Secure the NG tube to the patient's nose with hypoallergenic tape or another designated tube holder (as shown below). If the patient's skin is oily, wipe the bridge of the nose with an alcohol pad and allow to dry. You will need about 4″ (10 cm) of 1″ tape. Split one end of the tape up the center about 1½″ (3.8 cm). Make tabs on the split ends (by folding sticky sides together). Stick the uncut tape end on the patient's nose so that the split in the tape starts about ½″ (1.3 cm) to 1½″ from the tip of her nose. Crisscross the tabbed ends around the tube. Then apply another piece of tape over the bridge of the nose to secure the tube.

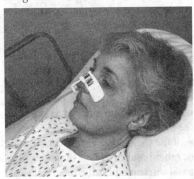

▶ Alternatively, stabilize the tube with a prepackaged product that secures and cushions it at the nose (as shown above).

▶ *To reduce discomfort from the weight of the tube,* tie a slipknot around the tube with a rubber band, and then secure the rubber band to the patient's gown

with a safety pin, or wrap another piece of tape around the end of the tube and leave a tab. Then fasten the tape tab to the patient's gown.

▶ Attach the tube to suction equipment, if ordered, and set the designated suction pressure.

Using an NG tube at home

If your patient will need to have a nasogastric (NG) tube in place at home—for short-term feeding or gastric decompression, for example—find out who will insert the tube. If the patient will have a home care nurse, identify her and, if possible, tell the patient when to expect her.

If the patient or a family member will perform the procedure, you'll need to provide additional instruction and supervision. Use the following checklist to prepare your teaching topics:

■ how and where to obtain equipment needed for home intubation

■ how to insert the tube

■ how to verify tube placement by aspirating stomach contents

■ how to correct tube misplacement

■ how to prepare formula for tube feeding

■ how to store formula, if appropriate

■ how to administer formula through the tube

■ how to remove and dispose of an NG tube

■ how to clean and store a reusable NG tube

■ how to use the NG tube for gastric decompression, if appropriate

■ how to set up and operate suctioning equipment

■ how to troubleshoot suctioning equipment

■ how to perform mouth care and other hygienic procedures.

Better charting

Documenting NG tube insertion and removal

Include the following information when documenting nasogastric (NG) tube insertion and removal:

- Document the date, time, and route of NG tube insertion and removal.
- Note how the patient tolerated the procedures.
- Include in your notes any signs and symptoms signaling complications, such as nausea, vomiting, and abdominal distention.
- Document any subsequent irrigation procedures and continuing problems after irrigation.
- Note any unusual events following NG removal, such as nausea, vomiting, abdominal distention, and food intolerance.

▶ Provide frequent nose and mouth care while the tube is in place.

Removing an NG tube

▶ Explain the procedure to the patient, informing her that it may cause some nasal discomfort and sneezing or gagging.

▶ Assess bowel function by auscultating for peristalsis or flatus.

▶ Help the patient into semi-Fowler's position. Then drape a towel or linen-saver pad across her chest *to protect her gown and bed linens from spills.*

▶ Wash your hands and put on gloves.

▶ Using a catheter-tip syringe, flush the tube with 10 ml of normal saline solution *to ensure that the tube doesn't contain stomach contents that could irritate tissues during tube removal.*

▶ Untape the tube from the patient's nose and then unpin it from her gown.

▶ Clamp the tube by folding it in your hand.

▶ Ask the patient to hold her breath *to close the epiglottis.* Then withdraw the tube gently and steadily. (When the distal end of the tube reaches the nasopharynx, you can pull it quickly.)

▶ When possible, immediately cover and remove the tube *because its sight and odor may nauseate the patient.*

▶ Assist the patient with thorough mouth care, and clean the tape residue from her nose with adhesive remover.

▶ For the next 48 hours, monitor the patient for signs of GI dysfunction, including nausea, vomiting, abdominal distention, and food intolerance. GI dysfunction may necessitate reinsertion of the tube.

Special considerations

▶ A helpful device for calculating the correct tube length is Ross-Hanson tape. Place the narrow end of this measuring tape at the tip of the patient's nose. Again, extend the tape to the patient's earlobe and down to the tip of the xiphoid process. Mark this distance on the edge of the tape labeled "nose to ear to xiphoid." The corresponding measurement on the opposite edge of the tape is the proper insertion length.

▶ If the patient has a deviated septum or other nasal condition that prevents nasal insertion, pass the tube orally after removing any dentures, if necessary. Sliding the tube over the tongue, proceed as you would for nasal insertion.

▶ When using the oral route, remember to coil the end of the tube around your hand. *This helps curve and direct the tube downward at the pharynx.*

▶ If your patient lies unconscious, tilt her chin toward her chest *to close the trachea.* Then advance the tube between respirations *to ensure that it doesn't enter the trachea.*

▶ While advancing the tube in an unconscious patient (or in a patient who can't swallow), stroke the patient's neck *to encourage the swallowing reflex and facilitate passage down the esophagus.*

▶ While advancing the tube, observe for signs that it has entered the trachea, such as choking or breathing difficulties in a conscious patient and cyanosis in an unconscious patient or a patient without a cough reflex. If these signs occur, remove the tube immediately. Allow the patient time to rest; then try to reinsert the tube.

▶ After tube placement, vomiting suggests tubal obstruction or incorrect position. Assess immediately to determine the cause.

Home care

An NG tube may be inserted or removed at home. Indications for insertion include gastric decompression and short-term feeding. A home care nurse or the patient may insert the tube, deliver the feeding, and remove the tube. (See *Using an NG tube at home,* page 555.)

Complications

Potential complications of prolonged intubation with an NG tube include skin erosion at the nostril, sinusitis, esophagitis, esophagotracheal fistula, gastric ulceration, and pulmonary and oral infection. Additional complications that may result from suction include electrolyte imbalances and dehydration.

Documentation

Record the type and size of the NG tube and the date, time, and route of insertion. Also, note the type and amount of suction, if used, and describe the drainage, including the amount, color, character, consistency, and odor. Note the patient's tolerance of the procedure. (See *Documenting NG tube insertion and removal.*)

When you remove the tube, record the date and time. Describe the color, consistency, and amount of gastric drainage. Again, note the patient's tolerance of the procedure.

NASOPHARYNGEAL AIRWAY INSERTION AND CARE

Insertion of a nasopharyngeal airway — soft rubber or latex uncuffed catheter — establishes or maintains a patent airway. This airway is the typical choice for patients who have had recent oral surgery or facial trauma and for patients with loose, cracked, or avulsed teeth. It's also used to protect the nasal mucosa from injury when the patient needs frequent nasotracheal suctioning.

The airway follows the curvature of the nasopharynx, passing through the nose and extending from the nostril to the posterior pharynx. The bevel-shaped pharyngeal end of the airway facilitates insertion, and its funnel-shaped nasal end helps prevent slippage.

Insertion of a nasopharyngeal airway is preferred when an oropharyngeal airway is contraindicated or fails to maintain a patent airway. A nasopharyngeal airway is contraindicated if the patient

Inserting a nasopharyngeal airway

First, hold the airway beside the patient's face to make sure it's the proper size (as shown below). It should be slightly smaller than the patient's nostril diameter and slightly longer than the distance from the tip of his nose to his earlobe.

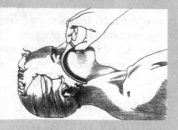

To insert the airway, hyperextend the patient's neck (unless contraindicated). Then push up the tip of his nose and pass the airway into his nostril (as shown below). Avoid pushing against any resistance to prevent tissue trauma and airway kinking.

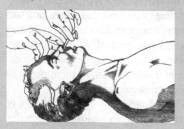

To check for correct airway placement, first close the patient's mouth. Then place your finger over the tube's opening to detect air exchange. Also, depress the patient's tongue with a tongue blade and look for the airway tip behind the uvula.

is receiving anticoagulant therapy or has a hemorrhagic disorder, sepsis, or pathologic nasopharyngeal deformity.

Key nursing diagnoses and patient outcomes

Ineffective breathing pattern related to alterations in normal gas exchange
The patient will:
▶ regain and maintain arterial blood gas values within normal limits
▶ regain baseline respiratory rate and maintain stable respirations.

Impaired spontaneous ventilation related to (specify)
The patient will:
▶ show no signs of dyspnea at rest within 24 hours
▶ have a chest X-ray that indicates full lung expansion within 24 hours.

Equipment
For insertion
Nasopharyngeal airway of proper size • tongue blade • water-soluble lubricant • gloves • optional: suction equipment

For cleaning
Hydrogen peroxide • water • basin • optional: pipe cleaner

Preparation of equipment
Measure the diameter of the patient's nostril and the distance from the tip of his nose to his earlobe. Select an airway of slightly smaller diameter than the nostril and of slightly longer length (1" [2.5 cm]) than measured. The sizes for this type of airway are labeled according to their internal diameter.

The recommended size for a large adult is 8 to 9 mm; for a medium adult, 7 to 8 mm; and for a small adult, 6 to 7 mm. Lubricate the distal half of the airway's surface with a water-soluble lubricant to prevent traumatic injury during insertion.

Implementation

▶ Put on gloves.
▶ In nonemergency situations, explain the procedure to the patient.
▶ Properly insert the airway. (See *Inserting a nasopharyngeal airway*.)
▶ After the airway is inserted, check it regularly *to detect dislodgment or obstruction.*
▶ When the patient's natural airway is patent, remove the airway in one smooth motion. If the airway sticks, apply lubricant around the nasal end of the tube and around the nostril; then gently rotate the airway until it's free.

Special considerations

▶ When you insert the airway, remember to use a chin-lift or jaw-thrust technique to anteriorly displace the patient's mandible. Immediately after insertion, assess the patient's respirations. If absent or inadequate, initiate artificial positive-pressure ventilation with a mouth-to-mask technique, a handheld resuscitation bag, or an oxygen-powered breathing device.
▶ If the patient coughs or gags, the tube may be too long. If so, remove the airway and insert a shorter one.
▶ At least once every 8 hours, remove the airway *to check nasal mucous membranes for irritation or ulceration.*
▶ Clean the airway by placing it in a basin and rinsing it with hydrogen peroxide and then with water. If secretions remain, use a pipe cleaner to remove them. Reinsert the clean airway into the other nostril (if it's patent) *to avoid skin breakdown.*

Complications

Sinus infection may result from obstruction of sinus drainage. Insertion of the airway may injure the nasal mucosa and cause bleeding and possibly aspiration of blood into the trachea. Suction as necessary to remove secretions or blood. If the tube is too long, it may enter the esophagus and cause gastric distention and hypoventilation during artificial ventilation. Although semiconscious patients usually tolerate nasopharyngeal airways better than conscious patients, they may still experience laryngospasm and vomiting.

Documentation

Record the date and time of the airway's insertion; size of the airway; removal and cleaning of the airway; shifts from one nostril to the other; condition of the mucous membranes; suctioning; complications and nursing action taken; and the patient's reaction to the procedure.

NEBULIZER THERAPY

An established component of respiratory care, nebulizer therapy aids bronchial hygiene by restoring and maintaining mucous blanket continuity; hydrating dried, retained secretions; promoting expectoration of secretions; humidifying inspired oxygen; and delivering medications. The therapy may be administered through nebulizers that have a large or small volume, are ultrasonic, or are placed inside ventilator tubing.

Ultrasonic nebulizers are electrically driven and use high-frequency vibrations to break up surface water into particles. The resultant dense mist can penetrate smaller airways and is useful for hydrating secretions and inducing a cough. Large-volume nebulizers are used to provide humidity for an artificial airway such as a tracheostomy, and small-volume nebulizers are used to deliver medications such as bronchodilators. In-line nebulizers are used to deliver medications to patients who are being mechanically ventilated. In this case, the nebulizer is placed in the inspiratory side of the ventilatory circuit as close to the endotracheal tube as possible.

Many questions still exist regarding aerosol therapy, including what type of fluid to use, the types of medications that can be delivered, and the effectiveness of therapy.

Key nursing diagnoses and patient outcomes

Ineffective breathing pattern related to (specify)
The patient will:
▶ maintain respiratory rate within 5 breaths/minute of baseline
▶ have normal arterial blood gas levels
▶ demonstrate correct use of the nebulizer
▶ report ability to breathe comfortably.

Deficient knowledge related to use of the nebulizer
The patient will:
▶ indicate a need to know how to use the nebulizer
▶ set realistic learning goals
▶ state and demonstrate an understanding of what has been taught.

Equipment
For an ultrasonic nebulizer
Ultrasonic gas-delivery device • large-bore oxygen tubing • nebulizer couplet compartment

For a large-volume nebulizer (such as a Venturi jet)
Pressurized gas source • flowmeter • large-bore oxygen tubing • nebulizer bottle • sterile distilled water • heater (if ordered) • in-line thermometer (if using heater)

For a small-volume nebulizer (such as a mininebulizer)
Pressurized gas source • flowmeter • oxygen tubing • nebulizer cup • mouthpiece or mask • normal saline solution • prescribed medication

For an in-line nebulizer
Pressurized gas source • flowmeter • nebulizer cup • normal saline solution • prescribed medication

Preparation of equipment
For an ultrasonic nebulizer
Fill the couplet compartment on the nebulizer to the level indicated.

For a large-volume nebulizer
Fill the water chamber to the indicated level with sterile distilled water. Avoid using saline solution *to prevent corrosion.* Add a heating device, if ordered, and place a thermometer in-line between the outlet port and the patient, as close to the patient as possible, *to monitor the actual temperature of the inhaled gas and to avoid burning the patient.* If the unit will supply oxygen, analyze the flow at the patient's end of the tubing *to ensure delivery of the prescribed oxygen percentage.*

For a small-volume nebulizer
Draw up the prescribed medication, inject it into the nebulizer cup, and add the prescribed amount of saline solu-

tion or water. Attach the mouthpiece, mask, or other gas-delivery device.

For an in-line nebulizer

Draw up the medication and diluent, remove the nebulizer cup, quickly inject the medication, and then replace the cup. If using an intermittent positive-pressure breathing machine, attach the mouthpiece and mask to the machine.

Implementation

▶ Explain the procedure to the patient and wash your hands.
▶ Take the patient's vital signs and auscultate his lung fields *to establish a baseline*. If possible, place the patient in a sitting or high Fowler's position *to encourage full lung expansion and promote aerosol dispersion*. Encourage the patient to take slow, even breaths during the treatment.

For an ultrasonic nebulizer

▶ Before beginning, administer an inhaled bronchodilator (metered-dose inhaler or small-volume nebulizer) *to prevent bronchospasm*.
▶ Turn on the machine and check the outflow port *to ensure proper misting*.
▶ Check the patient frequently during the procedure to observe for adverse reactions. Watch for labored respirations *because ultrasonic nebulizer therapy may hydrate retained secretions and obstruct airways*. Take the patient's vital signs and auscultate his lung fields.
▶ Encourage the patient to cough and expectorate, or suction as needed.

For a large-volume nebulizer

▶ Attach the delivery device to the patient.

▶ Encourage the patient to cough and expectorate, or suction as needed.
▶ Check the water level in the nebulizer at frequent intervals and refill or replace as indicated. When refilling a reusable container, discard the old water *to prevent infection from bacterial or fungal growth,* and refill the container to the indicator line with sterile distilled water.
▶ Change the nebulizer unit and tubing according to facility policy *to prevent bacterial contamination*.
▶ If the nebulizer is heated, tell the patient to report any warmth, discomfort, or hot tubing *because these may indicate a heater malfunction*. Use the in-line thermometer to monitor the temperature of the gas the patient is inhaling. If you turn off the flow for more than 5 minutes, unplug the heater *to avoid overheating the water and burning the patient when the aerosol is resumed*.

For a small-volume nebulizer

▶ After attaching the flowmeter to the gas source, attach the nebulizer to the flowmeter and then adjust the flow to at least 10 L/minute but no more than 14 L/minute *to ensure adequate functioning while preventing excess venting*.
▶ Check the outflow port *to ensure adequate misting*.
▶ Remain with the patient during the treatment, which lasts 15 to 20 minutes, and take his vital signs *to detect any adverse reaction to the medication*.
▶ Encourage the patient to cough and expectorate, or suction as necessary.
▶ Change the nebulizer cup and tubing according to your facility's policy *to prevent bacterial contamination*.

For an in-line nebulizer
▶ Turn on the machine and check the outflow port *to ensure proper misting.*
▶ Remain with the patient during the treatment, which lasts 15 to 20 minutes, and take his vital signs *to detect any adverse reaction to the medication.*
▶ Encourage the patient to cough and suction excess secretions as necessary.
▶ Auscultate the patient's lungs *to evaluate the effectiveness of therapy.*

Special considerations
▶ When using high-output nebulizers such as an ultrasonic nebulizer on pediatric patients or patients with a delicate fluid balance, be alert for signs of overhydration (exhibited by unexplained weight gain occurring over several days after the beginning of therapy), pulmonary edema, crackles, and electrolyte imbalance.
▶ If oxygen is being delivered concomitantly, the fraction of inspired oxygen (FIO_2) may be diluted if the flow isn't adequate. Therefore, if the mist disappears when the patient inhales, increase the gas flow.

Complications
Nebulized particulates can irritate the mucosa in some patients and cause bronchospasm and dyspnea. Other complications include airway burns (when heating elements are used), infection from contaminated equipment (although rare), and adverse reactions from medications.

Documentation
Record the date, time, and duration of therapy; type and amount of medication; FIO_2 or oxygen flow, if administered; baseline and subsequent vital signs and breath sounds; and the patient's response to treatment.

NEPHROSTOMY AND CYSTOSTOMY TUBE CARE

Two urinary diversion techniques—nephrostomy and cystostomy—ensure adequate drainage from the kidneys or bladder and help prevent urinary tract infection or kidney failure. (See *Urinary diversion techniques.*)

A nephrostomy tube drains urine directly from a kidney when a disorder inhibits the normal flow of urine. The tube is usually placed percutaneously, though sometimes it's surgically inserted through the renal cortex and medulla into the renal pelvis from a lateral incision in the flank. The usual indication is obstructive disease, such as calculi in the ureter or ureteropelvic junction, or an obstructing tumor. Draining urine with a nephrostomy tube also allows kidney tissue damaged by obstructive disease to heal.

A cystostomy tube drains urine from the bladder, diverting it from the urethra. This type of tube is used after certain gynecologic procedures, bladder surgery, prostatectomy, and for severe urethral strictures or traumatic injury. Inserted about 2″ (5 cm) above the symphysis pubis, a cystostomy tube may be used alone or with an indwelling urethral catheter.

Key nursing diagnoses and patient outcomes
Impaired urinary elimination related to the presence of a urinary diversion device
The patient will:
▶ maintain fluid balance (intake equals output)
▶ experience minimal complications
▶ describe feelings and concerns about indwelling urinary catheter.

Urinary diversion techniques

A cystostomy or a nephrostomy can be used to create a permanent diversion, to relieve obstruction from an inoperable tumor, or to provide an outlet for urine after cystectomy. A temporary diversion can relieve obstruction from a calculus or ureteral edema.

In a cystostomy, a catheter is inserted percutaneously through the suprapubic area into the bladder. In a nephrostomy, a catheter is inserted percutaneously through the flank into the renal pelvis.

Cystostomy

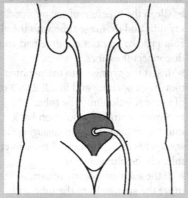

Nephrostomy

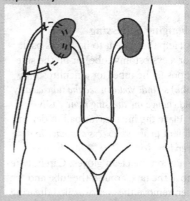

Risk for infection related to the presence of a nephrostomy or cystostomy tube
The patient will:
▶ have no pathogens in cultures
▶ remain afebrile
▶ show no evidence of urinary tract infections, such as cloudy, malodorous, or sediment-containing urine.

Equipment
Commercially prepared sterile dressing kits may be available.

For dressing changes
Povidone-iodine solution or povidone-iodine pads • 4″ × 4″ gauze pads • sterile cup or emesis basin • paper bag • linen-saver pad • clean gloves (for dressing removal) • sterile gloves (for

new dressing) • precut 4″ × 4″ drain dressings or transparent semipermeable dressings • adhesive tape (preferably hypoallergenic)

For nephrostomy-tube irrigation
3-ml syringe • alcohol pad or povidone-iodine pad • normal saline solution • optional: hemostat

Preparation of equipment
Wash your hands and assemble all equipment at the patient's bedside. Open several packages of gauze pads, place them in the sterile cup or emesis basin, and pour the povidone-iodine solution over them. Or, if available, open several packages of povidone-iodine pads. If you're using a commer-

cially packaged dressing kit, open it using aseptic technique. Fill the cup with antiseptic solution.

Open the paper bag and place it away from the other equipment *to avoid contaminating the sterile field.*

Implementation
▶ Wash your hands, provide privacy, and explain the procedure to the patient.

Changing a dressing
▶ Help the patient to lie on his back (for a cystostomy tube) or on the side opposite the tube (for a nephrostomy tube) *so that you can see the tube clearly and change the dressing more easily.*
▶ Place the linen-saver pad under the patient *to absorb excess drainage and keep him dry.*
▶ Put on the clean gloves. Carefully remove the tape around the tube and then remove the wet or soiled dressing. Discard the tape and dressing in the paper bag. Remove the gloves and discard them in the bag.
▶ Put on the sterile gloves. Pick up a saturated pad or dip a dry one into the cup of antiseptic solution.
▶ To clean the wound, wipe only once with each pad, moving from the insertion site outward. Discard the used pad in the paper bag. Don't touch the bag *to avoid contaminating your gloves.*
▶ Pick up a sterile 4″ × 4″ drain dressing and place it around the tube. If necessary, overlap two drain dressings *to provide maximum absorption.* Or, depending on your facility's policy, apply a transparent semipermeable dressing over the site and tubing *to allow observation of the site without removing the dressing.*

▶ Secure the dressing with hypoallergenic tape. Then tape the tube to the patient's lateral abdomen *to prevent tension on the tube.* (See *Taping a nephrostomy tube.*)
▶ Dispose of all equipment appropriately. Clean the patient as necessary.

Irrigating a nephrostomy tube
▶ Fill the 3-ml syringe with the normal saline solution.
▶ Clean the junction of the nephrostomy tube and drainage tube with the alcohol pad or povidone-iodine pad and disconnect the tubes.
▶ Insert the syringe into the nephrostomy tube opening and instill 2 to 3 ml of saline solution into the tube.
▶ Slowly aspirate the solution back into the syringe. *To avoid damaging the renal pelvis tissue,* never pull back forcefully on the plunger.
▶ If the solution doesn't return, remove the syringe from the tube and reattach it to the drainage tubing *to allow the solution to drain by gravity.*
▶ Dispose of all equipment appropriately.

Special considerations
▶ Change dressings once a day or more often, if needed.

Nursing alert Never irrigate a nephrostomy tube with more than 5 ml of solution *because the capacity of the renal pelvis is usually between 4 and 8 ml. (Remember: The purpose of irrigation is to keep the tube patent, not to lavage the renal pelvis.)*
▶ When necessary, irrigate a cystostomy tube as you would an indwelling urinary catheter. Perform the irrigation gently *to avoid damaging any suture lines.*

Taping a nephrostomy tube

To tape a nephrostomy tube directly to the skin, cut a wide piece of hypoallergenic adhesive tape twice lengthwise to its midpoint.

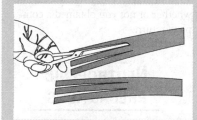

Apply the uncut end of the tape to the skin so that the midpoint meets the tube. Wrap the middle strip around the tube in a spiral fashion. Tape the other two strips to the patient's skin on both sides of the tube.

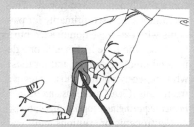

For greater security, repeat this step with a second piece of tape, applying it in the reverse direction. You may also apply two more strips of tape perpendicular to and over the first two pieces.

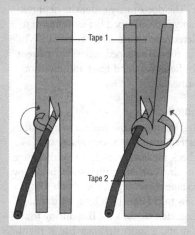

Always apply another strip of tape lower down on the tube in the direction of the drainage tube *to further anchor the tube*. Don't put tension on any sutures that prevent tube distention.

▶ Check a nephrostomy tube frequently for kinks or obstructions. Kinks are likely to occur if the patient lies on the insertion site. Suspect an obstruction when the amount of urine in the drainage bag decreases or the amount of urine around the insertion site increases. Pressure created by urine backing up in the tube can damage nephrons. Gently curve a cystostomy tube *to prevent kinks*.

▶ If a blood clot or mucus plug obstructs a nephrostomy or cystostomy tube, try milking the tube *to restore its*

patency. With your nondominant hand, hold the tube securely above the obstruction *to avoid pulling the tube out of the incision*. Then place the flat side of a closed hemostat under the tube, just above the obstruction, pinch the tube against the hemostat, and slide both your finger and the hemostat toward you, away from the patient.

▶ Typically, cystostomy tubes for postoperative urologic patients should be checked hourly for 24 hours *to ensure adequate drainage and tube patency*. To check tube patency, note the amount of urine in the drainage bag and check the patient's bladder for distention.

▶ Keep the drainage bag below the level of the kidney at all times *to prevent reflux of urine.*

▶ If the tube becomes dislodged, cover the site with a sterile dressing and notify the doctor immediately.

▶ The doctor may order the nephrostomy tube clamped before removal to determine readiness for removal. While the tube is clamped, assess the patient for flank pain and fever and monitor urine output.

Home care

Tell the home care patient to clean the insertion site with soap and water, check for skin breakdown, and change the dressing daily; then show him how to take these steps. Also, teach him how to change the leg bag or drainage bag. He can use a leg bag during the day and a larger drainage bag at night. Whether he uses a drainage bag or larger container, tell him to wash it daily with a 1:3 vinegar and water solution, rinse it with plain water, and dry it on a clothes hanger or over the towel rack. *This prevents crystalline buildup.*

Stress the importance of reporting to the doctor signs of infection (red skin or white, yellow, or green drainage at the insertion site) or tube displacement (drainage that smells like urine).

Complications

The patient has an increased risk of infection because nephrostomy and cystostomy tubes provide a direct opening to the kidneys and bladder.

Documentation

Describe the color and amount of drainage from the nephrostomy or cystostomy tube and record any color changes as they occur. Similarly, if the patient has more than one tube, describe the drainage (color, amount, and character) from each tube separately. If irrigation is necessary, record the amount and type of irrigant used and whether or not you obtained a complete return.

NEUTROPENIC PRECAUTIONS

Unlike other types of precaution procedures, neutropenic precautions (also known as protective precautions and reverse isolation) guard the patient who is at increased risk for infection against contact with potential pathogens. These precautions are used primarily for patients with extensive noninfected burns, for those who have leukopenia or a depressed immune system, and for those who are receiving immunosuppressive treatments. (See *Conditions and treatments requiring neutropenic precautions.*)

Neutropenic precautions require a single room equipped with positive air pressure, if possible, to force suspended particles down and out of the room. The degree of precautions may range from using a single room, thorough hand-washing technique, and limitation of traffic into the room to more extensive precautions requiring the use of gowns, gloves, and masks by facility staff and visitors. The extent of neutropenic precautions may vary from facility to facility, depending on the reason for and the degree of the patient's immunosuppression.

To care for patients who have temporarily increased susceptibility, such as

Conditions and treatments requiring neutropenic precautions

Condition and treatment	Precautionary period
Acquired immunodeficiency syndrome	Until white blood cell count reaches 1,000/µl or more, or according to facility guidelines
Agranulocytosis	Until remission
Burns, extensive noninfected	Until skin surface heals substantially
Dermatitis, noninfected vesicular, bullous, or eczematous	Until skin surface heals substantially
Immunosuppressive therapy	Until patient's immunity is adequate
Lymphomas and leukemia, especially late stages of Hodgkin's disease or acute leukemia	Until clinical improvement is substantial

those who have undergone bone marrow transplantation, neutropenic precautions may also require a patient isolator unit and the use of sterile linens, gowns, gloves, and head and shoe coverings. In such cases, all other items taken into the room should be sterilized or disinfected. The patient's diet also may be modified to eliminate raw fruits and vegetables and to allow only cooked foods and possibly only sterile beverages.

Key nursing diagnoses and patient outcomes

Risk for infection related to hospital admission
The patient will:
▶ remain free from all signs and symptoms of infection
▶ identify signs and symptoms of infection
▶ state factors that put him at risk for infection.

Equipment

Gloves • gowns • masks • shoe covers, if required • neutropenic precautions door card

Gather any additional supplies, such as a thermometer, stethoscope, and blood pressure cuff, so you don't have to leave the isolation room unnecessarily.

Preparation of equipment

Keep supplies in a clean enclosed cart or in an anteroom outside the room.

Implementation

▶ After placing the patient in a single room, explain isolation precautions to the patient and his family *to ease patient anxiety and promote cooperation.*
▶ Place a neutropenic precautions card on the door *to caution those entering the room.*
▶ Wash your hands with an antiseptic agent before putting on gloves, after removing gloves, and as indicated during patient care.

▶ Wear gloves and gown according to standard precautions, unless the patient's condition warrants sterile gown, gloves, and mask.

▶ Avoid transporting the patient out of the room; if he must be moved, make sure he wears a gown and mask. Notify the receiving department or area *so that the precautions will be maintained and the patient will be returned to the room promptly.*

▶ Don't allow visits by anyone known to be ill or infected.

Special considerations

▶ Don't perform invasive procedures such as urethral catheterization unless absolutely necessary *because these procedures risk serious infection in the patient with impaired resistance.*

▶ Instruct the housekeeping staff to put on gowns, gloves, and masks before entering the room; no ill or infected person should enter.

▶ Make sure that the room is cleaned with new or scrupulously clean equipment. Because the patient doesn't have a contagious disease, materials leaving the room need no special precautions beyond standard precautions.

Documentation

Document the need for neutropenic precautions on the nursing plan of care and as otherwise indicated by your facility.

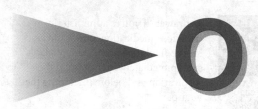

ORAL DRUG ADMINISTRATION

Because oral administration is usually the safest, most convenient, and least expensive method, most drugs are administered by this route. Drugs for oral administration are available in many forms: tablets, enteric-coated tablets, capsules, syrups, elixirs, oils, liquids, suspensions, powders, and granules. Some require special preparation before administration, such as mixing with juice to make them more palatable; oils, powders, and granules most often require such preparation.

Sometimes oral drugs are prescribed in higher dosages than their parenteral equivalents because after absorption through the GI system they are immediately broken down by the liver before they reach the systemic circulation.

 Age alert Oral dosages normally prescribed for adults may be dangerous for elderly patients.

Oral administration is contraindicated for unconscious patients; it may also be contraindicated in patients with nausea and vomiting and in those unable to swallow.

Key nursing diagnoses and patient outcomes

Deficient knowledge related to lack of exposure to information about oral drug administration
The patient will:
▶ state or demonstrate an understanding of what has been taught
▶ demonstrate the ability to perform new health-related behaviors as they are taught.

Risk for injury related to improper technique
The patient will:
▶ identify factors that increase the risk for injury
▶ assist in identifying and applying safety measures to prevent injury.

Equipment

Patient's medication record and chart • prescribed medication • medication cup • optional: appropriate vehicle, such as jelly or applesauce, for crushed pills commonly used with children or elderly patients, and juice, water, or milk for liquid medications; drinking straw; mortar and pestle for crushing pills

Implementation

▶ Verify the order on the patient's medication record by checking it against the doctor's order.

Measuring liquid medications

To pour liquids, hold the medication cup at eye level. Use your thumb to mark off the correct level on the cup (as shown below). Then set the cup down and read the bottom of the meniscus at eye level to ensure accuracy. If you've poured too much medication into the cup, discard the excess. Don't return it to the bottle.

Here are a few additional tips:

■ Hold the container so that the medication flows from the side opposite the label so it won't run down the container and stain or obscure the label. Remove drips from the lip of the bottle first and then from the sides, using a clean, damp paper towel.

■ For a liquid measured in drops, use only the dropper supplied with the medication.

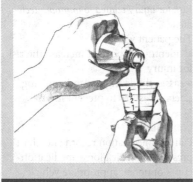

▶ Wash your hands.
▶ Check the label on the medication three times before administering it *to make sure you'll be giving the prescribed medication.* Check when you take the container from the shelf or drawer, again before you pour the medication into the medication cup, and again before returning the container to the shelf

or drawer. If you're administering a unit-dose medication, check the label for the final time at the patient's bedside immediately after pouring the medication and before discarding the wrapper.

▶ Confirm the patient's identity by asking his name and checking the name, room number, and bed number on his wristband.

▶ Assess the patient's condition, including level of consciousness and vital signs, as needed. *Changes in the patient's condition may warrant withholding medication.* For example, you may need to withhold a medication that will slow the patient's heart rate if his apical pulse rate is less than 60 beats/minute.

▶ Give the patient his medication and an appropriate vehicle or liquid, as needed, *to aid swallowing, minimize adverse effects, or promote absorption.* For example, cyclophosphamide is given with fluids to minimize adverse effects; antitussive cough syrup is given without a fluid to avoid diluting its soothing effect on the throat. If appropriate, crush the medication *to facilitate swallowing.*

▶ Stay with the patient until he has swallowed the drug. If he seems confused or disoriented, check his mouth *to make sure he has swallowed it.* Return and reassess the patient's response within 1 hour after giving the medication.

Special considerations

▶ Make sure you have a written order for every medication given. Verbal orders should be signed by the doctor within the specified time period. (Hospitals usually require a signature within 24 hours; long-term-care facilities, within 48 hours.)

▶ Use care in measuring out the prescribed dose of liquid oral medication. (See *Measuring liquid medications*.)

▶ Don't give medication from a poorly labeled or unlabeled container. Don't attempt to label or reinforce drug labels yourself. *This must be done by a pharmacist.*

▶ Never give a medication poured by someone else. Never allow your medication cart or tray out of your sight. *This prevents anyone from rearranging the medications or taking one without your knowledge.* Never return unwrapped or prepared medications to stock containers. Instead, dispose of them and notify the pharmacy. Keep in mind that the disposal of any narcotic drug must be cosigned by another nurse, as mandated by law.

▶ If the patient questions you about his medication or the dosage, check his medication record again. If the medication is correct, reassure him. Make sure you tell him about any changes in his medication or dosage. Instruct him, as appropriate, about possible adverse effects. Ask him to report anything he thinks may be an adverse effect.

▶ *To avoid damaging or staining the patient's teeth,* administer acid or iron preparations through a straw. An unpleasant-tasting liquid can usually be made more palatable if taken through a straw *because the liquid contacts fewer taste buds.*

▶ If the patient can't swallow a whole tablet or capsule, ask the pharmacist if the drug is available in liquid form or if it can be administered by another route. If not, ask him if you can crush the tablet or open the capsule and mix it with food. Keep in mind that many enteric-coated or time-release medications and gelatin capsules shouldn't be crushed. Remember to contact the doc-

tor for an order to change the administration route when necessary.

 Age alert **Oral medications are relatively easy to give to infants because of their natural sucking instinct and, in infants under 4 months old, their undeveloped sense of taste.**

Documentation

Note the drug administered, dose, date and time, and patient's reaction, if any. If the patient refuses a drug, document the refusal and notify the charge nurse and the patient's doctor, as needed. Also note if a drug was omitted or withheld for other reasons, such as radiology or laboratory tests, or if, in your judgment, the drug was contraindicated at the ordered time. Sign out all narcotics given on the appropriate narcotics central record.

ORONASOPHARYNGEAL SUCTION

Oronasopharyngeal suction removes secretions from the pharynx by a suction catheter inserted through the mouth or nostril. Used to maintain a patent airway, this procedure helps the patient who can't clear his airway effectively with coughing and expectoration, such as the unconscious or severely debilitated patient. The procedure should be done as often as necessary, depending on the patient's condition.

Because the catheter may inadvertently slip into the lower airway or esophagus, oronasopharyngeal suction is an aseptic procedure that requires sterile equipment. However, clean technique may be used for a tonsil tip suction device. In fact, an alert patient can use a tonsil tip suction device himself to remove secretions.

Nasopharyngeal suctioning should be used with caution in patients who have nasopharyngeal bleeding or spinal fluid leakage into the nasopharyngeal area, in trauma patients, in patients who are receiving anticoagulant therapy, and in those who have blood dyscrasias because these conditions increase the risk of bleeding.

Key nursing diagnoses and patient outcomes

Ineffective breathing pattern related to decreased energy
The patient will:
▶ achieve maximum lung expansion with adequate ventilation
▶ report feeling comfortable with breathing.

Impaired gas exchange related to altered oxygen supply
The patient will:
▶ cough effectively
▶ expectorate sputum.

Equipment

Wall suction or portable suction apparatus • collection bottle • connecting tubing • water-soluble lubricant • normal saline solution • disposable sterile container • sterile suction catheter (a #12 or #14 French catheter for an adult, #8 or #10 French catheter for a child, or pediatric feeding tube for an infant) • sterile gloves • clean gloves • nasopharyngeal or oropharyngeal airway (optional for frequent suctioning) • overbed table • waterproof trash bag • soap, water, and 70% alcohol for cleaning catheters • optional: tongue blade and tonsil tip suction device

A commercially prepared kit contains a sterile catheter, disposable container, and sterile gloves.

Preparation of equipment

Before beginning, check your facility's policy to determine whether a doctor's order is required for oropharyngeal suctioning. Also review the patient's blood gas and oxygen saturation values, and check vital signs. Evaluate the patient's ability to cough and deep-breathe *to determine his ability to move secretions up the tracheobronchial tree.* Check his history for a deviated septum, nasal polyps, nasal obstruction, traumatic injury, epistaxis, or mucosal swelling.

If no contraindications exist, gather and place the suction equipment on the patient's overbed table or bedside stand. Position the table or stand on your preferred side of the bed *to facilitate suctioning.* Attach the collection bottle to the suctioning unit, and attach the connecting tubing to it. Date and open the bottle of normal saline solution. Open the waterproof trash bag.

Implementation

▶ Explain the procedure to the patient even if he's unresponsive. Inform him that suctioning may stimulate transient coughing or gagging, but tell him that coughing helps to mobilize secretions. If he has been suctioned before, just summarize the reasons for the procedure. Reassure him throughout the procedure *to minimize anxiety and fear, which can increase oxygen consumption.* Also ask which nostril is more patent.
▶ Wash your hands.
▶ Place the patient in semi-Fowler's or high Fowler's position, if tolerated, *to*

promote lung expansion and effective coughing.

▶ Turn on the suction from the wall or portable unit, and set the pressure according to your facility's policy. The pressure is usually set between 80 and 120 mm Hg; *higher pressures cause excessive trauma without enhancing secretion removal.* Occlude the end of the connecting tubing to check suction pressure.

▶ Using strict sterile technique, open the suction catheter kit or the packages containing the sterile catheter, disposable container, and gloves. Put on the gloves; consider your dominant hand sterile and your nondominant hand nonsterile. Using your nondominant hand, pour the normal saline solution into the sterile container.

▶ With your nondominant hand, place a small amount of water-soluble lubricant on the sterile area. The lubricant is used *to facilitate passage of the catheter during nasopharyngeal suctioning.*

▶ Pick up the catheter with your dominant (sterile) hand, and attach it to the connecting tubing. Use your nondominant hand to control the suction valve while your dominant hand manipulates the catheter.

▶ Instruct the patient to cough and breathe slowly and deeply several times before beginning suction. *Coughing helps loosen secretions and may decrease the amount of suctioning necessary, while deep breathing helps minimize or prevent hypoxia.* (See *Tips on airway clearance,* page 574.)

For nasal insertion

▶ Raise the tip of the patient's nose with your nondominant hand to straighten the passageway and facilitate insertion of the catheter. Without ap-plying suction, gently insert the suction catheter into the patient's nares. Roll the catheter between your fingers to help it advance through the turbinates. Continue to advance the catheter approximately 5″ to 6″ (13 to 15 cm) until you reach the pool of secretions or the patient begins to cough.

For oral insertion

▶ Without applying suction, gently insert the catheter into the patient's mouth. Advance it 3″ to 4″ (7.5 to 10 cm) along the side of the patient's mouth until you reach the pool of secretions or the patient begins to cough. Suction both sides of the patient's mouth and pharyngeal area.

▶ Using intermittent suction, withdraw the catheter from either the mouth or the nose with a continuous rotating motion *to minimize invagination of the mucosa into the catheter's tip and side ports.* Apply suction for only 10 to 15 seconds at a time *to minimize tissue trauma.*

▶ Between passes, wrap the catheter around your dominant hand *to prevent contamination.*

▶ If secretions are thick, clear the lumen of the catheter by dipping it in normal saline solution and applying suction.

▶ Repeat the procedure until gurgling or bubbling sounds stop and respirations are quiet.

▶ After completing suctioning, pull your sterile glove off over the coiled catheter, and discard it and the nonsterile glove along with the container of water.

▶ Flush the connecting tubing with normal saline solution.

Tips on airway clearance

Deep breathing and coughing are vital for removing secretions from the lungs. Other techniques used to help clear the airways include diaphragmatic breathing and forced expiration. Here is how to teach these techniques to your patients.

Diaphragmatic breathing

First, tell the patient to lie in a supine position, with his head elevated 15 to 20 degrees on a pillow. Tell him to place one hand on his abdomen and then inhale so that he can feel his abdomen rise. Explain that this is known as "breathing with the diaphragm."

Next, instruct the patient to exhale slowly through his nose — or, better yet, through pursed lips — while letting his abdomen collapse. Explain that this action decreases his respiratory rate and increases his tidal volume.

Suggest that the patient perform this exercise for 30 minutes several times a day. After he becomes accustomed to the position and has learned to breathe using his diaphragm, he may apply abdominal weights of 8.8 to 11 lb (4 to 5 kg). The weights enhance the movement of the diaphragm toward the head during expiration.

To enhance the effectiveness of exercise, the patient may also manually compress the lower costal margins, perform straight leg lifts, and coordinate the breathing technique with a physical activity such as walking.

Forced expiration

Explain to the patient that forced expiration helps clear secretions while causing less traumatic injury than does a cough. To perform the technique, tell the patient to forcefully expire without closing his glottis, starting with a mid to low lung volume. Tell him to follow this expiration with a period of diaphragmatic breathing and relaxation.

Inform the patient that if his secretions are in the central airways, he may have to use a more forceful expiration or a cough to clear them.

▶ Replace the used items *so they're ready for the next suctioning* and wash your hands.

Special considerations

▶ If the patient has no history of nasal problems, alternate suctioning between nostrils *to minimize traumatic injury.* If repeated oronasopharyngeal suctioning is required, the use of a nasopharyngeal or oropharyngeal airway will help with catheter insertion, reduce traumatic injury, and promote a patent airway. *To facilitate catheter insertion for oropharyngeal suctioning,* depress the patient's tongue with a tongue blade, or ask another nurse to do so. *This helps you to*

visualize the back of the throat and also prevents the patient from biting the catheter.

▶ If the patient has excessive oral secretions, consider using a tonsil tip catheter *because this allows the patient to remove oral secretions independently.*

▶ Let the patient rest after suctioning while you continue to observe him. The frequency and duration of suctioning depends on the patient's tolerance for the procedure and on any complications.

Home care

Oronasopharyngeal suctioning may be performed in the home using a portable suction machine. Under these circumstances, suctioning is a clean rather than a sterile procedure. Properly cleaned catheters can be reused, putting less financial strain on patients.

Catheters should be cleaned by first washing them in soapy water and then boiling them for 10 minutes or soaking them in 70% alcohol for 3 to 5 minutes. The catheters should then be rinsed with normal saline solution or tap water.

Whether the patient requires disposable or reusable suction equipment, you should make sure that the patient and his caregivers have received proper teaching and support.

Complications
Increased dyspnea caused by hypoxia and anxiety may result from this procedure. Hypoxia can result because oxygen from the oronasopharynx is removed with the secretions. The amount of oxygen removed varies, depending upon the duration of the suctioning, suction flow and pressure, the size of the catheter in relation to the size of the patient's airway, and his physical condition.

In addition, bloody aspirate can result from prolonged or traumatic suctioning. Water-soluble lubricant can help to minimize traumatic injury.

Documentation
Record the date, time, reason for suctioning, and technique used; amount, color, consistency, and odor (if any) of the secretions; the patient's respiratory status before and after the procedure; any complications and the nursing action taken; and the patient's tolerance for the procedure.

OROPHARYNGEAL AIRWAY INSERTION AND CARE

An oropharyngeal airway, a curved rubber or plastic device, is inserted into the mouth to the posterior pharynx to establish or maintain a patent airway. In an unconscious patient, the tongue usually obstructs the posterior pharynx. The oropharyngeal airway conforms to the curvature of the palate, removing the obstruction and allowing air to pass around and through the tube. It also facilitates oropharyngeal suctioning. The oropharyngeal airway is intended for short-term use, as in the postanesthesia or postictal stage. It may be left in place longer as an airway adjunct to prevent the orally intubated patient from biting the endotracheal tube.

The oropharyngeal airway isn't the airway of choice for the patient with loose or avulsed teeth or recent oral surgery. Inserting this airway in the conscious or semiconscious patient may stimulate vomiting and laryngospasm; therefore, you'll usually insert the airway only in the unconscious patient.

Key nursing diagnoses and patient outcomes
Ineffective breathing pattern related to alterations in normal gas exchange
The patient will:
▶ regain and maintain arterial blood gas values within normal limits
▶ regain baseline respiratory rate and maintain stable respirations.

Impaired spontaneous ventilation related to (specify)
The patient will:

▶ show no signs of dyspnea at rest within 24 hours

▶ have a chest X-ray that indicates full lung expansion within 24 hours.

Equipment

For inserting

Oral airway of appropriate size • tongue blade • padded tongue blade •gloves • optional: suction equipment, handheld resuscitation bag or oxygen-powered breathing device

For cleaning

Hydrogen peroxide • water • basin • optional: pipe cleaner

For reflex testing

Cotton-tipped applicator

Preparation of equipment

Select an airway of appropriate size for your patient; an oversized airway can obstruct breathing by depressing the epiglottis into the laryngeal opening. Usually, you'll select a small size (size 1 or 2) for an infant or child, a medium size (size 4 or 5) for the average adult, and a large size (size 6) for the large adult. Be sure to confirm the correct size of the airway by placing the airway flange beside the patient's cheek, parallel to his front teeth. If the airway is the right size, the airway curve should reach to the angle of the jaw.

Implementation

▶ Explain the procedure to the patient even though he may not appear to be alert. Provide privacy and put on gloves *to prevent contact with body fluids.* If the patient is wearing dentures, remove them *so they don't cause further airway obstruction.*

▶ Suction the patient if necessary.

▶ Place the patient in the supine position with his neck hyperextended if this isn't contraindicated.

▶ Insert the airway using the cross-finger or tongue blade technique. (See *Inserting an oral airway.*)

▶ Auscultate the lungs *to ensure adequate ventilation.*

▶ After the airway is inserted, position the patient on his side *to decrease the risk of aspiration of vomitus.*

▶ Perform mouth care every 2 to 4 hours as needed. Begin by holding the patient's jaws open with a padded tongue blade and gently removing the airway. Place the airway in a basin, and rinse it with hydrogen peroxide and then water. If secretions remain, use a pipe cleaner to remove them. Complete standard mouth care and reinsert the airway.

▶ While the airway is removed for mouth care, observe the mouth's mucous membranes *because tissue irritation or ulceration can result from prolonged airway use.*

▶ Frequently check the position of the airway *to ensure correct placement.*

▶ When the patient regains consciousness and is able to swallow, remove the airway by pulling it outward and downward, following the mouth's natural curvature. After the airway is removed, test the patient's cough and gag reflexes *to ensure that removal of the airway wasn't premature and that the patient can maintain his own airway.*

▶ To test for the gag reflex, use a cotton-tipped applicator to touch both sides of the posterior pharynx. To test for the cough reflex, gently touch the posterior oropharynx with the cotton-tipped applicator.

Special considerations

▶ Clear breath sounds on auscultation indicate that the airway is the proper size and in the correct position.

▶ Avoid taping the airway in place *because untaping it could delay airway removal, thus increasing the patient's risk of aspiration.*

▶ Evaluate the patient's behavior *to provide the cue for airway removal.* The patient is likely to gag or cough as he becomes more alert, indicating that he no longer needs the airway.

Complications

Tooth damage or loss, tissue damage, and bleeding may result from insertion. If the airway is too long, it may press the epiglottis against the entrance of the larynx, producing complete airway obstruction. If the airway isn't inserted properly, it may push the tongue posteriorly, aggravating the problem of upper airway obstruction. To prevent traumatic injury, make sure that the patient's lips and tongue aren't between his teeth and the airway.

Immediately after inserting the airway, check for respirations. If respirations are absent or inadequate, initiate artificial positive pressure ventilation by using a mouth-to-mask technique, a handheld resuscitation bag, or an oxygen-powered breathing device. (See "Manual ventilation," page 508.)

Documentation

Record the date and time of the airway's insertion; size of the airway; removal and cleaning of the airway; condition of mucous membranes; any suctioning; any adverse reactions and the nursing action taken; and the patient's tolerance of the procedure.

Inserting an oral airway

Unless this position is contraindicated, hyperextend the patient's head (as shown below) before using either the cross-finger or tongue blade insertion method.

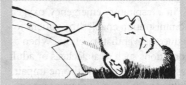

To insert an oral airway using the cross-finger method, place your thumb on the patient's lower teeth and your index finger on his upper teeth. Gently open his mouth by pushing his teeth apart (as shown below).

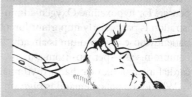

Insert the airway upside down to avoid pushing the tongue toward the pharynx, and slide it over the tongue toward the back of the mouth. Rotate the airway as it approaches the posterior wall of the pharynx so that it points downward (as shown below).

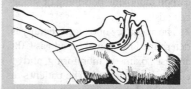

To use the tongue blade technique, open the patient's mouth and depress his tongue with the blade. Guide the airway over the back of the tongue as you did for the cross-finger technique.

OXYGEN ADMINISTRATION, ADULT

A patient will need oxygen therapy when hypoxemia results from a respiratory or cardiac emergency or an increase in metabolic function.

In a respiratory emergency, oxygen administration enables the patient to reduce his ventilatory effort. When conditions such as atelectasis or adult respiratory distress syndrome impair diffusion, or when lung volumes are decreased from alveolar hypoventilation, this procedure boosts alveolar oxygen levels.

In a cardiac emergency, oxygen therapy helps meet the increased myocardial workload as the heart tries to compensate for hypoxemia. Oxygen administration is particularly important for a patient whose myocardium is already compromised — perhaps from a myocardial infarction or cardiac arrhythmia.

When metabolic demand is high (in cases of massive trauma, burns, or high fever, for instance) oxygen administration supplies the body with enough oxygen to meet its cellular needs. This procedure also increases oxygenation in the patient with a reduced blood oxygen-carrying capacity, perhaps from carbon monoxide poisoning or sickle cell crisis.

The adequacy of oxygen therapy is determined by arterial blood gas (ABG) analysis, oximetry monitoring, and clinical examinations. The patient's disease, physical condition, and age will help determine the most appropriate method of administration.

Key nursing diagnoses and patient outcomes

Impaired gas exchange related to altered oxygen supply
The patient will:
▶ maintain a respiratory rate within 5 breaths/minute of baseline
▶ express feelings of comfort while maintaining air exchange
▶ have normal breath sounds
▶ restore baseline ABG levels: (specify) pH; (specify) partial pressure of arterial oxygen; and (specify) partial pressure of carbon dioxide.

Ineffective breathing pattern related to (specify)
The patient will:
▶ achieve maximum lung expansion with adequate ventilation.

Equipment

The equipment needed depends on the type of delivery system ordered. (See *Guide to oxygen delivery systems,* pages 580 to 583.) Equipment generally includes selections from the following list: oxygen source (wall unit, cylinder, liquid tank, or concentrator) • flowmeter • adapter, if using a wall unit, or a pressure-reduction gauge, if using a cylinder • sterile humidity bottle and adapters • sterile distilled water • OXYGEN PRECAUTION sign • appropriate oxygen delivery system (a nasal cannula, simple mask, partial rebreather mask, or nonrebreather mask for low-flow and variable oxygen concentrations; a Venturi mask, aerosol mask, T tube, tracheostomy collar, tent, or oxygen hood for high-flow and specific oxygen concentrations) • small-diameter and large-diameter connection tubing • flashlight (for nasal cannula) •

water-soluble lubricant • gauze pads and tape (for oxygen masks) • jet adapter for Venturi mask (if adding humidity) • optional: oxygen analyzer

Preparation of equipment

Although a respiratory therapist typically is responsible for setting up, maintaining, and managing the equipment, you'll need a working knowledge of the oxygen system being used.

Check the oxygen outlet port *to verify flow.* Pinch the tubing near the prongs *to ensure that an audible alarm will sound if the oxygen flow stops.*

Implementation

▶ Assess the patient's condition. In an emergency situation, verify that he has an open airway before administering oxygen.

▶ Explain the procedure to the patient, and let him know why he needs oxygen *to ensure his cooperation.*

▶ Check the patient's room *to make sure it's safe for oxygen administration.* Whenever possible, replace electrical devices with nonelectric ones.

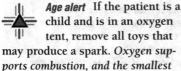 *Age alert* If the patient is a child and is in an oxygen tent, remove all toys that may produce a spark. *Oxygen supports combustion, and the smallest spark can cause a fire.*

▶ Place an OXYGEN PRECAUTION sign over the patient's bed and on the door to his room.

▶ Help place the oxygen delivery device on the patient. Make sure it fits properly and is stable.

▶ Monitor the patient's response to oxygen therapy. Check his ABG values during initial adjustments of oxygen flow. When the patient is stabilized, you may use pulse oximetry instead. Check the patient frequently for signs of hypoxia, such as decreased level of consciousness, increased heart rate, arrhythmias, restlessness, perspiration, dyspnea, use of accessory muscles, yawning or flared nostrils, cyanosis, and cool, clammy skin.

▶ Observe the patient's skin integrity *to prevent skin breakdown on pressure points from the oxygen delivery device.* Wipe moisture or perspiration from the patient's face and from the mask as needed.

▶ If the patient will be receiving oxygen at a concentration above 60% for more than 24 hours, watch carefully for signs of oxygen toxicity. Remind the patient to cough and deep-breathe frequently *to prevent atelectasis.* Also, *to prevent the development of serious lung damage,* measure ABG values repeatedly *to determine whether high oxygen concentrations are still necessary.*

Special considerations

⚡■⚡ *Nursing alert* Never administer oxygen by nasal cannula at more than 2 L/minute to a patient with chronic lung disease unless you have a specific order to do so. *That is because some patients with chronic lung disease become dependent on a state of hypercapnia and hypoxia to stimulate their respirations, and supplemental oxygen could cause them to stop breathing.* However, long-term oxygen therapy of 12 to 17 hours daily may help patients with chronic lung disease sleep better, survive longer, and experience a reduced incidence of pulmonary hypertension.

(Text continues on page 583.)

Guide to oxygen delivery systems

Patients may receive oxygen through one of several administration systems. Each has its own benefits, drawbacks, and indications for use. The advantages and disadvantages of each system are compared here.

Nasal cannula

Oxygen is delivered through plastic cannulas in the patient's nostrils.

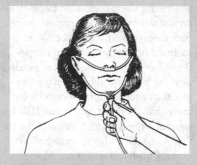

Simple mask

Oxygen flows through an entry port at the bottom of the mask and exits through large holes on the sides of the mask.

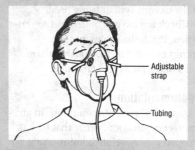

Adjustable strap

Tubing

Advantages

Safe and simple; comfortable and easily tolerated; nasal prongs can be shaped to fit any face; effective for low oxygen concentrations; allows movement, eating, and talking; inexpensive and disposable.

Disadvantages

Can't deliver concentrations higher than 40%; can't be used in complete nasal obstruction; may cause headaches or dry mucous membranes if flow rate exceeds 6 L/minute; can dislodge easily.

Administration guidelines

Ensure the patency of the patient's nostrils with a flashlight. If patent, hook the cannula tubing behind the patient's ears and under the chin. Slide the adjuster upward under the chin to secure the tubing. If using an elastic strap to secure the cannula, position it over the ears and around the back of the head. Avoid applying it too tightly, which can result in excess pressure on facial structures as well as cannula occlusion. With a nasal cannula, oral breathers achieve the same oxygen delivery as nasal breathers.

Advantages

Can deliver concentrations of 40% to 60%.

Disadvantages

Hot and confining; may irritate patient's skin; tight seal, which may cause discomfort, is required for higher oxygen concentration; interferes with talking and eating; impractical for long-term therapy because of imprecision.

Administration guidelines

Select the mask size that offers the best fit. Place the mask over the patient's nose, mouth, and chin, and mold the flexible metal edge to the bridge of the nose. Adjust the elastic band around the head to hold the mask firmly but comfortably over the cheeks, chin, and bridge of the nose. For elderly or cachectic patients with sunken cheeks, tape gauze pads to the mask over the cheek area to try to create an airtight seal. Without this seal, room air dilutes the oxygen, preventing delivery of the prescribed concentration. A minimum of 5 L/minute is required in all masks to flush expired carbon dioxide from the mask so that the patient doesn't rebreathe it.

Guide to oxygen delivery systems *(continued)*

Partial rebreather mask

The patient inspires oxygen from a reservoir bag along with atmospheric air and oxygen from the mask. The first third of exhaled tidal volume enters the bag; the rest exits the mask. Because air entering the reservoir bag comes from the trachea and bronchi, where no gas exchange occurs, the patient rebreathes the oxygenated air he just exhaled.

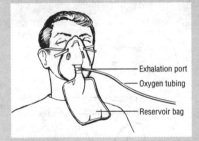

Exhalation port
Oxygen tubing
Reservoir bag

Advantages

Effectively delivers concentrations of 40% to 60%; openings in the mask allow patient to inhale room air if oxygen source fails.

Disadvantages

Tight seal required for accurate oxygen concentration may cause discomfort; interferes with eating and talking; hot and confining; may irritate skin; bag may twist or kink; impractical for long-term therapy.

Administration guidelines

Follow the procedures listed for the simple mask. If the reservoir bag collapses more than slightly during inspiration, raise the flow rate until you see only a slight deflation. Marked or complete deflation indicates insufficient oxygen flow, which could result in carbon dioxide accumulation in the mask and bag. Keep the reservoir bag from twisting or kinking. Ensure free expansion by making sure the bag lies outside the patient's gown and bedcovers.

Nonrebreather mask

On inhalation, the one-way inspiratory valve opens, directing oxygen from a reservoir bag into the mask. On exhalation, gas exits the mask through the one-way expiratory valves and enters the atmosphere. The patient breathes air only from the bag.

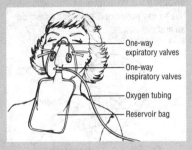

One-way expiratory valves
One-way inspiratory valves
Oxygen tubing
Reservoir bag

Advantages

Delivers the highest possible oxygen concentration (60% to 90%) short of intubation and mechanical ventilation; effective for short-term therapy; doesn't dry mucous membranes; can be converted to a partial rebreather mask, if necessary, by removing the one-way valve.

Disadvantages

Requires a tight seal, which may be difficult to maintain and may cause discomfort; may irritate the patient's skin; interferes with talking and eating; impractical for long-term therapy.

Administration guidelines

Follow procedures listed for the simple mask. Make sure that the mask fits very snugly and that the one-way valves are secure and functioning. Because the mask excludes room air, a valve malfunction could cause carbon dioxide buildup and suffocate an unconscious patient. If the reservoir bag collapses more than slightly during inspiration, raise the flow rate until you see only a slight deflation. Marked or complete deflation indicates an insufficient

(continued)

Guide to oxygen delivery systems *(continued)*

flow rate. Keep the reservoir bag from twisting or kinking. Ensure free expansion by making sure the bag lies outside the patient's gown and bedcovers.

CPAP mask

This system allows the spontaneously breathing patient to receive continuous positive airway pressure (CPAP) with or without an artificial airway.

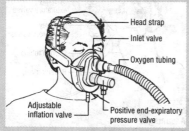

- Head strap
- Inlet valve
- Oxygen tubing
- Adjustable inflation valve
- Positive end-expiratory pressure valve

Advantages

Noninvasively improves arterial oxygenation by increasing functional residual capacity; allows the patient to avoid intubation; allows the patient to talk and cough without interrupting positive pressure.

Disadvantages

Requires a tight fit, which may cause discomfort; interferes with eating and talking; heightened risk of aspiration if the patient vomits; increased risk of pneumothorax, diminished cardiac output, and gastric distention; contraindicated in patients with chronic obstructive pulmonary disease, bullous lung disease, low cardiac output, or tension pneumothorax.

Administration guidelines

Place one strap behind the patient's head and the other strap over his head to ensure a snug fit. Attach one latex strap to the connector prong on one side of the mask. Then use one hand to position the mask on the patient's face while using the other hand to connect the strap to the other side of the mask.

After the mask is applied, assess the patient's respiratory, circulatory, and GI function every hour. Watch for signs of pneumothorax, decreased cardiac output, a drop in blood pressure, and gastric distention.

Transtracheal oxygen

The patient receives oxygen through a catheter inserted into the base of his neck in a simple outpatient procedure.

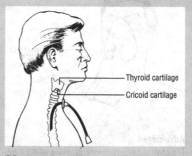

- Thyroid cartilage
- Cricoid cartilage

Advantages

Supplies oxygen to the lungs throughout the respiratory cycle; provides continuous oxygen without hindering mobility; doesn't interfere with eating or talking; doesn't dry mucous membranes; catheter can easily be concealed by a shirt or scarf.

Disadvantages

Not suitable for use in patients at risk for bleeding or those with severe bronchospasm, uncompensated respiratory acidosis, pleural herniation into the base of the neck, or high corticosteroid dosages.

Administration guidelines

After insertion, obtain a chest X-ray to confirm placement. Monitor the patient for bleeding, respiratory distress, pneumothorax, pain, coughing, or hoarseness. Don't use the catheter for about 1 week following insertion to decrease the risk of subcutaneous emphysema.

Guide to oxygen delivery systems *(continued)*

Venturi mask

The mask is connected to a Venturi device, which mixes a specific volume of air and oxygen.

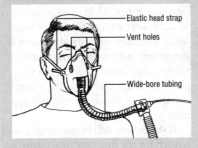

Elastic head strap
Vent holes
Wide-bore tubing

Advantages
Delivers highly accurate oxygen concentration despite the patient's respiratory pattern because the same amount of air is always entrained; dilute jets can be changed or dial turned to change oxygen concentration; doesn't dry mucous membranes; humidity or aerosol can be added.

Disadvantages
Confining and may irritate skin; oxygen concentration may be altered if mask fits loosely, tubing kinks, oxygen intake ports become blocked, flow is insufficient, or patient is hyperpneic; interferes with eating and talking; condensate may collect and drip on the patient if humidification is used.

Administration guidelines
Make sure that the oxygen flow rate is set at the amount specified on each mask and that the Venturi valve is set for the desired fraction of inspired oxygen.

Aerosols

A face mask, hood, tent, or tracheostomy tube or collar is connected to wide-bore tubing that receives aerosolized oxygen from a jet nebulizer. The jet nebulizer, which is attached near the oxygen source, adjusts air entrainment in a manner similar to the Venturi device.

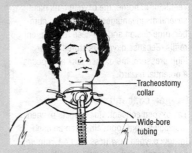

Tracheostomy collar
Wide-bore tubing

Advantages
Administers high humidity; gas can be heated (when delivered through artificial airway) or cooled (when delivered through a tent).

Disadvantages
Condensate collected in the tracheostomy collar or T tube may drain into the tracheostomy; the weight of the T tube can put stress on the tracheostomy tube.

Administration guidelines
Guidelines vary with the type of nebulizer used: ultrasonic, large-volume, small-volume, and in-line types. When using a high-output nebulizer, watch for signs of overhydration, pulmonary edema, crackles, and electrolyte imbalance.

▶ When monitoring a patient's response to a change in oxygen flow, check the pulse oximetry monitor or measure ABG values 20 to 30 minutes after adjusting the flow. In the interim, monitor the patient closely for any adverse response to the change in oxygen flow.

Home care
Before discharging a patient who will receive oxygen therapy at home, make

Types of home oxygen therapy

Oxygen therapy can be administered at home using an oxygen tank, an oxygen concentrator, or liquid oxygen.

Oxygen tank
Commonly used for patients who need oxygen on a standby basis or who need a ventilator at home, the oxygen tank has several disadvantages, including its cumbersome design and the need for frequent refills. Because oxygen is stored under high pressure, the oxygen tank also poses a potential hazard.

Oxygen concentrator
The oxygen concentrator extracts oxygen molecules from room air. It can be used for low oxygen flow (less than 4 L/minute) and doesn't need to be refilled with oxygen. However, because the oxygen concentrator runs on electricity, it won't function during a power failure.

Liquid oxygen
This option is commonly used by patients who are oxygen-dependent but still mobile. The liquid oxygen system includes a large liquid reservoir for home use. When the patient wants to leave the house, he fills a portable unit worn over the shoulder; this supplies oxygen for up to several hours, depending on the liter flow.

If the patient will be receiving transtracheal oxygen therapy, teach him how to properly clean and care for the catheter. Advise him to keep the skin surrounding the insertion site clean and dry *to prevent infection.*

No matter which device the patient uses, you'll need to evaluate his and his family members' ability and motivation to administer oxygen therapy at home. Make sure they understand the reason the patient is receiving oxygen and the safety issues involved in oxygen administration. Teach them how to properly use and clean the equipment and supplies.

If the patient will be discharged with oxygen for the first time, make sure his health insurance covers home oxygen. If it doesn't, find out what criteria he must meet to obtain coverage. Without a third-party payer, he may not be able to afford home oxygen therapy.

Documentation
Record the date and time of oxygen administration; the type of delivery device used; the oxygen flow rate; the patient's vital signs, skin color, respiratory effort, and breath sounds; the patient's response before and after initiation of therapy; and any patient or family teaching that you provided.

OXYGEN ADMINISTRATION, NEONATAL

The neonate with signs and symptoms of respiratory distress—such as cyanosis, pallor, tachypnea, nasal flaring, bradycardia, hypothermia, retractions, hypotonia, hyporeflexia, expiratory

sure you're familiar with the types of oxygen therapy, the kinds of services that are available, and the service schedules offered by local home suppliers. Together with the doctor and the patient, choose the device that is best-suited to the patient. (See *Types of home oxygen therapy.*)

grunting, and arterial blood gas (ABG) levels indicating hypoxia—will probably need oxygen. Because of his small size and special respiratory requirements, he'll also need special equipment and administration techniques.

In an emergency, for instance, a handheld resuscitation bag and a small oxygen mask may be sufficient until more permanent measures can be initiated. When the neonate requires additional oxygen above the ambient concentration, the oxygen can be delivered by means of an oxygen hood or nasal prongs. If he needs continuous positive airway pressure (CPAP) to prevent alveolar collapse at the end of a breath (as in respiratory distress syndrome), he may receive oxygen through a nasopharyngeal or an endotracheal (ET) tube. (Oxygenation typically improves with CPAP and any pulmonary shunting tends to decrease.) If the neonate can't breathe on his own or needs to conserve his energy, he may receive oxygen through a ventilator.

No matter which system delivers the oxygen, the therapy is potentially hazardous to the neonate. The gas must be warmed and humidified to prevent hypothermia and dehydration. In high concentrations over prolonged periods, oxygen can cause retrolental fibroplasia (which results in blindness). If the concentration is too low, hypoxia and central nervous system damage may occur. Also, depending on how it's delivered, oxygen can contribute to bronchopulmonary dysplasia.

In some cases, extracorporeal membrane oxygenation, an alternative to oxygen administration, may help neonates who have severe hypoxia. This technique also relies on a supplemental oxygen source. (See *Extracorporeal membrane oxygenation.*)

For neonates who require long-term oxygen therapy at home, special delivery systems are available. (See *Comparing home oxygen delivery systems,* page 586.)

Key nursing diagnoses and patient outcomes

Impaired gas exchange related to altered oxygen supply
The patient will:
▶ maintain a respiratory rate within 5 breaths/minute of baseline
▶ express feeling of comfort while maintaining air exchange
▶ have normal breath sounds
▶ restore baseline ABG levels: (specify) pH; (specify) partial pressure of arterial

Extracorporeal membrane oxygenation

Available in designated centers throughout the United States, extracorporeal membrane oxygenation (ECMO) was developed from cardiopulmonary bypass methods used during heart surgery. In this procedure, a machine circulates the patient's venous blood outside his body, passes the blood through a membrane oxygenator, and returns the newly oxygenated blood to the circulation. ECMO circuitry works by veno-arterial bypass or veno-venous bypass methods.

For neonates who meet stringent criteria, indications for ECMO include hyaline membrane disease, meconium aspiration, and congenital heart defects. Typically, the procedure is used as a last resort after maximum ventilatory support measures fail and when survival chances drop below 10%.

Comparing home oxygen delivery systems

If a neonate in your care is discharged on oxygen, the delivery system prescribed may depend on such factors as equipment availability and parental skill levels. Other factors to consider include the liter flow (or oxygen concentration) required and appropriate administration equipment, for example, nasal cannula or catheter, oxygen hood, tent, high-flow mask, or nebulizer.

The nasal cannula, which provides a direct flow of oxygen to the nostrils, is the most common oxygen delivery device for home use. It imposes the fewest restrictions on a child attempting to interact with the environment. For instance, attaching extension tubing (up to 50′ [15 m]) to the cannula allows the child to move freely from room to room. However, the cannula can become dislodged from the nostrils with extensive manipulation. Velcro straps or adhesive dressings can reduce this risk by securing the cannula in the proper position.

Common oxygen sources include the oxygen concentrator, cylinder oxygen, and liquid oxygen. When selecting the appropriate system for home care, the health care team looks at advantages and disadvantages, such as those that follow.

System	Advantages	Disadvantages
Oxygen concentrator Separates oxygen from ambient air and provides low-flow oxygen	■ Cost-effective for the neonate who needs continuous low-flow oxygen	■ Can't be used with a high-flow mask or nebulizer ■ Requires electricity ■ Requires an oxygen cylinder as a backup in case of malfunction or power failure ■ Bulky and noisy ■ Emits heat
Cylinder oxygen Uses oxygen stored as a gas in a cylinder with a valve	■ Cost-effective for the neonate who requires high-flow oxygen or intermittent oxygen for up to 12 hours daily ■ Can be used with a high-flow oxygen mask, a nasal cannula, a nasal catheter, or a nebulizer ■ Portable when a small cylinder is used	■ Requires a humidification source if the flow must exceed 0.75 L ■ Must be used with caution and kept in a stand or cart; safety cap must be fastened securely in case the neonate falls
Liquid oxygen Uses oxygen stored in a liquid state under high pressure in a cylinder with a valve	■ Cost-effective for the neonate who needs continuous low- to moderate-flow oxygen ■ Usually can be used with any oxygen delivery method ■ Smaller and more lightweight than other oxygen systems ■ Refillable, portable units available for when the neonate travels	■ Humidification source required if flow must exceed 0.75 L ■ May cause burns if oxygen comes into contact with skin during transfer from a stationary to a portable unit ■ Upright position required for cylinder

oxygen, and (specify) partial pressure of carbon dioxide.

Ineffective breathing pattern related to (specify)
The patient will:
▶ achieve maximum lung expansion with adequate ventilation.

Equipment

Oxygen source (wall, cylinder, or liquid unit) • compressed air source • flowmeters • nasal prongs • blender or Y-connector • large- and small-bore oxygen tubing (sterile) • warming-humidifying device • oxygen analyzer • thermometer • stethoscope • nasogastric (NG) tube

For handheld resuscitation bag and mask delivery

Specially sized mask with handheld resuscitation bag • manometer with connectors (resuscitation bag must have pressure-release valve)

For oxygen hood delivery

Appropriate-sized oxygen hood

For nasal prong delivery

Nasal prongs • water-soluble lubricant

For CPAP delivery

Manometer with connectors • nasopharyngeal or ET tube • hypoallergenic tape

For delivery with a ventilator

Ventilator unit with manometer and in-line thermometer • specimen tubes for ABG analyses • ET tube • optional: pulse oximeter or transcutaneous oxygen monitor

Preparation of equipment

Wash your hands. Gather the necessary equipment, and assemble it conveniently.

To calibrate the oxygen analyzer

Turn the analyzer on and read the results. Room air should be about 21% oxygen. Check the analyzer power or battery level. Expose the analyzer probe to 100% oxygen and adjust sensitivity as necessary. Then recheck the amount of oxygen in room air.

To set up a handheld resuscitation bag and mask

Place the resuscitation bag and mask in the crib. Connect the large-bore oxygen tubing to the mask outlet. Then use connectors and small-bore tubing to connect a manometer to the bag. Next, connect the free end of the oxygen tubing to the warming-humidifying device, and fill the device with sterile water. Turn on the device when you're ready to use it, or prepare it according to the manufacturer's instructions.

Connect another piece of small-bore tubing to the inlet of the warming-humidifying device. Attach a Y-connector to the opposite end of this tubing. Place a piece of small-bore tubing on each end of the Y-connector, and connect the pieces of tubing to the flowmeters. Place an in-line thermometer as close as possible to the delivery end of the apparatus.

To set up an oxygen hood

Bring a clean oxygen hood and tubing if needed to the neonate's bedside. If the neonate was receiving oxygen via bag and mask, remove them from the connecting tubing. Attach the oxygen hood to this tubing. Place an in-line thermometer as close to the neonate as possible whenever using warmed oxygen.

Implementation

▶ Always wash your hands before working with a neonate *to prevent cross-contamination from handling other neonates.*

Using a handheld resuscitation bag and mask

▶ Turn on the oxygen and compressed air flowmeters to the prescribed flow rates.

▶ Place the mask on the neonate's face. Don't cover the neonate's eyes. Check pressure settings and mask size *to ensure that air doesn't leak from the mask's edges.*

▶ As you work to stabilize the neonate, have another staff member notify the doctor immediately.

▶ Provide 40 to 60 breaths/minute. Use enough pressure to cause a visible rise and fall of the neonate's chest. Provide enough oxygen to maintain pink nail beds and mucous membranes. If you can't reach the doctor during the emergency, deliver the oxygen percentage defined by your facility's emergency policy.

▶ Continuously watch the neonate's chest movements and listen to breath sounds. Avoid overventilation, *which will blow off too much carbon dioxide and cause apnea.* If the neonate's heart rate falls below 100 beats/minute and fails to rise, continue to use the handheld resuscitation bag until the heart rate rises to 100 beats/minute or higher.

▶ Insert an NG tube *to vent air from the neonate's stomach.*

Using an oxygen hood

▶ Remove the connecting tubing from the face mask and connect it to the oxygen hood. Activate oxygen and a compressed air source, if needed, at ordered flow rates.

▶ Place the oxygen hood over the neonate's head.

▶ Measure the amount of oxygen the neonate is receiving with the oxygen analyzer. Be sure to place the analyzer probe close to the neonate's nose. Adjust the oxygen to the prescribed amount.

Using nasal prongs

▶ Match the prong size to the neonate's nose. Apply a small amount of water-soluble lubricant to the outside of the prongs. Turn on the oxygen and compressed air, if necessary. Connect the prongs to the oxygen tubing. Insert the prongs into the nose and steady them.

▶ Clean the prongs each shift *to ensure patency.*

Using CPAP

▶ Position the neonate on his back with a rolled towel under his neck *to keep the airway open without hyperextending the neck.*

▶ If you're administering oxygen through a nasopharyngeal or an ET tube, obtain the correct size tube. Turn on the oxygen and compressed air source. Then assist the doctor with inserting the ET tube, attaching the oxygen delivery system (as set up for mask and bag delivery), and taping the tube in place. Next, insert an NG or orogastric tube, and leave it in place *to keep the stomach decompressed,* if ordered. Leave it open unless the neonate is receiving gavage feedings. Suction the nasal passages and oropharynx every 2 hours or as needed *to maintain an open airway.* Apply suction only while removing the suction catheter.

Using a ventilator

▶ Turn on the ventilator and set the controls as ordered.

▶ Help the doctor insert the ET tube if appropriate.

▶ Connect the ET tube to the ventilator, and tape the tube securely.

▶ As with any delivery system, carefully watch the manometer *to maintain pressure at the prescribed level.* Also monitor the in-line thermometer *for correct temperature.*

▶ Monitor ABG levels every 15 to 20 minutes (or other reasonable interval) after any changes in oxygen concentration or pressure. Draw blood samples for ABG analysis from an umbilical artery catheter, radial artery catheter, or radial artery puncture. If desired, obtain capillary blood by warmed heel stick — this provides accurate levels of pH and carbon dioxide, but not oxygen. If ordered, monitor oxygen perfusion with transcutaneous oxygen monitoring, pulse oximetry, or mixed venous oxygen saturation monitoring.

▶ Keep the doctor aware of ABG levels *so he can order appropriate changes in oxygen concentration.* Usually, partial pressure of oxygen is maintained at 60 to 90 mm Hg for an arterial sample and at 40 to 60 mm Hg for a capillary sample.

▶ Auscultate the lungs for crackles, rhonchi, and bilateral breath sounds.

Special considerations

▶ When administering oxygen, always take safety precautions *to avoid fire or explosion.* As soon as possible, explain the situation and the procedures to the parents. Take measures to keep the neonate warm *because hypothermia impedes respiration.*

▶ Check ABG levels at least every hour whenever the unstable neonate receives high oxygen concentrations or experiences a clinical change. If he doesn't respond to oxygen administration, check for congenital anomalies.

▶ Perform neonatal chest auscultation carefully *to hear subtle respiratory changes.* Also be alert for respiratory distress signs, and be prepared to perform emergency procedures. If required, perform chest physiotherapy and percussion as ordered. Follow with suctioning *to remove secretions.* As ordered, discontinue oxygen when the neonate's fraction of inspired oxygen (FIO_2) reaches room air level and his arterial oxygen stabilizes at 60 to 90 mm Hg. Repeat ABG analysis 20 to 30 minutes after discontinuing oxygen and thereafter as ordered by the doctor or by facility policy.

▶ If the neonate will receive oxygen over a lengthy time span, prepare his parents or other caregivers to administer oxygen at home.

Complications

Infection or "drowning" can result from overhumidification, which allows water to collect in tubing and then provides a growth medium for bacteria or suffocates the neonate. Hypothermia and increased oxygen consumption can result from administering cool oxygen. Metabolic and respiratory acidosis may follow inadequate ventilation.

Pressure ulcers may develop on the neonate's head, face, and around the nose during prolonged oxygen therapy. A pulmonary air leak (pneumothorax, pneumomediastinum, pneumopericardium, interstitial emphysema) may develop spontaneously with respiratory distress or result from forced ventilation. Decreased cardiac output may come from excessive CPAP.

Documentation

Note any respiratory distress that requires oxygen administration, the oxygen concentration given, and the delivery method. Record each change in oxygen concentration and the neonate's FIO_2 as measured by the oxygen analyzer. Note all routine checks of oxygen concentration. Document all ABG values, the times that samples were obtained, the neonate's condition during therapy, times suctioned, the amount and consistency of mucus, the type of continuous oxygen monitoring (if any), and any complications. Note respiratory rate, and describe breath sounds and any signs of additional respiratory distress.

OXYTOCIN ADMINISTRATION

The hormone oxytocin stimulates the uterus to contract, thereby facilitating cervical dilation. The doctor may order synthetic oxytocin (Pitocin or Syntocinon) to induce or augment labor or to control bleeding and enhance uterine contraction after the placenta is delivered. Usually, the nurse administers oxytocin I.V. To regulate dosage and to help prevent uterine hyperstimulation, she always uses an infusion pump. Additional nursing responsibilities include managing the infusion and monitoring maternal and fetal responses.

Indications for oxytocin administration include pregnancy-induced hypertension, prolonged gestation, maternal diabetes, Rh sensitization, premature or prolonged rupture of membranes, incomplete or inevitable abortion, and evaluation of fetal distress after 31 weeks' gestation.

Contraindications include placenta previa, diagnosed cephalopelvic disproportion, fetal distress, prior classic uterine incision or uterine surgery, or active genital herpes. Oxytocin should be administered cautiously to a patient who has an overdistended uterus or a history of cervical surgery, uterine surgery, or grand multiparity.

Key nursing diagnoses and patient outcomes

Anxiety related to an unknown procedure
The patient will:
▶ express feelings of anxiety
▶ identify and use available emotional support systems
▶ show fewer signs of anxiety
▶ identify positive aspects of efforts to cope during childbirth.

Deficient knowledge related to lack of exposure to oxytocin administration
The patient will:
▶ state an understanding of the procedure
▶ demonstrate the ability to perform skills needed for coping with labor.

Equipment

Administration set for primary I.V. line • infusion pump and tubing • I.V. solution as ordered • external or internal fetal monitoring equipment • oxytocin • 20G 1″ needle • needleless adapter • label • venipuncture equipment with an 18G through-the-needle catheter • optional: autosyringe

Preparation of equipment

Prepare the oxytocin solution as ordered. Rotate the I.V. bag *to disperse the drug throughout the solution.* Label the I.V. container with the name of the medication. Attach the infusion pump tubing to the I.V. container and connect the tubing to the pump.

Because infusion pump features vary, review the operator's manual before proceeding. Attach the 20G 1″ needle to the tubing to piggyback it to the primary I.V. line. Or, if using a needleless system, attach the infusion pump tubing to a needleless adapter, then connect the adapter to the primary I.V. line, or use an autosyringe connected to the primary I.V. line. Then set up the equipment for internal or external fetal monitoring.

Implementation

▶ Explain the procedure to the patient and provide privacy. Wash your hands. Describe the equipment, and forewarn the patient that she may feel a pinch from the venipuncture.

Administering oxytocin during labor and delivery

▶ Help the patient to a lateral-tilt position, and support her hip with a pillow. Don't let her lie in a supine position. *In the supine position, the gravid uterus presses on the maternal great vessels, producing maternal hypotension and reduced uterine perfusion.*
▶ Identify and record the fetal heart rate (FHR), and assess uterine contractions occurring in a 20-minute span *to establish baseline fetal status and evaluate spontaneous maternal uterine activity.*
▶ Start the primary I.V. line using an 18G through-the-needle catheter. Use

this line to deliver oxytocin and fluids, blood, or other medications as needed.
▶ Piggyback the oxytocin solution (metered by the infusion pump) to the primary I.V. line at the Y injection site closest to the patient. *Piggybacking maintains I.V. line patency (which you'll need to preserve should you discontinue the oxytocin infusion). Also, using the Y injection site nearest the venipuncture ensures that the primary line holds the lowest concentration of oxytocin if you must stop the infusion.*
▶ Begin the oxytocin infusion as ordered. The typical recommended labor-starting dosage is 0.5 to 1.0 milliunit (mU)/minute. (The maximum dosage is 20 mU/minute.)
▶ *Because oxytocin begins acting immediately*, be prepared to start monitoring uterine contractions.
▶ Increase the oxytocin dosage as ordered. As a rule, each increase should range no more than 1 to 2 mU/minute infused once every 30 to 60 minutes. When induced labor simulates normal labor (contractions occurring every 2 to 3 minutes and lasting 40 to 60 seconds) and cervical dilation progresses at least 1 cm/hour in first-stage, active-phase labor, you can stop increases. However, continue the infusion at the dosage and rate that maintain the activity closest to normal labor.
▶ Before each increase, be sure to time the frequency and duration of contractions, palpate the uterus *to identify contraction intensity,* and assess maternal vital signs and fetal heart rhythm and rate *to ensure safety and to anticipate possible complications.* If you're using an external fetal monitor, the uterine activity strip or grid should show contractions occurring every 2 to 3 minutes. The contractions should last for about 60 sec-

Conversion formulas for oxytocin administration

To ensure that all members of the health care team speak the same language when administering oxytocin, use the following formulas, as needed, to convert milliliters (ml) per minute or drops (gtt) per minute to milliunits (mU) per minute. Conversion to mU per minute gives the actual drug dosage instead of the fluid dosage.

Which conversion formula you use may be dictated by the infusion pump you use.

Synthetic oxytocin for I.V. administration comes in a concentration of 10 units/ml in 10-ml vials, in 0.5- and 1-ml ampules, and in 1-ml disposable syringes.

To calculate oxytocin dilution (in mU/ml):

$$\frac{\text{\# of units oxytocin}}{\text{ml of fluid}} \times 1{,}000 = \frac{mU}{ml}$$

To convert ml/minute to mU/minute:

$$\frac{mU}{ml} \times \frac{ml}{minute} = \frac{mU}{minute}$$

To convert gtt/minute to mU/minute:

$$\frac{gtt}{minute} \times \frac{mU}{ml} \times \frac{ml}{gtt} = \frac{mU}{minute}$$

onds and be followed by uterine relaxation. If you're using an internal fetal monitor, look for an optimal baseline value ranging from 5 to 15 mm Hg. Your aim is to verify uterine relaxation between contractions.

▶ Assist with comfort measures, such as repositioning the patient on her other side, as needed.

▶ Continue assessing maternal and fetal responses to the oxytocin. For example, every 10 to 15 minutes, evaluate FHR, maternal response to increased contraction activity and subsequent discomfort, and maternal pulse rate and pattern, blood pressure, respiration rate and quality, and uterine contractions. Also, review the infusion rate *to prevent uterine hyperstimulation*. Signs of hyperstimulation include contractions less than 2 minutes apart and lasting 90 seconds or longer, uterine pressure that doesn't return to baseline between contractions, and intrauterine pressure that rises over 75 mm Hg.

▶ *To reduce uterine irritability*, try to increase uterine blood flow. Do this by changing the patient's position and increasing the infusion rate of the primary I.V. line. Avoid exceeding the maximum total infusion of 20 mU/minute.

▶ *To manage hyperstimulation*, discontinue the infusion, administer oxygen, and notify the doctor.

▶ After hyperstimulation resolves, resume the oxytocin infusion. Depending on maternal and fetal conditions, select one of the following methods: Resume the infusion beginning with oxytocin 0.5 mU/minute, increase the dosage to 1 mU/minute every 15 minutes, and increase the rate as before; or resume the infusion at one-half of the last dosage given and increase the rate as before; or resume the infusion at the dosage given before hyperstimulation signs occurred. Check your facility's policy for the appropriate method.

▶ Monitor and record intake and output. Output should be at least 30 ml/hour. Oxytocin has an antidiuretic effect at rates of 16 mU/minute and more, so you may need to administer an electrolyte-containing I.V. solution *to maintain electrolyte balance.*

Administering oxytocin after delivery

▶ As ordered after delivery, administer 10 to 40 units of oxytocin added to 1,000 ml of physiologic electrolyte solution. Infuse at a rate titrated to decrease postpartum bleeding or uterine atony after placental delivery. As an alternative, administer 10 units of oxytocin I.M. until you can establish the I.V. line.

Special considerations

▶ Most health care facilities require the use of an infusion pump to ensure accurate dosage and titration. (See *Conversion formulas for oxytocin administration.*)
▶ Without an infusion pump, administer oxytocin through a minidrop system (60 drops/ml) or an autosyringe, and observe the patient closely. Without an electronic fetal monitor, frequently palpate and assess contractions. Auscultate FHR every 5 to 15 minutes.

Complications

Oxytocin can cause uterine hyperstimulation that may progress to tetanic contractions, which last longer than 2 minutes. Other potential complications include fetal distress, abruptio placentae, and uterine rupture.

Watch for signs of oxytocin hypersensitivity such as elevated blood pressure. Rarely, oxytocin leads to maternal seizures or coma from water intoxication.

Documentation

Record maternal response to contractions, blood pressure, pulse rate and pattern, and respiratory rate and quality on the labor progression chart. Also document FHR, oxytocin infusion rate, and intake and output amounts. Describe uterine activity as well.

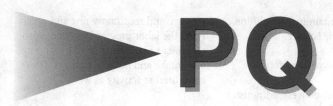

PACEMAKER INSERTION AND CARE, PERMANENT

Designed to operate for 3 to 20 years, a permanent pacemaker is a self-contained device surgically implanted in a pocket beneath the patient's skin. This is usually done in the operating room or cardiac catheterization laboratory. Nursing responsibilities involve monitoring the electrocardiogram (ECG) and maintaining sterile technique.

Today, permanent pacemakers function in the demand mode, allowing the patient's heart to beat on its own but preventing it from falling below a preset rate. Pacing electrodes can be placed in the atria, in the ventricles, or in both chambers (atrioventricular sequential, dual chamber). (See *Understanding pacemaker codes*.) The most common pacing codes are VVI for single-chamber pacing and DDD for dual-chamber pacing.

Candidates for permanent pacemakers include patients with myocardial infarction and persistent bradyarrhythmia and patients with complete heart block or slow ventricular rates stemming from congenital or degenerative heart disease or cardiac surgery. Patients who suffer Stokes-Adams syndrome, as well as those with Wolff-Parkinson-White syndrome or sick sinus syndrome, may also benefit from permanent pacemaker implantation.

Key nursing diagnoses and patient outcomes

Decreased cardiac output related to decreased stroke volume
The patient will:
▶ attain hemodynamic stability as evidenced by pulse not less than (specify) beats/minute and not greater than (specify) beats/minute and blood pressure no less than (specify) mm Hg and not greater than (specify) mm Hg
▶ have warm and dry skin
▶ perform specified activities with proper pacemaker functioning
▶ maintain adequate cardiac output.

Disturbed body image related to presence of pacemaker
The patient will:
▶ acknowledge change in body image
▶ participate in decision making about the pacemaker
▶ express positive feelings about self.

Equipment
Sphygmomanometer • stethoscope • ECG monitor and strip-chart recorder • sterile dressing tray • povidone-iodine ointment • shaving supplies • sterile gauze dressing • hypoallergenic tape • sedatives • alcohol pads • emergency resuscitation equipment • sterile gown

Understanding pacemaker codes

A permanent pacemaker's three-letter (or sometimes five-letter) code simply refers to how it's programmed. The first letter represents the chamber that is paced; the second letter, the chamber that is sensed; and the third letter, how the pulse generator responds.

First letter	Second letter	Third letter
A = atrium	A = atrium	I = inhibited
V = ventricle	V = ventricle	T = triggered
D = dual (both chambers)	D = dual (both chambers)	D = dual (inhibited and triggered)
O = not applicable	O = not applicable	O = not applicable

Examples of two common programming codes

DDD	VVI
Pace: atrium and ventricle	Pace: ventricle
Sense: atrium and ventricle	Sense: ventricle
Response: inhibited and triggered	Response: inhibited
This is a fully automatic, or universal, pacemaker.	This is a demand pacemaker, that is inhibited when ventricular activity is sensed.

and mask • optional: I.V. line for emergency medications

Implementation

▶ Explain the procedure to the patient. Provide and review literature from the manufacturer or the American Heart Association *so he can learn about the pacemaker and how it works.* Emphasize that the pacemaker merely augments his natural heart rate.

▶ Ensure that the patient or a responsible family member signs a consent form, and ask the patient if he's allergic to anesthetics or iodine.

Preoperative care

▶ For pacemaker insertion, shave the patient's chest from the axilla to the midline and from the clavicle to the nipple line on the side selected by the doctor.

▶ Establish an I.V. line at a keep-vein-open rate *so that you can administer emergency drugs if the patient experiences ventricular arrhythmia.*

▶ Obtain baseline vital signs and a baseline ECG.

▶ Provide sedation as ordered.

In the operating room

▶ If you'll be present to monitor arrhythmias during the procedure, put on a gown and mask.

▶ Connect the ECG monitor to the patient, and run a baseline rhythm strip. Make sure that the machine has enough paper to run additional rhythm strips during the procedure.

▶ In transvenous placement, the doctor, guided by a fluoroscope, passes the electrode catheter through the cephalic or external jugular vein and positions it in the right ventricle. He attaches the catheter to the pulse generator, inserts this into the chest wall, and sutures it

Teaching the patient who has a permanent pacemaker

If your patient is going home with a permanent pacemaker, teach him about daily care, safety and activity guidelines, and other precautions.

Daily care
■ Clean your pacemaker site gently with soap and water when you take a shower or a bath. Leave the incision exposed to the air.
■ Inspect your skin around the incision. A slight bulge is normal, but call your doctor if you feel discomfort or notice swelling, redness, a discharge, or other problems.
■ Check your pulse for 1 minute as your nurse or doctor showed you—on the side of your neck, inside your elbow, or on the thumb side of your wrist. Your pulse rate should be the same as your pacemaker rate or faster. Contact your doctor if you think your heart is beating too fast or too slow.
■ Take your medications, including those for pain, as prescribed. Even with a pacemaker, you still need the medication your doctor ordered.

Safety and activity
■ Keep your pacemaker instruction booklet handy, and carry your pacemaker identification card at all times. This card has your pacemaker model number and other information needed by health care personnel who treat you.
■ You can resume most of your usual activities when you feel comfortable doing so, but don't drive until the doctor gives you permission. Also avoid heavy lifting and stretching exercises for at least 4 weeks or as directed by your doctor.
■ Try to use both arms equally to prevent stiffness. Check with your doctor before you golf, swim, play tennis, or perform other strenuous activities.

Electromagnetic interference
■ Today pacemakers are designed and insulated to eliminate most electrical interference.

You can safely operate common household electrical devices, including microwave ovens, razors, and sewing machines. You can ride in or operate a motor vehicle without it affecting your pacemaker.
■ Take care to avoid direct contact with large running motors, high-powered citizen-band radios and other similar equipment, welding machinery, and radar devices.
■ If your pacemaker activates the metal detector in an airport, show your pacemaker identification card to the security official.
■ Because the metal in your pacemaker makes you ineligible for certain diagnostic studies, such as magnetic resonance imaging, be sure to inform your doctors, dentist, and other health care personnel that you have a pacemaker.

Special precautions
■ If you feel light-headed or dizzy when you're near any electrical equipment, moving away from the device should restore normal pacemaker function. Ask your doctor about particular electrical devices.
■ Notify your doctor if you experience any signs of pacemaker failure, such as palpitations, a fast heart rate, a slow heart rate (5 to 10 beats less than the pacemaker's setting), dizziness, fainting, shortness of breath, swollen ankles or feet, anxiety, forgetfulness, or confusion.

Checkups
■ Be sure to schedule and keep regular checkup appointments with your doctor.
■ If your doctor checks your pacemaker status by telephone, keep your transmission schedule and instructions in a handy place.

closed, leaving a small outlet for a drainage tube.

Postoperative care

▶ Monitor the patient's ECG *to check for arrhythmias and to ensure correct pacemaker functioning.*

▶ Monitor the I.V. flow rate; the I.V. line is usually kept in place for 24 to 48 hours postoperatively *to allow for possible emergency treatment of arrhythmias.*

▶ Check the dressing for signs of bleeding and infection (swelling, redness, or exudate). The doctor may order prophylactic antibiotics for up to 7 days after the implantation.

▶ Change the dressing and apply povidone-iodine ointment at least once every 24 to 48 hours, or according to doctor's orders and facility policy. If the dressing becomes soiled or the site is exposed to air, change the dressing immediately, regardless of when you last changed it.

▶ Check vital signs and level of consciousness (LOC) every 15 minutes for the first hour, every hour for the next 4 hours, every 4 hours for the next 48 hours, and then once every shift.

Age alert Confused, elderly patients with second-degree heart block won't show immediate improvement in LOC.

Nursing alert Watch for signs and symptoms of a perforated ventricle, with resultant cardiac tamponade: persistent hiccups, distant heart sounds, pulsus paradoxus, hypotension with narrow pulse pressure, increased venous pressure, cyanosis, distended neck veins, decreased urine output, restlessness, or complaints of fullness in the chest. If the patient develops any of these, notify the doctor immediately.

Special considerations

▶ If the patient wears a hearing aid, the pacemaker battery is placed on the opposite side accordingly.

▶ Provide the patient with an identification card that lists the pacemaker type and manufacturer, serial number, pacemaker rate setting, date implanted, and doctor's name. (See *Teaching the patient who has a permanent pacemaker.*)

▶ Watch for signs of pacemaker malfunction.

Complications

Insertion of a permanent pacemaker places the patient at risk for certain complications, such as infection, lead displacement, a perforated ventricle, cardiac tamponade, or lead fracture and disconnection.

Documentation

Document the type of pacemaker used, the serial number and the manufacturer's name, the pacing rate, the date of implantation, and the doctor's name. Note whether the pacemaker successfully treated the patient's arrhythmias and the condition of the incision site.

PACEMAKER INSERTION AND CARE, TEMPORARY

Usually inserted in an emergency, a temporary pacemaker consists of an external, battery-powered pulse generator and a lead or electrode system. Four types of temporary pacemakers exist: transcutaneous, transvenous, transthoracic, and epicardial.

In a life-threatening situation, when time is critical, a *transcutaneous pacemaker* is the best choice. This device works by sending an electrical impulse from the pulse generator to the patient's heart by way of two electrodes, which are placed on the front and back of the patient's chest. Transcutaneous pacing is quick and effective, but it's used only until the doctor can institute transvenous pacing.

In addition to being more comfortable for the patient, a *transvenous pacemaker* is more reliable than a transcutaneous pacemaker. Transvenous pacing involves threading an electrode catheter through a vein into the patient's right atrium or right ventricle. The electrode then attaches to an external pulse generator. As a result, the pulse generator can provide an electrical stimulus directly to the endocardium. This is the most common type of pacemaker.

As an elective surgical procedure or as an emergency measure during cardiopulmonary resuscitation (CPR), a doctor may choose to insert a *transthoracic pacemaker*. To insert this type of pacemaker, the doctor performs a procedure similar to pericardiocentesis, in which he uses a cardiac needle to pass an electrode through the chest wall and into the right ventricle. This procedure carries a significant risk of coronary artery laceration and cardiac tamponade.

During cardiac surgery, the surgeon may insert electrodes through the epicardium of the right ventricle and, if he wants to institute atrioventricular sequential pacing, the right atrium. From there, the electrodes pass through the chest wall, where they remain available if temporary pacing becomes necessary. This is called *epicardial pacing*.

In addition to helping to correct conduction disturbances, a temporary pacemaker may help diagnose conduction abnormalities. For example, during a cardiac catheterization or electrophysiology study, a doctor may use a temporary pacemaker to localize conduction defects. In the process, he may also learn whether the patient risks developing an arrhythmia.

Among the contraindications to pacemaker therapy are electromechanical dissociation and ventricular fibrillation.

Key nursing diagnoses and patient outcomes

Decreased cardiac output related to decreased stroke volume
The patient will:
▶ attain hemodynamic stability as evidenced by pulse not less than (specify) beats/minute and not greater than (specify) beats/minute and blood pressure not less than (specify) mm Hg and not greater than (specify) mm Hg
▶ have warm and dry skin
▶ perform specified activities with proper pacemaker functioning
▶ maintain adequate cardiac output.

Equipment
For transcutaneous pacing
Transcutaneous pacing generator • cardiac monitor • transcutaneous pacing electrodes

For all other types of temporary pacing
Temporary pacemaker generator with new battery • guide wire or introducer • electrode catheter • sterile gloves • sterile dressings • adhesive tape • povidone-iodine solution • nonconducting tape or rubber surgical glove • emergency cardiac drugs • intubation equipment • defibrillator • cardiac monitor with strip-chart recorder • equipment to start a peripheral I.V. line, if appropriate • I.V.

fluids • sedative • optional: elastic bandage or gauze strips, restraints

For transvenous pacing

All equipment listed for temporary pacing • bridging cable • percutaneous introducer tray or venous cutdown tray • sterile gowns • linen-saver pad • antimicrobial soap • alcohol pads • vial of 1% lidocaine • 5-ml syringe • fluoroscopy equipment, if necessary • fenestrated drape • prepackaged cutdown tray (for antecubital vein placement only) • sutures • receptacle for infectious wastes

For transthoracic pacing

All equipment listed for temporary pacing • transthoracic or cardiac needle

For epicardial pacing

All equipment listed for temporary pacing • atrial epicardial wires • ventricular epicardial wires • sterile rubber finger cot • sterile dressing materials (if the wires won't be connected to a pulse generator)

Implementation

▶ If applicable, explain the procedure to the patient.

For transcutaneous pacing

▶ If necessary, clip the hair over the areas of electrode placement. However, don't shave the area. *If you nick the skin, the current from the pulse generator could cause discomfort and the nicks could become irritated or infected after the electrodes are applied.*

▶ Attach monitoring electrodes to the patient in lead I, II, or III position. Do this even if the patient is already on telemetry monitoring *because you'll need to connect the electrodes to the pacemaker.*

If you select the lead II position, adjust the LL electrode placement to accommodate the anterior pacing electrode and the patient's anatomy.

▶ Plug the patient cable into the electrocardiogram (ECG) input connection on the front of the pacing generator. Set the selector switch to the MONITOR ON position.

▶ You should see the ECG waveform on the monitor. Adjust the R-wave beeper volume to a suitable level and activate the alarm by pressing the ALARM ON button. Set the alarm for 10 to 20 beats lower and 20 to 30 beats higher than the intrinsic rate.

▶ Press the START/STOP button for a printout of the waveform.

▶ Now you're ready to apply the two pacing electrodes. First, make sure the patient's skin is clean and dry *to ensure good skin contact.*

▶ Pull off the protective strip from the posterior electrode (marked BACK) and apply the electrode on the left side of the back, just below the scapula and to the left of the spine.

▶ The anterior pacing electrode (marked FRONT) has two protective strips — one covering the jellied area and one covering the outer rim. Expose the jellied area and apply it to the skin in the anterior position — to the left side of the precordium in the usual V_2 to V_5 position. Move this electrode around to get the best waveform. Then expose the electrode's outer rim and firmly press it to the skin. (See *Proper electrode placement,* page 600.)

▶ Now you're ready to pace the heart. After making sure the energy output in milliamperes (mA) is on 0, connect the electrode cable to the monitor output cable.

Proper electrode placement

Place the two pacing electrodes for a non-invasive temporary pacemaker at heart level on the patient's chest and back (as shown). This placement ensures that the electrical stimulus must travel only a short distance to the heart.

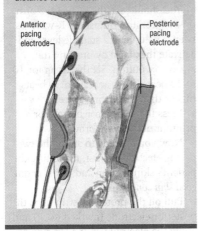

Anterior pacing electrode

Posterior pacing electrode

▶ Check the waveform, looking for a tall QRS complex in lead II.

▶ Next, turn the selector switch to PACER ON. Tell the patient that he may feel a thumping or twitching sensation. Reassure him that you'll give him medication if he can't tolerate the discomfort.

▶ Now set the rate dial to 10 to 20 beats higher than the patient's intrinsic rhythm. Look for pacer artifact or spikes, which will appear as you increase the rate. If the patient doesn't have an intrinsic rhythm, set the rate at 60.

▶ Slowly increase the amount of energy delivered to the heart by adjusting the OUTPUT mA dial. Do this until capture is achieved—you'll see a pacer spike followed by a widened QRS complex that resembles a premature ventricular contraction. This is the pacing threshold. To ensure consistent capture, increase output by 10%. Don't go any higher *because you could cause the patient needless discomfort.*

▶ With full capture, the patient's heart rate should be approximately the same as the pacemaker rate set on the machine. The usual pacing threshold is between 40 and 80 mA.

For transvenous pacing

▶ Check the patient's history for hypersensitivity to local anesthetics. Then attach the cardiac monitor to the patient and obtain a baseline assessment, including the patient's vital signs, skin color, level of consciousness (LOC), heart rate and rhythm, and emotional state. Next, insert a peripheral I.V. line if the patient doesn't already have one. Begin an I.V. infusion at a keep-vein-open rate.

▶ Insert a new battery into the external pacemaker generator, and test it to make sure it has a strong charge. Connect the bridging cable to the generator, and align the positive and negative poles. *This cable allows slack between the electrode catheter and the generator, reducing the risk of accidental catheter displacement.*

▶ Place the patient in the supine position. If necessary, clip the hair around the insertion site. Next, open the supply tray while maintaining a sterile field. Using sterile technique, clean the insertion site with antimicrobial soap and then wipe the area with povidone-iodine solution. Cover the insertion site with a fenestrated drape. *Because fluoroscopy may be used during the placement of leadwires, put on a protective apron.*

► Provide the doctor with the local anesthetic.

► After anesthetizing the insertion site, the doctor will puncture the brachial, femoral, subclavian, or jugular vein. Then he'll insert a guide wire or an introducer and advance the electrode catheter.

► As the catheter advances, watch the cardiac monitor. When the electrode catheter reaches the right atrium, you'll notice large P waves and small QRS complexes. Then, as the catheter reaches the right ventricle, the P waves will become smaller while the QRS complexes enlarge. When the catheter touches the right ventricular endocardium, expect to see elevated ST segments, premature ventricular contractions, or both.

► When the electrode catheter is in the right ventricle, it will send an impulse to the myocardium, causing depolarization. If the patient needs atrial pacing, either alone or with ventricular pacing, the doctor may place an electrode in the right atrium.

► Meanwhile, continuously monitor the patient's cardiac status and treat any arrhythmias, as appropriate. Also assess the patient for jaw pain and earache; *these symptoms indicate that the electrode catheter has missed the superior vena cava and has moved into the neck instead.*

► When the electrode catheter is in place, attach the catheter leads to the bridging cable, lining up the positive and negative poles.

► Check the battery's charge by pressing the BATTERY TEST button.

► Set the pacemaker as ordered.

► The doctor will then suture the catheter to the insertion site. Afterward, put on sterile gloves and apply a sterile dressing to the site. Label the dressing with the date and time of application.

For transthoracic pacing

► Clean the skin to the left of the xiphoid process with povidone-iodine solution. Work quickly *because CPR must be interrupted for the procedure.*

► After interrupting CPR, the doctor will insert a transthoracic needle through the patient's chest wall to the left of the xiphoid process into the right ventricle. He'll then follow the needle with the electrode catheter.

► Connect the electrode catheter to the generator, lining up the positive and negative poles. Watch the cardiac monitor for signs of ventricular pacing and capture.

► After the doctor sutures the electrode catheter into place, use sterile technique to apply a sterile 4″ × 4″ gauze dressing to the site. Tape the dressing securely, and label it with the date and time of application.

► Check the patient's peripheral pulses and vital signs *to assess cardiac output.* If you can't palpate a pulse, continue performing CPR.

► If the patient has a palpable pulse, assess the patient's vital signs, ECG, and LOC.

For epicardial pacing

► During your preoperative teaching, inform the patient that epicardial pacemaker wires may be placed during cardiac surgery.

► During cardiac surgery, the doctor will hook epicardial wires into the epicardium just before the end of the surgery. Depending on the patient's condition, the doctor may insert either atrial or ventricular wires, or both.

▶ If indicated, connect the electrode catheter to the generator, lining up the positive and negative poles. Set the pacemaker as ordered.

▶ If the wires won't be connected to an external pulse generator, place them in a sterile rubber finger cot. Then cover both the wires and the insertion site with a sterile, occlusive dressing. *This will help protect the patient from microshock as well as infection.*

Special considerations

▶ Take care to prevent microshock. This includes warning the patient not to use any electrical equipment that isn't grounded, such as telephones, electric shavers, televisions, or lamps.

▶ Other safety measures you'll want to take include placing a plastic cover supplied by the manufacturer over the pacemaker *controls to avoid an accidental setting change.* Also, insulate the pacemaker by covering all exposed metal parts, such as electrode connections and pacemaker terminals, with nonconducting tape, or place the pacing unit in a dry, rubber surgical glove. If the patient is disoriented or uncooperative, use restraints *to prevent accidental removal of pacemaker wires.* If the patient needs emergency defibrillation, make sure the pacemaker can withstand the procedure. If you're unsure, disconnect the pulse generator *to avoid damage.*

▶ When using a transcutaneous pacemaker, don't place the electrodes over a bony area *because bone conducts current poorly.* With female patients, place the anterior electrode under the patient's breast but not over her diaphragm. If the doctor inserts the electrode through the brachial or femoral vein, immobi-

lize the patient's arm or leg *to avoid putting stress on the pacing wires.*

▶ After insertion of any temporary pacemaker, assess the patient's vital signs, skin color, LOC, and peripheral pulses *to determine the effectiveness of the paced rhythm.* Perform a 12-lead ECG to serve as a baseline, and then perform additional ECGs daily or with clinical changes. Also, if possible, obtain a rhythm strip before, during, and after pacemaker placement; any time that pacemaker settings are changed; and whenever the patient receives treatment because of a complication due to the pacemaker.

▶ Continuously monitor the ECG reading, noting capture, sensing, rate, intrinsic beats, and competition of paced and intrinsic rhythms. If the pacemaker is sensing correctly, the sense indicator on the pulse generator should flash with each beat. (See *When a temporary pacemaker malfunctions.*)

▶ Record the date and time of pacemaker insertion, the type of pacemaker, the reason for insertion, and the patient's response. Note the pacemaker settings. Document any complications and the interventions taken.

▶ If the patient has epicardial pacing wires in place, clean the insertion site with povidone-iodine solution and change the dressing daily. At the same time, monitor the site for signs of infection. Always keep the pulse generator nearby in case pacing becomes necessary.

Complications

Complications associated with pacemaker therapy include microshock, equipment failure, and competitive or fatal arrhythmias. Transcutaneous pacemakers may also cause skin breakdown

Troubleshooting

When a temporary pacemaker malfunctions

Occasionally, a temporary pacemaker may fail to function appropriately. When this occurs, you'll need to take immediate action to correct the problem. Here you'll learn which steps to take when your patient's pacemaker fails to pace, capture, or sense intrinsic beats.

Failure to pace

Failure to pace occurs when the pacemaker doesn't fire or fires too often. The pulse generator may not be working properly, or it may not be conducting the impulse to the patient.

Nursing interventions

■ If the pacing or sensing indicator flashes, check the connections to the cable and the position of the pacing electrode in the patient (by X-ray). The cable may have come loose, or the electrode may have been dislodged, pulled out, or broken.

■ If the pulse generator is turned on but the indicators still aren't flashing, change the battery. If that doesn't help, use a different pulse generator.

■ Check the settings if the pacemaker is firing too rapidly. If they're correct, or if altering them (according to your facility's policy or the doctor's order) doesn't help, change the pulse generator.

Failure to capture

In failure to capture, you see pacemaker spikes but the heart isn't responding. This may be caused by changes in the pacing threshold from ischemia, an electrolyte imbalance (high or low potassium or magnesium levels), acidosis, an adverse reaction to a medication, a perforated ventricle, fibrosis, or the position of the electrode.

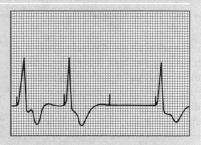

Nursing interventions

■ If the patient's condition has changed, notify the doctor and ask him for new settings.

■ If pacemaker settings are altered by the patient or another, return them to their correct positions. Then make sure the face of the pacemaker is covered with a plastic shield. Tell the patient or others not to touch the dials.

■ If the heart isn't responding, try any or all of these suggestions: Carefully check all connections; increase the milliamperes slowly (according to your facility's policy or the doctor's order); turn the patient on his left side, then on his right (if turning him to the left didn't help); reverse the cable in the pulse generator so the positive electrode wire is in the negative terminal and the negative electrode wire is in the positive terminal; schedule an anteroposterior or lateral chest X-ray to determine the position of the electrode.

(continued)

When a temporary pacemaker malfunctions *(continued)*

Failure to sense intrinsic beats

Failure to sense intrinsic beats could cause ventricular tachycardia or ventricular fibrillation if the pacemaker fires on the vulnerable T wave. This could be caused by the pacemaker sensing an external stimulus such as a QRS complex, which could lead to asystole, or by the pacemaker not being sensitive enough, which means it could fire anywhere within the cardiac cycle.

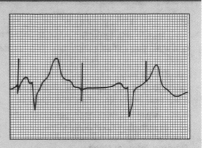

Nursing interventions

■ If the pacing is undersensing, turn the sensitivity control completely to the right. If it's oversensing, turn it slightly to the left.

■ If the pacemaker isn't functioning correctly, change the battery or the pulse generator.

■ Remove items in the room that could cause electromechanical interference (razors, radios, cautery devices, and so on). Check the ground wires on the bed and other equipment for obvious damage. Unplug each piece and see if the interference stops. When you locate the cause, notify the staff engineer and ask him to check it.

■ If the pacemaker is still firing on the T wave and all else has failed, turn off the pacemaker. Make sure atropine is available in case the patient's heart rate drops. Be prepared to call a code and institute cardiopulmonary resuscitation, if necessary.

and muscle pain and twitching when the pacemaker fires. Transvenous pacemakers may cause such complications as pneumothorax or hemothorax, cardiac perforation and tamponade, diaphragmatic stimulation, pulmonary embolism, thrombophlebitis, and infection. Also, if the doctor threads the electrode through the antecubital or femoral vein, venous spasm, thrombophlebitis, or lead displacement may result.

Complications associated with transthoracic pacemakers include pneumothorax, cardiac tamponade, emboli, sepsis, lacerations of the myocardium or coronary artery, and perforations of a cardiac chamber. Epicardial pacemakers carry a risk of infection, cardiac arrest, and diaphragmatic stimulation.

Documentation

Record the reason for pacing, the time it started, and the locations of the electrodes. For a transvenous or transthoracic pacemaker, note the date, the time, and reason for the temporary pacemaker.

For any temporary pacemaker, record the pacemaker settings. Note the patient's response to the procedure, along with any complications and the interventions taken. If possible, obtain rhythm strips before, during, and after pacemaker placement, and whenever pacemaker settings are changed or when the patient receives treatment for a complication caused by the pacemaker. As you monitor the patient, record his response to temporary pacing and note any changes in his condition.

PAIN MANAGEMENT

When a patient feels severe pain, he seeks medical help because he believes the pain signals a serious problem. This perception produces anxiety, which, in turn, increases the pain. To assess and manage pain properly, the nurse must depend on the patient's subjective description in addition to objective tools.

Several interventions can be used to manage pain. These include analgesic administration, emotional support, comfort measures, and cognitive techniques to distract the patient. Severe pain usually requires a narcotic analgesic. Invasive measures, such as epidural analgesia or patient-controlled analgesia, may also be required.

Key nursing diagnoses and patient outcomes

Chronic pain related to (specify)
The patient will:
▶ describe pain characteristics
▶ identify factors that intensify pain and modify behavior accordingly
▶ state and carry out appropriate interventions for pain relief
▶ express a feeling of comfort and relief from pain.

Ineffective individual coping related to pain
The patient will:
▶ communicate feelings about his current situation
▶ become involved in planning his care
▶ express feeling of greater control over the situation.

Equipment

Pain assessment tool or scale • oral hygiene supplies • water • nonnarcotic analgesic (such as acetaminophen or aspirin) • optional: patient-controlled analgesia (PCA) device, mild narcotic (such as oxycodone or codeine), strong narcotic (such as methadone, levorphanol, morphine, or hydromorphone)

Implementation

▶ Explain to the patient how pain medications work together with other pain management therapies to provide relief. Also explain that management aims to keep pain at a low level to permit optimal bodily function.

▶ Assess the patient's pain by using a pain assessment tool or scale or by asking key questions and noting his response to the pain. For instance, ask him to describe its duration, severity, and source. Look for physiologic or behavioral clues to the pain's severity. (See *How to assess pain*, page 606.)

▶ Develop nursing diagnoses. Appropriate nursing diagnostic categories include chronic pain, acute pain, anxiety, activity intolerance, fear, risk for injury, deficient knowledge, powerlessness, and self-care deficit.

▶ Work with the patient to develop a nursing plan of care using interventions appropriate to the patient's lifestyle. These may include prescribed medications, emotional support, comfort measures, cognitive techniques, and education about pain and its management. Emphasize the importance of maintaining good bowel habits, respiratory function, and mobility *because pain may exacerbate any problems in these areas.*

▶ Implement your plan of care. Because individuals respond to pain dif-

How to assess pain

To assess pain properly, you'll need to consider the patient's description and your observations of the patient's physical and behavioral responses. Start by asking the following series of key questions (keeping in mind that the patient's responses will be shaped by his prior experiences, self-image, and beliefs about his condition):

■ Where is the pain located? How long does it last? How often does it occur?

■ Can you describe the pain?

■ What relieves the pain or makes it worse?

Ask the patient to rank his pain on a scale of 0 to 10, with 0 denoting lack of pain and 10 denoting the worst pain level. This helps the patient verbally evaluate pain therapies.

Observe the patient's behavioral and physiologic responses to pain. Physiologic responses may be sympathetic or parasympathetic.

Behavioral responses

These include altered body position, moaning, sighing, grimacing, withdrawal, crying, restlessness, muscle twitching, and immobility.

Sympathetic responses

These are commonly associated with mild to moderate pain and include pallor, elevated blood pressure, dilated pupils, skeletal muscle tension, dyspnea, tachycardia, and diaphoresis.

Parasympathetic responses

These are commonly associated with severe, deep pain and include pallor, decreased blood pressure, bradycardia, nausea and vomiting, weakness, dizziness, and loss of consciousness.

ferently, you'll find that what works for one person may not work for another.

Giving medications

▶ If the patient is allowed oral intake, begin with a nonnarcotic analgesic, such as acetaminophen or aspirin, every 4 to 6 hours as ordered.

▶ If the patient needs more relief than a nonnarcotic analgesic provides, you may give a mild narcotic (such as oxycodone or codeine) as ordered.

▶ If the patient needs still more pain relief, you may administer a strong narcotic (such as methadone, levorphanol, morphine, or hydromorphone) as prescribed. Administer oral medications if possible. Check the appropriate drug information for each medication given.

▶ If ordered, teach the patient how to use a PCA device. *Such a device can help the patient manage his pain and decrease his anxiety.*

Providing emotional support

▶ Show your concern by spending time talking with the patient. Because of his pain and his inability to manage it, the patient may be anxious and frustrated. Such feelings can worsen his pain.

Performing comfort measures

▶ Periodically reposition the patient *to reduce muscle spasms and tension and to relieve pressure on bony prominences.* Increasing the angle of the bed can reduce pull on an abdominal incision, diminishing pain. If appropriate, elevate a limb *to reduce swelling, inflammation, and pain.*

▶ Give the patient a back massage *to help relax tense muscles.*

▶ Perform passive range-of-motion exercises *to prevent stiffness and further loss*

of mobility, relax tense muscles, and provide comfort.
▶ Provide oral hygiene. Keep a fresh water glass or cup at the bedside *because many pain medications tend to dry the mouth.*
▶ Wash the patient's face and hands.

Using cognitive therapy
▶ Help the patient enhance the effect of analgesics by using such techniques as distraction, guided imagery, deep breathing, and relaxation. You can easily use these "mind-over-pain" techniques at the bedside. Choose the method the patient prefers. If possible, start these techniques when the patient feels little or no pain. If he feels persistent pain, begin with short, simple exercises. Before beginning, dim the lights, remove the patient's restrictive clothing, and eliminate noise from the environment.
▶ For *distraction,* have the patient recall a pleasant experience or focus his attention on an enjoyable activity. For instance, he can use music as a distraction by turning on the radio when the pain begins. Have him close his eyes and concentrate on listening, raising or lowering the volume as his pain increases or subsides. Note, however, that distraction is usually effective only against brief pain episodes lasting less than 5 minutes.
▶ For *guided imagery,* help the patient concentrate on a peaceful, pleasant image, such as a walk on the beach. Encourage him to concentrate on the details of the image he has selected by asking about its sight, sound, smell, taste, and touch. The positive emotions evoked by this exercise minimize pain.
▶ For *deep breathing,* have the patient stare at an object and then slowly inhale and exhale as he counts aloud to maintain a comfortable rate and rhythm. Have him concentrate on the rise and fall of his abdomen. Encourage him to feel more and more weightless with each breath while he concentrates on the rhythm of his breathing or on any restful image.
▶ For *muscle relaxation,* have the patient focus on a particular muscle group. Then ask him to tense the muscles and note the sensation. After 5 to 7 seconds, tell him to relax the muscles and concentrate on the relaxed state. Have him note the difference between the tense and relaxed states. After he tenses and relaxes one muscle group, have him proceed to another and another until he's covered his entire body.

Special considerations
▶ Evaluate your patient's response to pain management. If he's still in pain, reassess him and alter your plan of care as appropriate.
▶ Remind the patient that results of cognitive therapy techniques improve with practice. Help him through the initial sessions.
▶ Remember that patients receiving narcotic analgesics are at risk for developing tolerance, dependence, or addiction. Patients with acute pain may have a smaller risk of dependence or addiction than patients with chronic pain.
▶ If a patient who is receiving a narcotic analgesic experiences abstinence syndrome when the drug is withdrawn abruptly, suspect physical dependence. The signs and symptoms include anxiety, irritability, chills and hot flashes, excessive salivation and tearing, rhinorrhea, sweating, nausea, vomiting, and seizures. These signs and symptoms are likely to begin in 6 to 12 hours and to

peak in 24 to 72 hours. *To reduce the risk of dependence,* discontinue a narcotic analgesic by decreasing the dose gradually each day. Also, you may switch to an oral narcotic and decrease its dose gradually.

▶ If a patient becomes addicted, his behavior will be characterized by compulsive drug use and a craving for the drug to experience effects other than pain relief. A patient demonstrating such behavior usually has a preexisting problem that is exacerbated by the narcotic use. Discuss the addicted patient's problem with supportive personnel, and make appropriate referrals to experts.

▶ During periods of intense pain, the patient's ability to concentrate diminishes. If your patient is in severe pain, help him select a cognitive technique that is simple to use. After he selects a technique, encourage him to use it consistently.

Complications

The most common adverse effects of analgesics include respiratory depression (the most serious), sedation, constipation, nausea, and vomiting.

Documentation

Document each step of the nursing process. Describe the subjective information you elicited from the patient, using his own words. Note the location, quality, and duration of the pain as well as any precipitating factors.

Record your nursing diagnoses, and include the pain relief method used. Summarize your interventions and the patient's response. If the patient's pain wasn't relieved, note alternative treatments to consider the next time pain

occurs. Also record any complications of drug therapy.

PAP AND PAWP
MONITORING

Continuous pulmonary artery pressure (PAP) and intermittent pulmonary artery wedge pressure (PAWP) measurements provide important information about left ventricular function and preload. You can use this information not only for monitoring but also for aiding diagnosis, refining your assessment, guiding interventions, and projecting patient outcomes.

Nearly all acutely ill patients are candidates for PAP monitoring—especially those who are hemodynamically unstable, who need fluid management or continuous cardiopulmonary assessment, or who are receiving multiple or frequently administered cardioactive drugs. PAP monitoring also is crucial for patients with shock, trauma, pulmonary or cardiac disease, or multiorgan disease.

The original PAP monitoring catheter, which had two lumens, was invented by two doctors, Swan and Ganz. The device still bears their name (Swan-Ganz catheter) but is commonly referred to as a pulmonary artery (PA) catheter. Current versions have up to six lumens, allowing more hemodynamic information to be gathered. In addition to distal and proximal lumens used to measure pressures, a PA catheter has a balloon inflation lumen that inflates the balloon for PAWP measurement and a thermistor connector lumen that allows cardiac output measurement. Some catheters also have a pacemaker wire lumen that provides a port for pacemaker electrodes and measures continuous mixed venous oxygen saturation. (See *PA catheter: From basic to complex,* page 610.)

Fluoroscopy usually isn't required during catheter insertion because the catheter is flow directed, following venous blood flow from the right heart chambers into the pulmonary artery. Also, the pulmonary artery, right atrium, and right ventricle produce characteristic pressures and waveforms that can be observed on the monitor to help track catheter-tip location. Marks on the catheter shaft, with 10-cm graduations, assist tracking by showing how far the catheter is inserted.

The PA catheter is inserted into the heart's right side with the distal tip lying in the pulmonary artery. Left-sided pressures can be assessed indirectly.

No specific contraindications for PAP monitoring exist. However, some patients undergoing it require special precautions. These include elderly patients with pulmonary hypertension, those with left bundle-branch heart block, and those for whom a systemic infection would be life-threatening.

Key nursing diagnoses and patient outcomes

Ineffective tissue perfusion (cardiopulmonary) related to decreased cellular exchange
The patient will:
▶ have warm and dry skin
▶ maintain adequate cardiac output
▶ not exhibit arrhythmias.

Decreased cardiac output related to decreased stroke volume
The patient will:
▶ attain hemodynamic stability as evidenced by pulse not less than (specify)

beats/minute and not greater than (specify) beats/minute and blood pressure not less than (specify) mm Hg and not greater than (specify) mm Hg
▶ exhibit PAP and PAWP measurements within normal limits
▶ have a diminished heart workload
▶ maintain adequate cardiac output.

Equipment
Balloon-tipped, flow-directed PA catheter • prepared pressure transducer system • I.V. solutions • sterile syringes • alcohol pads • medication-added label • monitor and monitor cable • I.V. pole with transducer mount • emergency resuscitation equipment • electrocardiogram (ECG) monitor • ECG electrodes • armboard (for antecubital insertion) • lead aprons (if fluoroscope is necessary) • sutures • sterile 4″ × 4″ gauze pads or other dry, occlusive dressing material • prepackaged introducer kit • optional: dextrose 5% in water, shaving materials (for femoral insertion site), small sterile basin, and sterile water

If a prepackaged introducer kit is unavailable, obtain the following: an introducer (one size larger than the catheter) • sterile tray containing instruments for procedure • masks • sterile gowns • sterile gloves • sterile drapes • povidone-iodine ointment and solution • sutures • two 10-ml syringes • local anesthetic (1% to 2% lidocaine) • one 5-ml syringe • 25G 1½″ needle • 1″ and 3″ tape

Preparation of equipment
To obtain reliable pressure values and clear waveforms, the pressure monitoring system and bedside monitor must be properly calibrated and zeroed. Make sure the monitor has the correct

PA catheter: From basic to complex

Depending on the intended uses, a pulmonary artery (PA) catheter may be simple or complex. The basic PA catheter has a distal and proximal lumen, a thermistor, and a balloon inflation gate valve. The distal lumen, which exits in the pulmonary artery, monitors PA pressure. Its hub usually is marked P DISTAL or is color-coded yellow. The proximal lumen exits in the right atrium or vena cava, depending on the size of the patient's heart. It monitors right atrial pressure and can be used as the injected solution lumen for cardiac output determination and infusing solutions. The proximal lumen hub usually is marked PROXIMAL or is color-coded blue.

The thermistor, located about 1½" (4 cm) from the distal tip, measures temperature (aiding core temperature evaluation) and allows cardiac output measurement. The thermistor connector attaches to a cardiac output connector cable, then to a cardiac output monitor. Typically, it's red.

The balloon inflation gate valve is used for inflating the balloon tip with air. A stopcock connection, typically color-coded red, may be used.

Additional lumens

Some PA catheters have additional lumens used to obtain other hemodynamic data or permit certain interventions. For instance, a proximal infusion port, which exits in the right atrium or vena cava, allows additional fluid administration. A right ventricular lumen, exiting in the right ventricle, allows fluid administration, right ventricular pressure measurement, or use of a temporary ventricular pacing lead.

Some catheters have additional right atrial and right ventricular lumens for atrioventricular pacing. A right ventricular ejection fraction test-response thermistor, with PA and right ventricular sensing electrodes, allows volumetric and ejection fraction measurements. Fiber-optic filaments, such as those used in pulse oximetry, exit into the pulmonary artery and permit measurement of continuous mixed venous oxygen saturation.

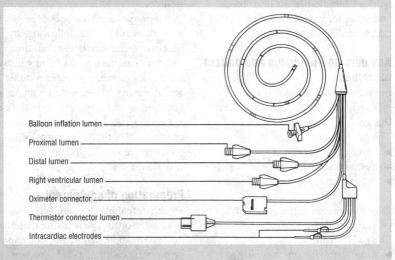

Balloon inflation lumen
Proximal lumen
Distal lumen
Right ventricular lumen
Oximeter connector
Thermistor connector lumen
Intracardiac electrodes

pressure modules; then calibrate it according to the manufacturer's instructions. (For instructions, see "Transducer system setup," page 854.)

Turn the monitor on before gathering the equipment to give it time to warm up. Be sure to check the operations manual for the monitor you're using; some older monitors may need 20 minutes to warm up.

Prepare the pressure monitoring system according to policy. Your facility's guidelines also may specify whether to mount the transducer on the I.V. pole or tape it to the patient and whether to add heparin to the flush. To manage any complications from catheter insertion, be sure to have emergency resuscitation equipment on hand (defibrillator, oxygen, and supplies for intubation and emergency drug administration).

Prepare a sterile field for insertion of the introducer and catheter. A bedside tray, placed on the same side as the insertion site for easier access, may be sufficient.

Implementation

▶ Check the patient's chart for heparin sensitivity, which contraindicates adding heparin to the flush solution. If the patient is alert, explain the procedure to him *to reduce his anxiety*. Mention that the catheter will monitor pressures from the pulmonary artery and heart. Reassure him that the catheter poses little danger and rarely causes pain. Tell him that if he feels pain at the introducer insertion site, the doctor will order an analgesic or a sedative.
▶ Be sure to tell the patient and his family not to be alarmed if they see the pressure waveform on the monitor "move around." Explain that the cause usually is artifact.

Positioning the patient for catheter placement
▶ Position the patient at the proper height and angle. If the doctor will use a superior approach for percutaneous insertion (most commonly using the internal jugular or subclavian vein), place the patient flat or in a slight Trendelenburg position. Remove the patient's pillow to help engorge the vessel and prevent air embolism. Turn his head to the side opposite the insertion site.
▶ If the doctor will use an inferior approach to access a femoral vein, position the patient flat. Be aware that with this approach, certain catheters are harder to insert and may require more manipulation.

Preparing the catheter
▶ Maintain sterile technique and use standard precautions throughout catheter preparation and insertion.
▶ Wash your hands. Clean the insertion site with a povidone-iodine solution and drape it.
▶ Put on a mask. Help the doctor put on a sterile mask, gown, and gloves.
▶ Open the outer packaging of the catheter, revealing the inner sterile wrapping. Using sterile technique, the doctor opens the inner wrapping and picks up the catheter. Take the catheter lumen hubs as he hands them to you.
▶ *To remove air from the catheter and verify its patency,* flush the catheter. In the more common flushing method, you connect the I.V. solutions aseptically to the appropriate pressure lines, and then flush them before insertion. *This method makes pressure waveforms easier to identify on the monitor during insertion.*
▶ Alternatively, you may flush the lumens with sterile I.V. solution from sterile syringes attached to the lumens.

Leave the filled syringes on during insertion.

▶ If the system has multiple pressure lines (such as a distal line to monitor PAP and a proximal line to monitor right atrial pressure), make sure the distal PA lumen hub is attached to the pressure line that will be observed on the monitor. *Inadvertently attaching the distal PA line to the proximal lumen hub will prevent the proper waveform from appearing during insertion.*

▶ Observe the diastolic values carefully during insertion. Make sure the scale is appropriate for lower pressures. A scale of 0 to 25 mm Hg or 0 to 50 mm Hg (more common) is preferred. (With a higher scale, such as 0 to 100 or 0 to 250 mm Hg, waveforms appear too small and the location of the catheter tip will be hard to identify.)

▶ *To verify the integrity of the balloon,* the doctor inflates it with air (usually 1.5 cc) before handing you the lumens to attach to the pressure monitoring system. He then observes the balloon for symmetrical shape. He also may submerge it in a small, sterile basin filled with sterile water and observe it for bubbles, which indicate a leak.

Inserting the catheter

▶ Assist the doctor as he inserts the introducer to access the vessel. He may perform a cutdown or (more commonly) insert the catheter percutaneously, as with a modified Seldinger technique.

▶ After the introducer is placed, and the catheter lumens are flushed, the doctor inserts the catheter through the introducer. In the internal jugular or subclavian approach, he inserts the catheter into the end of the introducer sheath with the balloon deflated, directing the curl of the catheter toward the patient's midline.

▶ As insertion begins, observe the bedside monitor for waveform variations. (See *Normal PA waveforms.*)

▶ When the catheter exits the end of the introducer sheath and reaches the junction of the superior vena cava and right atrium (at the 15- to 20-cm mark on the catheter shaft), the monitor shows oscillations that correspond to the patient's respirations. The balloon is then inflated with the recommended volume of air *to allow normal blood flow and aid catheter insertion.*

▶ Using a gentle, smooth motion, the doctor advances the catheter through the heart chambers, moving rapidly to the pulmonary artery *because prolonged manipulation here may reduce catheter stiffness.*

▶ When the mark on the catheter shaft reaches 15 to 20 cm, the catheter enters the right atrium. The waveform shows two small, upright waves; pressure is low (between 2 and 4 mm Hg). Read pressure values in the mean mode *because systolic and diastolic values are similar.*

▶ The doctor advances the catheter into the right ventricle, working quickly to minimize irritation. The waveform now shows sharp systolic upstrokes and lower diastolic dips. Depending on the size of the patient's heart, the catheter should reach the 30- to 35-cm mark. (The smaller the heart, the shorter the catheter length needed to reach the right ventricle.) Record both systolic and diastolic pressures. Systolic pressure normally ranges from 15 to 25 mm Hg; diastolic pressure, from 0 to 8 mm Hg.

▶ As the catheter floats into the pulmonary artery, note that the upstroke from right ventricular systole is smoother, and systolic pressure is nearly the same as right ventricular systolic

Normal PA waveforms

During pulmonary artery (PA) catheter insertion, the monitor shows various waveforms as the catheter advances through the heart chambers.

Right atrium

When the catheter tip enters the right atrium, the first heart chamber on its route, a waveform like the one shown below appears on the monitor. Note the two small upright waves. The *a* waves represent left atrial contraction; the *v* waves, increased pressure or volume in the left atrium during left ventricular systole.

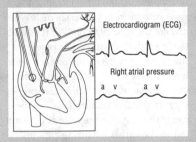

Right ventricle

As the catheter tip reaches the right ventricle, you'll see a waveform with sharp systolic upstrokes and lower diastolic dips.

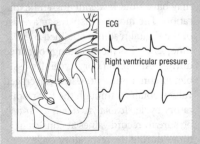

Pulmonary artery

The catheter then floats into the pulmonary artery, causing a waveform like the one shown below. Note that the upstroke is smoother than on the right ventricular waveform. The dicrotic notch indicates pulmonic valve closure.

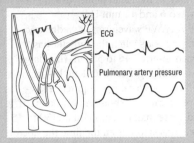

PAWP

Floating into a distal branch of the pulmonary artery, the balloon wedges where the vessel becomes too narrow for it to pass. The monitor now shows a pulmonary artery wedge pressure (PAWP) waveform, with two small uprises from left atrial systole and diastole. The balloon is then deflated and the catheter is left in the pulmonary artery.

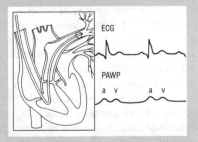

pressure. Record systolic, diastolic, and mean pressures (typically ranging from 8 to 15 mm Hg). A dicrotic notch on the diastolic portion of the waveform indicates pulmonic valve closure.

Wedging the catheter

▶ To obtain a wedge tracing, the doctor lets the inflated balloon float downstream with venous blood flow to a smaller, more distal branch of the pulmonary artery. Here, the catheter lodges, or wedges, causing occlusion of right ventricular and PA diastolic pressures. The tracing resembles the right atrial tracing because the catheter tip is recording left atrial pressure. The waveform shows two small uprises. Record PAWP in the mean mode (usually between 6 and 12 mm Hg).

▶ A PAWP waveform, or wedge tracing, appears when the catheter has been inserted 45 to 50 cm. (In a large heart, a longer catheter length — up to 55 cm — typically is required. However, a catheter should never be inserted more than 60 cm.) Usually, 30 to 45 seconds elapse from the time the doctor inserts the introducer until the wedge tracing appears.

▶ The doctor deflates the balloon, and the catheter drifts out of the wedge position and into the pulmonary artery, its normal resting place.

▶ If the appropriate waveforms don't appear at the expected times during catheter insertion, the catheter may be coiled in the right atrium and ventricle. To correct this problem, deflate the balloon. To do this, unlock the gate valve or turn the stopcock to the ON position and then detach the syringe from the balloon inflation port. Back pressure in the pulmonary artery causes the balloon to deflate on its own. (Active air withdrawal may compromise balloon integrity.) *To verify balloon deflation,* observe the monitor for return of the PA tracing.

▶ Typically, the doctor orders a portable chest X-ray to confirm catheter position.

▶ Apply a sterile occlusive dressing to the insertion site.

Obtaining intermittent PAP values

▶ After inserting the catheter and recording initial pressure readings, record subsequent PAP values and monitor waveforms. These values will be used to calculate other important hemodynamic indices. *To ensure accurate values,* make sure the transducer is properly leveled and zeroed.

▶ If possible, obtain PAP values at end expiration (when the patient completely exhales). *At this time, intrathoracic pressure approaches atmospheric pressure and has the least effect on PAP.* If you obtain a reading during other phases of the respiratory cycle, respiratory interference may occur. For instance, during inspiration, when intrathoracic pressure drops, PAP may be false-low because the negative pressure is transmitted to the catheter. During expiration, when intrathoracic pressure rises, PAP may be false-high.

▶ For patients with a rapid respiratory rate and subsequent variations, you may have trouble identifying end expiration. The monitor displays an average of the digital readings obtained over time, as well as those readings obtained during a full respiratory cycle. If possible, obtain a printout. Use the averaged values obtained through the full respiratory cycle. *To analyze trends accurately,* be sure to record values at consistent times during the respiratory cycle.

Taking a PAWP reading

▶ PAWP is recorded by inflating the balloon and letting it float in a distal artery. Some facilities allow only doctors or specially trained nurses to take a PAWP reading because of the risk of PA rupture — a rare but life-threatening complication. If your facility permits you to perform this procedure, do so with extreme caution and make sure you're thoroughly familiar with intracardiac waveform interpretation.

▶ To begin, verify that the transducer is properly leveled and zeroed. Detach the syringe from the balloon inflation hub. Draw 1.5 cc of air into the syringe, and then reattach the syringe to the hub. Watching the monitor, inject the air through the hub slowly and smoothly. When you see a wedge tracing on the monitor, immediately stop inflating the balloon. Never inflate the balloon beyond the volume needed to obtain a wedge tracing.

▶ Take the pressure reading at end expiration. Note the amount of air needed to change the PA tracing to a wedge tracing (normally, 1.25 to 1.5 cc). If the wedge tracing appeared with injection of less than 1.25 cc, suspect that the catheter has migrated into a more distal branch and requires repositioning. If the balloon is in a more distal branch, the tracings may move up the oscilloscope, indicating that the catheter tip is recording balloon pressure rather than PAWP. This may lead to PA rupture.

Removing the catheter

▶ To assist the doctor, inspect the chest X-ray for signs of catheter kinking or knotting. (In some states, you may be permitted to remove a PA catheter yourself under an advanced collaborative standard of practice.)

▶ Obtain the patient's baseline vital signs, and note the ECG pattern.

▶ Explain the procedure to the patient. Place the head of the bed flat, unless ordered otherwise. If the catheter was inserted using a superior approach, turn the patient's head to the side opposite the insertion site. Gently remove the dressing.

▶ The doctor will remove any sutures securing the catheter. However, if he wants to leave the introducer in place after catheter removal, he won't remove the sutures used to secure it.

▶ Turn all stopcocks off to the patient. (You may turn stopcocks on to the distal port if you wish to observe waveforms. However, use caution because this may cause an air embolism.)

▶ The doctor puts on sterile gloves. After verifying that the balloon is deflated, he withdraws the catheter slowly and smoothly. If he feels any resistance, he will stop immediately.

▶ Watch the ECG monitor for arrhythmias.

▶ If the introducer was removed, apply pressure to the site, and check it frequently for signs of bleeding. Dress the site again, as necessary. If the introducer is left in place, observe the diaphragm for any blood backflow, *which verifies the integrity of the hemostasis valve.*

▶ Return all equipment to the appropriate location. You may turn off the bedside pressure modules but leave the ECG module on.

▶ Reassure the patient and his family that he'll be observed closely. Make sure he understands that the catheter was removed because his condition has improved and he no longer needs it.

Special considerations

▶ Advise the patient to use caution when moving about in bed *to avoid dislodging the catheter.*

▶ Never leave the balloon inflated *because this may cause pulmonary infarction.* To determine if the balloon is inflated, check the monitor for a wedge tracing, which indicates inflation. (A PA tracing confirms balloon deflation.)

▶ Never inflate the balloon with more than the recommended air volume (specified on the catheter shaft) *because this may cause loss of elasticity or balloon rupture.* With appropriate inflation volume, the balloon floats easily through the heart chambers and rests in the main branch of the pulmonary artery, producing accurate waveforms. If the patient has a suspected left-to-right shunt, use carbon dioxide to inflate the balloon, as ordered, *because it diffuses more quickly than air.* Never inflate the balloon with fluids *because they may not be able to be retrieved from inside the balloon, preventing deflation.*

▶ Be aware that the catheter may slip back into the right ventricle. *Because the tip may irritate the ventricle,* check the monitor for a right ventricular waveform to detect this problem promptly.

▶ *To minimize valvular trauma,* make sure the balloon is deflated whenever the catheter is withdrawn from the pulmonary artery to the right ventricle or from the right ventricle to the right atrium.

▶ The Centers for Disease Control and Prevention (CDC) recommends changing the dressing whenever it's moist or every 24 to 48 hours, re-dressing the site according to your facility's policy, changing the catheter every 72 hours, changing the pressure tubing every 48 hours, and changing the flush solution every 24 hours. However, these recommendations were issued in 1982. Since then, some facilities have maintained closed-pressure monitoring systems for longer than the recommended times with no increase in infection rates. Nonetheless, before departing from CDC recommendations, determine your facility's policy.

Complications

Complications of PA catheter insertion include PA perforation, pulmonary infarction, catheter knotting, local or systemic infection, cardiac arrhythmias, and heparin-induced thrombocytopenia.

Documentation

Document the date and time of catheter insertion, the doctor who performed the procedure, the catheter insertion site, pressure waveforms and values for the various heart chambers, balloon inflation volume required to obtain a wedge tracing, any arrhythmias occurring during or after the procedure, type of flush solution used and its heparin concentration (if any), type of dressing applied, and the patient's tolerance of the procedure. Remember to initial and date the dressing.

After catheter removal, document the patient's tolerance for the removal procedure, and note any problems encountered during removal.

PAPANICOLAOU TESTING

Also known as the Pap test or Pap smear, the Papanicolaou test is a cytologic test that was developed in the 1920s by George N. Papanicolaou. It allows early detection of cervical cancer. The test involves scraping secretions from the cervix, spreading them on a slide, and immediately coating the slide with fixative spray or solution to preserve specimen cells for nuclear staining. Cytologic evaluation then outlines cell maturity, morphology, and metabolic activity. Although cervical scrapings are the most common test specimen, the Pap test also permits cytologic evaluation of the vaginal pool, prostatic secretions, urine, gastric secretions, cavity fluids, bronchial aspirations, and sputum.

Key nursing diagnoses and patient outcomes

Deficient knowledge related to lack of exposure to the papanicolaou testing
The patient will:
▶ express a need to increase knowledge
▶ state the intention to seek help from health care professionals when needed
▶ state or demonstrate an understanding of what has been taught.

Health-seeking behaviors (specify) related to potential for cervical cancer
The patient will:
▶ have regular scheduled tests
▶ express an understanding of the need for regular tests
▶ attend follow-up sessions with a health care professional when test results are abnormal.

Equipment

Bivalve vaginal speculum • gloves • Pap stick (wooden spatula) • long cotton-tipped applicator • three glass microscope slides • fixative (a commercial spray or 95% ethyl alcohol solution) • adjustable lamp • drape • laboratory request forms

Preparation of equipment

Select a speculum of the appropriate size, and gather the equipment in the examining room. Label each glass slide with the patient's name and the letter "E," "C," or "V" to differentiate endocervical, cervical, and vaginal specimens.

Implementation

▶ Explain the procedure to the patient and wash your hands.
▶ Instruct the patient to void *to relax the perineal muscles and facilitate bimanual examination of the uterus.*
▶ Provide privacy, and instruct the patient to undress below the waist but to wear her shoes, if desired, *to cushion her feet against the stirrups.* Then instruct her to sit on the examination table and to drape her genital region.
▶ Place the patient in the lithotomy position, with her feet in the stirrups and her buttocks extended slightly beyond the edge of the table. Adjust the drape.
▶ Adjust the lamp so that it fully illuminates the genital area. Then fold back the corner of the drape to expose the perineum.
▶ If you're performing the procedure, first put on gloves. Then take the speculum in your dominant hand and moisten it with warm water *to ease insertion.* Avoid using water-soluble lubricants, *which can interfere with accurate laboratory testing.*
▶ Warn the patient that you're about to touch her *to avoid startling her.* Then gently separate the labia with the thumb and forefinger of your nondominant hand.
▶ Instruct the patient to take several deep breaths, and insert the speculum into the vagina. Once it's in place, slowly open the blades to expose the cervix. Then lock the blades in place.
▶ Insert a cotton-tipped applicator through the speculum ¼" (5 mm) into the cervical os. Rotate the applicator 360 degrees to obtain an endocervical specimen. Then remove the applicator and gently roll it in a circle across the slide marked "E." Refrain from rubbing

the applicator on the slide *to prevent cell destruction.* Immediately place the slide in a fixative solution or spray it with a fixative *to prevent drying of the cells, which interferes with nuclear staining and cytologic interpretation.*

► Insert the small curved end of the Pap stick through the speculum, and place it directly over the cervical os. Rotate the stick gently but firmly *to scrape cells loose.* Remove the stick, spread the specimen across the slide marked "C," and fix it immediately, as before.

► Insert the opposite end of the Pap stick or a cotton-tipped applicator through the speculum, and scrape the posterior fornix or vaginal pool, an area that collects cells from the endometrium, vagina, and cervix. Remove the stick or applicator, spread the specimen across the slide marked "V," and fix it immediately.

► Unlock the speculum *to ease removal and avoid accidentally pinching the vaginal wall.* Then withdraw the speculum.

► Remove the glove from your nondominant hand to perform the bimanual examination, which usually follows the Pap test. Then remove your other glove, and discard both gloves.

► Gently remove the patient's feet from the stirrups, and assist her to a sitting position. Provide privacy for her to dress.

► Fill out the appropriate laboratory request forms, including the date of the patient's last menses.

Special considerations

► Many preventable factors can interfere with the Pap test's accuracy, so provide appropriate patient teaching beforehand. For example, use of a vaginal douche in the 48-hour period before

specimen collection washes away cellular deposits and prevents adequate sampling. Instillation of vaginal medications in the same period makes cytologic interpretation difficult. Collection of a specimen during menstruation prevents adequate sampling because menstrual flow washes away cells; ideally, such collection should take place 5 to 6 days before menses or 1 week after it. Application of topical antibiotics promotes rapid, heavy shedding of cells and requires postponement of the Pap test for at least 1 month.

► If the patient has had a complete hysterectomy, collect test specimens from the vaginal pool and cuff.

Complications

Failure to unlock the speculum blades before removal can pinch vaginal tissue. Slight cramping normally accompanies this examination, but rough handling of the speculum can cause severe cramping. Scraping an inflamed cervix with the Pap stick can cause slight bleeding.

Documentation

On the patient's chart, record the date and time of specimen collection, any complications, and the nursing action taken.

PERCUTANEOUS TRANSLUMINAL CORONARY ANGIOPLASTY

A nonsurgical approach to opening coronary vessels narrowed by arteriosclerosis, percutaneous transluminal coronary angioplasty (PTCA) uses a balloon-tipped catheter that is inserted

Performing PTCA

Percutaneous transluminal angio-plasty (PTCA) is a procedure that opens an occluded coronary artery without opening the chest. It's performed in the cardiac catheterization laboratory after coronary angiography confirms the presence and location of the occlusion. When the occlusion is located, the doctor threads a guide catheter through the patient's femoral artery and into the coronary artery under fluoroscopic guidance (as shown below).

When the guide catheter's position at the occlusion site is confirmed by angiography, the doctor carefully introduces into the catheter a double-lumen balloon that is smaller than the catheter lumen. He then directs the balloon through the lesion, where a marked pressure gradient will be obvious. The doctor alternately inflates (as shown below) and deflates the balloon until an angiogram verifies successful arterial dilation and the pressure gradient has decreased.

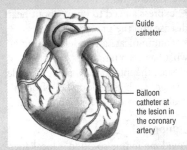

Guide catheter

Balloon catheter at the lesion in the coronary artery

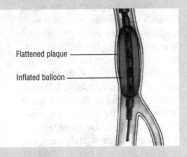

Flattened plaque

Inflated balloon

---

into a narrowed coronary artery. This procedure, performed in the cardiac catheterization laboratory under local anesthesia, relieves pain due to angina and myocardial ischemia.

Cardiac catheterization usually accompanies PTCA to assess the stenosis and the efficacy of the angioplasty. Catheterization is used as a visual tool to direct the balloon-tipped catheter through the vessel's area of stenosis. As the balloon is inflated, the plaque is compressed against the vessel wall, allowing coronary blood to flow more freely. (See *Performing PTCA*.)

PTCA provides an alternative for patients who are poor surgical risks because of chronic medical problems. It's also useful for patients who have total

coronary occlusion, unstable angina, and plaque buildup in several areas and for those with poor left ventricular function.

The ideal candidate for PTCA has single- or double-vessel disease excluding the left main coronary artery with at least 50% proximal stenosis. The lesion should be discrete, uncalcified, concentric, and not located near a bifurcation.

Your responsibilities in PTCA include teaching the patient and family about the procedure and assessing for complications afterward.

A newer procedure, laser-enhanced angioplasty, is showing promising results in vaporizing occlusions in atherosclerosis. (See *Laser-enhanced angioplasty*, page 620.)

Laser-enhanced angioplasty

Laser-enhanced angioplasty shows great potential for vaporizing occlusions in patients with atherosclerosis. The procedure achieves its best results with thrombotic occlusions, but it may also be used to remove calcified plaques. New lasers that deliver energy in brief pulses have helped solve the problem of thermal or acoustic damage to local tissues. Using the pulsed beam, doctors can dispatch the blockage without destroying the vessel wall.

To perform the procedure, the doctor threads a laser-containing catheter into the diseased artery. When the catheter nears the occlusion, the doctor triggers the laser to emit rapid bursts. Between bursts he rotates the catheter, advancing it until the occlusion is destroyed. The procedure takes about an hour and requires only a local anesthetic. Clearing a completely occluded coronary artery requires ten 1-second bursts of laser energy, followed by balloon angioplasty. After the procedure, angiography may be used to document vessel patency.

Cardiologists have successfully used laser techniques to open totally blocked right main coronary arteries, thereby avoiding bypass surgery. They have also used combinations of direct laser energy, fiber optics, and balloon angioplasty catheters to open totally blocked right main coronary arteries. These advances may make it possible to perform angioplasty in community hospitals in nonsurgical settings.

Key nursing diagnoses and patient outcomes

Activity intolerance related to decreased cardiac output
The patient will:

▶ maintain vital signs during prescribed activity including blood pressure not less than (specify) mm Hg and not greater than (specify) mm Hg; pulse not less than (specify) beats/minute and not greater than (specify) beats/minute; and respiratory rate within 5 breaths/minute from baseline

▶ demonstrate daily energy conservation skills at tolerance levels.

Deficient knowledge related to lack of information about heart disease and PTCA
The patient will:

▶ express a need to know about heart disease and the procedure

▶ communicate an understanding of what has been taught

▶ state the intention to make lifestyle changes such as seeking help from a health care professional when needed.

Equipment

Povidone-iodine solution • local anesthetic • I.V. solution and tubing • electrocardiogram (ECG) monitor and electrodes • oxygen • nasal cannula • shaving supplies or depilatory cream • sedative • pulmonary artery (PA) catheter • contrast medium • emergency medications • heparin for injection • 5-lb (2.3-kg) sandbag • introducer kit for PTCA catheter • sterile gown, gloves, and drapes • optional: nitroglycerin and soft restraints

Implementation

▶ Explain the procedure to the patient and family *to reduce the patient's fear and promote cooperation.*

▶ Inform the patient that the procedure lasts from 1 to 4 hours and that he may feel some discomfort from lying on a hard table for that long.

▶ Tell him that a catheter will be inserted into an artery or a vein in his groin and that he may feel pressure as the catheter moves along the vessel.

▶ Reassure him that although he'll be awake during the procedure, he'll be given a sedative. Explain that the doctor or nurse may ask him how he's feeling and that he should tell them if he experiences any angina.

▶ Explain that the doctor will inject a contrast medium *to outline the lesion's location.* Warn the patient that he may feel a hot, flushing sensation or transient nausea during the injection.

Before angioplasty

▶ Check the patient's history for allergies; if he's had allergic reactions to shellfish, iodine, or contrast media, notify the doctor.

▶ Give 650 mg of aspirin the evening before the procedure, as ordered, *to prevent platelet aggregation.*

▶ Make sure that the patient signs a consent form.

▶ Restrict food and fluids for at least 6 hours before the procedure or as ordered.

▶ Ensure that the results of coagulation studies, complete blood count, serum electrolyte studies, and blood typing and crossmatching are available.

▶ Insert an I.V. line *in case emergency medications are required.*

▶ Shave hair from the insertion site (groin or brachial area), or use a depilatory cream. Clean the area with povidone-iodine solution.

▶ Give the patient a sedative as ordered.

▶ Take baseline peripheral pulses in all extremities.

During angioplasty

▶ When the patient arrives at the cardiac catheterization laboratory, apply ECG electrodes and ensure I.V. line patency.

▶ Administer oxygen through a nasal cannula.

▶ The doctor will put on a sterile gown and gloves. Open the sterile supplies.

▶ The doctor prepares and drapes the site and injects a local anesthetic. If the patient doesn't have a PA catheter in place, the doctor may insert one now.

▶ The doctor inserts a large guide catheter into the artery and sutures it in place. Then he threads an angioplasty catheter through the guide catheter. An angioplasty catheter is thinner and longer and has a balloon at its tip. Using a thin, flexible guide wire, he then threads the catheter up through the aorta and into the coronary artery to the area of stenosis.

▶ He injects a contrast medium through the angioplasty catheter and into the obstructed coronary artery *to outline the lesion's location and help assess the blockage.* He also injects heparin *to prevent the catheter from clotting,* and intracoronary nitroglycerin *to dilate coronary vessels and prevent spasm, if needed.*

▶ He inflates the catheter's balloon for a gradually increasing amount of time and pressure. The expanding balloon compresses the atherosclerotic plaque against the arterial wall, expanding the arterial lumen. Because balloon inflation deprives the myocardium distal to the inflation area of blood, the patient may experience angina at this time. If balloon inflation fails to decrease the stenosis, a larger balloon may be used.

▶ After angioplasty, serial angiograms help determine the effectiveness of treatment.

Vascular stents

Two serious complications of percutaneous transluminal coronary angioplasty (PTCA) are acute vessel closure and late restenosis. To prevent these problems, doctors are performing a procedure called stenting. The stent currently used — the Palmaz balloon-expandable stent — consists of a stainless steel tube, the walls of which have a rectangular design. When the stent expands, each rectangle stretches to a diamond shape. The expanded stent supports the artery and helps prevent restenosis.

The stent is used in patients at risk for abrupt clotting after PTCA. Stents may also be inserted after failed PTCA to keep the patient stable until he can undergo coronary artery bypass surgery, or a stent may be used as an alternative to this surgery.

For insertion, the stent is put on a standard balloon angioplasty catheter and positioned over a guide wire (as shown below). Fluoroscopy verifies correct placement; then the stent is expanded and the catheter is removed.

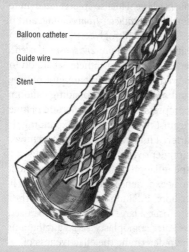

Balloon catheter

Guide wire

Stent

▶ The doctor removes the angioplasty catheter while leaving the guide catheter in place, *in case the procedure needs to be repeated because of vessel occlusion.* The guide catheter is usually removed 8 to 24 hours after the procedure.

After angioplasty

▶ When the patient returns to the unit, he may be receiving I.V. heparin or nitroglycerin. If he is bleeding at the catheter insertion site, he may also have a sandbag on it *to prevent a hematoma.*

▶ Assess the patient's vital signs every 15 minutes for the first hour, then every 30 minutes for 4 hours, unless his condition warrants more frequent checking.

▶ Assess peripheral pulses distal to the catheter insertion site as well as the color, sensation, temperature, and capillary refill of the affected extremity.

▶ Monitor ECG rhythm and arterial pressures.

Nursing alert Because coronary spasm may occur during or after PTCA, monitor the patient's ECG for ST-segment and T-wave changes, and take vital signs frequently. Coronary artery dissection may occur with no early symptoms, but it can cause restenosis of the vessel. Be alert for symptoms of ischemia, which requires emergency coronary revascularization.

▶ Instruct the patient to remain in bed for 8 hours and to keep the affected extremity straight; if the patient is restless and moving his extremities, apply soft restraints if necessary. Elevate the head of the bed 15 to 30 degrees.

▶ Assess the catheter site for hematoma, ecchymosis, and hemorrhage. If an area of expanding hematoma appears, mark the site and alert the doctor. If bleeding occurs, locate the artery and apply manual pressure; then notify the doctor.

▶ Administer I.V. fluids as ordered (usually 100 ml/hour) *to promote excretion of the contrast medium.* Be sure to assess for signs of fluid overload (distended neck veins, atrial and ventricular gallops, dyspnea, pulmonary congestion, tachycardia, hypertension, and hypoxemia).

▶ After the doctor removes the catheter, apply direct pressure for at least 10 minutes and monitor the site often.

Special considerations
PTCA is contraindicated in left main coronary artery disease, especially when the patient is a poor surgical risk; in patients with variant angina or critical valvular disease; and in patients with vessels that are occluded at the aortic wall orifice.

Complications
The most common complication of PTCA is prolonged angina. Others include coronary artery perforation, balloon rupture, reocclusion (necessitating a coronary artery bypass graft), myocardial infarction, pericardial tamponade, hematoma, hemorrhage, reperfusion arrhythmias, and closure of the vessel. Vascular stents may be inserted to prevent vessel closure. (See *Vascular stents.*)

Documentation
Note the patient's tolerance of the procedure and his condition after it, including vital signs and the condition of the extremity distal to the insertion site. Document any complications and interventions.

PERINEAL CARE

Perineal care, which includes care of the external genitalia and the anal area, should be performed during the daily bath and, if necessary, at bedtime and after urination and bowel movements. The procedure promotes cleanliness and prevents infection. It also removes irritating and odorous secretions, such as smegma, a cheeselike substance that collects under the foreskin of the penis and on the inner surface of the labia. For the patient with perineal skin breakdown, frequent bathing followed by application of an ointment or cream aids healing.

Standard precautions must be followed when providing perineal care, with due consideration given to the patient's privacy.

Key nursing diagnoses and patient outcomes
Bathing or hygiene self-care deficit related to (specify)
The patient will:
▶ meet self-care needs
▶ carry out self-care program daily
▶ communicate feelings and concerns.

Risk for infection
The patient will:
▶ state an understanding of signs and symptoms of infection, such as increased lochia, swelling, or malodorous lochia
▶ have no pathogens in cultures
▶ remain afebrile.

Equipment
Gloves • washcloths • clean basin • mild soap • bath towel • bath blanket • toilet tissue • linen-saver pad • trash

bag • optional: bedpan, peri bottle, antiseptic soap, petroleum jelly, zinc oxide cream, vitamin A and D ointment, and an ABD pad

Following genital or rectal surgery, you may need to use sterile supplies, including sterile gloves, gauze, and cotton balls.

Preparation of equipment

Obtain ointment or cream as needed. Fill the basin two-thirds full with warm water. Also fill the peri bottle with warm water if needed.

Implementation

▶ Assemble equipment at the patient's bedside and provide privacy.
▶ Wash your hands thoroughly, put on gloves, and explain to the patient what you're about to do.
▶ Adjust the bed to a comfortable working height *to prevent back strain,* and lower the head of the bed, if allowed.
▶ Provide privacy and help the patient to a supine position. Place a linen-saver pad under the patient's buttocks *to protect the bed from stains and moisture.*

Perineal care for the female patient

▶ *To minimize the patient's exposure and embarrassment,* place the bath blanket over her with corners head to foot and side to side. Wrap each leg with a side corner, tucking it under the hip. Then fold back the corner between the legs to expose the perineum.
▶ Ask the patient to bend her knees slightly and to spread her legs. Separate her labia with one hand and wash with the other, using gentle downward strokes from the front to the back of the perineum *to prevent intestinal organisms from contaminating the urethra or vagina.*

Avoid the area around the anus, and use a clean section of washcloth for each stroke by folding each used section inward. *This prevents the spread of contaminated secretions or discharge.*
▶ Using a clean washcloth, rinse thoroughly from front to back *because soap residue can cause skin irritation.* Pat the area dry with a bath towel *because moisture can also cause skin irritation and discomfort.*
▶ Apply ordered ointments or creams.
▶ Turn the patient on her side to Sims' position, if possible, *to expose the anal area.*
▶ Clean, rinse, and dry the anal area, starting at the posterior vaginal opening and wiping from front to back.

Perineal care for the male patient

▶ Drape the patient's legs *to minimize exposure and embarrassment* and expose the genital area.
▶ Hold the shaft of the penis with one hand and wash with the other, beginning at the tip and working in a circular motion from the center to the periphery *to avoid introducing microorganisms into the urethra.* Use a clean section of washcloth for each stroke *to prevent the spread of contaminated secretions or discharge.*
▶ Rinse thoroughly, using the same circular motion.
▶ For the uncircumcised patient, gently retract the foreskin and clean beneath it. Rinse well but don't dry *because moisture provides lubrication and prevents friction when replacing the foreskin.* Replace the foreskin to avoid constriction of the penis, *which causes edema and tissue damage.*
▶ Wash the rest of the penis, using downward strokes toward the scrotum. Rinse well and pat dry with a towel.

▶ Clean the top and sides of the scrotum; rinse thoroughly and pat dry. Handle the scrotum gently *to avoid causing discomfort.*

▶ Turn the patient on his side. Clean the bottom of the scrotum and the anal area. Rinse well and pat dry.

After providing perineal care

▶ Reposition the patient and make him comfortable. Remove the bath blanket and linen-saver pad; then replace the bed linens.

▶ Clean and return the basin and dispose of soiled articles, including gloves.

Special considerations

▶ Give perineal care in a matter-of-fact way *to minimize embarrassment.*

▶ If the patient is incontinent, first remove excess feces with toilet tissue. Position him on a bedpan and add a small amount of antiseptic soap to a peri bottle *to eliminate odor.* Irrigate the perineal area *to remove any remaining fecal matter.*

▶ After cleaning the perineum, apply ointment or cream (petroleum jelly, zinc oxide cream, or vitamin A and D ointment) *to prevent skin breakdown by providing a barrier between the skin and excretions.*

▶ To reduce the number of linen changes, tuck an ABD pad between the patient's buttocks *to absorb oozing feces.*

Documentation

Record perineal care and any special treatment in your notes. Document the need for continued treatment, if necessary, in your plan of care. Describe perineal skin condition and any odor or discharge.

PERIPHERAL I.V. LINE INSERTION

Peripheral I.V. line insertion involves selection of a venipuncture device and an insertion site, application of a tourniquet, preparation of the site, and venipuncture. Selection of a venipuncture device and site depends on the type of solution to be used; frequency and duration of infusion; patency and location of accessible veins; the patient's age, size, and condition; and, when possible, the patient's preference.

If possible, choose a vein in the nondominant arm or hand. Preferred venipuncture sites are the cephalic and basilic veins in the lower arm and the veins in the dorsum of the hand; least favorable are the leg and foot veins because of the increased risk of thrombophlebitis and infection. Antecubital veins can be used if no other venous access is available, to accommodate a large-bore needle, or to administer drugs that require large-volume dilution.

A peripheral line allows administration of fluids, medication, blood, and blood components and maintains I.V. access to the patient. Insertion is contraindicated in a sclerotic vein, an edematous or impaired arm or hand, or a postmastectomy arm and in patients with a mastectomy, burns, or an arteriovenous fistula. Subsequent venipunctures should be performed proximal to a previously used or injured vein.

Key nursing diagnoses and patient outcomes

Risk for infection related to the procedure
The patient will:

▶ have normal vital signs, temperature, and laboratory values

▶ have no pathogens in cultures
▶ show no signs or symptoms of infection, such as redness, swelling, or drainage at the infection site.

Risk for deficient fluid volume related to need for peripheral I.V. line
The patient will:
▶ maintain normal skin color and temperature
▶ exhibit no signs of dehydration
▶ maintain normal output of at least (specify) ml/hour
▶ have electrolyte values within normal range
▶ maintain fluid balance (intake will equal output).

Equipment

Alcohol pads or an approved antimicrobial solution, such as tincture of iodine 2% or 10% povidone-iodine • gloves • tourniquet (rubber tubing or a blood pressure cuff) • I.V. access devices • I.V. solution with attached and primed administration set • I.V. pole • sharps container • sterile 2″ × 2″ gauze pads or a transparent semipermeable dressing • 1″ hypoallergenic tape • optional: arm board, roller gauze, tube gauze, warm packs, scissors

Commercial venipuncture kits come with or without an I.V. access device. (See *Comparing venous access devices.*) In many facilities, venipuncture equipment is kept on a tray or cart, allowing choice of correct access devices and easy replacement of contaminated items.

Preparation of equipment

Check the information on the label of the I.V. solution container, including the patient's name and room number, type of solution, time and date of its preparation, preparer's name, and ordered infusion rate. Compare the doctor's orders with the solution label *to verify that the solution is the correct one.* Then select the smallest-gauge device that is appropriate for the infusion (unless subsequent therapy will require a larger one). *Smaller gauges cause less trauma to veins, allow greater blood flow around their tips, and reduce the clotting risk.*

If you're using a winged infusion set, connect the adapter to the administration set, and unclamp the line until fluid flows from the open end of the needle cover. Then close the clamp and place the needle on a sterile surface, such as the inside of its packaging. If you're using a catheter device, open its package *to allow easy access.*

Implementation

▶ Place the I.V. pole in the proper slot in the patient's bed frame. If you're using a portable I.V. pole, position it close to the patient.
▶ Hang the I.V. solution with attached primed administration set on the I.V. pole.
▶ Verify the patient's identity by comparing the information on the solution container with the patient's wristband.
▶ Wash your hands thoroughly. Then explain the procedure to the patient *to ensure his cooperation and reduce anxiety. Anxiety can cause a vasomotor response resulting in venous constriction.*

Selecting the site

▶ Select the puncture site. If long-term therapy is anticipated, start with a vein at the most distal site *so that you can move proximally as needed for subsequent I.V. insertion sites.* For infusion of an irritating medication, choose a large vein

Comparing venous access devices

Most I.V. infusions are delivered through one of three basic types of venous access devices: an over-the-needle cannula, a through-the-needle cannula, or a winged infusion set. To improve I.V. therapy and guard against accidental needle sticks, you can use a needle-free system.

Over-the-needle cannula
Purpose: Long-term therapy for an active or agitated patient

Advantages: Makes accidental puncture of the vein less likely than with a needle; more comfortable for the patient when it's in place; contains radiopaque thread for easy location. Some units come with a syringe that permits easy check of blood return; some units include wings.

Disadvantage: More difficult to insert than other devices

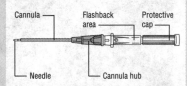

Through-the-needle cannula
Purpose: Long-term therapy for an active or agitated patient

Advantages: Makes accidental puncture of the vein less likely than with a needle; more comfortable for the patient when it's in place; available in many lengths; most plastic cannulas contain radiopaque thread for easy location. One variant, the peripherally inserted central catheter, is commonly inserted in the antecubital vein by a specially trained nurse.

Disadvantages: Leaking at the site, especially in an elderly patient. The cannula may be severed during insertion if pulled back through the needle.

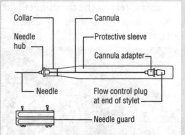

Winged infusion set
Purpose: Short-term therapy for cooperative adult patient; therapy of any duration for an infant or a child or for an elderly patient with fragile or sclerotic veins

Advantages: Less painful to insert; ideal for I.V. push drugs

Disadvantages: May easily cause infiltration if a rigid-needle winged infusion device is used

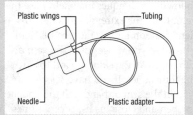

distal to any nearby joint. Make sure the intended vein can accommodate the cannula.

► Place the patient in a comfortable, reclining position, leaving the arm in a dependent position *to increase capillary fill of the lower arms and hands.* If the patient's skin is cold, warm it by rubbing and stroking the arm, or cover the entire arm with warm packs for 5 to 10 minutes.

Applying the tourniquet

▶ Apply a tourniquet about 4″ to 6″ (10 cm to 15 cm) above the intended puncture site *to dilate the vein* (as shown below). Check for a radial pulse. If it isn't present, release the tourniquet and reapply it with less tension *to prevent arterial occlusion.*

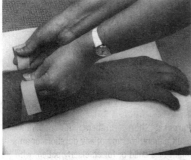

▶ Lightly palpate the vein with the index and middle fingers of your nondominant hand. Stretch the skin *to anchor the vein.* If the vein feels hard or ropelike, select another.
▶ If the vein is easily palpable but not sufficiently dilated, one or more of the following techniques may help raise the vein. Place the extremity in a dependent position for several seconds, and gently tap your finger over the vein or rub or stroke the skin upward toward the tourniquet. If you have selected a vein in the arm or hand, tell the patient to open and close his fist several times.
▶ Leave the tourniquet in place for no longer than 3 minutes. If you can't find a suitable vein and prepare the site in that time, release the tourniquet for a few minutes. Then reapply it and continue the procedure.

Preparing the site

▶ Put on gloves. Clip the hair around the insertion site if needed. Clean the site with alcohol pads or an approved antimicrobial solution, according to your facility's policy.

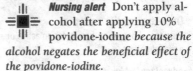 **Nursing alert** Don't apply alcohol after applying 10% povidone-iodine *because the alcohol negates the beneficial effect of the povidone-iodine.*

Work in a circular motion outward from the site to a diameter of 2″ to 4″ (5 to 10 cm) (as shown below) *to remove flora that would otherwise be introduced into the vascular system with the venipuncture.* Allow the antimicrobial solution to dry.

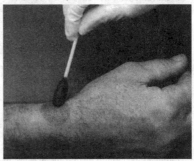

▶ If ordered, administer a local anesthetic. Make sure the patient isn't sensitive to lidocaine.
▶ Lightly press the vein with the thumb of your nondominant hand about 1½″ (4 cm) from the intended insertion site. The vein should feel round, firm, fully engorged, and resilient.
▶ Grasp the access cannula. If you're using a *winged infusion set,* hold the short edges of the wings (with the needle's bevel facing upward) between the thumb and forefinger of your dominant hand. Then squeeze the wings together. If you're using an *over-the-needle cannula,* grasp the plastic hub with your

dominant hand, remove the cover, and examine the cannula tip. If the edge isn't smooth, discard and replace the device. If you're using a *through-the-needle cannula,* grasp the needle hub with one hand, and unsnap the needle cover. Rotate the access device until the bevel faces upward.

▶ Using the thumb of your nondominant hand, stretch the skin taut below the puncture site *to stabilize the vein* (as shown below).

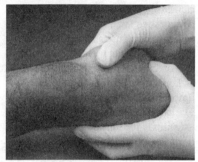

▶ Tell the patient that you are about to insert the device.

▶ Hold the needle bevel up and enter the skin directly over the vein at a 15- to 25-degree angle (as shown below).

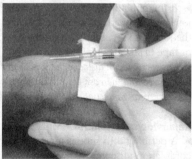

▶ Aggressively push the needle directly through the skin and into the vein in one motion. Check the flashback chamber behind the hub for blood return, signifying that the vein has been properly accessed. (You may not see a blood return in a small vein.)

▶ Then level the insertion device slightly by lifting the tip of the device up *to prevent puncturing the back wall of the vein with the access device.*

▶ If you're using a winged infusion set, advance the needle fully, if possible, and hold it in place. Release the tourniquet, open the administration set clamp slightly, and check for free flow or infiltration.

▶ If you're using an over-the-needle cannula, advance the device 2 to 3 mm to ensure that the cannula itself—not just the introducer needle—has entered the vein. Then remove the tourniquet.

▶ Grasp the cannula hub to hold it in the vein, and withdraw the needle. As you withdraw it, press lightly on the catheter tip to prevent bleeding (as shown below).

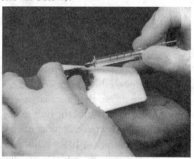

▶ Advance the cannula up to the hub or until you meet resistance.

▶ To advance the cannula while infusing I.V. solution, release the tourniquet and remove the inner needle. Using sterile technique, attach the I.V. tubing and begin the infusion. While stabilizing the vein with one hand, use the other to advance the catheter into the vein. When the catheter is advanced, decrease the I.V. flow rate. *This method reduces the risk of puncturing the vein's opposite wall because the catheter is ad-*

vanced without the steel needle and because the rapid flow dilates the vein.
▶ To advance the cannula before starting the infusion, first release the tourniquet. While stabilizing the vein with one hand, use the other to advance the catheter up to the hub (as shown).

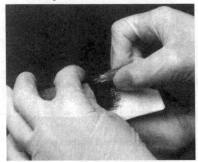

Next, remove the inner needle and, using sterile technique, quickly attach the I.V. tubing. *This method commonly results in less blood being spilled.*
▶ If you're using a through-the-needle cannula, remove the tourniquet, hold the needle in place with one hand and, with your opposite hand, grasp the cannula through the protective sleeve. Then slowly thread the cannula through the needle until the hub is within the needle collar. Never pull back on the cannula without pulling back on the needle *to avoid severing and releasing the cannula into the circulation, causing an embolus.* If you feel resistance from the valve, withdraw the cannula and needle slightly and reinsert them, rotating the cannula as you pass the valve. Then withdraw the metal needle, split the needle along the perforated edge (according to the manufacturer's instructions), and carefully remove it from around the cannula. Dispose of the needle pieces appropriately. Remove the stylet and protective sleeve, and attach the administration set to the can-

nula hub. Open the administration set clamp slightly, and check for free flow or infiltration.

Dressing the site
▶ After the venous access device has been inserted, clean the skin completely. If necessary, dispose of the stylet in a sharps container. Then regulate the flow rate.
▶ You may use a transparent semipermeable dressing *to secure the device.* (See *How to apply a transparent semipermeable dressing.*)
▶ If you don't use a transparent dressing, cover the site with a sterile gauze pad or small adhesive bandage.
▶ Loop the I.V. tubing on the patient's limb, and secure the tubing with tape. *The loop allows some slack to prevent dislodgment of the cannula from tension on the line.* (See *Methods of taping a venous access site,* page 632.)
▶ Label the last piece of tape with the type, gauge of needle, and length of cannula; date and time of insertion; and your initials. Adjust the flow rate as ordered.
▶ If the puncture site is near a movable joint, place a padded arm board under the joint and secure it with roller gauze or tape *to provide stability because excessive movement can dislodge the venous access device and increase the risk of thrombophlebitis and infection.*

Removing a peripheral I.V. line
▶ A peripheral I.V. line is removed on completion of therapy, for cannula site changes, and for suspected infection or infiltration; the procedure usually requires gloves, a sterile gauze pad, and an adhesive bandage.
▶ To remove the I.V. line, first clamp the I.V. *tubing to stop the flow of solution.*

Then gently remove the transparent dressing and all tape from the skin.

► Using sterile technique, open the gauze pad and adhesive bandage and place them within reach. Put on gloves. Hold the sterile gauze pad over the puncture site with one hand, and use your other hand to withdraw the cannula slowly and smoothly, keeping it parallel to the skin. (Inspect the cannula tip; if it isn't smooth, assess the patient immediately and notify the doctor.)

► Using the gauze pad, apply firm pressure over the puncture site for 1 to 2 minutes after removal or until bleeding has stopped.

► Clean the site and apply the adhesive bandage or, if blood oozes, apply a pressure bandage.

► If drainage appears at the puncture site, send the tip of the device and a sample of the drainage to the laboratory to be cultured according to your facility's policy. (A draining site may or may not be infected.) Then clean the area, apply a sterile dressing, and notify the doctor.

► Instruct the patient to restrict activity for about 10 minutes and to leave the dressing in place for at least 1 hour. If the patient experiences lingering tenderness at the site, apply warm packs and notify the doctor.

Special considerations

Age alert Apply the tourniquet carefully to avoid pinching the skin. If necessary, apply it over the patient's gown. Make sure skin preparation materials are at room temperature *to avoid vasoconstriction resulting from lower temperatures.*

How to apply a transparent semipermeable dressing

To secure the I.V. insertion site, you can apply a transparent semipermeable dressing as follows:
■ Make sure the insertion site is clean and dry.
■ Remove the dressing from the package and, using sterile technique, remove the protective seal. Avoid touching the sterile surface.
■ Place the dressing directly over the insertion site and the hub, as shown. Don't cover the tubing. Also, don't stretch the dressing; doing so may cause itching.
■ Tuck the dressing around and under the cannula hub to make the site impervious to microorganisms.
■ To remove the dressing, grasp one corner and then lift and stretch it. If removal is difficult, try loosening the edges with alcohol or water.

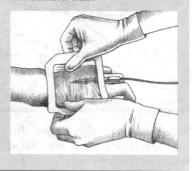

► If the patient is allergic to iodine-containing compounds, clean the skin with alcohol.

► If you fail to see blood flashback after the needle enters the vein, pull back slightly and rotate the device. If you still fail to see flashback, remove the cannula and try again or proceed according to your facility's policy.

Methods of taping a venous access site

When using tape to secure the access device to the insertion site, use one of the basic methods described below. Use only sterile tape under a transparent, semipermeable dressing.

Chevron method

- Cut a long strip of ½" tape and place it sticky side up under the cannula and parallel to the short strip of tape.
- Cross the ends of the tape over the cannula so that the tape sticks to the patient's skin (as shown below).
- Apply a piece of 1" tape across the two wings of the chevron.
- Loop the tubing and secure it with another piece of 1" tape. When the dressing is secured, apply a label. On the label, write the date and time of insertion, type and gauge of the needle, and your initials.

U method

- Cut a 2" (5-cm) strip of ½" tape. With the sticky side up, place it under the hub of the cannula.
- Bring each side of the tape up, folding it over the wings of the cannula in a U shape (as shown below). Press it down parallel to the hub.
- Apply tape to stabilize the catheter.
- When a dressing is secured, apply a label. On the label, write the date and time of insertion, type and gauge of the needle or cannula, and your initials.

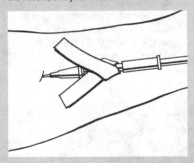

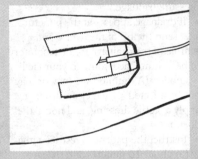

▶ Change a gauze or transparent dressing whenever you change the administration set (every 48 to 72 hours or according to your facility's policy).

▶ Be sure to rotate the I.V. site, usually every 48 to 72 hours or according to your facility's policy.

Home care

Most patients who receive I.V. therapy at home have a central venous line. But if you're caring for a patient going home with a peripheral line, you should teach him how to care for the I.V. site and identify certain complications. If the patient must observe movement restrictions, make sure he understands them.

Teach the patient how to examine the site, and instruct him to notify the doctor or home care nurse if redness, swelling, or discomfort develops; if the dressing becomes moist; or if blood appears in the tubing.

Also tell the patient to report any problems with the I.V. line, for instance, if the solution stops infusing or if an alarm goes off on an infusion

H method

- Cut three strips of 1″ tape.
- Place one strip of tape over each wing, keeping the tape parallel to the cannula (as shown below).
- Now place the other strip of tape perpendicular to the first two. Put it either directly on top of the wings or just below the wings, directly on top of the tubing.
- Make sure the cannula is secure; then apply a dressing and a label. On the label, write the date and time of insertion, type and gauge of needle or cannula, and your initials.

X method

- Place a transparent semipermeable dressing over the insertion site.
- Cut two 2 strips of ½″ tape.
- Place one strip diagonal over the hub of the cannula.
- Now place the second strip diagonal to the hub in the opposite direction, forming an X with the first strip (as shown below).

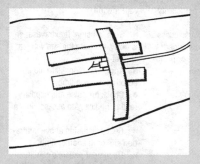

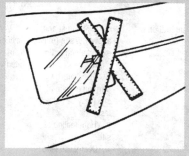

pump. Explain that the I.V. site will be changed at established intervals by a home care nurse.

If the patient is using an intermittent infusion device, teach him how and when to flush it. Finally, teach the patient to document daily whether the I.V. site is free from pain, swelling, and redness.

Complications

Peripheral line complications can result from the needle or catheter (infection, phlebitis, and embolism) or from the solution (circulatory overload, infiltration, sepsis, and allergic reaction). (See *Risks of peripheral I.V. therapy*, pages 634 to 639.)

Documentation

In your notes or on the appropriate I.V. sheets, record the date and time of the venipuncture; type, gauge, and length of the cannula or needle; anatomic location of the insertion site; and reason the site was changed.

(Text continues on page 639.)

Risks of peripheral I.V. therapy

Complication	Signs and symptoms	Possible causes	Nursing interventions
Local complications			
Phlebitis	■ Tenderness at tip of and proximal to venous access device ■ Redness at tip of cannula and along vein ■ Puffy area over vein ■ Vein hard on palpation ■ Elevated temperature	■ Poor blood flow around venous access device ■ Friction from cannula movement in vein ■ Venous access device left in vein too long ■ Clotting at cannula tip (thrombophlebitis) ■ Drug or solution with high or low pH or high osmolarity	■ Remove venous access device. ■ Apply warm soaks. ■ Notify doctor if patient has a fever. ■ Document patient's condition and your interventions. ***Prevention*** ■ Restart infusion using larger vein for irritating solution, or restart with smaller-gauge device to ensure adequate blood flow. ■ Use filter to reduce risk of phlebitis. ■ Tape device securely to prevent motion.
Infiltration	■ Swelling at and above I.V. site (may extend along entire limb) ■ Discomfort, burning or pain at site (may be painless) ■ Tight feeling at site ■ Decreased skin temperature around site ■ Blanching at site ■ Continuing fluid infusion even when vein is occluded (although rate may decrease) ■ Absent backflow of blood	■ Venous access device dislodged from vein, or perforated vein	■ Stop infusion. If extravasation is likely, infiltrate the site with an antidote. ■ Apply warm soaks to aid absorption. Elevate limb. ■ Check for pulse and capillary refill periodically to assess circulation. ■ Restart infusion above infiltration site or in another limb. ■ Document patient's condition and your interventions. ***Prevention*** ■ Check I.V. site frequently. ■ Don't obscure area above site with tape. ■ Teach patient to observe I.V. site and report pain or swelling.
Cannula dislodgment	■ Loose tape ■ Cannula partly backed out of vein ■ Solution infiltrating	■ Loosened tape, or tubing snagged in bed linens, resulting in partial retraction of cannula; pulled out by confused patient	■ If no infiltration occurs, retape without pushing cannula back into vein. If pulled out, apply pressure to I.V. site with sterile dressing. ***Prevention*** ■ Tape venipuncture device securely on insertion.

Risks of peripheral I.V. therapy (continued)

Complication	Signs and symptoms	Possible causes	Nursing interventions
Local complications (continued)			
Occlusion	■ No increase in flow rate when I.V. container is raised ■ Blood backflow in line ■ Discomfort at insertion site	■ I.V. flow interrupted ■ Heparin lock not flushed ■ Blood backflow in line when patient walks ■ Line clamped too long	■ Use mild flush injection. Don't force it. If unsuccessful, remove I.V. line and insert a new one. *Prevention* ■ Maintain I.V. flow rate. ■ Flush promptly after intermittent piggyback administration. ■ Have patient walk with his arm bent at the elbow *to reduce risk of blood backflow.*
Vein irritation or pain at I.V. site	■ Pain during infusion ■ Possible blanching if vasospasm occurs ■ Red skin over vein during infusion ■ Rapidly developing signs of phlebitis	■ Solution with high or low pH or high osmolarity, such as 40 mEq/L of potassium chloride, phenytoin, and some antibiotics (vancomycin, erythromycin, and nafcillin)	■ Decrease the flow rate. ■ Try using an electronic flow device *to achieve a steady flow.* *Prevention* ■ Dilute solutions before administration. For example, give antibiotics in 250-ml solution rather than 100-ml solution. If drug has low pH, ask pharmacist if drug can be buffered with sodium bicarbonate. (Refer to your facility's policy.) ■ If long-term therapy of irritating drug is planned, ask doctor to use central I.V. line.
Hematoma	■ Tenderness at venipuncture site ■ Bruised area around site ■ Inability to advance or flush I.V. line	■ Vein punctured through opposite wall at time of insertion ■ Leakage of blood from needle displacement ■ Inadequate pressure applied when cannula is discontinued	■ Remove venous access device. ■ Apply pressure and warm soaks to affected area. ■ Recheck for bleeding. ■ Document patient's condition and your interventions. *Prevention* ■ Choose a vein that can accommodate the size of venous access device. ■ Release tourniquet as soon as insertion is successful.
Severed cannula	■ Leakage from cannula shaft	■ Cannula inadvertently cut by scissors	■ If broken part is visible, attempt to retrieve it. If unsuccessful, notify the doctor.

(continued)

Risks of peripheral I.V. therapy *(continued)*

Complication	Signs and symptoms	Possible causes	Nursing interventions
Local complications *(continued)*			
Severed cannula *(continued)*		■ Reinsertion of needle into cannula	■ If portion of cannula enters bloodstream, place tourniquet above I.V. site *to prevent progression of broken part.* ■ Notify doctor and radiology department. ■ Document patient's condition and your interventions. ***Prevention*** ■ Don't use scissors around I.V. site. ■ Never reinsert needle into cannula. ■ Remove unsuccessfully inserted cannula and needle together.
Venous spasm	■ Pain along vein ■ Flow rate sluggish when clamp completely open ■ Blanched skin over vein	■ Severe vein irritation from irritating drugs or fluids ■ Administration of cold fluids or blood ■ Very rapid flow rate (with fluids at room temperature)	■ Apply warm soaks over vein and surrounding area. ■ Decrease flow rate. ***Prevention*** ■ Use a blood warmer for blood or packed red blood cells.
Thrombosis	■ Painful, reddened, and swollen vein ■ Sluggish or stopped I.V. flow	■ Injury to endothelial cells of vein wall, allowing platelets to adhere and thrombi to form	■ Remove venous access device; restart infusion in opposite limb if possible. ■ Apply warm soaks. ■ Watch for I.V. therapy–related infection; thrombi provide an excellent environment for bacterial growth. ***Prevention*** ■ Use proper venipuncture techniques *to reduce injury to vein.*
Thrombophlebitis	■ Severe discomfort ■ Reddened, swollen, and hardened vein	■ Thrombosis and inflammation	■ Same as for thrombosis. ***Prevention*** ■ Check site frequently. Remove venous access device at first sign of redness and tenderness.

Risks of peripheral I.V. therapy *(continued)*

Complication	Signs and symptoms	Possible causes	Nursing interventions
Local complications *(continued)*			
Nerve, tendon, or ligament damage	■ Extreme pain (similar to electrical shock when nerve is punctured) ■ Numbness and muscle contraction ■ Delayed effects, including paralysis, numbness, and deformity	■ Improper venipuncture technique, resulting in injury to surrounding nerves, tendons, or ligaments ■ Tight taping or improper splinting with arm board	■ Stop procedure. ***Prevention*** ■ Don't repeatedly penetrate tissues with venous access device. ■ Don't apply excessive pressure when taping; don't encircle limb with tape. ■ Pad arm boards and tape securing arm boards if possible.
Systemic complications			
Systemic infection (septicemia or bacteremia)	■ Fever, chills, and malaise for no apparent reason ■ Contaminated I.V. site, usually with no visible signs of infection at site	■ Failure to maintain aseptic technique during insertion or site care ■ Severe phlebitis, which can set up ideal conditions for organism growth ■ Poor taping that permits venous access device to move, which can introduce organisms into bloodstream ■ Prolonged indwelling time of device ■ Weak immune system	■ Notify the doctor. ■ Administer medications as prescribed. ■ Culture the site and device. ■ Monitor vital signs. ***Prevention*** ■ Use scrupulous aseptic technique when handling solutions and tubing, inserting venous access device, and discontinuing infusion. ■ Secure all connections. ■ Change I.V. solutions, tubing, and venous access device at recommended times. ■ Use I.V. filters.
Vasovagal reaction	■ Sudden collapse of vein during venipuncture ■ Sudden pallor, sweating, faintness, dizziness, and nausea ■ Decreased blood pressure	■ Vasospasm from anxiety or pain	■ Lower head of bed. ■ Have patient take deep breaths. ■ Check vital signs. ***Prevention*** ■ Prepare patient for therapy *to relieve his anxiety.* ■ Use local anesthetic *to prevent pain.*

(continued)

Risks of peripheral I.V. therapy *(continued)*

Complication	Signs and symptoms	Possible causes	Nursing interventions

Systemic complications *(continued)*

Complication	Signs and symptoms	Possible causes	Nursing interventions
Allergic reaction	■ Itching ■ Watery eyes and nose ■ Bronchospasm ■ Wheezing ■ Urticarial rash ■ Edema at I.V. site ■ Anaphylactic reaction (flushing, chills, anxiety, itching, palpitations, paresthesia, wheezing, seizures, cardiac arrest) up to 1 hour after exposure	■ Allergens such as medications	■ If reaction occurs, stop infusion immediately. ■ Maintain a patent airway. ■ Notify the doctor. ■ Administer antihistaminic steroid, anti-inflammatory, and antipyretic drugs, as prescribed. ■ Give 0.2 to 0.5 ml of 1:1,000 aqueous epinephrine S.C., as prescribed. Repeat at 3-minute intervals and as needed and prescribed. ***Prevention*** ■ Obtain patient's allergy history. Be aware of cross-allergies. ■ Assist with test dosing and document any new allergies. ■ Monitor patient carefully during first 15 minutes of administration of a new drug.
Circulatory overload	■ Discomfort ■ Neck vein engorgement ■ Respiratory distress ■ Increased blood pressure ■ Crackles ■ Increased difference between fluid intake and output	■ Roller clamp loosened to allow run-on infusion ■ Flow rate too rapid ■ Miscalculation of fluid requirements	■ Raise the head of the bed. ■ Administer oxygen as needed. ■ Notify the doctor. ■ Administer medications (probably furosemide) as prescribed. ***Prevention*** ■ Use pump, controller, or rate minder for elderly or compromised patients. ■ Recheck calculations of fluid requirements. ■ Monitor infusion frequently.
Air embolism	■ Respiratory distress ■ Unequal breath sounds ■ Weak pulse ■ Increased central venous pressure	■ Solution container empty ■ Solution container empties, and added container pushes air down the line (if line not purged first)	■ Discontinue infusion. ■ Place patient on his left side in Trendelenburg's position to allow air to enter right atrium and disperse by way of pulmonary artery. ■ Administer oxygen. ■ Notify the doctor. ■ Document patient's condition and your interventions.

Risks of peripheral I.V. therapy *(continued)*

Complication	Signs and symptoms	Possible causes	Nursing interventions
Systemic complications *(continued)*			
Air embolism *(continued)*	■ Decreased blood pressure ■ Loss of consciousness		***Prevention*** ■ Purge tubing of air completely before starting infusion. ■ Use air-detection device on pump or air-eliminating filter proximal to I.V. site. ■ Secure connections.

Also document the number of attempts at venipuncture (if you made more than one), type and flow rate of the I.V. solution, name and amount of medication in the solution (if any), any adverse reactions and actions taken to correct them, patient teaching and evidence of patient understanding, and your initials.

PERIPHERAL I.V. LINE MAINTENANCE

Routine maintenance of I.V. sites and systems includes regular assessment and rotation of the site and periodic changes of the dressing, tubing, and solution. These measures help prevent complications, such as thrombophlebitis and infection. They should be performed according to your facility's policy.

Typically, gauze I.V. dressings are changed every 48 hours and whenever the dressing becomes wet, soiled, or nonocclusive. Transparent semipermeable dressings are changed whenever I.V. tubing is changed every 48 to 72 hours or according to policy, and I.V.

solution is changed every 24 hours or as needed. The site should be assessed every 2 hours if a transparent semipermeable dressing is used or with every dressing change otherwise and should be rotated every 48 to 72 hours. Sometimes limited venous access prevents frequent site changes; if so, be sure to assess the site frequently.

Key nursing diagnoses and patient outcomes

Risk for infection related to the procedure
The patient will:
▶ have normal vital signs, temperature, and laboratory values
▶ have no pathogens appear in cultures
▶ show no signs or symptoms of infection, such as redness, swelling, or drainage at the infection site.

Risk for deficient fluid volume related to need for peripheral I.V. line
The patient will:
▶ maintain normal skin color and temperature
▶ exhibit no signs of dehydration
▶ maintain normal output of at least (specify) ml/hour

▶ have electrolyte values within normal range
▶ maintain fluid balance (intake will equal output).

Equipment

For dressing changes
Sterile gloves • povidone-iodine or alcohol pads • adhesive bandage, sterile 2″ × 2″ gauze pad, or transparent semipermeable dressing • 1″ adhesive tape

For solution changes
Solution container • alcohol pad

For tubing changes
I.V. administration set • sterile gloves • 2″ × 2″ gauze pad • adhesive tape for labeling • optional: hemostats

For I.V. site change
Commercial kits containing the equipment for dressing changes are available.

Preparation of equipment
If your facility keeps I.V. equipment and dressings in a tray or cart, have it nearby, if possible, *because you may have to select a new venipuncture site, depending on the current site's condition.* If you're changing both the solution and the tubing, attach and prime the I.V. administration set before entering the patient's room.

Implementation
▶ Wash your hands thoroughly *to prevent the spread of microorganisms.* Remember to wear sterile gloves whenever working near the venipuncture site.
▶ Explain the procedure to the patient *to allay his fears and ensure cooperation.*

Changing the dressing
▶ Remove the old dressing, open all supply packages, and put on sterile gloves.
▶ Hold the cannula in place with your nondominant hand *to prevent accidental movement or dislodgment, which could puncture the vein and cause infiltration.*
▶ Assess the venipuncture site for signs of infection (redness and pain at the puncture site), infiltration (coolness, blanching, and edema at the site), and thrombophlebitis (redness, firmness, pain along the path of the vein, and edema). If any such signs are present, cover the area with a sterile 2″ × 2″ gauze pad and remove the catheter or needle. Apply pressure to the area until the bleeding stops, and apply an adhesive bandage. Then, using fresh equipment and solution, start the I.V. in another appropriate site, preferably on the opposite extremity.
▶ If the venipuncture site is intact, stabilize the cannula and carefully clean around the puncture site with a povidone-iodine or alcohol pad. Work in a circular motion outward from the site *to avoid introducing bacteria into the clean area.* Allow the area to dry completely.
▶ Cover the site with a transparent semipermeable dressing. *The transparent dressing allows visualization of the insertion site and maintains sterility.* It's placed over the insertion site to halfway up the hub of the cannula.

Changing the solution
▶ Wash your hands.
▶ Inspect the new solution container for cracks, leaks, and other damage. Check the solution for discoloration, turbidity, and particulates. Note the date and time the solution was mixed and its expiration date.

▶ Clamp the tubing when inverting it *to prevent air from entering the tubing.* Keep the drip chamber half full.

▶ If you're replacing a bag, remove the seal or tab from the new bag and remove the old bag from the pole. Remove the spike, insert it into the new bag, and adjust the flow rate.

▶ If you're replacing a bottle, remove the cap and seal from the new bottle and wipe the rubber port with an alcohol pad. Clamp the line, remove the spike from the old bottle, and insert the spike into the new bottle. Then hang the new bottle and adjust the flow rate.

Changing the tubing

▶ Reduce the I.V. flow rate, remove the old spike from the container, and hang it on the I.V. pole. Place the cover of the new spike loosely over the old one.

▶ Keeping the old spike in an upright position above the patient's heart level, insert the new spike into the I.V. container.

▶ Prime the system. Hang the new I.V. container and primed set on the pole, and grasp the new adapter in one hand. Then stop the flow rate in the old tubing.

▶ Put on sterile gloves.

▶ Place a sterile gauze pad under the needle or cannula hub *to create a sterile field.* Press one of your fingers over the cannula to prevent bleeding.

▶ Gently disconnect the old tubing (as shown above right), being careful not to dislodge or move the I.V. device. (If you have trouble disconnecting the old tubing, use a hemostat to hold the hub securely while twisting the tubing to remove it. Or use one hemostat on the venipuncture device and another on the hard plastic end of the tubing. Then pull the hemostats in opposite directions. Don't clamp the hemostats shut;

this could crack the tubing adapter or the venipuncture device.)

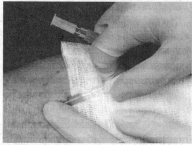

▶ Remove the protective cap from the new tubing, and connect the new adapter to the cannula. Hold the hub securely *to prevent dislodging the needle or cannula tip.*

▶ Observe for blood backflow into the new tubing *to verify that the needle or cannula is still in place.* (You may not be able to do this with small-gauge cannulas.)

▶ Adjust the clamp to maintain the appropriate flow rate.

▶ Retape the cannula hub and I.V. tubing, and recheck the I.V. flow rate *because taping may alter it.*

▶ Label the new tubing and container with the date and time. Label the solution container with a time strip (as shown below).

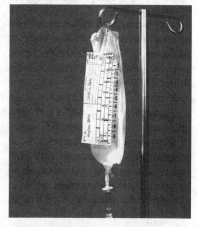

Special considerations

Check the prescribed I.V. flow rate before each solution change *to prevent errors*. If you crack the adapter or hub (or if you accidentally dislodge the cannula from the vein), remove the cannula. Apply pressure and an adhesive bandage to stop any bleeding. Perform a venipuncture at another site and restart the I.V.

Documentation

Record the time, date, and rate and type of solution (and any additives) on the I.V. flowchart. Also record this information, dressing or tubing changes, and appearance of the site in your notes.

PERITONEAL DIALYSIS

Peritoneal dialysis is indicated for patients with chronic renal failure who have cardiovascular instability, vascular access problems that prevent hemodialysis, fluid overload, or electrolyte imbalances. In this procedure, dialysate — the solution instilled into the peritoneal cavity by a catheter — draws waste products, excess fluid, and electrolytes from the blood across the semipermeable peritoneal membrane. (See *Principles of peritoneal dialysis*.) After a prescribed period, the dialysate is drained from the peritoneal cavity, removing impurities with it. The dialysis procedure is then repeated, using a new dialysate each time, until waste removal is complete and fluid, electrolyte, and acid-base balance has been restored.

The catheter is inserted in the operating room or at the patient's bedside with a nurse assisting. With special preparation, the nurse may perform dialysis, either manually or using an automatic or semiautomatic cycle machine.

Key nursing diagnoses and patient outcomes

Risk for infection related to invasive procedure
The patient will:
▶ maintain temperature within normal limits
▶ state risk factors for infection
▶ identify signs and symptoms of infection.

Impaired skin integrity related to presence of peritoneal catheter
The patient will:
▶ communicate an understanding of preventive skin care measures
▶ demonstrate preventive skin care measures.

Equipment

All equipment must be sterile. Commercially packaged dialysis kits or trays are available.

For catheter placement and dialysis

Prescribed dialysate (in 1- or 2-L bottles or bags, as ordered) • warmer, heating pad, or water bath • at least three face masks • medication, such as heparin, if ordered • dialysis administration set with drainage bag • two pairs of sterile gloves • I.V. pole • fenestrated sterile drape • vial of 1% or 2% lidocaine • povidone-iodine pads • 3-ml syringe with 25G 1″ needle • ordered type of multi-eyed, nylon, peritoneal catheter (see *Comparing peritoneal dialysis catheters,* pages 644 and 645) • scalpel (with #11 blade) • peritoneal stylet • sutures or hypoallergenic tape • povidone-iodine solution (to

Principles of peritoneal dialysis

Peritoneal dialysis works through a combination of diffusion and osmosis.

Diffusion

In diffusion, particles move through a semipermeable membrane from an area of high-solute concentration to an area of low-solute concentration.

In peritoneal dialysis, the water-based dialysate being infused contains glucose, sodium chloride, calcium, magnesium, acetate or lactate, and no waste products. Therefore, the waste products and excess electrolytes in the blood cross through the semipermeable peritoneal membrane into the dialysate. Removing the waste-filled dialysate and replacing it with fresh solution keeps the waste concentration low and encourages further diffusion.

Osmosis

In osmosis, fluids move through a semipermeable membrane from an area of low-solute concentration to an area of high-solute concentration. In peritoneal dialysis, dextrose is added to the dialysate to give it a higher solute concentration than the blood, creating a high osmotic gradient. Water migrates from the blood through the membrane at the beginning of each infusion, when the osmotic gradient is highest.

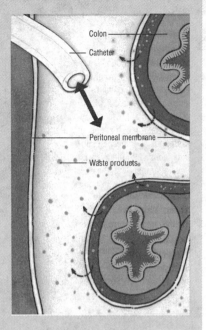

Colon

Catheter

Peritoneal membrane

Waste products

---

prepare abdomen) • precut drain dressings • protective cap for catheter • 4″ × 4″ gauze pads • small, sterile plastic clamp • optional: 10-ml syringe with 22G 1½″ needle, protein or potassium supplement, specimen container, label, and laboratory request form

For dressing changes

One pair of sterile gloves • 10 sterile cotton-tipped applicators or sterile 2″ × 2″ gauze pads • povidone-iodine ointment • two precut drain dressings • adhesive tape • povidone-iodine solution or normal saline solution • two sterile 4″ × 4″ gauze pads

Preparation of equipment

Bring all equipment to the patient's bedside. Make sure the dialysate is at body temperature. *This decreases patient discomfort during the procedure and reduces vasoconstriction of the peritoneal capillaries.* Dilated capillaries enhance

Comparing peritoneal dialysis catheters

The first step in any type of peritoneal dialysis is insertion of a catheter to allow instillation of dialyzing solution. The surgeon may insert one of the three different catheters described here.

Tenckhoff catheter

To implant a Tenckhoff catheter, the surgeon inserts the first 6¾" (17 cm) of the catheter into the patient's abdomen. The next 2¾" (7 cm) segment, which may have a Dacron cuff at one or both ends, is imbedded subcutaneously. Within a few days after insertion, the patient's tissues grow around the cuffs, forming a tight barrier against bacterial infiltration. The remaining 3⅞" (10 cm) of the catheter extends outside of the abdomen and is equipped with a metal adapter at the tip that connects to dialyzer tubing.

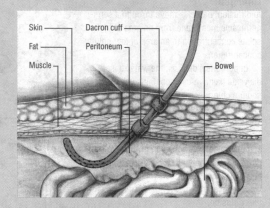

Flanged-collar catheter

To insert this kind of catheter, the surgeon positions its flanged collar just below the dermis so that the device extends through the abdominal wall. He keeps the distal end of the cuff from extending into the peritoneum, where it could cause adhesions.

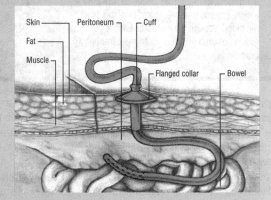

Column-disk peritoneal catheter

To insert a column-disk peritoneal catheter (CDPC), the surgeon rolls up the flexible disk section of the implant, inserts it into the peritoneal cavity, and retracts it against the abdominal wall. The implant's first cuff rests just outside the peritoneal membrane, while its second cuff rests just underneath the skin. Because the CDPC doesn't float freely in the peritoneal cavity, it keeps inflowing dialyzing solution from being directed at the sensitive organs, which increases patient comfort during dialysis.

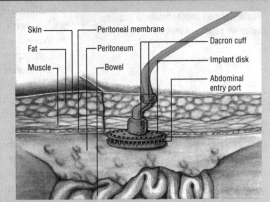

Skin — Fat — Muscle — Peritoneal membrane — Peritoneum — Bowel — Dacron cuff — Implant disk — Abdominal entry port

blood flow to the peritoneal membrane surface, increasing waste clearance into the peritoneal cavity. Place the container in a warmer or a water bath, or wrap it in a heating pad set at 98.6° F (37° C) for 30 to 60 minutes to warm the solution.

Implementation

▶ Explain the procedure to the patient. Assess and record vital signs, weight, and abdominal girth *to establish baseline levels*.

▶ Review recent laboratory values (blood urea nitrogen, serum creatinine, sodium, potassium, and complete blood count).

▶ Identify the patient's hepatitis B virus and human immunodeficiency virus status, if known.

Catheter placement and dialysis

▶ Have the patient try to urinate. *This reduces the risk of bladder perforation during insertion of the peritoneal catheter.* If he can't urinate and you suspect that his bladder isn't empty, obtain an order for straight catheterization *to empty his bladder.*

▶ Place the patient in the supine position, and have him put on one of the sterile face masks.

▶ Wash your hands.

▶ Inspect the warmed dialysate, which should appear clear and colorless.

▶ Put on a sterile face mask. Prepare to add any prescribed medication to the dialysate, using strict sterile technique *to avoid contaminating the solution.* Medications should be added immediately before the solution will be hung

Setup for peritoneal dialysis

The illustration below shows the proper setup for peritoneal dialysis.

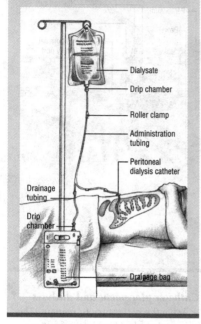

- Dialysate
- Drip chamber
- Roller clamp
- Administration tubing
- Peritoneal dialysis catheter
- Drainage tubing
- Drip chamber
- Drainage bag

and used. Disinfect multiple-dose vials by soaking them in povidone-iodine solution for 5 minutes. Heparin is typically added to the dialysate *to prevent accumulation of fibrin in the catheter.*

▶ Prepare the dialysis administration set. (See *Setup for peritoneal dialysis.*)

▶ Close the clamps on all lines. Place the drainage bag below the patient *to facilitate gravity drainage,* and connect the drainage line to it. Connect the dialysate infusion lines to the bottles or bags of dialysate. Hang the bottles or bags on the I.V. pole at the patient's bedside. *To prime the tubing,* open the infusion lines and allow the solution to flow until all lines are primed. Then close all clamps.

▶ At this point, the doctor puts on a mask and a pair of sterile gloves. He cleans the patient's abdomen with povidone-iodine solution and drapes it with a sterile drape.

▶ Wipe the stopper of the lidocaine vial with povidone-iodine and allow it to dry. Invert the vial and hand it to the doctor so he can withdraw the lidocaine, using the 3-ml syringe with the 25G 1″ needle.

▶ The doctor anesthetizes a small area of the patient's abdomen below the umbilicus. He then makes a small incision with the scalpel, inserts the catheter into the peritoneal cavity—using the stylet to guide the catheter—and sutures or tapes the catheter in place.

▶ If the catheter is already in place, clean the site with povidone-iodine solution in a circular outward motion, according to your facility's policy, before each dialysis treatment.

▶ Connect the catheter to the administration set, using strict aseptic technique *to prevent contamination of the catheter and the solution, which could cause peritonitis.*

▶ Open the drain dressing and the 4″ × 4″ gauze pad packages. Put on the other pair of sterile gloves. Apply the precut drain dressings around the catheter. Cover them with the gauze pads and tape them securely.

▶ Unclamp the lines to the patient. Rapidly instill 500 ml of dialysate into the peritoneal cavity *to test the catheter's patency.*

▶ Clamp the lines to the patient. Immediately unclamp the lines to the drainage bag *to allow fluid to drain into the bag.* Outflow should be brisk.

▶ Having established the catheter's patency, clamp the lines to the drainage bag and unclamp the lines to the patient *to infuse the prescribed volume of so-*

lution over a period of 5 to 10 minutes. As soon as the dialysate container empties, clamp the lines to the patient immediately *to prevent air from entering the tubing.*

▶ Allow the solution to dwell in the peritoneal cavity for the prescribed time (10 minutes to 4 hours). *This lets excess fluid, electrolytes, and accumulated wastes move from the blood through the peritoneal membrane and into the dialysate.*

▶ Warm the solution for the next infusion.

▶ At the end of the prescribed dwell time, unclamp the line to the drainage bag and allow the solution to drain from the peritoneal cavity into the drainage bag (normally 20 to 30 minutes).

▶ Repeat the infusion-dwell-drain cycle immediately after outflow until the prescribed number of fluid exchanges have been completed.

▶ If the doctor or your facility's policy requires a dialysate specimen, you'll usually collect one after every 10 infusion-dwell-drain cycles (*always* during the drain phase), after every 24-hour period, or as ordered. To do this, attach the 10-ml syringe to the 22G 1½″ needle and insert it into the injection port on the drainage line, using strict sterile technique, and aspirate the drainage sample. Transfer the sample to the specimen container, label it appropriately, and send it to the laboratory with a laboratory request form.

▶ After completing the prescribed number of exchanges, clamp the catheter and put on sterile gloves. Disconnect the administration set from the peritoneal catheter. Place the sterile protective cap over the catheter's distal end.

▶ Dispose of all used equipment appropriately.

Dressing changes

▶ Explain the procedure to the patient and wash your hands.

▶ If necessary, carefully remove the old dressings *to avoid putting tension on the catheter and accidentally dislodging it and to avoid introducing bacteria into the tract through movement of the catheter.*

▶ Put on the sterile gloves.

▶ Saturate the sterile applicators or the 2″ × 2″ gauze pads with povidone-iodine or normal saline solution, and clean the skin around the catheter, moving in concentric circles from the catheter site outward. Remove any crusted material carefully.

▶ Inspect the catheter site for drainage and the tissue around the site for redness and swelling.

▶ Apply povidone-iodine ointment to the catheter site with a sterile gauze pad.

▶ Place two precut drain dressings around the catheter site. Tape the 4″ × 4″ gauze pads over them *to secure the dressings.*

Special considerations

▶ During and after dialysis, monitor the patient and his response to treatment. Peritoneal dialysis is usually contraindicated in patients who have had extensive abdominal or bowel surgery or extensive abdominal trauma or who have severe vascular disease, obesity, or respiratory distress.

▶ Monitor the patient's vital signs every 10 to 15 minutes for the first 1 to 2 hours of exchanges, then every 2 to 4 hours, or more frequently if necessary. Notify the doctor of any abrupt changes in the patient's condition.

▶ *To reduce the risk of peritonitis,* use strict sterile technique during catheter insertion, dialysis, and dressing changes. Masks should be worn by all personnel in the room whenever the dialysis system is opened or entered. Change the dressing at least every 24 hours or whenever it becomes wet or soiled. Frequent dressing changes will also help prevent skin excoriation from any leakage.

▶ *To prevent respiratory distress,* position the patient for maximal lung expansion. Promote lung expansion through turning and deep-breathing exercises.

⫴ Nursing alert If the patient suffers severe respiratory distress during the dwell phase of dialysis, drain the peritoneal cavity and notify the doctor. Monitor any patient on peritoneal dialysis who is being weaned from a ventilator.

▶ *To prevent protein depletion,* the doctor may order a high-protein diet or a protein supplement. He will also monitor serum albumin levels.

▶ Dialysate is available in three concentrations—4.25% dextrose, 2.5% dextrose, and 1.5% dextrose. The 4.25% solution usually removes the largest amount of fluid from the blood because its glucose concentration is highest. If your patient receives this concentrated solution, monitor him carefully *to prevent excess fluid loss.* Also, some of the glucose in the 4.25% solution may enter the patient's bloodstream, causing hyperglycemia severe enough to require an insulin injection or an insulin addition to the dialysate.

▶ Patients with low serum potassium levels may require the addition of potassium to the dialysate solution *to prevent further losses.*

▶ Monitor fluid volume balance, blood pressure, and pulse *to help prevent fluid imbalance.* Assess fluid balance at the end of each infusion-dwell-drain cycle. Fluid balance is positive if less than the amount infused was recovered; it's negative if more than the amount infused was recovered. Notify the doctor if the patient retains 500 ml or more of fluid for three consecutive cycles or if he loses at least 1 L of fluid for three consecutive cycles.

▶ Weigh the patient daily *to help determine how much fluid is being removed during dialysis treatment.* Note the time and any variations in the weighing technique next to his weight on his chart.

▶ If inflow and outflow are slow or absent, check the tubing for kinks. You can also try raising the I.V. pole or repositioning the patient *to increase the inflow rate.* Repositioning the patient or applying manual pressure to the lateral aspects of the patient's abdomen may also help increase drainage. If these maneuvers fail, notify the doctor. Improper positioning of the catheter or an accumulation of fibrin may obstruct the catheter.

▶ Always examine outflow fluid (effluent) for color and clarity. Normally it's clear or pale yellow, but pink-tinged effluent may appear during the first three or four cycles. If the effluent remains pink-tinged, or if it's grossly bloody, suspect bleeding into the peritoneal cavity and notify the doctor. Also notify the doctor if the outflow contains feces, which suggests bowel perforation, or if it's cloudy, which suggests peritonitis. Obtain a sample for culture and Gram stain. Send the sample in a labeled specimen container to the laboratory with a laboratory request form.

▶ Patient discomfort at the start of the procedure is normal. If the patient experiences pain during the procedure, determine when it occurs, its quality and duration, and whether it radiates to other body parts. Then notify the doctor. Pain during infusion usually results from a dialysate that is too cool or acidic. Pain may also result from rapid inflow; slowing the inflow rate may reduce the pain. Severe, diffuse pain with rebound tenderness and cloudy effluent may indicate peritoneal infection. Pain that radiates to the shoulder often results from air accumulation under the diaphragm. Severe, persistent perineal or rectal pain can result from improper catheter placement.

▶ The patient undergoing peritoneal dialysis will require a great deal of assistance in his daily care. *To minimize his discomfort,* perform daily care during a drain phase in the cycle, when the patient's abdomen is less distended.

Complications

Peritonitis, the most common complication, usually follows contamination of the dialysate, but it may develop if solution leaks from the catheter exit site and flows back into the catheter tract. Respiratory distress may result when dialysate in the peritoneal cavity increases pressure on the diaphragm, which decreases lung expansion.

Protein depletion may result from the diffusion of protein in the blood into the dialysate solution through the peritoneal membrane. As much as ½ oz (14 g) of protein may be lost daily— more in patients with peritonitis.

Constipation is a major cause of inflow-outflow problems; therefore, *to ensure regular bowel movements,* give a laxative or stool softener as needed.

Excessive fluid loss from the use of 4.25% solution may cause hypovolemia, hypotension, and shock. Excessive

Better charting

Documenting peritoneal dialysis

- During and after dialysis, monitor and document the patient's response to treatment.
- Document any abrupt changes in the patient's condition, notify the doctor, and document doing so.
- Record each time that you notify the doctor of an abnormality.
- Document the amount of dialysate infused and drained and any medications added.
- Complete a peritoneal dialysis flowchart every 24 hours.
- Note the condition of the patient's skin at the dialysis catheter site, the patient's reports of unusual discomfort or pain, and your interventions.

fluid retention may lead to blood volume expansion, hypertension, peripheral edema, and even pulmonary edema and heart failure.

Other possible complications include electrolyte imbalance and hyperglycemia, which can be identified by frequent blood tests.

Documentation

Record the amount of dialysate infused and drained, any medications added to the solution, and the color and character of effluent. Also record the patient's daily weight and fluid balance. Use a peritoneal dialysis flowchart to compute total fluid balance after each exchange. Note the patient's vital signs and tolerance of the treatment as well as other pertinent observations. (See *Documenting peritoneal dialysis.*)

PERITONEAL LAVAGE

Used as a diagnostic procedure in a patient with blunt abdominal trauma, peritoneal lavage helps detect bleeding in the peritoneal cavity. The test may proceed through several steps. Initially, the doctor inserts a catheter through the abdominal wall into the peritoneal cavity and aspirates the peritoneal fluid with a syringe. If he can't see blood in the aspirated fluid, he then infuses a balanced saline solution and siphons the fluid from the cavity. He inspects the siphoned fluid for blood and also sends fluid samples to the laboratory for microscopic examination.

The medical team maintains strict sterile technique throughout this procedure to avoid introducing microorganisms into the peritoneum and causing peritonitis. (See *Tapping the peritoneal cavity*.)

Peritoneal lavage is contraindicated in a patient who has had multiple abdominal operations (adhesions), who has an abdominal wall hematoma, who is unstable and needs immediate surgery, or who can't be catheterized before the procedure. The procedure requires great caution and a different technique if the patient is pregnant.

Key nursing diagnoses and patient outcomes

Risk for injury related to the invasive procedure
The patient will:
▶ maintain effective breathing patterns
▶ maintain adequate cardiac output
▶ show no signs of bleeding from the incision site.

Risk for infection related to the invasive procedure
The patient will:
▶ maintain a normal body temperature
▶ remain free from signs and symptoms of infection.

Anxiety related to the procedure and its results
The patient will:
▶ communicate feelings of anxiety
▶ state an understanding of the need for the procedure.

Equipment

Indwelling urinary catheter, catheter insertion kit, and drainage bag • nasogastric (NG) tube • gastric suction machine • shaving kit • I.V. pole • macrodrip I.V. tubing • I.V. solutions (1 L of warmed, balanced saline solution, usually lactated Ringer's solution or normal saline solution) • peritoneal dialysis tray • sterile gloves • gown • goggles • antiseptic solution (such as povidone-iodine) • 3-ml syringe with 25G 1″ needle • bottle of 1% lidocaine with epinephrine • 8″ (20.3 cm) #14 intracatheter extension tubing and a small sterile hemostat (to clamp tubing) • 30-ml syringe • one 20G 1½″ needle • sterile towels • three containers for specimen collection, including one sterile tube for a culture and sensitivity specimen • labels • antiseptic ointment • 4″ × 4″ gauze pads • alcohol pads • 1″ hypoallergenic tape • 2-0 and 3-0 sutures

If using a commercially prepared peritoneal dialysis kit (containing a #15 peritoneal dialysis catheter, trocar, and extension tubing with roller clamp), make sure the macrodrip I.V. tubing doesn't have a reverse flow (or backcheck) valve that prevents infused fluid from draining out of the peritoneal cavity.

Implementation

▶ Provide privacy and wash your hands. Reinforce the doctor's explanation of the procedure.

▶ Put on the gown and goggles.

▶ Before the procedure, advise the patient to expect a sensation of abdominal fullness. Also inform him that he may experience a chill if the lavage solution isn't warmed or doesn't reach his body temperature.

▶ Then catheterize the patient with the indwelling urinary catheter, and connect this catheter to the drainage bag.

▶ Insert the NG tube. Attach this tube to the gastric suction machine (set for low intermittent suction) to drain the patient's stomach contents. *Decompressing the stomach prevents vomiting and subsequent aspiration and minimizes the possibility of bowel perforation during trocar or catheter insertion.*

▶ Using the shaving kit, clip or shave the hair, as ordered, from the area between the patient's umbilicus and pubis.

▶ Set up the I.V. pole. Attach the macrodrip tubing to the lavage solution container, and clear air from the tubing *to avoid introducing air into the peritoneal cavity during the lavage.*

▶ Using aseptic technique, open the peritoneal dialysis tray.

▶ The doctor will wipe the patient's abdomen from the costal margin to the pubic area and from flank to flank with the antiseptic solution. Then he'll drape the area with sterile towels from the dialysis tray *to create a sterile field.*

▶ Using aseptic technique, hand the doctor the 3-ml syringe and the 25G 1″ needle. If the peritoneal dialysis tray

Tapping the peritoneal cavity

After administering a local anesthetic to numb the area near the patient's navel, the surgeon will make a smaller incision (about ¾″ [2 cm]) through the skin and subcutaneous tissues of the abdominal wall. He'll retract the tissue, ligate several blood vessels, and use 4″ × 4″ gauze pads to absorb and keep incisional blood from entering the wound and producing a false-positive test result. Next, he'll direct the trocar through the incision into the pelvic midline until the instrument enters the peritoneum. Then he'll advance the peritoneal catheter (through the trocar) 6″ to 8″ (15 to 20 cm) into the pelvis.

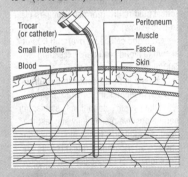

Using a syringe attached to the catheter, the surgeon will aspirate fluid from the peritoneal cavity and look for blood or other abnormal findings.

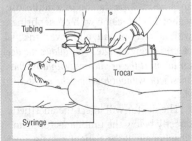

Interpreting peritoneal lavage results

If test findings in peritoneal lavage are abnormal, your patient may need laparotomy and further treatment. The most common abnormal findings include:
- unclotted blood, bile, or intestinal contents in aspirated peritoneal fluid (20 ml in an adult or 10 ml in a child)
- bloody or pinkish red fluid returned from lavage — dark enough to obscure reading newsprint through it (if you can read newsprint through the fluid, test results are considered negative, although the doctor may order more tests)
- green, cloudy, turbid, or milky peritoneal fluid return (normally appears clear to pale yellow)
- red blood cell count over 100,000/µl
- white blood cell count exceeding 500/µl
- bacteria in fluid (identified by culture and sensitivity testing or Gram stain).

If the patient's condition is stable, borderline positive results may suggest the need for additional tests, such as echography and arteriography. If test results are questionable or inconclusive, the doctor may leave the catheter in place to repeat the procedure.

trocar, withdraw fluid, and check the findings. If the findings are positive, the procedure ends and you'll prepare the patient for laparotomy and further measures. Even if retrieved fluid looks normal, lavage will continue. (See *Interpreting peritoneal lavage results.*)

▶ Wearing gloves, connect the catheter extension tubing to the I.V. tubing, if ordered, and instill 500 to 1,000 ml (10 ml/kg body weight) of the warmed I.V. solution into the peritoneal cavity over 5 to 10 minutes. Then clamp the tubing with the hemostat.

▶ Unless contraindicated by the patient's injuries (such as a spinal cord injury, fractured ribs, or an unstable pelvic fracture), gently tilt the patient from side to side *to distribute the fluid throughout the peritoneal cavity.* (If the patient's condition contraindicates tilting, the doctor may gently palpate the sides of the abdomen *to distribute the fluid.*)

▶ After 5 to 10 minutes, place the I.V. container below the level of the patient's body, and open the clamp on the I.V. tubing. *Lowering the container helps excess fluid to drain.* Gently drain as much of the fluid as possible from the peritoneal cavity to the container. Be careful not to disconnect the tubing from the catheter. The peritoneal cavity may take 20 to 30 minutes to drain completely.

▶ Although you don't need to vent a plastic bag container, be sure to vent glass I.V. containers with a needle to promote flow.

▶ To obtain a fluid specimen, put on gloves and use a 30-ml syringe and 20G 1½″ needle to withdraw between 25 and 30 ml of fluid from a port in the I.V. tubing. Clean the top of each specimen container with an alcohol pad.

doesn't contain a sterile ampule of anesthetic, wipe the top of a multidose vial of 1% lidocaine with epinephrine with an alcohol pad, and invert the vial at a 45-degree angle. *This allows the doctor to insert the needle and withdraw the anesthetic without touching the nonsterile vial.*

▶ The doctor will inject the anesthetic directly below the umbilicus (or at an adjacent site if the patient has a surgical scar). When the area is numb, he'll make an incision, insert the catheter or

Deposit fluid specimens in the containers, and send the specimens to the laboratory for culture and sensitivity analysis, Gram stain, red and white blood cell counts, amylase and bile level determinations, and spun-down sediment evaluation. *Note:* If you didn't obtain the culture and sensitivity specimen first, change the needle before drawing this fluid sample *to avoid contaminating the specimen.*

▶ Label the specimens, and send them to the laboratory immediately. With positive test results, the doctor will usually perform a laparotomy. If test results are normal, the doctor will close the incision with sutures.

▶ Wearing sterile gloves, apply antiseptic ointment to the site, and dress the incision with a 4″ × 4″ gauze pad secured with 1″ hypoallergenic tape.

▶ Discard disposable equipment. Return reusable equipment to the appropriate department for cleaning and sterilization.

Special considerations

▶ After lavage, monitor the patient's vital signs often. Report signs of shock (tachycardia, decreased blood pressure, diaphoresis, dyspnea or shortness of breath, and vertigo) at once. Assess the incisional site frequently for bleeding.

▶ If the doctor orders abdominal X-rays, they will probably precede peritoneal lavage. *X-ray films made after lavage may be unreliable because of air introduced into the peritoneal cavity.*

Complications

Bleeding from lacerated blood vessels may occur at the incisional site or intra-abdominally. A visceral perforation causes peritonitis and requires laparotomy for repair. If the patient has respiratory distress, infusion of a balanced saline solution may cause additional stress and trigger respiratory arrest.

The bladder may be lacerated or punctured if it isn't emptied completely before peritoneal lavage. Infection may develop at the incision site if strict aseptic technique hasn't been used.

Documentation

Record the type and size of the peritoneal dialysis catheter used, the type and amount of solution instilled and withdrawn from the peritoneal cavity, and the amount and color of fluid returned. Document whether the fluid flowed freely into and out of the abdomen. Note which specimens were obtained and sent to the laboratory. Also note any complications encountered, and the nursing actions taken to handle them.

PHOTOTHERAPY

Phototherapy involves exposing the neonate to high-intensity fluorescent light that breaks down bilirubin (a pigment of red blood cells [RBCs]) for transport to the GI system and excretion. The treatment is commonly given to neonates with hyperbilirubinemia — a symptom of physiologic jaundice, breast-milk jaundice, or hemolytic disease. Phototherapy continues until bilirubin drops to normal levels because unchecked hyperbilirubinemia can lead to kernicterus (deposits of unconjugated bilirubin in the brain cells), permanent brain damage, and even death.

Physiologic jaundice — resulting from the neonate's high RBC count and short RBC life span — develops 2 to 3 days after delivery in about 50% of full-term neonates and 3 to 5 days in about 80% of premature neonates.

Breast-milk jaundice typically develops 3 to 4 days after delivery in about 25% of breast-feeding neonates and 4 to 5 days after delivery in less than 5%. Experts think that this type of hyperbilirubinemia results from reduced calorie and fluid intake (before the mother develops an adequate milk supply) or from constituents in breast milk that reduce bilirubin decomposition. They encourage frequent breast-feeding to increase fluid and calorie intake until bilirubin levels reach about 15 mg/dl, then discontinuation of breast-feeding for 48 hours while bilirubin levels drop.

Treatment for hemolytic disease, a much more serious condition, includes phototherapy and exchange transfusions. In pathologic jaundice, which occurs within 24 hours of birth and raises serum bilirubin levels above 13 mg/dl, phototherapy may be used with appropriate treatment for the underlying cause.

Key nursing diagnoses and patient outcomes

Risk for deficient fluid volume related to phototherapy
The patient will:
▶ have normal skin color and temperature
▶ exhibit no signs of dehydration
▶ maintain urine output of at least (specify) ml/hour
▶ have normal bilirubin values
▶ maintain fluid balance (intake will equal output).

Risk for impaired parent, infant, and child attachment related to phototherapy

The family will:
▶ exhibit positive responses to the infant, such as making eye contact with him, caressing him, talking to him, calling him by name, and making positive remarks about him
▶ respond to the infant's behavioral cues, provide stimulation when he's alert and ready, avoid overstimulating him, and recognize when he needs to nap
▶ provide usual infant care with confidence
▶ express concerns and worries about the infant
▶ identify available resources for assistance.

Equipment

Phototherapy unit • photometer • opaque eye mask • thermometer • urinometer • surgical face mask or small diaper • optional: thermistor (if the phototherapy unit is combined with a temperature-controlled radiant heat warmer) or incubator (if the neonate is small for his gestational age); bilimeter; prepackaged eye coverings are available

Preparation of equipment

Set up the phototherapy unit about 18″ (46 cm) above the neonate's crib. Verify placement of the light-bulb shield *because this device filters ultraviolet rays and protects the neonate from broken bulbs*. If the neonate is in an incubator, place the phototherapy unit at least 3″ (7.5 cm) above the incubator *to promote sufficient air flow and prevent overheating*. Turn on the lights. Place a photometer probe in the middle of the crib *to measure the energy emitted by the lights*. The energy should range from 6 to 8 µw/cm^2/nanometer.

Implementation

▶ Explain the procedure to the parents *to reduce their anxiety and guilt and to ensure cooperation.*

▶ Record the neonate's initial bilirubin level and his axillary temperature *to establish baseline measurements.*

▶ Place the opaque eye mask over the neonate's closed eyes. Fasten the mask securely enough to stay in place and to prevent the neonate from opening his eyes, but loosely enough to ensure circulation and avoid pressure on the eyeballs. *This protects the eyes and prevents reflex bradycardia and head molding.*

▶ Clean the eyes periodically *to remove drainage and check circulation.*

▶ Undress the neonate *to expose the most skin to the most light.* Remember to place a diaper under him and to cover male genitalia with a surgical mask or a small diaper *to catch urine and to prevent possible testicular damage from the heat and light waves.*

▶ Take the neonate's axillary temperature every 2 hours *to make sure the neonate maintains a normal and stable body temperature.*

▶ If the neonate is in a servo-controlled incubator or a radiant warmer, place the thermistor on the neonate's side and cover it with opaque or reflective tape. *This prevents frequent sensor changes and protects the sensor from direct energy.*

▶ Provide additional warmth, if necessary, by adjusting the warming unit's thermostat.

▶ Monitor elimination. Note urine and stool amounts and frequency. Weigh the neonate twice daily, and watch for dehydration signs (dry skin, poor turgor, depressed fontanels) *because phototherapy increases fluid loss through stools and evaporation.*

▶ Clean the neonate carefully after each bowel movement *because the loose green stools that result from phototherapy can excoriate the skin.* Don't apply ointment *because this can cause burns under phototherapy lights.*

▶ Check urine specific gravity with a urinometer *to gauge the neonate's hydration status.*

▶ Feed the neonate every 3 to 4 hours and offer water between feedings *to ensure adequate hydration and to boost gastric motility.* Make sure water intake doesn't replace breast milk or formula. Take the neonate out of the crib, turn off the phototherapy lights, and unmask his eyes at least every 3 to 4 hours with feedings, if possible, *to provide visual stimulation and human contact.* Also assess his eyes for inflammation or injury.

▶ Reposition the neonate every 2 hours *to expose all body surfaces to the light and to prevent head molding and skin breakdown from pressure.*

▶ Check the bilirubin level at least once every 24 hours — more often if levels rise significantly. If you don't use a bilimeter, turn off the phototherapy unit before drawing venous blood for testing *because the lights may degrade bilirubin in the blood sample, resulting in inaccurate test results.*

▶ Notify the doctor if the bilirubin level nears 20 mg/dl in full-term neonates, or 15 mg/dl in premature neonates, *because these levels may lead to kernicterus.*

▶ Review the neonatal and maternal histories for clues to possible hyperbilirubinemia causes. Also watch for signs of infection and metabolic disorders, and check the neonate's hematocrit for polycythemia. Inspect the neonate for hematoma, bruising, petechiae, and cyanosis. If the photherapy unit has blue lights, turn them off for the examination *because these lights can mask cyanosis.*

Special considerations
▶ If the neonate cries excessively during phototherapy, place a blanket roll on each side of him *to give him a feeling of security.*
▶ If the doctor diagnoses breast-feeding jaundice (suspending breast-feeding temporarily), teach the mother to express milk manually or with a pump. Encourage continued breast-feeding when indicated. Reassure the parents by explaining that jaundice is transitory. If possible, give phototherapy treatment in the mother's room *to facilitate bonding and to decrease parental anxiety and guilt feelings.*

Home care
Home phototherapy programs are safe and effective alternatives for treating uncomplicated neonatal jaundice. Teach the parents how to perform the procedure, and encourage their compliance. Explain that testing will continue until results show serum bilirubin at acceptable levels. Provide written instructions at discharge.

Complications
Bronze baby syndrome (an idiopathic darkening of the skin, serum, and urine) may occur. Changes in feeding and activity patterns and hormonal secretions may follow prolonged therapy.

Documentation
At least once every 2 hours, note the progress of phototherapy and that the neonate's eyes remain protected. Record the time of all bilirubin testing, and plot results. Document eye covering

changes and eye care given. Keep records of measured radiant energy — initially and then every 8 hours. Document neonatal time away from lights, for example, for feeding or other procedures. Note fluid intake and the amount of urine and feces eliminated. Describe any changes in skin appearance and character, in feeding patterns, and in activity level.

PICC INSERTION AND REMOVAL

For a patient who needs central venous (CV) therapy for 1 to 6 months or who requires repeated venous access, a peripherally inserted central catheter (PICC) may be the best option. The doctor may order a PICC if the patient has suffered trauma or burns resulting in chest injury or if he has respiratory compromise due to chronic obstructive pulmonary disease, a mediastinal mass, cystic fibrosis, or pneumothorax. With any of these conditions, a PICC helps avoid complications that may occur with a CV line.

Made of silicone or polyurethane, a PICC is soft and flexible with increased biocompatibility. It may range from 16G to 23G in diameter and from 16″ to 24″ (40.6 to 61 cm) in length. PICCs are available in single- and double-lumen versions, with or without guide wires. A guide wire stiffens the catheter, easing its advancement through the vein, but can damage the vessel if used improperly.

PICCs are being used increasingly for patients receiving home care. The device is easier to insert than other CV devices and provides safe, reliable access for drug administration and blood sampling. A single catheter may be used for the entire course of therapy with greater convenience and at reduced cost.

Infusions commonly given by PICC include total parenteral nutrition, chemotherapy, antibiotics, narcotics, and analgesics. PICC therapy works best when introduced early in treatment; it shouldn't be considered a last resort for patients with sclerotic or repeatedly punctured veins.

The patient receiving PICC therapy must have a peripheral vein large enough to accept a 14G or 16G introducer needle and a 3.8G to 4.8G catheter. The doctor or nurse inserts a PICC by way of the basilic, median cubital, or cephalic vein. The PICC is then threaded to the superior vena cava or subclavian vein.

PICCs cost from $25 to $60. Insertion may cost from $50 to $300, compared with about $500 for insertion of short-term CV catheters and $1,200 for insertion of long-term CV catheters and implantable CV devices.

If your state nurse practice act permits, you may insert a PICC if you show sufficient knowledge of vascular access devices. To prove your competence in PICC insertion, it's recommended that you complete an 8-hour workshop and demonstrate three successful catheter insertions. You may have to demonstrate competence every year.

Key nursing diagnoses and patient outcomes

Risk for infection related to the procedure
The patient will:
▶ have normal vital signs, temperature, and laboratory values
▶ have no pathogens in cultures

▶ exhibit no signs or symptoms of infection at the PICC insertion site.

Risk for deficient fluid volume related to the need for a PICC line
The patient will:
▶ have normal skin color and temperature
▶ exhibit no signs of dehydration
▶ maintain urine output of at least (specify) ml/hour
▶ have normal electrolyte values
▶ maintain fluid balance (intake will equal output).

Equipment
Catheter insertion kit • three alcohol pads or an approved antimicrobial solution, such as 10% povidone-iodine or tincture of iodine 2% • povidone-iodine ointment • 3-ml vial of heparin (100 units/ml) • injection port with short extension tubing • sterile and clean measuring tape • vial of normal saline solution • sterile gauze pads • tape • linen-saver pad • sterile drapes • tourniquet • sterile transparent semipermeable dressing • two pairs of sterile gloves • sterile gown • mask • goggles • clean gloves

Preparation of equipment
Gather the necessary supplies. If you're administering PICC therapy in the patient's home, bring everything with you.

Implementation
▶ Describe the procedure to the patient and answer her questions.
▶ Wash your hands.

Inserting a PICC
▶ Place the tourniquet on the patient's arm and assess the antecubital fossa. Select the insertion site.
▶ Remove the tourniquet.

▶ Determine catheter tip placement or the spot at which the catheter tip will rest after insertion.

▶ For placement in the superior vena cava, measure the distance from the insertion site to the shoulder and from the shoulder to the sternal notch. Then add 3″ (7.6 cm) to the measurement (as shown below).

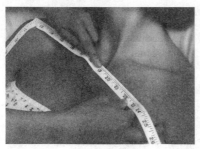

▶ Have the patient lie in a supine position with her arm at a 90-degree angle to her body. Place a linen-saver pad under her arm.

▶ Open the PICC tray and drop the rest of the sterile items onto the sterile field. Put on the sterile gown, mask, goggles, and gloves.

▶ Using the sterile measuring tape, cut the distal end of the catheter according to specific manufacturer's recommendations and guidelines, using the equipment provided by the manufacturer (as shown below).

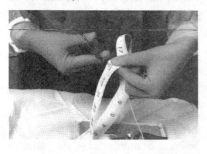

▶ Using sterile technique, withdraw 5 ml of the normal saline solution and flush the extension tubing and the cap.

▶ Remove the needle from the syringe. Attach the syringe to the hub of the catheter and flush (as shown below).

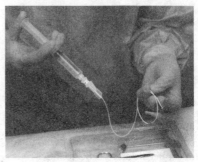

▶ Prepare the insertion site by rubbing it with three alcohol pads or other approved antimicrobial solution. Use a circular motion, working outward from the site about 6″ (15 cm). Allow the area to dry. Be sure not to touch the intended insertion site.

▶ Take your gloves off. Then apply the tourniquet about 4″ (10 cm) above the antecubital fossa.

▶ Put on a new pair of sterile gloves. Then place a sterile drape under the patient's arm and another on top of her arm. Drop a sterile 4″ × 4″ gauze pad over the tourniquet.

▶ Stabilize the patient's vein. Insert the catheter introducer at a 10-degree angle, directly into the vein (as shown below).

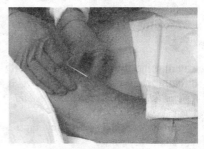

▶ After successful vein entry, you should see a blood return in the flash-back chamber. Without changing the needle's position, gently advance the plastic introducer sheath until you're sure the tip is well within the vein.

▶ Carefully withdraw the needle while holding the introducer still. *To minimize blood loss,* apply finger pressure on the vein just beyond the distal end of the introducer sheath (as shown below).

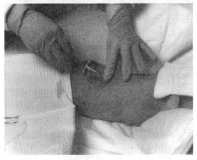

▶ Using sterile forceps, insert the catheter into the introducer sheath, and advance it 2″ to 4″ (5 to 10 cm) into the vein (as shown below).

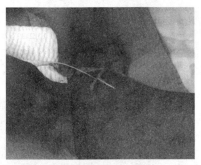

▶ Remove the tourniquet using the 4″ × 4″ gauze pad.

▶ When you have advanced the catheter to the shoulder, ask the patient to turn her head toward the affected arm and place her chin on her chest. *This will occlude the jugular vein and ease the*

catheter's advancement into the subclavian vein.

▶ Advance the catheter until about 4″ remain. Then pull the introducer sheath out of the vein and away from the venipuncture site (as shown below).

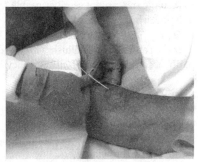

▶ Grasp the tabs of the introducer sheath, and flex them toward its distal end *to split the sheath.*

▶ Pull the tabs apart and away from the catheter until the sheath is completely split (as shown below). Discard the sheath.

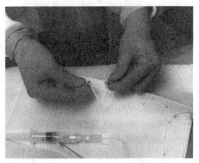

▶ Continue to advance the catheter until it's completely inserted. Flush with normal saline solution followed by heparin, according to your facility's policy.

▶ With the patient's arm below heart level, remove the syringe. Connect the capped extension set to the hub of the catheter.

▶ Apply a sterile 2" × 2" gauze pad directly over the site and a sterile transparent semipermeable dressing over that. Leave this dressing in place for 24 hours.

▶ After the initial 24 hours, apply a new sterile transparent semipermeable dressing. The gauze pad is no longer necessary. You can place Steri-Strips over the catheter wings. Flush with heparin, according to your facility's policy.

Administering drugs

▶ As with any CV line, be sure to check for blood return and flush with normal saline solution before administering a drug through a PICC line.

▶ Clamp the 7" (17.8 cm) extension tubing, and connect the empty syringe to the tubing. Release the clamp and aspirate slowly *to verify blood return.* Flush with 3 ml of normal saline solution in a 10-ml syringe, then administer the drug.

▶ After giving the drug, flush again with 3 ml of normal saline solution in a 10-ml syringe. (Remember to flush with normal saline solution between infusions of incompatible drugs or fluids.)

Changing the dressing

▶ Change the dressing every 3 to 7 days and more frequently if the integrity of the dressing becomes compromised. If possible, choose a transparent semipermeable dressing, *which has a high moisture-vapor transmission rate.* Use sterile technique.

▶ Wash your hands and assemble the necessary supplies. Position the patient with her arm extended away from her body at a 45- to 90-degree angle so that the insertion site is below heart level *to*

reduce the risk of air embolism. Put on a sterile mask.

▶ Open a package of sterile gloves, and use the inside of the package as a sterile field. Then open the transparent semipermeable dressing and drop it onto the field. Put on clean gloves, and remove the old dressing by holding your left thumb on the catheter and stretching the dressing parallel to the skin. Repeat the last step with your right thumb holding the catheter. Free the remaining section of the dressing from the catheter by peeling toward the insertion site from the distal end to the proximal end *to prevent catheter dislodgment.* Remove the clean gloves.

▶ Put on sterile gloves. Clean the area thoroughly with three alcohol swabs, starting at the insertion site and working outward from the site. Repeat the step three times with povidone-iodine swabs and allow to dry.

▶ Apply the dressing carefully. Secure the tubing to the edge of the dressing over the tape with ¼" adhesive tape.

Removing a PICC

▶ You'll remove a PICC when therapy is complete, if the catheter becomes damaged or broken and can't be repaired or, possibly, if the line becomes occluded. Measure the catheter after you remove it *to ensure that the line has been removed intact.*

▶ Assemble the necessary equipment at the patient's bedside.

▶ Explain the procedure to the patient. Wash your hands. Place a linen-saver pad under the patient's arm.

▶ Remove the tape holding the extension tubing. Open two sterile gauze pads on a clean, flat surface. Put on clean gloves. Stabilize the catheter at the hub with one hand. Without dislodging the catheter, use your other hand to gently remove the dressing by pulling it toward the insertion site.

▶ Next, withdraw the catheter with smooth, gentle pressure in small increments. It should come out easily. If you feel resistance, stop. Apply slight tension to the line by taping it down. Try to remove it again in a few minutes. If you still feel resistance after the second attempt, notify the doctor for further instructions.

▶ When you successfully remove the catheter, apply manual pressure to the site with a sterile gauze pad for 1 minute.

▶ Measure and inspect the catheter. If any part has broken off during removal, notify the doctor immediately and monitor the patient for signs of distress.

▶ Cover the site with povidone-iodine ointment, and tape a new folded gauze pad in place. Dispose of used items properly, and wash your hands.

Special considerations

▶ Be aware that the doctor or nurse probably will place the PICC in the superior vena cava if the patient will receive therapy in the facility.

▶ For a patient receiving intermittent PICC therapy, flush the catheter with 6 ml of normal saline solution and 3 ml of heparin (100 units/ml) after each use. For catheters that aren't being used routinely, flushing every 12 hours with 3 ml (100 units/ml) heparin will maintain patency.

▶ You can use a declotting agent to clear a clotted PICC, but make sure you read the manufacturer's recommendations first.

▶ Remember to add an extension set to all PICCs *so you can start and stop an infusion away from the insertion site.* An ex-

tension set will also make using a PICC easier for the patient who will be administering infusions herself.

▶ If a patient will be receiving blood or blood products through the PICC, use at least an 18G cannula.

▶ Assess the catheter insertion site through the transparent semipermeable dressing every 24 hours. Look at the catheter and cannula pathway, and check for bleeding, redness, drainage, and swelling. Ask your patient if she's having pain associated with therapy. Although oozing is common for the first 24 hours after insertion, excessive bleeding after that should be evaluated.

Nursing alert **If a portion of the catheter breaks during removal, immediately apply a tourniquet to the upper arm, close to the axilla,** *to prevent advancement of the catheter piece into the right atrium.* **Then check the patient's radial pulse. If you don't detect the radial pulse, the tourniquet is too tight. Keep the tourniquet in place until an X-ray can be obtained, the doctor is notified, and surgical retrieval is attempted.**

Complications

PICC therapy causes fewer and less severe complications than conventional CV therapy. Catheter breakage on removal is probably the most common complication. Catheter occlusion is also relatively common. Air embolism, always a potential risk of venipuncture, poses less danger in PICC therapy than in traditional CV therapy *because the line is inserted below heart level.*

Catheter tip migration may occur with vigorous flushing. Patients receiving chemotherapy are most vulnerable to this complication *because of frequent nausea and vomiting and subsequent changes in intrathoracic pressure.*

Documentation

Document the entire procedure, including any problems with catheter placement. Also document the size, length, and type of catheter as well as the insertion location.

POSTMORTEM CARE

After the patient dies, care includes preparing him for family viewing, arranging transportation to the morgue or funeral home, and determining the disposition of the patient's belongings. In addition, postmortem care entails comforting and supporting the patient's family and friends and providing for their privacy.

Postmortem care usually begins after a doctor certifies the patient's death. If the patient died violently or under suspicious circumstances, postmortem care may be postponed until the medical examiner completes an autopsy.

Key nursing diagnoses and patient outcomes

Anticipatory grieving related to the death of a family member
The family will:
▶ identify recent loss
▶ use coping mechanisms to deal with loss
▶ actively participate in discussions about loss with support groups or seek help from health care professionals
▶ communicate that grieving is an appropriate response to loss and come to terms with grief.

Equipment

Gauze or soft string ties • gloves • chin straps • ABD pads • cotton balls • plastic shroud or body wrap • three identification tags • adhesive bandages to cover wounds or punctures • plastic bag for patient's belongings • water-filled basin • soap • towels • washcloths • stretcher

A commercial morgue pack usually contains gauze or string ties, chin straps, a shroud, and identification tags.

Implementation

▶ Document any auxiliary equipment, such as a mechanical ventilator, still present. Put on gloves.
▶ Place the body in the supine position, arms at sides and head on a pillow. Elevate the head of the bed slightly *to prevent discoloration from blood settling in the face.*
▶ If the patient wore dentures and your facility's policy permits, gently insert them; then close the mouth. Close the eyes by gently pressing on the lids with your fingertips. If they don't stay closed, place moist cotton balls on the eyelids for a few minutes, and then try again to close them. Place a folded towel under the chin *to keep the jaw closed.*
▶ Remove all indwelling urinary catheters, tubes, and tape, and apply adhesive bandages to puncture sites. Replace soiled dressings.
▶ Collect all the patient's valuables to prevent loss. If you're unable to remove a ring, cover it with gauze, tape it in place, and tie the gauze to the wrist *to prevent slippage and subsequent loss.*
▶ Clean the body thoroughly, using soap, a basin, and washcloths. Place one or more ABD pads between the buttocks *to absorb rectal discharge or drainage.*

▶ Cover the body up to the chin with a clean sheet.

▶ Offer comfort and emotional support to the family and intimate friends. Ask if they wish to see the body. If they do, allow them to do so in privacy. Ask if they would prefer to leave the patient's jewelry on the body.

▶ After the family leaves, remove the towel from under the chin of the deceased patient. Pad the chin, and wrap chin straps under the chin and tie them loosely on top of the head. Then, pad the wrists and ankles to prevent bruises, and tie them together with gauze or soft string ties.

▶ Fill out the three identification tags. Each tag should include the deceased patient's name, room and bed numbers, date and time of death, and doctor's name. Tie one tag to the deceased patient's hand or foot, but don't remove his identification bracelet *to ensure correct identification.*

▶ Place the shroud or body wrap on the morgue stretcher and, after obtaining assistance, transfer the body to the stretcher. Wrap the body, and tie the shroud or wrap with the string provided. Attach another identification tag, and cover the shroud or wrap with a clean sheet. If a shroud or wrap isn't available, dress the deceased patient in a clean gown and cover the body with a sheet.

▶ Place the deceased patient's personal belongings, including valuables, in a bag and attach the third identification tag to it.

▶ If the patient died of an infectious disease, label the body according to your facility's policy.

▶ Close the doors of adjoining rooms if possible. Then take the body to the morgue. Use corridors that aren't crowded and, if possible, use a service elevator.

Special considerations

▶ Give the deceased patient's personal belongings to his family or bring them to the morgue. If you give the family jewelry or money, make sure a coworker is present as a witness. Obtain the signature of an adult family member *to verify receipt of valuables or to state their preference that jewelry remain on the patient.*

▶ Offer emotional support to the deceased patient's family and friends, and to the patient's facility roommate, if appropriate.

Documentation

Although the extent of documentation varies among facilities, always record the disposition of the patient's possessions, especially jewelry and money. Also note the date and time the patient was transported to the morgue.

POSTOPERATIVE CARE

Postoperative care begins when the patient arrives in the postanesthesia care unit (PACU) and continues as he moves on to the short procedure unit, medical-surgical unit, or critical care area. Postoperative care aims to minimize postoperative complications by early detection and prompt treatment. After anesthesia a patient may experience pain, inadequate oxygenation, or adverse physiologic effects of sudden movement.

Recovery from general anesthesia takes longer than induction because the anesthetic is retained in fat and muscle. Fat has a meager blood supply; thus, it releases the anesthetic slowly, providing enough anesthesia to maintain adequate blood and brain levels during surgery. The patient's recovery time varies with his amount of body fat, his overall condition, his premedication regimen, and the type, dosage, and duration of anesthesia.

Key nursing diagnoses and patient outcomes

Risk for infection related to the procedure
The patient will:
▶ have normal vital signs, temperature, and laboratory values
▶ have no pathogens in cultures
▶ show no signs or symptoms of infection at the surgical site.

Equipment

Thermometer • watch with second hand • stethoscope • sphygmomanometer • postoperative flowchart or other documentation tool

Implementation

▶ Assemble the equipment at the patient's bedside.
▶ Obtain the patient's record from the PACU nurse. This should include a summary of operative procedures and pertinent findings; type of anesthesia; vital signs (preoperative, intraoperative and postoperative); medical history; medication history, including preoperative, intraoperative, and postoperative medications; fluid therapy, including estimated blood loss, type and number of drains, catheters, and characteristics of drainage; and notes on the condition of the surgical wound. *If the patient had vascular surgery, for example, knowing the location and duration of blood vessel clamping can prevent postoperative complications.*

▶ Transfer the patient from the PACU stretcher to the bed, and position him properly. Get a coworker to help if necessary. When moving the patient, keep transfer movements smooth *to minimize pain and postoperative complications and avoid back strain among team members.*
▶ If the patient has had orthopedic surgery, always get a coworker to help transfer him. Ask the coworker to move only the affected extremity.
▶ If the patient is in skeletal traction, you may receive special orders for moving him. If you must move him, have a coworker move the weights as you and another coworker move the patient.
▶ Make the patient comfortable and raise the bed's side rails *to ensure the patient's safety.*
▶ Assess the patient's level of consciousness, skin color, and mucous membranes.
▶ Monitor the patient's respiratory status by assessing his airway. Note breathing rate and depth, and auscultate for breath sounds. Administer oxygen and initiate oximetry *to monitor oxygen saturation if ordered.*
▶ Monitor the patient's pulse rate. It should be strong and easily palpable. The heart rate should be within 20% of the preoperative heart rate.
▶ Compare postoperative blood pressure to preoperative blood pressure. It should be within 20% of the preoperative level unless the patient suffered a hypotensive episode during surgery.
▶ Assess the patient's temperature *because anesthesia lowers body temperature.* Body temperature should be at least 95° F (35° C). If it's lower, apply blankets to warm the patient.
▶ Assess the patient's infusion sites for redness, pain, swelling, or drainage.

▶ Assess surgical wound dressings; they should be clean and dry. If they're soiled, assess the characteristics of the drainage and outline the soiled area. Note the date and time of assessment on the dressing. Assess the soiled area frequently; if it enlarges, reinforce the dressing and alert the doctor.

▶ Note the presence and condition of any drains and tubes. Note the color, type, odor, and amount of drainage. Make sure all drains are properly connected and free of kinks and obstructions.

▶ If the patient has had vascular or orthopedic surgery, assess the appropriate extremity — or all extremities, depending on the surgical procedure. Assess color, temperature, sensation, movement, and presence and quality of pulses, and notify the doctor of any abnormalities.

▶ As the patient recovers from anesthesia, monitor his respiratory and cardiovascular status closely. Be alert for signs of airway obstruction and hypoventilation caused by laryngospasm, or for sedation, which can lead to hypoxemia. Cardiovascular complications — such as arrhythmias and hypotension — may result from the anesthetic agent or the operative procedure.

▶ Encourage coughing and deep-breathing exercises. Don't encourage them if the patient has just had nasal, ophthalmic, or neurologic surgery, *to avoid increasing intracranial pressure.*

▶ Administer postoperative medications, such as antibiotics, analgesics, antiemetics, or reversal agents, as ordered and appropriate.

▶ Remove all fluids from the patient's bedside until he's alert enough to eat and drink. Before giving him liquids, assess his gag reflex to prevent aspiration. To do this, lightly touch the back of his throat with a cotton swab — the patient will gag if the reflex has returned. Do this test quickly *to prevent a vagal reaction.*

Special considerations

▶ Fear, pain, anxiety, hypothermia, confusion, and immobility can upset the patient and jeopardize his safety and postoperative status. Offer emotional support to the patient and his family. Keep in mind that the patient who has lost a body part or who has been diagnosed with an incurable disease will need ongoing emotional support. Refer him and his family for counseling as needed.

▶ As the patient recovers from general anesthesia, reflexes appear in reverse order to that in which they disappeared. Hearing recovers first, so avoid holding inappropriate conversations.

▶ The patient under general anesthesia can't protect his own airway because of muscle relaxation. As he recovers, his cough and gag reflexes reappear. If he can lift his head without assistance, he's usually able to breathe on his own.

▶ If the patient received spinal anesthesia, he will need to remain supine with the bed adjusted to between 0 degrees and 20 degrees for at least 6 hours *to reduce the risk of spinal headache from leakage of cerebrospinal fluid.* The patient won't be able to move his legs so be sure to reassure him that sensation and mobility will return.

▶ If the patient has had epidural anesthesia for postoperative pain control, monitor his respiratory status closely. *Respiratory arrest may result from paralysis of the diaphragm by the anesthetic.* He may also suffer nausea, vomiting, or itching.

▶ If the patient will be using a patient-controlled anesthesia (PCA) unit, make sure he understands how to use it. Caution him to activate it only when he has pain, not when he feels sleepy or is pain-free. Review your facility's criteria for PCA use.

Complications

Postoperative complications may include arrhythmias, hypotension, hypovolemia, septicemia, septic shock, atelectasis, pneumonia, thrombophlebitis, pulmonary embolism, urine retention, wound infection, wound dehiscence, evisceration, abdominal distention, paralytic ileus, constipation, altered body image, and postoperative psychosis.

Documentation

Document vital signs on the appropriate flowchart. Record the condition of dressings and drains, and characteristics of drainage. Document all interventions taken to alleviate pain and anxiety and the patient's responses to them. Document any complications and interventions taken.

PREOPERATIVE CARE

Preoperative care begins when surgery is first planned and ends with the administration of anesthesia. This phase of care includes a preoperative interview and assessment to collect baseline subjective and objective data from the patient and his family; diagnostic tests such as urinalysis, electrocardiogram, and chest radiography; preoperative teaching; securing informed consent from the patient; and physical preparation.

Key nursing diagnoses and patient outcomes

Deficient knowledge related to lack of exposure to the procedure
The patient will:
▶ communicate a need to increase knowledge
▶ state or demonstrate an understanding of what has been taught
▶ state the intention to make needed lifestyle changes, including seeking help from health care professionals when needed.

Anxiety related to a situational crisis
The patient will:
▶ identify factors that elicit anxious behaviors
▶ practice progressive relaxation techniques during the procedure
▶ cope with current medical situation (specify) without demonstrating signs of severe anxiety (specify for individual).

Equipment

Thermometer • sphygmomanometer • stethoscope • watch with second hand • weight scale • tape measure

Preparation of equipment

Assemble all equipment needed at the patient's bedside or in the admission area.

Implementation

▶ If the patient is having same-day surgery, make sure he knows ahead of time not to eat or drink anything for 8 hours prior to surgery. Confirm with him what time he's scheduled to arrive at the facility, and tell him to leave all jewelry and valuables at home. Also make sure the patient has arranged for someone to accompany him home after surgery.

▶ Obtain a health history and assess the patient's knowledge, perceptions, and expectations about his surgery. Ask about previous medical and surgical interventions. Also determine the patient's psychosocial needs; ask about occupational well-being, financial matters, support systems, mental status, and cultural beliefs. Use your facility's preoperative surgical assessment database, if available, to gather this information. Obtain a drug history. Ask about current prescription and over-the-counter medications and about known allergies to foods, drugs, and latex.

▶ Measure the patient's height, weight, and vital signs.

▶ Identify risk factors that may interfere with a positive expected outcome. Be sure to consider age, general health, medications, mobility, nutritional status, fluid and electrolyte disturbances, and lifestyle. Also consider the primary disorder's duration, location, and nature and the extent of the surgical procedure.

▶ Explain preoperative procedures to the patient. Include typical events that the patient can expect. Discuss equipment that may be used postoperatively, such as nasogastric tubes and I.V. equipment. Explain the typical incision, dressings, and staples or sutures that will be used. *Preoperative teaching can help reduce postoperative anxiety and pain, increase patient compliance, hasten recovery, and decrease length of stay.*

▶ Talk the patient through the sequence of events from operating room to recovery room (postanesthesia care unit [PACU]) back to patient's room. Some patients may be transferred from the PACU to an intensive care unit or surgical care unit. Your patient may also benefit from a tour of the areas he'll see during the perioperative events.

▶ Tell the patient that when he goes to the operating room, he may have to wait a short time in the holding area. Explain that the doctors and nurses will wear surgical dress, and even though they'll be observing him closely, they'll refrain from talking to him very much. Explain that *minimal conversation will help the preoperative medication take effect.*

▶ When discussing transfer procedures and techniques, describe sensations that the patient will experience. Tell him that he'll be taken to the operating room on a stretcher and transferred from the stretcher to the operating room table. *For his own safety,* he'll be held securely to the table with soft restraints. The operating room nurses will check his vital signs frequently.

▶ Warn the patient that the operating room may feel cool. Electrodes may be put on his chest to monitor his heart rate during surgery. Describe the drowsy floating sensation he'll feel as the anesthetic takes effect. Tell him it's important that he relax at this time.

▶ Tell the patient about exercises that he may be expected to perform after surgery, such as deep-breathing, coughing (while splinting the incision if necessary), extremity exercises, and movement and ambulation to minimize respiratory and circulatory complications. If the patient will undergo ophthalmic or neurologic surgery, he won't be asked to cough because coughing increases intracranial pressure.

▶ On the day of surgery, important interventions include giving morning care, verifying that the patient has signed an informed consent form (see *Obtaining informed consent,* page 668), administering ordered preoperative

Obtaining informed consent

Informed consent means that the patient has consented to a procedure after receiving a full explanation of the procedure, its risks and complications, and the risk if the procedure isn't performed at this time. Although obtaining informed consent is the doctor's responsibility, the nurse is responsible for verifying that this step has been taken.

You may be asked to witness the patient's signature. However, if you didn't hear the doctor's explanation to the patient, you must sign that you are witnessing the patient's signature only.

Consent forms must be signed before the patient receives preoperative medication because forms signed after sedatives are given are legally invalid. Adults and emancipated minors can sign their own consent forms. Consent forms of children or of adults with impaired mental status must be signed by a parent or guardian.

medications, completing the preoperative checklist and chart, and providing support to the patient and his family.

▶ Other immediate preoperative interventions may include preparing the GI tract (restricting food and fluids for about 8 hours before surgery) *to reduce vomiting and the risk of aspiration,* cleaning the lower GI tract of fecal material by enemas before abdominal or GI surgery, and giving antibiotics for 2 or 3 days preoperatively *to prevent contamination of the peritoneal cavity by GI bacteria.*

▶ Just before the patient is moved to the surgical area, make sure he is wearing a hospital gown, has his identification band in place, and has his vital signs recorded. Check to see that hairpins, nail polish, and jewelry have been removed. Note whether dentures, contact lenses, or prosthetic devices have been removed or left in place.

Special considerations

▶ Preoperative medications must be given on time *to enhance the effect of ordered anesthesia.* The patient should take nothing by mouth preoperatively. Don't give oral medications unless ordered. Be sure to raise the bed's side rails immediately after giving preoperative medications.

▶ If family members or others are present, direct them to the appropriate waiting area and offer support as needed.

Documentation

Complete the preoperative checklist used by your facility. Record all nursing care measures and preoperative medications, results of diagnostic tests, and the time the patient is transferred to the surgical area. The chart and the surgical checklist must accompany the patient to surgery.

PRESSURE DRESSING APPLICATION

For effective control of capillary or small-vein bleeding, temporary application of pressure directly over a wound may be achieved with a bulk dressing held by a glove-protected hand, bound into place with a pressure bandage, or held under pressure by an inflated air splint. A pressure dressing requires frequent checks for wound drainage to determine its effectiveness in controlling bleeding.

Pressure dressing may be prescribed for patients with fluid volume deficit, impaired skin integrity, impaired tissue integrity, or altered tissue perfusion.

Key nursing diagnoses and patient outcomes

Risk for deficient fluid volume related to excessive losses
The patient will:
▶ exhibit vital signs that remain stable
▶ have normal electrolyte values.

Equipment

Two or more sterile gauze pads • roller gauze • adhesive tape • gloves • metric ruler

Preparation of equipment

Obtain the pressure dressing quickly *to avoid excessive blood loss.* Use clean cloth for the dressing if sterile gauze pads are unavailable.

Implementation

▶ Quickly explain the procedure to the patient *to help decrease his anxiety,* and put on gloves.
▶ Elevate the injured body part *to help reduce bleeding.*
▶ Place enough gauze pads over the wound to cover it. Don't clean the wound until the bleeding stops.
▶ For an extremity or a trunk wound, hold the dressing firmly over the wound and wrap the roller gauze tightly across it and around the body part *to provide pressure on the wound.* Secure the bandage with adhesive tape.
▶ To apply a dressing to the neck, the shoulder, or another location that can't be tightly wrapped, don't use roller gauze. Instead, apply tape directly over the dressings *to provide the necessary pressure at the wound site.*
▶ Check pulse, temperature, and skin condition distal to the wound site *because excessive pressure can obstruct normal circulation.*
▶ Check the dressing frequently *to monitor wound drainage.* Use the metric

standard of measurement to determine the amount of drainage, and document these serial measurements for later reference. Don't circle a potentially wet dressing with ink *because this provides no permanent documentation in the medical record and also runs the risk of contaminating the dressing.*
▶ If the dressing becomes saturated, don't remove it *because this will interfere with the pressure.* Instead, apply an additional dressing over the saturated one and continue to monitor and record drainage.
▶ Obtain additional medical care as soon as possible.

Special considerations

▶ Apply pressure directly to the wound with your gloved hand if sterile gauze pads and clean cloth are unavailable.
▶ Avoid using an elastic bandage to bind the dressing *because it can't be wrapped tightly enough to create pressure on the wound site.*

Complications

A pressure dressing that is applied too tightly can impair circulation.

Documentation

When the bleeding is controlled, record the date and time of dressing application, presence or absence of distal pulses, integrity of distal skin, amount of wound drainage, and complications.

PRESSURE ULCER CARE

As their name implies, pressure ulcers result when pressure — applied with great force for a short period or with less force over a longer period — impairs circulation, depriving tissues of oxygen and other life-sustaining nutri-

Assessing pressure ulcers

To select the most effective treatment for a pressure ulcer, you first need to assess its characteristics. The pressure ulcer staging system described below, used by the National Pressure Ulcer Advisory Panel and the Agency for Health Care Policy and Research, reflects the anatomic depth of exposed tissue. Keep in mind that if the wound contains necrotic tissue, you won't be able to determine the stage until you can see the wound base.

Stage 1
The heralding lesion of a pressure ulcer is persistent redness in lightly pigmented skin and persistent red, blue, or purple hues on darker skin. Other indicators include changes in temperature, consistency, or sensation.

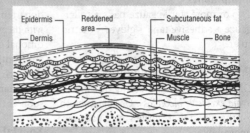

Stage 2
This stage is marked by partial-thickness skin loss involving the epidermis, the dermis, or both. The ulcer is superficial and appears as an abrasion, a blister, or a shallow crater.

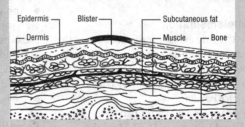

Stage 3
The ulcer constitutes a full-thickness wound penetrating the subcutaneous tissue, which may extend to — but not through — underlying fascia. The ulcer resembles a deep crater and may or may not undermine adjacent tissue.

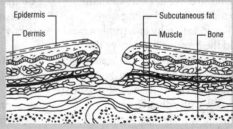

Stage 4
The ulcer extends through the skin, accompanied by extensive destruction, tissue necrosis, or damage to muscle, bone, or supporting structures (such as tendons and joint capsules).

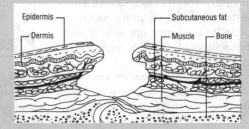

ents. This process damages skin and underlying structures. Untreated, the ischemic lesions that result can lead to serious infection.

Most pressure ulcers develop over bony prominences, where friction and shearing force combine with pressure to break down skin and underlying tissues. Common sites include the sacrum, coccyx, ischial tuberosities, and greater trochanters. Other common sites include the skin over the vertebrae, scapulae, elbows, knees, and heels in bedridden and relatively immobile patients.

Successful pressure ulcer treatment involves relieving pressure, restoring circulation and, if possible, resolving or managing related disorders. Typically, the effectiveness and duration of treatment depend on the pressure ulcer's characteristics. (See *Assessing pressure ulcers*.)

Ideally, prevention is the key to avoiding extensive therapy. Preventive measures include ensuring adequate nourishment and mobility to relieve pressure and promote circulation. (See *Braden scale for predicting pressure ulcer risk,* pages 672 and 673.)

When a pressure ulcer develops despite preventive efforts, treatment includes methods to decrease pressure, such as frequent repositioning to shorten pressure duration and the use of special equipment to reduce pressure intensity. Treatment also may involve special pressure-reducing devices, such as beds, mattresses, mattress overlays, and chair cushions. Other therapeutic measures include risk factor reduction and the use of topical treatments, wound cleansing, debridement, and dressings to support moist wound heal-

ing. (See *Guide to topical agents for pressure ulcers,* page 674.)

Nurses usually perform or coordinate treatments according to facility policy. The procedures detailed below address cleaning and dressing the pressure ulcer. Always follow the standard precautions guidelines of the Centers for Disease Control and Prevention.

Key nursing diagnoses and patient outcomes

Impaired skin integrity related to a pressure ulcer
The patient will:
▶ exhibit no evidence of further skin breakdown
▶ show normal skin turgor
▶ regain skin integrity (the pressure ulcer will heal)
▶ communicate an understanding of skin protection measures
▶ demonstrate skill in caring for the wound or incision.

Risk for infection related to a pressure ulcer
The patient will:
▶ have normal vital signs, temperature, and laboratory values
▶ have no pathogens in cultures
▶ show no signs or symptoms of worsening infection at the pressure ulcer site.

Equipment

Hypoallergenic tape or elastic netting • overbed table • piston-type irrigating system • two pairs of gloves • normal saline solution as ordered • sterile 4″ × 4″ gauze pads • sterile cotton swabs • selected topical dressing • linen-saver pads • disposable wound-measuring device • impervious plastic trash bag

Braden scale for predicting pressure ulcer risk

The Braden scale, shown below, is the most reliable of several instruments for assessing the older patient's risk of developing pressure ulcers. The lower the score, the greater the risk.

Sensory perception
Ability to respond meaningfully to pressure-related discomfort
1. Completely limited: Is unresponsive (doesn't moan, flinch, or grasp in response) to painful stimuli because of diminished level of consciousness or sedation
OR
Has a limited ability to feel pain over most of body surface
2. Very limited: Responds only to painful stimuli; can't communicate discomfort except through moaning or restlessness
OR
Has a sensory impairment that limits ability to feel pain or discomfort over half of body
3. Slightly limited: Responds to verbal commands but can't always communicate discomfort or need to be turned
OR
Has some sensory impairment that limits ability to feel pain or discomfort in one or two extremities
4. No impairment: Responds to verbal commands; has no sensory deficit that would limit ability to feel or voice pain or discomfort

Moisture
Degree to which skin is exposed to moisture
1. Constantly moist: Skin is kept moist almost constantly by perspiration, urine, or other fluid; dampness is detected every time patient is moved or turned
2. Very moist: Skin is often but not always moist; linen must be changed at least once per shift
3. Occasionally moist: Skin is occasionally moist; linen requires an extra change approximately once per day
4. Rarely moist: Skin is usually dry; linen requires changing only at routine intervals.

Activity
Degree of physical activity
1. Bedridden: Confined to bed
2. Confined to chair: Ability to walk severely limited or nonexistent; can't bear own weight and must be assisted into chair or wheelchair
3. Walks occasionally: Walks occasionally during day, but for very short distances, with or without assistance; spends majority of each shift in bed or chair
4. Walks frequently: Walks outside room at least twice per day and inside room at least once every 2 hours during waking hours

Mobility
Ability to change and control body position
1. Completely immobile: Doesn't make even slight changes in body or extremity position without assistance
2. Very limited: Makes occasional slight changes in body or extremity position but is unable to make frequent or significant changes independently
3. Slightly limited: Makes frequent though slight changes in body or extremity position independently
4. No limitations: Makes major and frequent changes in body or extremity position without assistance

Nutrition
Usual food intake pattern
1. Very poor: Never eats a complete meal; rarely eats more than one-third of any food offered; eats two servings or less of protein (meat or dairy products) per day; takes fluids poorly; doesn't take a liquid dietary supplement
OR
Is nothing-by-mouth status or maintained on clear liquids or I.V. fluids for more than 5 days

Braden scale for predicting pressure ulcer risk *(continued)*

2. Probably inadequate: Rarely eats a complete meal and generally eats only about half of any food offered; protein intake includes only three servings of meat or dairy products per day; occasionally will take a dietary supplement

OR

Receives less than optimum amount of liquid diet or tube feeding

3. Adequate: Eats more than half of most meals; eats four servings of protein (meat and dairy products) per day; occasionally refuses a meal but will usually take a supplement if offered

OR

Is on a tube feeding or total parenteral nutrition regimen that probably meets most nutritional needs

4. Excellent: Eats most of every meal and never refuses a meal; usually eats four or more servings of meat and dairy products per day; occasionally eats between meals; doesn't require supplementation

Friction and shear

Ability to assist with movement or to be moved in a way that prevents skin contact with bedding or other surface

1. Problem: Requires moderate to maximum assistance in moving; complete lifting without sliding against sheets is impossible; frequently slides down in bed or chair, requiring frequent repositioning with maximum assistance; spasticity, contractures, or agitation leads to almost constant friction

2. Potential problem: Moves feebly or requires minimum assistance during a move; skin probably slides to some extent against sheets, chair restraints, or other devices; maintains relatively good position in chair or bed most of the time but occasionally slides down

3. No apparent problem: Moves in bed and in chair independently and has sufficient muscle strength to lift up completely during move; maintains good position in bed or chair at all times

Total score: 6 to 23

Preparation of equipment

Assemble equipment at the patient's bedside. Cut tape into strips for securing dressings. Loosen lids on cleaning solutions and medications for easy removal. Loosen existing dressing edges and tapes before putting on gloves. Attach an impervious plastic trash bag to the overbed table to hold used dressings and refuse.

Implementation

▶ Before any dressing change, wash your hands and review the principles of standard precautions.

Cleaning the pressure ulcer

▶ Provide privacy, and explain the procedure to the patient *to allay his fears and promote cooperation.*

▶ Position the patient in a way that maximizes his comfort while allowing easy access to the pressure ulcer site.

▶ Cover bed linens with a linen-saver pad *to prevent soiling.*

▶ Open the normal saline solution container and the piston syringe. Carefully pour normal saline solution into an irrigation container *to avoid splashing.* (The container may be clean or sterile, depending on facility policy.)

Guide to topical agents for pressure ulcers

Topical agents	Nursing considerations
Antibiotics silver sulfadiazine, triple antibiotics	■ Consider a 2-week trial of topical antibiotics for clean or exudated pressure ulcers that aren't responding to moist-wound healing therapy.
Circulatory stimulants (Granulex, Proderm)	■ Use these agents to promote blood flow. Both contain balsam of Peru and castor oil, but Granulex also contains trypsin, an enzyme that facilitates debridement.
Enzymes collagenase (Santyl), sutilains (Travase)	■ Apply collagenase in thin layers after cleaning the wound with normal saline solution. ■ Avoid concurrent use of collagenase with agents that decrease enzymatic activity, including detergents, hexachlorophene, antiseptics with heavy-metal ions, iodine, and such acid solutions as Burow's solution. ■ Use collagenase cautiously near the patient's eyes. If contact occurs, flush the eyes repeatedly with normal saline solution or sterile water. ■ If using sutilains and topical antibacterials, apply sutilains ointment first. ■ Avoid applying sutilains to ulcers in major body cavities, areas with exposed nerve tissue, or fungating neoplastic lesions. Don't use sutilains in women of childbearing age or in patients with limited cardiopulmonary reserve. ■ Store sutilains at a cool temperature: 35.6° to 50° F (2° to 10° C). ■ Use sutilains cautiously near the patient's eyes. If contact occurs, flush the eyes repeatedly with normal saline solution or sterile water.
Exudate absorbers dextranomer beads (Debrisan)	■ Use dextranomer beads on secreting ulcers. Discontinue use when secretions stop. ■ Clean—but don't dry—the ulcer before applying dextranomer beads. Don't use in tunneling ulcers. ■ Remove gray-yellow beads (which indicate saturation) by irrigating with sterile water or normal saline solution. ■ Use cautiously near the eyes. If contact occurs, flush the eyes repeatedly with normal saline solution or sterile water.
Isotonic solutions normal saline solution	■ This agent moisturizes tissue without injuring cells.

Put the piston syringe into the opening provided in the irrigation container.
▶ Open the packages of supplies.
▶ Put on gloves to remove the old dressing and expose the pressure ulcer. Discard the soiled dressing in the impervious plastic trash bag *to avoid contaminating the sterile field and spreading infection.*
▶ Inspect the wound. Note the color, amount, and odor of drainage and necrotic debris. Measure the wound perimeter with the disposable wound-measuring device (a square, transparent card with concentric circles arranged in

Understanding pressure ulcer debridement

Because moist necrotic tissue promotes the growth of pathologic organisms, removing such tissue aids pressure ulcer healing. A pressure ulcer can be debrided using various methods. The patient's condition and the goals of care determine which method to use. Sharp debridement is indicated for patients with an urgent need for debridement, such as those with sepsis or cellulitis. Otherwise, another method, such as mechanical, enzymatic, or autolytic debridement, may be used. Sometimes, several methods are used in combination.

Sharp debridement
The most rapid method, sharp debridement removes thick, adherent eschar and devitalized tissue through the use of a scalpel, scissors, or another sharp instrument. Small amounts of necrotic tissue can be debrided at the bedside; extensive amounts must be debrided in the operating room.

Mechanical debridement
Typically, this method involves the use of wet-to-dry dressings. Gauze moistened with normal saline solution is applied to the wound and then removed after it dries and adheres to the wound bed. The goal is to debride the wound as the dressing is removed. Mechanical debridement has certain disadvantages; for example, it is often painful and it may take a long time to completely debride the ulcer.

Enzymatic debridement
This method removes necrotic tissue by breaking down tissue elements. Topical enzymatic debriding agents are placed on the necrotic tissue. If eschar is present, it must be crosshatched to allow the enzyme to penetrate the tissue.

Autolytic debridement
This technique involves the use of moisture-retentive dressings to cover the wound bed. Necrotic tissue is then removed through self-digestion of enzymes in the wound fluid. Although autolytic debridement takes longer than other debridement methods, it's appropriate for patients who can't tolerate any other method. If the ulcer is infected, autolytic debridement isn't the treatment of choice.

---

bull's-eye fashion and bordered with a straight-edge ruler).

▶ Using the piston syringe, apply full force to irrigate the pressure ulcer *to remove necrotic debris and help decrease bacteria in the wound.*

▶ Remove and discard your soiled gloves, and put on a fresh pair.

▶ Insert a gloved finger or sterile cotton swab into the wound to assess wound tunneling or undermining. *Tunneling usually signals wound extension along fascial planes.* Gauge tunnel depth by determining how far you can insert your finger or the cotton swab.

▶ Next, reassess the condition of the skin and the ulcer. Note the character of the clean wound bed and the surrounding skin.

▶ If you observe adherent necrotic material, notify a wound care specialist or a doctor *to ensure appropriate debridement.* (See *Understanding pressure ulcer debridement.*)

▶ Prepare to apply the appropriate topical dressing. Directions for typical moist saline gauze, hydrocolloid, transparent, alginate, foam, and hydrogel dressings follow. For other dressings or

Choosing a pressure ulcer dressing

The patient's needs and the ulcer's characteristics determine which type of dressing to use on a pressure ulcer.

Gauze dressings
Made of absorptive cotton or synthetic fabric, these dressings are permeable to water, water vapor, and oxygen and may be impregnated with petroleum jelly or another agent. When uncertain about which dressing to use, you may apply a gauze dressing moistened in saline solution until a wound specialist recommends definitive treatment.

Hydrocolloid dressings
These adhesive, moldable wafers are made of a carbohydrate-based material and usually have waterproof backings. They are impermeable to oxygen, water, and water vapor, and most have some absorptive properties.

Transparent film dressings
Clear, adherent, and nonabsorptive, these polymer-based dressings are permeable to oxygen and water vapor but not to water. Their transparency allows visual inspection. Because they can't absorb drainage, transparent film dressings are used on partial-thickness wounds with minimal exudate.

Alginate dressings
Made from seaweed, these nonwoven, absorptive dressings are available as soft white sterile pads or ropes. They absorb excessive exudate and may be used on infected wounds. As these dressings absorb exudate, they turn into a gel that keeps the wound bed moist and promotes healing. When exudate is no longer excessive, switch to another type of dressing.

Foam dressings
These spongelike polymer dressings may be impregnated or coated with other materials. Somewhat absorptive, they may or may not be adherent. Foam dressings promote moist wound healing and are useful when a nonadherent surface is desired.

Hydrogel dressings
Water-based and nonadherent, these polymer-based dressings have some absorptive properties. They're available as a gel in a tube, as flexible sheets, and as saturated gauze packing strips. They may have a cooling effect, which eases pain.

---

topical agents, follow your facility's protocol or the supplier's instructions.

Applying a moist saline gauze dressing
▶ Irrigate the pressure ulcer with normal saline solution. Blot the surrounding skin dry.
▶ Moisten the gauze dressing with normal saline solution.
▶ Gently place the dressing over the surface of the ulcer. *To separate surfaces within the wound*, gently place a dressing

between opposing wound surfaces. *To avoid damage to tissues*, don't pack the gauze tightly.
▶ Change the dressing often enough to keep the wound moist. (See *Choosing a pressure ulcer dressing*.)

Applying a hydrocolloid dressing
▶ Irrigate the pressure ulcer with normal saline solution. Blot the surrounding skin dry.
▶ Choose a clean, dry, presized dressing, or cut one to overlap the pressure

ulcer by about 1″ (2.5 cm). Remove the dressing from its package, pull the release paper from the adherent side of the dressing, and apply the dressing to the wound. *To minimize irritation,* carefully smooth out wrinkles as you apply the dressing.

▶ If the dressing's edges need to be secured with tape, apply a skin sealant to the intact skin around the ulcer. After the area dries, tape the dressing to the skin. *The sealant protects the skin and promotes tape adherence.* Avoid using tension or pressure when applying the tape.

▶ Remove your gloves and discard them in the impervious plastic trash bag. Dispose of refuse according to facility policy, and wash your hands.

▶ Change a hydrocolloid dressing every 2 to 7 days as necessary — for example, if the patient complains of pain, the dressing no longer adheres, or leakage occurs.

Applying a transparent dressing

▶ Irrigate the pressure ulcer with normal saline solution. Blot the surrounding skin dry.

▶ Clean and dry the wound as described above.

▶ Select a dressing to overlap the ulcer by 2″ (5 cm).

▶ Gently lay the dressing over the ulcer. *To prevent shearing force,* don't stretch the dressing. Press firmly on the edges of the dressing *to promote adherence.* Although this type of dressing is self-adhesive, you may have to tape the edges *to prevent them from curling.*

▶ If necessary, aspirate accumulated fluid with a 21G needle and syringe. After aspirating the pocket of fluid, clean the aspiration site with an alcohol pad and cover it with another strip of transparent dressing.

▶ Change the dressing every 3 to 7 days, depending on the amount of drainage.

Applying an alginate dressing

▶ Irrigate the pressure ulcer with normal saline solution. Blot the surrounding skin dry.

▶ Apply the alginate dressing to the ulcer surface. Cover the area with a secondary dressing (such as gauze pads) as ordered. Secure the dressing with tape or elastic netting.

▶ If the wound is draining heavily, change the dressing once or twice daily for the first 3 to 5 days. As drainage decreases, change the dressing less frequently — every 2 to 4 days or as ordered. When the drainage stops or the wound bed looks dry, stop using alginate dressing.

Applying a foam dressing

▶ Irrigate the pressure ulcer with normal saline solution. Blot the surrounding skin dry.

▶ Gently lay the foam dressing over the ulcer.

▶ Use tape, elastic netting, or gauze to hold the dressing in place.

▶ Change the dressing when the foam no longer absorbs the exudate.

Applying a hydrogel dressing

▶ Irrigate the pressure ulcer with normal saline solution. Blot the surrounding skin dry.

▶ Apply gel to the wound bed.

▶ Cover the area with a secondary dressing.

▶ Change the dressing daily or as needed *to keep the wound bed moist.*

▶ If the dressing you select comes in sheet form, cut the dressing to match the wound base; *otherwise, the intact surrounding skin can become macerated.*

▶ Hydrogel dressings also come in a prepackaged, saturated gauze for wounds that require "dead space" to be filled. Follow the manufacturer's directions for usage.

Preventing pressure ulcers

▶ Turn and reposition the patient every 1 to 2 hours unless contraindicated. For a patient who can't turn himself or who is turned on a schedule, use a pressure-reducing device, such as air, gel, or a 4″ foam mattress overlay. Low- or high-air-loss therapy may be indicated *to reduce excessive pressure and promote evaporation of excess moisture.* As appropriate, implement active or passive range-of-motion exercises *to relieve pressure and promote circulation. To save time,* combine these exercises with bathing if applicable.

▶ When turning the patient, lift him rather than slide him *because sliding increases friction and shear.* Use a turning sheet and get help from coworkers if necessary.

▶ Use pillows *to position your patient and increase his comfort.* Be sure to eliminate sheet wrinkles that could increase pressure and cause discomfort.

▶ Post a turning schedule at the patient's bedside. Adapt position changes to his situation. Emphasize the importance of regular position changes to the patient and his family, and encourage their participation in treatment and prevention of pressure ulcers by having them perform a position change correctly after you have demonstrated how.

▶ Avoid placing the patient directly on the trochanter. Instead, place him on his side, at about a 30-degree angle.

▶ Except for brief periods, avoid raising the head of the bed more than 30 degrees *to prevent shearing pressure.*

▶ Direct the patient confined to a chair or wheelchair to shift his weight every 15 minutes *to promote blood flow to compressed tissues.* Show a paraplegic patient how to shift his weight by doing push-ups in the wheelchair. If the patient needs your help, sit next to him and help him shift his weight to one buttock for 60 seconds; then repeat the procedure on the other side. Provide him with pressure-relieving cushions as appropriate. However, avoid seating the patient on a rubber or plastic doughnut, *which can increase localized pressure at vulnerable points.*

▶ Adjust or pad appliances, casts, or splints as needed *to ensure proper fit and avoid increased pressure and impaired circulation.*

▶ Tell the patient to avoid heat lamps and harsh soaps *because they dry the skin.* Applying lotion after bathing will help keep his skin moist. Also tell him to avoid vigorous massage *because it can damage capillaries.*

▶ If the patient's condition permits, recommend a diet that includes adequate calories, protein, and vitamins. Dietary therapy may involve nutritional consultation, food supplements, enteral feeding, or total parenteral nutrition.

▶ If diarrhea develops or if the patient is incontinent, clean and dry soiled skin. Then apply a protective moisture barrier *to prevent skin maceration.*

▶ Make sure the patient, family members, and caregivers learn pressure ulcer prevention and treatment strategies so that they understand the importance of care, the choices that are available, the rationales for treatments, and their own role in selecting goals and shaping the plan of care.

Special considerations

▶ Avoid using elbow and heel protectors that fasten with a single narrow strap. *The strap may impair neurovascular function in the involved hand or foot.*

▶ Avoid using artificial sheepskin. *It doesn't reduce pressure, and it may create a false sense of security.*

▶ Repair of stage 3 and stage 4 ulcers may require surgical intervention — such as direct closure, skin grafting, and flaps — depending on the patient's needs.

Complications

Infection may cause foul-smelling drainage, persistent pain, severe erythema, induration, and elevated skin and body temperatures. Advancing infection or cellulitis can lead to septicemia. Severe erythema may signal worsening cellulitis, which indicates that the offending organisms have invaded the tissue and are no longer localized.

Documentation

Record the date and time of initial and subsequent treatments. Note the specific treatment given. Detail preventive strategies performed. Document the pressure ulcer's location and size (length, width, and depth); color and appearance of the wound bed; amount, odor, color, and consistency of drainage; and condition of the surrounding skin. Reassess pressure ulcers at least weekly.

Update the plan of care as required. Note any change in the condition or size of the pressure ulcer and any elevation of skin temperature on the clinical record. Document when the doctor was notified of any pertinent abnormal observations. Record the patient's temperature daily on the graphic sheet to allow easy assessment of body temperature patterns.

PULSE AMPLITUDE MONITORING

Determining the presence and strength of peripheral pulses, an essential part of cardiovascular assessment, helps you to evaluate the adequacy of peripheral perfusion. A pulse amplitude monitor simplifies this procedure. A sensor taped to the patient's skin over a pulse point sends signals to a monitor, which measures the amplitude of the pulse and displays it as a waveform on a screen. The system continuously monitors the patient's peripheral pulse so you can perform other patient care duties.

The pulse amplitude monitor can be used after peripheral vascular reconstruction on the upper or lower extremities or after percutaneous transluminal peripheral or coronary angioplasty (either with the sheaths in place or after they've been removed).

Because the sensor monitors only relatively flat pulse points, it can't be used for the posterior tibial pulse point. Also, movement distorts the waveform, so the patient must stay as still as possible during monitoring. The patient shouldn't have lesions on the skin where the pulse will be monitored because the sensor must be placed directly on this site. The sensor and tape could irritate the lesion, or the lesion could impair transmission of the pulse amplitude. If the patient has a strong peripheral pulse, you'll see an adequate waveform.

Key nursing diagnoses and patient outcomes

Ineffective tissue perfusion (peripheral) related to (specify)
The patient will:
▶ express a feeling of comfort or absence of pain at rest
▶ have strong peripheral pulses
▶ show no evidence of pressure ulcers
▶ maintain tissue perfusion and cellular oxygenation.

Decreased cardiac output related to decreased stroke volume
The patient will:
▶ attain hemodynamic stability, as evidenced by pulse not less than (specify) beats/minute and not more than (specify) beats/minute and blood pressure not less than (specify) mm Hg and not greater than (specify) mm Hg
▶ have warm and dry skin
▶ maintain adequate cardiac output.

Equipment

Pulse amplitude display monitor with sensor

Preparation of equipment

Plug the monitor into a grounded outlet. Although the monitor has battery power for up to 24 hours, it should be plugged in when the battery isn't needed.

Turn on the monitor and allow it to warm up, which may take up to 10 seconds. Plug the sensor cable into the monitor; then tap the sensor gently. If tapping causes interference on the display screen, you can assume that the sensor-monitor connection is functioning properly.

Implementation

▶ Explain to the patient how the pulse amplitude monitor works.

▶ Locate the pulse you want to monitor. Mention that you'll tape the sensor to a selected site, usually the foot.
▶ Place the sensor over the strongest point of the pulse you're going to monitor. While observing the display screen, move the sensor until you see a strong upright waveform.
▶ Without moving the sensor from this site, peel off the adhesive strips and affix the sensor securely to the patient's foot. The sensor must maintain proper skin contact, so be sure to tape it firmly.
▶ Adjust the height of the pulse wave signal to half the height of the display screen. *This will give the waveform room to fluctuate as the pulse amplitude increases and decreases.*
▶ Set the low and high waveform amplitude alarms *so you'll be alerted to any waveform changes.*

Discontinuing monitor use

▶ Peel the sensor tapes from the patient's skin.
▶ Turn the machine off but keep it plugged in.
▶ Discard the sensor and, if necessary, wipe the monitor with a mild soap solution.

Special considerations

▶ Be aware that although the waveform displayed by a pulse amplitude monitor may resemble an electrocardiogram or blood pressure waveform, it isn't the same.
▶ Don't apply much pressure on the pulse sensor film or press on it with a sharp object *because such stress may warp or destroy the sensor.*
▶ Never place the sensor over an open wound or ulcerated skin.
▶ If waveform amplitude decreases, assess the patient's leg for capillary refill

time, temperature, color, and sensation. The amplitude change may stem from a malfunction in the monitor itself (such as a low battery) or from a thrombus, a hematoma, or a significant change in the patient's hemodynamic status.

▶ If the display screen is blank when you turn on the machine, make sure that the monitor is plugged in. If it's plugged in but the screen remains blank, the screen may need repair.

▶ If the screen is functioning but no waveform appears on it, first check the sensor-monitor connection. Then check the sensor by gently tapping it to see if interference appears on the screen. If the sensor is working properly, relocate the peripheral pulse on the patient's foot, and reapply the sensor. If your interventions don't work, the screen may need servicing.

Documentation

Print out a strip of the patient's waveform, and place the strip in the patient's medical record during every shift and whenever you note a change in the waveform or the patient's condition. Along the left side of the strip, you'll see a reference scale used to measure pulse amplitude height. Include this scale in your documentation.

PULSE OXIMETRY

Performed intermittently or continuously, oximetry is a relatively simple procedure used to monitor arterial oxygen saturation noninvasively. Pulse oximeters usually denote arterial oxygen saturation values with the symbol SpO_2, whereas invasively measured arterial oxygen saturation values are denoted by the symbol SaO_2. (See *How oximetry works*.)

How oximetry works

The pulse oximeter allows noninvasive monitoring of a patient's arterial oxygen saturation (SaO_2) levels by measuring the absorption (amplitude) of light waves as they pass through areas of the body that are highly perfused by arterial blood. Oximetry also monitors pulse rate and amplitude.

Light-emitting diodes in a transducer (photodetector) attached to the patient's body (shown below on the index finger) send red and infrared light beams through tissue. The photodetector records the relative amount of each color absorbed by arterial blood and transmits the data to a monitor, which displays the information with each heartbeat. If the SaO_2 level or pulse rate varies from preset limits, the monitor triggers visual and audible alarms.

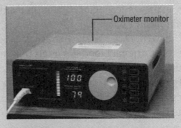

Oximeter monitor

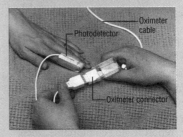

Oximeter cable

Photodetector

Oximeter connector

In this procedure, two diodes send red and infrared light through a pulsating arterial vascular bed, like the one in the fingertip. A photodetector slipped over the finger measures the transmitted light as it passes through the vascular bed, detects the relative amount of color absorbed by arterial blood, and calculates the exact mixed venous oxygen saturation without interference from surrounding venous blood, skin, connective tissue, or bone. Ear oximetry works by monitoring the transmission of light waves through the vascular bed of a patient's earlobe. Results will be inaccurate if the patient's earlobe is poorly perfused, as from a low cardiac output.

Key nursing diagnoses and patient outcomes

Impaired gas exchange related to altered oxygen supply
The patient will:
▶ maintain a respiratory rate within 5 breaths/minute of baseline
▶ express a feeling of comfort in maintaining air exchange
▶ have normal breath sounds
▶ have arterial blood gas levels that return to baseline, as evidenced by (specify) pH; (specify) partial pressure of arterial oxygen; and (specify) partial pressure of arterial carbon dioxide.

Ineffective breathing pattern related to (specify)
The patient will:
▶ have pulse and ear oximetry levels that remain between 95% and 100% (if an adult) or between 93.8% and 100% by 1 hour after birth (if a healthy, full-term neonate)
▶ report feeling comfortable when breathing
▶ achieve maximum lung expansion with adequate ventilation.

Equipment

Oximeter • finger or ear probe • alcohol pads • nail polish remover, if necessary

Preparation of equipment

Review the manufacturer's instructions for assembly of the oximeter.

Implementation

▶ Explain the procedure to the patient.

For pulse oximetry

▶ Select a finger for the test. Although the index finger is commonly used, a smaller finger may be selected if the patient's fingers are too large for the equipment. Make sure the patient isn't wearing false fingernails, and remove any nail polish from the test finger. Place the transducer (photodetector) probe over the patient's finger so that light beams and sensors oppose each other. If the patient has long fingernails, position the probe perpendicular to the finger, if possible, or clip the fingernail. Always position the patient's hand at heart level *to eliminate venous pulsations and to promote accurate readings.*

Age alert If you're testing a neonate or a small infant, wrap the probe around the foot so that light beams and detectors oppose each other. For a large infant, use a probe that fits on the great toe and secure it to the foot.
▶ Turn on the power switch. If the device is working properly, a beep will sound, a display will light momentarily, and the pulse searchlight will flash. The SpO_2 and pulse rate displays will show stationary zeros. After four to six heartbeats, the SpO_2 and pulse rate displays will supply information with each beat, and the pulse amplitude indicator will begin tracking the pulse.

For ear oximetry

▶ Using an alcohol pad, massage the patient's earlobe for 10 to 20 seconds. Mild erythema indicates adequate vascularization. Following the manufacturer's instructions, attach the ear probe to the patient's earlobe or pinna. Use the ear probe stabilizer for prolonged or exercise testing. Be sure to establish good contact on the ear; *an unstable probe may set off the low-perfusion alarm.* After the probe has been attached for a few seconds, a saturation reading and pulse waveform will appear on the oximeter's screen.

▶ Leave the ear probe in place for 3 or more minutes until readings stabilize at the highest point, or take three separate readings and average them. Make sure you revascularize the patient's earlobe each time.

▶ After the procedure, remove the probe, turn off and unplug the unit, and clean the probe by gently rubbing it with an alcohol sponge.

Special considerations

▶ If oximetry has been performed properly, readings are typically accurate. However, certain factors may interfere with accuracy. For example, an elevated bilirubin level may falsely lower SpO_2 readings, while elevated carboxyhemoglobin or methemoglobin levels, such as occur in heavy smokers and urban dwellers, can cause a falsely elevated SpO_2 reading.

▶ If light is a problem, cover the probes; if patient movement is a problem, move the probe or select a different probe; and if ear pigment is a problem, reposition the probe, revascularize the site, or use a finger probe. (See *Diagnosing pulse oximeter problems.*)

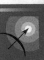

Troubleshooting

Diagnosing pulse oximeter problems

To maintain a continuous display of arterial oxygen saturation levels, you'll need to keep the monitoring site clean and dry. Make sure the skin doesn't become irritated from adhesives used to keep disposable probes in place. You may need to change the site if this happens. Disposable probes that irritate the skin also can be replaced by nondisposable models that don't need tape.

Another common problem with pulse oximeters is the failure of the devices to obtain a signal. Your first reaction if this happens should be to check the patient's vital signs. If they're sufficient to produce a signal, check for the following problems.

Poor connection

See if the sensors are properly aligned. Make sure that wires are intact and securely fastened and that the pulse oximeter is plugged into a power source.

Inadequate or intermittent blood flow to site

Check the patient's pulse rate and capillary refill time, and take corrective action if blood flow to the site is decreased. This may mean loosening restraints, removing tight-fitting clothes, taking off a blood pressure cuff, or checking arterial and I.V. lines. If none of these interventions works, you may need to find an alternate site. Finding a site with proper circulation may also prove challenging when a patient is receiving vasoconstrictive drugs.

Equipment malfunctions

Remove the pulse oximeter from the patient, set the alarm limits at 85% and 100%, and try the instrument on yourself or another healthy person. This will tell you if the equipment is working correctly.

▶ Certain intravascular substances, such as lipid emulsions and dyes, can also prevent accurate readings. Other factors that may interfere with accurate results include excessive light (for example, from phototherapy, surgical lamps, direct sunlight, and excessive ambient lighting), excessive patient movement, excessive ear pigment, hypothermia, hypotension, and vasoconstriction.

▶ If the patient has compromised circulation in his extremities, you can place a photodetector across the bridge of his nose.

▶ If SpO_2 is used to guide weaning the patient from forced inspiratory oxygen, obtain arterial blood gas analysis occasionally to correlate SpO_2 readings with SaO_2 levels.

▶ If an automatic blood pressure cuff is used on the same extremity that is used for measuring SpO_2, the cuff will interfere with SpO_2 readings during inflation.

▶ Normal SpO_2 levels for ear and pulse oximetry are 95% to 100% for adults and 93.8% to 100% by 1 hour after birth for healthy, full-term neonates. Lower levels may indicate hypoxemia that warrants intervention. For such patients, follow your facility's policy or the doctor's orders, which may include increasing oxygen therapy. If SaO_2 levels decrease suddenly, you may need to resuscitate the patient immediately. Notify the doctor of any significant change in the patient's condition.

Documentation

Document the procedure, including the date, time, procedure type, oximetric measurement, and any action taken. Record reading on appropriate flowcharts if indicated.

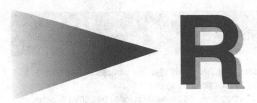

RADIATION IMPLANT THERAPY

In radiation implant therapy, also called brachytherapy, the doctor uses implants of radioactive isotopes (encapsulated in seeds, needles, or sutures) to deliver ionizing radiation within a body cavity or interstitially to a tumor site. Implants can deliver a continuous radiation dose over several hours or days to a specific site while minimizing exposure to adjacent tissues. The implants may be permanent or temporary. Isotopes, such as cesium 137, gold 198, iodine 125, iridium 192, palladium 103, and phosphorus 32 (^{32}P) are used to treat cancers. (See *Radioisotopes and their uses,* pages 686 and 687.)

Common implant sites include the brain, breast, cervix, endometrium, lung, neck, oral cavity, prostate, and vagina. Radiation implant therapy is commonly combined with external radiation therapy (teletherapy) for increased effectiveness.

For treatment, the patient is usually placed in a private room (with its own bathroom) located as far away from high-traffic areas as practical. If monitoring shows an increased radiation hazard, adjacent rooms and hallways may also need to be restricted. Consult your facility's radiation safety policy for specific guidelines.

Key nursing diagnoses and patient outcomes

Disturbed body image related to the presence of implants
The patient will:
▶ acknowledge change in body image
▶ participate in decision making about radiation implant therapy
▶ express positive feelings about self.

Decisional conflict related to perceived threat to value system
The patient will:
▶ state feelings about the current situation
▶ identify desirable and undesirable consequences of available options
▶ accept assistance from family, friends, clergy, and other support persons.

Equipment

Film badge or pocket dosimeter • RADI-ATION PRECAUTION sign for door • RADI-ATION PRECAUTION warning labels • masking tape • lead-lined container • long-handled forceps • optional: lead shield and lead strip

For implants inserted in the oral cavity or neck
Emergency tracheotomy tray

Radioisotopes and their uses

Radioisotopes are unstable elements and emit three kinds of energy particles as they decay to a stable state. These particles are ranked by their penetrating power.

Alpha particles possess the lowest energy level and are easily stopped by a sheet of paper. More powerful beta particles can be stopped by the skin's surface. Gamma rays, the most powerful, can be stopped only by dense shielding such as lead. Some isotopes commonly used in cancer treatments are described below.

Isotope and indications	Description	Nursing considerations
Cesium 137 (^{137}Cs) Gynecologic cancers	■ 30-year half-life ■ Emits gamma particles ■ Encased in steel capsules that are placed temporarily in the patient in the operating room	■ Elevate the head of the bed no more than 45 degrees. ■ Encourage fluids and implement a low-residue diet. ■ Encourage quiet activities and enforce strict bed rest as ordered.
Iodine 125 (^{125}I) Localized or unresectable tumors; slow-growing tumors; recurrent disease	■ 60-day half-life ■ Emits gamma particles ■ Permanently implanted as tiny seeds or sutures directly into the tumor or tumor bed	■ Because a seed may become dislodged, no linens, body fluids, instruments, or utensils may leave the patient's room until they're monitored. ■ If a seed is dislodged and found, call the radiation oncology department; use long-handled forceps to put it in a lead-linen container in the room. ■ Monitor body fluids to detect displaced seeds. Give the patient a 24-hour urine container that can be closed.
Iridium 192 (^{192}Ir) Localized or unresectable tumors	■ 74-day half-life ■ Emits gamma particles ■ Temporarily implanted as seeds strung inside special catheters that are implanted around the tumor	■ If a catheter is dislodged, call the radiation oncology department; use long-handled forceps to put the implant in a lead-lined container in the room.
Palladium 103 (^{103}Pd) Superficial, localized, or unresectable intrathoracic or intra-abdominal tumors	■ 17-day half-life ■ Emits beta particles ■ Permanently implanted as seeds in the tumor or tumor bed	■ See iodine 125.
Phosphorus 32 (^{32}P) Polycythemia, leukemia, bone metastasis, and malignant ascites	■ 14-day half-life ■ Emits beta particles ■ Used as an I.V. solution rather than an implant because of its low energy level	■ No shielding is required other than a Lucite syringe shield. ■ Patients receiving ^{32}P are placed in a private room with a separate bathroom.

Radioisotopes and their uses (continued)

Isotope and indications	Description	Nursing considerations
Gold 198 (^{198}Au) Localized male genitourinary tumors	■ 3-day half-life ■ Emits gamma particles ■ Permanently implanted as tiny seeds directly into the tumor or tumor bed	■ If a seed is dislodged and found, call the radiation oncology department for disposal.

For implants inserted in the anal cavity or vagina

Male T-binder • two sanitary napkins with safety pins

Preparation of equipment

Place the lead-lined container and long-handled forceps in a corner of the patient's room. Mark a "safe line" on the floor with masking tape 6' (1.8 m) from the patient's bed *to warn visitors to keep clear of the patient to minimize their radiation exposure.* If desired, place a portable lead shield in the back of the room to use when providing care.

Place an emergency tracheotomy tray in the room if an implant will be inserted in the oral cavity or neck.

Implementation

▶ Explain the treatment and its goals to the patient. Before treatment begins, review radiation safety procedures, visitation policies, potential adverse effects, and interventions for those effects. Also, review long-term concerns and home care issues.

▶ Place the RADIATION PRECAUTION sign on the door.

▶ Check to see that informed consent has been obtained.

▶ Ensure that all laboratory tests are performed before beginning treatment. If laboratory work is required during treatment, the badged technician obtains the specimen, labels the collection tube with a RADIOACTIVE PRECAUTION label, and alerts the laboratory personnel before transporting it. If urine tests are needed for ^{32}P therapy, ask the radiation oncology department or laboratory technician how to transport the specimens safely.

▶ Affix a RADIATION PRECAUTION warning label to the patient's identification wristband.

▶ Affix warning labels to the patient's chart and Kardex *to ensure staff awareness of the patient's radioactive status.*

▶ Wear a film badge or dosimeter at waist level during the entire shift. Turn in the radiation badge monthly or according to your facility's protocol. Pocket dosimeters measure immediate exposures. In many centers, these measurements aren't part of the permanent exposure record but are used to ensure that nurses receive the lowest possible exposure.

▶ Each nurse must have a personal, nontransferable film badge or ring badge. *Badges document each person's cumulative lifetime radiation exposure.* Only primary caregivers are badged and allowed into the patient's room.

▶ To minimize exposure to radiation, use the three principles of time, distance, and shielding. For time, plan to give care in the shortest time possible. *Less time equals less exposure.* For distance, work as far away from the radiation source as possible. Give care from the side opposite the implant or from a position allowing the greatest working distance possible. *The intensity of radiation exposure varies inversely as the square of the distance from the source.* For shielding, use a portable shield, if needed and desired.

▶ Provide essential nursing care only; omit bed baths. If ordered, provide perineal care, making sure that wipes, sanitary pads, and similar items are bagged correctly and monitored. (Refer to your facility's radiation policy.)

▶ Dressing changes over an implanted area must be supervised by the radiation technician or another designated caregiver.

▶ Before discharge, a patient's temporary implant must be removed and properly stored by the radiation oncology department. A patient with a permanent implant may not be released until his radioactivity level is less than 5 millirems/hour at $3\frac{1}{4}'$ (1 m).

Special considerations

▶ Nurses and visitors who are pregnant or trying to conceive or father a child must not attend patients receiving radiation implant therapy *because the gonads and developing embryo and fetus are highly susceptible to the damaging effects of ionizing radiation.*

▶ If the patient must be moved out of his room, notify the appropriate department of the patient's status *to give re-ceiving personnel time to make appropriate preparations to receive the patient.* When moving the patient, ensure that the route is clear of equipment and other people and that the elevator, if there is one, is keyed and ready to receive the patient. Move the patient in a bed or wheelchair, accompanied by two badged caregivers. If the patient is delayed along the way, stand as far away from the bed as possible until you can continue.

▶ The patient's room must be monitored daily by the radiation oncology department, and disposables must be monitored and removed according to facility guidelines.

▶ If a code is called on a patient with an implant, follow your facility's code procedures as well as these steps: Notify the code team of the patient's radioactive status *to exclude any team member who is pregnant or trying to conceive or father a child.* Also, notify the radiation oncology department. Cover the implant site with a strip of lead shielding, if possible. Don't allow anything to leave the patient's room until it's monitored for radiation. The primary care nurse must remain in the room (as far from the patient as possible) *to act as a resource person for the patient and to provide film badges or dosimeters to code team members.*

▶ If an implant becomes dislodged, notify the radiation oncology department staff and follow their instructions. Typically, the dislodged implant is collected with long-handled forceps and placed in a lead-shielded container.

▶ Tell the patient who has had a cervical implant to expect slight to moderate vaginal bleeding after being discharged. This flow normally changes color from pink to brown to white. Instruct her to notify the doctor if bleeding increases, persists for more than 48 hours, or has a foul odor. Explain to the patient that she may resume most normal activities but should avoid sexual intercourse and the use of tampons until after her follow-up visit to the doctor (about 6 weeks after discharge). Instruct her to take showers rather than baths for 2 weeks, avoid douching unless allowed by the doctor, and avoid activities that cause abdominal strain for 6 weeks.

▶ Refer the patient for sexual or psychological counseling, if needed.

▶ If a patient with an implant dies on the unit, notify the radiation oncology department *so they can remove a temporary implant and store it properly.* If the implant was permanent, radiation oncology staff members will determine which precautions to follow before postmortem care can be provided and before the body can be moved to the morgue.

Complications

Depending on the implant site and total radiation dose, complications of implant therapy may include dislodgment of the radiation source or applicator, tissue fibrosis, xerostomia, radiation pneumonitis, muscle atrophy, sterility, vaginal dryness or stenosis, fistulas, hypothyroidism, altered bowel habits, infection, airway obstruction, diarrhea, cystitis, myelosuppression, neurotoxicity, and secondary cancers. Encourage the patient and family members to keep in contact with the radiation oncology department and to call them if concerns or physical changes occur.

Documentation

Record radiation precautions taken during treatment, adverse effects of therapy, any teaching given to the pa-

tient and his family and their responses to it, patient's tolerance of isolation procedures and the family's compliance with procedures, and referrals to local cancer services.

RADIOACTIVE IODINE THERAPY

Because the thyroid gland concentrates iodine, radioactive iodine 131 (^{131}I) can be used to treat thyroid cancer. Usually administered orally, this isotope is used to treat postoperative residual cancer, recurrent disease, inoperable primary thyroid tumors, invasion of the thyroid capsule, and thyroid ablation as well as cancers that have metastasized to cervical or mediastinal lymph nodes or other distant sites.

Because ^{131}I is absorbed systemically, all body secretions, especially urine, must be considered radioactive. For ^{131}I treatments, the patient usually is placed in a private room (with its own bathroom) located as far away from high-traffic areas as practical. Adjacent rooms and hallways may also need to be restricted. Consult your facility's radiation safety policy for specific guidelines.

In lower doses, ^{131}I also may be used to treat hyperthyroidism. Most patients receive this treatment on an outpatient basis and are sent home with appropriate home care instructions.

Key nursing diagnoses and patient outcomes

Disturbed body image related to the presence of implants
The patient will:

▶ acknowledge change in body image

▶ participate in decision making about radiation implant therapy
▶ express positive feelings about self.

Decisional conflict related to perceived threat to value system
The patient will:
▶ state feelings about the current situation
▶ identify desirable and undesirable consequences of available options
▶ accept assistance from family, friends, clergy, and other support persons.

Equipment
Film badges, pocket dosimeters, or ring badges • RADIATION PRECAUTION sign for door • RADIATION PRECAUTION warning labels • waterproof gowns • clear and red plastic bags for contaminated articles • plastic wrap • absorbent plastic-lined pads • masking tape • radioresistant gloves • trash cans • emergency tracheotomy tray • optional: portable lead shield

Preparation of equipment
Assemble all necessary equipment in the patient's room. Keep an emergency tracheotomy tray just outside the room or in a handy place at the nurses' station. Place the RADIATION PRECAUTION sign on the door. Affix warning labels to the patient's chart and Kardex *to ensure staff awareness of the patient's radioactive status.*

Place an absorbent plastic-lined pad on the bathroom floor and under the sink; if the patient's room is carpeted, cover it with such a pad as well. Place an additional pad over the bedside table. Secure plastic wrap over the telephone, television controls, bed controls, mattress, call button, and toilet.

These measures prevent radioactive contamination of working surfaces.

Keep large trash cans in the room lined with plastic bags (two clear bags inserted inside an outer red bag). Monitor all objects before they leave the room.

Notify the dietitian to supply foods and beverages only in disposable containers and with disposable utensils.

Implementation
▶ Explain the procedure and review treatment goals with the patient and his family. Before treatment begins, review the facility's radiation safety procedures and visitation policies, potential adverse effects, interventions, and home care procedures. (See *What to do after* ^{131}I *treatment.*)
▶ Verify that the doctor has obtained informed consent.
▶ Check for allergies to iodine-containing substances, such as contrast media and shellfish. Review the medication history for thyroid-containing or thyroid-altering drugs and for lithium carbonate, *which may increase* ^{131}I *uptake.*
▶ Review the patient's health history for vomiting, diarrhea, productive cough, and sinus drainage, *which could increase the risk of radioactive secretions.*
▶ If necessary, remove the patient's dentures *to avoid contaminating them and to reduce radioactive secretions.* Tell him that they'll be replaced 48 hours after treatment.
▶ Affix a RADIATION PRECAUTION warning label to the patient's identification wristband.
▶ Encourage the patient to use the toilet rather than a bedpan or urinal and to flush it three times after each use *to reduce radiation levels.*

▶ Tell the patient to remain in his room except for tests or procedures. Allow him to ambulate.

▶ Unless contraindicated, instruct the patient to increase his daily fluid intake to 3 qt (2.8 L).

▶ Encourage the patient to chew or suck on hard candy *to keep salivary glands stimulated and prevent them from becoming inflamed (which may develop in the first 24 hours).*

▶ Ensure that all laboratory tests are performed before beginning treatment. If laboratory work is required, the badged laboratory technician obtains the specimen, labels the collection tube with a RADIATION PRECAUTION warning label, and alerts the laboratory personnel before transporting it. If urine tests are needed, ask the radiation oncology department or laboratory technician how to transport the specimens safely.

▶ Wear a film badge or dosimeter at waist level during the entire shift. Turn in the radiation badge monthly or according to your facility's protocol and record your exposures accurately. *Pocket dosimeters measure immediate exposures. These measurements may not be part of the permanent exposure record but help to ensure that nurses receive the lowest possible exposure.*

▶ Each nurse must have a personal, nontransferable film badge or ring badge. *Badges document each person's cumulative lifetime radiation exposure.* Only primary caregivers are badged and allowed into the patient's room.

▶ Wear gloves to touch the patient or objects in his room.

▶ Wear a waterproof gown and gloves when handling the patient's body secretions (for example, when moving his emesis basin).

What to do after ^{131}I treatment

■ Instruct the patient to report long-term adverse reactions. In particular, review signs and symptoms of hypothyroidism and hyperthyroidism. Also ask him to report signs and symptoms of thyroid cancer, such as enlarged lymph nodes, dyspnea, bone pain, nausea, vomiting, and abdominal discomfort.

■ Although the patient's radiation level at discharge will be safe, suggest that he take extra precautions during the 1st week, such as using separate eating utensils, sleeping in a separate bedroom, and avoiding bodily contact, especially with infants and children.

■ Sexual intercourse may be resumed 1 week after iodine 131 (^{131}I) treatment. However, urge a female patient to avoid pregnancy for 6 months after treatment and tell a male patient to avoid impregnating his partner for 3 months after treatment.

▶ Allow visitors to stay no longer than 30 minutes every 24 hours with the patient. Stress that no visitors will be allowed who are pregnant or trying to conceive or father a child.

Age alert **Visitors under age 18 aren't allowed.**

▶ Restrict direct contact to no longer than 30 minutes or 20 millirems per day. If the patient is receiving 200 millicuries of ^{131}I, remain with him only 2 to 4 minutes and stand no closer than 1′ (30.5 cm) away. If standing 3′ (.9 m) away, the time limit is 20 minutes; if standing 5′ (1.5 m) away, the limit is 30 minutes.

▶ Give essential nursing care only; omit bed baths. If ordered, provide perineal care, making sure that wipes, sanitary pads, and similar items are bagged correctly.

▶ If the patient vomits or urinates on the floor, notify the nuclear medicine department and use nondisposable radioresistant gloves when cleaning the floor. After cleanup, wash your gloved hands, remove the gloves and leave them in the room, and then rewash your hands.

▶ If the patient must be moved from his room, notify the appropriate department of his status *so that receiving personnel can make appropriate arrangements to receive him.* When moving the patient, ensure that the route is clear of equipment and other people and that the elevator, if there is one, is keyed and ready to receive the patient. Move the patient in a bed or wheelchair, accompanied by two badged caregivers. If delayed, stand as far away from him as possible until you can continue.

▶ The patient's room must be cleaned by the radiation oncology department, not by housekeeping. The room must be monitored daily, and disposables must be monitored and removed according to facility guidelines.

▶ At discharge, schedule the patient for a follow-up examination. Also, arrange for a whole-body scan about 7 to 10 days after ^{131}I treatment.

▶ Inform the patient and his family of community support services for cancer patients.

Special considerations

▶ Nurses and visitors who are pregnant or trying to conceive or father a child must not attend or visit patients receiving ^{131}I therapy *because the gonads and developing embryo and fetus are highly susceptible to the damaging effects of ionizing radiation.*

▶ If a code is called on a patient undergoing ^{131}I therapy, follow your facility's code procedures as well as the following steps: Notify the code team of the patient's radioactive status *to exclude any team member who is pregnant or trying to conceive or father a child.* Also, notify the radiation oncology department. Don't allow anything out of the patient's room until it's monitored. The primary care nurse must remain in the room (as far as possible from the patient) *to act as a resource person and to provide film badges or dosimeters to code team members.*

▶ If the patient dies on the unit, notify the radiology safety officer, who will determine which precautions to follow before postmortem care is provided and before the body can be removed to the morgue.

Complications

Myelosuppression is common in patients who undergo repeated ^{131}I treatments. Radiation pulmonary fibrosis may develop if extensive lung metastasis was present when ^{131}I was administered.

Other complications may include nausea, vomiting, headache, radiation thyroiditis, fever, sialadenitis, and pain and swelling at metastatic sites.

Documentation

Record radiation precautions taken during treatment, any teaching given to the patient and his family, the patient's tolerance of (and the family's compliance with) isolation procedures, and referrals to local cancer counseling services.

RANGE-OF-MOTION EXERCISES, PASSIVE

Used to move the patient's joints through as full a range of motion as possible, passive range-of-motion (ROM) exercises improve or maintain joint mobility and help prevent contractures. Performed by a nurse, a physical therapist, or a caregiver of the patient's choosing, these exercises are indicated for the patient with temporary or permanent loss of mobility, sensation, or consciousness. Performed properly, passive ROM exercises require recognition of the patient's limits of motion and support of all joints during movement.

Passive ROM exercises are contraindicated in patients with septic joints, acute thrombophlebitis, severe arthritic joint inflammation, or recent trauma with possible hidden fractures or internal injuries.

Key nursing diagnoses and patient outcomes

Risk for disuse syndrome related to prolonged inactivity
The patient will:
▶ display no evidence of altered mental, sensory, or motor ability
▶ maintain muscle strength and tone and joint range of motion
▶ maintain normal neurologic, cardiovascular, respiratory, musculoskeletal, gastrointestinal, and integumentary function during periods of inactivity.

Impaired physical mobility related to neuromuscular impairment
The patient will:
▶ show no evidence of complications, such as contractures, venous stasis, thrombus formation, or skin breakdown
▶ have mobility regimen carried out by self or caregiver.

Implementation

▶ Determine the joints that need ROM exercises and consult the doctor or physical therapist about limitations or precautions for specific exercises. The exercises below treat all joints, but they don't have to be performed in the order given or all at once. You can schedule them over the course of a day, whenever the patient is in the most convenient position. Remember to perform all exercises slowly, gently, and to the end of the normal ROM or to the point of pain but no further. (See *Glossary of joint movements,* page 694.)
▶ Before you begin, raise the bed to a comfortable working height.

Exercising the neck

▶ Support the patient's head with your hands and extend the neck, flex the chin to the chest, and tilt the head laterally toward each shoulder.
▶ Rotate the head from right to left.

Exercising the shoulders

▶ Support the patient's arm in an extended, neutral position; then extend the forearm and flex it back. Abduct the arm outward from the side of the body and adduct it back to the side.
▶ Rotate the shoulder so that the arm crosses the midline and bend the elbow so that the hand touches the opposite shoulder, then touches the mattress of the bed for complete internal rotation.
▶ Return the shoulder to a neutral position and, with elbow bent, push the arm backward so that the back of the

Glossary of joint movements

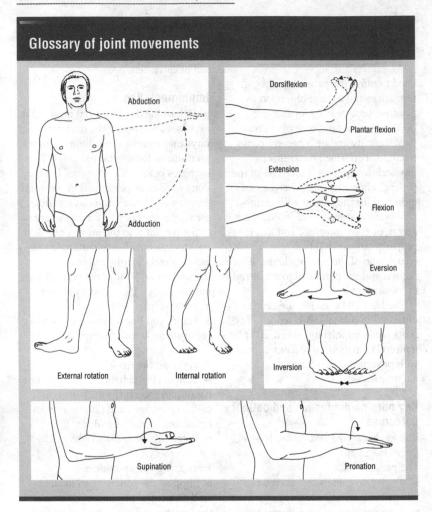

hand touches the mattress for complete external rotation.

Exercising the elbow
▶ Place the patient's arm at his side with his palm facing up.
▶ Flex and extend the arm at the elbow.

Exercising the forearm
▶ Stabilize the patient's elbow and then twist the hand to bring the palm up (supination).
▶ Twist it back again to bring the palm down (pronation).

Exercising the wrist
▶ Stabilize the forearm and flex and extend the wrist. Then rock the hand

Learning about isometric exercises

Patients can strengthen and increase muscle tone by contracting muscles against resistance (from other muscles or from a stationary object, such as a bed or a wall) without joint movement. These exercises require only a comfortable position—standing, sitting, or lying down—and proper body alignment. For each exercise, instruct the patient to hold each contraction for 2 to 5 seconds and to repeat it three to four times daily, below peak contraction level for the first week and at peak level thereafter.

Neck rotators
The patient places the heel of his hand above one ear. Then he pushes his head toward the hand as forcefully as possible, without moving the head, neck, or arm. He repeats the exercise on the other side.

Neck flexors
The patient places both palms on his forehead. Without moving his neck, he pushes the head forward while resisting with the palms.

Neck extensors
The patient clasps his fingers behind his head, then pushes the head against the clasped hands without moving his neck.

Shoulder elevators
Holding the right arm straight down at the side, the patient grasps his right wrist with his left hand. He then tries to shrug his right shoulder but prevents it from moving by holding his arm in place. He repeats this exercise, alternating arms.

Shoulder, chest, and scapular musculature
The patient places his right fist in his left palm and raises both arms to shoulder height. He pushes the fist into the palm as forcefully as possible without moving either arm. Then with his arms in the same position, he clasps the fingers and tries to pull the hands apart. He repeats the pattern, beginning with the left fist in the right palm.

Elbow flexors and extensors
With his right elbow bent 90 degrees and his right palm facing upward, the patient places his left fist against his right palm. He tries to bend the right elbow further while resisting with the left fist. He repeats the pattern, bending the left elbow.

Abdomen
The patient assumes a sitting position and bends slightly forward with his hands in front of the middle of his thighs. He tries to bend forward further, resisting by pressing the palms against the thighs.

Alternatively, in the supine position, he clasps his hands behind his head. Then he raises his shoulders about 1″ (2.5 cm), holding this position for a few seconds.

Back extensors
In a sitting position, the patient bends forward and places his hands under his buttocks. He tries to stand up, resisting with both hands.

Hip abductors
While standing, the patient squeezes his inner thighs together as tightly as possible. Placing a pillow between the knees supplies resistance and increases the effectiveness of this exercise.

Hip extensors
The patient squeezes his buttocks together as tightly as possible.

(continued)

Learning about isometric exercises (*continued*)

Knee extensors
The patient straightens his knee fully. Then he vigorously tightens the muscle above the knee so that it moves the kneecap upward. He repeats this exercise, alternating legs.

Ankle flexors and extensors
The patient pulls his toes upward, holding briefly. Then he pushes them down as far as possible, again holding briefly.

---

sideways for lateral flexion and rotate the hand in a circular motion.

Exercising the fingers and thumb
▶ Extend the patient's fingers and then flex the hand into a fist; repeat extension and flexion of each joint of each finger and thumb separately.
▶ Spread two adjoining fingers apart (abduction) and then bring them together (adduction).
▶ Oppose each fingertip to the thumb and rotate the thumb and each finger in a circle.

Exercising the hip and knee
▶ Fully extend the patient's leg and then bend the hip and knee toward the chest, allowing full joint flexion.
▶ Next, move the straight leg sideways, out and away from the other leg (abduction), and then back, over, and across it (adduction).
▶ Rotate the straight leg internally toward the midline, then externally away from the midline.

Exercising the ankle
▶ Bend the patient's foot so that the toes push upward (dorsiflexion) and then bend the foot so that the toes push downward (plantar flexion).
▶ Rotate the ankle in a circular motion.

▶ Invert the ankle so that the sole of the foot faces the midline and evert the ankle so that the sole faces away from the midline.

Exercising the toes
▶ Flex the patient's toes toward the sole and then extend them back toward the top of the foot.
▶ Spread two adjoining toes apart (abduction) and bring them together (adduction).

Special considerations
▶ Because joints begin to stiffen within 24 hours of disuse, start passive ROM exercises as soon as possible and perform them at least once a shift, particularly while bathing or turning the patient. Use proper body mechanics and repeat each exercise at least three times.
▶ Patients who experience prolonged bed rest or limited activity without profound weakness can also be taught to perform ROM exercises on their own (called active ROM), or they may benefit from isometric exercises. (See *Learning about isometric exercises,* pages 695 and 696.)
▶ If the disabled patient requires long-term rehabilitation after discharge, consult with a physical therapist and teach a family member or caregiver to perform passive ROM exercises.

Documentation

Record which joints were exercised, the presence of edema or pressure areas, any pain resulting from the exercises, any limitation of ROM, and the patient's tolerance of the exercises.

RECTAL SUPPOSITORY AND OINTMENT ADMINISTRATION

A rectal suppository is a small, solid, medicated mass, usually cone-shaped, with a cocoa butter or glycerin base. It may be inserted to stimulate peristalsis and defecation or to relieve pain, vomiting, and local irritation. Rectal suppositories commonly contain drugs that reduce fever, induce relaxation, interact poorly with digestive enzymes, or have a taste too offensive for oral use. Rectal suppositories melt at body temperature and are absorbed slowly.

Because insertion of a rectal suppository may stimulate the vagus nerve, this procedure is contraindicated in patients with potential cardiac arrhythmias. It may have to be avoided in patients with recent rectal or prostate surgery because of the risk of local trauma or discomfort during insertion.

An ointment is a semisolid medication used to produce local effects. It may be applied externally to the anus or internally to the rectum. Rectal ointments commonly contain drugs that reduce inflammation or relieve pain and itching.

Key nursing diagnoses and patient outcomes

Constipation related to (specify)
The patient will:

▶ have elimination pattern return to normal
▶ state an understanding of the causes of constipation
▶ move bowels every (specify) days without the use of suppositories.

Impaired tissue integrity related to (specify)
The patient will:
▶ express feelings of rectal comfort
▶ show symptoms of rectal tissue healing without evidence of infection.

Equipment

Rectal suppository or tube of ointment and applicator • patient's medication record and chart • gloves • water-soluble lubricant • 4″ × 4″ gauze pads • optional: bedpan

Preparation of equipment

Store rectal suppositories in the refrigerator until needed *to prevent softening and, possibly, decreased effectiveness of the medication.* A softened suppository is also difficult to handle and insert. To harden it again, hold the suppository (in its wrapper) under cold running water.

Implementation

▶ Verify the order on the patient's medication record by checking it against the doctor's order.
▶ Make sure the label on the medication package agrees with the medication order. Read the label again before you open the wrapper and again as you remove the medication. Check the expiration date.
▶ Wash your hands with warm soap and water.
▶ Confirm the patient's identity by asking his name and checking the name,

How to administer a rectal suppository or ointment

When inserting a suppository, direct its tapered end toward the side of the rectum so that it contacts the membranes (as shown below); doing so encourages absorption of the medication.

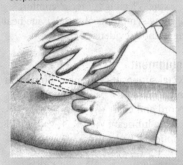

When applying a rectal ointment internally, lubricate the applicator to minimize pain on insertion (as shown below). Then direct the applicator tip toward the patient's umbilicus.

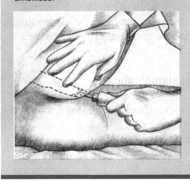

Inserting a rectal suppository

▶ Place the patient on his left side in Sims' position. Drape him with the bedcovers to expose only the buttocks.

▶ Put on gloves. Remove the suppository from its wrapper and lubricate it with water-soluble lubricant.

▶ Lift the patient's upper buttock with your nondominant hand *to expose the anus.*

▶ Instruct the patient to take several deep breaths through his mouth *to help relax the anal sphincters and reduce anxiety or discomfort during insertion.*

▶ Using the index finger of your dominant hand, insert the suppository — tapered end first — about 3″ (7.5 cm), until you feel it pass the internal anal sphincter. Try to direct the tapered end toward the side of the rectum so that it contacts the membranes. (See *How to administer a rectal suppository or ointment.*)

▶ Ensure the patient's comfort. Encourage him to lie quietly and, if applicable, retain the suppository for the appropriate length of time. A suppository administered to relieve constipation should be retained as long as possible (at least 20 minutes) to be effective. Press on the anus with a gauze pad, if necessary, until the urge to defecate passes.

▶ Remove and discard your gloves.

Applying rectal ointment

▶ Put on gloves.

▶ To apply externally, use gloves or a gauze pad to spread medication over the anal area.

▶ To apply internally, attach the applicator to the tube of ointment and coat the applicator with water-soluble lubricant.

▶ Expect to use about 1″ (2.5 cm) of ointment. *To gauge how much pressure to*

room number, and bed number on his wristband.

▶ Explain the procedure and the purpose of the medication to the patient.

▶ Provide privacy.

use during application, squeeze a small amount from the tube before you attach the applicator.

▶ Lift the patient's upper buttock with your nondominant hand *to expose the anus.*

▶ Instruct the patient to take several deep breaths through his mouth *to relax the anal sphincters and reduce anxiety or discomfort during insertion.*

▶ Gently insert the applicator, directing it toward the umbilicus.

▶ Slowly squeeze the tube *to eject the medication.*

▶ Remove the applicator and place a folded 4″ × 4″ gauze pad between the patient's buttocks *to absorb excess ointment.*

▶ Detach the applicator from the tube and recap the tube. Then clean the applicator thoroughly with soap and warm water.

Special considerations

▶ Because the intake of food and fluid stimulates peristalsis, a suppository for relieving constipation should be inserted about 30 minutes before mealtime *to help soften the feces in the rectum and facilitate defecation.* A medicated retention suppository should be inserted between meals.

▶ Instruct the patient to avoid expelling the suppository. If he has difficulty retaining it, place him on a bedpan.

▶ Make sure the patient's call button is handy and watch for his signal *because he may be unable to suppress the urge to defecate.* For example, a patient with proctitis has a highly sensitive rectum and may not be able to retain a suppository for long.

▶ Inform the patient that the suppository may discolor his next bowel movement. Anusol suppositories, for example, can give feces a silver-gray pasty appearance.

Documentation
Record the administration time, dose, and patient's response.

RECTAL TUBE INSERTION AND REMOVAL

Whether GI hypomotility simply slows the normal release of gas and feces or results in paralytic ileus, inserting a rectal tube may relieve the discomfort of distention and flatus. Decreased motility may result from various medical or surgical conditions, certain medications (such as atropine sulfate), or even swallowed air. Conditions that contraindicate using a rectal tube include recent rectal or prostatic surgery, recent myocardial infarction, and diseases of the rectal mucosa.

Key nursing diagnoses and patient outcomes
Acute pain or chronic pain related to abdominal distention
The patient will:
▶ have GI motility return to normal
▶ express feelings of comfort and relief from pain
▶ have abdominal distention reduced.

Deficient knowledge related to lack of exposure to rectal tube
The patient will:
▶ state an understanding of the need for a rectal tube
▶ state an understanding of what has been taught.

Equipment

Stethoscope • linen-saver pads • drape • water-soluble lubricant • commercial kit or #22 to #32 French rectal tube of soft rubber or plastic • container (such as an emesis basin, a plastic bag, or a water bottle with vent) • tape • gloves • linens

Implementation

▶ Bring all equipment to the patient's bedside, provide privacy, and wash your hands.

▶ Explain the procedure and encourage the patient to relax.

▶ Check for abdominal distention. Using the stethoscope, auscultate for bowel sounds.

▶ Place the linen-saver pads under the patient's buttocks *to absorb any drainage that may leak from the tube.*

▶ Position the patient in the left-lateral Sims' position *to facilitate rectal tube insertion.*

▶ Put on gloves.

▶ Drape the patient's exposed buttocks.

▶ Lubricate the rectal tube tip with water-soluble lubricant *to ease insertion and prevent rectal irritation.*

▶ Lift the patient's right buttock *to expose the anus.*

▶ Insert the rectal tube tip into the anus, advancing the tube 2″ to 4″ (5 to 10 cm) into the rectum. Direct the tube toward the umbilicus along the anatomic course of the large intestine.

▶ As you insert the tube, tell the patient to breathe slowly and deeply, or suggest that he bear down as he would for a bowel movement *to relax the anal sphincter and ease insertion.*

▶ Using tape, secure the rectal tube to the buttocks. Then attach the tube to

the container to collect possible leakage.

▶ Remove the tube after 15 to 20 minutes. If the patient reports continued discomfort or if gas wasn't expelled, you can repeat the procedure in 2 or 3 hours, if ordered.

▶ Clean the patient and replace soiled linens and the linen-saver pad. Make sure the patient feels as comfortable as possible. Again, check for abdominal distention and listen for bowel sounds.

▶ If you'll reuse the equipment, clean it and store it in the bedside cabinet; otherwise discard the tube.

Special considerations

▶ Inform the patient about each step and reassure him throughout the procedure *to encourage cooperation and promote relaxation.*

▶ Fastening a plastic bag (like a balloon) to the external end of the tube lets you observe gas expulsion. Leaving a rectal tube in place indefinitely does little to promote peristalsis, can reduce sphincter responsiveness, and may lead to permanent sphincter damage or pressure necrosis of the mucosa.

▶ Repeat insertion periodically *to stimulate GI activity.* If the tube fails to relieve distention, notify the doctor.

Documentation

Record the date and time that you insert the tube. Jot down the amount, color, and consistency of any evacuated matter. Describe the patient's abdomen: hard, distended, soft, or drumlike on percussion. Note bowel sounds before and after insertion.

Checklist of reportable diseases

Because reporting laws vary from state to state, this list isn't conclusive and may be changed periodically. Local agencies report certain diseases to their state health departments, which in turn determine which diseases are reported to the Centers for Disease Control and Prevention.

Acquired immunodeficiency syndrome
Anthrax
Botulism, foodborne
Botulism, infant
Botulism, unspecified
Botulism, wound
Brucellosis
Chancroid
Chlamydia trachomatis genital infections
Cholera
Coccidioidomycosis
Cryptosporidiosis
Diptheria
Encephalitis, arboviral (California, eastern equine, St. Louis, western equine, West Nile)
Escherichia coli O157:H7
Gonorrhea
Haemophilus influenzae (invasive disease)

Hansen's disease (leprosy)
Hantavirus pulmonary syndrome
Hemolytic uremic syndrome, post diarrheal
Hepatitis, viral, acute
Hepatitis, viral, perinatal hepatitis B virus infection
Human immunodeficiency virus infection, pediatric
Legionellosis
Lyme disease
Malaria
Measles
Meningococcal disease
Mumps
Neurosyphilis
Pertussis
Plague
Poliomyelitis, paralytic
Psittacosis
Rabies, animal
Rabies, human

Rocky Mountain spotted fever
Rubella
Rubella, congenital syndrome
Salmonellosis
Shigellosis
Streptococcal disease, invasive group A
Streptococcal toxic-shock syndrome
Streptococcus pneumoniae, drug-resistant invasive disease
Syphilis, all stages
Syphilis, congenital
Syphilis, primary and secondary
Syphilitic stillbirth
Tetanus
Toxic shock syndrome
Trichinosis
Tuberculosis
Typhoid fever
Yellow fever

REPORTABLE DISEASES SURVEILLANCE

Certain contagious diseases must be reported to local and state public health officials and, ultimately, to the Centers for Disease Control and Prevention. Typically, these diseases fit one of two categories: those reported individually based on a definitive or suspected diagnosis and those reported by the number of cases per week. The most commonly reported diseases include hepatitis, measles, salmonellosis, shigellosis, syphilis, and gonorrhea. (See *Checklist of reportable diseases* for an extensive listing.)

In most states, the patient's doctor must report communicable diseases to health officials. In hospitals, the infection control practitioner or epidemiologist reports them. However, you should know the reporting requirements and procedure. Fast, accurate reporting helps identify and control infection sources, prevent epidemics, and guide public health planning and policy.

Key nursing diagnoses and patient outcomes

Risk for infection related to external factors
The patient will:
▶ have temperature remain within normal limits
▶ have white blood cell count and differential stay within normal range
▶ have no pathogens in cultures.

Equipment

Nursing procedure or infection control manual • disease reporting form, if available

Implementation

▶ Make sure reportable diseases are listed and that the list is available to all shifts.
▶ Know your facility's protocol for reporting diseases. Typically, you'll contact the infection control practitioner or epidemiologist. If this person isn't available, contact your supervisor or the infectious disease doctor on call.

Documentation

Document any diseases reported to the infection control practitioner, the practitioner's name, and the date and time of the report.

Restraint application

Restraints are used only when other less restrictive measures have been found to be ineffective to protect the patient and others from harm. Various soft restraints limit movement to prevent the confused, disoriented, or combative patient from injuring himself or others. Vest and belt restraints, which are used to prevent falls from a bed or a chair, permit full movement of arms

and legs. Limb restraints, which are used to prevent removal of supportive equipment — such as I.V. lines, indwelling catheters, and nasogastric tubes — allow only slight limb motion. Like limb restraints, mitts prevent removal of supportive equipment, keep the patient from scratching rashes or sores, and prevent the combative patient from injuring himself or others. Body restraints, which are used to control the combative or hysterical patient, immobilize all or most of the body.

When soft restraints aren't sufficient and sedation is dangerous or ineffective, leather restraints can be used. Depending on the patient's behavior, leather restraints may be applied to all limbs (four-point restraints) or to one arm and one leg (two-point restraints). The duration of such restraint is governed by state law and by facility policy.

Restraints must be used cautiously in seizure-prone patients because they increase the risk of fracture and trauma. Restraints can cause skin irritation and restrict blood flow, so they shouldn't be applied directly over wounds or I.V. catheters. Vest restraints should be used with caution in patients who have heart failure or respiratory disorders. Such restraints can tighten with movement, further limiting circulation and respiratory function.

Key nursing diagnoses and patient outcomes

Risk for injury related to neural disorders
The patient will:
▶ identify factors that increase the potential for injury
▶ assist in identifying and applying safety measures to prevent injury
▶ perform activities of daily living optimally, within sensorimotor limitations.

Impaired memory related to (specify)
The patient will:
▶ remain free from injury
▶ have family members or other care-givers contact appropriate resources as needed.

Equipment
For soft restraints
Restraint (such as a vest, limb, mitt, belt, or body as needed) • gauze pads, if needed

For leather restraints
Two wrist and two ankle leather re-straints • four straps • key • large gauze pads to cushion each extremity

Preparation of equipment
Before entering the patient's room, make sure the restraints are the correct size, using the patient's build and weight as a guide. If you use leather re-straints, make sure that the straps are unlocked and the key fits the locks.

 Age alert For children, who typically are too small for standard restraints, use a child restraint. (See *Types of child re-straints,* page 704.)

Implementation
▶ Obtain a doctor's order for the re-straint. Keep in mind that the doctor's order must be time limited — 4 hours for adults, 2 hours for children and ado-lescents ages 9 to 17, and 1 hour for pa-tients under age 9. The original order may only be renewed for a total of 24 hours. After the original order expires, the doctor must see and evaluate the pa-tient before a new order can be written.
▶ If necessary, obtain adequate assis-tance to restrain the patient before en-tering his room. Enlist the aid of several

coworkers and organize their effort, giving each person a specific task; for example, one person explains the pro-cedure to the patient and applies the restraints while the others immobilize the patient's arms and legs.
▶ Tell the patient what you're about to do and describe the restraints to him. Assure him that they're being used to protect him from injury rather than to punish him.

Applying a vest restraint
▶ Assist the patient to a sitting posi-tion, if his condition permits. Then slip the vest over his gown. Crisscross the cloth flaps at the front, placing the V-shaped opening at the patient's throat. Never crisscross the flaps in the back *because this may cause the patient to choke if he tries to squirm out of the vest.*
▶ Pass the tab on one flap through the slot on the opposite flap. Then adjust the vest for the patient's comfort. You should be able to slip your fist between the vest and the patient. Avoid wrap-ping the vest too tightly *because it may restrict respiration.*
▶ Tie all restraints securely to the frame of the bed, chair, or wheelchair and out of the patient's reach. Use a bow or a knot that can be released quickly and easily in an emergency. (See *Knots for securing soft restraints,* page 705.) Never tie a regular knot to secure the straps. Leave 1″ to 2″ (2.5 to 5 cm) of slack in the straps *to allow room for movement.*
▶ After applying the vest, check the patient's respiratory rate and breath sounds regularly. Be alert for signs of respiratory distress. Also, make sure the vest hasn't tightened with the patient's movement. Loosen the vest frequently,

Types of child restraints

You may need to restrain an infant or a child to prevent injury or to facilitate examination, diagnostic tests, or treatment. If so, take the following steps:

- Provide a simple explanation, reassurance, and constant observation to minimize the child's fear.
- Explain the restraint to the parents and enlist their help.
- Reassure them that it won't hurt the child.

- Make sure restraint ties or safety pins are secured outside the child's reach to prevent injury.
- When using a mummy restraint, secure the infant's arms in proper alignment with the body to avoid dislocation and other injuries.

Vest

Elbow

Mummy

Belt

Limb

Crib with net

Mitt

Restraining board

if possible, *so the patient can stretch, turn, and breathe deeply.*

Applying a limb restraint

▶ Wrap the patient's wrist or ankle with gauze pads *to reduce friction between the patient's skin and the restraint, helping to prevent irritation and skin breakdown.* Then wrap the restraint around the gauze pads.

▶ Pass the strap on the narrow end of the restraint through the slot in the broad end and adjust for a snug fit. Or fasten the buckle or Velcro cuffs to fit the restraint. You should be able to slip one or two fingers between the restraint and the patient's skin. Avoid applying the restraint too tightly *because it may impair circulation distal to the restraint.*

▶ Tie the restraint as above.

▶ After applying limb restraints, be alert for signs of impaired circulation in the extremity distal to the restraint. If the skin appears blue or feels cold, or if the patient complains of a tingling sensation or numbness, loosen the restraint. Perform range-of-motion (ROM) exercises regularly *to stimulate circulation and prevent contractures and resultant loss of mobility.*

Applying a mitt restraint

▶ Wash and dry the patient's hands.

▶ Roll up a washcloth or gauze pad and place it in the patient's palm. Have him form a loose fist, if possible; then pull the mitt over it and secure the closure.

▶ *To restrict the patient's arm movement,* attach the strap to the mitt and tie it securely, using a bow or a knot that can be released quickly and easily in an emergency.

▶ When using mitts made of transparent mesh, check hand movement and

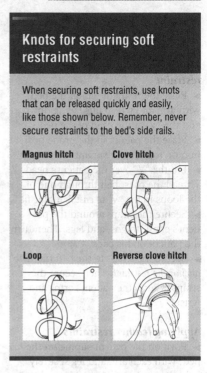

Knots for securing soft restraints

When securing soft restraints, use knots that can be released quickly and easily, like those shown below. Remember, never secure restraints to the bed's side rails.

Magnus hitch

Clove hitch

Loop

Reverse clove hitch

skin color frequently *to assess circulation.* Remove the mitts regularly *to stimulate circulation,* and perform passive ROM exercises *to prevent contractures.*

Applying a belt restraint

▶ Center the flannel pad of the belt on the bed. Then wrap the short strap of the belt around the bed frame and fasten it under the bed.

▶ Position the patient on the pad. Then have him roll slightly to one side while you guide the long strap around his waist and through the slot in the pad.

▶ Wrap the long strap around the bed frame and fasten it under the bed.

▶ After applying the belt, slip your hand between the patient and the belt *to ensure a secure but comfortable fit. A loose belt can be raised to chest level; a tight one can cause abdominal discomfort.*

Applying a body (Posey net) restraint

▶ Place the restraint flat on the bed, with arm and wrist cuffs facing down and the "V" at the head of the bed.

▶ Place the patient in the prone position on top of the restraint.

▶ Lift the "V" over the patient's head. Thread the chest belt through one of the loops in the "V" *to ensure a snug fit.*

▶ Secure the straps around the patient's chest, thighs, and legs. Then turn the patient on his back.

▶ Secure the straps to the bed frame *to anchor the restraint.* Then secure the straps around the patient's arms and wrists.

Applying leather restraints

▶ Position the patient supine on the bed, with each arm and leg securely held down *to minimize combative behavior and to prevent injury to the patient and others.* Immobilize the patient's arms and legs at the joints—knee, ankle, shoulder, and wrist—*to minimize his movement without exerting excessive force.*

▶ Apply pads to the patient's wrists and ankles *to reduce friction between his skin and the leather, preventing skin irritation and breakdown.*

▶ Wrap the restraint around the gauze pads. Then insert the metal loop through the hole that gives the best fit. Apply the restraints securely but not too tightly. You should be able to slip one or two fingers between the restraint and the patient's skin. *A tight restraint can compromise circulation; a loose one can slip off or move up the patient's arm or leg, causing skin irritation and breakdown.*

▶ Thread the strap through the metal loop on the restraint, close the metal loop, and secure the strap to the bed frame, out of the patient's reach.

▶ Lock the restraint by pushing in the button on the side of the metal loop and tug it gently to make sure it's secure. Once the restraint is secure, a coworker can release the arm or leg. Flex the patient's arm or leg slightly before locking the strap *to allow room for movement and to prevent frozen joints and dislocations.*

▶ Place the key in an accessible location at the nurse's station.

▶ After applying leather restraints, observe the patient regularly *to give emotional support and to reassess the need for continued use of the restraint.* Check his pulse rate and vital signs at least every 2 hours. Remove or loosen the restraints one at a time, every 2 hours, and perform passive ROM exercises, if possible. Watch for signs of impaired peripheral circulation such as cool, cyanotic skin. To unlock the restraint, insert the key into the metal loop, opposite the locking button. This releases the lock, and the metal loop can be opened.

Special considerations

▶ Some facilities may require that a consent form be signed by the family indicating that they agree to the application of restraints, if they're absolutely necessary.

▶ When the patient is at high risk for aspiration, restrain him on his side. Never secure all four restraints to one side of the bed *because the patient may fall out of bed.*

▶ When loosening restraints, have a coworker on hand to assist in restraining the patient, if necessary.

▶ After assessing the patient's behavior and condition, you may decide to use a two-point restraint, which should restrain one arm and the opposite leg—for example, the right arm and the left leg. Never restrain the arm and leg on the same side *because the patient may fall out of bed.*

▶ Don't apply a limb restraint above an I.V. site because the constriction may occlude the infusion or cause infiltration into surrounding tissue.

▶ Never secure restraints to the side rails *because someone might inadvertently lower the rail before noticing the attached restraint. This may jerk the patient's limb or body, causing him discomfort and trauma.* Never secure restraints to the fixed frame of the bed if the patient's position is to be changed.

▶ Don't restrain a patient in the prone position. This position limits his field of vision, intensifies feelings of helplessness and vulnerability, and impairs respiration, especially if the patient has been sedated.

▶ Because the restrained patient has limited mobility, his nutrition, elimination, and positioning become your responsibility. To prevent pressure ulcers, reposition the patient regularly and massage and pad bony prominences and other vulnerable areas.

▶ Continually monitor, assess, and evaluate the condition of the restrained patient. Document restraint use hourly on a Restraint Flow Sheet. Release the restraints every 2 hours; assess the patient's pulse and skin condition, and perform ROM exercises..

Complications

Excessively tight limb restraints can reduce peripheral circulation; tight vest restraints can impair respiration. Apply restraints carefully and check them regularly.

Skin breakdown can also occur under limb restraints. To prevent this, pad the patient's wrists and ankles, loosen or remove the restraints frequently, and provide regular skin care.

Long periods of immobility can predispose the patient to pneumonia, urine retention, constipation, and sensory deprivation. Reposition the patient and attend to his elimination requirements as needed.

Some patients resist restraints by biting, kicking, scratching, or head butting, in the course of which they may injure themselves or others.

Documentation

Record the behavior that necessitated restraints, when the restraints were applied and removed, and the type of restraints used.

Record vital signs, skin condition, respiratory status, peripheral circulation, and mental status.

Rotation bed use

Because of their constant motion, rotation beds—such as the Roto Rest—promote postural drainage and peristalsis and help prevent the complications of immobility. The bed rotates from side to side in a cradlelike motion, achieving a maximum elevation of 62 degrees and full side-to-side turning approximately every 4½ minutes.

Because the bed holds the patient motionless, it's especially helpful for patients with spinal cord injury, multiple trauma, cerebrovascular accident, multiple sclerosis, coma, severe burns, hypostatic pneumonia, and atelectasis or

Understanding the Roto Rest bed

Driven by a silent motor, this bed turns the immobilized patient slowly and continuously, more than 300 times daily. The motion provides constant passive exercise and peristaltic stimulation without depriving the patient of sleep or risking further injury. The bed is radiolucent, permitting X-rays to be taken through it without moving the patient. It also has a built-in cooling fan and allows access for surgery on multiple-trauma patients without disrupting spinal alignment or traction.

The bed's hatches provide access to various parts of the patient's body. Arm hatches permit full range of motion and have holes for chest tubes. Leg hatches allow full hip extension. The perineal hatch provides access for bowel and bladder care, the thoracic hatch for chest auscultation and lumbar puncture, and the cervical hatch for wound care, bathing, and shampooing.

Top view

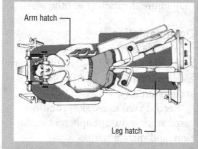

Back view

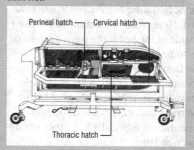

other unilateral lung involvement causing poor ventilation and perfusion.

Rotation beds, such as the Roto Rest bed, can accommodate cervical traction devices and tongs. One type of Roto Rest bed has an access hatch underneath for the perineal area; another type has access hatches for the perineal, cervical, and thoracic areas. Both have arm and leg hatches that fold down to allow range-of-motion exercises. Other features include variable angles of rotation, a fan, access for X-rays, and supports and clips for chest tubes, catheters, and drains. Racks beneath the bed hold X-ray plates in place for chest

and spinal films. (See *Understanding the Roto Rest bed*.)

Rotation beds are contraindicated for the patient who has severe claustrophobia or who has an unstable cervical fracture without neurologic deficit and the complications of immobility. Patient transfer and positioning on the bed should be performed by at least two persons to ensure the patient's safety.

The instructions given below apply to the Roto Rest bed.

Key nursing diagnoses and patient outcomes

Impaired physical mobility related to neuromuscular impairment

The patient will:
▶ show no evidence of complications, such as contractures, venous stasis, thrombus formation, or skin breakdown
▶ have mobility regimen carried out by caregiver.

Risk for disuse syndrome related to prolonged inactivity
The patient will:
▶ display no evidence of altered mental, sensory, or motor activity
▶ maintain muscle strength and tone and range of motion
▶ maintain normal neurologic, cardiovascular, respiratory, musculoskeletal, GI, and integumentary function during periods of inactivity.

Equipment
Rotation bed with appropriate accessories • pillowcases or linen-saver pads • flat sheet or padding

Preparation of equipment
When using the Roto Rest bed, carefully inspect the bed and run it through a complete cycle in both automatic and manual modes *to ensure that it's working properly.* If you're using the Mark I model, check the tightness of the set screws at the head of the bed.

To prepare the bed for the patient, remove the counterbalance weights from the keel and place them in the base frame's storage area. Release the connecting arm by pulling down on the cam handle and depressing the lower side of the footboard. Next, lock the table in the horizontal position and place all side supports in the extreme lateral position by loosening the cam handles on the underside of the table. Slide the supports off the bed. Note

that all supports and packs are labeled RIGHT or LEFT on the bottom *to facilitate reassembly.*

Remove the knee packs by depressing the snap button and rotating and pulling the packs from the tube. Then remove the abductor packs (the Mark III model has only one) by depressing and sliding them toward the head of the bed. Next, loosen the foot and knee assemblies by lifting the cam handle at its base and slide them to the foot of the bed. Finally, loosen the shoulder clamp assembly and knobs; swing the shoulder clamps to the vertical position and retighten them.

If you're using the Mark I model, remove the cervical, thoracic, and perineal packs. Cover them with pillowcases or linen-saver pads, smooth all wrinkles, and replace the packs. If you're using the Mark III model, remove the perineal pack, cover the pack, and replace it. Cover the upper half of the bed, which is a solid unit, with padding or a sheet. Install new disposable foam cushions for the patient's head, shoulders, and feet.

Implementation
▶ If possible, show the patient the bed before use. Explain and demonstrate its operation and reassure the patient that the bed will hold him securely.
▶ Before positioning the patient on the bed, make sure it's turned off. Then place and lock the bed in horizontal position, out of gear. Latch all hatches and lock the wheels.
▶ Obtain assistance and transfer the patient. Move him gently to the center of the bed to prevent contact with the pillar posts and to ensure proper balance during bed operation. Smooth the pillowcase or linen-saver pad beneath

his hips. Then place any tubes through the appropriate notches in the hatches and ensure that any traction weights hang freely.

▶ Insert the thoracic side supports in their posts. Adjust the patient's longitudinal position to allow a 1″ (2.5 cm) space between the axillae and the supports, *thereby avoiding pressure on the axillary blood vessels and the brachial plexus.* Push the supports against his chest and lock the cam arms securely *to provide support and ensure patient safety.*

▶ Place the disposable supports under his legs *to remove pressure from his heels and prevent pressure ulcers.*

▶ Install and adjust the foot supports so that the patient's feet lie in the normal anatomic position, *thereby helping to prevent footdrop.* The foot supports should be in position for only 2 hours of every shift *to prevent excessive pressure on the soles and toes.*

▶ Place the abductor packs in the appropriate supports, allowing a 6″ (15.2 cm) space between the packs and the patient's groin. Tighten the knobs on the bed's underside at the base of the support tubes.

▶ Install the leg side supports snugly against the patient's hips and tighten the cam arms. Position the knee assemblies slightly above his knees and tighten the cam arms. Then place your hand on the patient's knee and move the knee pack until it rests lightly on the top of your hand. Repeat for the other knee.

▶ Loosen the retaining rings on the crossbar and slide the head and shoulder assembly laterally. *The retaining rings maintain correct lateral position of the shoulder clamp assembly and head support pack.*

▶ Carefully lower the head and shoulder assembly into place and slide it to touch the patient's head.

▶ Place your hand on the patient's shoulder and move the shoulder pack until it touches your hand. Tighten it in place. Repeat for the other shoulder. *The 1″ clearance between the shoulders and the packs prevents excess pressure, which can lead to pressure ulcers.*

▶ Place the head pack close to, but not touching, the patient's ears or tongs.

▶ Tighten the head and shoulder assembly securely *so it won't lift off the bed.* Position the restraining rings next to the shoulder assembly bracket and tighten them.

▶ Place the patient's arms on the disposable supports. Install the side arm supports and secure the safety straps, placing one across the shoulder assembly and the other over the thoracic supports. If necessary, cover the patient with a flat sheet.

Balancing the bed

▶ Place one hand on the footboard *to prevent the bed from turning rapidly if it's unbalanced.* Then remove the locking pin. If the bed rotates to one side, reposition the patient in its center; if it tilts to the right, gently turn it slightly to the left and slide the packs on the right side toward the patient; if it tilts to the left, reverse the process. If a large imbalance exists, you may have to adjust the packs on both sides.

▶ After the patient is centered, gently turn the bed to the 62-degree position.

▶ Measure the space between the patient's chest, hip, and thighs and the inside of the packs. If this space exceeds ½″ (1.3 cm) for the Mark III model or 1″ for the Mark I, return the bed to the horizontal position, lock it in place, and slide the packs inward on both sides. If the space appears too tight, proceed as above but slide both packs outward. *Excessively loose packs cause the patient to slide from side to side during turning, possibly resulting in unnecessary movement at fracture sites, skin irritation from shearing force, and bed imbalance. Overly tight packs can place pressure on the patient during turning.*

▶ After adjusting the packs, check the bed; balance it and make any necessary adjustments.

▶ If you're using the Mark III model bed and the patient weighs more than 160 lb (72.6 kg), the bed may become top-heavy. To correct this, place counterbalance weights in the appropriate slots in the keel of the bed. Add one weight for every 20 lb (9.1 kg) over 160 lb, but remember that placement of weights doesn't replace correct patient positioning.

▶ If you're using the Mark I model, it may be necessary to add weights for the patient weighing less than 160 lb. Place one weight for each 20 lb less than 160 lb in the proper bracket at the foot of the bed.

Initiating automatic bed rotation

▶ Ensure that all packs are securely in place. Then hold the footboard firmly and remove the locking pin *to start the bed's motor*. The bed will continue to rotate until the pin is reinserted.

▶ Raise the connecting arm cam handle until the connecting assembly snaps into place, locking the bed into automatic rotation.

▶ Remain with the patient for at least three complete turns from side to side *to evaluate his comfort and safety*. Observe his response and offer him emotional support.

Special considerations

▶ If the patient develops cardiac arrest while on the bed, perform cardiopulmonary resuscitation after taking the bed out of gear, locking it in the horizontal position, removing the side arm support and the thoracic pack, lifting the shoulder assembly, and dropping the arm pack. Doing all these steps takes only 5 to 10 seconds. You won't need a cardiac board because of the bed's firm surface.

▶ If the electricity fails, lock the bed in the horizontal or lateral position and rotate it manually every 30 minutes *to prevent pressure ulcers*. If cervical traction causes the patient to slide upward, place the bed in reverse Trendelenburg's position; if extremity traction causes the patient to migrate toward the foot of the bed, use Trendelenburg's position.

▶ Lock the bed in the extreme lateral position for access to the back of the head, thorax, and buttocks through the appropriate hatches. Clean the mattress and nondisposable packs during patient care and rinse them thoroughly *to remove all soap residue*. When replacing the packs and hatches, take care not to pinch the patient's skin between the packs. *This can cause pain and tissue necrosis.*

▶ Expect increased drainage from any pressure ulcers for the first few days the patient is on the bed *because the motion helps debride necrotic tissue and improves local circulation.*

▶ Perform or schedule daily range-of-motion exercises as ordered *because the bed allows full access to all extremities without disturbing spinal alignment.* Drop the arm hatch for shoulder rotation, remove the thoracic packs for shoulder abduction, and drop the leg hatch and remove leg and knee packs for hip rotation and full leg motion.

▶ For female patients, tape an indwelling urinary catheter to the thigh before bringing it through the perineal hatch. For the male patient with spinal cord lesions, tape the catheter to the abdomen and then to the thigh *to facilitate gravity drainage.* Hang the drainage bag on the clips provided and make sure it doesn't become caught between the bed frames during rotation.

▶ If the patient has a tracheal or endotracheal tube and is on mechanical ventilation, attach the tube support bracket between the cervical pack and the arm packs. Tape the connecting T tubing to the support and run it beside the patient's head and off the center of the table *to help prevent reflux of condensation.*

▶ For a patient with pulmonary congestion or pneumonia, suction secretions more often during the first 12 to 24 hours on the bed *because the motion will increase drainage.* A vibrator is available for use under the thoracic hatch of the Mark I to help mobilize pulmonary secretions more quickly.

Documentation

Record changes in the patient's condition and his response to therapy in your progress notes. Note turning times and ongoing care on the flowchart.

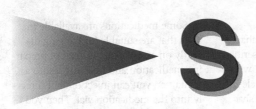

SECONDARY I.V. LINE USE

A secondary I.V. line is a complete I.V. set — container, tubing, and microdrip or macrodrip system — connected to the lower Y-port (secondary port) of a primary line instead of to the I.V. catheter or needle. It can be used for continuous or intermittent drug infusion. When used continuously, a secondary I.V. line permits drug infusion and titration while the primary line maintains a constant total infusion rate.

When used intermittently, a secondary I.V. line is commonly called a piggyback set. In this case, the primary line maintains venous access between drug doses. Typically, a piggyback set includes a small I.V. container, short tubing, and a macrodrip system. This set connects to the primary line's upper Y-port, also called a piggyback port. Antibiotics are most commonly administered by intermittent (piggyback) infusion. To make this set work, the primary I.V. container must be positioned below the piggyback container. (The manufacturer provides an extension hook for this purpose.)

Most drugs can be piggybacked with a needle-free system, which consists of a blunt-tipped plastic insertion device and a rubber injection port. The port may be part of a special administration set or an adapter for existing administration sets. The rubber injection port has a preestablished slit that can open and reseal immediately. The needle-free system aims to reduce the risk of accidental needle-stick injuries.

I.V. pumps may be used to maintain constant infusion rates, especially with a drug such as lidocaine. A pump allows more accurate titration of drug dosage and helps maintain venous access because the drug is delivered under sufficient pressure to prevent clot formation in the I.V. cannula.

Key nursing diagnoses and patient outcomes

Deficient knowledge related to lack of exposure to secondary I.V. line use
The patient will:
▶ state or demonstrate an understanding of what has been taught
▶ demonstrate the ability to perform new health-related behaviors as taught.

Risk for injury related to improper technique
The patient will:
▶ identify factors that increase risk of injury
▶ assist in identifying and applying safety measures to prevent injury.

Equipment

Patient's medication record and chart • prescribed I.V. medication • prescribed I.V. solution • administration set with secondary injection port • needleless adapter • alcohol pads • 1″ adhesive tape • time tape • labels • infusion pump • extension hook and appropriate solution for intermittent piggyback infusion • optional: normal saline solution for infusion with incompatible solutions

For intermittent infusion, the primary line typically has a piggyback port with a backcheck valve that stops the flow from the primary line during drug infusion and returns to the primary flow after infusion. A volume-control set can also be used with an intermittent infusion line.

Preparation of equipment

Verify the order on the patient's medication record by checking it against the doctor's order. Wash your hands. Inspect the I.V. container for cracks, leaks, and contamination, and check drug compatibility with the primary solution. Verify the expiration date. Check to see whether the primary line has a secondary injection port. If it doesn't and the medication is to be given regularly, replace the I.V. set with one that has a secondary injection port.

If necessary, add the drug to the secondary I.V. solution. To do so, remove any seals from the secondary container and wipe the main port with an alcohol pad. Inject the prescribed medication and gently agitate the solution to mix the medication thoroughly. Properly label the I.V. mixture. Insert the administration set spike and attach the needle. Open the flow clamp and prime the line. Then close the flow clamp.

Some medications are available in vials that are suitable for hanging directly on an I.V. pole. Instead of preparing medication and injecting it into a container, you can inject diluent directly into the medication vial. Then you can spike the vial, prime the tubing, and hang the set as directed.

Implementation

▶ Confirm the patient's identity by asking his name and checking the name, room number, and bed number on his wristband.

▶ If the drug is incompatible with the primary I.V. solution, replace the primary solution with a fluid that is compatible with both solutions, such as normal saline solution, and flush the line before starting the drug infusion. Many facility protocols require that the primary I.V. solution be removed and that a sterile I.V. plug be inserted into the container until it's ready to be rehung. *This maintains the sterility of the solution and prevents someone else from inadvertently restarting the incompatible solution before the line is flushed with normal saline solution.*

▶ Hang the secondary set's container and wipe the injection port of the primary line with an alcohol pad.

▶ Insert the needleless adapter from the secondary line into the injection port and secure it to the primary line.

▶ To run the secondary set's container by itself, lower the primary set's container with an extension hook. To run both containers simultaneously, place them at the same height. (See *Assembling a piggyback set.*)

▶ Open the clamp and adjust the drip rate. For continuous infusion, set the secondary solution to the desired drip rate; then adjust the primary solution *to achieve the desired total infusion rate.*

▶ For intermittent infusion, adjust the primary drip rate as required on completion of the secondary solution. If the secondary solution tubing is being reused, close the clamp on the tubing and follow your facility's policy: Either remove the needleless adapter and replace it with a new one or leave it securely taped in the injection port and label it with the time it was first used. Also, in this case, leave the empty container in place until you replace it with a new dose of medication at the prescribed time. If the tubing won't be reused, discard it appropriately with the I.V. container.

Special considerations

▶ If policy allows, use a pump for drug infusion. Put a time tape on the secondary container *to help prevent an inaccurate administration rate.*

▶ When reusing secondary tubing, change it according to your facility's policy, usually every 48 to 72 hours. Similarly, inspect the injection port for leakage with each use and change it more often, if needed.

▶ Unless you're piggybacking lipids, don't piggyback a secondary I.V. line to a total parenteral nutrition line *because of the risk of contamination.* Check your facility's policy for possible exceptions.

Complications

The patient may experience an adverse reaction to the infused drug. In addition, repeated punctures of the secondary injection port can damage the seal, possibly allowing leakage or contamination.

Assembling a piggyback set

A piggyback set is useful for intermittent drug infusion. To work properly, the secondary set's container must be positioned higher than the primary set's container.

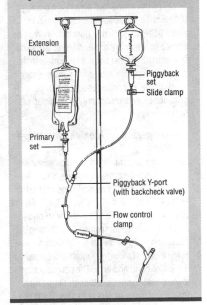

Extension hook

Piggyback set

Slide clamp

Primary set

Piggyback Y-port (with backcheck valve)

Flow control clamp

Documentation

Record the amount and type of drug and the amount of I.V. solution on the intake and output and medication records. Note the date, duration and rate of infusion, and patient's response, where applicable.

SEIZURE MANAGEMENT

Seizures are paroxysmal events associated with abnormal electrical discharges of neurons in the brain. Partial seizures are usually unilateral, involving a localized or focal area of the

Differentiating among seizure types

The hallmark of epilepsy is recurring seizures, which can be classified as partial or generalized. Some patients may be affected by more than one type.

Partial seizures

Arising from a localized area in the brain, partial seizures cause specific symptoms. In some patients, partial seizure activity may be spread to the entire brain, causing a generalized seizure. Partial seizures include simple partial (jacksonian motor-type and sensory type), complex partial (psychomotor or temporal lobe), and secondarily generalized partial seizures.

Simple partial jacksonian motor-type seizure

The simple jacksonian motor-type seizure begins as a localized motor seizure, which is characterized by a spread of abnormal activity to adjacent areas of the brain. Typically, the patient experiences a stiffening or jerking in one extremity, accompanied by a tingling sensation in the same area. For example, the seizure may start in the thumb and spread to the entire hand and arm. The patient seldom loses consciousness, although the seizure may secondarily progress to a generalized tonic-clonic seizure.

Simple partial sensory-type seizure

Perception is distorted in the simple partial sensory-type seizure. Symptoms can include hallucinations, flashing lights, tingling sensations, vertigo, or déjà vu (the feeling of having experienced something before).

Complex partial seizure

Symptoms of the complex partial seizure are variable but usually include purposeless behavior. The patient may experience an aura and exhibit overt signs, including a glassy stare, picking at his clothes, aimless wandering, lip smacking or chewing motions, and unintelligible speech. The seizure may last for a few seconds or as long as 20 minutes. Afterward, mental confusion may last for several minutes; as a result, an observer may mistakenly suspect psychosis or intoxication with alcohol or drugs. The patient has no memory of his actions during the seizure.

Secondarily generalized partial seizure

The secondarily generalized partial seizure can be either simple or complex and can progress to a generalized seizure. An aura may precede the progression. Loss of consciousness occurs immediately or within 1 to 2 minutes of the start of the progression.

Generalized seizures

As the term suggests, generalized seizures cause a general electrical abnormality within the brain. They include several distinct types.

Absence (petit mal) seizure

The absence seizure occurs most commonly in children, but it also may affect adults. It usually begins with a brief change in the level of consciousness, indicated by blinking or rolling of the eyes, or a blank stare, and slight mouth movements. The patient retains his posture and continues preseizure activity without difficulty. Typically, the seizure lasts 1 to 10 seconds. The impairment is so brief that the patient is sometimes unaware of it. If not properly treated, these seizures can recur as often as 100 times a day. An absence seizure may progress to a generalized tonic-clonic seizure.

Myoclonic seizure

Also called bilateral massive epileptic monoclonus, the myoclonic seizure is marked by brief, involuntary muscular jerks of the body or extremities, which may occur in a rhythmic manner, and a brief loss of consciousness.

Differentiating among seizure types *(continued)*

Generalized tonic-clonic (grand mal) seizure

Typically, the generalized tonic-clonic seizure begins with a loud cry, precipitated by air rushing from the lungs through the vocal cords. The patient falls to the ground, losing consciousness. The body stiffens (tonic phase) and then alternates between episodes of muscle spasm and relaxation (clonic phase). Tongue biting, incontinence, labored breathing, apnea, and subsequent cyanosis may also occur. The seizure stops in 2 to 5 minutes, after abnormal electrical conduction of the neurons is completed. The patient then regains consciousness but is somewhat confused and may have difficulty talking. If he can talk, he may complain of drowsiness, fatigue, headache, muscle soreness, and arm or leg weakness. He may fall into a deep sleep after the seizure.

Akinetic seizure

Characterized by a general loss of postural tone and a temporary loss of consciousness, the akinetic seizure occurs in young children. It's sometimes called a "drop attack" because it causes the child to fall.

brain. Generalized seizures involve the entire brain. (See *Differentiating among seizure types.*) When a patient has a generalized seizure, nursing care aims to protect him from injury and prevent serious complications. Appropriate care also includes observation of seizure characteristics to help determine the area of the brain involved.

Patients considered at risk for seizures are those with a history of seizures and those with conditions that predispose them to seizures. These conditions include metabolic abnormalities, such as hypocalcemia, hypoglycemia, and pyridoxine deficiency; brain tumors or other space-occupying lesions; infections, such as meningitis, encephalitis, and brain abscess; traumatic injury, especially if the dura mater was penetrated; ingestion of toxins, such as mercury, lead, or carbon monoxide; genetic abnormalities, such as tuberous sclerosis and phenylketonuria; perinatal injuries; and cerebrovascular accident. Patients at risk for seizures need precautionary measures to help prevent injury if a seizure occurs. (See *Precautions for generalized seizures,* page 718.)

Key nursing diagnoses and patient outcomes

Risk for injury related to external factors
The patient will:
▶ remain free from injury
▶ identify and eliminate safety hazards in environment
▶ describe safety measures.

Ineffective airway clearance related to presence of tracheobronchial obstruction or secretions
The patient will:
▶ expectorate sputum
▶ reveal no crackles, rhonchi, wheezes or stridor during auscultation of lung fields
▶ have no abnormality on chest X-ray.

Equipment

Oral airway • suction equipment • side rail pads • seizure activity record • additional equipment: I.V., normal saline

Precautions for generalized seizures

By taking appropriate precautions, you can help protect a patient from injury, aspiration, and airway obstruction should he have a seizure. Plan your precautions using information obtained from the patient's history. What kind of seizure has the patient previously had? Is he aware of exacerbating factors? Sleep deprivation, missed doses of anticonvulsants, and even upper respiratory infections can increase seizure frequency in some people who have had seizures. Was his previous seizure an acute episode, or did it result from a chronic condition?

Gather the equipment

Based on answers provided in the patient's history, you can tailor your precautions to his needs. Start by gathering the appropriate equipment, including a hospital bed with full-length side rails, commercial side rail pads or six bath blankets (four for a crib), adhesive tape, an oral airway, and oral or nasal suction equipment.

Bedside preparations

Now carry out the precautions you think appropriate for the patient. Remember that a patient with preexisting seizures who is being admitted for a change in medication, treatment for an infection, or detoxification may have an increased risk of seizures.

■ Explain the reasons for the precautions to the patient.

■ *To protect the patient's limbs, head, and feet from injury if he has a seizure while in bed,* cover the side rails, headboard, and footboard with side rail pads or bath blankets. If you use blankets, keep them in place with adhesive tape. Keep the side rails raised while the patient is in bed *to prevent falls.* Keep the bed in a low position *to minimize any injuries that may occur if the patient climbs over the rails.*

■ Place an airway at the patient's bedside, or tape it to the wall above the bed according to your facility's protocol. Keep suction equipment nearby in case you need to establish a patent airway. Explain to the patient how the airway will be used.

■ If the patient has frequent or prolonged seizures, prepare an I.V. heparin lock *to facilitate administration of emergency medications.*

solution, oxygen, and endotracheal intubation equipment

Implementation

▶ If you're with a patient when he experiences an aura, help him into bed, raise the side rails, and adjust the bed flat. If he's away from his room, lower him to the floor and place a pillow, blanket, or other soft material under his head *to keep it from hitting the floor.*

▶ Stay with the patient during the seizure and be ready to intervene if complications such as airway obstruc-

tion develop. If necessary, have another staff member obtain the appropriate equipment and notify the doctor of the obstruction.

▶ Provide privacy, if possible.

▶ Depending on your facility's policy, if the patient is in the beginning of the tonic phase of the seizure, you may insert an oral airway into his mouth *so that his tongue doesn't block his airway.* If an oral airway isn't available, don't try to hold his mouth open or place your hands inside *because you may be bitten.* After the patient's jaw becomes rigid, don't force the airway into place *because you could break his teeth or cause another injury.* Some clinicians advocate waiting until the seizure subsides before inserting the airway.

▶ Move hard or sharp objects out of the patient's way and loosen his clothing.

▶ Don't forcibly restrain the patient or restrict his movements during the seizure *because the force of the patient's movements against restraints could cause muscle strain or even joint dislocation.*

▶ Continually assess the patient during the seizure. Observe the earliest symptom, such as head or eye deviation, as well as how the seizure progresses, what form it takes, and how long it lasts. *Your description may help determine the seizure's type and cause.*

▶ If this is the patient's first seizure, notify the doctor immediately. If the patient has had seizures before, notify the doctor only if the seizure activity is prolonged or if the patient fails to regain consciousness. (See *Understanding status epilepticus.*)

▶ If ordered, establish an I.V. line and infuse normal saline solution at a keep-vein-open rate.

▶ If the seizure is prolonged and the patient becomes hypoxemic, administer oxygen as ordered. Some patients may require endotracheal intubation.

▶ For a patient known to be diabetic, administer 50 ml of dextrose 50% in water by I.V. push as ordered. For a patient known to be an alcoholic, a 100-mg bolus of thiamine may be ordered to stop the seizure.

▶ After the seizure, turn the patient on his side and apply suction, if necessary, *to facilitate drainage of secretions and maintain a patent airway.* Insert an oral airway, if needed.

Understanding status epilepticus

A continuous seizures state unless interrupted by emergency interventions, status epilepticus can occur in all seizure types. The most life-threatening example is generalized tonic-clonic status epilepticus, which is a continuous generalized tonic-clonic seizure without intervening return of consciousness.

Status epilepticus, always an emergency, is accompanied by respiratory distress. It can result from abrupt withdrawal of anticonvulsant medications, hypoxic or metabolic encephalopathy, acute head trauma, or septicemia secondary to encephalitis or meningitis.

Emergency treatment of status epilepticus usually consists of diazepam, phenytoin, or phenobarbital; dextrose 50% I.V. (when seizures are secondary to hypoglycemia); and thiamine I.V. (in the presence of chronic alcoholism or withdrawal).

▶ Check for injuries.

▶ Reorient and reassure the patient as necessary.

▶ When the patient is comfortable and safe, document what happened during the seizure.

▶ Place side rail pads on the bed in case the patient experiences another seizure.

▶ After the seizure, monitor vital signs and mental status every 15 to 20 minutes for 2 hours.

▶ Ask the patient about his aura and activities preceding the seizure. The type of aura (such as auditory, visual, olfactory, gustatory, or somatic) helps pinpoint the site in the brain where the seizure originated.

Special considerations

▶ Because a seizure commonly indicates an underlying disorder, such as meningitis or a metabolic or electrolyte imbalance, a complete diagnostic workup will be ordered if the cause of the seizure isn't evident.

Complications

The patient who experiences a seizure may experience an injury, respiratory difficulty, and decreased mental capability. Common injuries include scrapes and bruises suffered when the patient hits objects during the seizure and traumatic injury to the tongue caused by biting. If you suspect a serious injury, such as a fracture or deep laceration, notify the doctor and arrange for appropriate evaluation and treatment.

Changes in respiratory function may include aspiration, airway obstruction, and hypoxemia. After the seizure, complete a respiratory assessment and notify the doctor if you suspect a problem. Expect most patients to experience a postictal period of decreased mental status lasting 30 minutes to 24 hours. Reassure the patient that this doesn't indicate incipient brain damage.

Documentation

Document that the patient requires seizure precautions and record all precautions taken. Record the date and the time the seizure began as well as its duration and any precipitating factors. Identify any sensation that may be considered an aura. If the seizure was preceded by an aura, have the patient describe what he experienced.

Record any involuntary behavior that occurred at the onset, such as lip smacking, chewing movements, or hand and eye movements. Describe where the movement began and the parts of the body involved. Note any progression or pattern to the activity. Document whether the patient's eyes deviated to one side and whether the pupils changed in size, shape, equality, or reaction to light. Note if the patient's teeth were clenched or open. Record any incontinence, vomiting, or salivation that occurred during the seizure.

Note the patient's response to the seizure. Was the patient aware of what happened? Did he fall into a deep sleep following the seizure? Was he upset or ashamed? Also, document any medications given, any complications experienced during the seizure, and any interventions performed. Finally, record the patient's postseizure mental status.

SELF-CATHETERIZATION

A patient with impaired or absent bladder function may catheterize himself for routine bladder drainage. Self-catheterization requires thorough and careful teaching by the nurse. The patient will probably use clean technique for self-catheterization at home, but he must use sterile technique in the facility because of the increased risk of infection.

Key nursing diagnoses and patient outcomes

Risk for infection related to self-catheterization
The patient will:
▶ have vital signs, temperature, and laboratory values that remain within normal limits
▶ have no pathogens in cultures

► show no evidence of urinary tract infection, such as urine that is cloudy, malodorous, or with sediment.

Deficient knowledge related to lack of exposure to self-catheterization
The patient will:
► verbalize or demonstrate knowledge of what has been taught
► verbalize an understanding of the need for the procedure.

Urinary retention related to sensory or neuromuscular impairment
The patient will:
► express a feeling of increased comfort
► maintain fluid balance so intake equals output
► demonstrate skill in performing self-catheterization
► identify resources to assist with care following discharge.

Equipment

Rubber catheter • washcloth • soap and water • small packet of water-soluble lubricant • plastic storage bag • optional: drainage container, paper towels, cornstarch, rubber or plastic sheets, gooseneck lamp, catheterization record, and mirror

Preparation of equipment

Instruct the patient to keep a supply of catheters at home and to use each catheter only once before cleaning it. Advise him to wash the used catheter in warm, soapy water, rinse it inside and out, and then dry it with a clean towel and store it in a plastic bag until the next time it's needed. *Because catheters become brittle with repeated use,* tell the patient to check them often and to order a new supply well in advance.

Implementation

► Tell the patient to begin by trying to urinate into the toilet or, if a toilet isn't available or he needs to measure urine quantity, into a drainage container. Then he should wash his hands thoroughly with soap and water and dry them.
► Demonstrate how the patient should perform the catheterization, explaining each step clearly and carefully. Position a gooseneck lamp nearby if room lighting is inadequate *to make the urinary meatus clearly visible.* Arrange the patient's clothing so that it's out of the way.

Teaching a woman

► Demonstrate and explain to the female patient that she should separate the vaginal folds as widely as possible with the fingers of her nondominant hand *to obtain a full view of the urinary meatus.* She may need to use a mirror to visualize the meatus. Ask if she's right- or left-handed and then tell her which is her nondominant hand. While holding her labia open with the nondominant hand, she should use the dominant hand to wash the perineal area thoroughly with a soapy washcloth, using downward strokes. Tell her to rinse the area with the washcloth, using downward strokes as well.
► Show her how to squeeze some lubricant onto the first 3″ (7.6 cm) of the catheter and then how to insert the catheter. (See *Teaching self-catheterization,* page 722.)
► When the urine stops draining, tell her to remove the catheter slowly, get dressed, and wash the catheter with warm, soapy water. Then she should rinse it inside and out and dry it with a paper towel.

Teaching self-catheterization

Teach a woman to hold the catheter in her dominant hand as if it were a pencil or a dart, about ½″ (1.5 cm) from its tip. Keeping the vaginal folds separated, she should slowly insert the lubricated catheter about 3″ (7.5 cm) into the urethra. Tell her to press down with her abdominal muscles to empty the bladder, allowing all urine to drain through the catheter and into the toilet or drainage container.

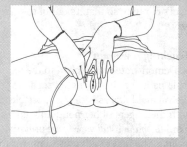

Teach a man to hold his penis in his nondominant hand, at a right angle to his body. He should hold the catheter in his dominant hand as if it were a pencil or a dart and slowly insert it 7″ to 10″ (18 to 25.5 cm) into the urethra until urine begins flowing. Then he should gently advance the catheter about 1″ (2.5 cm) farther, allowing all urine to drain into the toilet or drainage container.

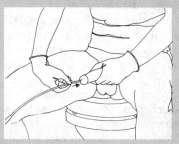

Teaching a man

▶ Tell a male patient to wash and rinse the end of his penis thoroughly with soap and water, pulling back the foreskin, if appropriate. He should keep the foreskin pulled back during the procedure.

▶ Show him how to squeeze lubricant onto a paper towel and have him roll the first 7″ to 10″ (18 to 25.5 cm) of the catheter in the lubricant. Tell him that copious lubricant will make the procedure more comfortable for him. Then show him how to insert the catheter.

▶ When the urine stops draining, tell him to remove the catheter slowly and, if necessary, pull the foreskin forward again. Have him get dressed and have him wash and dry the catheter as described above.

Special considerations

▶ Impress upon the patient that the timing of catheterization is critical *to prevent overdistention of the bladder, which can lead to infection.* Self-catheterization is usually performed every 4 to 6 hours around the clock (or more often at first).

▶ Female patients should be able to identify the body parts involved in self-catheterization, such as the labia majora, labia minora, vagina, and urinary meatus.

▶ Keep in mind the difference between boiling and sterilization. Boiling kills bacteria, viruses, and fungi but doesn't kill spores, whereas sterilization does. However, for catheter cleaning done in the patient's home, boiling is a sufficient safeguard against spreading infections.

▶ Advise the patient to hold off storing the cleaned catheters in a plastic bag until after they're completely dry *to prevent growth of gram-negative organisms.*

▶ Stress the importance of regulating fluid intake as ordered *to prevent incontinence while maintaining adequate hydration.* However, explain that incontinent episodes may occur occasionally. For managing incontinence, the doctor or a home health care nurse can help develop a plan such as more frequent catheterizations. After an incontinent episode, tell the patient to wash with soap and water, pat himself dry with a towel, and expose the skin to the air for as long as possible. He can reduce urine odor by putting methylbenzethonium (Diaparene) or cornstarch on his skin. Bedding and furniture can be protected by covering them with rubber or plastic sheets and then covering the rubber or plastic with fabric.

▶ Also, stress the importance of taking medications as ordered *to increase urine retention and help prevent incontinence.* Advise the patient to avoid calcium-rich and phosphorus-rich foods as ordered *to reduce the chance of renal calculus formation.*

Complications

Overdistention of the bladder can lead to urinary tract infection and urine leakage. Improper hand washing or equipment cleaning can also cause urinary tract infection. Incorrect catheter insertion can injure the urethral or bladder mucosa.

Documentation

Record the date and times of catheterization, character of the urine (such as color, odor, clarity, and presence of particles or blood), the amount of urine (such as increase, decrease, or no change), and any problems encountered during the procedure. Note whether the patient has difficulty performing a return demonstration.

SEQUENTIAL COMPRESSION THERAPY

Safe, effective, and noninvasive, sequential compression therapy helps prevent deep vein thrombosis (DVT) in surgical patients. This therapy massages the legs in a wavelike, milking motion that promotes blood flow and deters thrombosis.

Typically, sequential compression therapy complements other preventive measures, such as antiembolism stockings and anticoagulant medications. Although patients at low risk for DVT may require only antiembolism stockings, those at moderate to high risk may require both antiembolism stockings and sequential compression therapy. These preventive measures are continued for as long as the patient remains at risk.

Both antiembolism stockings and sequential compression sleeves are commonly used preoperatively and postoperatively because blood clots tend to form during surgery. About 20% of blood clots form in the femoral vein. Sequential compression therapy counteracts blood stasis and coagulation changes: two of the three major factors that promote DVT. It reduces stasis by increasing peak blood flow velocity, helping to empty the femoral vein's valve cusps of pooled or static blood. Also, the compressions cause an anti-clotting effect by increasing fibrinolytic activity, which stimulates the release of a plasminogen activator.

Key nursing diagnoses and patient outcomes

Impaired physical mobility related to (specify)

The patient will:

▶ maintain muscle strength and joint range of motion

▶ show no evidence of complications, such as contractures, venous stasis, thrombus formation, or skin breakdown

▶ have mobility regimen carried out by family member or other caregiver.

Risk for peripheral neurovascular dysfunction

The patient will:

▶ maintain circulation in extremities

▶ demonstrate correct body positioning techniques

▶ have no symptoms of neurovascular compromise.

Equipment

Measuring tape and sizing chart for the brand of sleeves you're using • pair of compression sleeves in correct size • connecting tubing • compression controller

Implementation

▶ Explain the procedure to the patient *to increase her cooperation.*

Determining proper sleeve size

▶ Before applying the compression sleeve, determine the proper size of sleeve that you need. Begin by washing your hands.

▶ Then measure the circumference of the upper thigh while the patient rests in bed. Do this by placing the measuring tape under the thigh at the gluteal furrow (as shown at top of next column).

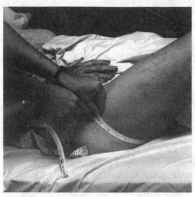

▶ Hold the tape snugly, but not tightly, around the patient's leg. Note the exact circumference.

▶ Find the patient's thigh measurement on the sizing chart and locate the corresponding size of the compression sleeve.

▶ Remove the compression sleeves from the package and unfold them.

▶ Lay the unfolded sleeves on a flat surface with the cotton lining facing up (as shown below).

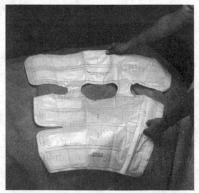

▶ Notice the markings on the lining denoting the ankle and the area behind the knee at the popliteal pulse point. Use these markings to position the sleeve at the appropriate landmarks.

Applying the sleeves

▶ Place the patient's leg on the sleeve lining. Position the back of the knee over the popliteal opening.

▶ Make sure that the back of the ankle is over the ankle marking.

▶ Starting at the side opposite the clear plastic tubing, wrap the sleeve snugly around the patient's leg.

▶ Fasten the sleeve securely with the Velcro fasteners. For the best fit, first secure the ankle and calf sections and then the thigh.

▶ The sleeve should fit snugly but not tightly. Check the fit by inserting two fingers between the sleeve and the patient's leg at the knee opening. Loosen or tighten the sleeve by readjusting the Velcro fastener.

▶ Using the same procedure, apply the second sleeve (as shown below).

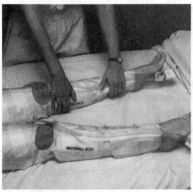

Operating the system

▶ Connect each sleeve to the tubing leading to the controller. Both sleeves must be connected to the compression controller for the system to operate. Line up the blue arrows on the sleeve connector with the arrows on the tubing connectors and push the ends together firmly. Listen for a click, signal-ing a firm connection. Make sure that the tubing isn't kinked.

▶ Plug the compression controller into the proper wall outlet. Turn on the power.

▶ The controller automatically sets the compression sleeve pressure at 45 mm Hg, which is the midpoint of the normal range (35 to 55 mm Hg).

▶ Observe the patient to see how well she tolerates the therapy and the controller as the system completes its first cycle. With the instrument, each cycle lasts 71 seconds — 11 seconds of compression and 60 seconds of decompression.

▶ Check the AUDIBLE ALARM key. The green light should be lit, indicating that the alarm is working.

▶ The compression sleeves should function continuously (24 hours daily) until the patient is fully ambulatory. Check the sleeves at least once each shift *to ensure proper fit and inflation.*

Removing the sleeves

▶ You may remove the sleeves when the patient is walking, bathing, or leaving the room for tests or other procedures. Reapply them immediately after any of these activities. To disconnect the sleeves from the tubing, press the latches on each side of the connectors and pull the connectors apart.

▶ Store the tubing and compression controller according to facility protocol. This equipment isn't disposable.

Special considerations

▶ The compression controller also has a mechanism to help cool the patient.

▶ If you're applying only one sleeve — for example, if the patient has a cast — leave the unused sleeve folded in the plastic bag. Cut a small hole in the bag's sealed bottom edge and pull the sleeve connector (the part that holds the connecting tubing) through the hole. Then you can join both sleeves to the compression controller.

▶ If a malfunction triggers the instrument's alarm, you'll hear beeping. The system shuts off whenever the alarm is activated.

▶ To respond to the alarm, remove the operator's card from the slot on the top of the compression controller.

▶ Follow the instructions printed on the card next to the matching code.

Complications

Don't use this therapy in patients with any of the following conditions:

▶ acute DVT (or DVT diagnosed within the past 6 months)

▶ severe arteriosclerosis or any other ischemic vascular disease

▶ massive edema of the legs resulting from pulmonary edema or heart failure

▶ any local condition that the compression sleeves would aggravate, such as dermatitis, vein ligation, gangrene, and recent skin grafting. A patient with a pronounced leg deformity also would be unlikely to benefit from the compression sleeves.

Documentation

Document the procedure, the patient's response to and understanding of the procedure, and the status of the alarm and cooling settings.

SITZ BATH

Also known as a hip bath, a sitz bath involves immersion of the pelvic area in warm or hot water. It's used to relieve discomfort, especially after perineal or rectal surgery or childbirth. The bath promotes wound healing by cleaning the perineum and anus, increasing circulation, and reducing inflammation. It also helps relax local muscles.

To be performed correctly, the sitz bath requires frequent checks of water temperature to ensure therapeutic effects as well as correct draping of the patient during the bath and prompt dressing afterward to prevent vasoconstriction.

Key nursing diagnoses and patient outcomes

Impaired skin integrity related to (specify)
The patient will:

▶ show no evidence of skin breakdown

▶ have normal skin turgor

▶ regain skin integrity, exhibiting wound site healing.

Risk for infection related to altered skin integrity
The patient will:

▶ have vital signs, temperature, and laboratory values remain within normal limits

▶ show no signs or symptoms of infection at the wound site, such as redness, pus, drainage, or odor

▶ have no pathogens in cultures.

Equipment

Sitz tub, portable sitz bath, or regular bathtub • bath mat • rubber mat • bath (utility) thermometer • two bath blankets • towels • patient gown • gloves, if the patient has an open lesion or has been incontinent • optional: rubber ring, footstool, overbed table, I.V. pole (to hold irrigation bag), wheelchair or cart, and dressings

A disposable sitz bath kit is available for single-patient use. It includes a plastic basin that fits over a commode and an irrigation bag with tubing and clamp.

Preparation of equipment

Make sure the sitz tub, portable sitz bath, or regular bathtub is clean and disinfected. Or, obtain a disposable sitz bath kit from the central supply department.

Position the bath mat next to the bathtub, sitz tub, or commode. If you're using a tub, place a rubber mat on its surface *to prevent falls.* Place the rubber ring on the bottom of the tub *to serve as a seat for the patient* and cover the ring with a towel *for comfort. Keeping the patient elevated improves water flow over the wound site and avoids unnecessary pressure on tender tissues.*

If you're using a commercial kit, open the package and familiarize yourself with the equipment.

Fill the sitz tub or bathtub one-third to one-half full, so that the water will reach the seated patient's umbilicus. Use warm water (94° to 98° F [34.4° to 36.7° C]) for relaxation or wound cleaning and healing and hot water (110° to 115° F [43.3° to 46.1° C]) for heat application. Run the water slightly warmer than desired *because it will cool while the patient prepares for the bath.* Measure the water temperature using the bath thermometer.

If you're using a commercial kit, fill the basin to the specified line with water at the prescribed temperature. Place the basin under the commode seat, clamp the irrigation tubing to block water flow, and fill the irrigation bag with water of the same temperature as that in the basin. To create flow pressure, hang the bag above the patient's head on a hook, towel rack, or I.V. pole.

Implementation

▶ Check the doctor's order and assess the patient's condition.
▶ Explain the procedure to the patient. Wash your hands thoroughly and put on gloves, if necessary.
▶ Have the patient void.
▶ Assist the patient to the bath area, provide privacy, and make sure the area is warm and free from drafts. Help the patient undress as needed.
▶ Remove and dispose of any soiled dressings. If a dressing adheres to a wound, allow it to soak off in the tub.
▶ Assist the patient into the tub or onto the commode as needed. Instruct him to use the safety rail for balance. Explain that the sensation may be unpleasant initially *because the wound area is already tender.* Assure him that this discomfort will soon be relieved by the warm water.
▶ For any apparatus except a regular bathtub, if the patient's feet don't reach the floor and the weight of his legs presses against the edge of the equipment, place a small stool under the patient's feet. *This decreases pressure on local blood vessels.* Also, place a folded towel against the patient's lower back *to prevent discomfort and promote correct body alignment.*
▶ Drape the patient's shoulders and knees with bath blankets *to avoid chills that cause vasoconstriction.*
▶ If you're using the sitz bath kit, open the clamp on the irrigation tubing *to allow a stream of water to flow continuously over the wound site.* Refill the bag with water of the correct temperature as needed and encourage the patient to regulate the flow himself. Place the patient's overbed table in front of him *to provide support and comfort.*
▶ If you're using a tub, check the water temperature frequently with the bath

thermometer. If the temperature drops significantly, add warm water. For maximum safety, first help the patient stand up slowly *to prevent dizziness and loss of balance*. Then, with the patient holding the safety rail for support, run warm water into the tub. Check the water temperature. When the water reaches the correct temperature, help the patient sit down again to resume the bath.

▶ If necessary, stay with the patient during the bath. If you must leave, show him how to use the call button and ensure his privacy.

▶ Check the patient's color and general condition frequently. If he complains of feeling weak, faint, or nauseated or shows signs of cardiovascular distress, discontinue the bath, check the patient's pulse and blood pressure, and assist him back to bed. Use a wheelchair or cart to transport the patient to his room, if necessary. Notify the doctor.

▶ When the prescribed bath time has elapsed — usually 15 to 20 minutes — tell the patient to use the safety rail *for balance,* and help him to a standing position slowly *to prevent dizziness and to allow him to regain his equilibrium.*

▶ If necessary, help the patient to dry himself. Re-dress the wound as needed, provide a clean gown, and assist the patient to dress and return to bed or back to his room.

▶ Dispose of soiled materials properly. Empty, clean, and disinfect the sitz tub, bathtub, or portable sitz bath. Return the commercial kit to the patient's bedside for later use.

Special considerations
▶ Use a regular bathtub only if a special sitz tub, portable sitz bath, or commercial sitz bath kit is unavailable. *Because the application of heat to the ex-* *tremities causes vasodilation and draws blood away from the perineal area,* a regular bathtub is less effective for local treatment than a sitz device.

▶ If the patient will be sitting in a bathtub with his extremities immersed in the hot water, check his pulse before, during, and after the bath *to help detect vasodilation that could make him feel faint when he stands up.*

▶ Tell the patient never to touch an open wound *because of the risk of infection.*

Home care
Instruct the patient to adhere to the manufacturer's guidelines for disposable equipment.

Complications
Weakness or faintness can result from heat or the exertion of changing position. Irregular or accelerated pulse may indicate cardiovascular distress.

Documentation
Record the date, time, duration, and temperature of the bath; wound condition before and after treatment, including color, odor, and amount of drainage; any complications; and the patient's response to treatment.

Skin biopsy

Skin biopsy is a diagnostic test in which a small piece of tissue is removed, under local anesthesia, from a lesion that is suspected of being malignant or from another dermatosis.

One of three techniques may be used: shave biopsy, punch biopsy, or excisional biopsy. Shave biopsy cuts the lesion above the skin line, which allows further biopsy of the site. Punch biopsy removes an oval core from the center of the lesion. Excisional biopsy removes the entire lesion and is indicated for rapidly expanding lesions; for sclerotic, bullous, or atrophic lesions; and for examination of the border of a lesion surrounding normal skin.

Lesions suspected of being malignant usually have changed color, size, or appearance or have failed to heal properly after injury. Fully developed lesions should be selected for biopsy whenever possible because they provide more diagnostic information than lesions that are resolving or in early stages of development. For example, if the skin shows blisters, the biopsy should include the most mature ones.

Normal skin consists of squamous epithelium (epidermis) and fibrous connective tissue (dermis). Histologic examination of the tissue specimen obtained during biopsy may reveal a benign or malignant lesion. Benign growths include cysts, seborrheic keratoses, warts, pigmented nevi (moles), keloids, dermatofibromas, and neurofibromas. Malignant tumors include basal cell carcinoma, squamous cell carcinoma, and malignant melanoma.

Key nursing diagnoses and patient outcomes

Impaired skin integrity related to lesion
The patient will:
▶ exhibit improved or healed lesions
▶ have few or no complications
▶ explain skin care regimen.

Anxiety related to possible medical diagnoses
The patient will:
▶ state a feeling of anxiety

▶ cope with the threat of anxiety by being involved in decisions about his care
▶ use support systems to assist with coping.

Equipment

Gloves • #15 scalpel for shave or excisional biopsy • local anesthetic • specimen bottle containing 10% formaldehyde solution • 4-0 sutures for punch or excisional biopsy • adhesive bandage • forceps • adhesive strips

Implementation

▶ Explain to the patient that the biopsy provides a skin specimen for microscopic study. Describe the procedure and tell him who will perform it. Answer any questions he may have *to ease anxiety and ensure cooperation.*
▶ Inform the patient that he need not restrict food or fluids.
▶ Tell him that he'll receive a local anesthetic for pain.
▶ Inform him that the biopsy will take about 15 minutes and that the test results are usually available in 1 day.
▶ Have the patient or an appropriate family member sign a consent form.
▶ Check the patient's history for hypersensitivity to the local anesthetic.
▶ Position the patient comfortably and clean the biopsy site before the local anesthetic is administered.
▶ For a shave biopsy, the protruding growth is cut off at the skin line with a #15 scalpel. The tissue is placed immediately in a properly labeled specimen bottle containing 10% formaldehyde solution. Apply pressure to the area to stop the bleeding. Apply an adhesive bandage.
▶ For a punch biopsy, the skin surrounding the lesion is pulled taut, and

the punch is firmly introduced into the lesion and rotated to obtain a tissue specimen. The plug is lifted with forceps or a needle and is severed as deeply into the fat layer as possible. The specimen is placed in a properly labeled specimen bottle containing 10% formaldehyde solution or in a sterile container, if indicated. Closing the wound depends on the size of the punch: A 3-mm punch requires only an adhesive bandage, a 4-mm punch requires one suture, and a 6-mm punch requires two sutures.

▶ For an excisional biopsy, a #15 scalpel is used to excise the lesion; the incision is made as wide and as deep as necessary. The tissue specimen is removed and placed immediately in a properly labeled specimen bottle containing 10% formaldehyde solution. Apply pressure to the site *to stop the bleeding*. The wound is closed using a 4-0 suture. If the incision is large, a skin graft may be required. If the incision is small, adhesive strips may be applied.

▶ Check the biopsy site for bleeding.

▶ Send the specimen to the laboratory immediately.

▶ If the patient experiences pain, administer analgesics.

Special considerations

▶ Advise the patient going home with sutures to keep the area clean and as dry as possible. Tell him that facial sutures will be removed in 3 to 5 days and trunk sutures, in 7 to 14 days.

▶ Instruct the patient with adhesive strips to leave them in place for 14 to 21 days.

Complications

Possible complications include bleeding and infection of the surrounding tissue.

Documentation

Document the time and location where the specimen was obtained, the appearance of the specimen and site, and whether bleeding occurred at the biopsy site.

SKIN GRAFT CARE

A skin graft consists of healthy skin taken either from the patient (autograft) or a donor (allograft) and applied to a part of the patient's body. There the graft resurfaces an area damaged by burns, traumatic injury, or surgery. Care procedures for an autograft or an allograft are essentially the same. However, an autograft requires care for two sites: the graft site and the donor site.

The graft itself may be one of several types: split-thickness, full-thickness, or pedicle-flap. (See *Understanding types of grafts*.) Successful grafting depends on various factors, including clean wound granulation with adequate vascularization, complete contact of the graft with the wound bed, aseptic technique to prevent infection, adequate graft immobilization, and skilled care.

The size and depth of the patient's burns determine whether the burns will require grafting. Grafting usually occurs at the completion of wound debridement. The goal is to cover all wounds with an autograft or allograft within 2 weeks. With enzymatic debridement, grafting may be performed 5 to 7 days after debridement is complete; with surgical debridement, grafting can occur the same day as the surgery.

Depending on your facility's policy, a doctor or a specially trained nurse may change graft dressings. The dressings usually stay in place for 3 to 5 days after surgery *to avoid disturbing the graft site.* Meanwhile, the donor graft site needs diligent care. (See *How to care for a donor graft site,* page 732.)

Key nursing diagnoses and patient outcomes

Impaired skin integrity related to surgery
The patient will:
▶ exhibit no evidence of skin breakdown
▶ show normal skin turgor
▶ regain skin integrity, exhibiting graft site healing with no evidence of rejection
▶ communicate an understanding of skin care protection measures.

Risk for infection related to presence of graft
The patient will:
▶ have vital signs, temperature, and laboratory values remain within normal limits
▶ have no pathogens in cultures
▶ show no signs or symptoms of infection at graft site.

Equipment

Ordered analgesic • clean and sterile gloves • sterile gown • cap • mask • sterile forceps • sterile scissors • sterile scalpel • sterile 4″ × 4″ gauze pads • Xeroflo gauze • elastic gauze dressing • warm normal saline solution • moisturizing cream • topical medication (such as micronized silver sulfadiazine cream) • optional: sterile cotton-tipped applicators

Understanding types of grafts

A burn patient may receive one or more of the graft types described below.

Split-thickness
The type used most commonly for covering open burns, a split-thickness graft includes the epidermis and part of the dermis. It may be applied as a sheet (usually on the face or neck *to preserve the cosmetic result*) or as a mesh. A mesh graft has tiny slits cut in it, which allow the graft to expand up to nine times its original size. Mesh grafts prevent fluids from collecting under the graft and typically are used over extensive full-thickness burns.

Full-thickness
This graft type includes the epidermis and the entire dermis. Consequently, the graft contains hair follicles, sweat glands, and sebaceous glands, which typically aren't included in split-thickness grafts. Full-thickness grafts usually are used for small burns that cause deep wounds.

Pedicle-flap
This full-thickness graft includes not only skin and subcutaneous tissue but also subcutaneous blood vessels *to ensure a continued blood supply to the graft.* Pedicle-flap grafts may be used during reconstructive surgery *to cover previous defects.*

Preparation of equipment
Assemble the equipment on the dressing cart.

Implementation
▶ Explain the procedure to the patient and provide privacy.

How to care for a donor graft site

Autografts are usually taken from another area of the patient's body with a dermatome, an instrument that cuts uniform, split-thickness skin portions — typically about 0.013 to 0.05 cm thick. Autografting makes the donor site a partial-thickness wound, which may bleed, drain, and cause pain.

This site needs scrupulous care to prevent infection, which could convert the site to a full-thickness wound. Depending on the graft's thickness, tissue may be obtained from the donor site again in as few as 10 days.

Usually, Xeroflo gauze is applied postoperatively. The outer gauze dressing can be taken off on the first postoperative day; the Xeroflo will protect the new epithelial proliferation.

Dressing the wound

Care for the donor site as you care for the autograft, using dressing changes at the initial stages *to prevent infection and promote healing.* Use the following guidelines:

■ Wash your hands and put on sterile gloves.

■ Remove the outer gauze dressings within 24 hours. Inspect the Xeroflo for signs of infection; then leave it open to the air *to speed drying and healing.*

■ Leave small amounts of fluid accumulation alone. Using aseptic technique, aspirate larger amounts through the dressing with a small-gauge needle and syringe.

■ Apply a lanolin-based cream daily to completely healed donor sites *to keep skin tissue pliable and to remove crusts.*

▶ Administer an analgesic as ordered 20 to 30 minutes before beginning the procedure. Alternatively, give an I.V.

analgesic immediately before the procedure.
▶ Wash your hands.
▶ Put on the sterile gown, sterile gloves, mask, and cap.
▶ Gently lift off all outer dressings. Soak the middle dressings with warm saline solution. Remove these carefully and slowly *to avoid disturbing the graft site.* Leave the Xeroflo intact *to avoid dislodging the graft.*
▶ Remove and discard the gloves, wash your hands, and put on the sterile gloves.
▶ Assess the condition of the graft. If you see purulent drainage, notify the doctor.
▶ Remove the Xeroflo with sterile forceps and clean the area gently. If necessary, soak the Xeroflo with warm saline solution *to facilitate removal.*
▶ Inspect an allograft for signs of rejection, such as infection and delayed healing. Inspect a sheet graft frequently for blebs. If ordered, evacuate them carefully with a sterile scalpel. (See *Evacuating fluid from a sheet graft.*)
▶ Apply topical medication, if ordered.
▶ Place fresh Xeroflo over the site *to promote wound healing and prevent infection.* Use sterile scissors to cut the appropriate size. Cover this with 4″ × 4″ gauze and elastic gauze dressing.
▶ Clean any completely healed areas and apply a moisturizing cream to them *to keep the skin pliable and to retard scarring.*

Special considerations

▶ *To avoid dislodging the graft,* hydrotherapy is usually discontinued as ordered for 3 to 4 days after grafting. Avoid using a blood pressure cuff over the graft. Don't tug or pull dressings

Evacuating fluid from a sheet graft

When small pockets of fluid (called blebs) accumulate beneath a sheet graft, you'll need to evacuate the fluid using a sterile scalpel and sterile cotton-tipped applicators. First, carefully perforate the center of the bleb with the scalpel.

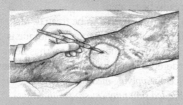

Gently express the fluid with the cotton-tipped applicators.

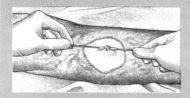

Never express fluid by rolling the bleb to the edge of the graft. *This disturbs healing in other areas.*

during dressing changes. Keep the patient from lying on the graft.

▶ If the graft dislodges, apply sterile skin compresses *to keep the area moist until the surgeon reapplies the graft.* If the graft affects an arm or a leg, elevate the affected extremity *to reduce postoperative edema.* Check for bleeding and signs or symptoms of neurovascular impairment, such as increasing pain, numbness or tingling, coolness, and pallor.

Home care
Teach the patient how to apply moisturizing cream. Stress the importance of using a sunscreen containing titanium dioxide or oxybenzone that has a sun protection factor of 20 or higher on all grafted areas *to avoid sunburn and discoloration.*

Complications
Graft failure may result from traumatic injury, hematoma or seroma formation, infection, an inadequate graft bed, rejection, or compromised nutritional status.

Documentation
Record the time and date of all dressing changes. Document all medications used, and note the patient's response to the medications. Describe the condition of the graft and note any signs of infection or rejection. Record any additional treatment and note the patient's reaction to the graft.

SKIN MEDICATION ADMINISTRATION

Topical drugs are applied directly to the skin surface. They include lotions, pastes, ointments, creams, powders, shampoos, patches, and aerosol sprays. Topical medications are absorbed through the epidermal layer into the dermis. The extent of absorption depends on the vascularity of the region.

Nitroglycerin, fentanyl, nicotine, and certain supplemental hormone replacements are used for systemic effects. Most other topical medications are used for local effects. Ointments have a fatty base, which is an ideal vehicle for such drugs as antimicrobials and antiseptics.

Typically, topical medications should be applied two or three times per day to achieve their therapeutic effect.

Key nursing diagnoses and patient outcomes

Deficient knowledge related to lack of exposure to skin medication administration
The patient will:
▶ state or demonstrate an understanding of what has been taught
▶ demonstrate the ability to perform new health-related behaviors as taught.

Risk for injury related to improper technique
The patient will:
▶ identify factors that increase the risk of injury
▶ assist in identifying and applying safety measures to prevent injury.

Equipment

Patient's medication record and chart • prescribed medication • gloves • sterile tongue blades • sterile 4″ × 4″ gauze pads • transparent semipermeable dressing • adhesive tape • solvent (such as cottonseed oil)

Implementation

▶ Verify the order on the patient's medication record by checking it against the doctor's order in the chart.
▶ Make sure the label on the medication agrees with the medication order. Read the label again before you open the container and as you remove the medication from the container. Check the expiration date.
▶ Confirm the patient's identity by asking his name and checking the name, room number, and bed number on his wristband.
▶ Provide privacy.

▶ Explain the procedure thoroughly to the patient *because he may have to apply the medication by himself after discharge.*
▶ Wash your hands *to prevent cross-contamination* and put a glove on your dominant hand. Use gloves on both hands if exposure to body fluids is likely.
▶ Help the patient assume a comfortable position that provides access to the area to be treated.
▶ Expose the area to be treated. Make sure the skin or mucous membrane is intact (unless the medication has been ordered to treat a skin lesion such as an ulcer). *Applying medication to broken or abraded skin may cause unwanted systemic absorption and result in further irritation.*
▶ If necessary, clean the skin of debris, including crusts, epidermal scales, and old medication. You may have to change the glove if it becomes soiled.

Applying paste, cream, or ointment
▶ Open the container. Place the lid or cap upside down *to prevent contamination of the inside surface.*
▶ Remove a tongue blade from its sterile wrapper and cover one end with medication from the tube or jar. Then transfer the medication from the tongue blade to your gloved hand.
▶ Apply the medication to the affected area with long, smooth strokes that follow the direction of hair growth. *This technique avoids forcing medication into hair follicles, which can cause irritation and lead to folliculitis.* Avoid excessive pressure when applying the medication *because it could abrade the skin.*
▶ *To prevent contamination of the medication,* use a new tongue blade each time you remove medication from the container.

Removing ointment

▶ Wash your hands and apply gloves. Then rub solvent on them and apply it liberally to the ointment-treated area in the direction of hair growth. Alternatively, saturate a sterile gauze pad with the solvent and use the pad to gently remove the ointment. Remove excess oil by gently wiping the area with a sterile gauze pad. Don't rub too hard to remove the medication *because you could irritate the skin.*

Applying other topical medications

▶ To apply shampoos, follow package directions. (See *Using medicated shampoos.*)

▶ To apply aerosol sprays, shake the container, if indicated, *to completely mix the medication.* Hold the container 6″ to 12″ (15 to 30.5 cm) from the skin, or follow the manufacturer's recommendation. Spray a thin film of the medication evenly over the treatment area.

▶ To apply powders, dry the skin surface, making sure to spread skin folds where moisture collects. Then apply a thin layer of powder over the treatment area.

▶ *To protect applied medications and prevent them from soiling the patient's clothes,* tape an appropriate amount of sterile gauze pad or a transparent semipermeable dressing over the treated area. With certain medications (such as topical steroids), semipermeable dressings may be contraindicated. Check medication information and cautions. If you're applying a topical medication to the patient's hands or feet, cover the site with white cotton gloves for the hands or terry cloth scuffs for the feet.

 Age alert In children, topical medications (such as steroids) should be covered only

Using medicated shampoos

Medicated shampoos include keratolytic and cytostatic agents, coal tar preparations, and lindane (gamma benzene hexachloride) solutions. They can be used to treat such conditions as dandruff, psoriasis, and head lice. However, they're contraindicated in patients with broken or abraded skin.

Because application instructions may vary among brands, check the label on the shampoo before starting the procedure *to ensure use of the correct amount.* Keep the shampoo away from the patient's eyes. If any shampoo should accidentally get in his eyes, irrigate them promptly with water. Selenium sulfide, used in cytostatic agents is extremely toxic if ingested.

To apply medicated shampoo, take the following steps:
■ Prepare the patient for shampoo treatment.
■ Shake the bottle of shampoo well *to mix the solution evenly.*
■ Wet the patient's hair thoroughly and wring out excess water.
■ Apply the proper amount of shampoo as directed on the label.
■ Work the shampoo into a lather, adding water as necessary. Part the hair and work the shampoo into the scalp, taking care not to use your fingernails.
■ Leave the shampoo on the scalp and hair for as long as instructed (usually 5 to 10 minutes). Then rinse the hair thoroughly.
■ Towel-dry the patient's hair.
■ After the hair is dry, comb or brush it. Use a fine-tooth comb to remove nits, if necessary.

loosely with a diaper. Don't use plastic pants.

▶ Assess the patient's skin for signs of irritation, allergic reaction, or breakdown.

Special considerations

▶ Never apply medication without first removing previous applications *to prevent skin irritation from an accumulation of medication.*

▶ Wear gloves *to prevent absorption by your own skin.* If the patient has an infectious skin condition, use sterile gloves and dispose of old dressings according to your facility's policy.

▶ Don't apply ointments to mucous membranes as liberally as you would to skin *because mucous membranes are usually moist and absorb ointment more quickly than skin does.* Also, don't apply too much ointment to any skin area *because it might cause irritation and discomfort, stain clothing and bedding, and make removal difficult.*

▶ Never apply ointment to the eyelids or ear canal unless ordered. *The ointment might congeal and occlude the tear duct or ear canal.*

▶ Inspect the treated area frequently for adverse effects such as signs of an allergic reaction.

Complications

Skin irritation, a rash, or an allergic reaction may occur.

Documentation

Record the medication applied; time, date, and site of application; and condition of the patient's skin at the time of application. Note subsequent effects of the medication, if any.

SKIN PREPARATION, PREOPERATIVE

Proper preparation of the patient's skin for surgery renders it as free as possible from microorganisms, thereby reducing the risk of infection at the incision site. It doesn't duplicate or replace the full sterile preparation that immediately precedes surgery. Rather, it may involve a bath, shower, or local scrub with an antiseptic detergent solution, followed by hair removal. (See *Where to remove hair for surgery.*)

The Association of Operating Room Nurses recommends that hair not be removed from the area surrounding the operative site unless it's thick enough to interfere with surgery because hair removal may increase the risk of infection. Each facility has a hair removal policy.

The area of preparation always exceeds that of the expected incision to minimize the number of microorganisms in the areas adjacent to the proposed incision and to allow surgical draping of the patient without contamination.

Key nursing diagnoses and patient outcomes

Disturbed body image
The patient will:

▶ acknowledge a change in body image

▶ communicate feelings about change in body image

▶ express positive feelings about self.

Impaired skin integrity related to surgery
The patient will:

▶ exhibit no evidence of skin breakdown

▶ show normal skin turgor

▶ regain skin integrity, exhibiting surgical incision site healing with no evidence of infection

▶ communicate an understanding of skin care protection measures.

(Text continues on page 740.)

Where to remove hair for surgery

Shoulder and upper arm

On operative side, remove hair from finger-tips to hairline and center chest to center spine, extending to iliac crest and including the axilla.

Chest

Remove hair from chin to iliac crests and side to midline of back on operative side (2″ [5 cm] beyond midline of back for thoracotomy). Include axilla and entire arm to elbow on operative side.

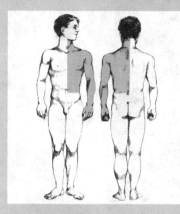

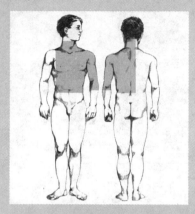

Forearm, elbow, and hand

On operative side, remove hair from finger-tips to shoulder. Include the axilla unless surgery is for hand. Trim and clean fingernails.

Abdomen

Remove hair from 3″ (7.6 cm) above nipples to upper thighs, including pubic area.

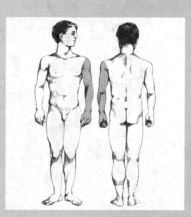

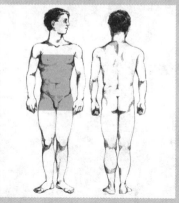

(continued)

Where to remove hair for surgery *(continued)*

Thigh

On operative side, remove hair from toes to 3″ (7.6 cm) above umbilicus and from midline front to midline back, including pubis. Clean and trim toenails.

Lower abdomen

Remove hair from 2″ (5 cm) above umbilicus to midthigh, including pubic area; for femoral ligation, to midline of thigh in back; and for hernioplasty and embolectomy, to costal margin and down to knee.

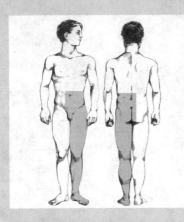

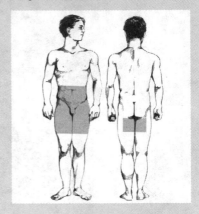

Ankle and foot

On operative side, remove hair from toes to 3″ above the knee. Clean and trim toenails.

Spine

Remove all hair from the axillae and back, including the shoulders and neck to the hairline, down to both knees.

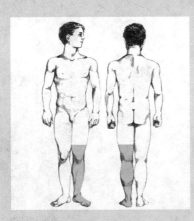

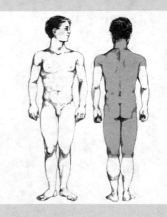

Where to remove hair for surgery *(continued)*

Knees and lower leg
On operative side, remove hair from toes to groin. Clean and trim toenails.

Perineum
Remove hair from pubis, perineum, and perianal area and from the waist to at least 3″ below the groin in front and at least 3″ below the buttocks in back.

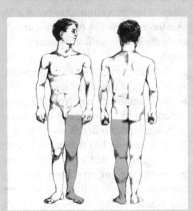

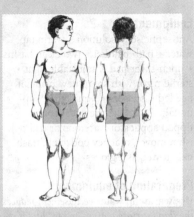

Hip
On operative side, remove hair from toes to nipples and at least 3″ (7.6 cm) beyond midline back and front, including the pubis. Clean and trim toenails.

Flank
On operative side, remove hair from nipples to pubis, 3″ beyond midline in back and 2″ (5 cm) past abdominal midline. Include pubic area and, on affected side, upper thigh and axilla.

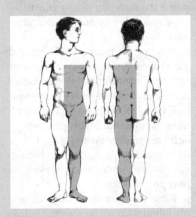

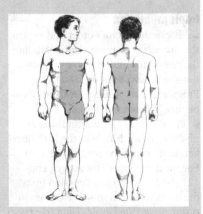

Risk for infection related to presence of graft
The patient will:
▶ have vital signs, temperature, and laboratory values remain within normal limits
▶ have no pathogens in cultures
▶ show no signs or symptoms of infection at surgical incision site.

Equipment
Antiseptic soap solution • warm tap water • bath blanket • two clean basins • linen-saver pad • adjustable light • sterile razor with sharp new blade, if needed • scissors • liquid soap •optional: 4″ × 4″ gauze pads, cotton-tipped applicators, acetone or nail polish remover, orangewood stick, trash bag, towel, and gloves

Preparation of equipment
Use warm tap water *because heat reduces the skin's surface tension and facilitates removal of soil and hair.* Dilute the antiseptic soap solution with warm tap water in one basin *for washing,* and pour plain warm water into the second basin *for rinsing.*

Implementation
▶ Check the doctor's order and explain the procedure to the patient, including the reason for the extensive preparations *to avoid causing undue anxiety.* Provide privacy, wash your hands thoroughly, and put on gloves.
▶ Place the patient in a comfortable position, drape him with the bath blanket, and expose the preparation area. For most surgeries, this area extends 12″ (30.5 cm) in each direction from the expected incision site. However, *to ensure privacy and avoid chilling the patient,* expose only one small area at a time while performing skin preparation.
▶ Position a linen-saver pad beneath the patient *to catch spills and avoid linen changes.* Adjust the light to illuminate the preparation area.
▶ Assess skin condition in the preparation area and report any rash, abrasion, or laceration to the doctor before beginning the procedure. *Any break in the skin increases the risk of infection and could cause cancellation of planned surgery.*
▶ Have the patient remove all jewelry in or near the operative site.
▶ Begin removing hair from the preparation area by clipping any long hairs with scissors. If ordered, shave all remaining hair within the area *to remove microorganisms.* Perform the procedure as near to the time of surgery as possible *so that microorganisms will have minimal time to proliferate.* Use only a sterilized or sterile disposable razor with a sharp new blade *to avoid the risk of infection from a contaminated razor.*
▶ Use a gauze pad to spread liquid soap over the shave site.
▶ Pull the skin taut in the direction opposite the direction of hair growth *because this makes the hair rise and facilitates shaving.*
▶ Holding the razor at a 45-degree angle, shave with short strokes in the direction of hair growth *to avoid skin irritation and achieve a smooth clean shave.*
▶ If possible, avoid lifting the razor from the skin and placing it down again *to minimize the risk of lacerations.* Also, avoid applying pressure *because this can cause abrasions, particularly over bony prominences.*
▶ Rinse the razor frequently and reapply liquid soap to the skin as needed *to keep the area moist.*

▶ Change the rinse water, if necessary. Then rinse the soap solution and loose hair from the preparation area and inspect the skin. Immediately notify the doctor of any new nicks, lacerations, or abrasions, and file a report if your facility requires it.

▶ Proceed with a 10-minute scrub *to ensure a clean preparation area.* Wash the area with a gauze pad dipped in the antiseptic soap solution. Using a circular motion, start at the expected incision site and work outward toward the periphery of the area *to avoid recontaminating the clean area.* Apply light friction while washing *to improve the antiseptic effect of the solution.* Replace the gauze pad as necessary.

▶ Carefully clean skin folds and crevices *because they harbor greater numbers of microorganisms.* Scrub the perineal area last, if it's part of the preparation area, for the same reason. Pull loose skin taut. If necessary, use cotton-tipped applicators to clean the umbilicus and an orangewood stick to clean under nails. Remove any nail polish with acetone or nail polish remover *because the anesthetist uses nail bed color to determine adequate oxygenation and may place a probe on the nail to measure oxygen saturation.*

▶ Dry the area with a clean towel and remove the linen-saver pad.

▶ Give the patient any special instructions for care of the prepared area and remind him to keep the area clean for surgery. Make sure the patient is comfortable.

▶ Properly dispose of solutions and the trash bag and clean or dispose of soiled equipment and supplies according to your facility's policy.

Special considerations

▶ Avoid shaving facial or neck hair on women and children unless ordered. Never shave eyebrows *because this disrupts normal hair growth and the new growth may prove unsightly.* Scalp shaving is usually performed in the operating room, but if you're required to prepare the patient's scalp, put all hair in a plastic or paper bag and store it with the patient's possessions.

▶ If the patient won't hold still for shaving, remove hair with a depilatory cream. Although this method produces clean, intact skin without risking lacerations or abrasions, it can cause skin irritation or rash, especially in the groin area. If possible, cut long hairs with scissors before applying the cream *because removal of remaining hair then requires less cream.* Then use a glove to apply the cream in a layer ½″ (1.3 cm) thick. After about 10 minutes, remove the cream with moist gauze pads. Next, wash the area with antiseptic soap solution, rinse, and pat dry.

Complications

Rashes, nicks, lacerations, and abrasions are the most common complications of skin preparation. They also increase the risk of postoperative infection.

Documentation

Record the date, time, and area of preparation; skin condition before and after preparation; any complications; and the patient's tolerance. If your facility requires it, complete an incident report if the patient suffers nicks, lacerations, or abrasions during skin preparation.

SKIN STAPLE AND CLIP REMOVAL

Skin staples or clips may be used instead of standard sutures to close lacerations or surgical wounds. Because they can secure a wound more quickly than sutures, they may substitute for surface sutures when cosmetic results aren't a prime consideration such as in abdominal closure. When properly placed, staples and clips distribute tension evenly along the suture line with minimal tissue trauma and compression, facilitating healing and minimizing scarring. Because staples and clips are made from surgical stainless steel, tissue reaction to them is minimal. Usually, doctors remove skin staples and clips, but some facilities permit qualified nurses to perform this procedure.

Skin staples and clips are contraindicated when wound location requires cosmetically superior results or when the incision site makes it impossible to maintain at least a 5-mm distance between the staple and underlying bone, vessels, or internal organs.

Key nursing diagnoses and patient outcomes

Risk for infection related to surgical incision
The patient will:
▶ have vital signs, temperature, and laboratory values within normal limits
▶ remain free from signs and symptoms of infection at incision site.

Anxiety related to situational crisis
The patient will:
▶ state at least two ways to eliminate or minimize anxious behaviors

▶ report the ability to cope with the current situation without experiencing severe anxiety.

Equipment

Waterproof trash bag • adjustable light • clean gloves, if needed • sterile gloves • sterile gauze pads • sterile staple or clip extractor • povidone-iodine solution or other antiseptic cleaning agent • sterile cotton-tipped applicators • optional: butterfly adhesive strips or Steri-Strips and compound benzoin tincture or other skin protectant

Prepackaged, sterile, disposable staple or clip extractors are available.

Preparation of equipment

Assemble all equipment in the patient's room. Check the expiration date on each sterile package and inspect for tears. Open the waterproof trash bag and place it near the patient's bed. Position the bag properly *to avoid reaching across the sterile field or the wound when disposing of soiled articles.* Form a cuff by turning down the top of the bag *to provide a wide opening and prevent contamination of instruments or gloves by touching the bag's edge.*

Implementation

▶ If your facility allows you to remove skin staples and clips, check the doctor's order *to confirm the exact timing and details for this procedure.*
▶ Check for patient allergies, especially to adhesive tape and povidone-iodine or other topical solutions or medications.
▶ Explain the procedure to the patient. Tell him that he may feel a slight pulling or tickling sensation but little discomfort during staple removal. Reassure him that because his incision is

healing properly, removing the supporting staples or clips won't weaken the incision line.

▶ Provide privacy and place the patient in a comfortable position that doesn't place undue tension on the incision. *Because some patients experience nausea or dizziness during the procedure,* have the patient recline, if possible. Adjust the light to shine directly on the incision.

▶ Wash your hands thoroughly.

▶ If the patient's wound has a dressing, put on clean gloves and carefully remove it. Discard the dressing and the gloves in the waterproof trash bag.

▶ Assess the patient's incision. Notify the doctor of gaping, drainage, inflammation, and other signs of infection.

▶ Establish a sterile work area with all the equipment and supplies you'll need for removing staples or clips and for cleaning and dressing the incision. Open the package containing the sterile staple or clip extractor, maintaining asepsis. Put on sterile gloves.

▶ Wipe the incision gently with sterile gauze pads soaked in an antiseptic cleaning agent or with sterile cotton-tipped applicators *to remove surface encrustations.*

▶ Pick up the sterile staple or clip extractor. Then, starting at one end of the incision, remove the staple or clip. (See *Removing a staple.*) Hold the extractor over the trash bag and release the handle to discard the staple or clip.

▶ Repeat the procedure for each staple or clip until all are removed.

▶ Apply a sterile gauze dressing, if needed, *to prevent infection and irritation from clothing.* Then discard your gloves.

▶ Make sure the patient is comfortable. According to the doctor's preference, inform the patient that he may shower

Removing a staple

Position the extractor's lower jaws beneath the span of the first staple (as shown below).

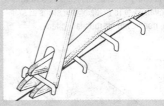

Squeeze the handles until they're completely closed; then lift the staple away from the skin (as shown below). The extractor changes the shape of the staple and pulls the prongs out of the intradermal tissue.

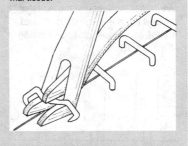

in 1 or 2 days if the incision is dry and healing well.

▶ Properly dispose of solutions and the trash bag and clean or dispose of soiled equipment and supplies according to facility policy.

Special considerations

▶ Carefully check the doctor's order for the time and extent of staple or clip removal. The doctor may want you to remove only alternate staples or clips initially and to leave the others in place

Types of adhesive skin closures

Steri-Strips are used as a primary means of keeping a wound closed after suture removal. They're made of thin strips of sterile, nonwoven, porous fabric tape.

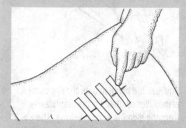

Butterfly closures consist of sterile, waterproof adhesive strips. A narrow, nonadhesive "bridge" connects the two expanded adhesive portions. These strips are used to close small wounds and assist healing after suture removal.

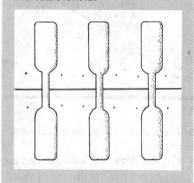

skin or left in place too long may resist removal.

► If the wound dehisces after staples or clips are removed, apply butterfly adhesive strips or Steri-Strips to approximate and support the edges and call the doctor immediately to repair the wound. (See *Types of adhesive skin closures*.)

► You may also apply butterfly adhesive strips or Steri-Strips after removing staples or clips even if the wound is healing normally *to give added support to the incision and prevent lateral tension from forming a wide scar.* Use a small amount of compound benzoin tincture or other skin protectant *to ensure adherence.* Leave the strips in place for 3 to 5 days.

Home care

If the patient is being discharged, teach him how to remove the dressing and care for the wound. Instruct him to call the doctor immediately if he observes wound discharge or any other abnormal change. Tell him that the redness surrounding the incision should gradually disappear and that, after a few weeks, only a thin line should be visible.

Documentation

Record the date and time of staple or clip removal, number of staples or clips removed, appearance of the incision, dressings or butterfly strips applied, signs of wound complications, and patient's tolerance of the procedure.

SKULL TONGS SITE CARE

Applying skeletal traction with skull tongs immobilizes the cervical spine after a fracture or dislocation, invasion by

for an additional day or two *to support the incision.*

► When removing a staple or clip, place the extractor's jaws carefully between the patient's skin and the staple or clip *to avoid patient discomfort.* If extraction is difficult, notify the doctor; *staples or clips placed too deeply within the* tumor or infection, or surgery. Three types of skull tongs are commonly used: Crutchfield, Gardner-Wells, and Vinke. (See *Types of skull tongs,* pages 746 and 747.) Crutchfield tongs are applied by incising the skin with a scalpel, drilling a hole in the exposed skull, and inserting the pins on the tongs into the hole. Gardner-Wells tongs and Vinke tongs are applied less invasively. Gardner-Wells tongs have spring-loaded pins attached to the tongs. These pins are advanced gently into the scalp. Then the tongs are tightened to secure the apparatus.

When any tong device is in place, traction is created by extending a rope from the center of the tongs over a pulley and attaching weights to it. With the help of X-ray monitoring, the weights are adjusted to establish reduction, if necessary, and to maintain alignment. Meticulous pin-site care (three times per day to prevent infection) and frequent observation of the traction apparatus to make sure it's working properly are required.

Key nursing diagnoses and patient outcomes

Risk for infection related to presence of invasive appliance
The patient will:
▶ have vital signs, temperature, and laboratory values within normal limits
▶ have no pathogens in cultures
▶ remain free from signs or symptoms of infection at insertion site.

Impaired physical mobility related to skeletal traction
The patient will:
▶ maintain muscle strength and joint range of motion

▶ show no evidence of complications, such as contractures, venous stasis, thrombus formation, or skin breakdown.

Equipment
Three sterile specimen containers • one bottle each of ordered cleaning solution, normal saline solution, and povidone-iodine solution • sterile, cotton-tipped applicators • sandbags or cervical collar (hard or soft) • fine mesh gauze strips • 4″ × 4″ gauze pads • sterile gloves • sterile basin • sterile scissors • hair clippers • optional: turning frame and antibacterial ointment

Preparation of equipment
Bring the equipment to the patient's room. Place the sterile specimen containers on the bedside table. Fill one with a small amount of cleaning solution, one with normal saline solution, and one with povidone-iodine solution. Then set out the cotton-tipped applicators. Keep the sandbags or cervical collar handy for emergency immobilization of the head and neck if the pins in the tongs should slip.

Implementation
▶ Explain the procedure to the patient and wash your hands. Inform the patient that pin sites usually feel tender for several days after the tongs are applied. Tell him that he'll also feel some muscular discomfort in the injured area.
▶ Before providing care, observe each pin site carefully for signs of infection, such as loose pins, swelling or redness, or purulent drainage. Use hair clippers to trim the patient's hair around the pin sites, when necessary, *to facilitate assessment.*

Types of skull tongs

Skull (or cervical) tongs consist of a stainless steel body with a pin at the end of each arm. Each pin is about ⅛″ (0.3 cm) in diameter and has a sharp tip.

On Crutchfield tongs, the pins are placed about 5″ (12.5 cm) apart in line with the long axis of the cervical spine.

On Gardner-Wells tongs, the pins are farther apart. They're inserted slightly above the patient's ears.

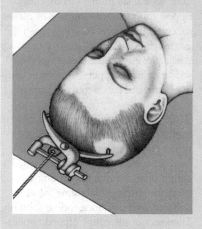

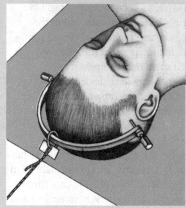

▶ Put on gloves and gently wipe each pin site with a cotton-tipped applicator dipped in cleaning solution *to loosen and remove crusty drainage.* Repeat with a fresh applicator as needed for thorough cleaning. Use a separate applicator for each site *to avoid cross-contamination.* Next, wipe each site with normal saline solution *to remove excess cleaning solution.* Finally, wipe with povidone-iodine solution *to provide asepsis at the site and prevent infection.*

▶ After providing care, discard all pin-site cleaning materials.

▶ If the pin sites are infected, apply a povidone-iodine wrap as ordered. First, obtain strips of fine mesh gauze or cut a 4″ × 4″ gauze pad into strips (using sterile scissors and wearing sterile gloves). Soak the strips in a sterile basin of povidone-iodine solution or normal saline solution as ordered and squeeze out the excess solution. Wrap one strip securely around each pin site. Leave the strip in place to dry until you provide care again. *Removing the dried strip aids in debridement and helps clear the infection.*

▶ Check the traction apparatus — rope, weights, and pulleys — at the start of each shift, every 4 hours, and as necessary (for example, after position changes). Make sure the rope hangs freely and that the weights never rest on the floor or become caught under the bed.

On Vinke tongs, the pins are placed at the parietal bones, near the widest transverse diameter of the skull, about 1″ (2.5 cm) above the helix.

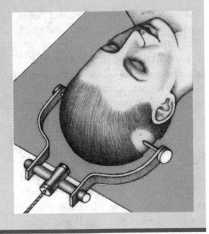

Special considerations

▶ Occasionally, the doctor may prefer an antibacterial ointment for pin-site care instead of povidone-iodine solution. *To remove old ointment,* wrap a cotton-tipped applicator with a 4″ × 4″ gauze pad, moisten it with cleaning solution, and gently clean each site. Keep a box of sterile gauze pads handy at the patient's bedside.

▶ Watch for signs and symptoms of loose pins, such as persistent pain or tenderness at pin sites, redness, and drainage. The patient may also report feeling or hearing the pins move.

▶ If you suspect a pin has loosened or slipped, don't turn the patient until the doctor examines the skull tongs and fixes them as needed.

▶ If the pins pull out, immobilize the patient's head and neck with sandbags or apply a cervical collar. Then carefully remove the traction weights. Apply manual traction to the patient's head by placing your hands on each side of the mandible and pulling very gently while maintaining proper alignment. After you stabilize the alignment, have someone send for the doctor immediately. Remain calm and reassure the patient. When traction is reestablished, take neurologic vital signs.

Nursing alert Never add or subtract weights to the traction apparatus without an order from the doctor. *Doing so can cause neurologic impairment.*

▶ Take neurologic vital signs at the beginning of each shift, every 4 hours, and as necessary (for example, after turning or transporting the patient). Carefully assess the function of cranial nerves, *which may be impaired by pin placement.* Note any asymmetry, deviation, or atrophy. Review the patient's chart to determine baseline neurologic vital signs on admission to the facility and immediately after the tongs were applied.

▶ Monitor respirations closely and keep suction equipment handy. Remember, injury to the cervical spine may affect respiration. Be alert for signs of respiratory distress, such as unequal chest expansion and an irregular or altered respiratory rate or pattern.

▶ Patients with skull tongs may be placed on a turning frame *to facilitate turning without disrupting vertebral alignment.* Establish a turning schedule for the patient (usually a supine position for 2 hours and then a prone position for 1 hour) *to help prevent complications of immobility.*

▶ Never remove a patient from the bed or turning frame when transporting him to another department.

Complications

Infection, excessive tractive force, or osteoporosis can cause the skull pins to slip or pull out. Because this interrupts traction, the patient must receive immediate attention to prevent further injury.

Documentation

Record the date, time, and type of pin-site care and the patient's response to the procedure in your notes. Describe any signs of infection. Also, note whether any weights were added or removed. Record neurologic vital signs, the patient's respiratory status, and the turning schedule on the Kardex.

SOAK APPLICATION

A soak application involves immersion of a body part in warm water or a medicated solution. This treatment helps to soften exudates, facilitate debridement, enhance suppuration, clean wounds or burns, rehydrate wounds, apply medication to infected areas, and increase local blood supply and circulation.

Most soaks are applied with clean tap water and clean technique. Sterile solution and sterile equipment are required for treating wounds, burns, and other breaks in the skin.

Key nursing diagnoses and patient outcomes

Impaired skin integrity related to (specify)
The patient will:

▶ show no evidence of skin breakdown

▶ have normal skin turgor

▶ regain skin integrity, exhibiting wound site healing

▶ communicate an understanding of skin protection measures

▶ demonstrate skill in care of wound site.

Risk for infection related to altered skin integrity
The patient will:

▶ have vital signs, temperature and laboratory values within normal limits

▶ have no pathogens in cultures

▶ remain free from signs or symptoms of infection at wound site.

Equipment

Basin or arm or foot tub • bath thermometer • hot tap water or prescribed solution • cup • pitcher • linen-saver pad • overbed table • footstool • pillows • towels • gauze pads and other dressing materials • clean and sterile gloves, if necessary

Preparation of equipment

Clean and disinfect the basin or tub. Run hot tap water into a pitcher or heat the prescribed solution as applicable. Measure the water or solution temperature with a bath thermometer. If the temperature isn't within the prescribed range (usually 105° to 110° F [40.6° to 43.3° C]), add hot or cold water or reheat or cool the solution as needed.

If you're preparing the soak outside the patient's room, heat the liquid slightly above the correct temperature to allow for cooling during transport. If the solution for a medicated soak isn't premixed, prepare the solution and heat it.

Implementation

▶ Check the doctor's order and assess the patient's condition.

▶ Explain the procedure to the patient and, if necessary, check his history for a previous allergic reaction to the medicated solution. Provide privacy. Wash your hands thoroughly.

▶ If the soak basin or tub will be placed in bed, make sure the bed is flat beneath it *to prevent spills.* For an arm soak, have the patient sit erect. For a leg or foot soak, ask him to lie down and bend the appropriate knee. For a foot soak in the sitting position, let him sit on the edge of the bed or transfer him to a chair.

▶ Place a linen-saver pad under the treatment site and, if necessary, cover the pad with a towel *to absorb spillage.*

▶ Expose the treatment site. Put on gloves before removing any dressing; dispose of the soiled dressing properly. If the dressing is encrusted and stuck to the wound, leave it in place and proceed with the soak. Remove the dressing several minutes later when it has begun to soak free.

▶ Position the soak basin under the treatment site on the bed, overbed table, footstool, or floor as appropriate. Pour the heated liquid into the soak basin or tub. Then lower the arm or leg into the basin gradually *to allow adjustment to the temperature change.* Make sure the soak solution covers the treatment site.

▶ Support other body parts with pillows or towels as needed *to prevent discomfort and muscle strain.* Make the patient comfortable and ensure proper body alignment.

▶ Check the temperature of the soak solution with the bath thermometer every 5 minutes. If the temperature drops below the prescribed range, remove some of the cooled solution with a cup. Then lift the patient's arm or leg from the basin *to avoid burns* and add hot water or solution to the basin. Mix the liquid thoroughly and then check its temperature. If the temperature is within the prescribed range, lower the patient's affected part back into the basin.

▶ Observe the patient for signs of tissue intolerance, such as extreme redness at the treatment site, excessive drainage, bleeding, or maceration. If such signs develop or the patient complains of pain, discontinue the treatment and notify the doctor.

▶ After 15 to 20 minutes or as ordered, lift the patient's arm or leg from the basin and remove the basin.

▶ Dry the arm or leg thoroughly with a towel. If the patient has a wound, dry the skin around it without touching the wound.

▶ While the skin is hydrated from the soak, use gauze pads to remove loose scales or crusts.

▶ Observe the treatment area for general appearance, degree of swelling, debridement, suppuration, and healing. Put on sterile gloves and re-dress the wound, if appropriate.

▶ Remove the towel and linen-saver pad and make the patient comfortable in bed.

▶ Discard the soak solution, dispose of soiled materials properly, and clean and disinfect the basin. Remove and discard your gloves. If the treatment is to be repeated, store the equipment in the patient's room, out of his reach; otherwise, return it to the central supply department.

Special considerations

To treat large areas, particularly burns, a soak may be administered in a whirlpool or Hubbard tank.

Documentation

Record the date, time, and duration of the soak; treatment site; solution and its temperature; skin and wound appearance before, during, and after treatment; and the patient's tolerance for treatment.

SPLINT APPLICATION

By immobilizing the site of an injury, a splint alleviates pain and allows the injury to heal in proper alignment. It also minimizes possible complications, such as excessive bleeding into tissues, restricted blood flow caused by bone pressing against vessels, and possible paralysis from an unstable spinal cord injury. In cases of multiple serious injuries, a splint or spine board allows caretakers to move the patient without risking further damage to bones, muscles, nerves, blood vessels, and skin.

A splint can be applied to immobilize a simple or compound fracture, a dislocation, or a subluxation. (See *Types of splints.*) During an emergency, any injury suspected of being a fracture, dislocation, or subluxation should be splinted. No contraindications exist for rigid splints; don't use traction splints for upper extremity injuries and open fractures.

Key nursing diagnoses and patient outcomes

Impaired physical mobility related to neuromuscular impairment
The patient will:

▶ maintain muscle strength and joint range of motion
▶ show no evidence of complications, such as contractures, venous stasis, thrombus formation, or skin breakdown.

Acute pain related to physical agents
The patient will:
▶ express feelings of comfort and relief from pain
▶ state and carry out appropriate interventions for pain relief.

Equipment

Rigid splint, spine board, traction splint or Velcro support splint • bindings • padding • sandbags or rolled towels or clothing • optional: roller gauze, cloth strips, sterile compress, and ice bag

Several commercial splints are widely available. Consult the manufacturer's instructions before applying the device. In an emergency, any long, sturdy object, such as a tree limb, mop handle, or broom — even a magazine — can be used to make a rigid splint for an extremity; a door can be used as a spine board.

An inflatable semirigid splint, called an air splint, sometimes can be used to secure an injured extremity. (See *Using an air splint,* page 752.) Velcro straps, 2″ roller gauze, or 2″ cloth strips can be used as bindings. When improvising, avoid using twine or rope, if possible, *because they can restrict circulation.*

Implementation

▶ Obtain a complete history of the injury, if possible, and begin a thorough head-to-toe assessment, inspecting for obvious deformities, swelling, or bleeding.

Types of splints

Three kinds of splints are commonly used to help provide support for injured or weakened limbs or to help correct deformities.

A rigid splint can be used to immobilize a fracture or dislocation in an extremity. Ideally, two people should apply a rigid splint to an extremity.

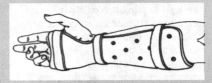

A traction splint immobilizes a fracture and exerts a longitudinal pull that reduces muscle spasms, pain, and arterial and neural damage. Used primarily for femoral fractures, a traction splint may also be applied for a fractured hip or tibia. Two trained people should apply a traction splint.

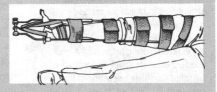

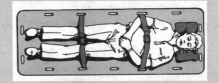

A spine board, applied for a suspected spinal fracture, is a rigid splint that supports the injured person's entire body. Three people should apply a spine board.

▶ Ask the patient if he can move the injured area (typically an extremity). Compare it bilaterally with the uninjured extremity, where applicable. Gently palpate the injured area; inspect for swelling, obvious deformities, bleeding, discoloration, and evidence of fracture or dislocation.

▶ Remove or cut away clothing from the injury site, if necessary. Check neurovascular integrity distal to the site. Explain the procedure to the patient *to allay his fears*.

▶ If an obvious bone misalignment causes the patient acute distress or severe neurovascular problems, align the extremity in its normal anatomic position, if possible. Stop, however, if this causes further neurovascular deterioration. Don't try to straighten a dislocation *to avoid damaging displaced vessels and nerves*. Also, don't attempt reduction of a contaminated bone end *because this may cause additional laceration of soft tissues, vessels, and nerves as well as gross contamination of deep tissues*.

▶ Apply a sterile compress to any open wound.

▶ Choose a splint that will immobilize the joints above and below the fracture; pad the splint as necessary *to protect bony prominences*.

Using an air splint

In an emergency, an air splint can be applied to immobilize a fracture or control bleeding, especially from a forearm or lower leg. This compact, comfortable splint is made of double-walled plastic and provides gentle, diffuse pressure over an injured area. The appropriate splint is chosen, wrapped around the affected extremity, secured with Velcro or other strips, and then inflated. The fit should be snug enough to immobilize the extremity without impairing circulation.

An air splint (shown below) may actually control bleeding better than a local pressure bandage. Its clear plastic construction simplifies inspection of the affected site for bleeding, pallor, or cyanosis. An air splint also allows the patient to be moved without further damage to the injured limb.

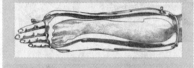

Applying a rigid splint

▶ Support the injured extremity above and below the fracture site while applying firm, gentle traction.
▶ Have an assistant place the splint under, beside, or on top of the extremity as ordered.
▶ Tell the assistant to apply the bindings *to secure the splint.*
▶ Assess the neurovascular status of the extremity; if it's impaired by the bindings, reapply them.

Applying a spine board

▶ Pad the spine board (or door) carefully, especially the areas that will support the lumbar region and knees, *to prevent uneven pressure and discomfort.*
▶ If the patient is lying on his back, place one hand on each side of his head and apply gentle traction to the head and neck, keeping the head aligned with the body. Have one assistant logroll the patient onto his side while another slides the spine board under the patient. Then instruct the assistants to roll the patient onto the board while you maintain traction and alignment.
▶ If the patient is prone, logroll him onto the board so he ends up in a supine position.
▶ *To maintain body alignment,* use strips of cloth to secure the patient on the spine board; *to keep head and neck aligned,* place sandbags or rolled towels or clothing on both sides of his head.

Applying a traction splint

▶ Specialized training is required before applying a traction splint.
▶ Place the splint beside the injured leg. (Never use a traction splint on an arm *because the major axillary plexus of nerves and blood vessels can't tolerate countertraction.*) Adjust the splint to the correct length and then open and adjust the Velcro straps.
▶ Have an assistant keep the leg motionless while you pad the ankle and foot and fasten the ankle hitch around them. (You may leave the shoe on.)
▶ Tell the assistant to lift and support the leg at the injury site as you apply firm, gentle traction.
▶ While you maintain traction, tell the assistant to slide the splint under the leg, pad the groin *to avoid excessive pressure on external genitalia,* and gently apply the ischial strap.

▶ Have the assistant connect the loops of the ankle hitch to the end of the splint.

▶ Adjust the splint to apply enough traction *to secure the leg comfortably in the corrected position.*

▶ After applying traction, fasten the Velcro support splints *to secure the leg closely to the splint.*

 Nursing alert Don't use a traction splint for a severely angulated femur or knee fracture.

Special considerations

▶ At the scene of an accident, always examine the patient completely for other injuries. Avoid unnecessary movement or manipulation, *which might cause additional pain or injury.*

▶ Always consider the possibility of cervical injury in an unconscious patient. If possible, apply the splint before repositioning the patient.

▶ If the patient requires a rigid splint but one isn't available, use another body part as a splint. To splint a leg in this manner, pad its inner aspect and secure it to the other leg with roller gauze or cloth strips.

▶ After applying any type of splint, monitor vital signs frequently *because bleeding in fractured bones and surrounding tissues may cause shock.* Also, monitor the neurovascular status of the fractured limb by assessing skin color, taking the patient's temperature, and checking for pain and numbness in the fingers or toes. *Numbness or paralysis distal to the injury indicates pressure on nerves.*

▶ Transport the patient as soon as possible to a health care facility. Apply ice to the injury. Regardless of the apparent extent of the injury, don't allow the pa-

tient to eat or drink anything until the doctor evaluates him.

▶ Indications for removing a splint include evidence of improper application or vascular impairment. Apply gentle traction and remove the splint carefully under a doctor's direct supervision.

Complications

Multiple transfers and repeated manipulation of a fracture may result in fat embolism, indicated by shortness of breath, agitation, and irrational behavior. This complication usually occurs 24 to 72 hours after injury or manipulation.

Documentation

Record the circumstances and cause of the injury. Document the patient's complaints, noting whether symptoms are localized. Also, record neurovascular status before and after applying the splint. Note the type of wound and the amount and type of drainage, if any. Document the time of splint application. If the bone end should slip into surrounding tissue or if transportation causes any change in the degree of dislocation, be sure to note it.

SPONGE BATH

A sponge bath with tepid water reduces fever by dilating superficial blood vessels, thus releasing heat and lowering body temperature. A tepid-water sponge bath may lower systemic temperature when routine fever treatments fail, particularly for infants and children, whose temperatures tend to rise very high, very quickly.

Key nursing diagnoses and patient outcomes

Ineffective thermoregulation related to trauma or illness

The patient will:

▶ maintain body temperature at normothermic levels

▶ demonstrate no signs of shivering

▶ have warm, dry skin

▶ maintain heart rate and blood pressure within normal range

▶ exhibit no signs of impaired neurologic status

▶ express a feeling of comfort.

Equipment

Basin of tepid water, about 80° to 93° F (26.7° to 33.9° C) • bath (utility) thermometer • bath blanket • linen-saver pad • washcloths • patient thermometer • hot-water bottle and cover • ice bag and cover • towel • patient gown • gloves, if the patient has open lesions or has been incontinent

Preparation of equipment

Prepare a hot-water bottle and an ice bag. Then place the bath thermometer in a basin and run water over it until the temperature reaches the high end of the tepid range (93° F) *because the water will cool during the bath*. Immerse the washcloths in the tepid solution until saturated.

Implementation

▶ Check the doctor's order and assess the patient's condition.

▶ Check the medication Kardex for recent administration of an antipyretic *because this can affect patient response to the bath*.

▶ Explain the procedure to the patient, provide privacy, and make sure the room is warm and free from drafts.

Wash your hands thoroughly and put on gloves, if necessary.

▶ Place a linen-saver pad under the patient *to catch any spills* and a bath blanket over him *for privacy*. Then remove his pajamas. Also remove the top bed linen *to avoid wetting it*.

▶ Take the patient's temperature, pulse, and respirations *to serve as a baseline*.

▶ Place the hot-water bottle with protective covering on the patient's feet *to reduce the sensation of chilliness*. Place the covered ice bag on his head *to prevent headache and nasal congestion that occur as the rest of the body cools*.

▶ Wring out each washcloth before sponging the patient *so they don't drip and cause discomfort*.

▶ Place moist washcloths over the major superficial blood vessels in the axillae, groin, and popliteal areas *to accelerate cooling*. Change the washcloths as they warm.

▶ Bathe each extremity separately for about 5 minutes; then sponge the chest and abdomen for 5 minutes. Turn the patient and bathe his back and buttocks for 5 to 10 minutes. Keep the patient covered except for the body part you're sponging.

▶ Pat each area dry after sponging but avoid rubbing with the towel *because rubbing increases cell metabolism and produces heat*.

▶ Add warm water to the basin as necessary *to maintain the desired water temperature*.

▶ Check the patient's temperature, pulse, and respirations every 10 minutes. Notify the doctor if the patient's temperature doesn't fall within 30 minutes. Stop the bath when the patient's temperature reaches 1° to 2° F (0.6° to 1.1° C) above the desired level *because his temperature will continue to fall natu-*

rally. Continue to monitor his temperature until it stabilizes.

▶ Observe the patient for chills, shivering, pallor, mottling, cyanosis of the lips or nail beds, and vital sign changes—especially a rapid, weak, or irregular pulse *because such signs may indicate an emergency.* If any of these signs occur, discontinue the bath, cover the patient lightly, and notify the doctor.

▶ If no adverse effects occur, bathe the patient for at least 30 minutes *to reduce his temperature.*

▶ After the bath, make sure the patient is dry and comfortable. Dress him in a fresh gown and cover him lightly.

▶ Dispose of liquids and soiled materials properly. If the treatment will be repeated, clean and store the equipment in the patient's room, out of his reach; otherwise, return the items to storage.

▶ Check the patient's temperature, pulse, and respirations 30 minutes after the bath *to determine the treatment's effectiveness.*

Special considerations

▶ If ordered, administer an antipyretic 15 to 20 minutes before the sponge bath *to achieve more rapid fever reduction.* Consider covering the patient's trunk with a wet towel for 15 minutes *to speed cooling.* Resaturate the towel as necessary.

▶ Refrain from bathing the breasts of a postpartum patient because they could become overly dry or fissures could develop on the nipples.

▶ Take a rectal or tympanic temperature, unless contraindicated, *for accuracy.* Axillary temperatures are unreliable *because the cool compresses applied to these areas alter the readings.* If you must take an oral temperature, do so cautiously *because chills may cause the pa-*

tient to bite down and shatter the thermometer. If possible, use an electronic thermometer to take a tympanic temperature *because it gives the temperature reading more quickly.*

Home care

Sponge baths to reduce fever are used most commonly in nonfacility settings; febrile patients in a health care facility usually receive antibiotics or antipyretics and, if needed, treatment with hypothermia blankets, which can lower and maintain body temperature more effectively than sponge baths.

Complications

Accelerated temperature reduction can provoke seizure activity.

Documentation

Record the date, time, and duration of the bath; the temperature of the solution; the patient's temperature, pulse, and respirations before, during, and after the procedure; any complications that arise; and the patient's tolerance for treatment.

Sputum collection

Secreted by mucous membranes lining the bronchioles, bronchi, and trachea, sputum helps protect the respiratory tract from infection. When expelled from the respiratory tract, sputum carries saliva, nasal and sinus secretions, dead cells, and normal oral bacteria from the respiratory tract. Sputum specimens may be cultured for identification of respiratory pathogens.

The usual method of sputum specimen collection, expectoration, may require ultrasonic nebulization, hydra-

Attaching a specimen trap to a suction catheter

Wearing gloves, push the suction tubing onto the male adapter of the in-line trap.

Insert the suction catheter into the rubber tubing of the trap.

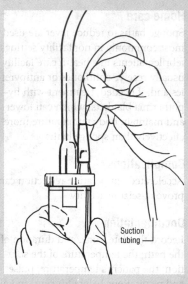

Suction tubing

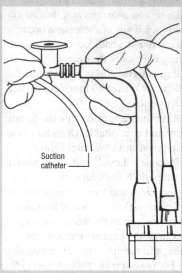

Suction catheter

tion, or chest percussion and postural drainage. Less common methods include tracheal suctioning and, rarely, bronchoscopy. Tracheal suctioning is contraindicated within 1 hour of eating and in patients with esophageal varices, nausea, facial or basilar skull fractures, laryngospasm, or bronchospasm. It should be performed cautiously in patients with heart disease because it may precipitate arrhythmias.

Key nursing diagnoses and patient outcomes

Ineffective breathing pattern related to decreased energy
The patient will:
▶ achieve maximum lung expansion with adequate ventilation

▶ report feeling comfortable with breathing.

Impaired gas exchange related to altered oxygen supply
The patient will:
▶ cough effectively
▶ expectorate sputum.

Equipment

For expectoration
Sterile specimen container with tight-fitting cap • gloves, if necessary • label • laboratory request form • aerosol (such as 10% sodium chloride, propylene glycol, acetylcysteine, or sterile or distilled water) as ordered

Implementation

▶ Tell the patient that you'll collect a specimen of sputum (not saliva) and explain the procedure to promote co-operation. If possible, collect the specimen early in the morning, before breakfast, *to obtain an overnight accumulation of secretions.*

Collection by expectoration

▶ Instruct the patient to sit in a chair or at the edge of the bed. If he can't sit up, place him in high Fowler's position.
▶ Ask the patient to rinse his mouth with water *to reduce specimen contamination.* (Avoid mouthwash or toothpaste *because they may affect the mobility of organisms in the sputum sample.*) Then tell him to cough deeply and expectorate directly into the specimen container. Ask him to produce at least 15 ml of sputum, if possible.
▶ Put on gloves.
▶ Cap the container and, if necessary, clean its exterior. Remove and discard your gloves, and wash your hands thoroughly. Label the container with the patient's name and room number, doctor's name, date and time of collection, and initial diagnosis. Also, include on the laboratory request form whether the patient was febrile or taking antibiotics and whether sputum was induced (*because such specimens commonly appear watery and may resemble saliva*). Send the specimen to the laboratory immediately.

Collection by tracheal suctioning

▶ If the patient can't produce an adequate specimen by coughing, prepare to suction him to obtain the specimen. Explain the suctioning procedure to him and tell him that he may cough, gag, or feel short of breath during the procedure.

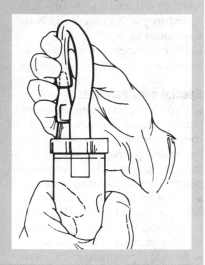

After suctioning, disconnect the in-line trap from the suction tubing and catheter. To seal the container, connect the rubber tubing to the male adapter of the trap.

For tracheal suctioning

#12 to #14 French sterile suction catheter • water-soluble lubricant • label • laboratory request form • sterile gloves • mask • sterile in-line specimen trap (Lukens trap) • normal saline solution • portable suction machine, if wall suction is unavailable • oxygen therapy equipment

Commercial suction kits have all equipment except the suction machine and an in-line specimen container.

Preparation of equipment

Equipment and preparation depend on the method of collection. Gather the appropriate equipment for the task.

► Check the suction equipment *to make sure it's functioning properly.* Then place the patient in high Fowler's or semi-Fowler's position.

► Administer oxygen to the patient before beginning the procedure.

► Wash your hands thoroughly.

► Position a mask over your face.

► Put on sterile gloves. Consider one hand sterile and the other hand clean *to prevent cross-contamination.*

► Connect the suction tubing to the male adapter of the in-line specimen trap. Attach the sterile suction catheter to the rubber tubing of the trap. (See *Attaching a specimen trap to a suction catheter,* pages 756 and 757.)

► Tell the patient to tilt his head back slightly. Then lubricate the catheter with normal saline solution and or water-soluble lubricant and gently pass it through the patient's nostril without suction.

► When the catheter reaches the larynx, the patient will cough. As he does, quickly advance the catheter into the trachea. Tell him to take several deep breaths through his mouth *to ease insertion.*

► To obtain the specimen, apply suction for 5 to 10 seconds but never longer than 15 seconds *because prolonged suction can cause hypoxia.* If the procedure must be repeated, let the patient rest for four to six breaths. When collection is completed, discontinue the suction, gently remove the catheter, and administer oxygen.

► Detach the catheter from the in-line trap, gather it up in your dominant hand, and pull the glove cuff inside out and down around the used catheter to enclose it for disposal. Remove and discard the other glove and your mask.

► Detach the trap from the tubing connected to the suction machine. Seal the trap tightly by connecting the rubber tubing to the male adapter of the trap. Examine the specimen *to make sure it's actually sputum, not saliva.* Label the trap's container as an expectorated specimen and send it to the laboratory immediately with a completed laboratory request form.

► Offer the patient a glass of water or mouthwash.

Special considerations

► If you can't obtain a sputum specimen through tracheal suctioning, perform chest percussion *to loosen and mobilize secretions,* and position the patient for optimal drainage. After 20 to 30 minutes, repeat the tracheal suctioning procedure.

► Before sending the specimen to the laboratory, examine it to make sure it's actually sputum, not saliva, *because saliva will produce inaccurate test results.*

► Because expectorated sputum is contaminated by normal mouth flora, tracheal suctioning provides a more reliable specimen for diagnosis.

► If the patient becomes hypoxic or cyanotic during suctioning, remove the catheter immediately and administer oxygen.

► If the patient has asthma or chronic bronchitis, watch for aggravated bronchospasms with the use of more than a 10% concentration of sodium chloride or acetylcysteine in an aerosol. If he's suspected of having tuberculosis, don't use more than 20% propylene glycol with water when inducing a sputum specimen *because a higher concentration inhibits growth of the pathogen and causes erroneous test results.* If propylene glycol isn't available, use 10% to 20% acetylcysteine with water or sodium chloride.

Complications

Patients with cardiac disease may develop arrhythmias during the procedure as a result of coughing, especially when the specimen is obtained by suctioning. Other potential complications include tracheal trauma or bleeding, vomiting, aspiration, and hypoxemia.

Documentation

In your notes, record the collection method used, time and date of collection, how the patient tolerated the procedure, color and consistency of the specimen, and its proper disposition.

STANDARD PRECAUTIONS

Standard precautions were developed by the Centers for Disease Control and Prevention (CDC) to provide the widest possible protection against the transmission of infection. CDC officials recommend that health care workers handle all blood, body fluids (including secretions, excretions, and drainage), tissues, and contact with mucous membranes and broken skin as if they contain infectious agents, regardless of the patient's diagnosis.

Standard precautions encompass much of the isolation precautions previously recommended by the CDC for patients with known or suspected blood-borne pathogens as well as the precautions previously known as body substance isolation. They're to be used in conjunction with other transmission-based precautions, including airborne, droplet, and contact precautions.

Standard precautions recommend wearing gloves for any known or anticipated contact with blood, body fluids, tissue, mucous membrane, and nonin-

tact skin. (See *Choosing the right glove,* page 760.) If the task or procedure being performed may result in splashing or splattering of blood or body fluids to the face, a mask and goggles or a face shield should be worn. If the task or procedure being performed may result in splashing or splattering of blood or body fluids to the body, a fluid-resistant gown or apron should be worn. Additional protective clothing, such as shoe covers, may be appropriate to protect the caregiver's feet in situations that may expose him to large amounts of blood or body fluids (or both) such as care of a trauma patient in the operating room or emergency department.

Airborne precautions are initiated in situations of suspected or known infections spread by the airborne route. The causative organisms are coughed, talked, or sneezed into the air by the infected person in droplets of moisture. The moisture evaporates, leaving the microorganisms suspended in the air to be breathed in by susceptible persons who enter the shared air space. Airborne precautions recommend placing the infected patient in a negative-pressure isolation room and the wearing of respiratory protection by all persons entering the patient's room.

Droplet precautions are used to protect health care workers and visitors from mucous membrane contact with oral and nasal secretions of the infected individual.

Contact precautions use barrier precautions to interrupt the transmission of specific epidemiologically important organisms by direct or indirect contact. Each institution must establish an infection control policy that lists specific barrier precautions.

Choosing the right glove

Health care workers may develop allergic reactions as a result of their exposure to latex gloves and other products containing natural rubber latex. Patients also may have latex sensitivity.

Take the following steps to protect yourself and your patient from allergic reactions to latex:

■ Use nonlatex (for example, vinyl or synthetic) gloves for activities that aren't likely to involve contact with infectious materials (such as food preparation, routine cleaning, and so forth).

■ Use appropriate barrier protection when handling infectious materials. If you choose latex gloves, use powder-free gloves with reduced protein content.

■ After wearing and removing gloves, wash your hands with soap and dry them thoroughly.

■ When wearing latex gloves, don't use oil-based hand creams or lotions (which can cause gloves to deteriorate) unless they have been shown to maintain glove barrier protection.

■ Refer to the material safety data sheet for the appropriate glove to wear when handling chemicals.

■ Learn procedures for preventing latex allergy, and learn how to recognize the following signs of latex allergy: skin rashes; hives; flushing; itching; nasal, eye, or sinus symptoms; asthma; and shock.

■ If you have (or suspect you have) a latex sensitivity, use nonlatex gloves, avoid contact with latex gloves and other latex-containing products, and consult a physician experienced in treating latex allergy.

For latex allergy

If you have latex allergy, consider the following precautions:

■ Avoid contact with latex gloves and other products that contain latex.

■ Avoid areas where you might inhale the powder from latex gloves worn by other workers.

■ Inform your employers and your health care providers (such as doctors, nurses, dentists, and others).

■ Wear a medical alert bracelet.

■ Follow your doctor's instructions for dealing with allergic reactions to latex.

Key nursing diagnoses and patient outcomes

Risk for infection related to hospital admission

The patient will:

▶ have vital signs, temperature, and laboratory values within normal limits

▶ remain free from all signs and symptoms of infection

▶ state factors that put him at risk for infection

▶ identify signs and symptoms of infection.

Equipment

Gloves • face shields or masks and goggles or glasses • gowns or aprons • resuscitation bag • bags for specimens • Environmental Protection Agency (EPA)–registered tuberculocidal disinfectant or diluted bleach solution (diluted between 1:10 and 1:100, mixed fresh daily), or both, or EPA-registered disinfectant labeled effective against hepatitis B virus (HBV) and human immunodeficiency virus (HIV)

Implementation

▶ Wash your hands immediately if they become contaminated with blood or body fluids, excretions, secretions, or drainage; also, wash your hands before and after patient care and after removing gloves. *Hand washing removes microorganisms from your skin.*

▶ Wear gloves if you will or could come in contact with blood, specimens, tissue, body fluids, secretions or excretions, mucous membrane, broken skin, or contaminated surfaces or objects.

▶ Change your gloves and wash your hands between patient contacts *to avoid cross-contamination.*

▶ Wear a fluid-resistant gown or apron and face shield or a mask and glasses or goggles during procedures likely to generate splashing or splattering of blood or body fluids, such as surgery, endoscopic procedures, dialysis, assisting with intubation or manipulation of arterial lines, or any other procedure with potential for splashing or splattering of body fluids.

▶ Handle used needles and other sharp instruments carefully. Don't bend, break, reinsert them into their original sheaths, remove needles from syringes, or unnecessarily handle them. Discard them intact immediately after use into a puncture-resistant disposal box. Use tools to pick up broken glass or other sharp objects. *These measures reduce the risk of accidental injury or infection.*

▶ Immediately notify your employer health care provider of all needle-stick or other sharp object injuries, mucosal splashes, or contamination of open wounds or nonintact skin with blood or body fluids *to allow investigation of the incident and appropriate care and documentation.*

▶ Properly label all specimens collected from patients and place them in plastic bags at the collection site. Attach requisition slips to the outside of the bag.

▶ Place all items that have come in direct contact with the patient's secretions, excretions, blood, drainage, or body fluids — such as nondisposable utensils or instruments — in a single impervious bag or container before removal from the room. Place linens and trash in single bags of sufficient thickness to contain the contents.

▶ While wearing the appropriate personal protective equipment, promptly clean all blood and body fluid spills with detergent and water followed by an EPA-registered tuberculocidal disinfectant or diluted bleach solution (diluted between 1:10 and 1:100, mixed daily), or both, or an EPA-registered disinfectant labeled effective against HBV and HIV, provided that the surface hasn't been contaminated with agents or volumes of or concentrations of agents for which higher-level disinfection is recommended.

▶ Disposable food trays and dishes aren't necessary.

▶ If you have an exudative lesion, avoid all direct patient contact until the condition has resolved and you've been cleared by the employer health care provider.

▶ If you have dermatitis or other conditions resulting in broken skin on your hands, avoid situations where you may have contact with blood and body fluids (even though gloves could be worn) until the condition has resolved and you've been cleared by the employee health provider.

Special considerations

▶ Standard precautions, such as hand washing and appropriate use of personal protective equipment, should be routine infection control practices.

▶ Keep mouthpieces, resuscitation bags, and other ventilation devices nearby *to minimize the need for emergency mouth-to-mouth resuscitation, thus reducing the risk of exposure to body fluids.*

**ɪ|ɪ   *Nursing alert* Because you may
≡■≡   not always know what or-
ɪ|ɪ   ganisms may be present in
every clinical situation, you must use
standard precautions for every contact with blood, body fluids, secretions, excretions, drainage, mucous membranes, and nonintact skin. Use your judgment in individual cases about whether to implement additional isolation precautions, such as airborne, droplet, or contact precautions or a combination of them. In addition, if your work requires you to be exposed to blood, you should receive the HBV vaccine series.**

Complications

Failure to follow standard precautions may lead to exposure to blood-borne diseases or other infections and to all the complications they may cause.

Documentation

Record any special needs for isolation precautions on the nursing plan of care and as otherwise indicated by your facility.

STOOL COLLECTION

Stool specimens are collected to determine the presence of blood, ova and parasites, bile, fat, pathogens, or such substances as ingested drugs. Gross examination of stool characteristics, such as color, consistency, and odor, can reveal such conditions as GI bleeding and steatorrhea.

Stool specimens are collected randomly or for specific periods such as 72 hours. Because stool specimens can't be obtained on demand, proper collection requires careful instructions to the patient to ensure an uncontaminated specimen.

Key nursing diagnoses and patient outcomes

Diarrhea related to irritation of bowel
The patient will:
▶ have elimination pattern return to normal
▶ regain and maintain fluid and electrolyte balance.

Equipment

Specimen container with lid • gloves • two tongue blades • paper towel • bedpan or portable commode • two patient-care reminders (for timed specimens) • laboratory request form • optional: enema

Implementation

▶ Explain the procedure to the patient and to the family members, if possible, *to ensure their cooperation and prevent inadvertent disposal of timed stool specimens.*

Collecting a random specimen

▶ Tell the patient to notify you when he has the urge to defecate. Have him defecate into a clean, dry bedpan or commode. Instruct him not to contaminate the specimen with urine or toilet tissue *because urine inhibits fecal bacterial growth and toilet tissue contains bismuth, which interferes with test results.*

▶ Put on gloves.

▶ Using a tongue blade, transfer the most representative stool specimen from the bedpan to the container and cap the container. If the patient passes blood, mucus, or pus with the stool, include this with the specimen.

▶ Wrap the tongue blade in a paper towel and discard it. Remove and discard your gloves and wash your hands thoroughly *to prevent cross-contamination.*

Collecting a timed specimen

▶ Place a patient-care reminder stating SAVE ALL STOOLS over the patient's bed, in his bathroom, and in the utility room.

▶ After putting on gloves, collect the first specimen, and include this in the total specimen.

▶ Obtain the timed specimen as you would a random specimen, but remember to transfer all stools to the specimen container.

▶ If a stool specimen must be obtained with an enema, use only tap water or normal saline solution.

▶ As ordered, send each specimen to the laboratory immediately with a laboratory request form or, if permitted, refrigerate the specimens collected during the test period and send them when collection is complete. Remove and discard gloves.

▶ Make sure the patient is comfortable after the procedure and that he has the opportunity to thoroughly clean his hands and perianal area. Perineal care may be necessary for some patients.

Special considerations

▶ Never place a stool specimen in a refrigerator that contains food or medication *to prevent contamination.*

▶ Notify the doctor if the stool specimen looks unusual.

Home care

If the patient is to collect a specimen at home, instruct him to collect it in a clean container with a tight-fitting lid, wrap the container in a brown paper bag, and keep it in the refrigerator (separate from any food items) until it can be transported.

Documentation

Record the time of the specimen collection and transport to the laboratory. Note stool color, odor, and consistency, and any unusual characteristics; also, note whether the patient had difficulty passing the stool.

STUMP AND PROSTHESIS CARE

Patient care directly after limb amputation includes monitoring drainage from the stump, positioning the affected limb, assisting with exercises prescribed by a physical therapist, and wrapping and conditioning the stump. Postoperative care of the stump will vary slightly, depending on the amputation site (arm or leg) and the type of dressing applied to the stump (elastic bandage or plaster cast).

After the stump heals, it requires only routine daily care, such as proper hygiene and continued muscle-strengthening exercises. The prosthesis, when in use, also requires daily care. Typically, a plastic prosthesis, the most common type, must be cleaned and lubricated and checked for proper fit. As the patient recovers from the physical and psychological trauma of amputation, he'll need to learn correct procedures for routine daily care of the stump and the prosthesis.

Key nursing diagnoses and patient outcomes

Impaired physical mobility related to neuromuscular impairment
The patient will:
▶ maintain muscle strength and joint range of motion (ROM)
▶ show no evidence of complications, such as contractures, venous stasis, thrombus formation, or skin breakdown.

Chronic pain related to medical condition
The patient will:
▶ state feelings of comfort and relief from pain
▶ state and carry out appropriate interventions for pain relief.

Equipment

For postoperative stump care
Pressure dressing • abdominal (ABD) pad • suction equipment, if ordered • overhead trapeze • 1″ adhesive tape, bandage clips or safety pins • sandbags or trochanter roll (for a leg) • elastic stump shrinker or 4″ elastic bandage • optional: tourniquet (as a last resort to control bleeding)

For stump and prosthesis care
Mild soap or alcohol pads • stump socks or athletic tube socks • two washcloths • two towels • appropriate lubricating oil

Implementation

▶ Perform routine postoperative care. Frequently assess respiratory status and level of consciousness, monitor vital signs and I.V. infusions, check tube patency, and provide for the patient's comfort and safety.

Monitoring stump drainage

▶ *Because gravity causes fluid to accumulate at the stump,* frequently check the amount of blood and drainage on the dressing. Notify the doctor if accumulations of drainage or blood increase rapidly. If excessive bleeding occurs, notify the doctor immediately and apply a pressure dressing or compress the appropriate pressure points. If this doesn't control bleeding, use a tourniquet only as a last resort. Keep a tourniquet available, if needed.
▶ Tape the ABD pad over the moist part of the dressing as needed. *Providing a dry area helps prevent bacterial infection.*
▶ Monitor the suction drainage equipment and note the amount and type of drainage.

Positioning the extremity

▶ Elevate the extremity for the first 24 hours *to reduce swelling and promote venous return.*
▶ *To prevent contractures,* position an arm with the elbow extended and the shoulder abducted.
▶ *To correctly position a leg,* elevate the foot of the bed slightly and place sandbags or a trochanter roll against the hip *to prevent external rotation.*

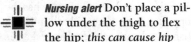 **Nursing alert** Don't place a pillow under the thigh to flex the hip; *this can cause hip flexion contracture.* For the same reason, tell the patient to avoid prolonged sitting.
▶ After a below-the-knee amputation, maintain knee extension *to prevent hamstring muscle contractures.*

▶ After any leg amputation, place the patient on a firm surface in the prone position for at least 2 hours per day with his legs close together and without pillows under his stomach, hips, knees, or stump, unless this position is contraindicated. *This position helps prevent hip flexion, contractures, and abduction; it also stretches the flexor muscles.*

Assisting with prescribed exercises

▶ After arm amputation, encourage the patient to exercise the remaining arm *to prevent muscle contractures.* Help the patient perform isometric and ROM exercises for both shoulders as prescribed by the physical therapist *because use of the prosthesis requires both shoulders.*

▶ After leg amputation, stand behind the patient and, if necessary, support him with your hands at his waist during balancing exercises.

▶ Instruct the patient to exercise the affected and unaffected limbs *to maintain muscle tone and increase muscle strength.* A patient with a leg amputation may perform push-ups as ordered (in the sitting position, arms at his sides) or pull-ups on the overhead trapeze *to strengthen his arms, shoulders, and back in preparation for using crutches.*

Wrapping and conditioning the stump

▶ If the patient doesn't have a rigid cast, apply an elastic stump shrinker *to prevent edema* and shape the limb in preparation for the prosthesis. Wrap the stump so that it narrows toward the distal end. *This helps to ensure comfort when the patient wears the prosthesis.*

▶ If an elastic stump shrinker isn't available, you can wrap the stump in a 4″ elastic bandage. To do this, stretch the bandage to about two-thirds its

maximum length as you wrap it diagonally around the stump, with the greatest pressure distally. (Depending on the size of the leg, you may need to use two 4″ bandages.) Secure the bandage with clips, safety pins, or adhesive tape. Make sure the bandage covers all portions of the stump smoothly *because wrinkles or exposed areas encourage skin breakdown.* (See *Wrapping a stump*, page 766.)

▶ If the patient experiences throbbing after the stump is wrapped, the bandage may be too tight; remove the bandage immediately and reapply it less tightly. *Throbbing indicates impaired circulation.*

▶ Check the bandage regularly. Rewrap it when it begins to bunch up at the end (usually about every 12 hours for a moderately active patient) or as necessary.

▶ After removing the bandage to rewrap it, massage the stump gently, always pushing toward the suture line rather than away from it. *This stimulates circulation and prevents scar tissue from adhering to the bone.*

▶ When healing begins, instruct the patient to push the stump against a pillow. Then have him progress gradually to pushing against harder surfaces, such as a padded chair, then a hard chair. *These conditioning exercises will help the patient adjust to experiencing pressure and sensation in the stump.*

Caring for the healed stump

▶ Bathe the stump but never shave it *to prevent infection.* If possible, bathe the stump at the end of the day *because the warm water may cause swelling, making reapplication of the prosthesis difficult.* Don't soak the stump for long periods of time.

Wrapping a stump

Proper stump care helps protect the limb, reduces swelling, and prepares the limb for a prosthesis. As you perform the procedure, teach it to the patient.

Start by obtaining two 4″ elastic bandages. Center the end of the first 4″ bandage at the top of the patient's thigh. Unroll the bandage downward over the stump and to the back of the leg.

Make three figure-eight turns to adequately cover the ends of the stump. As you wrap, include the roll of flesh in the groin area. Use enough pressure to ensure that the stump narrows toward the end so that it fits comfortably into the prosthesis.

Use the second 4″ bandage to anchor the first bandage around the waist. For a below-the-knee amputation, use the knee to anchor the bandage in place. Secure the bandage with clips, safety pins, or adhesive tape. Check the stump bandage regularly and rewrap it if it bunches at the end.

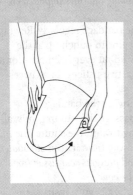 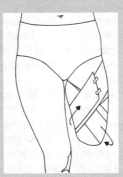 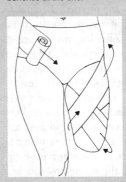

▶ Don't apply lotion to the stump; this may clog hair follicles, which increases the risk of infection.

▶ Inspect the stump for redness, swelling, irritation, and calluses. Report any of these to the doctor. Tell the patient to avoid putting weight on the stump. (The skin should be firm but not taut over the bony end of the limb.)

▶ Continue muscle-strengthening exercises *so the patient can build the strength he'll need to control the prosthesis.*

▶ Change and wash the patient's elastic bandages every day *to avoid exposing the*

skin to excessive perspiration, which can be irritating. Wash the elastic bandages in warm water and gentle, nondetergent soap; lay them flat on a towel to dry. Machine washing or drying may shrink the elastic bandages. *To shape the stump,* an elastic bandage should be worn 24 hours per day except while bathing.

Caring for the plastic prosthesis

▶ Wipe the plastic socket of the prosthesis with a damp washcloth and mild soap or alcohol *to prevent bacterial accumulation*.

▶ Wipe the insert (if the prosthesis has one) with a dry washcloth.

▶ Dry the prosthesis thoroughly; if possible, allow it to dry overnight.

▶ Maintain and lubricate the prosthesis as instructed by the manufacturer.

▶ Check for malfunctions and adjust or repair the prosthesis as necessary *to prevent further damage*.

▶ Check the condition of the shoe on a foot prosthesis frequently and change it as necessary.

Applying the prosthesis

▶ Apply a stump sock. Keep the seams away from bony prominences.

▶ If the prosthesis has an insert, remove it from the socket, place it over the stump, and insert the stump into the prosthesis.

▶ If it has no insert, merely slide the prosthesis over the stump. Secure the prosthesis onto the stump according to the manufacturer's directions.

Special considerations

▶ If a patient arrives at the facility with a traumatic amputation, the amputated part may be saved for possible reimplantation. (See *Caring for an amputated body part,* page 768.)

▶ Teach the patient how to care for his stump and prosthesis properly. Make sure he knows signs and symptoms that indicate problems in the stump. Explain that a 10-lb (4.5-kg) change in body weight will alter his stump size and require a new prosthesis socket *to ensure a correct fit*.

▶ Exercise of the remaining muscles in an amputated limb must begin the day after surgery. A physical therapist will direct these exercises. For example, arm exercises progress from isometrics to assisted ROM to active ROM. Leg exercises include rising from a chair, balancing on one leg, and ROM exercises of the knees and hips.

▶ For a below-the-knee amputation, you may substitute an athletic tube sock for a stump sock by cutting off the elastic band. If the patient has a rigid plaster of paris dressing, perform normal cast care. Check the cast frequently to make sure it doesn't slip off. If it does, apply an elastic bandage immediately and notify the doctor *because edema will develop rapidly*.

Home care

Emphasize to the patient that proper care of his stump can speed healing. Tell him to inspect his stump carefully every day using a mirror and to continue proper daily stump care. Instruct him to call the doctor if the incision appears to be opening, looks red or swollen, feels warm, is painful to touch, or is seeping drainage.

Tell the patient to massage the stump toward the suture line *to mobilize the scar and prevent its adherence to bone*. Advise him to avoid exposing the skin around the stump to excessive perspiration, which can be irritating. Tell him to change his elastic bandages or stump socks daily to avoid this.

Tell the patient that he may experience twitching, spasms, or phantom limb pain as his stump muscles adjust to amputation. Advise him that he can decrease these symptoms with heat, massage, or gentle pressure. If his stump is sensitive to touch, tell him to rub it with a dry washcloth for 4 minutes three times per day.

Stress the importance of performing prescribed exercises *to help minimize*

Caring for an amputated body part

After traumatic amputation, a surgeon may be able to reimplant the severed body part through microsurgery. The chance of successful reimplantation is much greater if the amputated part has received proper care.

If a patient arrives at the hospital with a severed body part, first make sure that bleeding at the amputation site has been controlled. Then use the following guidelines for preserving the body part.

■ Put on sterile gloves. Place several sterile gauze pads and an appropriate amount of sterile roller gauze in a sterile basin, and pour sterile normal saline or sterile lactated Ringer's solution over them. *Note:* Never use any other solution and don't try to scrub or debride the part.

■ Holding the body part in one gloved hand, carefully pat it dry with sterile gauze. Place saline-soaked gauze pads over the stump; then wrap the whole body part with saline-soaked roller gauze. Wrap the gauze with a sterile towel, if available. Then put this package in a watertight container or bag and seal it.

■ Fill another plastic bag with ice and place the part, still in its watertight container, inside. Seal the outer bag. (Always protect the part from direct contact with ice — and never use dry ice — *to prevent irreversible tissue damage, which would make the part unsuit-*

able for reimplantation.) Keep this bag ice-cold until the doctor is ready to do the reimplantation surgery.

■ Label the bag with the patient's name, identification number, identification of the amputated part, the facility's identification number, and the date and time when cooling began.

Note: The body part must be wrapped and cooled quickly. *Irreversible tissue damage occurs after only 6 hours at ambient temperature.* However, hypothermic management seldom preserves tissues for more than 24 hours.

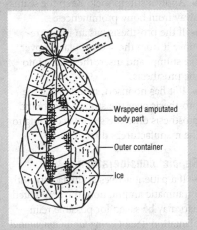

Wrapped amputated body part
Outer container
Ice

---

complications, maintain muscle strength and tone, prevent contractures, and promote independence. Also, stress the importance of positioning *to prevent contractures and edema.*

Complications

The most common postoperative complications include hemorrhage, stump infection, contractures, and a swollen

or flabby stump. Complications that may develop at any time after an amputation include skin breakdown or irritation from lack of ventilation; friction from an irritant in the prosthesis; a sebaceous cyst or boil from tight socks; psychological problems, such as denial, depression, or withdrawal; and phantom limb pain caused by stimulation of nerves that once carried sensations from the distal part of the extremity.

Documentation

Record the date, time, and specific procedures of all postoperative care, including amount and type of drainage, condition of the dressing, need for dressing reinforcement, and appearance of the suture line and surrounding tissue. Also, note any signs of skin irritation or infection, any complications and the nursing action taken, the patient's tolerance of exercises, and his psychological reaction to the amputation.

During routine daily care, document the date, time, type of care given, and condition of the skin and suture line, noting any signs or symptoms of irritation, such as redness or tenderness. Also, note the patient's progress in caring for the stump or prosthesis.

SUBCUTANEOUS INJECTION

When injected into the adipose (fatty) tissues beneath the skin, a drug moves into the bloodstream more rapidly than if given by mouth. Subcutaneous (S.C.) injection allows slower, more sustained drug administration than I.M. injection; it also causes minimal tissue trauma and carries little risk of striking large blood vessels and nerves.

Absorbed mainly through the capillaries, drugs recommended for S.C. injection include nonirritating aqueous solutions and suspensions contained in 0.5 to 2 ml of fluid. Heparin and insulin, for example, are usually administered S.C. (Some diabetic patients,

however, may benefit from an insulin infusion pump.)

Drugs and solutions for S.C. injection are injected through a relatively short needle, using meticulous sterile technique. The most common S.C. injection sites are the outer aspect of the upper arm, anterior thigh, loose tissue of the lower abdomen, upper hips, buttocks, and upper back. (See *Locating subcutaneous injection sites,* page 770.) Injection is contraindicated in sites that are inflamed, edematous, scarred, or covered by a mole, birthmark, or other lesion. It may also be contraindicated in patients with impaired coagulation mechanisms.

Key nursing diagnoses and patient outcomes

Deficient knowledge related to lack of exposure to subcutaneous injection
The patient will:
▶ state or demonstrate an understanding of what has been taught
▶ demonstrate the ability to perform new health-related behaviors as taught.

Risk for injury related to improper technique
The patient will:
▶ identify factors that increase the risk of injury
▶ assist in identifying safety measures to prevent injury.

Equipment

Prescribed medication • patient's medication record and chart • 25G to 27G ⅝" to ½" needle • gloves • 1- or 3-ml syringe • alcohol pads • optional: antiseptic cleaning agent, filter needle, and insulin syringe

Locating subcutaneous injection sites

Subcutaneous (S.C.) injection sites (as indicated by the dotted areas shown at right) include the fat pads on the abdomen, upper hips, upper back, and lateral upper arms and thighs. For S.C. injections administered repeatedly, such as insulin, rotate sites. Choose one injection site in one area, move to a corresponding injection site in the next area, and so on.

When returning to an area, choose a new site in that area. Preferred injection sites for insulin are the arms, abdomen, thighs, and buttocks. The preferred injection site for heparin is the lower abdominal fat pad just below the umbilicus.

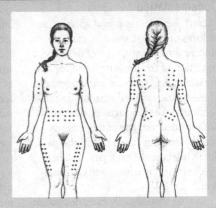

Preparation of equipment

Verify the order on the patient's medication record by checking it against the doctor's order. Also, note whether the patient has any allergies, especially before the first dose.

Inspect the medication *to make sure it isn't abnormally discolored or cloudy and doesn't contain precipitates* (unless the manufacturer's instructions allow it).

Wash your hands. Choose equipment appropriate to the prescribed medication and injection site and make sure it works properly.

Check the medication label against the patient's medication record. Read the label again as you draw up the medication for injection.

For single-dose ampules

Wrap an alcohol pad around the ampule's neck and snap off the top, directing the force away from your body. Attach a filter needle to the needle and withdraw the medication, keeping the needle's bevel tip below the level of the solution. Tap the syringe *to clear any air from it.* Cover the needle with the needle sheath.

Before discarding the ampule, check the medication label against the patient's medication record. Discard the filter needle and the ampule. Attach the appropriate needle to the syringe.

For single-dose or multidose vials

Reconstitute powdered drugs according to instructions. Make sure all crystals have dissolved in the solution. Warm the vial by rolling it between your palms to help the drug dissolve faster.

Clean the vial's rubber stopper with an alcohol pad. Pull the syringe plunger back until the volume of air in the syringe equals the volume of drug to be withdrawn from the vial.

Without inverting the vial, insert the needle into the vial. Inject the air, invert the vial, and keep the needle's bevel tip below the level of the solution as you withdraw the prescribed amount of medication. Cover the needle with the needle sheath. Tap the syringe *to clear any air from it.*

Check the medication label against the patient's medication record before discarding the single-dose vial or returning the multidose vial to the shelf.

Implementation

▶ Confirm the patient's identity by asking his name and checking the name, room number, and bed number on his wristband.

▶ Explain the procedure to the patient and provide privacy.

▶ Select an appropriate injection site. Rotate sites according to a schedule for repeated injections, using different areas of the body unless contraindicated. (Heparin, for example, should be injected only in the abdomen, if possible.)

▶ Put on gloves.

▶ Position the patient and expose the injection site.

▶ Clean the injection site with an alcohol pad, beginning at the center of the site and moving outward in a circular motion. Allow the skin to dry before injecting the drug *to avoid a stinging sensation from introducing alcohol into subcutaneous tissues.*

▶ Loosen the protective needle sheath.

▶ With your nondominant hand, grasp the skin around the injection site firmly to elevate the subcutaneous tissue, forming a 1″ (2.5-cm) fat fold.

▶ Holding the syringe in your dominant hand, insert the loosened needle sheath between the fourth and fifth fingers of your other hand while still pinching the skin around the injection site. Pull back the syringe with your dominant hand *to uncover the needle by*

Technique for subcutaneous injections

Before giving the injection, elevate the subcutaneous tissue at the site by grasping it firmly.

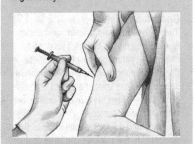

Insert the needle at a 45- or 90-degree angle to the skin surface, depending on needle length and the amount of subcutaneous tissue at the site. Some medications, such as heparin, should always be injected at a 90-degree angle.

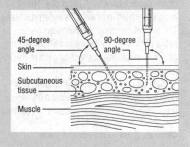

grasping the syringe like a pencil. Don't touch the needle.

▶ Position the needle with its bevel up.

▶ Tell the patient he'll feel a needle prick.

▶ Insert the needle quickly in one motion at a 45- or 90-degree angle. (See *Technique for subcutaneous injections.*) Release the patient's skin *to avoid injecting the drug into compressed tissue and irritating nerve fibers.*

Types of insulin infusion pumps

A subcutaneous insulin infusion pump provides continuous, long-term insulin therapy for patients with type 1 diabetes mellitus. Complications include infection at the injection site, catheter clogging, and insulin loss from loose reservoir-catheter connections. Insulin pumps work on either an open-loop or a closed-loop system.

Open-loop system

The open-loop pump is used most commonly. It infuses insulin but can't respond to changes in serum glucose levels. These portable, self-contained, programmable insulin pumps are smaller and less obtrusive than ever—about the size of a credit card—and have fewer buttons.

The pump delivers insulin in small (basal) doses every few minutes and large (bolus) doses that the patient sets manually. The system consists of a reservoir containing the insulin syringe, a small pump, an infusion-rate selector that allows insulin release adjustments, a battery, and a plastic catheter with an attached needle leading from the syringe to the subcutaneous injection site. The needle is typically held in place with waterproof tape. The patient can wear the pump on his belt or in his pocket—practically anywhere as long as the infusion line has a clear path to the injection site.

The infusion-rate selector automatically releases about one-half the total daily insulin requirement. The patient releases the remain-

der in bolus doses before meals and snacks. The patient must change the syringe daily; he must change the needle, catheter, and injection site every other day.

Closed-loop system

The self-contained closed-loop system detects and responds to changing serum glucose levels. The typical closed-loop system includes a glucose sensor, a programmable computer, a power supply, a pump, and an insulin reservoir. The computer triggers continuous insulin delivery in appropriate amounts from the reservoir.

Nonneedle catheter system

In the nonneedle delivery system, a tiny plastic catheter is inserted into the skin over a needle using a special insertion device (shown below). The needle is then withdrawn, leaving the catheter in place (shown in inset). This catheter can be placed in the abdomen, thigh, or flank and should be changed every 2 to 3 days.

Close-up of open-loop infusion pump

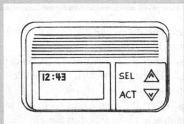

Nonneedle catheter insertion system

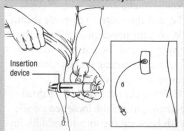

▶ Pull back the plunger slightly *to check for blood return*. If none appears, begin injecting the drug slowly. If blood appears on aspiration, withdraw the needle, prepare another syringe, and repeat the procedure.

▶ Don't aspirate for blood return when giving insulin or heparin. *It isn't necessary with insulin and may cause a hematoma with heparin.*

▶ After injection, remove the needle gently but quickly at the same angle used for insertion.

▶ Cover the site with an alcohol pad and massage the site gently (unless contraindicated as with heparin and insulin) *to distribute the drug and facilitate absorption.*

▶ Remove the alcohol pad and check the injection site for bleeding and bruising.

▶ Dispose of injection equipment according to your facility's policy. *To avoid needle-stick injuries,* don't resheath the needle.

Special considerations
▶ When using prefilled syringes, adjust the angle and depth of insertion according to needle length.

For insulin injections
▶ *To establish more consistent blood insulin levels,* rotate insulin injection sites within anatomic regions. Preferred insulin injection sites are the arms, abdomen, thighs, and buttocks.

▶ Make sure the type of insulin, unit dosage, and syringe are correct.

▶ When combining insulins in a syringe, make sure they're compatible. Regular insulin can be mixed with all other types. Prompt insulin zinc suspension (semilente insulin) can't be mixed with NPH insulin. Follow your facility's policy regarding which insulin to draw up first.

▶ Before drawing up insulin suspension, gently roll and invert the bottle. Don't shake the bottle *because this can cause foam or bubbles to develop in the syringe.*

▶ Insulin may be administered through an inserted insulin pump. However, before administering the drug, make sure the patient doesn't already have a pump in place. (See *Types of insulin infusion pumps.*)

For heparin injections
▶ The preferred site for a heparin injection is the lower abdominal fat pad, 2″ (5 cm) beneath the umbilicus, between the right and left iliac crests. *Injecting heparin into this area, which isn't involved in muscle activity, reduces the risk of local capillary bleeding.* Always rotate the sites from one side to the other.

▶ Inject the drug slowly into the fat pad. Leave the needle in place for 10 seconds after injection; then withdraw it.

▶ Don't administer an injection within 2″ of a scar, a bruise, or the umbilicus.

▶ Don't aspirate to check for blood return *because this can cause bleeding into the tissues at the site.*

▶ Don't rub or massage the site after the injection. *Rubbing can cause localized minute hemorrhages or bruises.*

▶ If the patient bruises easily, apply ice to the site for the first 5 minutes after the injection *to minimize local hemorrhage and then apply pressure.*

Complications
Concentrated or irritating solutions may cause sterile abscesses to form. Repeated injections in the same site can cause lipodystrophy. A natural immune

Better charting
Guidelines for documenting medication administration

When using the medication administration record (MAR), use the following guidelines:
- Know and follow your facility's policies and procedures for recording drug orders and charting drug administration.
- Make sure that all drug orders include the patient's full name, the date, and the drug's name, dose, administration route or method, and frequency.
- When appropriate, include the specific number of doses given or the stop date.
- When administering a drug dose immediately, or stat, record the time.
- Include drug allergy information.
- Write legibly.
- Use only standard abbreviations approved by the facility.
- When doubtful about an abbreviation, write out the word or phrase.

- After administering the first dose, sign your full name, licensure status, and initials in the appropriate space on the MAR.
- Record drugs immediately after administration *so that another nurse doesn't give the drug again.*
- If you document medication administration by computer, chart your information for each drug immediately after you give it. This is particularly important if you don't use printouts as a backup. By keying in information immediately, you ensure that all health care team members have access to the latest drug administration data for the patient.
- Document the reason the drug wasn't given (for example, if the patient is having a test that requires him not to take the drug).

response, lipodystrophy can be minimized by rotating injection sites. (See *Guidelines for documenting medication administration*.)

Documentation
Record the time and date of the injection, medication and dose administered, injection site and route, and patient's reaction.

SURGICAL WOUND MANAGEMENT

When caring for a surgical wound, you carry out procedures that help prevent infection by stopping pathogens from entering the wound. In addition to promoting patient comfort, such procedures protect the skin surface from maceration and excoriation caused by contact with irritating drainage. They also allow you to measure wound drainage to monitor healing and fluid and electrolyte balance.

The two primary methods used to manage a draining surgical wound are dressing and pouching. Dressing is preferred unless caustic or excessive drainage is compromising your patient's skin integrity. Usually, lightly seeping wounds with drains and wounds with minimal purulent drainage can be managed with packing and gauze dressings. Some wounds, such as those that become chronic, may require an occlusive dressing.

A wound with copious, excoriating drainage calls for pouching to protect the surrounding skin. If your patient

Tailoring wound care to wound color

With any wound, promote healing by keeping it moist, clean, and free from debris. For open wounds, use the wound color to guide the specific management approach and to assess how well the wound is healing.

Red wounds

Red, the color of healthy granulation tissue, indicates normal healing. When a wound begins to heal, a layer of pale pink granulation tissue covers the wound bed. As this layer thickens, it becomes beefy red. Cover a red wound, keep it moist and clean, and protect it from trauma. Use a transparent dressing (such as Tegaderm or Op-site), a hydrocolloidal dressing (such as DuoDerm), or a gauze dressing moistened with sterile normal saline solution or impregnated with petroleum jelly or an antibiotic.

Yellow wounds

Yellow is the color of exudate produced by microorganisms in an open wound. When a wound heals without complications, the immune system removes microorganisms. However, if there are too many microorganisms to remove, exudate accumulates and becomes visible. Exudate usually appears whitish yellow, creamy yellow, yellowish green, or beige. Dry exudate appears darker.

If your patient has a yellow wound, clean it and remove exudate, using high-pressure irrigation; then cover it with a moist dressing.

Use absorptive products (for example, Debrisan beads and paste) or a moist gauze dressing with or without an antibiotic. You may also use hydrotherapy with whirlpool or high-pressure irrigation.

Black wounds

Black, the least healthy color, signals necrosis. Dead, avascular tissue slows healing and provides a site for microorganisms to proliferate.

You should debride a black wound. After removing dead tissue, apply a dressing to keep the wound moist and guard against external contamination. As ordered, use enzyme products (such as Elase or Travase), surgical debridement, hydrotherapy with whirlpool or high-pressure irrigation, or a moist gauze dressing.

Multicolored wounds

You may note two or even all three colors in a wound. In this case, you'd classify the wound according to the least healthy color present. For example, if your patient's wound is both red and yellow, classify it as a yellow wound.

---

has a surgical wound, you must monitor him and choose the appropriate dressing.

Dressing a wound calls for sterile technique and sterile supplies to prevent contamination. You may use the color of the wound to help determine which type of dressing to apply. (See *Tailoring wound care to wound color.*) Change the dressing often enough to keep the skin dry. Always follow standard precautions set by the Centers for Disease Control and Prevention (CDC).

Key nursing diagnoses and patient outcomes

Risk for infection related to surgical incision

The patient will:

▶ have vital signs, temperature, and laboratory values within normal limits

▶ have incision site free from signs of infection, such as redness, swelling, or malodorous drainage.

Anxiety related to situational crisis
The patient will:
▶ state at least two ways to eliminate or minimize anxious behaviors
▶ report the ability to cope with the current situation without experiencing severe anxiety.

Equipment

Waterproof trash bag • clean gloves • sterile gloves • gown and face shield or goggles, if indicated • sterile 4″ × 4″ gauze pads • large absorbent dressings, if indicated • povidone-iodine swabs • sterile cotton-tipped applicators • sterile dressing set • topical medication, if ordered • adhesive or other tape • soap and water • optional: forceps; skin protectant; nonadherent pads; collodion spray or acetone-free adhesive remover; sterile normal saline solution; graduated biohazard container; and fishnet tube elasticized dressing support, Montgomery straps, or T-binder

For a wound with a drain

Sterile scissors • sterile 4″ × 4″ gauze pads without cotton lining • sump drain • ostomy pouch or another collection bag • sterile precut tracheostomy pads or drain dressings • adhesive tape (paper or silk tape if the patient is hypersensitive) • surgical mask

For pouching a wound

Collection pouch with drainage port • sterile gloves • skin protectant • sterile gauze pads

Preparation of equipment

Ask the patient about allergies to tapes and dressings. Assemble all equipment in the patient's room. Check the expiration date on each sterile package and inspect for tears.

Open the waterproof trash bag and place it near the patient's bed. Position the bag properly *to avoid reaching across the sterile field or the wound when disposing of soiled articles.* Form a cuff by turning down the top of the trash bag *to provide a wide opening and prevent contamination of instruments or gloves by touching the bag's edge.*

Implementation

▶ Explain the procedure to the patient *to allay his fears and ensure his cooperation.*

Removing the old dressing

▶ Check the doctor's order for specific wound care and medication instructions. Note the location of surgical drains *to avoid dislodging them during the procedure.*
▶ Assess the patient's condition.
▶ Identify the patient's allergies, especially to adhesive tape, povidone-iodine or other topical solutions, or medications.
▶ Provide privacy and position the patient as necessary. *To avoid chilling him,* expose only the wound site.
▶ Wash your hands thoroughly. Put on a gown and a face shield, if necessary. Then put on clean gloves.
▶ Loosen the soiled dressing by holding the patient's skin and pulling the tape or dressing toward the wound. *This protects the newly formed tissue and prevents stress on the incision.* Moisten the tape with acetone-free adhesive re-

mover, if necessary, *to make the tape removal less painful (particularly if the skin is hairy).* Don't apply solvents to the incision *because they could contaminate the wound.*

▶ Slowly remove the soiled dressing. If the gauze adheres to the wound, loosen the gauze by moistening it with sterile normal saline solution.

▶ Observe the dressing for the amount, type, color, and odor of drainage.

▶ Discard the dressing and gloves in the waterproof trash bag.

Caring for the wound

▶ Wash your hands. Establish a sterile field with all the equipment and supplies you'll need for suture-line care and the dressing change, including a sterile dressing set and povidone-iodine swabs. If the doctor has ordered ointment, squeeze the needed amount onto the sterile field. If you're using an antiseptic from a nonsterile bottle, pour the antiseptic cleaning agent into a sterile container *so you won't contaminate your gloves.* Then put on sterile gloves. (See *How to put on sterile gloves,* page 778.)

▶ Saturate the sterile gauze pads with the prescribed cleaning agent. Avoid using cotton balls *because they may shed fibers in the wound, causing irritation, infection, or adhesion.*

▶ If ordered, obtain a wound culture; then proceed to clean the wound.

▶ Pick up the moistened gauze pad or swab and squeeze out the excess solution.

▶ Working from the top of the incision, wipe once to the bottom and then discard the gauze pad. With a second moistened pad, wipe from top to bottom in a vertical path next to the incision (as shown below).

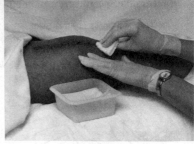

▶ Continue to work outward from the incision in lines running parallel to it. Always wipe from the clean area toward the less clean area (usually from top to bottom). Use each gauze pad or swab for only one stroke *to avoid tracking wound exudate and normal body flora from surrounding skin to the clean areas.* Remember that the suture line is cleaner than the adjacent skin and the top of the suture line is usually cleaner than the bottom *because more drainage collects at the bottom of the wound.*

▶ Use sterile, cotton-tipped applicators for efficient cleaning of tight-fitting wire sutures, deep and narrow wounds, and wounds with pockets. *Because the cotton on the swab is tightly wrapped,* it's less likely than a cotton ball to leave fibers in the wound. Remember to wipe only once with each applicator.

▶ If the patient has a surgical drain, clean the drain's surface last. *Because moist drainage promotes bacterial growth,* the drain is considered the most contaminated area. Clean the skin around the drain by wiping in half or full circles from the drain site outward.

▶ Clean all areas of the wound to wash away debris, pus, blood, and necrotic material. Try not to disturb sutures or irritate the incision. Clean to at least 1"

How to put on sterile gloves

Using your nondominant hand, pick up the opposite glove by grasping the exposed inside of the cuff.

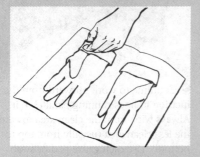

Slip the gloved fingers of your dominant hand under the glove of the loose glove to pick it up.

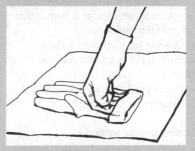

Pull the glove onto your dominant hand. Keep your thumb folded inward to avoid touching the sterile part of the glove. Allow the glove to come uncuffed as you finish inserting your hand, but don't touch the outside of the glove.

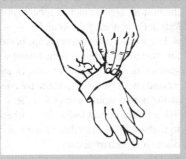

Slide your nondominant hand into the glove, holding your dominant thumb as far away as possible to avoid brushing against your arm. Allow the glove to come uncuffed as you finish putting it on, but don't touch the skin side of the cuff with your other gloved hand.

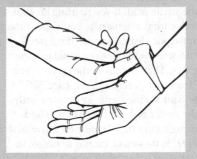

(2.5 cm) beyond the end of the new dressing. If you aren't applying a new dressing, clean to at least 2″ (5 cm) beyond the incision.
▶ Check to make sure that the edges of the incision are lined up properly and check for signs of infection (such as heat, redness, swelling, induration, and odor), dehiscence, and evisceration. If you observe such signs or if the patient reports pain at the wound site, notify the doctor.
▶ Irrigate the wound as ordered.
▶ Wash skin surrounding the wound with soap and water and pat dry using a sterile 4″ × 4″ gauze pad. Avoid oil-based soap *because it may interfere with pouch adherence.* Apply any prescribed topical medication.

▶ Apply a skin protectant, if needed.
▶ If ordered, pack the wound with gauze pads or strips folded to fit, using a sterile forceps. Avoid using cotton-lined gauze pads *because cotton fibers can adhere to the wound surface and cause complications.* Pack the wound, using the wet-to-damp method. Soaking the packing material in solution and wringing it out so that it's slightly moist provides a moist wound environment that absorbs debris and drainage. However, removing the packing won't disrupt new tissue. Don't pack the wound tightly; doing so will exert pressure and may damage the wound.

Applying a fresh gauze dressing

▶ Gently place sterile 4″ × 4″ gauze pads at the center of the wound and move progressively outward to the edges of the wound site. Extend the gauze at least 1″ (2.5 cm) beyond the incision in each direction and cover the wound evenly with enough sterile dressings (usually two or three layers) to absorb all drainage until the next dressing change. Use large absorbent dressings to form outer layers, if needed, *to provide greater absorbency.*
▶ Secure the dressing's edges to the patient's skin with strips of tape *to maintain the sterility of the wound site* (as shown below).

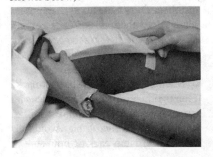

Or secure the dressing with a T-binder or Montgomery straps to prevent skin excoriation, which may occur with repeated tape removal necessitated by frequent dressing changes. (See *How to make Montgomery straps,* page 781.) If the wound is on a limb, secure the dressing with a fishnet tube elasticized dressing support.
▶ Make sure that the patient is comfortable.
▶ Properly dispose of the solutions and trash bag and clean or discard soiled equipment and supplies according to your facility's policy. If your patient's wound has purulent drainage, don't return unopened sterile supplies to the sterile supply cabinet *because this could cause cross-contamination of other equipment.*

Dressing a wound with a drain

▶ Prepare a drain dressing by using sterile scissors to cut a slit in a sterile 4″ × 4″ gauze pad. Fold the pad in half; then cut inward from the center of the folded edge. Don't use a cotton-lined gauze pad *because cutting the gauze opens the lining and releases cotton fibers into the wound.* Prepare a second pad the same way, or use commercially pre-cut gauze.
▶ Gently press one folded pad close to the skin around the drain so that the tubing fits into the slit. Press the second folded pad around the drain from the opposite direction so that the two pads encircle the tubing.
▶ Layer as many uncut sterile 4″ × 4″ gauze pads or large absorbent dressings around the tubing as needed *to absorb expected drainage.* Tape the dressing in place, or use a T-binder or Montgomery straps.

Pouching a wound

▶ If your patient's wound is draining heavily or if drainage may damage surrounding skin, you'll need to apply a pouch.

▶ Measure the wound. Cut an opening ³⁄₈″ (1 cm) larger than the wound in the facing of the collection pouch (as shown below).

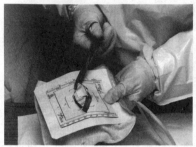

▶ Apply a skin protectant as needed. (Some protectants are incorporated within the collection pouch and also provide adhesion.)

▶ Before you apply the pouch, keep in mind the patient's usual position. Then plan to position the pouch's drainage port so that gravity facilitates drainage.

▶ Make sure that the drainage port at the bottom of the pouch is closed firmly *to prevent leaks*. Then gently press the contoured pouch opening around the wound, starting at its lower edge *to catch any drainage* (as shown below).

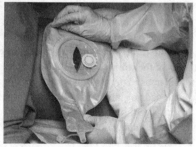

▶ To empty the pouch, put on clean gloves and a face shield or mask and goggles to avoid any splashing. Then insert the pouch's bottom half into a graduated biohazard container and open the drainage port (as shown below). Note the color, consistency, odor, and amount of fluid. If ordered, obtain a culture specimen and send it to the laboratory immediately. Remember to follow the CDC's standard precautions when handling infectious drainage.

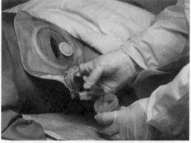

▶ Wipe the bottom of the pouch and the drainage port with a sterile gauze pad *to remove any drainage that could irritate the patient's skin or cause an odor.* Then reseal the port. Change the pouch only if it leaks or fails to adhere. *More frequent changes are unnecessary and only irritate the patient's skin.*

Special considerations

▶ If the patient has two wounds in the same area, cover each wound separately with layers of sterile 4″ × 4″ gauze pads. Then cover each site with a large absorbent dressing secured to the patient's skin with tape. Don't use a single large absorbent dressing to cover both sites *because drainage quickly saturates a pad, promoting cross-contamination.*

▶ When packing a wound, don't pack it too tightly *because this compresses adjacent capillaries and may prevent the wound edges from contracting.* Avoid overlapping damp packing onto sur-

How to make Montgomery straps

An abdominal dressing requiring frequent changes can be secured with Montgomery straps to promote the patient's comfort. If ready-made straps aren't available, take the following steps to make your own:

■ Cut four to six strips of 2″- or 3″-wide hypoallergenic tape of sufficient length to allow the tape to extend about 6″ (15.5 cm) beyond the wound on each side. (The length of the tape varies, depending on the patient's size and the type and amount of dressing.)

■ Fold one of each strip 2″ to 3″ back on itself (sticky sides together) to form a nonadhesive tab. Then cut a small hole in the folded tab's center, close to its top edge. Make as many pairs of straps as you'll need to snugly secure the dressing.

■ Clean the patient's skin to prevent irritation. After the skin dries, apply a skin protectant. Then apply the sticky side of each tape to a skin barrier sheet composed of opaque hydrocolloidal or nonhydrocolloidal materials and apply the sheet directly to the skin near the dressing. Next, thread a separate piece of gauze tie, umbilical tape, or twill tape (about 12″ [30.5 cm]) through each pair of holes in the straps and fasten each tie as you would a shoelace. Don't stress the surrounding skin by securing the ties too tightly.

■ Repeat this procedure according to the number of Montgomery straps needed.

■ Replace Montgomery straps whenever they become soiled (every 2 to 3 days). If skin maceration occurs, place new tapes about 1″ (2.5 cm) away from any irritation.

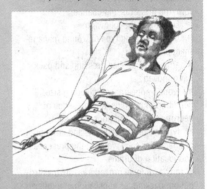

rounding skin *because it macerates the intact tissue.*

▶ To save time when dressing a wound with a drain, use sterile precut tracheostomy pads or drain dressings instead of custom-cutting gauze pads to fit around the drain. If your patient is sensitive to adhesive tape, use paper or silk tape *because it's less likely to cause a skin reaction and peels off more easily than adhesive tape.* Use a surgical mask to cradle a chin or jawline dressing; *this provides a secure dressing and avoids the need to shave the patient's hair.*

▶ If ordered, use a collodion spray or similar topical protectant instead of a gauze dressing. Moisture- and contaminant-proof, this covering dries in a clear, impermeable film that leaves the wound visible for observation and avoids the friction caused by a dressing.

▶ If a sump drain isn't adequately collecting wound secretions, reinforce it with an ostomy pouch or another collection bag. Use waterproof tape to strengthen a spot on the front of the pouch near the adhesive opening; then cut a small "X" in the tape. Feed the drain catheter into the pouch through the "X" cut. Seal the cut around the tubing with more waterproof tape; then connect the tubing to the suction pump. *This method frees the drainage port at the bottom of the pouch so you*

Better charting

Documenting surgical incision care

In addition to documenting vital signs and the level of consciousness when the patient returns from surgery, pay particular attention to maintaining records pertaining to the surgical incision and drains and the care you provide. Read the records that travel with the patient from the postanesthesia care unit. Look for a doctor's order directing whether you or the doctor perform the first dressing change.

Document the following:
■ date, time, and type of wound management procedure
■ amount of spoiled dressing and packing removed
■ wound appearance (including size, condition of margins, and presence of necrotic tissue) and odor (if present)
■ type, color, consistency, and amount of drainage (for each wound); the presence and location of drains
■ any additional procedures, such as irrigation, packing, or application of a topical medication
■ type and amount of new dressing or pouch applied
■ patient's tolerance of the procedure.

don't have to remove the tubing to empty the pouch. If you use more than one collection pouch for a wound or wounds, record drainage volume separately for each pouch. Avoid using waterproof material over the dressing *because it reduces air circulation and promotes infection from accumulated heat and moisture.*
▶ Because many doctors prefer to change the first postoperative dressing themselves to check the incision, don't change the first dressing unless you

have specific instructions to do so. If you have no such order and drainage comes through the dressings, reinforce the dressing with fresh sterile gauze. Request an order to change the dressing, or ask the doctor to change it as soon as possible. A reinforced dressing shouldn't remain in place longer than 24 hours *because it's an excellent medium for bacterial growth.*
▶ For the recent postoperative patient or a patient with complications, check the dressing every 15 to 30 minutes or as ordered. For the patient with a properly healing wound, check the dressing at least once every 8 hours.
▶ If the dressing becomes wet from the outside (for example, from spilled drinking water), replace it as soon as possible *to prevent wound contamination.*
▶ If your patient will need wound care after discharge, provide appropriate teaching. If he'll be caring for the wound himself, stress the importance of using aseptic technique and teach him how to examine the wound for signs of infection and other complications. Also, show him how to change dressings and give him written instructions for all procedures to be performed at home.

Complications

A major complication of a dressing change is an allergic reaction to an antiseptic cleaning agent, a prescribed topical medication, or an adhesive tape. This reaction may lead to skin redness, rash, excoriation, or infection.

Documentation

Document the date, time, and type of wound management procedure; amount of soiled dressing and packing removed; wound appearance (size, condition of margins, presence of necrotic tissue) and odor (if present); type, color, consistency, and amount of drainage (for each wound); presence and location of drains; additional procedures, such as irrigation, packing, or application of a topical medication; type and amount of new dressing or pouch applied; and patient's tolerance of the procedure.

Document special or detailed wound care instructions and pain management steps on the plan of care. Record the color and amount of drainage on the intake and output sheet. (See *Documenting surgical incision care*.)

Suture removal

The goal of suture removal is to remove skin sutures from a healed wound without damaging newly formed tissue. The timing of suture removal depends on the shape, size, and location of the sutured incision; the absence of inflammation, drainage, and infection; and the patient's general condition. Usually, for a sufficiently healed wound, sutures are removed 7 to 10 days after insertion. Techniques for removal depend on the method of suturing, but all require sterile procedure to prevent contamination. Although sutures usually are removed by a doctor, in many facilities, a nurse may remove them on the doctor's order.

Key nursing diagnoses and patient outcomes

Risk for infection related to surgical incision
The patient will:
▶ have vital signs, temperature, and laboratory values within normal limits

▶ remain free from signs and symptoms of infection at incision site.

Anxiety related to situational crisis
The patient will:
▶ state at least two ways to eliminate or minimize anxious behaviors
▶ report the ability to cope with the current situation without experiencing severe anxiety.

Equipment

Waterproof trash bag • adjustable light • clean gloves, if the wound is dressed • sterile gloves • sterile forceps or sterile hemostat • normal saline solution • sterile gauze pads • antiseptic cleaning agent • sterile curve-tipped suture scissors • povidone-iodine pads • optional: adhesive butterfly strips or Steri-Strips and compound benzoin tincture or other skin protectant

Prepackaged, sterile suture-removal trays are available.

Preparation of equipment

Assemble all equipment in the patient's room. Check the expiration date on each sterile package and inspect for tears. Open the waterproof trash bag and place it near the patient's bed. Position the bag properly *to avoid reaching across the sterile field or the suture line when disposing of soiled articles.* Form a cuff by turning down the top of the trash bag *to provide a wide opening and prevent contamination of instruments or gloves by touching the bag's edge.*

Implementation

▶ If your facility allows you to remove sutures, check the doctor's order *to confirm the details for this procedure.*
▶ Check for patient allergies, especially to adhesive tape and povidone-iodine

or another topical solution or medication.

▶ Tell the patient that you're going to remove the stitches from his wound. Assure him that this procedure typically is painless but that he may feel a tickling sensation as the stitches come out. Reassure him that because his wound is healing properly, removing the stitches won't weaken the incision.

▶ Provide privacy and position the patient so he's comfortable without placing undue tension on the suture line. *Because some patients experience nausea or dizziness during the procedure,* have the patient recline, if possible. Adjust the light to have it shine directly on the suture line.

▶ Wash your hands thoroughly. If the patient's wound has a dressing, put on clean gloves and carefully remove the dressing. Discard the dressing and the gloves in the waterproof trash bag.

▶ Observe the patient's wound for possible gaping, drainage, inflammation, signs of infection, and embedded sutures. Notify the doctor if the wound has failed to heal properly. The absence of a healing ridge under the suture line 5 to 7 days after insertion indicates that the line needs continued support and protection during the healing process.

▶ Establish a sterile work area with all the equipment and supplies you'll need for suture removal and wound care. Put on sterile gloves and open the sterile suture-removal tray if you're using one.

▶ Using sterile technique, clean the suture line *to decrease the number of microorganisms present and reduce the risk of infection.* The cleaning process should also moisten the sutures sufficiently *to ease removal.* Soften them further, if needed, with normal saline solution.

▶ Then proceed according to the type of suture you're removing. (See *Methods for removing sutures.) Because the visible part of a suture is exposed to skin bacteria and considered contaminated,* cut sutures at the skin surface on one side of the visible part of the suture. Remove the suture by lifting and pulling the visible end off the skin *to avoid drawing this contaminated portion back through subcutaneous tissue.*

▶ If ordered, remove every other suture *to maintain some support for the incision.* Then go back and remove the remaining sutures.

▶ After removing sutures, wipe the incision gently with sterile gauze pads soaked in an antiseptic cleaning agent or with a povidone-iodine pad. Apply a light sterile gauze dressing, if needed, *to prevent infection and irritation from clothing.* Then discard your gloves.

▶ Make sure the patient is comfortable. According to the doctor's preference, inform the patient that he may shower in 1 or 2 days if the incision is dry and heals well.

▶ Properly dispose of the solutions and trash bag and clean or dispose of soiled equipment and supplies according to your facility's policy.

Special considerations

▶ Check the doctor's order for the time of suture removal. Usually, you'll remove sutures on the head and neck 3 to 5 days after insertion; on the chest and abdomen, 5 to 7 days after insertion; and on the lower extremities, 7 to 10 days after insertion.

▶ If the patient has interrupted sutures or an incompletely healed suture line, remove only those sutures specified by the doctor. He may want to leave some

Methods for removing sutures

Removal techniques depend in large part on the type of sutures to be removed. The illustrations here show removal steps for four common suture types. Keep in mind that for all suture types, it's important to grasp and cut sutures in the correct place to avoid pulling the exposed (thus contaminated) suture material through subcutaneous tissue.

Plain interrupted sutures

Using sterile forceps, grasp the knot of the first suture and raise it off the skin. This will expose a small portion of the suture that was below skin level. Place the rounded tip of sterile curved-tip suture scissors against the skin and cut through the exposed portion of the suture. Then, still holding the knot with the forceps, pull the cut suture up and out of the skin in a smooth continuous motion to avoid causing the patient pain. Discard the suture. Repeat the process for every other suture initially; if the wound doesn't gape, you can then remove the remaining sutures as ordered.

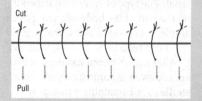

Mattress interrupted sutures

If possible, remove the small, visible portion of the suture opposite the knot by cutting it at each visible end and lifting the small piece away from the skin to prevent pulling it through and contaminating subcutaneous tissue. Then remove the rest of the suture by pulling it out in the direction of the knot. If the visible portion is too small to cut twice, cut it once and pull the entire suture out in the opposite direction. Repeat these steps for the remaining sutures and monitor the incision carefully for infection.

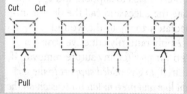

Plain continuous sutures

Cut the first suture on the side opposite the knot. Next, cut the same side of the next suture in line. Then lift the first suture out in the direction of the knot. Proceed along the suture line, grasping each suture where you grasped the knot on the first one.

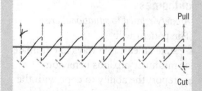

Mattress continuous sutures

Follow the procedure for removing mattress interrupted sutures, first removing the small visible portion of the suture, if possible, to prevent pulling it through and contaminating subcutaneous tissue. Then extract the rest of the suture in the direction of the knot.

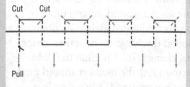

sutures in place for an additional day or two *to support the suture line.*

▶ If the patient has both retention and regular sutures in place, check the doctor's order for the sequence in which they're to be removed. *Because retention sutures link underlying fat and muscle tissue and give added support to the obese or slow-healing patient,* they usually remain in place for 14 to 21 days.

▶ Be particularly careful to clean the suture line before attempting to remove mattress sutures. *This decreases the risk of infection when the visible, contaminated part of the stitch is too small to cut twice for sterile removal and must be pulled through tissue.* After you have removed mattress sutures this way, monitor the suture line carefully *for subsequent infection.*

▶ If the wound dehisces during suture removal, apply butterfly adhesive strips or Steri-Strips to support and approximate the edges and call the doctor immediately to repair the wound.

▶ Apply butterfly adhesive strips or Steri-Strips after any suture removal, if desired, *to give added support to the incision line and prevent lateral tension on the wound from forming a wide scar.* Use a small amount of compound benzoin tincture or other skin protectant *to ensure adherence.* Leave the strips in place for 3 to 5 days as ordered.

Home care

If the patient is being discharged, teach him how to remove the dressing and care for the wound. Instruct him to call the doctor immediately if he observes wound discharge or any other abnormal change. Tell him that the redness surrounding the incision should gradually disappear and only a thin line should show after a few weeks.

Documentation

Record the date and time of suture removal, type and number of sutures, appearance of the suture line, signs of wound complications, dressings or butterfly strips applied, and patient's tolerance of the procedure.

SWAB SPECIMEN COLLECTION

Correct collection and handling of swab specimens helps the laboratory staff identify pathogens accurately with a minimum of contamination from normal bacterial flora. Collection normally involves sampling inflamed tissues and exudates from the throat, nasopharynx, wounds, eye, ear, or rectum with sterile swabs of cotton or other absorbent material. The type of swab used depends on the part of the body affected. For example, collection of a nasopharyngeal specimen requires a cotton-tipped swab.

After the specimen has been collected, the swab is immediately placed in a sterile tube containing a transport medium and, in the case of sampling for anaerobes, an inert gas. Swab specimens are usually collected to identify pathogens and sometimes to identify asymptomatic carriers of certain easily transmitted disease organisms.

Key nursing diagnoses and patient outcomes

Anxiety related to situational crisis
The patient will:
▶ state at least two ways to eliminate or minimize anxious behaviors
▶ report the ability to cope with the current situation without experiencing severe anxiety.

Deficient knowledge related to lack of exposure

The patient will:

▶ communicate a need to know about the procedure

▶ state or demonstrate an understanding of the procedure.

Equipment

For a throat specimen

Gloves • tongue blade • penlight • sterile cotton-tipped swab • sterile culture tube with transport medium (or commercial collection kit) • label • laboratory request form

For a nasopharyngeal specimen

Gloves • penlight • sterile, flexible cotton-tipped swab • tongue blade • sterile culture tube with transport medium • label • laboratory request form • optional: nasal speculum

For a wound specimen

Sterile gloves • sterile forceps • alcohol or povidone-iodine pads • sterile cotton-tipped swabs • sterile 10-ml syringe • sterile 21G needle • sterile culture tube with transport medium (or commercial collection kit for aerobic culture) • labels • special anaerobic culture tube containing carbon dioxide or nitrogen • fresh dressings for the wound • laboratory request form • optional: rubber stopper for needle

For an ear specimen

Gloves • normal saline solution • two 2″ × 2″ gauze pads • sterile swabs • sterile culture tube with transport medium • label • 10-ml syringe and 22G 1″ needle (for tympanocentesis) • laboratory request form

For an eye specimen

Sterile gloves • sterile normal saline solution • two 2″ × 2″ gauze pads • sterile swabs • sterile wire culture loop (for corneal scraping) • sterile culture tube with transport medium • label • laboratory request form

For a rectal specimen

Gloves • soap and water • washcloth • sterile swab • normal saline solution or sterile broth medium • sterile culture tube with transport medium • label • laboratory request form

Implementation

▶ Explain the procedure to the patient *to ease his anxiety and ensure cooperation.*

Collecting a throat specimen

▶ Tell the patient that he may gag during the swabbing but that the procedure will probably take less than 1 minute.

▶ Instruct the patient to sit erect at the edge of the bed or in a chair, facing you. Then wash your hands and put on gloves.

▶ Ask the patient to tilt his head back. Depress his tongue with the tongue blade and illuminate his throat with the penlight *to check for inflamed areas.*

▶ If the patient starts to gag, withdraw the tongue blade and tell him to breathe deeply. When he's relaxed, reinsert the tongue blade but not as deeply as before.

▶ Using the sterile cotton-tipped swab, wipe the tonsillar areas from side to side, including any inflamed or purulent sites. Make sure you don't touch the tongue, cheeks, or teeth with the swab *to avoid contaminating it with oral bacteria.*

Obtaining a nasopharyngeal specimen

After you've passed the swab into the nasopharynx, quickly but gently rotate the swab to collect the specimen. Then remove the swab, taking care not to injure the nasal mucous membrane.

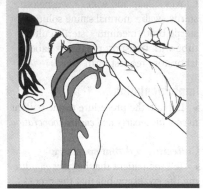

▶ Withdraw the swab and immediately place it in the sterile culture tube. If you're using a commercial kit, crush the ampule of culture medium at the bottom of the tube and then push the swab into the medium *to keep the swab moist.*

▶ Remove and discard your gloves and wash your hands.

▶ Label the specimen with the patient's name and room number, the doctor's name, and the date, time, and site of collection.

▶ On the laboratory request form, indicate whether any organism is strongly suspected, especially *Corynebacterium diphtheriae* (requires two swabs and special growth medium), *Bordetella pertussis* (requires a nasopharyngeal culture and special growth medium), and *Neisseria meningitidis* (requires enriched selective media).

▶ Send the specimen to the laboratory immediately *to prevent growth or deterioration of microbes.*

Collecting a nasopharyngeal specimen

▶ Tell the patient that he may gag or feel the urge to sneeze during the swabbing but that the procedure takes less than 1 minute.

▶ Have the patient sit erect at the edge of the bed or in a chair, facing you. Then wash your hands and put on gloves.

▶ Ask the patient to blow his nose *to clear his nasal passages.* Then check his nostrils for patency with a penlight.

▶ If the nostril appears narrow, use a nasal speculum *to have better access to the specimen.*

▶ Tell the patient to occlude one nostril first and then the other as he exhales. Listen for the more patent nostril *because you'll insert the swab through it.*

▶ Ask the patient to cough *to bring organisms to the nasopharynx for a better specimen.*

▶ While it's still in the package, bend the sterile cotton-tipped swab in a curve and then open the package without contaminating the swab.

▶ Ask the patient to tilt his head back and gently pass the swab through the more patent nostril about 3″ to 4″ (7.5 to 10 cm) into the nasopharynx, keeping the swab near the septum and floor of the nose. Rotate the swab quickly and remove it. (See *Obtaining a nasopharyngeal specimen.*)

▶ Alternatively, depress the patient's tongue with a tongue blade and pass the bent swab up behind the uvula. Rotate the swab and withdraw it.

▶ Remove the cap from the sterile culture tube, insert the swab, and break off the contaminated end. Then close the tube tightly.

► Remove and discard your gloves and wash your hands.

► Label the specimen for culture, complete a laboratory request form, and send the specimen to the laboratory immediately. If you're collecting a specimen to isolate a possible virus, check with the laboratory for the recommended collection technique.

Collecting a wound specimen

► Wash your hands, prepare a sterile field, and put on sterile gloves. With sterile forceps, remove the dressing to expose the wound. Dispose of the soiled dressings properly.

► Clean the area around the wound with an alcohol or a povidone-iodine pad *to reduce the risk of contaminating the specimen with skin bacteria.* Then allow the area to dry.

► For an aerobic culture, use a sterile cotton-tipped swab to collect as much exudate as possible, or insert the swab deeply into the wound and gently rotate it. Remove the swab from the wound and immediately place it in the aerobic culture tube. Label the tube and send it to the laboratory immediately with a completed laboratory request form. Never collect exudate from the skin and then insert the same swab into the wound; *this could contaminate the wound with skin bacteria.*

► For an anaerobic culture, insert the sterile cotton-tipped swab deeply into the wound, rotate it gently, remove it, and immediately place it in the anaerobic culture tube (see *Anaerobic specimen collection*). Alternatively, insert a sterile 10-ml syringe, without a needle, into the wound and aspirate 1 to 5 ml of exudate into the syringe. Then attach the

Anaerobic specimen collection

Because most anaerobes die when exposed to oxygen, they must be transported in tubes filled with carbon dioxide or nitrogen. The anaerobic specimen collector shown here includes a rubber-stoppered tube filled with carbon dioxide, a small inner tube, and a swab attached to a plastic plunger.

Before specimen collection, the small inner tube containing the swab is held in place with the rubber stopper (as shown on the left). After collecting the specimen, quickly replace the swab in the inner tube and depress the plunger to separate the inner tube from the stopper (as shown on the right), forcing it into the larger tube and exposing the specimen to a carbon dioxide–rich environment.

Before   **After**

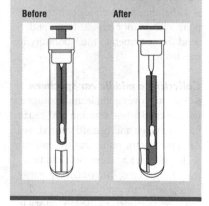

21G needle to the syringe and immediately inject the aspirate into the anaerobic culture tube. If an anaerobic culture tube is unavailable, obtain a rubber stopper, attach the needle to the syringe, and gently push all the air out of the syringe by pressing on the plunger. Stick the needle tip into the rubber stopper, remove and discard your

gloves, and send the syringe of aspirate to the laboratory immediately with a completed laboratory request form.
► Put on sterile gloves.
► Apply a new dressing to the wound.

Collecting an ear specimen
► Wash your hands and put on gloves.
► Gently clean excess debris from the patient's ear with normal saline solution and gauze pads.
► Insert the sterile swab into the ear canal and rotate it gently along the walls of the canal *to avoid damaging the eardrum.*
► Withdraw the swab, being careful not to touch other surfaces *to avoid contaminating the specimen.*
► Place the swab in the sterile culture tube with transport medium.
► Remove and discard your gloves and wash your hands.
► Label the specimen for culture, complete a laboratory request form, and send the specimen to the laboratory immediately.

Collecting a middle ear specimen
► Put on gloves and clean the outer ear with normal saline solution and gauze pads. Remove and discard your gloves. After the doctor punctures the eardrum with a needle and aspirates fluid into the syringe, label the container, complete a laboratory request form, and send the specimen to the laboratory immediately.

Collecting an eye specimen
► Wash your hands and put on sterile gloves.
► Gently clean excess debris from the outside of the eye with sterile normal saline solution and gauze pads, wiping from the inner to the outer canthus.

► Retract the lower eyelid to expose the conjunctival sac. Gently rub the sterile swab over the conjunctiva, being careful not to touch other surfaces. Hold the swab parallel to the eye, rather than pointed directly at it, *to prevent corneal irritation or trauma due to sudden movement.* (If a corneal scraping is required, this procedure is performed by a doctor, using a wire culture loop.)
► Immediately place the swab or wire loop in the culture tube with transport medium.
► Remove and discard your gloves and wash your hands.
► Label the specimen for culture, complete a laboratory request form, and send the specimen to the laboratory immediately.

Collecting a rectal specimen
► Wash your hands and put on gloves.
► Clean the area around the patient's anus using a washcloth and soap and water.
► Insert the sterile swab, moistened with normal saline solution or sterile broth medium, through the anus and advance it about ⅜″ (1 cm) for infants or 1½″ (4 cm) for adults. While withdrawing the swab, gently rotate it against the walls of the lower rectum to sample a large area of the rectal mucosa.
► Place the swab in a culture tube with transport medium.
► Remove and discard your gloves and wash your hands.
► Label the specimen for culture, complete a laboratory request form, and send the specimen to the laboratory immediately.

Special considerations
▶ Note recent antibiotic therapy on the laboratory request form.

For a wound specimen
Although you would normally clean the area around a wound to prevent contamination by normal skin flora, don't clean a perineal wound with alcohol *because this could irritate sensitive tissues.* Also, make sure that the antiseptic doesn't enter the wound.

For an eye specimen
Don't use an antiseptic before culturing *to avoid irritating the eye and inhibiting growth of organisms in the culture.* If the patient is a child or an uncooperative adult, ask a coworker to restrain the patient's head *to prevent eye trauma resulting from sudden movement.*

Documentation
Record the time, date, and site of specimen collection and any recent or current antibiotic therapy. Also, note whether the specimen has an unusual appearance or odor.

SYNCHRONIZED CARDIOVERSION

Used to treat tachyarrhythmias, synchronized cardioversion delivers an electric charge to the myocardium at the peak of the R wave. This causes immediate depolarization, interrupting reentry circuits, and allowing the sinoatrial node to resume control. Synchronizing the electric charge with the R wave ensures that the current won't be delivered on the vulnerable T wave and thus disrupt repolarization.

Synchronized cardioversion is the treatment of choice for arrhythmias that don't respond to vagal massage or drug therapy, such as atrial tachycardia, atrial flutter, atrial fibrillation, and symptomatic ventricular tachycardia.

Cardioversion may be an elective or urgent procedure, depending on how well the patient tolerates the arrhythmia. For example, if the patient is hemodynamically unstable, he'd require urgent cardioversion. Remember that, when preparing for cardioversion, the patient's condition can deteriorate quickly, necessitating immediate defibrillation.

Indications for cardioversion include stable paroxysmal atrial tachycardia, unstable paroxysmal supraventricular tachycardia, atrial fibrillation, atrial flutter, and ventricular tachycardia.

Key nursing diagnoses and patient outcomes
Ineffective tissue perfusion (cardiopulmonary) related to decreased cellular exchange
The patient will:
▶ attain hemodynamic stability, with pulse not less than (specify) beats/minute and not greater than (specify) beats/minute and blood pressure not less than (specify) mm Hg and not greater than (specify) mm Hg
▶ exhibit no arrhythmias
▶ maintain adequate cardiac output.

Decreased cardiac output related to arrhythmias
The patient will:
▶ achieve activity within limits of prescribed heart rate
▶ have heart's workload diminished
▶ have a balanced intake and output.

Equipment

Cardioverter-defibrillator • conductive gel pads • anterior, posterior, or transverse paddles • electrocardiogram (ECG) monitor with recorder • sedative • oxygen therapy equipment • airway • handheld resuscitation bag • emergency pacing equipment • emergency cardiac medications • automatic blood pressure cuff (if available) • pulse oximeter (if available)

Implementation

▶ Explain the procedure to the patient and make sure he has signed a consent form.

▶ Check the patient's recent serum potassium and magnesium levels and arterial blood gas results. Also, check recent digoxin levels. Although digitalized patients may undergo cardioversion, they tend to require lower energy levels to convert. If the patient takes digoxin, withhold the dose on the day of the procedure.

▶ Withhold all food and fluids for 6 to 12 hours before the procedure. If the cardioversion is urgent, withhold the previous meal.

▶ Obtain a 12-lead ECG to serve as a baseline.

▶ Check to see if the doctor has ordered administration of any cardiac drugs before the procedure. Also, verify that the patient has a patent I.V. site in case drug administration becomes necessary.

▶ Connect the patient to a pulse oximeter and automatic blood pressure cuff, if available.

▶ Consider administering oxygen for 5 to 10 minutes before the cardioversion *to promote myocardial oxygenation.* If the patient wears dentures, evaluate whether they support his airway or might cause an airway obstruction. If they might cause an obstruction, remove them.

▶ Place the patient in the supine position and assess his vital signs, level of consciousness (LOC), cardiac rhythm, and peripheral pulses.

▶ Remove any oxygen delivery device just before cardioversion *to avoid possible combustion.*

▶ Have epinephrine, lidocaine, and atropine at the patient's bedside.

▶ Make sure the resuscitation bag is at the patient's bedside.

▶ Administer a sedative as ordered. The patient should be heavily sedated but still able to breathe adequately.

▶ Carefully monitor the patient's blood pressure and respiratory rate until he recovers.

▶ Press the POWER button to turn on the defibrillator. Next, push the SYNC button *to synchronize the machine with the patient's QRS complexes.* Make sure the SYNC button flashes with each of the patient's QRS complexes. You should also see a bright green flag flash on the monitor.

▶ Turn the ENERGY SELECT dial to the ordered amount of energy. Advanced Cardiac Life Support protocols call for 50 to 360 joules for a patient with stable paroxysmal atrial tachycardia, 75 to 360 joules for a patient with unstable paroxysmal supraventricular tachycardia, 100 joules for a patient with atrial fibrillation, 50 joules for a patient with atrial flutter, 100 to 360 joules for a patient who has ventricular tachycardia with a pulse, and 200 to 360 joules for a patient with pulseless ventricular tachycardia.

▶ Remove the paddles from the machine and prepare them as you would if you were defibrillating the patient.

Place the conductive gel pads or paddles in the same positions as you would to defibrillate.

▶ Make sure everyone stands away from the bed; then push the discharge buttons. Hold the paddles in place and wait for the energy to be discharged — the machine has to synchronize the discharge with the QRS complex.

▶ Check the waveform on the monitor. If the arrhythmia fails to convert, repeat the procedure two or three more times at 3-minute intervals. Gradually increase the energy level with each additional countershock.

▶ After the cardioversion, frequently assess the patient's LOC and respiratory status, including airway patency, respiratory rate and depth, and the need for supplemental oxygen. *Because the patient will be heavily sedated,* he may require airway support.

▶ Record a postcardioversion 12-lead ECG and monitor the patient's ECG rhythm for 2 hours. Check the patient's chest for electrical burns.

Special considerations

▶ If the patient is attached to a bedside or telemetry monitor, disconnect the unit before cardioversion. *The electric current it generates could damage the equipment.*

▶ Be aware that improper synchronization may result if the patient's ECG tracing contains artifact-like spikes, such as peaked T waves or bundle-branch heart blocks when the R′ wave may be taller than the R wave.

▶ Although the electric shock of cardioversion won't usually damage an implanted pacemaker, avoid placing the paddles directly over the pacemaker.

Complications

Common complications following cardioversion include transient, harmless arrhythmias such as atrial, ventricular, and junctional premature beats. Serious ventricular arrhythmias such as ventricular fibrillation may also occur. However, this type of arrhythmia is more likely to result from high amounts of electrical energy, digitalis toxicity, severe heart disease, electrolyte imbalance, or improper synchronization with the R wave.

Documentation

Document the procedure, including the voltage delivered with each attempt, rhythm strips before and after the procedure, and how the patient tolerated the procedure.

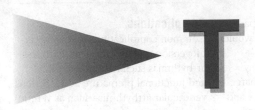

THERMOREGULATION, NEONATAL

Thermoregulation provides a neutral thermal environment that helps the neonate maintain a normal core temperature with minimal oxygen consumption and caloric expenditure. Although it varies with the neonate, the average core temperature is 97.7° F (36.5° C).

Two kinds of thermoregulators are common in a hospital nursery: radiant warmers and incubators. The radiant warmer controls environmental temperature while the nurse gives initial care in the delivery room. Then, when the neonate arrives in the nursery, another radiant warmer may be used until his temperature stabilizes and he can occupy a bassinet. If the temperature doesn't stabilize or if the neonate has a condition that affects thermoregulation, a temperature-controlled incubator will house him. (See *Understanding thermoregulators.*)

Key nursing diagnoses and patient outcomes

Ineffective tissue perfusion (peripheral) related to decreased arterial blood flow
The neonate will:
▶ have no arrhythmias
▶ have skin color and temperature within normal limits.

Ineffective thermoregulation related to trauma or illness
The neonate will:
▶ maintain body temperature at normothermic levels
▶ demonstrate no signs of shivering
▶ express feelings of comfort.

Equipment

Radiant warmer or incubator (if necessary) • blankets • washcloths or towels • skin probe • adhesive pad • water-soluble lubricant • thermometer • clothing (including a cap) • optional: stockinette gauze

Preparation of equipment

Turn on the radiant warmer in the delivery room and set the desired temperature. Warm the blankets, washcloths, or towels under a heat source.

Implementation

▶ Continue nursing measures to conserve neonatal body warmth until the patient is discharged.

In the delivery room

▶ Place the neonate under the radiant warmer and dry him with the warm washcloths or towels *to prevent heat loss by evaporation.*
▶ Pay special attention to drying his scalp and hair. Then, if you take him off the warmer, make sure you cover

Understanding thermoregulators

Thermoregulators preserve neonatal body warmth in various ways. A radiant warmer maintains the neonate's temperature by *radiation*. An incubator maintains the neonate's temperature by *conduction* and *convection*.

Temperature settings
Radiant warmers and incubators have two operating modes: *nonservo* and *servo*. The nurse manually sets temperature controls on nonservo equipment; a probe on the neonate's skin controls temperature settings on servo models.

Other features
Most thermoregulators come with alarms. Incubators have the added advantage of providing a stable, enclosed environment, which protects the neonate from evaporative heat loss.

Radiant warmer

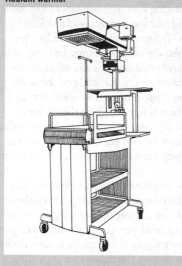

Incubator

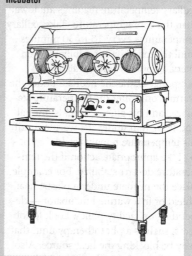

his head (which makes up about 25% of neonatal body surface) with a ready-made cap *to prevent heat loss.*
▶ Perform required procedures quickly *to reduce the neonate's exposure to cool delivery room air.*
▶ Wrap him in the warmed blankets. If his condition permits, give him to his parents *to promote bonding.*
▶ Transport the neonate to the nursery in the warmed blankets. Use a trans-

port incubator when the nursery is far from the delivery room.

In the nursery
▶ Remove the blankets and cap and place the neonate under the radiant warmer.
▶ Use the adhesive pad to attach the temperature control probe to his skin in the upper-right abdominal quadrant. *This lets the servo control maintain neonatal skin temperature between 96.8° and*

97.7° F (36° and 36.5° C). If the neonate will lie prone, put the skin probe on his back *to ensure accurate temperature control and avoid false-high readings from the neonate lying on the probe.* Don't cover the device with anything *because this could interfere with the servo control.* Be sure to raise the warmer's side panels *to prevent accidents.*

▶ Lubricate the thermometer and take the neonate's rectal temperature on admission *to identify core temperature.* Take axillary temperatures thereafter *to avoid injuring delicate rectal mucosa.* Usually, axillary temperature readings are lower than the core temperature. Take axillary temperatures every 15 to 30 minutes until the temperature stabilizes, then every 4 hours *to ensure stability.*

▶ Sponge-bathe the neonate under the warmer only after his temperature stabilizes and his glucose level is normal and leave him under the warmer until his temperature remains stable.

▶ Take appropriate action if the temperature doesn't stabilize. For example, place the neonate under a plastic heat shield or in a warmed incubator — depending on facility policy. Look for objects, such as a phototherapy unit, that may be blocking the heat source. Also check for signs of infection, which can cause hypothermia.

▶ Apply a skin probe to the neonate in an incubator as you would for a neonate in a radiant warmer. Move the incubator away from cold walls or objects.

▶ Perform all required procedures quickly *to maintain a neutral thermal environment and to minimize heat loss.* Close portholes in the hood immediately after completing any procedure, *also to reduce heat loss.* If procedures must be performed outside the incubator, do them under a radiant warmer.

▶ To leave the facility or to move to a bassinet, the neonate must be weaned from the incubator. Slowly reduce the incubator's temperature to that of the nursery. Check periodically for hypothermia. *To ensure temperature stability,* never discharge the neonate to home directly from an incubator.

▶ When the neonate's temperature stabilizes, dress him, put him in a bassinet, and cover him with a blanket.

Special considerations

▶ Always warm oxygen before administering it to the neonate *to avoid initiating heat loss from his head and face.*

▶ *To prevent conductive heat loss,* preheat the radiant warmer bed and linen; warm stethoscopes and other instruments before use; and pad the scale with paper or a preweighed, warmed sheet before weighing the neonate.

▶ *To avoid convective heat loss,* place the neonate's bed out of direct line with an open window, fan, or an air-conditioning vent.

▶ *To control evaporative heat loss,* dry the neonate immediately after delivery. When bathing the neonate, expose only one body part at a time; wash each part thoroughly and then dry it immediately.

▶ Review the reasons for regulating body temperature with the neonate's family. Instruct them to keep him wrapped in a blanket and out of drafts when he isn't in the bassinet, both in the facility and at home. In a warm place, guard against overheating the neonate.

Complications

Hypothermia from ineffective natural or external thermoregulation can inhibit weight gain because the neonate must use caloric energy to maintain his temperature. Hyperthermia can cause increased oxygen consumption and apnea. Both conditions can result from equipment failures or insufficient monitoring.

Documentation

Name the heat source and record its temperature and the neonate's temperature, whenever taken. Document any complications that result from using thermoregulatory equipment.

THORACENTESIS

Thoracentesis involves the aspiration of fluid or air from the pleural space. It relieves pulmonary compression and respiratory distress by removing accumulated air or fluid that results from injury or such conditions as tuberculosis or cancer. It also provides a specimen of pleural fluid or tissue for analysis and allows instillation of chemotherapeutic agents or other medications into the pleural space. Thoracentesis is contraindicated in patients with bleeding disorders.

Key nursing diagnoses and patient outcomes

Ineffective breathing pattern related to decreased energy
The patient will:
▶ achieve maximum lung expansion with adequate ventilation
▶ report feeling comfortable with breathing.

Impaired gas exchange related to altered oxygen supply
The patient will:
▶ cough effectively
▶ expectorate sputum.

Equipment

Most facilities use a prepackaged thoracentesis tray that typically includes: sterile gloves • sterile drapes • 70% isopropyl alcohol or povidone-iodine solution • 1% or 2% lidocaine • 5-ml syringe with 21G and 25G needles for anesthetic injection • 17G thoracentesis needle for aspiration • 50-ml syringe • three-way stopcock and tubing • sterile specimen containers • sterile hemostat • sterile 4″ × 4″ gauze pads.

You'll also need: adhesive tape • sphygmomanometer • gloves • stethoscope • laboratory request slips • drainage bottles • optional: Teflon catheter, shaving supplies, biopsy needle, prescribed sedative with 3-ml syringe and 21G needle, and drainage bottles (if the doctor expects a large amount of drainage).

Preparation of equipment

Assemble all equipment at the patient's bedside or in the treatment area. Check the expiration date on each sterile package and inspect for tears. Prepare the necessary laboratory request form. Be sure to list current antibiotic therapy on the laboratory forms *because this will be considered in analyzing the specimens.* Make sure the patient has signed an appropriate consent form. Note any drug allergies, especially to the local anesthetic. Have the patient's chest X-rays available.

Implementation

▶ Explain the procedure to the patient. Inform him that he may feel some discomfort and a sensation of pressure during the needle insertion. Provide privacy and emotional support. Wash your hands.

▶ Obtain baseline vital signs and assess respiratory function.

▶ Administer the prescribed sedative as ordered.

▶ Position the patient. Make sure he's firmly supported and comfortable. Although the choice of position varies, you'll usually seat the patient on the edge of the bed with his legs supported and his head and folded arms resting on a pillow on the overbed table. Or have him straddle a chair backward and rest his head and folded arms on the back of the chair. If the patient is unable to sit, turn him on the unaffected side with the arm of the affected side raised above his head. Elevate the head of the bed 30 to 45 degrees if such elevation isn't contraindicated. *Proper positioning stretches the chest or back and allows easier access to the intercostal spaces.*

▶ Remind the patient not to cough, breathe deeply, or move suddenly during the procedure *to avoid puncture of the visceral pleura or lung.* If the patient coughs, the doctor will briefly halt the procedure and withdraw the needle slightly *to prevent puncture.*

▶ Expose the patient's entire chest or back as appropriate.

▶ Shave the aspiration site as ordered.

▶ Wash your hands again before touching the sterile equipment. Then, using sterile technique, open the thoracentesis tray and assist the doctor as necessary in disinfecting the site.

▶ If an ampule of local anesthetic isn't included in the sterile tray and a multidose vial of local anesthetic is to be used, assist the doctor by wiping the rubber stopper with an alcohol pad and holding the inverted vial while the doctor withdraws the anesthetic solution.

▶ After draping the patient and injecting the anesthetic, the doctor attaches a three-way stopcock with tubing to the aspirating needle and turns the stopcock to prevent air from entering the pleural space through the needle.

▶ Attach the other end of the tubing to the drainage bottle.

▶ The doctor then inserts the needle into the pleural space and attaches a 50-ml syringe to the needle's stopcock. A hemostat may be *used to hold the needle in place and prevent pleural tear or lung puncture.* As an alternative, the doctor may introduce a Teflon catheter into the needle, remove the needle, and attach a stopcock and syringe or drainage tubing to the catheter *to reduce the risk of pleural puncture by the needle.*

▶ Support the patient verbally throughout the procedure and keep him informed of each step. Assess him for signs of anxiety and provide reassurance as necessary.

▶ Check vital signs regularly during the procedure. Continually observe the patient for such signs of distress as pallor, vertigo, faintness, weak and rapid pulse, decreased blood pressure, dyspnea, tachypnea, diaphoresis, chest pain, blood-tinged mucus, and excessive coughing. Alert the doctor if such signs develop *because they may indicate complications, such as hypovolemic shock and tension pneumothorax.*

▶ Put on gloves and assist the doctor as necessary in specimen collection, fluid drainage, and dressing the site.

▶ After the doctor withdraws the needle or catheter, apply pressure to the puncture site using a sterile 4″ × 4″ gauze pad. Then apply a new sterile gauze pad and secure it with tape.

▶ Place the patient in a comfortable position, take his vital signs, and assess his respiratory status.

▶ Label the specimens properly and send them to the laboratory.
▶ Discard disposable equipment. Clean nondisposable items and return them for sterilization.
▶ Check the patient's vital signs and the dressing for drainage every 15 minutes for 1 hour. Continue to assess the patient's vital signs and respiratory status as indicated by his condition.

Special considerations
▶ To prevent pulmonary edema and hypovolemic shock after thoracentesis, fluid is removed slowly, and no more than 1,000 ml of fluid is removed during the first 30 minutes. *Removing the fluid increases the negative intrapleural pressure, which can lead to edema if the lung doesn't reexpand to fill the space.*
▶ Pleuritic or shoulder pain may indicate pleural irritation by the needle point.
▶ A chest X-ray is usually ordered after the procedure *to detect pneumothorax and evaluate the results of the procedure.*

Complications
Pneumothorax (possibly leading to mediastinal shift and requiring chest tube insertion) can occur if the needle punctures the lung and allows air to enter the pleural cavity. Pyogenic infection can result from contamination during the procedure. Other potential difficulties include pain, cough, anxiety, dry taps, and subcutaneous hematoma.

Documentation
Record the date and time of thoracentesis; location of the puncture site; volume and description (color, viscosity, odor) of the fluid withdrawn; specimens sent to the laboratory; vital signs and respiratory assessment before, dur-

Better charting

Documenting thoracentesis

When documenting thoracentesis, remember to note the following:
■ date, time, and name of the doctor performing the procedure
■ amount and quality of fluid aspirated
■ patient's response to the procedure
■ whether a fluid specimen was sent to the laboratory for analysis.
  If later symptoms of pneumothorax, subcutaneous emphysema, or infection occur, notify the doctor immediately and document your observations and interventions on the chart.

ing, and after the procedure; any postprocedural tests such as a chest X-ray; any complications and the nursing action taken; and the patient's reaction to the procedure. (See *Documenting thoracentesis.*)

THORACIC DRAINAGE

Thoracic drainage uses gravity and possibly suction to restore negative pressure and remove any material that collects in the pleural cavity. The disposable drainage system combines drainage collection, a water seal, and suction control into a single unit. The underwater seal in the drainage system allows air and fluid to escape from the pleural cavity but doesn't allow air to reenter. (See *Disposable drainage systems,* page 800.)
  Specifically, thoracic drainage may be ordered to remove accumulated air, fluids (blood, pus, chyle, and serous fluids), or solids (blood clots) from the

Disposable drainage systems

Commercially prepared disposable drainage systems combine drainage collection, water seal, and suction control in one unit (as shown here). These systems ensure patient safety with positive- and negative-pressure relief valves and have a prominent air-leak indicator. Some systems produce no bubbling sound.

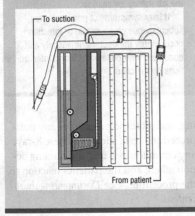

To suction

From patient

pleural cavity; to restore negative pressure in the pleural cavity; or to reexpand a partially or totally collapsed lung.

Key nursing diagnoses and patient outcomes

Ineffective breathing pattern related to physical condition
The patient will:
▶ have a respiratory rate within _____ breaths of baseline
▶ have arterial blood gas levels remain normal.

Acute pain related to physical condition
The patient will:

▶ express feelings of comfort and relief from pain
▶ state and carry out appropriate interventions for pain relief.

Equipment

Thoracic drainage system (Pleur-evac, Argyle, Ohio, or Thora-Klex system, which can function as gravity draining systems or be connected to suction to enhance chest drainage) • sterile distilled water (usually 1 L) • adhesive tape • sterile clear plastic tubing • two rubber-tipped Kelly clamps • sterile 50-ml catheter-tip syringe • suction source, if ordered • rubber band or safety pin.

Preparation of equipment

Check the doctor's order to determine the type of drainage system to be used and specific procedural details. If appropriate, request the drainage system and suction system from the central supply department. Collect the appropriate equipment and take it to the patient's bedside.

Implementation

▶ Explain the procedure to the patient and wash your hands.
▶ Maintain sterile technique throughout the entire procedure and whenever you make changes in the system or alter any of the connections *to avoid introducing pathogens into the pleural space.*

Setting up a commercially prepared disposable system

▶ Open the packaged system and place it on the floor in the rack supplied by the manufacturer *to avoid accidentally knocking it over or dislodging the components.* After the system is prepared, it may be hung from the side of the patient's bed.

▶ Remove the plastic connector from the short tube that is attached to the water-seal chamber. Using a 50-ml catheter-tip syringe, instill sterile distilled water into the water-seal chamber until it reaches the 2-cm mark or the mark specified by the manufacturer. The Ohio and Thora-Klex systems are ready to use, but with the Thora-Klex system, 15 ml of sterile water may be added to help detect air leaks. Replace the plastic connector.

▶ If suction is ordered, remove the cap (also called the muffler or atmosphere vent cover) on the suction-control chamber *to open the vent*. Next, instill sterile distilled water until it reaches the 20-cm mark or the ordered level and recap the suction-control chamber.

▶ Using the long tube, connect the patient's chest tube to the closed drainage collection chamber. Secure the connection with tape.

▶ Connect the short tube on the drainage system to the suction source and turn on the suction. Gentle bubbling should begin in the suction chamber, *indicating that the correct suction level has been reached.*

Managing closed-chest underwater seal drainage

▶ Repeatedly note the character, consistency, and amount of drainage in the drainage collection chamber.

▶ Mark the drainage level in the drainage collection chamber by noting the time and date at the drainage level on the chamber every 8 hours (or more often if there is a large amount of drainage).

▶ Check the water level in the water-seal chamber every 8 hours. If necessary, carefully add sterile distilled water until the level reaches the 2-cm mark indicated on the water-seal chamber of the commercial system.

▶ Check for fluctuation in the water-seal chamber as the patient breathes. Normal fluctuations of 2″ to 4″ (5 to 10 cm) reflect pressure changes in the pleural space during respiration. To check for fluctuation when a suction system is being used, momentarily disconnect the suction system so the air vent is opened and observe for fluctuation.

▶ Check for intermittent bubbling in the water-seal chamber. This occurs normally when the system is removing air from the pleural cavity. If bubbling isn't readily apparent during quiet breathing, have the patient take a deep breath or cough. Absence of bubbling indicates that the pleural space has sealed.

▶ Check the water level in the suction-control chamber. Detach the chamber or bottle from the suction source; when bubbling ceases, observe the water level. If necessary, add sterile distilled water to bring the level to the −20-cm line or as ordered.

▶ Check for gentle bubbling in the suction control chamber *because it indicates that the proper suction level has been reached.* Vigorous bubbling in this chamber increases the rate of water evaporation.

▶ Periodically check that the air vent in the system is working properly. *Occlusion of the air vent results in a buildup of pressure in the system that could cause the patient to develop a tension pneumothorax.*

▶ Coil the system's tubing and secure it to the edge of the bed with a rubber band or tape and a safety pin. Avoid creating dependent loops, kinks, or pressure on the tubing. Avoid lifting the drainage system above the patient's chest *because fluid may flow back into the pleural space.*

▶ Be sure to keep two rubber-tipped clamps at the bedside *to clamp the chest tube if the system cracks or to locate an air leak in the system.*

▶ Encourage the patient to cough frequently and breathe deeply *to help drain the pleural space and expand the lungs.*

▶ Tell him to sit upright *for optimal lung expansion* and to splint the insertion site while coughing *to minimize pain.*

▶ Check the rate and quality of the patient's respirations and auscultate his lungs periodically *to assess air exchange in the affected lung.* Diminished or absent breath sounds may indicate that the lung hasn't reexpanded.

▶ Tell the patient to report any breathing difficulty immediately. Notify the doctor immediately if the patient develops cyanosis, rapid or shallow breathing, subcutaneous emphysema, chest pain, or excessive bleeding.

▶ Check the chest tube dressing at least every 8 hours. Palpate the area surrounding the dressing for crepitus or subcutaneous emphysema, which indicates that air is leaking into the subcutaneous tissue surrounding the insertion site. Change the dressing if necessary or according to policy.

▶ Encourage active or passive range-of-motion (ROM) exercises for the patient's arm or the affected side if he has been splinting the arm. Usually, the thoracotomy patient will splint his arm to decrease his discomfort.

▶ Give ordered pain medication as needed *for comfort and to help with deep breathing, coughing, and ROM exercises.*

▶ Remind the ambulatory patient to keep the drainage system below chest level and to be careful not to disconnect the tubing *to maintain the water seal.* With a suction system, the patient must stay within range of the length of tubing attached to a wall outlet or portable pump.

Special considerations

▶ Instruct staff and visitors to avoid touching the equipment *to prevent complications from separated connections.*

▶ If excessive continuous bubbling is present in the water-seal chamber, especially if suction is being used, rule out a leak in the drainage system. Try to locate the leak by clamping the tube momentarily at various points along its length. Begin clamping at the tube's proximal end and work down toward the drainage system, paying special attention to the seal around the connections. If any connection is loose, push it back together and tape it securely. *The bubbling will stop when a clamp is placed between the air leak and the water seal.* If you clamp along the tube's entire length and the bubbling doesn't stop, the drainage unit may be cracked and need replacement.

▶ If the drainage collection chamber fills, replace it. To do this, double-clamp the tube close to the insertion site (use two clamps facing in opposite directions), exchange the system, remove the clamps, and retape the connection.

Nursing alert Never leave the tubes clamped for more than a minute to prevent a tension pneumothorax, which may occur when clamping stops air and fluid from escaping.

▶ If the system cracks, clamp the chest tube momentarily with the two rubber-tipped clamps at the bedside (placed there at the time of tube insertion). Place the clamps close to each other near the insertion site; they should face in opposite directions to provide a more complete seal. Observe the patient for altered respirations while the tube is clamped. Then replace the damaged equipment. (Prepare the new unit before clamping the tube.)

▶ Instead of clamping the tube, you can submerge the distal end of the tube in a container of normal saline solution *to create a temporary water seal while you replace the drainage system.* Check your facility's policy for the proper procedure.

Complications

Tension pneumothorax may result from excessive accumulation of air, drainage, or both and eventually may exert pressure on the heart and aorta, causing a precipitous fall in cardiac output.

Documentation

Record the date and time thoracic drainage began, type of system used, amount of suction applied to the pleural cavity, presence or absence of bubbling or fluctuation in the water-seal chamber, initial amount and type of drainage, and the patient's respiratory status.

At the end of each shift, record the frequency of system inspection; amount, color, and consistency of drainage; presence or absence of bubbling or fluctuation in the water-seal chamber; the patient's respiratory status; condition of the chest dressings; pain medication, if given; and any complications and the nursing action taken.

THORACIC ELECTRICAL BIOIMPEDANCE MONITORING

A noninvasive alternative for tracking hemodynamic status, thoracic electrical bioimpedance monitoring provides information about a patient's cardiac index, preload, afterload, contractibility, cardiac output, and blood flow. In this procedure, electrodes are placed on the patient's thorax. The electrodes have two purposes: to send harmless low-level electricity through the patient's body and to detect return electrical signals. These signals, which are interruptions in the electrical flow, come from changes in the volume and velocity of blood as it flows through the aorta. The bioimpedance monitor interprets the signals as a waveform. Cardiac output is then computed from this waveform and the electrocardiogram (ECG).

Key nursing diagnoses and patient outcomes

Deficient knowledge related to lack of exposure to procedure
The patient will:
▶ communicate a need to know reasons for doing the procedure
▶ state an understanding of the procedure and the reasons for it.

Decreased cardiac output related to reduced stroke volume
The patient will:
▶ maintain hemodynamic stability — pulse not less than (specify) beats/minute and not greater than (specify) beats/minute; blood pressure not less than (specify) mm Hg and not greater than (specify) mm Hg

▶ exhibit no signs of arrhythmias
▶ not complain of chest pain, dizziness, or syncope.

Ineffective tissue perfusion (cardiopulmonary) related to decreased cellular exchange
The patient will:
▶ maintain adequate cardiac output
▶ have clear breath sounds on auscultation
▶ have arterial blood gas results within normal limits.

Equipment
Thoracic electrical bioimpedance unit • patient harness with color-coded leadwires • connecting cable • four sets of thoracic electrical bioimpedance electrodes • three ECG electrodes • 3″ × 3″ or 4″ × 4″ gauze pads • tape measure • gloves

Preparation of equipment
▶ Explain the procedure to the patient; wash your hands and put on gloves. Plug the thoracic electrical bioimpedance unit into a power supply.
▶ Press the POWER button. The initial display screen will appear.
▶ Press the RUN key on the display screen. The patient data screen will appear.
▶ Enter the patient data by pressing each patient data block on the screen. Choose METRIC or ENGLISH for numbers, MALE or FEMALE, and ADULT or PED-NEO. When you press the appropriate block on the screen, a dot will appear beside your choice.
▶ To enter data for the patient's identification number, thoracic length, height, and weight, press the block that identifies the index you wish to include. Afterward, the numeric keypad screen will appear.

▶ Enter the actual value for the chosen index by pressing the smaller blocks on the keypad. When you've entered all the data for the chosen index, press ENTER. This will return you to the patient data screen. Now repeat the process for each index you wish to include.
▶ When you've entered your data, press the > block on the patient data screen to call up the waveform screen.
▶ You'll routinely use this screen to monitor the patient's status. It displays ECG and a pulmonary artery pressure waveform as well as six parameters that you choose. To select a parameter, press the block labeled PARAMETERS.
▶ The parameter screen will appear. Press the blocks labeled with the parameters you wish to display on the waveform screen. Press the > at the bottom of the parameter screen to return to the waveform screen. All of the selected parameters will now appear on the waveform screen.

Implementation
▶ Assist the patient onto his back. Provide privacy and expose his chest. Wet some 4″ × 4″ or 3″ × 3″ gauze pads with warm water and clean the skin on each side of his neck from the base of the neck to 2″ (5 cm) above the base. Also clean the skin on both sides of the chest at the midaxillary line directly across the xyphoid process. *To ensure that you've cleaned a large enough area for electrode placement,* clean at least two fingerbreadths above and below the site.
▶ Place one electrode set vertically at the neck base below the ear with the arrow end (containing the round electrode) pointing down. Place the bar electrode at least 2″ above the round electrode. If the two electrodes are an

attached set, place the bar electrode directly above the round one.

▶ Place the second set of electrodes on the opposite side of the neck in line with the ear and about 180 degrees from the first set.

▶ Place the remaining two sets of electrodes on either side of the patient's chest. *To determine the correct location,* draw a line with your finger from the xyphoid process to the midaxillary line on one side of the chest. This is the site for the first chest electrode. Place the round electrode here with the arrow pointing up.

▶ Place the second (bar) electrode at least 2″ (5.1 cm) below the first. Or, if you're using an attached set of electrodes, place the bar electrode directly below the round one.

▶ Next, place the final set of electrodes on the midaxillary line directly opposite the first set of electrodes.

▶ Attach ECG electrodes and try different lead selections until you obtain a consistent QRS signal. Don't remove the patient from the primary monitor. *The regular system must be maintained to ensure monitoring at the central station and to keep the alarms intact.*

▶ Now attach the leadwires of the bioimpedance harness to the thoracic electrical bioimpedance electrodes and the ECG electrodes.

▶ Attach the harness cable to the cable from the bioimpedance monitor.

▶ Next, measure the distance between the round electrode on one side of the patient's neck and the round electrode on the same side of his chest. This distance, the thorax length, is the numeric value required by the monitor's computer to calculate accurate stroke volume. Enter this value by calling up the patient data screen and entering the value. Return to the waveform screen.

Special considerations

▶ Baseline bioimpedance values may be reduced in patients who have conditions characterized by increased fluid in the chest, such as pulmonary edema and pleural effusion.

▶ Bioimpedance values may be lower than thermodilution values in patients with tachycardia and other arrhythmias.

▶ If you fail to get a clear waveform, place the bar electrode on each side of the patient's forehead, *which increases the distance between the electrodes and often improves the waveform quality.*

Documentation

Note the waveforms and values on the monitor and document the values by pressing PRINT on the waveform screen to print a strip containing all the values monitored. Place the strip on the patient's chart.

TILT TABLE USE

The tilt table, a padded table or bed-length board that can be raised gradually from a horizontal to a vertical position, can help prevent the complications of prolonged bed rest. Used for the patient with a spinal cord injury, brain damage, orthostatic hypotension, or any other condition that prevents free standing, the tilt table increases tolerance of the upright position, conditions the cardiovascular system, stretches muscles, and helps prevent contractures, bone demineralization, and urinary calculi formation.

Key nursing diagnoses and patient outcomes

Impaired physical mobility related to neuromuscular impairment
The patient will:
▶ show no evidence of such complications as contractures, venous stasis, thrombus formation, and skin breakdown
▶ have mobility regimen carried out by caregiver.

Risk for disuse syndrome related to prolonged inactivity
The patient will:
▶ display no evidence of altered mental, sensory, or motor activity
▶ maintain muscle strength and tone and range of motion
▶ maintain normal neurologic, cardiovascular, respiratory, musculoskeletal, GI, and integumentary function during period of inactivity.

Equipment

Tilt table with footboard and restraining straps • sphygmomanometer • stethoscope • antiembolism stockings or elastic bandages • optional: abdominal binder

Preparation of equipment

Common types of tilt tables include the electric table, which moves at a slow, steady rate; the manual table, which is raised by a handle; and the spring-assisted table, which is raised by a pedal. Familiarize yourself with operating instructions for the model you'll be using.

Implementation

▶ Explain the use and benefits of the tilt table to the patient.
▶ Apply antiembolism stockings *to restrict vessel walls and help prevent blood*

pooling and edema. If necessary, apply an abdominal binder *to avoid pooling of blood in the splanchnic region, which contributes to insufficient cerebral circulation and orthostatic hypotension.*
▶ Make sure the tilt table is locked in the horizontal position. Then summon assistance and transfer the patient to the table, placing him in the supine position with his feet flat against the footboard.
▶ If the patient can't bear weight on one leg, place a wooden block between the footboard and the weight-bearing foot, permitting the non-weight-bearing leg to dangle freely.
▶ Fasten the safety straps, then take the patient's blood pressure and pulse rate.
▶ Tilt the table slowly in 15- to 30-degree increments, evaluating the patient constantly. Take his blood pressure every 3 to 5 minutes *because movement from the supine to the upright position decreases systolic pressure.* Be alert for signs and symptoms of insufficient cerebral circulation: dizziness, nausea, pallor, diaphoresis, tachycardia, or a change in mental status. If the patient experiences any of these signs or symptoms, or hypotension or seizures, return the table immediately to the horizontal position.
▶ If the patient tolerates the position shift, continue to tilt the table until reaching the desired angle, usually between 45 degrees and 80 degrees. A 60-degree tilt gives the patient the physiologic effects and sensations of standing upright.
▶ Gradually return the patient to the horizontal position and check his vital signs. Then obtain assistance and transfer the patient onto the stretcher for transport back to his room.

Special considerations

Let the patient's response determine the angle of tilt and duration of elevation but avoid prolonged upright positioning because it may lead to venous stasis.

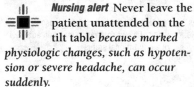 **Nursing alert** Never leave the patient unattended on the tilt table *because marked physiologic changes, such as hypotension or severe headache, can occur suddenly.*

Complications

Use of a tilt table can lead to sudden hypotension, severe headache, and other dramatic physiologic changes.

Documentation

Record the angle and duration of elevation; changes in the patient's pulse rate, blood pressure, and physical and mental status; and his response to treatment.

TOTAL PARENTERAL NUTRITION

When a patient can't meet his nutritional needs by oral or enteral feedings, he may require I.V. nutritional support, or parenteral nutrition. The patient's diagnosis, history, and prognosis determine the need for parenteral nutrition. Generally, this treatment is prescribed for any patient who can't absorb nutrients through the GI tract for more than 10 days. More specific indications include:
▶ debilitating illness lasting longer than 2 weeks
▶ loss of 10% or more of preillness weight
▶ serum albumin level below 3.5 g/dl
▶ excessive nitrogen loss from wound infection, fistulas, or abscesses

▶ renal or hepatic failure
▶ a nonfunctioning GI tract for 5 to 7 days in a severely catabolic patient.

Parenteral nutrition may be given through a peripheral or central venous (CV) line. Depending on the solution, it may be used to boost the patient's caloric intake, to supply full caloric needs, or to surpass the patient's caloric requirements.

The type of parenteral solution prescribed depends on the patient's condition and metabolic needs and on the administration route. The solution usually contains protein, carbohydrates, electrolytes, vitamins, and trace minerals. A lipid emulsion provides the necessary fat. (See *Types of parenteral nutrition,* pages 808 and 809.)

Total parenteral nutrition (TPN) refers to any nutrient solution, including lipids, given through a CV line. Peripheral parenteral nutrition (PPN), which is given through a peripheral line, supplies full caloric needs while avoiding the risks that accompany a CV line. To keep from sclerosing the vein through which it's administered, the dextrose in PPN solution must be limited to 10% or less. Therefore, the success of PPN depends on the patient's tolerance for the large volume of fluid necessary to supply his nutritional needs.

Often, you'll need to increase the glucose content beyond the level a peripheral vein can handle. For example, most TPN solutions are six times more concentrated than blood. As a result, they must be delivered into a vein with a high rate of blood flow to dilute the solution.

The most common delivery route for TPN is through a central venous catheter (CVC) into the superior vena cava.

(Text continues on page 810.)

Types of parenteral nutrition

Type	Solution components/liter	Special considerations
Standard I.V. therapy	■ Dextrose, water, electrolytes in varying amounts, for example: – dextrose 5% in water (D_5W) = 170 calories/L – $D_{10}W$ = 340 calories/L – normal saline = 0 calories ■ Vitamins as ordered	■ Nutritionally incomplete; doesn't provide sufficient calories to maintain adequate nutritional status
Total parenteral nutrition (TPN) by way of central venous (CV) line	■ $D_{15}W$ to $D_{25}W$ (1 L dextrose 25% = 850 nonprotein calories) ■ Crystalline amino acids 2.5% to 8.5% ■ Electrolytes, vitamins, trace elements, and insulin, as ordered ■ Lipid emulsion 10% to 20% (usually infused as a separate solution)	*Basic solution* ■ Nutritionally complete ■ Requires minor surgical procedure for CV line insertion (can be done at bedside by the doctor) ■ Highly hypertonic solution ■ May cause metabolic complications (glucose intolerance, electrolyte imbalance, essential fatty acid deficiency) *I.V. lipid emulsion* ■ May not be used effectively in severely stressed patients (especially burn patients) ■ May interfere with immune mechanisms; in patients suffering respiratory compromise, reduces carbon dioxide buildup ■ Given by way of CV line; irritates peripheral vein in long-term use
Protein-sparing therapy	■ Crystalline amino acids in same amounts as TPN ■ Electrolytes, vitamins, minerals, and trace elements as ordered	■ Nutritionally complete ■ Requires little mixing ■ May be started or stopped any time during the hospital stay ■ Other I.V. fluids, medications, and blood by-products may be administered through the same I.V. line ■ Not as likely to cause phlebitis as peripheral parenteral nutrition ■ Adds a major expense; has limited benefits
Total nutrient admixture	■ One day's nutrients are contained in a single, 3-L bag (also called 3:1 solution)	■ See TPN (above) ■ Reduces need to handle bag, cutting risk of contamination

Types of parenteral nutrition *(continued)*

Type	Solution components/liter	Special considerations
Total nutrient admixture *(continued)*	■ Combines lipid emulsion with other parenteral solution components	■ Decreases nursing time and reduces need for infusion sets and electronic devices, lowering facility costs, increasing patient mobility, and allowing easier adjustment to home care ■ Has limited use because not all types and amounts of components are compatible ■ Precludes use of certain infusion pumps because they can't accurately deliver large volumes of solution; precludes use of standard I.V. tubing filters because a 0.22-micron filter blocks lipid and albumin molecules
Peripheral parenteral nutrition (PPN)	■ D_5W to $D_{10}W$ ■ Crystalline amino acids 2.5% to 5% ■ Electrolytes, minerals, vitamins, and trace elements as ordered ■ Lipid emulsion 10% or 20% (1 L of dextrose 10% and amino acids 3.5% infused at the same time as 1 L of lipid emulsion = 1,440 nonprotein calories) ■ Heparin or hydrocortisone as ordered	***Basic solution*** ■ Nutritionally complete for a short time ■ Can't be used in nutritionally depleted patients ■ Can't be used in volume-restricted patients because PPN requires large fluid volume ■ Doesn't cause weight gain ■ Avoids insertion and care of CV line but requires adequate venous access; site must be changed every 72 hours ■ Delivers less hypertonic solutions than CV line TPN ■ May cause phlebitis and increases risk of metabolic complications ■ Less chance of metabolic complications than with CV line TPN ***I.V. lipid emulsion*** ■ As effective as dextrose for caloric source ■ Diminishes phlebitis if infused at the same time as basic nutrient solution ■ Irritates vein in long-term use ■ Reduces carbon dioxide buildup when pulmonary compromise is present

The catheter may also be placed through the infraclavicular approach or, less commonly, through the supraclavicular, internal jugular, or antecubital fossa approach.

Key nursing diagnoses and patient outcomes

Imbalanced nutrition: Less than body requirements related to inability to digest or absorb nutrients
The patient will:
▶ tolerate oral, tube, or I.V. feedings without adverse effects
▶ show no evidence of further weight loss.

Risk for fluid volume imbalance related to active loss
The patient will:
▶ have fluid volume remain adequate
▶ have electrolyte levels stay within normal range.

Equipment

Bag or bottle of prescribed parenteral nutrition solution • sterile I.V. tubing with attached extension tubing • 0.22-micron filter (or 1.2-micron filter if solution contains lipids or albumin) • reflux valve • time tape • alcohol pads • electronic infusion pump • portable glucose monitor • scale • intake and output record • sterile gloves • optional: mask

Preparation of equipment

Make sure the solution, the patient, and the equipment are ready. Remove the solution from the refrigerator at least 1 hour before use *to avoid pain, hypothermia, venous spasm, and venous constriction, which can result from delivery of a chilled solution.* Check the solution against the doctor's order for correct patient name, expiration date, and formula components. Observe the container for cracks and the solution for cloudiness, turbidity, and particles. If any of these is present, return the solution to the pharmacy. If you'll be administering a total nutrient admixture solution, look for a brown layer on the solution, which indicates that the lipid emulsion has "cracked," or separated from the solution. If you see a brown layer, return the solution to the pharmacy.

When you're ready to administer the solution, explain the procedure to the patient. Check the name on the solution container against the name on the patient's wristband. Then put on gloves and, if specified by facility policy, a mask. Throughout the procedure, use strict sterile technique.

In sequence, connect the pump tubing, the micron filter with attached extension tubing (if the tubing doesn't contain an in-line filter), and the reflux valve. Insert the filter as close to the catheter site as possible. If the tubing doesn't have luer-lock connections, tape all connections *to prevent accidental separation, which could lead to air embolism, exsanguination, or sepsis.* Next, squeeze the I.V. drip chamber and, holding it upright, insert the tubing spike into the I.V. bag or bottle. Then release the drip chamber. Squeeze the drip chamber before spiking an I.V. bottle *to prevent accidental dripping of the parenteral nutrition solution.* An I.V. bag, however, shouldn't drip.

Next, prime the tubing. Invert the filter at the distal end of the tubing and open the roller clamp. Let the solution fill the tubing and the filter. Gently tap it *to dislodge air bubbles trapped in the Y-ports.* If indicated, attach a time tape to the parenteral nutrition container *for* accurate measurement of fluid intake. Record the date and time you hung the fluid and initial the parenteral nutrition solution container. Next, attach the set-up to the infusion pump and prepare it according to the manufacturer's instructions. Remove and discard your gloves.

With the patient in the supine position, flush the catheter with normal saline solution, according to your facility's policy. Then put on gloves and clean the catheter injection cap with an alcohol pad.

Implementation

▶ If you'll be attaching the container of parenteral nutrition solution to a CV line, clamp the CV line before disconnecting it *to prevent air from entering the catheter.* If a clamp isn't available, ask the patient to perform Valsalva's maneuver just as you change the tubing, if possible. Or, if the patient is being mechanically ventilated, change the I.V. tubing immediately after the machine delivers a breath at peak inspiration. *Both of these measures increase intrathoracic pressure and prevent air embolism.*
▶ Using sterile technique, attach the tubing to the designated luer-locking port. After connecting the tubing, remove the clamp, if applicable.
▶ Make sure the catheter junction is secure. Set the infusion pump at the ordered flow rate and start the infusion.
▶ Tag the tubing with the date and time of change.

Starting the infusion
▶ *Because parenteral nutrition solution often contains a large amount of glucose,* you may need to start the infusion slowly to allow the patient's pancreatic beta cells time to increase their output of insulin. Depending on the patient's

tolerance, parenteral nutrition is usually initiated at a rate of 40 to 50 ml/hour and then advanced by 25 ml/hour every 6 hours (as tolerated) until the desired infusion rate is achieved. However, when the glucose concentration is low, as occurs in most PPN formulas, you can initiate the rate necessary to infuse the complete 24-hour volume and discontinue the solution without tapering.
▶ You may allow a container of parenteral nutrition solution to hang for 24 hours.

Changing solutions
▶ Prepare the new solution and I.V. tubing as described earlier. Put on gloves. Remove the protective caps from the solution containers and wipe the tops of the containers with alcohol pads.
▶ Turn off the infusion pump and close the flow clamps. Using strict sterile technique, remove the spike from the solution container that is hanging and insert it into the new container.
▶ Hang the new container and tubing alongside the old. Turn on the infusion pump, set the flow rate, and open the flow clamp completely.
▶ If you'll be attaching the solution to a peripheral line, examine the skin above the insertion site for redness and warmth and assess for pain. If you suspect phlebitis, remove the existing I.V. line and start a line in a different vein. Also insert a new line if the I.V. catheter has been in place for 72 hours or more *to reduce the risk of phlebitis and infiltration.*
▶ Next, turn off the infusion pump and close the flow clamp on the old tubing. Disconnect the tubing from the catheter hub and connect the new tub-

ing. Open the flow clamp on the new container to a moderately slow rate.

▶ Remove the old tubing from the infusion pump and insert the new tubing according to the manufacturer's instructions. Then turn on the infusion pump, set it to the desired flow rate, and open the flow clamp completely. Remove the old equipment and dispose of it properly.

Special considerations

▶ Always infuse a parenteral nutrition solution at a constant rate without interruption *to avoid blood glucose fluctuations.* If the infusion slows, consult the doctor before changing the infusion rate.

▶ Monitor the patient's vital signs every 4 hours or more often if necessary. Watch for an increased temperature, *an early sign of catheter-related sepsis.* (See *Correcting common parenteral nutrition problems.*)

▶ Check the patient's blood glucose level every 6 hours. Some patients may require supplementary insulin, which the pharmacist may add directly to the solution. The patient may require additional subcutaneous doses.

▶ *Because most patients receiving PPN are in a protein-wasted state,* the therapy causes marked changes in fluid and electrolyte status and in levels of glucose, amino acids, minerals, and vitamins. Therefore, record daily intake and output accurately. Specify the volume and type of each fluid and calculate the daily caloric intake.

▶ Monitor the results of routine laboratory tests and report abnormal findings to the doctor *to allow for appropriate changes in the parenteral nutrition solution.* Such tests typically include measurement of serum electrolyte, calcium, blood urea nitrogen, and creatinine at

least three times weekly; serum magnesium and phosphorus levels twice weekly; liver function studies, complete blood count and differential, and serum albumin and transferrin levels weekly; and urine nitrogen balance and creatinine-height index studies weekly. A serum zinc level is obtained at the start of parenteral nutrition therapy. The doctor may also order serum prealbumin levels, total lymphocyte count, amino acid levels, fatty acid-phospholipid fraction, skin testing, and expired gas analysis. (Also see "Total Parenteral Nutrition Monitoring," page 814.)

▶ Physically assess the patient daily. If ordered, measure arm circumference and skin-fold thickness over the triceps. Weigh him at the same time each morning after he voids; he should be weighed in similar clothing and on the same scale. Suspect fluid imbalance if he gains more than 1 lb (0.5 kg) daily.

▶ Change the dressing over the catheter according to your facility's policy or whenever the dressing becomes wet, soiled, or nonocclusive. Always use strict sterile technique. When performing dressing changes, watch for signs of phlebitis and catheter retraction from the vein. Measure the catheter length from the insertion site to the hub for verification.

▶ Change the tubing and filters every 24 hours or according to your facility's policy.

▶ Closely monitor the catheter site for swelling, which may indicate infiltration. Extravasation of parenteral nutrition solution can lead to tissue necrosis.

▶ Use caution when using the parenteral nutrition line for other functions. Don't use a single-lumen CVC to infuse blood or blood products, to give a bolus injection, to administer simultaneous

Correcting common parenteral nutrition problems

Complications	Signs and symptoms	Interventions
Hepatic dysfunction	Elevated serum aspartate amino-transferase, alkaline phosphatase, and bilirubin levels	Reduce total caloric intake and dextrose intake, making up lost calories by administering lipid emulsion. Change to cyclical infusion. Use specific hepatic formulations only if the patient has encephalopathy.
Hypercapnia	Heightened oxygen consumption, increased carbon dioxide production, measured respiratory quotient of 1 or greater	Reduce total caloric and dextrose intake and balance dextrose and fat calories.
Hyperglycemia	Fatigue, restlessness, confusion, anxiety, weakness, polyuria, dehydration, elevated serum glucose levels and, in severe hyperglycemia, delirium or coma	Restrict dextrose intake by decreasing either the rate of infusion or the dextrose concentration. Compensate for calorie loss by administering lipid emulsion. Begin insulin therapy.
Hyperosmolarity	Confusion, lethargy, seizures, hyperosmolar hyperglycemic nonketotic syndrome, hyperglycemia, dehydration, and glycosuria	Discontinue dextrose infusion. Administer insulin and half-normal saline solution with 10 to 20 mEq/L of potassium to rehydrate the patient.
Hypocalcemia	Polyuria, dehydration, and elevated blood and urine glucose levels	Increase calcium supplements.
Hypoglycemia	Sweating, shaking, and irritability after infusion has stopped	Increase dextrose intake or decrease exogenous insulin intake.
Hypokalemia	Muscle weakness, paralysis, paresthesia, and arrhythmias	Increase potassium supplements.
Hypomagnesemia	Tingling around mouth, paresthesia in fingers, mental changes, and hyperreflexia	Increase magnesium supplements.
Hypophosphatemia	Irritability, weakness, paresthesia, coma, and respiratory arrest	Increase phosphate supplements.
Metabolic acidosis	Elevated serum chloride level, reduced serum bicarbonate level	Increase acetate and decrease chloride in parenteral nutrition solution.
Metabolic alkalosis	Reduced serum chloride level, elevated serum bicarbonate level	Decrease acetate and increase chloride in parenteral nutrition solution.
Zinc deficiency	Dermatitis, alopecia, apathy, depression, taste changes, confusion, poor wound healing, and diarrhea	Increase zinc supplements.

Better charting

Documenting TPN

If a patient is receiving total parenteral nutrition (TPN), document the following:
- type and location of the central line
- condition of the insertion site
- volume and rate of the solution infused
- your observations of any adverse reactions and your interventions
- when you discontinue a central or peripheral I.V. line for TPN
- date and time and the type of dressing applied after it was discontinued
- the appearance of the administration site.

I.V. solutions, to measure CV pressure, or to draw blood for laboratory tests.
▶ Provide regular mouth care. Also provide emotional support. Keep in mind that patients commonly associate eating with positive feelings and become disturbed when they can't eat.
▶ Teach the patient the potential adverse effects and complications of parenteral nutrition. Encourage the patient to inspect his mouth regularly for signs of parotitis, glossitis, and oral lesions. Tell him that he may have fewer bowel movements while receiving parenteral nutrition therapy. Encourage him to remain physically active *to help his body use the nutrients more fully.*

Home care
Patients who require prolonged or indefinite parenteral nutrition may be able to receive therapy at home. Home parenteral nutrition reduces the need for long hospitalizations and allows the patient to resume many of his normal activities. Meet with a home care patient before discharge *to make sure he knows*

how to perform the administration procedure and how to handle complications.

Complications
Catheter-related sepsis is the most serious complication of parenteral nutrition. Although rare, a malpositioned subclavian or jugular vein catheter may lead to thrombosis or sepsis.

An air embolism, a potentially fatal complication, can occur during I.V. tubing changes if the tubing is inadvertently disconnected. It may also result from undetected hairline cracks in the tubing. Extravasation of parenteral nutrition solution can cause necrosis and then sloughing of the epidermis and dermis.

Documentation
Document the times of the dressing, filter, and solution changes; the condition of the catheter insertion site; your observations of the patient's condition; and any complications and interventions. (See *Documenting TPN.*)

TOTAL PARENTERAL NUTRITION MONITORING

Total parenteral nutrition (TPN) requires careful monitoring. Because the typical patient is in a protein-wasting state, TPN therapy causes marked changes in fluid and electrolyte status and in glucose, amino acid, mineral, and vitamin levels. If the patient displays an adverse reaction or signs of complications, the TPN regimen can be changed as needed.

Assessment of the patient's nutritional status includes a physical examination, anthropometric measurements, biochemical determinations, and tests of cell-mediated immunity. Assessment of the patient's condition to detect complications requires recognition of the signs and symptoms of possible complications, understanding of laboratory test results, and careful record keeping.

Because the TPN solution is high in glucose content, the infusion must start slowly to allow the patient's pancreatic beta cells to adapt to it by increasing insulin output. Within the first 3 to 5 days of TPN, the typical adult patient can tolerate 3 L of solution daily without adverse reactions. Lipid emulsions also require monitoring.

Key nursing diagnoses and patient outcomes

Imbalanced nutrition: Less than body requirements related to inability to digest or absorb nutrients
The patient will:
▶ tolerate oral, tube, or I.V. feedings without adverse effects
▶ show no evidence of further weight loss.

Risk for fluid volume imbalance related to active loss
The patient will:
▶ have fluid volume remain adequate
▶ have electrolyte levels stay within normal range.

Equipment
TPN solution and administration equipment • blood glucose meter • stethoscope • sphygmomanometer • watch with second hand • thermometer • scale • input and output chart • time tape • additional equipment for nutritional assessment as ordered

Preparation of equipment
Attach a time tape to the TPN container to allow approximate measurement of fluid intake. Make sure each bag or bottle has a label listing the expiration date, glucose concentration, and total volume of solution. (If the bag or bottle is damaged and you don't have an immediate replacement, hang a bag of dextrose 10% in water until the new container is ready.)

Implementation
▶ Explain the procedure to the patient *to diminish his anxiety and encourage cooperation.* Instruct him to inform you if he experiences any unusual sensations during the infusion.
▶ Record vital signs every 4 hours or more often if necessary *because increased temperature is one of the earliest signs of catheter-related sepsis.*
▶ Perform I.V. site care and dressing changes at least three times a week (once a week for transparent semipermeable dressings) or whenever the dressing becomes wet, soiled, or nonocclusive. Use strict sterile technique.
▶ Physically assess the patient daily. If ordered, measure arm circumference and skin-fold thickness over the triceps.
▶ Weigh the patient at the same time each morning (after voiding), in similar clothing, and on the same scale. Compare this data with his fluid intake and output record. Weight gain, especially early in treatment, may indicate fluid overload rather than increasing fat and protein stores. A patient shouldn't gain more than 3 lb (1.5 kg) a week; a gain of 1 lb (0.5 kg) a week is a reasonable goal for most patients. Suspect fluid imbalance if the patient gains more than 1 lb daily. Assess for peripheral and pulmonary edema.

► Monitor the patient for signs and symptoms of glucose metabolism disturbance, fluid and electrolyte imbalances, and nutritional aberrations. Remember that some patients may require supplemental insulin for the duration of TPN; the pharmacy usually adds insulin directly to the TPN solution.

► Monitor levels of electrolytes and protein frequently — daily at first for electrolytes and twice weekly for serum albumin. Later, as the patient's condition stabilizes, you won't need to monitor these values quite as closely. (Be aware that in a severely dehydrated patient, albumin levels may drop initially as treatment restores hydration.)

Pay close attention to magnesium and calcium levels. If these electrolytes have been added to the TPN solution, the dose may need adjusting to maintain normal serum levels. Assess the patient for signs and symptoms of magnesium and calcium imbalances.

► Monitor serum glucose levels every 6 hours initially and then once a day and stay alert for signs and symptoms of hyperglycemia, such as thirst and polyuria. Periodically confirm blood glucose meter readings with laboratory tests.

► Check kidney function by monitoring blood urea nitrogen and creatinine levels; *increases can indicate excess amino acid intake.* Also assess nitrogen balance with 24-hour urine collection.

► Assess liver function by periodically monitoring liver enzyme, bilirubin, triglyceride, and cholesterol levels. *Abnormal values may indicate an intolerance or excess of lipid emulsions or a problem with metabolizing the protein or glucose in the TPN formula.*

► Change I.V. administration sets every 24 hours using sterile technique. Because the risk of contamination is so high with TPN, each facility should continuously evaluate protocols based on quality-control findings.

► Monitor for signs of inflammation, infection, and sepsis, the most common complications of TPN. Microbial contamination of the venous access device is the usual cause. Watch for redness and drainage at the venous access site and monitor the patient for fever and other signs and symptoms of sepsis.

► Provide emotional support. Keep in mind that patients often associate eating with positive feelings and become disturbed when eating is prohibited.

► Provide frequent mouth care.

► Keep the patient active *to enable him to use nutrients more fully.*

► When discontinuing TPN, decrease the infusion rate slowly, depending on the patient's current glucose intake, *to minimize the risk of hyperinsulinemia and resulting hypoglycemia.* Weaning usually takes place over 24 to 48 hours but can be completed in 4 to 6 hours if the patient receives sufficient oral or I.V. carbohydrates.

Special considerations

► Always maintain strict sterile technique when handling the equipment used to administer therapy. *Because the TPN solution serves as a medium for bacterial growth and the central venous (CV) line provides systemic access, the patient risks infection and sepsis.*

► When using a filter, position it as close to the access site as possible. Check the filter's porosity and pounds-per-square-inch (psi) capacity *to make sure it exceeds the number of pounds per square inch exerted by the infusion pump.*

► Don't let TPN solutions hang for more than 24 hours.

▶ Be careful when using the TPN line for other functions. If using a single-lumen CV catheter, don't use the line to infuse blood or blood products, to give a bolus injection, to administer simultaneous I.V. solutions, to measure CV pressure, or to draw blood for laboratory tests. Never add medication to a TPN solution container. Also, don't use a three-way stopcock, if possible, *because add-on devices increase the risk of infection.*

Complications

Catheter-related, metabolic, and mechanical complications can occur during TPN administration.

Documentation

Record serial monitoring indexes on the appropriate flowchart to determine the patient's progress and response. Note any abnormal, adverse, or altered responses. While weaning from TPN, document his dietary intake.

TRACHEAL CUFF–PRESSURE MEASUREMENT

An endotracheal (ET) or tracheostomy cuff provides a closed system for mechanical ventilation, allowing a desired tidal volume to be delivered to the patient's lungs. To function properly, the cuff must exert enough pressure on the tracheal wall to seal the airway without compromising the blood supply to the tracheal mucosa.

The ideal pressure (known as minimal occlusive volume) is the lowest amount needed to seal the airway. Many authorities recommend maintaining a cuff pressure lower than venous perfusion pressure — usually 16 to 24 cm H_2O. (More than 24 cm H_2O may exceed venous perfusion pressure.) Actual cuff pressure will vary with each patient, however.

Key nursing diagnoses and patient outcomes

Ineffective breathing pattern related to decreased energy
The patient will:
▶ achieve maximum lung expansion with adequate ventilation
▶ report feeling comfortable with breathing.

Impaired gas exchange related to altered oxygen supply
The patient will:
▶ cough effectively
▶ expectorate sputum.

Equipment

10-ml syringe • three-way stopcock • cuff pressure manometer • stethoscope • suction equipment • gloves

Preparation of equipment

Assemble all equipment at the patient's bedside. If measuring with a blood pressure manometer, attach the syringe to one stopcock port; then attach the tubing from the manometer to another port of the stopcock. Turn off the stopcock port where you'll be connecting the pilot balloon cuff *so that air can't escape from the cuff.* Use the syringe to instill air into the manometer tubing until the pressure reading reaches 10 mm Hg. *This will prevent sudden cuff deflation when you open the stopcock to the cuff and the manometer.*

Implementation

▶ Explain the procedure to the patient. Put on gloves and suction the ET or tracheostomy tube and the patient's oropharynx to remove accumulated secretions above the cuff. Then attach the cuff pressure manometer to the pilot balloon port.

▶ Place the diaphragm of the stethoscope over the trachea and listen for an air leak (as shown below). Keep in mind that a smooth, hollow sound indicates a sealed airway; a loud, gurgling sound indicates an air leak.

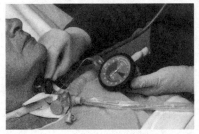

▶ If you don't hear an air leak, press the red button under the dial of the cuff pressure manometer to slowly release air from the balloon on the tracheal tube (as shown below). Auscultate for an air leak.

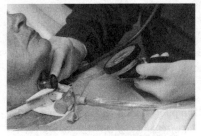

▶ As soon as you hear an air leak, release the red button and gently squeeze the handle of the cuff pressure manometer to inflate the cuff (as shown at top of next column). Continue to add air to the cuff until you no longer hear an air leak.

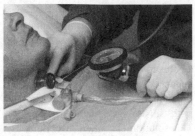

▶ When the air leak ceases, read the dial on the cuff pressure manometer (as shown below). This is the minimal pressure required to effectively occlude the trachea around the tracheal tube. In many cases, this pressure will fall within the green area (16 to 24 cm H_2O) on the manometer dial.

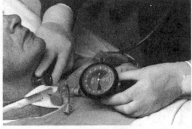

▶ Disconnect the cuff pressure manometer from the pilot balloon port. Document the pressure value.

Special considerations

▶ Measure cuff pressure at least every 8 hours *to avoid overinflation.*

▶ Keep in mind that some patients require less pressure, whereas others — for example, those with tracheal malacia (an abnormal softening of the tracheal tissue) — require more pressure. Maintaining the cuff pressure at the lowest possible level will minimize cuff-related problems.

▶ When measuring cuff pressure, keep the connection between the measuring device and the pilot balloon port tight *to avoid an air leak that could compromise* cuff pressure. If you're using a stopcock, don't leave the manometer in the OFF position *because air will leak from the cuff if the syringe accidentally comes off.* Also note the volume of air needed to inflate the cuff. A gradual increase in this volume indicates tracheal dilation or erosion. A sudden increase in volume indicates rupture of the cuff and requires immediate reintubation if the patient is being ventilated.

Complications

Aspiration of upper airway secretions, underventilation, or coughing spasms may occur if a leak is created during cuff pressure measurement.

Documentation

After cuff pressure measurement, record the date and time of the procedure, cuff pressure, total amount of air in the cuff after the procedure, any complications and the nursing action taken, and the patient's tolerance of the procedure.

TRACHEAL SUCTION

Tracheal suction involves the removal of secretions from the trachea or bronchi by means of a catheter inserted through the mouth or nose, a tracheal stoma, a tracheostomy tube, or an endotracheal (ET) tube. In addition to removing secretions, tracheal suctioning also stimulates the cough reflex. This procedure helps maintain a patent airway to promote optimal exchange of oxygen and carbon dioxide and to prevent pneumonia that results from pooling of secretions. Performed as frequently as the patient's condition warrants, tracheal suction calls for strict aseptic technique.

Key nursing diagnoses and patient outcomes

Ineffective breathing pattern related to decreased energy
The patient will:
▶ achieve maximum lung expansion with adequate ventilation
▶ report feeling comfortable with breathing.

Impaired gas exchange related to altered oxygen supply
The patient will:
▶ cough effectively
▶ expectorate sputum.

Equipment

Oxygen source (wall or portable unit and handheld resuscitation bag with a mask, 15-mm adapter, or a positive end-expiratory pressure [PEEP] valve, if indicated) • wall or portable suction apparatus • collection container • connecting tube • suction catheter kit, or a sterile suction catheter, one sterile glove, one clean glove, and a disposable sterile solution container • 1-L bottle of sterile water or normal saline solution • sterile water-soluble lubricant (for nasal insertion) • syringe for deflating cuff of ET or tracheostomy tube • waterproof trash bag • optional: sterile towel

Preparation of equipment

Choose a suction catheter of appropriate size. The diameter should be no larger than half the inside diameter of the tracheostomy or ET tube *to minimize hypoxia during suctioning.* (A #12 or #14 French catheter may be used for an 8-mm or larger tube.) Place the suction apparatus on the patient's overbed table or bedside stand. Position the table or stand on your preferred side of the bed *to facilitate suctioning.*

Attach the collection container to the suction unit and the connecting tube to the collection container. Label and date the normal saline solution or sterile water. Open the waterproof trash bag.

Implementation

▶ Before suctioning, determine whether your facility requires a doctor's order and obtain one, if necessary.
▶ Assess the patient's vital signs, breath sounds, and general appearance *to establish a baseline for comparison after suctioning.* Review the patient's arterial blood gas values and oxygen saturation levels if they're available. Evaluate the patient's ability to cough and deep-breathe *because this will help move secretions up the tracheobronchial tree.* If you'll be performing nasotracheal suctioning, check the patient's history for a deviated septum, nasal polyps, nasal obstruction, nasal trauma, epistaxis, or mucosal swelling.
▶ Wash your hands. Explain the procedure to the patient even if he's unresponsive. Tell him that suctioning usually causes transient coughing or gagging but that coughing is helpful for removal of secretions. If the patient has been suctioned previously, summarize the reasons for suctioning. Continue to reassure the patient throughout the procedure *to minimize anxiety, promote relaxation, and decrease oxygen demand.*
▶ Unless contraindicated, place the patient in semi-Fowler's or high Fowler's position *to promote lung expansion and productive coughing.*
▶ Remove the top from the normal saline solution or water bottle.
▶ Open the package containing the sterile solution container.
▶ Using sterile technique, open the suction catheter kit and put on the gloves. If using individual supplies, open the suction catheter and the gloves, placing the nonsterile glove on your nondominant hand and then the sterile glove on your dominant hand.
▶ Using your nondominant (nonsterile) hand, pour the normal saline solution or sterile water into the solution container.
▶ Place a small amount of water-soluble lubricant on the sterile area. Lubricant may be used to facilitate passage of the catheter during nasotracheal suctioning.
▶ Place a sterile towel over the patient's chest, if desired, *to provide an additional sterile area.*
▶ Using your dominant (sterile) hand, remove the catheter from its wrapper. Keep it coiled so it can't touch a nonsterile object. Using your other hand to manipulate the connecting tubing, attach the catheter to the tubing (as shown below).

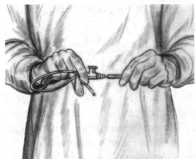

▶ Using your nondominant hand, set the suction pressure according to facility policy. Typically, pressure may be set between 80 and 120 mm Hg. *Higher pressures don't enhance secretion removal and may cause traumatic injury.* Occlude the suction port to assess suction pressure (as shown at top of next page).

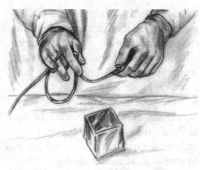

▶ Dip the catheter tip in the saline solution *to lubricate the outside of the catheter and reduce tissue trauma during insertion.*

▶ With the catheter tip in the sterile solution, occlude the control valve with the thumb of your nondominant hand. Suction a small amount of solution through the catheter (as shown below) *to lubricate the inside of the catheter, thus facilitating passage of secretions through it.*

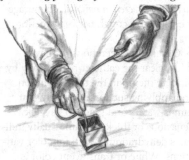

▶ For nasal insertion of the catheter, lubricate the tip of the catheter with the sterile, water-soluble lubricant *to reduce tissue trauma during insertion.*

▶ If the patient isn't intubated or is intubated but isn't receiving supplemental oxygen or aerosol, instruct him to take three to six deep breaths *to help minimize or prevent hypoxia during suctioning.*

▶ If the patient isn't intubated but is receiving oxygen, evaluate his need for

preoxygenation. If indicated, instruct him to take three to six deep breaths while using his supplemental oxygen. (If needed, the patient may continue to receive supplemental oxygen during suctioning by leaving his nasal cannula in one nostril or by keeping the oxygen mask over his mouth.)

▶ If the patient is being mechanically ventilated, preoxygenate him using either a handheld resuscitation bag or the sigh mode on the ventilator. To use the resuscitation bag, set the oxygen flow meter at 15 L/minute, disconnect the patient from the ventilator, and deliver three to six breaths with the resuscitation bag (as shown below).

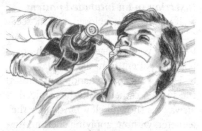

▶ If the patient is being maintained on PEEP, use a resuscitation bag with a PEEP valve.

▶ To preoxygenate using the ventilator, first adjust the fraction of inspired oxygen (FIO_2) and tidal volume according to facility policy and patient need. Then, either use the sigh mode or manually deliver three to six breaths. If you have an assistant for the procedure, the assistant can manage the patient's oxygen needs while you perform the suctioning.

Nasotracheal insertion in a nonintubated patient
▶ Disconnect the oxygen from the patient, if applicable.

► Using your nondominant hand, raise the tip of the patient's nose *to straighten the passageway and facilitate insertion of the catheter.*

► Insert the catheter into the patient's nostril while gently rolling it between your fingers *to help it advance through the turbinates.*

► As the patient inhales, quickly advance the catheter as far as possible. *To avoid oxygen loss and tissue trauma,* don't apply suction during insertion.

► If the patient coughs as the catheter passes through the larynx, briefly hold the catheter still and then resume advancement when the patient inhales.

Insertion in an intubated patient

► If you're using a closed system, see *Closed tracheal suctioning.*

► Using your nonsterile hand, disconnect the patient from the ventilator.

► Using your sterile hand, gently insert the suction catheter into the artificial airway (as shown below). Advance the catheter, without applying suction, until you meet resistance. If the patient coughs, pause briefly and then resume advancement.

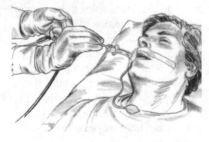

Suctioning the patient

► After inserting the catheter, apply suction intermittently by removing and replacing the thumb of your nondominant hand over the control valve. Simultaneously use your dominant hand to withdraw the catheter as you

roll it between your thumb and forefinger. *This rotating motion prevents the catheter from pulling tissue into the tube as it exits, thus avoiding tissue trauma.* Never suction more than 10 seconds at a time *to prevent hypoxia.*

► If the patient is intubated, use your nondominant hand to stabilize the tip of the ET tube as you withdraw the catheter *to prevent mucous membrane irritation or accidental extubation.*

► If applicable, resume oxygen delivery by reconnecting the source of oxygen or ventilation and hyperoxygenating the patient's lungs before continuing *to prevent or relieve hypoxia.*

► Observe the patient and allow him to rest for a few minutes before the next suctioning. The timing of each suctioning and the length of each rest period depend on his tolerance of the procedure and the absence of complications. *To enhance secretion removal,* encourage the patient to cough between suctioning attempts.

► Observe the secretions. If they're thick, clear the catheter periodically by dipping the tip in the saline solution and applying suction. Normally, sputum is watery and tends to be sticky. Tenacious or thick sputum usually indicates dehydration. Watch for color variations. White or translucent color is normal; yellow indicates pus; green indicates retained secretions or *Pseudomonas* infection; brown usually indicates old blood; red indicates fresh blood; and a "red currant jelly" appearance indicates *Klebsiella* infection. When sputum contains blood, note whether it is streaked or well mixed. Also indicate how often blood appeared. If the patient's heart rate and rhythm are being monitored, observe for arrhythmias. If they occur, stop suctioning and ventilate the patient.

Closed tracheal suctioning

The closed tracheal suction system can ease removal of secretions and reduce patient complications. Consisting of a sterile suction catheter in a clear plastic sleeve, the system permits the patient to remain connected to the ventilator during suctioning.

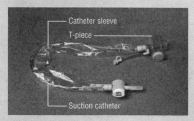

Catheter sleeve
T-piece
Suction catheter

As a result, the patient can maintain the tidal volume, oxygen concentration, and positive end-expiratory pressure delivered by the ventilator while being suctioned. In turn, this reduces the occurrence of suction-induced hypoxemia.

Another advantage of this system is a reduced risk of infection, even when the same catheter is used many times. The caregiver doesn't need to touch the catheter and the ventilator circuit remains closed.

Implementation

To perform the procedure, gather a closed suction control valve, a T-piece to connect the artificial airway to the ventilator breathing circuit, and a catheter sleeve that encloses the catheter and has connections at each end for the control valve and the T-piece. Then follow these steps:

■ Remove the closed suction system from its wrapping. Attach the control valve to the connecting tubing.

■ Depress the thumb suction control valve, and keep it depressed while setting the suction pressure to the desired level.

■ Connect the T-piece to the ventilator breathing circuit, making sure that the irrigation port is closed; then connect the T-piece

to the patient's endotracheal or tracheostomy tube (as shown below).

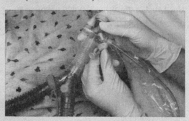

■ With one hand keeping the T-piece parallel to the patient's chin, use the thumb and index finger of the other hand to advance the catheter through the tube and into the patient's tracheobronchial tree (as shown below).

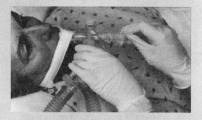

It may be necessary to gently retract the catheter sleeve as you advance the catheter.

■ While continuing to hold the T-piece and control valve, apply intermittent suction and withdraw the catheter until it reaches its fully extended length in the sleeve. Repeat the procedure as necessary.

■ After you've finished suctioning, flush the catheter by maintaining suction while slowly introducing normal saline solution or sterile water into the irrigation port.

■ Place the thumb control valve in the off position.

■ Dispose of and replace the suction equipment and supplies according to your facility's policy.

■ Change the closed suction system every 24 hours to minimize the risk of infection.

Tracheal suctioning at home

If a patient can't mobilize secretions effectively by coughing, he may have to perform tracheal suctioning at home using either clean or sterile technique. Most patients use clean technique, which consists of thorough hand washing and possibly wearing a clean glove. However, a patient with poor hand-washing technique, recurrent respiratory infections, or a compromised immune system or a patient who has had recent surgery may need to use sterile technique.

Clean technique

Because the cost of disposable catheters can be prohibitive, many patients reuse disposable catheters, but the practice remains controversial. If the catheter has thick secretions adhering to it, the patient may clean it with Control III, a quaternary compound.

An alternative to disposable catheters is to use nondisposable, red rubber catheters. However, these catheters contain latex, so use with caution. Consult your facility's policy regarding the care and cleaning of suction catheters in the home setting. Some protocols recommend soaking such catheters in soapy water and then placing them in boiling water for 10 minutes or, alternately, soaking them in 70% alcohol for 3 to 5 minutes and then rinsing in normal saline solution.

Supplies needed

Obviously, the supplies needed will vary with the technique used. If the patient will be using clean technique, he'll need suction catheter kits (or clean gloves, suction catheters, and basin) and distilled water. If he'll be using sterile technique, everything will need to be sterile: the suction catheters, gloves, basin, and water (or normal saline solution).

The type of suction machine necessary will depend on the patient's needs. You'll need to evaluate the amount of suction the machine provides, how easy it is to clean, how much it costs, the volume of the collection bottles, and whether the machine has an overflow safety device to prevent secretions from entering the compressor. You'll also need to determine whether the patient needs a machine that operates on batteries and, if so, how long the batteries will last and whether and how they can be recharged.

Nursing goals

Before discharge, the patient and his family should demonstrate the suctioning procedure. They also need to recognize the indications for suctioning, the signs and symptoms of infection, the importance of adequate hydration, and when to use adjunct therapy, such as aerosol therapy, chest physiotherapy, oxygen therapy, or a handheld resuscitation bag. At discharge, arrange for a home health care provider and a durable medical equipment vendor to follow up with the patient.

▶ Patients who can't mobilize secretions effectively may need to perform tracheal suctioning after discharge. (See *Tracheal suctioning at home.*)

After suctioning

▶ After suctioning, hyperoxygenate the patient being maintained on a ventilator with the handheld resuscitation bag or by using the ventilator's sigh mode, as described earlier.

▶ Readjust the FIO_2 and, for ventilated patients, the tidal volume to the ordered settings.

▶ After suctioning the lower airway, assess the patient's need for upper airway suctioning. If the cuff of the ET or tracheostomy tube is inflated, suction the upper airway before deflating the cuff with a syringe. (See "Oronasopharyngeal suction," page 571, and "Endotracheal tube care," page 282.) Always change the catheter and sterile glove before resuctioning the lower airway *to avoid introducing microorganisms into the lower airway.*

▶ Discard the gloves and catheter in the waterproof trash bag. Clear the connecting tubing by aspirating the remaining saline solution or water. Discard and replace suction equipment and supplies according to your facility's policy. Wash your hands.

▶ Auscultate the lungs bilaterally and take vital signs, if indicated, *to assess the procedure's effectiveness.*

Special considerations

▶ Raising the patient's nose into the sniffing position helps align the larynx and pharynx and may facilitate passing the catheter during nasotracheal suctioning. If the patient's condition permits, have an assistant extend the patient's head and neck above his shoulders. The patient's lower jaw may need to be moved up and forward. If the patient is responsive, ask him to stick out his tongue *so he won't be able to swallow the catheter during insertion.*

▶ During suctioning, the catheter typically is advanced as far as the mainstem bronchi. However, because of tracheobronchial anatomy, the catheter tends to enter the right mainstem bronchi instead of the left. Using an angled catheter (such as a coudé) may help you guide the catheter into the left mainstem bronchus. Rotating the patient's head to the right seems to have a limited effect.

▶ Don't allow the collection container on the suction machine to become more than three-quarters full *to keep from damaging the machine.*

Complications

Because oxygen is removed along with secretions, the patient may experience hypoxemia and dyspnea. Anxiety may alter respiratory patterns. Cardiac arrhythmias can result from hypoxia and stimulation of the vagus nerve in the tracheobronchial tree. Tracheal or bronchial trauma can result from traumatic or prolonged suctioning.

Patients with compromised cardiovascular or pulmonary status are at risk for hypoxemia, arrhythmias, hypertension, or hypotension. Patients with a history of nasopharyngeal bleeding, those who are taking anticoagulants, those who have undergone a tracheostomy recently, and those who have a blood dyscrasia are at increased risk for bleeding as a result of suctioning. Use caution when suctioning patients who have increased intracranial pressure because suction may increase pressure further.

If the patient experiences laryngospasm or bronchospasm (rare complications) during suctioning, discuss with the patient's doctor the use of bronchodilators or lidocaine to reduce the risk of this complication.

Documentation

Record the date and time of the procedure; the technique used; the reason for suctioning; the amount, color, consistency, and odor (if any) of the secretions; any complications and the nursing action taken; and any pertinent data regarding the patient's subjective response to the procedure.

Tracheostomy and Ventilator Speaking Valve

Patients with a tracheostomy tube can't speak because the cuffed tracheostomy tube that directs air into the lungs on inspiration expels air through the tracheostomy tube rather than the vocal cords, mouth, and nose on expiration.

Now, a positive-closure, one-way speaking valve is available. Developed by a ventilator-dependent patient, David Muir, the Passy-Muir Tracheostomy and Ventilator Speaking Valve (PMV) opens upon inspiration to allow the patient to inspire through the tracheostomy tube. It closes after inspiration, redirecting the exhaled air around the tube, through the vocal cords, and out the mouth, allowing the patient to speak.

To function safely, the tracheostomy cuff must be *completely* deflated to enable the patient to exhale, or the tracheostomy tube must be cuffless. For maximum airflow around the tube, the tube should be no larger than two-thirds the size of the tracheal lumen.

The PMV 005 is most commonly used by nonventilated tracheostomy patients, but it can be used by ventilator patients with rubber, nondisposable ventilator tubing. The PMV 007 fits easily into the ventilator tubing by mechanically ventilated tracheostomy patients. Both valves fit the 15-mm hub of adult, pediatric, and neonatal tracheostomy tubes and can be used by patients either on or off the ventilator.

Two new PMV valves have recently been introduced: the PMV 2000 and the PMV 2001. Both of these valves are low-profile and low-resistance, feature the positive closure design, and can be used on or off the ventilator. The PMV 2000 is clear in color and is used readily in the home care setting because it's less noticeable. The PMV 2001 is bright purple and is used more commonly in health care facilities because the color is more noticeable. These new valves also include safety ties that prevent valve loss if the patient inadvertently coughs the PMV out of the tracheostomy tube.

A PMV O_2 adapter is now available for use with the PMV 2000 series speaking valves. This adapter allows improved mobility and comfort for patients who require a tracheostomy tube, speaking valve, and low-flow supplemental oxygen.

Indications and contraindications

Short- and long-term adult, pediatric, and infant tracheostomy and ventilator-dependent patients may benefit from the use of a PMV. PMV use is contraindicated in patients with severe tracheal or laryngeal stenosis, laryngectomy, or excessive oral secretions and in patients who are unconscious or at risk for gross aspiration.

Initial trial required

An initial trial assesses the patient's tolerance. Make sure he understands how the PMV functions and what to expect during the trial. If he's anxious, especially during cuff deflation, he may be unwilling to use the valve, so provide emotional support.

If the patient can't tolerate the PMV initially, the health care team should troubleshoot to determine the cause. The problem often can be remedied easily (for example, by repositioning the patient, downsizing the tracheostomy tube, changing to a cuffless tube, or correcting an airway obstruction).

Some patients will only be able to wear the PMV for a few minutes at a time, building up time gradually, as tolerated.

If repeated trials fail, a speech-language pathologist should assess the patient for other communication options.

Key nursing diagnoses and patient outcomes

Impaired verbal communication related to physical barriers
The patient will:
▶ communicate needs and desires without undue frustration
▶ demonstrate use of adaptive equipment
▶ express plans to use appropriate resources to maximize communication skills.

Equipment

Appropriate size PMV • gloves • suction equipment • a 10-ml luer-lock syringe • PMV instruction booklet

Note: The PMV 005 is for the more ambulatory tracheostomy patient and can be used with flexible rubber tubing. The PMV 007 is more convenient to use with disposable ventilator tubing. Its aqua color makes it easier to identify when it's in position in the ventilator circuitry.

Preparing the patient

Explain the procedure to the patient and make sure that he's comfortable with the procedure before beginning. Provide him with written instructions included in the PMV booklet. Allay any fear and anxiety he might feel before proceeding. If this is the patient's first wearing experience, the trial should be coordinated with the respiratory therapist and the speech-language pathologist.

Implementation

▶ Elevate the head of the patient's bed about 45 degrees. The tracheostomy cuff *must* be completely deflated before the PMV is placed.
▶ Put on gloves. Deflate the cuff slowly *so the patient can become accustomed to using his upper airways again.* Do this by attaching a 10-ml syringe to the tracheostomy tube's pilot balloon (as shown below) and removing the air until air can no longer be extracted and a vacuum is created. Suction the trachea and oral cavity as needed.

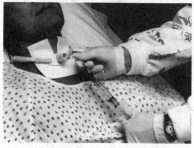

▶ Hold the PMV between your fingers. For a patient who isn't ventilator-dependent, attach the PMV to the hub of the existing tracheostomy hub with a quarter-turn twist (as shown below).

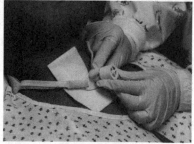

▶ Once the PMV is in place, encourage the patient to relax and concentrate on exhaling through his mouth and nose as he becomes accustomed to using his upper airways. Then have him slowly count aloud to 10 or ask him to speak

as he becomes comfortable breathing with the PMV in place. The speech language pathologist can facilitate voice production and speech.

► The aqua-colored PMV 007 is more convenient to use on patients who are ventilator-dependent because it's tapered to fit into disposable ventilator tubing. Insert the PMV into the end of the wide-mouth, short flex tubing (as shown below).

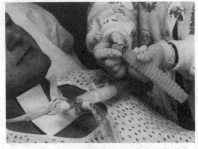

► Connect the other end of the short flex tubing to the ventilator tubing. Then attach the PMV (connected to the short flex tubing) and the ventilator tubing to the closed-suction system (as shown below).

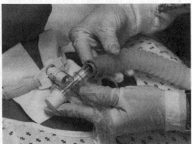

► The PMV can also be attached between the swivel adapter and the short flex tubing and ventilator tubing.

► Post cuff-deflation warning signs in the room. Also, label the tracheostomy pilot balloon *to remind health care providers to reinflate the pilot balloon after removing the PMV.*

► Gently twist the PMV to remove it. Only when it's removed and the original setup is in place should you return the ventilator settings to their original levels and reinflate the pilot balloon cuff. Always remember to reinflate the tracheostomy cuff *after* removing the PMV.

Special considerations

► *Never* place the PMV on the tracheostomy tube before deflating the cuff *because the patient won't be able to breathe.*

► The nurse and the respiratory therapist are responsible for monitoring the patient's response to the PMV during both the trial and ongoing use. They should evaluate blood pressure, heart rate, and respiratory status.

► *Caution:* Remove the PMV immediately if the patient shows signs and symptoms of distress, such as a significant change in blood pressure or heart rate, increased respiratory rate, dyspnea, diaphoresis, anxiety, uncontrollable coughing, or arterial oxygen saturation less than 90%. Reassess the patient before trying the valve again.

Documentation

Document the patient's response to the procedure, including how long the PMV has been in place, respiratory and hemodynamic status, secretion management, and ability to vocalize.

TRACHEOSTOMY CARE

Whether a tracheotomy is performed in an emergency situation or after careful preparation, as a permanent measure or as temporary therapy, tracheostomy care has identical goals: to ensure airway patency by keeping the tube free from mucus buildup, to maintain mucous membrane and skin integrity, to prevent infection, and to provide psychological support.

The patient may have one of three types of tracheostomy tube — uncuffed, cuffed, or fenestrated. Tube selection depends on the patient's condition and the doctor's preference.

An *uncuffed* tube, which may be plastic or metal, allows air to flow freely around the tracheostomy tube and through the larynx, reducing the risk of tracheal damage. A *cuffed* tube, made of plastic, is disposable. The cuff and the tube won't separate accidentally inside the trachea because the cuff is bonded to the tube. Also, it doesn't require periodic deflating to lower pressure because cuff pressure is low and evenly distributed against the tracheal wall. Although cuffed tubes may cost more than other tubes, they reduce the risk of tracheal damage. A plastic *fenestrated* tube permits speech through the upper airway when the external opening is capped and the cuff is deflated. It also allows easy removal of the inner cannula for cleaning. However, a fenestrated tube may become occluded.

Whichever tube is used, tracheostomy care should be performed using aseptic technique until the stoma has healed to prevent infection. For recently performed tracheotomies, use sterile gloves for all manipulations at the tracheostomy site. When the stoma has healed, clean gloves may be substituted for sterile ones.

Key nursing diagnoses and patient outcomes

Ineffective breathing pattern related to decreased energy
The patient will:
▶ achieve maximum lung expansion with adequate ventilation
▶ report feeling comfortable with breathing.

Impaired gas exchange related to altered oxygen supply
The patient will:
▶ cough effectively
▶ expectorate sputum.

Equipment
For aseptic stoma and outer-cannula care
Waterproof trash bag • two sterile solution containers • normal saline solution • hydrogen peroxide • sterile cotton-tipped applicators • sterile 4″ × 4″ gauze pads • sterile gloves • prepackaged sterile tracheostomy dressing (or 4″ × 4″ gauze pad) • equipment and supplies for suctioning and for mouth care • water-soluble lubricant or topical antibiotic cream • materials as needed for cuff procedures and for changing tracheostomy ties (see below)

For aseptic inner-cannula care
All of the preceding equipment plus a prepackaged commercial tracheostomy-care set, or sterile forceps • sterile nylon brush • sterile 6″ (15 cm) pipe cleaners • clean gloves • a third sterile solution container • disposable temporary inner cannula (for a patient on a ventilator)

For changing tracheostomy ties
30″ (76-cm) length of tracheostomy twill tape • bandage scissors • sterile gloves • hemostat

For emergency tracheostomy tube replacement
Sterile tracheal dilator or sterile hemostat • sterile obturator that fits the tracheostomy tube in use • extra sterile tracheostomy tube and obturator in appropriate size • suction equipment and supplies (Keep these supplies in full view in the patient's room at all times

for easy access in case of emergency. Consider taping an emergency sterile tracheostomy tube in a sterile wrapper to the head of the bed for easy access in an emergency.)

For cuff procedures
5- or 10-ml syringe • padded hemostat • stethoscope

Preparation of equipment
Wash your hands and assemble all equipment and supplies in the patient's room. Check the expiration date on each sterile package and inspect the package for tears. Open the waterproof trash bag and place it next to you *so that you can avoid reaching across the sterile field or the patient's stoma when discarding soiled items.*

Establish a sterile field near the patient's bed (usually on the overbed table) and place equipment and supplies on it. Pour normal saline solution, hydrogen peroxide, or a mixture of equal parts of both solutions into one of the sterile solution containers; then pour normal saline solution into the second sterile container for rinsing. For inner-cannula care, you may use a third sterile solution container to hold the gauze pads and cotton-tipped applicators saturated with cleaning solution. If you'll be replacing the disposable inner cannula, open the package containing the new inner cannula while maintaining sterile technique. Obtain or prepare new tracheostomy ties, if indicated.

Implementation
▶ Assess the patient's condition *to determine his need for care.*
▶ Explain the procedure to the patient even if he's unresponsive. Provide privacy.

▶ Place the patient in semi-Fowler's position (unless it's contraindicated) *to decrease abdominal pressure on the diaphragm and promote lung expansion.*
▶ Remove any humidification or ventilation device.
▶ Using sterile technique, suction the entire length of the tracheostomy *tube to clear the airway of any secretions that may hinder oxygenation.* (See "Tracheal suction," page 819.)
▶ Reconnect the patient to the humidifier or ventilator, if necessary.

Cleaning a stoma and outer cannula
▶ Put on sterile gloves if you aren't already wearing them.
▶ With your dominant hand, saturate a sterile gauze pad with the cleaning solution. Squeeze out the excess liquid *to prevent accidental aspiration.* Wipe the patient's neck under the tracheostomy tube flanges and twill tapes.
▶ Saturate a second pad and wipe until the skin around the tracheostomy is cleaned. Use more pads or cotton-tipped applicators to clean the stoma site and the tube's flanges. Wipe only once with each pad and then discard it *to prevent contamination of a clean area with a soiled pad.*
▶ Rinse debris and peroxide (if used) with one or more sterile 4" × 4" gauze pads dampened in normal saline solution. Dry the area thoroughly with additional sterile gauze pads; then apply a new sterile tracheostomy dressing.
▶ Remove and discard your gloves.

Cleaning a nondisposable inner cannula
▶ Put on sterile gloves.
▶ Using your nondominant hand, remove and discard the patient's tracheostomy dressing. Then, with the same hand, disconnect the ventilator or

humidification device and unlock the tracheostomy tube's inner cannula by rotating it counterclockwise. Place the inner cannula in the container of hydrogen peroxide.

► Working quickly, use your dominant hand to scrub the cannula with the sterile nylon brush. If the brush doesn't slide easily into the cannula, use a sterile pipe cleaner.

► Immerse the cannula in the container of normal saline solution and agitate it for about 10 seconds to rinse it thoroughly.

► Inspect the cannula for cleanliness. Repeat the cleaning process if necessary. If it's clean, tap it gently against the inside edge of the sterile container *to remove excess liquid and prevent aspiration.* Don't dry the outer surface *because a thin film of moisture acts as a lubricant during insertion.*

► Reinsert the inner cannula into the patient's tracheostomy tube. Lock it in place and then gently pull on it *to make sure it's positioned securely.* Reconnect the mechanical ventilator. Apply a new sterile tracheostomy dressing.

► If the patient can't tolerate being disconnected from the ventilator for the time it takes to clean the inner cannula, replace the existing inner cannula with a clean one and reattach the mechanical ventilator. Then clean the cannula just removed from the patient and store it in a sterile container the next time.

Caring for a disposable inner cannula

► Put on clean gloves.

► Using your dominant hand, remove the patient's inner cannula. After evaluating the secretions in the cannula, discard it properly.

► Pick up the new inner cannula, touching only the outer locking portion. Insert the cannula into the tracheostomy and, following the manufacturer's instructions, lock it securely.

Changing tracheostomy ties

► Obtain assistance from another nurse or a respiratory *therapist because of the risk of accidental tube expulsion during this procedure.* Patient movement or coughing can dislodge the tube.

► Wash your hands thoroughly and put on sterile gloves if you aren't already wearing them.

► If you aren't using commercially packaged tracheostomy ties, prepare new ties from a 30″ (76-cm) length of twill tape by folding one end back 1″ (2.5 cm) on itself. Then, with the bandage scissors, cut a ½″ (1.5-cm) slit down the center of the tape from the folded edge.

► Prepare the other end of the tape the same way.

► Hold both ends together and, using scissors, cut the resulting circle of tape so that one piece is approximately 10″ (25.5 cm) long and the other is about 20″ (51 cm) long.

► Help the patient into semi-Fowler's position if possible.

► After your assistant puts on gloves, instruct her to hold the tracheostomy tube in place *to prevent its expulsion during replacement of the ties.* If you must perform the procedure without assistance, fasten the clean ties in place before removing the old ties *to prevent tube expulsion.*

► With the assistant's gloved fingers holding the tracheostomy tube in place, cut the soiled tracheostomy ties with the bandage scissors or untie them and discard the ties. Be careful not to cut the tube of the pilot balloon.

► Thread the slit end of one new tie a short distance through the eye of one tracheostomy tube flange from the underside; use the hemostat, if needed, to pull the tie through. Then thread the other end of the tie completely through the slit end and pull it taut so it loops firmly through the flange. *This avoids knots that can cause throat discomfort, tissue irritation, pressure, and necrosis at the patient's throat.*

▶ Fasten the second tie to the opposite flange in the same manner.

▶ Instruct the patient to flex his neck while you bring the ties around to the side and tie them together with a square knot. *Flexion produces the same neck circumference as coughing and helps prevent an overly tight tie.* Instruct your assistant to place one finger under the tapes as you tie them *to ensure that they're tight enough to avoid slippage but loose enough to prevent choking or jugular vein constriction.* Placing the closure on the side allows easy access and prevents pressure necrosis at the back of the neck when the patient is recumbent.

▶ After securing the ties, cut off the excess tape with the scissors and instruct your assistant to release the tracheostomy tube.

▶ Make sure the patient is comfortable and can reach the call button easily.

▶ Check tracheostomy-tie tension often on patients with traumatic injury, radical neck dissection, or cardiac failure *because neck diameter can increase from swelling and cause constriction;* also check neonatal or restless patients frequently *because ties can loosen and cause tube dislodgment.*

Concluding tracheostomy care
▶ Replace any humidification device.
▶ Provide mouth care as needed *because the oral cavity can become dry and malodorous or develop sores from encrusted secretions.*

▶ Observe soiled dressings and any suctioned secretions for amount, color, consistency, and odor.

▶ Properly clean or dispose of all equipment, supplies, solutions, and trash according to policy.

▶ Take off and discard your gloves.

▶ Make sure that the patient is comfortable and that he can easily reach the call button.

▶ Make sure all necessary supplies are readily available at the bedside.

▶ Repeat the procedure at least once every 8 hours or as needed. Change the dressing as often as necessary regardless of whether you also perform the entire cleaning procedure, *because a wet dressing with exudate or secretions predisposes the patient to skin excoriation, breakdown, and infection.*

Deflating and inflating a tracheostomy cuff
▶ Read the cuff manufacturer's instructions *because cuff types and procedures vary widely.*

▶ Assess the patient's condition, explain the procedure to him, and reassure him. Wash your hands thoroughly.

▶ Help the patient into semi-Fowler's position, if possible, or place him in a supine position *so secretions above the cuff site will be pushed up into his mouth if he's receiving positive-pressure ventilation.*

▶ Suction the oropharyngeal cavity *to prevent pooled secretions from descending into the trachea after cuff deflation.*

▶ Release the padded hemostat clamping the cuff inflation tubing, if a hemostat is present.

▶ Insert a 5- or 10-ml syringe into the cuff pilot balloon and very slowly withdraw all air from the cuff. Leave the syringe attached to the tubing for later reinflation of the cuff. *Slow deflation allows positive lung pressure to push secretions upward from the bronchi. Cuff deflation may also stimulate the patient's cough reflex, producing additional secretions.*

▶ Remove any ventilation device. Suction the lower airway through any existing tube to remove all secretions. Then reconnect the patient to the ventilation device.

▶ Maintain cuff deflation for the prescribed time. Observe the patient for adequate ventilation, and suction as necessary. If the patient has difficulty breathing, reinflate the cuff immediately by depressing the syringe plunger very slowly. Use a stethoscope to listen over the trachea for the air leak, then inject the least amount of air needed to achieve an adequate tracheal seal.

▶ When inflating the cuff, you may use the minimal-leak technique or the minimal occlusive volume technique *to help gauge the proper inflation point.* (For more information, see "Endotracheal intubation," page 274, and "Endotracheal tube care," page 282.)

▶ If you're inflating the cuff using cuff pressure measurement, be careful not to exceed 25 mm Hg. If pressure exceeds 25 mm Hg, notify the doctor *because you may need to change to a larger size tube, use higher inflation pressures, or permit a larger air leak.* Recommended cuff pressure is about 18 mm Hg.

▶ After you've inflated the cuff, if the tubing doesn't have a one-way valve at the end, clamp the inflation line with a padded hemostat (to protect the tubing) and remove the syringe.

▶ Check for a minimal-leak cuff seal. You shouldn't feel air coming from the patient's mouth, nose, or tracheostomy site, and a conscious patient shouldn't be able to speak.

▶ Be alert for air leaks from the cuff itself. Suspect a leak if injection of air fails to inflate the cuff or increase cuff pressure, if you're unable to inject the amount of air you withdrew, if the patient can speak, if ventilation fails to maintain adequate respiratory movement with pressures or volumes previously considered adequate, or if air escapes during the ventilator's inspiratory cycle.

▶ Note the exact amount of air used to inflate the cuff *to detect tracheal malacia if more air is consistently needed.*

▶ Make sure the patient is comfortable and can easily reach the call button and communication aids.

▶ Properly clean or dispose of all equipment, supplies, and trash according to facility policy.

▶ Replenish any used supplies and make sure all necessary emergency supplies are at the bedside.

Special considerations

▶ Keep appropriate equipment at the patient's bedside for immediate use in an emergency. (For a list, see "Tracheotomy," page 834.)

▶ Consult the doctor about first-aid measures you can use for your tracheostomy patient should an emergency occur. Follow facility policy regarding procedure if a tracheostomy tube is expelled or if the outer cannula becomes blocked. If the patient's breathing is obstructed—for example, when the tube is blocked with mucus that can't be removed by suctioning or by withdrawing the inner cannula—call the appropriate code and provide manual resuscitation with a handheld resuscitation bag or reconnect the patient to the ventilator. *Don't remove the tracheostomy tube entirely because this may allow the airway to close completely.* Use extreme caution when attempting to reinsert an expelled tracheostomy tube *because of the risk of tracheal trauma, perforation, compression, and asphyxiation.* Reassure the patient until the doctor arrives (usually a minute or less in this type of code or emergency).

▶ Refrain from changing tracheostomy ties unnecessarily during the immediate postoperative period before the stoma track is well formed (usually 4 days) *to avoid accidental dislodgment and expulsion of the tube.* Unless secretions or drainage is a problem, ties can be changed once per day.

▶ Refrain from changing a single-cannula tracheostomy tube or the outer cannula of a double-cannula tube. Because of the risk of tracheal complications, the doctor usually changes the cannula, with the frequency of change depending on the patient's condition.

▶ If the patient's neck or stoma is excoriated or infected, apply a water-soluble lubricant or topical antibiotic cream as ordered. Remember not to use a powder or an oil-based substance on or around a stoma *because aspiration can cause infection and abscess.*

▶ Replace all equipment, including solutions, regularly according to policy *to reduce the risk of nosocomial infections.*

Home care

If the patient is being discharged with a tracheostomy, start self-care teaching as soon as he's receptive. Teach the patient how to change and clean the tube. If he's being discharged with suction equipment (a few patients are), make sure he and his family feel knowledgeable and comfortable about using this equipment.

Complications

The following complications can occur within the first 48 hours after tracheostomy tube insertion: hemorrhage at the operative site, causing drowning; bleeding or edema in tracheal tissue, causing airway obstruction; aspiration of secretions; introduction of air into the pleural cavity, causing pneumothorax; hypoxia or acidosis, triggering cardiac arrest; and introduction of air into surrounding tissues, causing subcutaneous emphysema.

Secretions collecting under dressings and twill tape can encourage skin excoriation and infection. Hardened mucus or a slipped cuff can occlude the cannula opening and obstruct the airway. Tube displacement can stimulate the cough reflex if the tip rests on the carina, or it can cause blood vessel erosion and hemorrhage. Just the presence of the tube or cuff pressure can produce tracheal erosion and necrosis.

Documentation

Record the date and time of the procedure; type of procedure; the amount, consistency, color, and odor of secretions; stoma and skin condition; the patient's respiratory status; change of the tracheostomy tube by the doctor; the duration of any cuff deflation; the amount of any cuff inflation; and cuff pressure readings and specific body position. Note any complications and the nursing action taken; any patient or family teaching and their comprehension and progress; and the patient's tolerance of the treatment.

TRACHEOTOMY

A tracheotomy involves the surgical creation of an external opening—called a tracheostomy—into the trachea and insertion of an indwelling tube to maintain the airway's patency. If all other attempts to establish an airway have failed, a doctor may perform a tracheotomy at a patient's bedside. This procedure may be necessary when an airway obstruction results from laryngeal edema, foreign body obstruction, or a tumor. An emergency tracheotomy also may be performed when endotracheal intubation is contraindicated.

Use of a cuffed tracheostomy tube provides and maintains a patent airway, prevents the unconscious or paralyzed patient from aspirating food or secretions, allows removal of tracheobronchial secretions from the patient unable to cough, replaces an endotracheal tube, and permits the use of positive-pressure ventilation.

Although tracheostomy tubes come in plastic and metal, plastic tubes are commonly used in emergencies because they have a universal adapter for respiratory support equipment, such as a mechanical ventilator, and a cuff to allow positive-pressure ventilation.

Key nursing diagnoses and patient outcomes

Ineffective breathing pattern related to decreased energy
The patient will:
▶ achieve maximum lung expansion with adequate ventilation
▶ report feeling comfortable with breathing.

Impaired gas exchange related to altered oxygen supply
The patient will:
▶ cough effectively
▶ expectorate sputum.

Equipment

Tracheostomy tube of the proper size (usually #13 to #38 French or #00 to #9

Jackson) with obturator • tracheostomy tape • sterile tracheal dilator • vein retractor • sutures and needles • 4″ × 4″ gauze pads • sterile drapes, gloves, mask, and gown • sterile bowls • stethoscope • sterile tracheostomy dressing • pillow • tracheostomy ties • suction apparatus • alcohol pad • povidone-iodine solution • sterile water • 5-ml syringe with 22G needle • local anesthetic such as lidocaine • oxygen therapy device • oxygen source • emergency equipment to be kept at bedside, including suctioning equipment, sterile obturator, sterile tracheostomy tube, sterile inner cannula, sterile tracheostomy tube and inner cannula one size smaller than tubes in use, sterile tracheal dilator or sterile hemostat (many hospitals use prepackaged sterile tracheotomy trays)

Preparation of equipment

Have one person stay with the patient while another obtains the necessary equipment. Wash your hands; then, maintaining sterile technique, open the tray and the packages containing the solution. Take the tracheostomy tube from its container and place it on the sterile field. Set up the suction equipment and make sure it works. When the doctor opens the sterile bowls, pour in the povidone-iodine solution.

Implementation

▶ Explain the procedure to the patient even if he's unresponsive.
▶ Assess his condition and provide privacy. Maintain ventilation until the tracheotomy is performed.
▶ Wipe the top of the local anesthetic vial with an alcohol pad. Invert the vial so that the doctor can withdraw the anesthetic using the 22G needle attached to the 5-ml syringe.

► Before the doctor begins, place a pillow under the patient's shoulders and neck and hyperextend his neck.

► The doctor will put on a sterile gown, gloves, and mask.

► Help the doctor with the tube insertion as needed. (See *Assisting with a tracheotomy*.)

► When the tube is in position, attach it to the appropriate oxygen therapy device, which is connected to an oxygen source.

► Inject air into the distal cuff port *to inflate the cuff*.

► Auscultate the patient's lungs using a stethoscope.

► The doctor will suture the corners of the incision and secure the tracheostomy tube with tape.

► Put on sterile gloves.

► Apply the sterile tracheostomy dressing under the tracheostomy tube flange. Place the tracheostomy ties through the openings of the tube flanges and tie them on the side of the patient's neck. *This allows easy access and prevents pressure necrosis at the back of the neck.*

► Clean or dispose of the used equipment according to policy. Replenish all supplies as needed.

► Make sure that a chest X-ray is ordered *to confirm tube placement*.

Special considerations

► Assess the patient's vital signs and respiratory status every 15 minutes for 1 hour, then every 30 minutes for 2 hours, and then every 2 hours until his condition is stable.

► Monitor the patient carefully for signs of infection. Ideally, the tracheotomy should be performed using sterile technique as described. But, in an emergency, this may not be possible.

► Make sure the following equipment is always at the patient's bedside:

– suctioning equipment *because the patient may need his airway cleared at any time*

– the sterile obturator used to insert the tracheostomy tube *in case the tube is expelled*

– a sterile tracheostomy tube and obturator (the same size as the one used) *in case the tube must be replaced quickly*

– a spare, sterile inner cannula *that can be used if the cannula is expelled*

– a sterile tracheostomy tube and obturator one size smaller than the one used, *which may be needed if the tube is expelled and the trachea begins to close*

– a sterile tracheal dilator or sterile hemostat *to maintain an open airway before inserting a new tracheostomy tube.*

► Review emergency first-aid measures and always follow your facility's policy concerning an expelled or blocked tracheostomy tube. When a blocked tube can't be cleared by suctioning or withdrawing the inner cannula, policy may require you to stay with the patient while someone else calls the doctor or the appropriate code. You should continue trying to ventilate the patient with whatever method works, for example, a handheld resuscitation bag. Don't remove the tracheostomy tube entirely; *doing so may close the airway completely.*

► Use extreme caution if you try to reinsert an expelled tracheostomy tube *to avoid tracheal trauma, perforation, compression, and asphyxiation.*

Complications

A tracheotomy can cause an airway obstruction (from improper tube placement), hemorrhage, edema, a perforated esophagus, subcutaneous or medi-

Assisting with a tracheotomy

To perform a tracheotomy, the doctor will first clean the area from the chin to the nipples with povidone-iodine solution. Next, he'll place sterile drapes on the patient and locate the area for the incision—usually 1 to 2 cm below the cricoid cartilage. Then he'll inject a local anesthetic.

He'll make a horizontal or vertical incision in the skin. (A vertical incision helps avoid arteries, veins, and nerves on the lateral borders of the trachea.) Then he'll dissect subcutaneous fat and muscle and move the muscle aside with vein retractors to locate the tracheal rings. He'll make an incision between the second and third tracheal rings (as shown above right) and use a hemostat to control bleeding.

He'll inject a local anesthetic into the tracheal lumen to suppress the cough reflex and then he'll create a stoma in the trachea. When this is done, carefully apply suction to remove blood and secretions that may obstruct the airway or be aspirated into the lungs. The doctor then will insert the tracheostomy tube and obturator into the stoma (as shown in center). After inserting the tube, he'll remove the obturator.

Apply a sterile tracheostomy dressing and anchor the tube with tracheostomy ties (as shown below right). Check for air movement through the tube and auscultate the lungs to ensure proper placement.

An alternative approach

In a newer approach, the doctor inserts the tracheostomy tube percutaneously at the bedside. After the skin is prepared and anesthetized, the doctor makes a 1-cm midline incision.

Using either a series of dilators or a pair of forceps, he creates a stoma for tube insertion. When the stoma reaches the desired size, the doctor inserts the tracheostomy tube. When the tube is in place, inflate the cuff, secure the tube, and check the patient's breath sounds. Obtain a portable chest X-ray. Unlike the surgical technique, this method dilates rather than cuts the tissue structures. z

Incision site

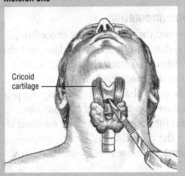

Cricoid cartilage

Tube insertion

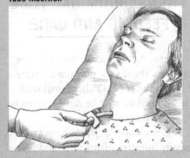

Sterile dressing

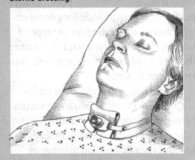

astinal emphysema, aspiration of secretions, tracheal necrosis (from cuff pressure), infection, or lacerations of arteries, veins, or nerves.

Documentation

Record the reason for the procedure, the date and time it took place, and the patient's respiratory status before and after the procedure. Include any complications that occurred during the procedure, the amount of cuff pressure, and the respiratory therapy initiated after the procedure. Also note the patient's response to respiratory therapy.

TRANSABDOMINAL TUBE FEEDING AND CARE

To access the stomach, duodenum, or jejunum, the doctor may place a tube through the patient's abdominal wall. This procedure may be done surgically or percutaneously.

A gastrostomy or jejunostomy tube is usually inserted during intra-abdominal surgery. The tube may be used for feeding during the immediate postoperative period or it may provide long-term enteral access, depending on the type of surgery. Typically, the doctor will suture the tube in place to prevent gastric contents from leaking.

In contrast, a percutaneous endoscopic gastrostomy (PEG) or a percutaneous endoscopic jejunostomy (PEJ) tube can be inserted endoscopically without the need for laparotomy or general anesthesia. Typically, the insertion is done in the endoscopy suite or at the patient's bedside. A PEG or PEJ tube may be used for nutrition, drainage, and decompression. Contraindications to endoscopic placement include obstruction (such as an esophageal stricture or duodenal blockage), previous gastric surgery, morbid obesity, and ascites. These conditions would necessitate surgical placement.

With either type of tube placement, feedings may begin after 24 hours (or when peristalsis resumes).

After a time, the tube may need replacement, and the doctor may recommend a similar tube, such as an indwelling urinary catheter or a mushroom catheter, or a gastrostomy button—a skin-level feeding tube. (See "Gastrostomy feeding button care," page 362.)

Key nursing diagnoses and patient outcomes

Imbalanced nutrition: Less than body requirements related to inability to absorb nutrients
The patient will:
▶ tolerate tube feedings without adverse reactions
▶ show no further evidence of weight loss.

Risk for fluid volume imbalance related to active loss
The patient will:
▶ have fluid volume remain adequate
▶ have electrolyte levels stay within normal range.

Equipment
For feeding
Feeding formula • 120 ml of water • large-bulb or catheter-tip syringe • 4″ × 4″ gauze pads • soap • skin protectant • hypoallergenic tape • gravity-drip administration bags • mouthwash, toothpaste, or mild salt solution • gloves • stethoscope • optional: enteral infusion pump

For decompression
Suction apparatus with tubing and straight drainage collection set

Preparation of equipment

Always check the expiration date on commercially prepared feeding formulas. If the formula has been prepared by the dietitian or pharmacist, check the preparation time and date. Discard any opened formula that is more than 1 day old.

Commercially prepared administration sets and enteral pumps allow continuous formula administration. Place the desired amount of formula into the gavage container and purge air from the tubing. To avoid contamination, hang only a 4- to 6-hour supply of formula at a time.

Implementation

▶ Provide privacy and wash your hands.
▶ Explain the procedure to the patient. Tell him, for example, that feedings usually start at a slow rate and increase as tolerated. After he tolerates continuous feedings, he may progress to intermittent feedings as ordered.
▶ Assess for bowel sounds before feeding and monitor for abdominal distention.
▶ Ask the patient to sit, or assist him into semi-Fowler's position, for the entire feeding. *This helps to prevent esophageal reflux and pulmonary aspiration of the formula.* For an intermittent feeding, have him maintain this position throughout the feeding and for 30 minutes to 1 hour afterward.
▶ Put on gloves. Before starting the feeding, measure residual gastric contents. Attach the syringe to the feeding tube and aspirate. If the contents measure more than twice the amount in-

fused, hold the feeding and recheck in 1 hour. If residual contents still remain too high, notify the doctor. Chances are the formula isn't being absorbed properly. Keep in mind that residual contents will be minimal with PEJ tube feedings.
▶ Allow 30 ml of water to flow into the feeding tube *to establish patency.*
▶ Be sure to administer formula at room temperature. *Cold formula may cause cramping.*

Intermittent feedings

▶ Allow gravity to help the formula flow over 30 to 45 minutes. *Faster infusions may cause bloating, cramps, or diarrhea.*
▶ Begin intermittent feeding with a low volume (200 ml) daily. According to the patient's tolerance, increase the volume per feeding as needed *to reach the desired calorie intake.*
▶ When the feeding finishes, flush the feeding tube with 30 to 60 ml of water. *This maintains patency and provides hydration.*
▶ Cap the tube *to prevent leakage.*
▶ Rinse the feeding administration set thoroughly with hot water *to avoid contaminating subsequent feedings.* Allow it to dry between feedings.

Continuous feedings

▶ Measure residual gastric contents every 4 hours.
▶ To administer the feeding with a pump, set up the equipment according to the manufacturer's guidelines, and fill the feeding bag. To administer the feeding by gravity, fill the container with formula and purge air from the tubing.
▶ Monitor the gravity drip rate or pump infusion rate frequently *to ensure accurate delivery of formula.*

Caring for a PEG or PEJ site

The exit site of a percutaneous endoscopic gastrostomy (PEG) or percutaneous endoscopic jejunostomy (PEJ) tube requires routine observation and care. Follow these care guidelines:

■ Change the dressing daily while the tube is in place.

■ After removing the dressing, carefully slide the tube's outer bumper away from the skin (as shown below) about ½″ (1.5 cm).

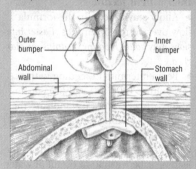

■ Examine the skin around the tube. Look for redness and other signs of infection or erosion.

■ Gently depress the skin surrounding the tube and inspect for drainage (as shown above right). Expect minimal wound drainage initially after implantation. This should subside in about 1 week.

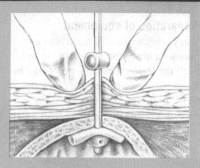

■ Inspect the tube for wear and tear. (A tube that wears out will need replacement.)

■ Clean the site with the prescribed cleaning solution. Then apply povidone-iodine ointment over the exit site according to your facility's guidelines.

■ Rotate the outer bumper 90 degrees *(to avoid repeating the same tension on the same skin area)*, and slide the outer bumper back over the exit site.

■ If leakage appears at the PEG site, or if the patient risks dislodging the tube, apply a sterile gauze dressing over the site. Don't put sterile gauze underneath the outer bumper. *Loosening the anchor this way allows the feeding tube free play, which could lead to wound abscess.*

■ Write the date and time of the dressing change on the tape.

▶ Flush the feeding tube with 30 to 60 ml of water every 4 hours *to maintain patency and to provide hydration.*

▶ Monitor intake and output *to anticipate and detect fluid or electrolyte imbalances.*

Decompression

▶ To decompress the stomach, connect the PEG port to the suction device with tubing or straight gravity drainage tubing. Jejunostomy feeding may be given

simultaneously via the PEJ port of the dual-lumen tube.

Tube exit site care

▶ Provide daily skin care.

▶ Gently remove the dressing by hand. Never cut away the dressing over the catheter *because you might cut the tube or the sutures holding the tube in place.*

▶ At least daily and as needed, clean the skin around the tube's exit site using a 4″ × 4″ gauze pad soaked in the prescribed cleaning solution. When healed, wash the skin around the exit site daily with soap. Rinse the area with water and pat dry. Apply skin protectant, if necessary.

▶ Anchor a gastrostomy or jejunostomy tube to the skin with hypoallergenic tape *to prevent peristaltic migration of the tube. This also prevents tension on the suture anchoring the tube in place.*

▶ Coil the tube, if necessary, and tape it to the *abdomen to prevent pulling and contamination of the tube.* PEG and PEJ tubes have toggle-bolt-like internal and external bumpers that make tape anchors unnecessary. (See *Caring for a PEG or PEJ site.*)

Special considerations

▶ If the patient vomits or complains of nausea, feeling too full, or regurgitation, stop the feeding immediately and assess his condition. Flush the feeding tube and attempt to restart the feeding in 1 hour (measure residual gastric contents first). You may have to decrease the volume or rate of feedings. If the patient develops dumping syndrome, which includes nausea, vomiting, cramps, pallor, and diarrhea, the feedings may have been given too quickly.

▶ Provide oral hygiene frequently. Brush all surfaces of the teeth, gums, and tongue at least twice daily using mouthwash, toothpaste, or a mild salt solution.

▶ You can administer most tablets and pills through the tube by crushing them and diluting as necessary. (However, don't crush enteric-coated or sustained-release drugs, *which lose their effectiveness when crushed.*) Medications should be in liquid form for administration.

▶ Control diarrhea resulting from dumping syndrome by using continuous pump or gravity-drip infusions, di-

luting the feeding formula, or adding antidiarrheal medications.

Home care

Instruct the patient and family members or other caregivers in all aspects of enteral feedings, including tube maintenance and site care. Specify signs and symptoms to report to the doctor, define emergency situations and review actions to take.

When the tube needs replacement, advise the patient that the doctor may insert a replacement gastrostomy button or a latex, indwelling, or mushroom catheter after removing the initial feeding tube. The procedure may be done in the doctor's office or your facility's endoscopy suite.

As the patient's tolerance of tube feeding improves, he may wish to try syringe feedings rather than intermittent feedings. If appropriate, teach him how to feed himself by the syringe method. (See *Teaching the patient about syringe feeding,* page 842.)

Complications

Common complications related to transabdominal tubes include GI or other systemic problems, mechanical malfunction, and metabolic disturbances. Cramping, nausea, vomiting, bloating, and diarrhea may be related to medication; rapid infusion rate; formula contamination, osmolarity, or temperature (too cold or too warm); fat malabsorption; or intestinal atrophy from malnutrition. Constipation may result from inadequate hydration or insufficient exercise.

Systemic problems may be caused by pulmonary aspiration, infection at the tube exit site, or contaminated formula. Proper positioning during feeding, verification of tube placement, meticulous

Teaching the patient about syringe feeding

If the patient plans to feed himself by syringe when he returns home, you'll need to teach him how to do this before he's discharged. Here are some points to emphasize.

Initial instructions

First, show the patient how to clamp the feeding tube, remove the syringe's bulb or plunger, and place the tip of the syringe into the feeding tube (as shown below). Then tell him to instill between 30 and 60 ml of water into the feeding tube *to make sure it stays open and patent.*

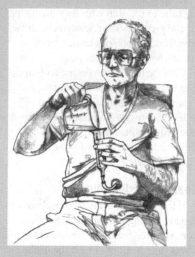

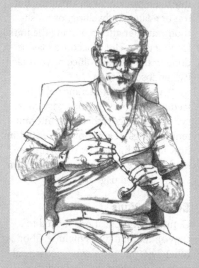

Next, tell him to pour the feeding solution into the syringe and begin the feeding (as shown above right). As the solution flows into the stomach, show him how to tilt the syringe *to allow air bubbles to escape.* Describe the discomfort that air bubbles may cause.

Tips for free flow

When about one-fourth of the feeding solution remains, direct the patient to refill the syringe. Caution him to avoid letting the syringe empty completely. *Doing so may result in abdominal cramping and gas.*

Show the patient how to increase and decrease the solution's flow rate by raising or lowering the syringe. Explain that he may need to dilute a thick solution *to promote free flow.*

Finishing up

Inform the patient that the feeding infusion process should take at least 15 minutes. If the process takes less than 15 minutes, dumping syndrome may result.

Show the patient the steps needed to finish the feeding, including how to flush the tube with water, clamp the tube, and clean the equipment for later use. If he's using disposable gear, urge him to discard it properly. Review how to store unused feeding solution as appropriate.

skin care, and aseptic formula preparation are ways to prevent these complications.

Typical mechanical problems include tube dislodgment, obstruction, or impairment. For example, a PEG or PEJ tube may migrate if the external bumper loosens. Occlusion may result from incompletely crushed and liquefied medication particles or inadequate tube flushing. Further, the tube may rupture or crack from age, drying, or frequent manipulation.

Monitor the patient for vitamin and mineral deficiencies, glucose tolerance, and fluid and electrolyte imbalances, which may follow bouts of diarrhea or constipation.

Documentation

On the intake and output record, note the date, time, and amount of each feeding and the water volume instilled. Maintain total volumes for nutrients and water separately to allow calculation of nutrient intake. In your notes, document the type of formula, the infusion method and rate, the patient's tolerance of the procedure and formula, and the amount of residual gastric contents. Also record complications and abdominal assessment findings. Note patient-teaching topics covered and the patient's progress in self-care.

TRANSCRANIAL DOPPLER MONITORING

Transcranial Doppler ultrasonography is a noninvasive method of monitoring blood flow in the intracranial vessels, specifically the circle of Willis. This procedure is used in the intensive care unit to monitor patients who have experienced cerebrovascular disorders, such as stroke, head trauma, or subarachnoid hemorrhage. It can help detect intracranial stenosis, vasospasm, and arteriovenous malformations as well as assess collateral pathways. Because it has the advantage of monitoring a continuous waveform, it can be used in intraoperative monitoring of cerebral circulation.

Transcranial Doppler ultrasonography is also used to monitor the effect of intracranial pressure changes on the cerebral circulation, to monitor patient response to various medications, and to evaluate carbon dioxide reactivity, which may be impaired or lost from arterial obstruction or trauma. In addition, it has been used to confirm brain death.

The transcranial Doppler unit transmits pulses of high-frequency ultrasound, which are then reflected back to the transducer by the red blood cells moving in the vessel being monitored. This information is then processed by the instrument into an audible signal and a velocity waveform, which is displayed on the monitor. The displayed waveform is actually a moving graph of blood flow velocities with TIME displayed along the horizontal axis, VELOCITY displayed along the vertical axis, and AMPLITUDE represented by various colors or intensities within the waveform. The heart's contractions speed up the movement of blood cells during systole and slow it down during diastole, resulting in a waveform that varies in velocity over the cardiac cycle.

The major benefits of transcranial Doppler monitoring are that it provides instantaneous, real-time information about cerebral blood flow and that it's noninvasive and painless for the patient. Also, the unit itself is portable and easy to use. The major disadvantage is that it relies on the ability of ultrasound waves to penetrate thin areas of the cranium; this is difficult if the patient has thickening of the temporal bone, which increases with age.

The transcranial Doppler unit should always be used with its power set at the lowest level needed to provide an adequate waveform. This procedure requires specialized training to ensure accurate vessel identification and correct interpretation of the signals.

Key nursing diagnoses and patient outcomes

Anxiety related to situational crisis
The patient will:
▶ state at least two ways to eliminate or minimize anxious behaviors
▶ report being able to cope with current situation without experiencing severe anxiety.

Deficient knowledge related to lack of exposure to procedure
The patient will:
▶ communicate a need to know about transcranial Doppler monitoring
▶ state or demonstrate understanding of procedure.

Equipment

Transcranial Doppler unit • transducer with an attachment system • terry cloth headband • ultrasonic coupling gel • marker

Implementation

▶ Explain the procedure to the patient and answer any questions he has about the procedure as thoroughly as possible.

▶ Place the patient in the proper position—usually the supine position.
▶ Turn the Doppler unit on and observe as it performs a self-test. The screen should show six parameters: PEAK (CM/S), MEAN (CM/S), DEPTH (M/M), DELTA (%), EMBOLI (AGR), and PIL.
▶ Enter the patient's name and identification number in the appropriate place on the Doppler unit. Depending on the unit you're using, you may need to enter additional information, such as the patient's diagnosis or the doctor's name.
▶ Indicate the vessel that you wish to monitor (usually the right or left middle cerebral artery [MCA]). You'll also need to set the approximate depth of the vessel within the skull (50 mm for the MCA).
▶ Next, use the keypad to increase the power level to 100% to initially locate the signal. You can later decrease the level as needed, depending on the thickness of the patient's skull.
▶ Examine the temporal region of the patient's head, and mentally identify the three windows of the transtemporal access route: posterior, middle, and anterior (as shown below).

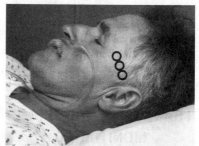

▶ Apply a generous amount of ultrasonic gel at the level of the temporal bone between the tragus of the ear and the end of the eyebrow, and over the area of the three windows.

▶ Next, place the transducer on the posterior window. Angle the transducer slightly in an anterior direction and slowly move it in a narrow circle. This movement is commonly called the "flashlighting" technique. As you hold the transducer at an angle and perform flashlighting, also begin to very slowly move the transducer forward across the temporal area. As you do this, listen for the audible signal with the highest pitch. This sound corresponds to the highest velocity signal, which corresponds to the signal of the vessel you are assessing. You can also use headphones *to let you better evaluate the audible signal and provide patient privacy.*

▶ After you've located the highest-pitched signal, use a marker to draw a circle around the transducer head on the patient's temple (as shown below). Note the angle of the transducer *so that you can duplicate it after the transducer attachment system is in place.*

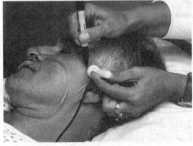

▶ Next, place the transducer system on the patient. To do this, first place the plate of the transducer attachment system over the patient's temporal area; match the circular opening in the plate exactly with the circle drawn on the patient's head. Then, holding the plate in place, encircle the patient's head with the straps attached to the system. Finally, tighten the straps so that the

transducer attachment system will stay in place on the patient's head.

▶ Fill the circular opening in the plate with the ultrasonic gel.

▶ Place the transducer in the gel-filled opening in the attachment system plate. Using the plastic screws provided, loosely secure the two plates together. *This will hold the transducer in place but allow it to rotate for the best angle.*

▶ Adjust the position and angle of the transducer until you again hear the highest-pitched audible signal. When you hear this signal, look at the waveform on the monitor screen. You should see a clear waveform with a bright white line (called an envelope) at the upper edge of the waveform. The envelope exactly follows the contours of the waveform itself.

▶ If the envelope doesn't follow the waveform's contours, adjust the GAIN setting. If the signal is wrapping around the screen, use the SCALE key to increase the scale and the BASELINE key to drop the baseline.

▶ When you've determined that you have the strongest, highest-pitched signal and the best waveform, lock the transducer in place by tightening the plastic screws (as shown below). The tightened plates will hold the transducer at the angle you've chosen. Disconnect the transducer handle.

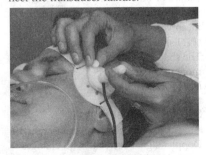

Comparing velocity waveforms

A normal transcranial Doppler signal is usually characterized by mean velocities that fall within the normal reported values. Additional information can be gathered by evaluating the shape of the velocity waveform.

Effect of significant proximal vessel obstruction

A delayed systolic upstroke can be seen in a waveform when significant proximal vessel obstruction is present.

Normal

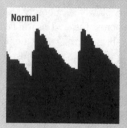

Proximal vessel obstruction

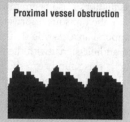

Effect of increased cerebrovascular resistance

Changes in cerebrovascular resistance, as occur with increased intracranial pressure, cause a decrease in diastolic flow.

Normal

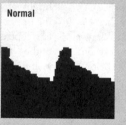

Increased resistance

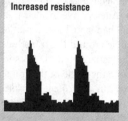

▶ Place a wide terry cloth headband over the transducer attachment system and secure it around the patient's head *to provide additional stability for the transducer.*

▶ Look at the monitor screen. You should be able to see a waveform and read the numeric values of the peak, mean velocities, and pulsatility index (PI1) above the displayed waveform. The shape of the waveform reveals more information. (See *Comparing velocity waveforms.*)

Special considerations

▶ Velocity changes in the transcranial Doppler signal correlate with changes in cerebral blood flow. The parameter that most clearly reflects this change is the mean velocity. First, establish a baseline for the mean velocity. Then, as the patient's velocity increases or decreases, the value (%) will change negatively or positively from the baseline.

▶ Emboli appear as high-intensity transients that occur randomly during the cardiac cycle. Emboli make a distinctive "clicking," "chirping," or "plunking" sound. You can set up an emboli counter to count either the total number of emboli aggregates or the number of embolic events per minute.

▶ Various screens can be stored on the system's hard drive and can be recalled or printed.

▶ Before using the transcranial Doppler system, be sure to remove turban head dressings or thick dressings over the test site.

Documentation

Record the date and the time that the monitoring began and which artery is being monitored. Document any patient teaching as well as the patient's tolerance of the procedure.

TRANSCUTANEOUS ELECTRICAL NERVE STIMULATION

Transcutaneous electrical nerve stimulation (TENS) is based on the gate control theory of pain, which proposes that painful impulses pass through a "gate" in the brain. TENS is performed with a portable, battery-powered device that transmits painless electrical current to peripheral nerves or directly to a painful area over relatively large nerve fibers. This treatment effectively alters the patient's perception of pain by blocking painful stimuli traveling over smaller fibers.

Used for postoperative patients and those with chronic pain, TENS reduces the need for analgesic drugs and may allow the patient to resume normal activities. Typically, a course of TENS treatments lasts 3 to 5 days. Some conditions such as phantom limb pain may require continuous stimulation; other conditions such as a painful arthritic joint require shorter periods (3 to 4 hours). (See *Current uses of TENS*.)

TENS is contraindicated for patients with cardiac pacemakers because it can interfere with pacemaker function. The

Current uses of TENS

Transcutaneous electrical nerve stimulation (TENS), which must be prescribed by a doctor, is most successful if administered and taught to the patient by a therapist skilled in its use. TENS has been used for temporary relief of acute pain, such as postoperative pain, and for ongoing relief of chronic pain such as that associated with sciatica.

Types of pain that respond to TENS include:
- arthritis pain
- bone fracture pain
- bursitis pain
- cancer-related pain
- musculoskeletal pain
- myofascial pain
- pain from neuralgias and neuropathies
- phantom limb pain
- postoperative incision pain
- pain from sciatica
- whiplash pain.

procedure is also contraindicated for pregnant patients because its effect on the fetus is unknown. It's also contraindicated in patients with dementia. TENS should be used cautiously in all patients with cardiac disorders. TENS electrodes shouldn't be placed on the head or neck of patients with vascular disorders or seizure disorders.

Key nursing diagnoses and patient outcomes

Impaired physical mobility related to neuromuscular impairment
The patient will:
▶ maintain muscle strength and joint range-of-motion
▶ show no evidence of complications such as skin breakdown.

Chronic pain related to physical agents
The patient will:
► express a feeling of comfort and relief from pain
► state and carry out appropriate interventions for pain relief.

Equipment

TENS device • alcohol pads • electrodes • electrode gel • warm water and soap • leadwires • charged battery pack • battery recharger • adhesive patch or hypoallergenic tape

Commercial TENS kits are available. They include the stimulator, leadwires, electrodes, spare battery pack, battery recharger and, sometimes, the adhesive patch.

Preparation of equipment

Before beginning the procedure, always test the battery pack to make sure it's fully charged.

Implementation

► Wash your hands and provide privacy. If the patient has never seen a TENS unit, show him the device and explain the procedure.

Before TENS treatment

► With an alcohol pad, thoroughly clean the skin where the electrode will be applied. Then dry the skin.
► Apply electrode gel to the bottom of each electrode.
► Place the ordered number of electrodes on the proper skin area, leaving at least 2″ (5.1 cm) between them. (See *Positioning TENS electrodes.*) Then secure them with the adhesive patch or hypoallergenic tape. Tape all sides evenly *so that the electrodes are firmly attached to the skin.*

► Plug the pin connectors into the electrode sockets. *To protect the cords,* hold the connectors—not the cords themselves—during insertion.
► Turn the channel controls to the OFF position or as recommended in the operator's manual.
► Plug the leadwires into the jacks in the control box.
► Turn the amplitude and rate dials slowly as the manual directs. (The patient should feel a tingling sensation.) Then adjust the controls on this device to the prescribed settings or to settings that are most comfortable. Most patients select stimulation frequencies of 60 to 100 Hz.
► Attach the TENS control box to part of the patient's clothing, such as a belt, pocket, or bra.
► *To make sure the device is working effectively,* monitor the patient for signs of excessive stimulation, such as muscular twitches, and for signs of inadequate stimulation, signaled by the patient's inability to feel any mild tingling sensation.

After TENS treatment

► Turn off the controls and unplug the electrode leadwires from the control box.
► If another treatment will be given soon, leave the electrodes in place; if not, remove them.
► Clean the electrodes with soap and water and clean the patient's skin with alcohol pads. (Don't soak the electrodes in alcohol *because it will damage the rubber.*)
► Remove the battery pack from the unit and replace it with a charged battery pack.
► Recharge the used battery pack *so that it's always ready for use.*

Positioning TENS electrodes

In transcutaneous electrical nerve stimulation (TENS), electrodes placed around peripheral nerves (or an incisional site) transmit mild electrical pulses to the brain. The current is thought to block pain impulses. The patient can influence the level and frequency of his pain relief by adjusting the controls on the device.

Typically, electrode placement varies even though patients may have similar complaints. Electrodes can be placed in several ways:

■ to cover the painful area or surround it, as with muscle tenderness or spasm or painful joints

■ to "capture" the painful area between electrodes, as with incisional pain.

In peripheral nerve injury, electrodes should be placed proximal to the injury (between the brain and the injury site) to avoid increasing pain. Placing electrodes in a hypersensitive area also increases pain. In an area lacking sensation, electrodes should be placed on adjacent dermatomes.

The illustrations below show combinations of electrode placement (dark squares) and areas of nerve stimulation (shaded strips) for low back and leg pain.

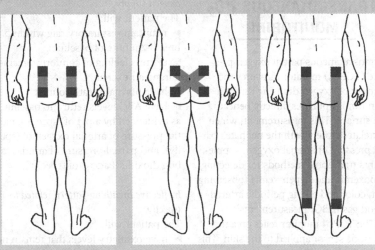

Special considerations

▶ If you must move the electrodes during the procedure, turn off the controls first. Follow the doctor's orders regarding electrode placement and control settings. *Incorrect placement of the electrodes will result in inappropriate pain control. Setting the controls too high can cause pain; setting them too low will fail to relieve pain.*

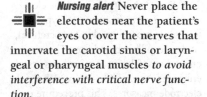

Nursing alert Never place the electrodes near the patient's eyes or over the nerves that innervate the carotid sinus or laryngeal or pharyngeal muscles *to avoid interference with critical nerve function.*

▶ If TENS is used continuously for postoperative pain, remove the elec-

trodes at least daily *to check for skin irritation and provide skin care.*
▶ If appropriate, let the patient study the operator's manual. Teach him how to place the electrodes properly and how to take care of the TENS unit.

Documentation
On the patient's medical record and the nursing plan of care, record the electrode sites and the control settings. Document the patient's tolerance to treatment. Also evaluate and record pain control.

TRANSCUTANEOUS PO₂ MONITORING

A transcutaneous partial oxygen pressure ($TCPO_2$) monitor measures the amount of oxygen diffusing through skin from capillaries directly beneath the surface. This measurement, which correlates closely with the neonate's partial pressure of arterial oxygen, supplements traditional methods for detecting hypoxemia and hyperoxemia (observing skin color and taking periodic arterial blood gas [ABG] measurements).

The $TCPO_2$ monitor relies on a tiny electrode sensor applied to the skin. This sensor — a metallic, oxygen-sensitive device — warms to between 107.6° and 115° F (42° and 46.1° C). As the electrode's temperature increases (typically, to slightly more than skin temperature), so does capillary blood flow. The increased vasodilation in cutaneous vessels enhances oxygen diffusion, which the electrode measures. This procedure is sometimes used in neonatal intensive care units by staff nurses trained to use the monitor. However, it has been widely replaced by pulse oximetry.

Because neonatal skin is thin with little subcutaneous fat, $TCPO_2$ monitoring produces accurate findings. However, in neonates with shock or hypoperfusion, the results seldom accurately reflect arterial oxygen levels. In these neonates, peripheral blood flow decreases as blood is shunted to the heart, brain, and lungs.

Another device for monitoring arterial oxygen levels is the pulse oximeter. (See *Neonatal pulse oximetry.*)

Key nursing diagnoses and patient outcomes
Impaired gas exchange related to altered oxygen supply
The patient will:
▶ maintain respiratory rate within 5 breaths/minute of baseline
▶ express feeling of comfort in maintaining air exchange
▶ have normal breath sounds
▶ have ABG levels return to baseline, as evidenced by a pH of (specify); partial pressure of arterial oxygen of (specify); and partial pressure of arterial carbon dioxide ($PaCO_2$) of (specify).

Ineffective breathing pattern related to (specify)
The patient will:
▶ have oximetry levels that remain no lower than (specify) and no higher than (specify)
▶ report feeling comfortable when breathing
▶ achieve maximum lung expansion with adequate ventilation.

Equipment
$TCPO_2$ monitor and electrode • cotton balls • soap and water • alcohol pad • adhesive ring for electrode

Preparation of equipment

Set up the monitor and calibrate it, if necessary, following the manufacturer's instructions. Ensure that the strip chart recorder works properly.

Implementation

► Wash your hands and decide where to place the electrode. Choose a flat site, with good capillary blood flow, few fatty deposits, and no bony prominences. Common sites include the neonate's upper chest, abdomen, and inner thigh.
► Clean the site first with a cotton ball and soap and water. Then wipe the site with an alcohol pad *to remove dirt and oils and to ensure good electrode contact.*
► Dry the skin, attach the adhesive ring to the electrode, and moisten the skin site with a drop of water, according to the manufacturer's instructions, *to seal out all air.*
► Place the electrode on the site and make sure that the adhesive ring is tight.
► Set the alarm switches and the electrode temperature according to the manufacturer's instructions or your facility's policy.
► Expect the monitor reading to stabilize in 10 to 20 minutes. Normal oxygen pressures vary with the neonate and the equipment but usually range from 50 to 80 mm Hg. TCPO_2 monitors usually have digital readouts and strip chart recorders to show trends.
► Rotate the electrode site every 4 hours *to prevent skin irritation, breakdown, and burns.*

Special considerations

► Expect TCPO_2 values to vary with neonatal movement and treatment. Also expect them to drop markedly whenever the neonate cries vigorously.

Neonatal pulse oximetry

Another noninvasive technique for monitoring oxygenation is pulse oximetry. The sensor of the pulse oximeter, which is attached to the neonate's foot, measures beat-to-beat arterial oxygen saturation. Normally, oxygenation values should drop no lower than 90%.

Don't be guided only by oximetric findings. Every 3 to 4 hours, you'll need to correlate laboratory values (from arterial blood gas analyses) with oximetric values for a reliable overview of neonatal status.

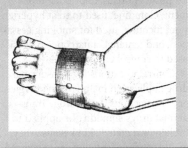

However, be prepared to start resuscitation if a sudden, significant drop in TCPO_2 pressure occurs.
► Remember that TCPO_2 monitoring doesn't replace ABG measurements because it doesn't give information about the PaCO_2 and pH.

Complications

Be alert for burns and blisters from the electrode and for skin reactions to the adhesive ring.

Documentation

Place graphic or printout results on the neonate's chart. Record the range of values observed during monitoring in your notes. Also record any skin disorders related to the electrode.

TRANSDERMAL DRUG THERAPY

Through an adhesive patch or a measured dose of ointment applied to the skin, transdermal drugs deliver constant, controlled medication directly into the bloodstream for a prolonged systemic effect.

Medications available in transdermal form include nitroglycerin, used to control angina; scopolamine, used to treat motion sickness; estradiol, used for postmenopausal hormone replacement; clonidine, used to treat hypertension; nicotine, used for smoking cessation; and fentanyl, a narcotic analgesic used to control chronic pain.

Contraindications for transdermal drug application include skin allergies or skin reactions to the drug. Transdermal drugs shouldn't be applied to broken or irritated skin because they would increase irritation, or to scarred or callused skin, which might impair absorption.

Key nursing diagnoses and patient outcomes

Deficient knowledge related to lack of exposure to procedure
The patient will:
▶ state or demonstrate understanding of what has been taught
▶ demonstrate ability to perform new health-related behaviors as they're taught.

Risk for injury related to improper technique
The patient will:
▶ identify factors that increase risk for injury

▶ assist in identifying and applying safety measures to prevent injury.

Equipment
Patient's medication record and chart • gloves • prescribed medication (patch or ointment) • application strip or measuring paper (for nitroglycerin ointment) • adhesive tape • plastic wrap (optional for nitroglycerin ointment) or semipermeable dressing

Implementation
▶ Verify the order on the patient's medication record by checking it against the doctor's order.
▶ Wash your hands and, if necessary, put on gloves.
▶ Check the label on the medication *to make sure you're giving the correct drug in the correct dose.* Note the expiration date.
▶ Confirm the patient's identity by asking his name and checking the name, room number, and bed number on his wristband.
▶ Explain the procedure to the patient and provide privacy.
▶ Remove any previously applied medication.

Applying transdermal ointment
▶ Place the prescribed amount of ointment on the application strip or measuring paper, taking care not to get any on your skin. (See *Applying nitroglycerin ointment.*)
▶ Apply the strip to any dry, hairless area of the body. Don't rub the ointment into the skin.
▶ Tape the ointment-filled strip to the skin.
▶ If desired, cover the application strip with the plastic wrap and tape the wrap in place.

Applying nitroglycerin ointment

Unlike most topical medications, nitroglycerin ointment is used for its transdermal systemic effect. It's used to dilate the veins and arteries, thus improving cardiac perfusion in a patient with cardiac ischemia or angina pectoris.

To apply nitroglycerin ointment, start by taking the patient's baseline blood pressure so that you can compare it with later readings. Gather your equipment. Nitroglycerin ointment, which is prescribed by the inch, comes with a rectangular piece of ruled paper to be used in applying the medication. Squeeze the prescribed amount of ointment onto the ruled paper (as shown below). Put on gloves, if desired, to avoid contact with the medication. Nitroglycerin ointment also comes in premeasured single-dose packages.

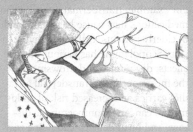

After applying the correct amount of ointment, tape the paper—drug side down—di-

rectly to the skin (as shown below). (Some facilities require you to use the paper to apply the medication to the patient's skin, usually on the chest or arm. Spread a thin layer of the ointment over a 3″ [7.5-cm] area.) For increased absorption, the doctor may request that you cover the site with plastic wrap or a transparent semipermeable dressing.

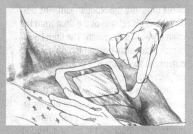

After 5 minutes, record the patient's blood pressure. If it has dropped significantly and he has a headache (from vasodilation of blood vessels in his head), notify the doctor immediately. He may reduce the dose. If the patient's blood pressure has dropped but he has no symptoms, instruct him to lie still until it returns to normal.

Transdermal nitroglycerin should be removed at bedtime to provide a 10- to 12-hour nitrate-free interval, thereby preventing drug tolerance.

Applying a transdermal patch
▶ Open the package and remove the patch.
▶ Without touching the adhesive surface, remove the clear plastic backing.
▶ Apply the patch to a dry, hairless area—behind the ear, for example, as with scopolamine. (See *Applying a transdermal medication patch,* page 854.)
▶ Write the date, time, and your initials on the patch.

After applying transdermal medications
▶ Store the medication as ordered.
▶ Instruct the patient to keep the area around the patch or strip as dry as possible.
▶ If you didn't wear gloves, wash your hands immediately after applying the patch or ointment *to avoid absorbing the drug yourself.*

Applying a transdermal medication patch

If the patient will be receiving medication by transdermal patch, instruct him in its proper use, as described here:

■ Explain to the patient that the patch consists of several layers. The layer closest to his skin contains a small amount of the drug and allows prompt introduction of the drug into the bloodstream. The next layer controls release of the drug from the main portion of the patch. The third layer contains the main dose of the drug. The outermost layer consists of an aluminized polyester barrier.

■ Teach the patient to apply the patch to appropriate skin areas, such as the upper arm or chest and behind the ear. Warn him to avoid touching the gel or surrounding tape. Tell him to use a different site for each application to avoid skin irritation. If necessary, he can shave the site. Tell him to avoid any area that may cause uneven absorption, such as skin folds, scars, and calluses, or any irritated or damaged skin areas. Also, tell him not to apply the patch below the elbow or knee.

■ Instruct the patient to wash his hands after application to remove any medication that may have rubbed off.

■ Warn the patient not to get the patch wet. Tell him to discard it if it leaks or falls off and then to clean the site and apply a new patch at a different site.

■ Instruct the patient to apply the patch at the same time at the prescribed interval to ensure continuous drug delivery. Bedtime application is ideal for some transdermal medication patches because body movement is reduced during the night. Finally, tell him to apply a new patch about 30 minutes before removing the old one.

Special considerations

► Reapply daily transdermal medications at the same time every day *to ensure a continuous effect,* but alternate the application sites *to avoid skin irritation.*

► When applying a scopolamine or fentanyl patch, instruct the patient not to drive or operate machinery until his response to the drug has been determined.

► Warn a patient using a clonidine patch to check with his doctor before taking an over-the-counter cough preparation *because such drugs may counteract clonidine's effects.*

Complications

Topical medications may cause skin irritation, such as pruritus and a rash. The patient may also suffer adverse effects of the specific drug administered. For example, transdermal nitroglycerin medications may cause headaches and, in elderly patients, orthostatic hypotension. Scopolamine has various adverse effects; dry mouth and drowsiness are the most common. Transdermal estradiol carries an increased risk of endometrial cancer, thromboembolic disease, and birth defects. Clonidine may cause severe rebound hypertension, especially if withdrawn suddenly.

Documentation

Record the type of medication; date, time, and site of application; and dose. Also note any adverse effects and the patient's response.

TRANSDUCER SYSTEM SETUP

The exact type of transducer system used depends on the patient's needs and the doctor's preference. Some systems monitor pressure continuously, whereas others monitor pressure intermittently. Single-pressure transducers monitor only one type of pressure — for example, pulmonary artery pressure (PAP). Multiple-pressure transducers can monitor two or more types of pressure, such as PAP and central venous pressure.

Key nursing diagnoses and patient outcomes

Ineffective tissue perfusion (cardiopulmonary) related to decreased cellular exchange
The patient will:
▶ have warm, dry skin
▶ maintain adequate cardiac output
▶ not exhibit arrhythmias.

Decreased cardiac output related to decreased stroke volume
The patient will:
▶ attain hemodynamic stability as evidenced by pulse not less than (specify) beats/minute and not more than (specify) beats/minute, blood pressure not less than (specify) mm Hg and not greater than (specify) mm Hg
▶ exhibit PAP and pulmonary artery wedge pressure measurements within normal limits
▶ have a diminished heart workload
▶ maintain adequate cardiac output.

Equipment

Bag of heparin flush solution (usually 500 ml normal saline solution with 500 or 1,000 units heparin) • pressure infusion bag • medication-added label • preassembled disposable pressure tubing with flush device and disposable transducer • monitor and monitor cable • I.V. pole with transducer mount • carpenter's level

Preparation of equipment

Turn the monitor on before gathering the equipment to give it sufficient time to warm up. Gather the equipment you'll need. Wash your hands.

Implementation

To set up and zero a single-pressure transducer system, perform the following steps.

Setting up the system

▶ Follow your facility's policy on adding heparin to the flush solution. If your patient has a history of bleeding or clotting problems, use heparin with caution. Add the ordered amount of heparin to the solution — usually, 1 to 2 units of heparin/ml of solution — and then label the bag.
▶ Put the pressure module into the monitor, if necessary, and connect the transducer cable to the monitor.
▶ Remove the preassembled pressure tubing from the package. If necessary, connect the pressure tubing to the transducer. Tighten all tubing connections.
▶ Position all stopcocks so the flush solution can flow through the entire system. Then roll the tubing's flow regulator to the OFF position.
▶ Spike the flush solution bag with the tubing, invert the bag, open the roller clamp, and squeeze all the air through the drip chamber. Then, compress the tubing's drip chamber, filling it no more than halfway with the flush solution.
▶ Place the flush solution bag into the pressure infuser bag. To do this, hang the pressure infuser bag on the I.V. pole and then position the flush solution bag inside the pressure infuser bag.
▶ Open the tubing's flow regulator, uncoil the tube if you haven't already

done so, and remove the protective cap at the end of the pressure tubing. Squeeze the continuous flush device slowly to prime the entire system, including the stopcock ports, with the flush solution.

▶ As the solution nears the disposable transducer, hold the transducer at a 45-degree angle (as shown below). *This forces the solution to flow upward to the transducer. In doing so, the solution forces any air out of the system.*

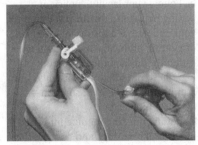

▶ When the solution nears a stopcock, open the stopcock to air, allowing the solution to flow into the stopcock (as shown below). When the stopcock fills, close it to air and turn it open to the remainder of the tubing. Do this for each stopcock.

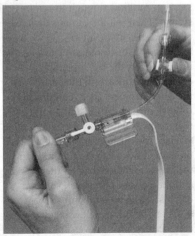

▶ After you've completely primed the system, replace the protective cap at the end of the tubing.

▶ Inflate the pressure infuser bag to 300 mm Hg. *This bag keeps the pressure in the arterial line higher than the patient's systolic pressure, preventing blood backflow into the tubing and ensuring a continuous flow rate.* When you inflate the pressure bag, take care that the drip chamber doesn't completely fill with fluid. Afterward, flush the system again *to remove all air bubbles.*

▶ Replace the vented caps on the stopcocks with sterile nonvented caps. If you're going to mount the transducer on an I.V. pole, insert the device into its holder.

Zeroing the system
▶ Now you're ready for a preliminary zeroing of the transducer. To ensure accuracy, position the patient and the transducer on the same level each time you zero the transducer or record a pressure. Typically, the patient lies flat in bed, if he can tolerate that position.

▶ Next, use the carpenter's level to position the air-reference stopcock or the air-fluid interface of the transducer level with the phlebostatic axis (midway between the posterior chest and the sternum at the fourth intercostal space; midaxillary line). Alternatively, you may level the air-reference stopcock or the air-fluid interface to the same position as the catheter tip.

▶ After leveling the transducer, turn the stopcock next to the transducer off to the patient and open to air. Remove the cap to the stopcock port. Place the cap inside an opened sterile gauze package *to prevent contamination.*

▶ Now zero the transducer. To do so, follow the manufacturer's directions for zeroing.

▶ When you've finished zeroing, turn the stopcock on the transducer so that it's open to air and open to the patient. This is the monitoring position. Replace the cap on the stopcock. You're now ready to attach the single-pressure transducer to the patient's catheter. Now you've assembled a single-pressure transducer system. The photograph below shows how the system will look.

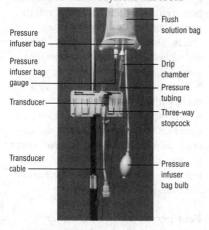

Pressure infuser bag

Pressure infuser bag gauge

Transducer

Transducer cable

Flush solution bag

Drip chamber

Pressure tubing

Three-way stopcock

Pressure infuser bag bulb

Special considerations
▶ You may use any of several methods to set up a multiple-pressure transducer system. The easiest way is to add to the single-pressure system. You'll also need another bag of heparin flush solution in a second pressure infuser bag. Then you'll prime the tubing, mount the second transducer, and connect an additional cable to the monitor. Finally, you'll zero the second transducer.

Documentation
Document the patient's position for zeroing so that other health care team members can replicate the placement.

TRANSFER FROM BED TO STRETCHER

Transfer from bed to stretcher, one of the most common transfers, can require the help of one or more coworkers, depending on the patient's size and condition and the primary nurse's physical abilities. Techniques for achieving this transfer include the straight lift, carry lift, lift sheet, and sliding board.

Key nursing diagnoses and patient outcomes
Impaired physical mobility related to neuromuscular impairment
The patient will:
▶ maintain muscle strength and joint range-of-motion
▶ show no evidence of such complications as contractures, venous stasis, thrombus formation, or skin breakdown
▶ have mobility regimen carried out by significant other.

Risk for injury related to sensory deficits
The patient will:
▶ identify factors that increase potential for injury
▶ identify and apply safety measures to prevent injury
▶ optimize activities of daily living within sensorimotor limitations.

Equipment
Stretcher • sliding board or lift sheet, if necessary

Preparation of equipment
Adjust the bed to the same height as the stretcher.

Implementation

▶ Tell the patient that you're going to move him from the bed to the stretcher and place him in the supine position.

▶ Ask team members to remove watches and rings *to avoid scratching the patient during transfer.*

Four-person straight lift

▶ Place the stretcher parallel to the bed and lock the wheels of both *to ensure the patient's safety.*

▶ Stand at the center of the stretcher and have another team member stand at the patient's head. The two other team members should stand next to the bed, on the other side—one at the center and the other at the patient's feet.

▶ Slide your arms, palms up, beneath the patient, while the other team members do the same. In this position, you and the team member directly opposite support the patient's buttocks and hips; the team member at the head of the bed supports the patient's head and shoulders; the one at the foot supports the patient's legs and feet.

▶ On a count of three, the team members lift the patient several inches, move him onto the stretcher, and slide their arms out from under him. Keep movements smooth *to minimize patient discomfort and avoid muscle strain by team members.*

Four-person carry lift

▶ Place the stretcher perpendicular to the bed, with the head of the stretcher at the foot of the bed. Lock the bed and stretcher wheels *to ensure the patient's safety.*

▶ Raise the bed to a comfortable working height.

▶ Line up all four team members on the same side of the bed as the stretcher, with the tallest member at the patient's head and the shortest at his feet. The member at the patient's head is the leader of the team and gives the lift signals.

▶ Tell the team members to flex their knees and slide their hands, palms up, under the patient until he rests securely on their upper arms. Make sure the patient is adequately supported at the head and shoulders, buttocks and hips, and legs and feet.

▶ On a count of three, the team members straighten their knees and roll the patient onto his side, against their chests. *This reduces strain on the lifters and allows them to hold the patient for several minutes if necessary.*

▶ Together, the team members step back, with the member supporting the feet moving the farthest. The team members move forward to the stretcher's edge and, on a count of three, lower the patient onto the stretcher by bending at the knees and sliding their arms out from under the patient.

Four-person lift sheet transfer

▶ Position the bed, stretcher, and team members for the straight lift. Instruct the team to hold the edges of the sheet under the patient, grasping them close to the patient *to obtain a firm grip, provide stability, and spare the patient undue feelings of instability.*

▶ On a count of three, the team members lift or slide the patient onto the stretcher in a smooth, continuous motion *to avoid muscle strain and minimize patient discomfort.*

Sliding-board transfer

▶ Place the stretcher parallel to the bed and lock the wheels of both *to ensure the patient's safety.*

▶ Stand next to the bed and instruct a coworker to stand next to the stretcher.
▶ Reach over the patient and pull the far side of the bedsheet toward you to turn the patient slightly on his side. Your coworker then places the sliding board beneath the patient, making sure the board bridges the gap between stretcher and bed.
▶ Ease the patient onto the sliding board and release the sheet. Your coworker then grasps the near side of the sheet at the patient's hips and shoulders and pulls him onto the stretcher in a smooth, continuous motion. She then reaches over the patient, grasps the far side of the sheet, and logrolls him toward her.
▶ Remove the sliding board as your coworker returns the patient to the supine position.

After all transfers
▶ Position the patient comfortably on the stretcher, apply safety straps, and raise and secure the side rails.

Special considerations

When transferring a helpless or markedly obese patient from bed to stretcher, first lift and move him, in increments, to the edge of the bed. Rest for a few seconds, repositioning the patient if necessary, and lift him onto the stretcher. If the patient can bear weight on his arms or legs, two or three coworkers can perform this transfer: One can support the buttocks and guide the patient, another can stabilize the stretcher by leaning over it and guiding the patient into position, and a third can transfer any attached equipment. One team member must stabilize the patient's head if he can't support it himself, has cervical instability or injury, or has undergone surgery.

Documentation

Record the time and, if necessary, the type of transfer in your notes. Complete other required forms as necessary.

TRANSFER FROM BED TO WHEELCHAIR

For the patient with diminished or absent lower-body sensation or one-sided weakness, immobility, or injury, transfer from bed to wheelchair may require partial support to full assistance — initially by at least two persons. Subsequent transfer of the patient with generalized weakness may be performed by one nurse. After transfer, proper positioning helps prevent excessive pressure on bony prominences, which predisposes the patient to skin breakdown.

Key nursing diagnoses and patient outcomes

Impaired physical mobility related to neuromuscular impairment
The patient will:
▶ maintain muscle strength and joint range of motion
▶ show no evidence of such complications as contractures, venous stasis, thrombus formation, and skin breakdown
▶ have mobility regimen carried out by significant other.

Risk for injury related to sensory deficits
The patient will:
▶ identify factors that increase potential for injury
▶ identify and apply safety measures to prevent injury
▶ optimize activities of daily living within sensorimotor limitations.

Equipment

Wheelchair with locks (or sturdy chair) • pajama bottoms (or robe) • shoes or slippers with nonslip soles • watch with a second had • stethoscope • sphygmomanometer • optional: transfer board if appropriate (see *Teaching the patient to use a transfer board*)

Implementation

▶ Explain the procedure to the patient and demonstrate his role.

▶ Place the wheelchair parallel to the bed, facing the foot of the bed, and lock its wheels. Make sure the bed wheels are also locked. Raise the footrests *to avoid interfering with the transfer.*

▶ Check pulse rate and blood pressure with the patient supine *to obtain a baseline.* Help him put on the pajama bottoms and slippers or shoes with nonslip soles to prevent falls.

▶ Raise the head of the bed and allow the patient to rest briefly *to adjust to posture changes.* Then bring him to the dangling position (see "Ambulation, progressive," page 8). Recheck pulse rate and blood pressure if you suspect cardiovascular instability. Don't proceed until the patient's pulse rate and blood pressure are stabilized *to prevent falls.*

▶ Tell the patient to move toward the edge of the bed and, if possible, to place his feet flat on the floor. Stand in front of the patient, blocking his toes with your feet and his knees with yours *to prevent his knees from buckling.*

▶ Flex your knees slightly, place your arms around the patient's waist, and tell him to place his hands on the edge of the bed. Avoid bending at your waist *to prevent back strain.*

▶ Ask the patient to push himself off the bed and to support as much of his own weight as possible. At the same time, straighten your knees and hips, raising the patient as you straighten your body.

▶ Supporting the patient as needed, pivot toward the wheelchair, keeping your knees next to his. Tell the patient to grasp the farthest armrest of the wheelchair with his closest hand.

▶ Help the patient lower himself into the wheelchair by flexing your hips and knees, but not your back. Instruct him to reach back and grasp the other wheelchair armrest as he sits *to avoid abrupt contact with the seat.* Fasten the seat belt *to prevent falls* and, if necessary, check pulse rate and blood pressure *to assess cardiovascular stability.* If the pulse rate is 20 beats or more above baseline, stay with the patient and monitor him closely until it returns to normal *because he is experiencing orthostatic hypotension.*

▶ If the patient can't position himself correctly, help him move his buttocks against the back of the chair *so that the ischial tuberosities, not the sacrum, provide the base of support.*

▶ Place the patient's feet flat on the footrests, pointed straight ahead. Position the knees and hips with the correct amount of flexion and in appropriate alignment. If appropriate, use elevating leg rests to flex the patient's hips at more than 90 degrees; *this position relieves pressure on the popliteal space and places more weight on the ischial tuberosities.*

▶ Position the patient's arms on the wheelchair's armrests with shoulders abducted, elbows slightly flexed, forearms pronated, and wrists and hands in the neutral position. If necessary, support or elevate the patient's hands and forearms with a pillow *to prevent dependent edema.*

Teaching the patient to use a transfer board

For the patient who can't stand, a transfer board allows safe transfer from bed to wheelchair. To perform this transfer, take the following steps:

■ First, explain and demonstrate the procedure. Eventually, the patient may become proficient enough to transfer himself independently or with some supervision.

■ Help the patient put on pajama bottoms or a robe and shoes or slippers.

■ Place the wheelchair angled slightly and facing the foot of the bed. Lock the wheels and remove the armrest closest to the patient. Make sure the bed is flat and adjust its height so that it's level with the wheelchair seat.

■ Assist the patient to a sitting position on the edge of the bed, with his feet resting on the floor. Make sure the front edge of the wheelchair seat is aligned with the back of the patient's knees (as shown below left). Although it's important that the patient have an even surface on which to transfer, he may find it easier to transfer to a slightly lower surface.

■ Ask the patient to lean away from the wheelchair while you slide one end of the transfer board under him.

■ Now place the other end of the transfer board on the wheelchair seat and help the patient return to the upright position.

■ Stand in front of the patient to prevent him from sliding forward. Tell him to push down with both arms, lifting the buttocks up and onto the transfer board. The patient then repeats this maneuver, edging along the board, until he's seated in the wheelchair. If the patient can't use his arms to assist with the transfer, stand in front of him, put your arms around him and, if he's able, have him put his arms around you. Gradually slide him across the board until he's safely in the chair (as shown below right).

■ When the patient is in the chair, fasten a seat belt, if necessary, to prevent falls.

■ Then remove the transfer board, replace the wheelchair armrest, and reposition the patient in the chair.

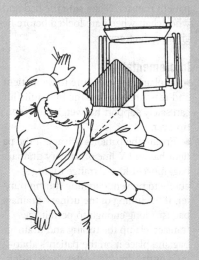

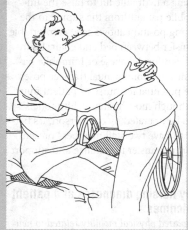

Special considerations

▶ If the patient starts to fall during transfer, ease him to the closest surface — bed, floor, or chair. Never stretch to finish the transfer. *Doing so can cause loss of balance, falls, muscle strain, and other injuries to you and the patient.*

▶ If the patient has one-sided weakness, follow the preceding steps, but place the wheelchair on the patient's unaffected side. Instruct the patient to pivot and bear as much weight as possible on the unaffected side. Support the affected side *because the patient will tend to lean to this side.* Use pillows to support the hemiplegic patient's affected side *to prevent slumping in the wheelchair.*

Documentation

If necessary, record the time of transfer and the extent of assistance. Also note how the patient tolerated the transfer.

TRANSFER WITH A HYDRAULIC LIFT

Using a hydraulic lift to raise the immobile patient from the supine to the sitting position allows safe, comfortable transfer between bed and chair. It's indicated for the obese or immobile patient for whom manual transfer poses the potential for nurse or patient injury. Although most hydraulic lift models can be operated by one person, it's better to have two staff members present during transfer to stabilize and support the patient.

Key nursing diagnoses and patient outcomes

Impaired physical mobility related to neuromuscular impairment

The patient will:
▶ maintain muscle strength and joint range of motion
▶ show no evidence of such complications as contractures, venous stasis, thrombus formation, and skin breakdown
▶ have mobility regimen carried out by significant other.

Risk for injury related to sensory deficits
The patient will:
▶ identify factors that increase potential for injury
▶ identify and apply safety measures to prevent injury
▶ optimize activities of daily living within sensorimotor limitations.

Equipment

Hydraulic lift, with sling, chains or straps, and hooks • chair or wheelchair

Preparation of equipment

Because hydraulic lift models may vary in weight capacity, check the manufacturer's specifications before attempting patient transfer. Make sure the bed and wheelchair wheels are locked before beginning the transfer.

Implementation

▶ Explain the procedure to the patient and reassure him that the hydraulic lift can safely support his weight and won't tip over.
▶ Ensure the patient's privacy. If the patient has an I.V. line or urinary drainage bag, move it first. Arrange tubing securely to prevent dangling during transfer. If the tubing of the urinary drainage bag isn't long enough to permit the transfer, clamp the tubing and drainage bag and place it on the patient's abdomen during transfer. After the transfer,

Using a hydraulic lift

After placing the patient in a supine position in the center of the sling, position the hydraulic lift above him (as shown below). Attach the chains to the hooks on the sling.

Turn the lift handle clockwise to raise the patient to the sitting position (as shown below). If he's positioned properly, continue to raise him until he's suspended just above the bed.

After positioning the patient above the wheelchair, turn the lift handle counterclockwise to lower him onto the seat (as shown below). When the chains become slack, stop turning and unhook the sling from the lift.

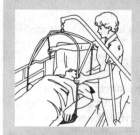
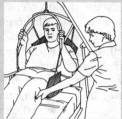
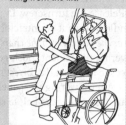

place the drainage bag in a dependent position and unclamp the tubing.

▶ Make sure the side rail opposite you is raised and secure. Roll the patient toward you, onto his side, and raise the side rail. Walk to the opposite side of the bed and lower the side rail.

▶ Place the sling under the patient's buttocks with its lower edge below the greater trochanter. Fanfold the far side of the sling against the back and buttocks.

▶ Roll the patient toward you onto the sling and raise the side rail. Lower the opposite side rail.

▶ Slide your hands under the patient and pull the sling from beneath him, smoothing out all wrinkles. Then roll the patient onto his back and center him on the sling.

▶ Place the appropriate chair next to the head of the bed, facing the foot.

▶ Lower the side rail next to the chair and raise the bed only until the base of the lift can extend under the bed. *To avoid alarming and endangering the patient,* don't raise the bed completely.

▶ Set the lift's adjustable base to its widest position *to ensure optimal stability.* Move the lift so that its arm lies perpendicular to the bed, directly over the patient.

▶ Connect one end of the chains (or straps) to the side arms on the lift; connect the other, hooked end to the sling. Face the hooks away from the patient *to prevent them from slipping and to avoid the risk of their pointed edges injuring the patient.* The patient may place his arms inside or outside the chains (or straps) or he may grasp them once the slack is gone (to avoid injury). (See *Using a hydraulic lift.*)

▶ Tighten the turnscrew on the lift. Then, depending on the type of lift you're using, pump the handle or turn it clockwise until the patient has assumed a sitting position and his buttocks clear the bed surface by at least 1″ (2.5 cm). Momentarily suspend him above the bed until he feels secure in the lift and sees that it can bear his weight.

▶ Steady the patient as you move the lift or, preferably, have another coworker guide the patient's body while you move the lift. Depending on the type of lift you're using, the arm should now rest in front or to one side of the chair.

▶ Release the turnscrew. Depress the handle or turn it counterclockwise *to lower the patient into the chair*. While lowering the patient, push gently on his knees *to maintain the correct sitting posture*. After lowering the patient into the chair, fasten the seat belt *to ensure his safety*.

▶ Remove the hooks or straps from the sling, but leave the sling in place under the patient so you'll be able to transfer him back to the bed from the chair. Move the lift away from the patient.

▶ To return the patient to bed, reverse the procedure.

Special considerations

▶ If the patient has an altered center of gravity (caused by a halo vest or a lower-extremity cast, for example), obtain help from a coworker before transferring him with a hydraulic lift.

▶ If the patient will require use of a hydraulic lift for transfers after discharge, teach his family how to use this device correctly and allow them to practice with supervision.

Documentation

If necessary, record the time of transfer in your notes.

TRANSFUSION OF AUTOLOGOUS BLOOD

Also called autotransfusion, transfusion of autologous blood is the collection, filtration, and reinfusion of the patient's own blood. Today, with the concern over acquired immunodeficiency syndrome and other blood-borne diseases, the use of autologous transfusion is on the rise.

Indications for autologous transfusion include:

▶ elective surgery (blood donated over time)

▶ nonelective surgery (blood withdrawn immediately before surgery)

▶ perioperative and emergency blood salvage during and after thoracic or cardiovascular surgery and hip, knee, or liver resection and during surgery for ruptured ectopic pregnancy and hemothorax

▶ perioperative and emergency blood salvage for traumatic injury of the lungs, liver, chest wall, heart, pulmonary vessels, spleen, kidneys, inferior vena cava, and iliac, portal, or subclavian veins.

Autologous transfusion is performed before, during, or after surgery and after traumatic injury. The three techniques used are preoperative blood donation, perioperative blood donation, and acute normovolemic hemodilution.

Preoperative blood donation is commonly recommended for patients scheduled for orthopedic surgery, which causes large blood loss. The donation period begins 4 to 6 weeks before surgery.

Perioperative blood donation (sometimes called intraoperative or postoperative) is used in vascular and orthopedic surgery and in treatment of traumatic injury. Blood may be collected during surgery or up to 12 hours afterward. (Considerable bleeding may follow vascular and orthopedic surgery.) The blood is transfused immediately after collection or processed (washed) before infusion. Blood obtained postoperatively may be collected from chest tubes, mediastinal drains, or wound drains (placed in the surgical wound during surgery). Commonly inserted during orthopedic surgery, wound drains can be used when enough uncontaminated blood is recovered from a closed wound to be reinfused.

Acute normovolemic hemodilution is used mainly in open-heart surgery. One or 2 units of blood are drawn immediately before or after anesthesia induction. The blood is replaced with a crystalloid or colloid solution, such as lactated Ringer's solution or dextran 40, to produce normovolemic anemia. The blood is reinfused right after surgery. The combination of reduced hemoglobin and the replacement solution causes the patient to lose fewer red blood cells during surgery.

The equipment and procedures presented here are for preoperative and perioperative blood donation only. Acute normovolemic hemodilution is performed the same way as preoperative blood donation, and blood collected this way is reinfused the same way as any other transfusion.

Key nursing diagnoses and patient outcomes

Deficient fluid volume related to blood loss
The patient will:
▶ maintain stable vital signs
▶ have fluid and blood volume return to normal
▶ produce adequate urine output.

Equipment
For preoperative blood donation
Ferrous sulfate • povidone-iodine solution • alcohol • tourniquet • rubber ball • large-bore needle for venipuncture • collection bags • I.V. line • in-line filter for reinfusion

For perioperative blood donation
Autologous transfusion system, such as the Davol or Pleur-evac system • ACD or CPD • collection bags • vacuum source regulator • suction tubing • 18G needle • blood administration set with in-line filter • 500 ml of normal saline solution • optional: Hemovac and another autologous transfusion system

Implementation
The steps to take depend on the circumstances of the autologous transfusion.

For preoperative blood donation
▶ Explain autologous transfusion to the patient, including what it is, how it's performed, how often he can donate blood (every 7 days), and how much he can donate (1 unit every week until 3 to 7 days before surgery).
▶ At least 1 week before the first donation, give the patient ferrous sulfate or another iron preparation to take three times a day, as ordered.
▶ To prevent hypovolemia, tell the patient to drink plenty of fluids before donating blood.
▶ Warn him that he may feel lightheaded during the donation but that the problem can be treated without further compromise.
▶ Check the patient's hemoglobin level, which must be 11 g/dl or higher to donate blood.
▶ Check vital signs before blood donation.

▶ Help the patient into a supine position.

▶ Clean the needle insertion site (usually the antecubital fossa) with alcohol or povidone-iodine solution.

▶ Apply a tourniquet.

▶ Insert the large-bore needle into the antecubital vein. Have the patient squeeze a rubber ball while you collect blood.

▶ Recheck vital signs after the collection.

▶ If ordered, provide replacement I.V. fluids immediately after the collection.

▶ Send a blood sample to the laboratory to be tested.

For perioperative blood donation

▶ If you know that the patient will leave surgery with a drain to the autologous transfusion device, tell him this beforehand.

For perioperative blood donation using a Davol system

▶ Open the transfusion unit onto the sterile field. The doctor inserts the drain tube (from the patient) to the connecting tube of the unit.

▶ The doctor injects 25 to 35 ml of ACD or CPD into the injection port on top of the filter and wets the filter with anticoagulant to keep the blood from clotting.

▶ Label the collection bag with the patient's name and the time the transfusion was started *so that the reinfusion time is within guidelines.*

After patient arrival in postanesthesia care unit or medical-surgical unit

▶ Note the amount of blood in the bag and on the postoperative sheet.

▶ Attach the tube from the suction source to the port on the suction control module.

▶ Adjust the suction source to between 80 and 100 mm Hg on the wall regulator. Pinch the suction tube. If the regulator exceeds 100 mm Hg, turn the suction down. Suction set at more than 100 mm Hg may cause the collection bag to collapse, resulting in lysis of blood cells. The potential for renal damage renders this blood unsafe. If the collection bag collapses, change the entire collection setup.

▶ If the doctor orders it, start reinfusing the blood when 500 ml has been collected or 4 hours have passed, whichever comes first. Blood reinfusion must be completed within 6 hours of initiating the collection in the operating room.

▶ If less than 200 ml is collected in 4 hours, record the amount on the intake and output sheet and the postoperative sheet. Discard the drainage appropriately because the proportion of anticoagulant (inserted in the operating room) to blood is too great to infuse. If this happens, switch from the container to a closed-wound suction unit. First remove the suction tube from the suction control unit. Clamp the connecting tubing above the filter. Detach the connecting tubing from the patient's tube and cap the patient's tube. Connect a closed-wound suction unit, such as a Hemovac, if you aren't going to collect more blood for reinfusion. If more than 500 ml of blood is collected in the first 4 hours, connect a new autologous transfusion unit to the patient. Then reconnect the unit to suction. Monitor and record the drainage on the intake and output sheet.

For blood reinfusion

▶ Prime the blood filter with 500 ml of normal saline solution.

▶ Twist the suction control module to remove it.

▶ Remove the hanger assembly from the collection bag.

▶ Pull the clear cap from the top of the bag and discard the cap and filter.

▶ Insert a spike adapter into the large port on top of the bottle.

▶ Remove the protective seal to expose the filtered vent.

▶ Attach the blood to the Y-connector of the blood filter.

▶ Invert the bag and hang it.

● Obtain vital signs and document them.

▶ Begin the infusion, following your facility's policy.

▶ Be sure to complete the infusion within 2 hours.

For perioperative blood donation using the Pleur-evac system connected to a chest tube

▶ Establish underwater seal drainage. Following the steps printed on the Pleur-evac unit, connect the patient's chest tube. Inspect the blood collection bag and tubing, making sure that all clamps are open and all connections are airtight.

▶ Before collection, add an anticoagulant, such as heparin or CPD, if prescribed. With CPD, add one part CPD to seven parts blood. Using an 18G (or smaller) needle, inject the anticoagulant through the red self-sealing port on the autologous transfusion connector. The system is now ready to use. You should see chest cavity blood begin to collect in the bag.

▶ To collect more than one bag of blood, open a replacement bag when the first one is nearly full. Close the clamps on top of the second bag. Before removing the first collection bag from the drainage unit, reduce excess negativity by using the high-negativity relief valve. Depress the button; release it when negativity drops to the desired level (watch the water seal manometer).

▶ Close the white clamp on the patient tubing. Then close the two white clamps on top of the collection bag.

▶ Disconnect all connectors on the first bag. Attach the red (female) and blue (male) connector sections on top of the autologous transfusion bag.

▶ Remove the protective cap from the collection tubing on the replacement bag. Connect the collection tubing to the patient's chest drainage tube, using the red connectors.

▶ Remove the protective cap from the replacement bag's suction tube and attach the tube to the Pleur-evac unit, using the blue connectors. Make sure all connections are tight. Open all clamps and inspect the system for airtight connections.

▶ Spread the metal support arms and disconnect them. Remove the first bag from the drainage unit by disconnecting the foot hook.

▶ Use the foot hook and support arm to attach the replacement bag.

▶ To reinfuse blood from the original collection bag, slide the bag off the support frame; then invert it so that the spike points upward. Reinfuse blood within 6 hours of the start of collection. Never store collected blood.

▶ Remove the protective cap from the spike port and insert a microaggregate filter into the port, using a twisting motion. Prime the filter by gently squeezing the inverted bag. A new filter should be used with each bag.

Managing problems of autologous transfusion

Problem	Cause	Intervention
Coagulation	■ Not enough anticoagulant ■ Blood not defibrinated in mediastinum	■ Add CPD or another regional anticoagulant at a ratio of 7 parts blood to 1 part anticoagulant. Keep blood and CPD mixed by shaking collection bottle regularly. ■ Check for anticoagulant reversal.
Coagulopathies	■ Reduced platelet and fibrinogen levels ■ Platelets caught in filters ■ Enhanced levels of fibrin split products	■ Transfuse fresh frozen plasma or platelet concentrate as ordered for patients receiving autologous transfusions of more than 4,000 ml of blood.
Emboli	■ Microaggregate debris ■ Air	■ Don't use equipment with roller pumps or pressure infusion systems. Before reinfusion, remove air from blood bags. ■ Reinfuse with a 20- to 40-unit microaggregate filter.
Hemolysis	■ Trauma to blood caused by turbulence or roller pumps	■ Don't skim operative field or use equipment with roller pumps. When collecting blood from chest tubes, keep vacuum below 30 mm Hg; when aspirating from a surgical site, keep vacuum below 60 mm Hg.
Sepsis	■ Lack of sterile technique ■ Contaminated blood	■ Give broad-spectrum antibiotics. Use strict sterile technique. Reinfuse patient within 4 hours. ■ Don't infuse blood from infected areas or blood that contains feces, urine, or other contaminants.

▶ Continue squeezing until the filter is saturated and the drip chamber is half full. Then close the clamp on the reinfusion line and remove residual air from the bag. Invert the bag and suspend it from an I.V. pole. After carefully flushing the I.V. line to remove all air, infuse blood according to your facility's policy.

Special considerations

Autologous transfusion is contraindicated in patients with malignant neoplasms, coagulopathies, excessive hemolysis, and active infections. It's also contraindicated in patients taking antibiotics and in those whose blood becomes contaminated by bowel contents. In addition, patients who have recently lost weight because of illness or malnutrition shouldn't donate blood.

For preoperative blood donation
▶ Monitor the patient closely during and after donation and autologous transfusion. Although vasovagal reac-

tions are usually mild and easy to treat, they can quickly progress to severe reactions, such as loss of consciousness and seizures. Also, make sure the patient isn't bacteremic when he donates blood. *Bacteria can proliferate in the collection bag and cause sepsis when reinfused.*

▶ Clearly label the collection bag autologous use only. *This way the blood won't be subjected to rigorous blood bank testing or be accidentally given to another patient.*

▶ Caution the patient to remain in a supine position for at least 10 minutes after donating blood.

▶ Encourage him to drink more fluids than usual for a few hours after blood donation and to eat heartily at his next meal.

▶ Tell him to keep an eye on the needle wound in his arm for a few hours after blood donation. If some bleeding occurs, he should apply firm pressure for 5 to 10 minutes. If the bleeding doesn't stop, he should notify the blood bank or his doctor.

▶ If the patient feels light-headed or dizzy, advise him to sit down immediately and to lower his head between his knees. Or he can lie down with his head lower than the rest of his body until the feeling subsides.

▶ Tell him that he can resume normal activities after resting 15 minutes.

For all donation methods

▶ Check the patient's laboratory data (coagulation profile, hemoglobin and calcium levels, and hematocrit) after he donates blood and again after reinfusion. Before reinfusion, identify the patient and make sure that the collection bag is clearly marked with his name, his identification number, and an autologous blood label.

▶ Be alert for signs and symptoms of a hemolytic reaction: pain at the I.V. site, fever, chills, back pain, hypotension, and anxiety. If any occurs, stop the transfusion and call the blood bank and doctor. The patient may have received the wrong unit of blood.

▶ Check the patient's laboratory data again after reinfusion.

Complications

Autologous transfusion may cause hemolysis, air and particulate emboli, coagulation, thrombocytopenia, vasovagal reactions (from transient hypotension and bradycardia), and hypovolemia (especially in elderly patients). (See *Managing problems of autologous transfusion.*)

Documentation

Document the amount of blood the patient donated and had reinfused and how he tolerated each procedure.

TRANSFUSION OF WHOLE BLOOD AND PACKED CELLS

Whole blood transfusion replenishes both the volume and the oxygen-carrying capacity of the circulatory system by increasing the mass of circulating red cells. Transfusion of packed red blood cells (RBCs), from which 80% of the plasma has been removed, restores only the oxygen-carrying capacity. After plasma is removed, the resulting component has a hematocrit of 65% to 80% and a usual volume of 300 to 350 ml. (Whole blood without the plasma removed has a hematocrit of about 38%). Each unit of whole blood or RBCs contains enough hemogloblin to raise the hemoglobin concentration in an average-sized adult 1 g/dL or by 3%. Both types of transfusion treat decreased hemoglobin levels and hematocrit. Whole blood is usually used only when decreased levels result from hemorrhage; packed RBCs are used when such depressed levels accompany normal blood volume to avoid possible fluid and circulatory overload. (See *Transfusing blood and selected components,* pages 872 and 873.) Both whole blood and packed RBCs contain cellular debris, requiring in-line filtration during administration. (Washed packed RBCs, commonly used for patients previously sensitized to transfusions, are rinsed with a special solution that removes white blood cells and platelets, thus decreasing the chance of transfusion reaction.)

If the patient is a Jehovah's Witness, a transfusion requires a court order.

Key nursing diagnoses and patient outcomes

Deficient fluid volume related to active loss
The patient will:
▶ have vital signs remain stable
▶ have fluid and blood volume return to normal.

Ineffective tissue perfusion (specify) related to decreased cellular exchange
The patient will:
▶ attain hemodynamic stability as evidenced by pulse not less than (specify) beats/minute and not more than (specify) beats/minute, blood pressure not less than (specify) mm Hg and not greater than (specify) mm Hg
▶ not exhibit arrhythmias.

Equipment

Blood recipient set (170 to 260 micron filter and tubing with drip chamber for blood, or combined set) • I.V. pole • gloves • gown • face shield • multiple-lead tubing • whole blood or packed RBCs • 250 ml of normal saline solution • venipuncture equipment, if necessary (should include 20G or larger catheter) • optional: ice bag, warm compresses

Straight-line and Y-type blood administration sets are commonly used. The use of these filters can postpone sensitization to transfusion therapy.

Administer packed RBCs with a Y-type set. Using a straight-line set forces you to piggyback the tubing so you can stop the transfusion if necessary but still keep the vein open. Piggybacking increases the chance of harmful microorganisms entering the tubing as you're connecting the blood line to the established line.

Multiple-lead tubing minimizes the risk of contamination, especially when transfusing multiple units of blood (a straight-line set would require multiple piggybacking). A Y-type set gives you the option of adding normal saline solution to packed cells — decreasing their viscosity — if the patient can tolerate the added fluid volume.

Preparation of equipment

Avoid obtaining either whole blood or packed RBCs until you're ready to begin the transfusion. Prepare the equipment when you're ready to start the infusion.

Implementation

▶ Explain the procedure to the patient. Make sure he has signed an informed consent form before transfusion therapy is initiated.
▶ Record the patient's baseline vital signs.

▶ If the patient doesn't have an I.V. line in place, perform a venipuncture, using a 20G or larger-diameter catheter. Avoid using an existing line if the needle or catheter lumen is smaller than 20G. Central venous access devices also may be used for transfusion therapy.

▶ Obtain whole blood or packed RBCs from the blood bank within 30 minutes of the transfusion start time. Check the expiration date on the blood bag and observe for abnormal color, RBC clumping, gas bubbles, and extraneous material. Return outdated or abnormal blood to the blood bank.

▶ Compare the name and number on the patient's wristband with those on the blood bag label. Check the blood bag identification number, ABO blood group, and Rh compatibility. Also, compare the patient's blood bank identification number, if present, with the number on the blood bag. Identification of blood and blood products is performed at the patient's bedside by two licensed professionals, according to the facility's policy.

▶ Put on gloves, a gown, and a face shield. Using a Y-type set, close all the clamps on the set. Then insert the spike of the line you're using for the normal saline solution into the bag of saline solution. Next, open the port on the blood bag and insert the spike of the line you're using to administer the blood or cellular component into the port. Hang the bag of normal saline solution and blood or cellular component on the I.V. pole, open the clamp on the line of saline solution, and squeeze the drip chamber until it's half full. Then remove the adapter cover at the tip of the blood administration set, open the main flow clamp, and prime the tubing with saline solution.

▶ If you're administering packed RBCs with a Y-type set, you can add saline solution to the bag to dilute the cells by closing the clamp between the patient and the drip chamber and opening the clamp from the blood. Then lower the blood bag below the saline container and let 30 to 50 ml of saline solution flow into the packed cells. Finally, close the clamp to the blood bag, rehang the bag, rotate it gently *to mix the cells and saline solution,* and close the clamp to the saline container.

▶ If you're administering whole blood, gently invert the bag several times *to mix the cells.*

▶ Attach the prepared blood administration set to the venipuncture device and flush it with normal saline solution. Then close the clamp to the saline solution and open the clamp between the blood bag and the patient. Adjust the flow rate to no greater than 5 ml/minute for the first 15 minutes of the transfusion to observe for a possible transfusion reaction.

▶ Remain with the patient and watch for signs of a transfusion reaction. If such signs develop, record vital signs and stop the transfusion. Infuse saline solution at a moderately slow infusion rate and notify the doctor at once. If no signs of a reaction appear within 15 minutes, you'll need to adjust the flow clamp to the ordered infusion rate. The rate of infusion should be as rapid as the patient's circulatory system can tolerate. It's undesirable for RBC preparations to remain at room temperature for more than 4 hours. If the infusion rate must be so slow that the entire unit can't be infused within 4 hours, it may be appropriate to divide the unit and keep one portion refrigerated until it can be safely administered.

(*Text continues on page 874.*)

Transfusing blood and selected components

Blood component	Indications	Crossmatching
Whole blood Complete (pure) blood *Volume: 450 or 500 ml*	■ To restore blood volume lost from hemorrhaging, trauma, or burns	■ ABO identical: Type A receives A; type B receives B; type AB receives AB; type O receives O ■ Rh match necessary
Packed red blood cells (RBCs) Same RBC mass as whole blood but with 80% of the plasma removed *Volume: 250 ml*	■ To restore or maintain oxygen-carrying capacity ■ To correct anemia and blood loss that occurs during surgery ■ To increase RBC mass	■ Type A receives A or O ■ Type B receives B or O ■ Type AB receives AB, A, B, or O ■ Type O receives O ■ Rh match necessary
Platelets Platelet sediment from RBCs or plasma *Volume: 35 to 50 ml/unit; 1 unit of platelets = 7×10^7 platelets*	■ To treat thrombocytopenia caused by decreased platelet production, increased platelet destruction, or massive transfusion of stored blood ■ To treat acute leukemia and marrow aplasia ■ To improve platelet count preoperatively in a patient whose count is 100,000/µl or less	■ ABO compatibility unnecessary but preferable with repeated platelet transfusions ■ Rh match preferred
Fresh frozen plasma (FFP) Uncoagulated plasma separated from RBCs and rich in coagulation factors V, VIII, and IX *Volume: 180 to 300 ml*	■ To expand plasma volume ■ To treat postoperative hemorrhage or shock ■ To correct an undetermined coagulation factor deficiency ■ To replace a specific factor when that factor alone isn't available ■ To correct factor deficiencies resulting from hepatic disease	■ ABO compatibility unnecessary but preferable with repeated platelet transfusions ■ Rh match preferred
Albumin 5% (buffered saline); albumin 25% (salt poor) A small plasma protein prepared by fractionating pooled plasma *Volume: 5% = 12.5 g/ 250 ml; 25% = 12.5 g/50 ml*	■ To replace volume lost because of shock from burns, trauma, surgery, or infections ■ To replace volume and prevent marked hemoconcentration ■ To treat hypoproteinemia (with or without edema)	■ Unnecessary
Factor VIII (cryoprecipitate) Insoluble portion of plasma recovered from FFP *Volume: approximately 30 ml (freeze-dried)*	■ To treat a patient with hemophilia A ■ To control bleeding associated with factor VIII deficiency ■ To replace fibrinogen or deficient factor VIII	■ ABO compatibility unnecessary but preferable

Nursing considerations

- Use a straight-line or Y-type I.V. set to infuse blood over 2 to 4 hours.
- Avoid giving whole blood when the patient can't tolerate the circulatory volume.
- Reduce the risk of a transfusion reaction by adding a microfilter to the administration set to remove platelets.
- Warm blood if giving a large quantity.

- Use a straight-line or Y-type I.V. set to infuse blood over 2 to 4 hours.
- Bear in mind that packed RBCs provide the same oxygen-carrying capacity as whole blood with less risk of volume overload.
- Give packed RBCs, as ordered, to prevent potassium and ammonia buildup, which may occur in stored plasma.
- Avoid administering packed RBCs for anemic conditions correctable by nutritional or drug therapy.

- Use a component drip administration set to infuse 100 ml over 15 minutes.
- As prescribed, premedicate with antipyretics and antihistamines if the patient's history includes a platelet transfusion reaction.
- Avoid administering platelets when the patient has a fever.
- Prepare to draw blood for a platelet count, as ordered, 1 hour after the platelet transfusion to determine platelet transfusion increments.
- Keep in mind that the doctor seldom orders a platelet transfusion for conditions in which platelet destruction is accelerated, such as idiopathic thrombocytopenic purpura and drug-induced thrombocytopenia.

- Use a straight-line I.V. set and administer the infusion rapidly.
- Keep in mind that large-volume transfusions of FFP may require correction for hypocalcemia because citric acid in FFP binds calcium.

- Use a straight-line I.V. set with rate and volume dictated by the patient's condition and response.
- Remember that reactions to albumin (fever, chills, nausea) are rare.
- Avoid mixing albumin with protein hydrolysates and alcohol solutions.
- Consider delivering albumin as a volume expander until the laboratory completes crossmatching for a whole blood transfusion.
- Keep in mind that albumin is contraindicated in severe anemia and administered cautiously in cardiac and pulmonary disease because heart failure may result from circulatory overload.

- Use the administration set supplied by the manufacturer. Administer factor VIII with a filter. Standard dose recommended for treatment of acute bleeding episodes in hemophilia is 15 to 20 units/kg.
- Half-life of factor VIII (8 to 10 hours) necessitates repeated transfusions at specified intervals to maintain normal levels.

Better charting

Documenting blood transfusions

Whether you administer blood or blood components, you must use proper identification and crossmatching procedures.

After matching the patient's name, medical record number, blood group (or type) and Rh factor (the patient's and the donor's), the cross-match data, and the blood bank identification number with the label on the blood bag, you'll need to clearly document that you did so. The blood or blood component must be identified and documented properly by two health care professionals as well.

On the transfusion record, document:
■ date and time the transfusion was started and completed
■ name of the health care professional who verified the information
■ type and gauge of the catheter
■ total amount of the transfusion
■ patient's vital signs before, during, and after the transfusion
■ any infusion device used
■ flow rate any blood warming unit used.

If the patient receives his own blood, document in the intake and output records:
■ amount of autologous blood retrieved
■ reinfused in the intake and output records
■ laboratory data during and after the autotransfusion
■ patient's pre- and post-transfusion vital signs.

Pay particular attention to:
■ patient's coagulation profile
■ hemoglobin level
■ hematocrit values
■ arterial blood gas levels
■ calcium levels.

▶ After completing the transfusion, you'll need to put on gloves and remove and discard the used infusion equipment. Then remember to reconnect the original I.V. fluid, if necessary, or discontinue the I.V. infusion.
▶ Return the empty blood bag to the blood bank, if facility policy dictates, and discard the tubing and filter.
▶ Record the patient's vital signs.

Special considerations

▶ Although some microaggregate filters can be used for up to 10 units of blood, always replace the filter and tubing if more than 1 hour elapses between transfusions. When administering multiple units of blood under pressure, use a blood warmer *to avoid hypothermia.* Blood components may be warmed to no more than 107.6° F (42° C).
▶ For rapid blood replacement, you may need to use a pressure bag. Be aware that excessive pressure may develop, leading to broken blood vessels and extravasation, with hematoma and hemolysis of the infusing RBCs.
▶ If the transfusion stops, take these steps as needed:
– Check that the I.V. container is at least 3′ (1 m) above the level of the I.V. site.
– Make sure the flow clamp is open and that the blood completely covers the filter. If it doesn't, squeeze the drip chamber until it does.
– Gently rock the bag back and forth, agitating blood cells that may have settled.
– Untape the dressing over the I.V. site to check cannula placement. Reposition the cannula if necessary.
– Flush the line with saline solution and restart the transfusion. Using a Y-type set, close the flow clamp to the patient and lower the blood bag. Next,

open the saline clamp and allow some saline solution to flow into the blood bag. Rehang the blood bag, open the flow clamp to the patient, and reset the flow rate.

– If a hematoma develops at the I.V. site, immediately stop the infusion. Remove the I.V. cannula. Notify the doctor and expect to place ice on the site intermittently for 8 hours; then apply warm compresses. Follow your facility's policy.

– If the blood bag empties before the next one arrives, administer normal saline solution slowly. If you're using a Y-type set, close the blood-line clamp, open the saline clamp, and let the saline run slowly until the new blood arrives. Decrease the flow rate or clamp the line before attaching the new unit of blood.

Complications

Despite improvements in crossmatching precautions, transfusion reactions can still occur. Unlike a transfusion reaction, an infectious disease transmitted during a transfusion may go undetected until days, weeks, or even months later, when it produces signs and symptoms. Measures to prevent disease transmission include laboratory testing of blood products and careful screening of potential donors, neither of which is guaranteed.

Hepatitis C accounts for most posttransfusion hepatitis cases. The tests that detect hepatitis B and hepatitis C can produce false-negative results and may allow some hepatitis cases to go undetected.

When testing for antibodies to human immunodeficiency virus (HIV), keep in mind that antibodies don't appear until 6 to 12 weeks after exposure.

The estimated risk of acquiring HIV from blood products varies from 1 in 40,000 to 1 in 153,000.

Many blood banks screen blood for cytomegalovirus (CMV). Blood with CMV is especially dangerous for an immunosuppressed, seronegative patient. Blood banks also test blood for syphilis, but refrigerating blood virtually eliminates the risk of transfusion-related syphilis.

Circulatory overload and hemolytic, allergic, febrile, and pyogenic reactions can result from any transfusion. Coagulation disturbances, citrate intoxication, hyperkalemia, acid-base imbalance, loss of 2,3-diphosphoglycerate, ammonia intoxication, and hypothermia can result from massive transfusion.

Documentation

Record the date and time of the transfusion, the type and amount of transfusion product, the patient's vital signs, your check of all identification data, and the patient's response. Document any transfusion reaction and treatment. (See *Documenting blood transfusions*.)

TRANSFUSION REACTION MANAGEMENT

A transfusion reaction typically stems from a major antigen-antibody reaction and can result from a single or massive transfusion of blood or blood products. Although many reactions occur during transfusion or within 96 hours afterward, infectious diseases transmitted during a transfusion may go undetected until days, weeks, or months later, when signs and symptoms appear.

Guide to transfusion reactions

Any patient receiving a transfusion of processed blood products can experience a transfusion reaction. Transfusion reactions typically occur from antigen-antibody reactions; however, they may also occur as a result of bacterial contamination.

Reaction and causes	Signs and symptoms	Nursing interventions
Allergic ■ Allergen in donor blood ■ Donor blood hypersensitive to certain drugs	■ Anaphylaxis (chills, facial swelling, laryngeal edema, pruritus, urticaria, wheezing), fever, nausea, and vomiting	■ Administer antihistamines as prescribed. ■ Monitor patient for anaphylactic reaction and administer epinephrine and corticosteroids if indicated.
Bacterial contamination ■ Organisms that can survive cold, such as *Pseudomonas* and *Staphylococcus*	■ Chills, fever, vomiting, abdominal cramping, diarrhea, shock, signs of renal failure	■ Provide broad-spectrum antibiotics, corticosteroids, or epinephrine as prescribed. ■ Maintain strict blood storage control. ■ Change blood administration set and filter every 4 hours or after every 2 units. ■ Infuse each unit of blood over 2 to 4 hours; stop the infusion if the time span exceeds 4 hours. ■ Maintain sterile technique when administering blood products.
Febrile ■ Bacterial lipopolysaccharides ■ Antileukocyte recipient antibodies directed against donor white blood cells	■ Temperature up to 104° F (40° C), chills, headache, facial flushing, palpitations, cough, chest tightness, increased pulse rate, flank pain	■ Relieve symptoms with an antipyretic, an antihistamine, or meperidine, as prescribed. ■ If the patient requires further transfusions, use frozen RBCs, add a special leukocyte removal filter to the blood line, or premedicate him with acetaminophen, as prescribed, before starting another transfusion.
Hemolytic ■ ABO or Rh incompatibility ■ Intradonor incompatibility ■ Improper cross-matching ■ Improperly stored blood	■ Chest pain, dyspnea, facial flushing, fever, chills, shaking, hypotension, flank pain, hemoglobinuria, oliguria, bloody oozing at the infusion site or surgical incision site, burning sensation along vein receiving blood, shock, renal failure	■ Monitor blood pressure. ■ Manage shock with I.V. fluids, oxygen, epinephrine, a diuretic, and a vasopressor, as prescribed. ■ Obtain posttransfusion-reaction blood samples and urine specimens for analysis. ■ Observe for signs of hemorrhage resulting from disseminated intravascular coagulation.
Plasma protein incompatibility ■ Immunoglobulin-A incompatibility	■ Abdominal pain, diarrhea, dyspnea, chills, fever, flushing, hypotension	■ Administer oxygen, fluids, epinephrine, or a corticosteroid as prescribed.

A transfusion reaction requires immediate recognition and prompt nursing action to prevent further complications and, possibly, death — particularly if the patient is unconscious or so heavily sedated that he can't report the common symptoms. (See *Guide to transfusion reactions.*)

Key nursing diagnoses and patient outcomes

Deficient fluid volume related to active loss
The patient will:
▶ have vital signs remain stable
▶ have fluid and blood volume return to normal.

Equipment

Normal saline solution • I.V. administration set • sterile urine specimen container • needle, syringe, and tubes for blood samples • transfusion reaction report form • optional: oxygen, epinephrine, hypothermia blanket, leukocyte removal filter

Implementation

▶ As soon as you suspect an adverse reaction, stop the transfusion and start the saline infusion (using a new I.V. administration set) at a keep-vein-open rate *to maintain venous access.* Don't discard the blood bag or administration set.
▶ Notify the doctor.
▶ Monitor vital signs every 15 minutes or as indicated by the severity and type of reaction.
▶ Compare the labels on all blood containers with corresponding patient identification forms *to verify that the transfusion was the correct blood or blood product.*
▶ Notify the blood bank of a possible transfusion reaction and collect blood

samples, as ordered. Immediately send the samples, all transfusion containers (even if empty), and the administration set to the blood bank. *The blood bank will test these materials to further evaluate the reaction.*
▶ Collect the first posttransfusion urine specimen, mark the collection slip "Possible transfusion reaction," and send it to the laboratory immediately. *The laboratory tests this urine specimen for the presence of hemoglobin (Hb), which indicates a hemolytic reaction.*
▶ Closely monitor intake and output. Note evidence of oliguria or anuria *because Hb deposition in the renal tubules can cause renal damage.*
▶ If prescribed, administer oxygen, epinephrine, or other drugs and apply a hypothermia blanket *to reduce fever.*
▶ Make the patient as comfortable as possible and provide reassurance as necessary.

Special considerations

▶ Treat all transfusion reactions as serious until proven otherwise. If the doctor anticipates a transfusion reaction, such as one that may occur in a leukemia patient, he may order prophylactic treatment with antihistamines or antipyretics to precede blood administration.
▶ *To avoid a possible febrile reaction,* the doctor may order the blood washed to remove as many leukocytes as possible, or a leukocyte removal filter may be used during the transfusion.

Documentation

Record the time and date of the transfusion reaction, type and amount of infused blood or blood products, clinical signs of the transfusion reaction in order of occurrence, patient's vital signs, specimens sent to the laboratory for analysis, treatment given, and patient's response to treatment. If required by your facility's policy, complete the transfusion reaction form.

TRAUMATIC WOUND MANAGEMENT

Traumatic wounds include abrasions, lacerations, puncture wounds, and amputations. In an abrasion, the skin is scraped, with partial loss of the skin surface. In a laceration, the skin is torn, causing jagged, irregular edges; the severity of a laceration depends on its size, depth, and location. A puncture wound occurs when a pointed object, such as a knife or glass fragment, penetrates the skin. Traumatic amputation refers to removal of part of the body, a limb, or part of a limb.

Initial management concentrates on controlling bleeding, usually by applying firm, direct pressure and elevating the extremity. If bleeding continues, you may need to compress a pressure point. Assess the condition of the wound. Management and cleaning technique usually depend on the specific type of wound and degree of contamination.

Key nursing diagnoses and patient outcomes

Deficient fluid volume related to active blood loss
The patient will:
▶ have vital signs remain stable
▶ have fluid and blood volume return to normal.

Ineffective tissue perfusion (specify) related to decreased cellular exchange
The patient will:

▶ attain hemodynamic stability as evidenced by pulse not less than (specify) beats/minute and not more than (specify) beats/minute, blood pressure not less than (specify) mm Hg and not greater than (specify) mm Hg
▶ not exhibit arrhythmias.

Equipment

Sterile basin • normal saline solution • sterile 4″ × 4″ gauze pads • sterile gloves • clean gloves • dry sterile dressing, nonadherent pad, or petroleum gauze • linen-saver pad • optional: scissors, towel, goggles, mask, gown, 50-ml catheter-tip syringe, surgical scrub brush, antibacterial ointment, porous tape, sterile forceps, sutures and suture set, hydrogen peroxide

Preparation of equipment

Place a linen-saver pad under the area to be cleaned. Remove any clothing covering the wound. If necessary, cut hair around the wound with scissors to promote cleaning and treatment.

Assemble needed equipment at the patient's bedside. Fill a sterile basin with normal saline solution. Make sure the treatment area has enough light to allow close observation of the wound. Depending on the nature and location of the wound, wear sterile or clean gloves *to avoid spreading infection.*

Implementation

▶ Check the patient's medical history for previous tetanus immunization and, if needed and ordered, arrange for immunization.
▶ Administer pain medication, if ordered.
▶ Wash your hands.
▶ Use appropriate protective equipment, such as a gown, mask, and gog-

gles, if spraying or splashing of body fluids is possible.

For an abrasion

▶ Flush the scraped skin with normal saline solution.

▶ Remove dirt or gravel with a sterile 4″ × 4″ gauze pad moistened with normal saline solution. Rub in the opposite direction from which the dirt or gravel became embedded.

▶ If the wound is extremely dirty, you may use a surgical brush to scrub it.

▶ With a small wound, allow it to dry and form a scab. With a larger wound, you may need to cover it with a nonadherent pad or petroleum gauze and a light dressing. Apply antibacterial ointment if ordered.

For a laceration

▶ Moisten a sterile 4″ × 4″ gauze pad with normal saline solution. Clean the wound gently, working outward from its center to about 2″ (5 cm) beyond its edges. Discard the soiled gauze pad and use a fresh one as necessary. Continue until the wound appears clean.

▶ If the wound is dirty, you may irrigate it with a 50-ml catheter-tip syringe and normal saline solution.

▶ Assist the doctor in suturing the wound edges using the suture kit, or apply sterile strips of porous tape.

▶ Apply the prescribed antibacterial ointment *to help prevent infection.*

▶ Apply a dry sterile dressing over the wound *to absorb drainage and help prevent bacterial contamination.*

For a puncture wound

▶ If the wound is minor, allow it to bleed for a few minutes before cleaning it.

▶ For a larger puncture wound, you may need to irrigate it before applying a dry dressing.

▶ Stabilize any embedded foreign object until the doctor can remove it. After he removes the object and bleeding is stabilized, clean the wound as you'd clean a laceration or deep puncture wound.

For an amputation

▶ Apply a gauze pad moistened with normal saline solution to the amputation site. Elevate the affected part and immobilize it for surgery.

▶ Recover the amputated part and prepare it for transport to a facility where microvascular surgery is performed.

Special considerations

▶ When irrigating a traumatic wound, avoid using more than 8 psi of pressure. *High-pressure irrigation can seriously interfere with healing, kill cells, and allow bacteria to infiltrate the tissue.*

▶ To clean the wound, you may use hydrogen peroxide; *its foaming action facilitates debris removal.* However, peroxide should never be instilled into a deep wound *because of the risk of embolism from the evolving gases.* Be sure to rinse your hands well after using hydrogen peroxide.

▶ After a wound has been cleaned, the doctor may want to debride it *to remove dead tissue and reduce the risk of infection and scarring.* If this is necessary, pack the wound with gauze pads soaked in normal saline solution until debridement.

▶ Observe for signs and symptoms of infection, such as warm red skin at the site or purulent discharge. Be aware that infection of a traumatic wound can delay healing, increase scar formation, and trigger systemic infection such as septicemia.

▶ Observe all dressings. If edema is present, adjust the dressing *to avoid impairing circulation to the area.*

Complications

Cleaning and care of traumatic wounds may temporarily increase the patient's pain. Excessive, vigorous cleaning may further disrupt tissue integrity.

Documentation

Document the date and time of the procedure, wound size and condition, medication administration, specific wound care measures, and patient teaching.

TRIANGULAR SLING APPLICATION

Made from a triangular piece of muslin, canvas, or cotton, a sling supports and immobilizes an injured arm, wrist, or hand, and thereby facilitates healing. It may be applied to restrict movement of a fracture or dislocation or to support a muscle sprain. A sling can also support the weight of a splint or help secure dressings.

Key nursing diagnoses and patient outcomes

Impaired physical mobility related to musculoskeletal injury
The patient will:
▶ maintain muscle strength and joint range of motion
▶ show no evidence of such complications as contractures, venous stasis, thrombus formation, and skin breakdown.

Dressing or grooming self-care deficit related to need for triangular sling
The patient will:
▶ have self-care needs met daily
▶ have minimal or no complications
▶ identify resources to help cope with problems after discharge.

Equipment

Triangular bandage or commercial sling • gauze (for padding) • safety pins (tape for children under age 7)

Implementation

▶ Explain the procedure to the patient and wash your hands.

 Age alert If the patient is a child, fold the bandage in half *to make a smaller triangle.* Then follow the steps shown in *Making a sling.*

▶ If you anticipate prolonged use of a sling, pad the area under the knot with gauze *to prevent skin irritation.* Place the sling outside the shirt collar *to reduce direct pressure on the neck and shoulder.*

▶ If the arm requires complete immobilization, apply a swathe after placing the arm in a sling. (See *Applying a swathe,* page 882.) At regular intervals, check to be sure that the sling is in proper position. Also assess patient comfort and circulation to the fingers.

Special considerations

▶ Before the patient leaves the hospital, provide an extra triangular bandage. Teach him and a family member or friend how to change the sling. If appropriate, instruct him to change the sling regularly *because a soiled sling can cause irritation and infection.* Also teach him how to check periodically for axillary and cervical skin breakdown.

Making a sling

Place the apex of a triangular bandage behind the patient's elbow on the injured side. Hold one end of the bandage so it extends up toward the patient's neck on the uninjured side and let the other end hang straight down. The bandage's long side should parallel the midline of the patient's body.

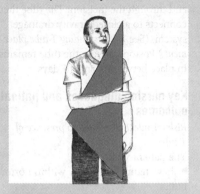

Loop the top corner of the bandage over the shoulder on the uninjured side and around the back of the patient's neck. Then bring the lower end of the bandage over the flexed forearm and up to the shoulder on the injured side.

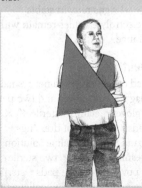

Adjust the bandage so that the forearm and upper arm form an angle of slightly less than 90 degrees *to increase venous return from the hand and forearm* and *to facilitate drainage from swelling.* Then tie the two bandage ends at the side of the patient's neck, rather than at the back, *to prevent neck flexion and avoid irritation and pressure over a cervical vertebra.*

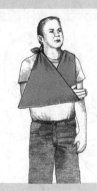

Carefully secure the sling with a safety pin above and behind the elbow. For a child under age 7, use tape instead of a pin *to avoid the chance of an injury.*

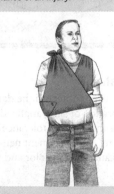

Applying a swathe

To further immobilize an arm after applying a sling, wrap a folded triangular bandage or wide elastic bandage around the patient's upper torso and the upper arm on the injured side. Don't cover the patient's uninjured arm. Make the swathe just tight enough to secure the injured arm to the body. Pin the ends of the bandage just in front of the axilla on the uninjured side.

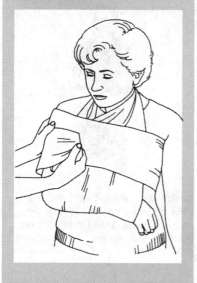

Documentation
In the patient's chart, record the date, time, and location of sling application and describe the patient's tolerance of the procedure. Also document neurovascular status, noting color and temperature.

T-TUBE CARE

The T tube (or biliary drainage tube) may be placed in the common bile duct after cholecystectomy or choledochostomy. This tube facilitates biliary drainage during healing. The surgeon inserts the short end (crossbar) of the T tube in the common bile duct and draws the long end through the incision. The tube then connects to a closed gravity drainage system. (See *Understanding T-tube placement.*) Postoperatively, the tube remains in place between 7 and 14 days.

Key nursing diagnoses and patient outcomes
Risk for infection related to presence of T tube
The patient will:
▶ have temperature stay within normal limits
▶ have white blood cell count and differential stay within normal range.

Risk for deficient fluid volume related to excessive loss through indwelling tube
The patient will:
▶ have vital signs remain stable
▶ have electrolyte values remain within normal range.

Equipment
Graduated collection container • small plastic bag • sterile gloves and two pair of clean gloves • clamp • sterile 4″ × 4″ gauze pads • transparent dressings • rubber band • normal saline solution • sterile cleaning solution • two sterile basins • povidone-iodine pads • sterile precut drain dressings • hypoallergenic paper tape • skin protectant, such as petroleum jelly, zinc oxide, or aluminum-based gel • optional: Montgomery straps

Understanding T-tube placement

The T tube is placed in the common bile duct, anchored to the abdominal wall, and connected to a closed drainage system.

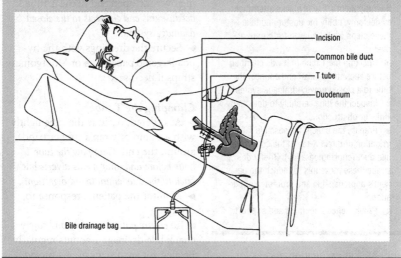

Incision

Common bile duct

T tube

Duodenum

Bile drainage bag

Preparation of equipment

Assemble equipment at the bedside. Open all sterile equipment. Place one sterile 4″ × 4″ gauze pad in each sterile basin. Using sterile technique, pour 50 ml of cleaning solution into one basin and 50 ml of normal saline solution into the other basin. Tape a small plastic bag on the table to use for refuse.

Implementation

▶ Provide privacy and explain the procedure to the patient. Wash your hands thoroughly.

Emptying drainage

▶ Put on clean gloves.
▶ Place the graduated collection container under the outlet valve of the drainage bag. Without contaminating the clamp, valve, or outlet valve, empty

the bag's contents completely into the container and reseal the outlet valve. Carefully measure and record the character, color, and amount of drainage. Discard your gloves.

Re-dressing the T tube

▶ Wash your hands thoroughly *to prevent bacterial contamination of the incision*. Put on clean gloves.
▶ Without dislodging the T tube, remove old dressings and dispose of them in the small plastic bag. Remove the gloves.
▶ Wash your hands again and put on sterile gloves. From this point on, follow strict sterile technique *to prevent bacterial contamination of the incision*.
▶ Inspect the incision and tube site for signs of infection, including redness, edema, warmth, tenderness, indura-

Troubleshooting

Managing T-tube obstruction

If your patient's T tube blocks after chole-cystectomy, notify the doctor and take these steps while you wait for him to arrive:

■ Unclamp the T tube (if it was clamped before and after a meal) and connect the tube to a closed gravity-drainage system.

■ Inspect the tube carefully to detect any kinks or obstructions.

■ Prepare the patient for possible T-tube irrigation or direct X-ray of the common bile duct (cholangiography). Briefly describe these measures to reduce the patient's apprehension and promote cooperation.

■ Provide encouragement and support.

tion, or skin excoriation. Assess for wound dehiscence or evisceration.

▶ Use sterile cleaning solution as prescribed to clean and remove dried matter or drainage from around the tube. Always start at the tube site and gently wipe outward in a continuous motion *to prevent recontamination of the incision.*

▶ Use normal saline solution to rinse off the prescribed cleaning solution. Dry the area with a sterile 4″ × 4″ gauze pad and discard all used materials.

▶ Using a povidone-iodine pad, wipe the incision site in a circular motion. Allow the area to dry thoroughly.

▶ Lightly apply a skin protectant, such as petroleum jelly, zinc oxide, or aluminum-based gel, *to protect the skin from injury caused by draining bile.*

▶ Apply a sterile precut drain dressing on each side of the T tube *to absorb drainage.*

▶ Apply a sterile 4″ × 4″ gauze pad or transparent dressing over the T tube and the drain dressings. Be careful not to kink the tubing, *which might block the drainage.* Also avoid putting the dressing over the open end of the T tube *because this end connects to the closed drainage system.*

▶ Secure the dressings with the hypoallergenic paper tape or Montgomery straps if necessary.

Clamping the T tube

▶ As ordered, occlude the tube lightly with a clamp or wrap a rubber band around the end. *Clamping the tube 1 hour before and after meals diverts bile back to the duodenum to aid digestion.*

▶ Monitor the patient's response to clamping.

▶ *To ensure patient comfort and safety,* check bile drainage amounts regularly. Be alert for such signs of obstructed bile flow as chills, fever, tachycardia, nausea, right-upper-quadrant fullness and pain, jaundice, dark foamy urine, and clay-colored stools. Report them immediately. (See *Managing T-tube obstruction.*)

Special considerations

▶ The T tube usually drains 300 to 500 ml of blood-tinged bile in the first 24 hours after surgery. Report drainage that exceeds 500 ml in the first 24 hours after surgery; if it's 50 ml or less, notify the doctor because the tube may be obstructed. Drainage typically declines to 200 ml or less after 4 days and the color changes to green-brown. Monitor fluid, electrolyte, and acid-base status carefully.

▶ To prevent excessive bile loss (over 500 ml in first 24 hours) or backflow contamination, secure the T-tube drainage system at abdominal level. Bile will flow into the bag only when biliary pressure increases.

▶ Provide meticulous skin care and frequent dressing changes. Observe for bile leakage, which may indicate obstruction. Assess tube patency and site condition hourly for the first 8 hours and then every 4 hours until the doctor removes the tube. Protect the skin edges and avoid excessive taping to prevent shearing the skin.

▶ Monitor all urine and stools for color changes. Assess for icteric skin and sclera, which may signal jaundice.

Home care

Loose bowels occur commonly in the first few weeks after surgery. Teach the patient about signs and symptoms of T-tube and biliary obstruction, which he should report to the doctor. Teach him how to care for the tube at home. In addition, caution him that bile stains clothing.

Complications

Obstructed bile flow, skin excoriation or breakdown, tube dislodgment, drainage reflux, and infection are the most common complications related to a biliary T tube.

Documentation

Record the date and time of each dressing change. Note the appearance of the wound and surrounding skin. Write down the color, character, and volume of bile collected. Also record the color of skin and mucous membranes around the T tube. Keep a precise record of temperature trends and the amount and frequency of urination and bowel movements.

TUBE FEEDINGS

Tube feeding involves delivery of a liquid feeding formula directly to the stomach (known as gastric gavage), duodenum, or jejunum. Gastric gavage typically is indicated for a patient who can't eat normally because of dysphagia or oral or esophageal obstruction or injury. Gastric feedings also may be given to an unconscious or intubated patient or to a patient recovering from GI tract surgery who can't ingest food orally.

Duodenal or jejunal feedings decrease the risk of aspiration because the formula bypasses the pylorus. Jejunal feedings result in reduced pancreatic stimulation; thus, the patient may require an elemental diet.

Patients usually receive gastric feedings on an intermittent schedule. For duodenal or jejunal feedings, however, most patients seem to better tolerate a continuous slow drip.

Liquid nutrient solutions come in various formulas for administration through a nasogastric tube, small-bore feeding tube, gastrostomy or jejunostomy tube, percutaneous endoscopic gastrostomy or jejunostomy tube, or gastrostomy feeding button. (For more information, see "Transabdominal tube feeding and care," page 838.) Tube feeding is contraindicated in patients who have no bowel sounds or a suspected intestinal obstruction.

Key nursing diagnoses and patient outcomes

Imbalanced nutrition: Less than body requirements
The patient will:
▶ show no further evidence of weight loss

▶ tolerate (specify) ml of tube feedings
▶ gain (specify) lb weekly.

Equipment

For gastric feedings

Feeding formula • graduated container • 120 ml of water • gavage bag with tubing and flow regulator clamp • towel or linen-saver pad • 60-ml syringe • stethoscope • optional: infusion controller and tubing set (for continuous administration), adapter to connect gavage tubing to feeding tube

For duodenal or jejunal feedings

Feeding formula • enteral administration set containing a gavage container, drip chamber, roller clamp or flow regulator, and tube connector • I.V. pole • 60-ml syringe with adapter tip • water • optional: pump administration set (for an enteral infusion pump), Y-connector

For nasal and oral care

Cotton-tipped applicators • water-soluble lubricant • sponge-tipped swabs • petroleum jelly

A bulb syringe or large catheter-tip syringe may be substituted for a gavage bag after the patient demonstrates tolerance for a gravity drip infusion. The doctor may order an infusion pump to ensure accurate delivery of the prescribed formula.

Preparation of equipment

Be sure to refrigerate formulas prepared in the dietary department or pharmacy. Refrigerate commercial formulas only after opening them. Check the date on all formula containers. Discard expired commercial formula. Use powdered formula within 24 hours of mixing. Always shake the container well to mix the solution thoroughly.

Allow the formula to warm to room temperature before administration. *Cold formula can increase the chance of diarrhea.* Never warm it over direct heat or in a microwave *because heat may curdle the formula or change its chemical composition. Also, hot formula may injure the patient.*

Pour 60 ml of water into the graduated container. After closing the flow clamp on the administration set, pour the appropriate amount of formula into the gavage bag. Hang no more than a 4- to 6-hour supply at one time *to prevent bacterial growth.*

Open the flow clamp on the administration set to remove air from the lines. *This keeps air from entering the patient's stomach and causing distention and discomfort.*

Implementation

▶ Provide privacy and wash your hands.
▶ Inform the patient that he'll receive nourishment through the tube and explain the procedure to him. If possible, give him a schedule of subsequent feedings.
▶ If the patient has a nasal or oral tube, cover his chest with a towel or linen-saver pad *to protect him and the bed linens from spills.*
▶ Assess the patient's abdomen for bowel sounds and distention.

Delivering a gastric feeding

▶ Elevate the bed to semi-Fowler's or high Fowler's position *to prevent aspiration by gastroesophageal reflux and to promote digestion.*
▶ Check placement of the feeding tube *to be sure it hasn't slipped out since the last feeding.*

‖‖
≡■≡ ***Nursing alert*** Never give a
‖‖ tube feeding until you're
sure the tube is properly
positioned in the patient's stomach.
*Administering a feeding through a
misplaced tube can cause formula to
enter the patient's lungs.*

▶ *To check tube patency and position,* remove the cap or plug from the feeding
tube and use the syringe to inject 5 to
10 cc of air through the tube. At the
same time, auscultate the patient's
stomach with the stethoscope. Listen
for a whooshing sound to confirm tube
positioning in the stomach. Also aspirate stomach contents to confirm tube
patency and placement.

▶ *To assess gastric emptying,* aspirate
and measure residual gastric contents.
Hold feedings if residual volume is
greater then the predetermined amount
specified in the doctor's order (usually
50 to 100 ml). Reinstill any aspirate obtained.

▶ Connect the gavage bag tubing to
the feeding tube. Depending on the
type of tube used, you may need to use
an adapter to connect the two.

▶ If you're using a bulb or catheter-tip
syringe, remove the bulb or plunger
and attach the syringe to the pinched-
off feeding tube *to prevent excess air
from entering the patient's stomach, causing distention.* If you're using an infusion
controller, thread the tube from the formula container through the controller
according to the manufacturer's directions. Blue food dye can be added to
the feeding *to quickly identify aspiration.*
Purge the tubing of air and attach it to
the feeding tube.

▶ Open the regulator clamp on the
gavage bag tubing and adjust the flow
rate appropriately. When using a bulb
syringe, fill the syringe with formula

and release the feeding tube *to allow
formula to flow through it.* The height at
which you hold the syringe will determine the flow rate. When the syringe is
three-quarters empty, pour more formula into it.

▶ *To prevent air from entering the tube
and the patient's stomach,* never allow the
syringe to empty completely. If you're
using an infusion controller, set the
flow rate according to the manufacturer's directions. Always administer a
tube feeding slowly — typically 200 to
350 ml over 15 to 30 minutes, depending on the patient's tolerance and the
doctor's order — *to prevent sudden stomach distention, which can cause nausea,
vomiting, cramps, or diarrhea.*

▶ After administering the appropriate
amount of formula, flush the tubing by
adding about 60 ml of water to the gavage bag or bulb syringe, or manually
flush it using a barrel syringe. *This
maintains the tube's patency by removing
excess formula, which could occlude the
tube.*

▶ If you're administering a continuous
feeding, flush the feeding tube every 4
hours *to help prevent tube occlusion.*
Monitor gastric emptying every 4 hours.

▶ To discontinue gastric feeding (depending on the equipment you're using), close the regulator clamp on the
gavage bag tubing, disconnect the syringe from the feeding tube, or turn off
the infusion controller.

▶ Cover the end of the feeding tube
with its plug or cap *to prevent leakage
and contamination of the tube.*

▶ Leave the patient in semi-Fowler's or
high Fowler's position for at least 30
minutes.

▶ Rinse all reusable equipment with
warm water. Dry it and store it in a
convenient place for the next feeding.

Change equipment every 24 hours or according to your facility's policy.

Delivering a duodenal or jejunal feeding

▶ Elevate the head of the bed and place the patient in low Fowler's position.

▶ Open the enteral administration set and hang the gavage container on the I.V. pole.

▶ If you're using a nasoduodenal tube, measure its length *to check tube placement*. Remember that you may not get any residual when you aspirate the tube.

▶ Open the flow clamp and regulate the flow to the desired rate. To regulate the rate using a volumetric infusion pump, follow the manufacturer's directions for setting up the equipment. Most patients receive small amounts initially, with volumes increasing gradually once tolerance is established.

▶ Flush the tube every 4 hours with water *to maintain patency and provide hydration*. A needle catheter jejunostomy tube may require flushing every 2 hours *to prevent formula buildup inside the tube*. A Y connector may be useful for frequent flushing. Attach the continuous feeding to the main port and use the side port for flushes.

▶ Change equipment every 24 hours or according to facility policy.

Special considerations

▶ If the feeding solution doesn't initially flow through a bulb syringe, attach the bulb and squeeze it gently to start the flow. Then remove the bulb. Never use the bulb to force the formula through the tube.

▶ If the patient becomes nauseated or vomits, stop the feeding immediately.

The patient may vomit if the stomach becomes distended from overfeeding or delayed gastric emptying.

▶ *To reduce oropharyngeal discomfort from the tube*, allow the patient to brush his teeth or care for his dentures regularly and encourage frequent gargling. If the patient is unconscious, administer oral care with wet sponge-tipped swabs every 4 hours. Use petroleum jelly on dry, cracked lips. (Note: Dry mucous membranes may indicate dehydration, which requires increased fluid intake.) Clean the patient's nostrils with cotton-tipped applicators, apply lubricant along the mucosa, and assess the skin for signs of breakdown.

▶ During continuous feedings, assess the patient frequently for abdominal distention. Flush the tubing by adding about 50 ml of water to the gavage bag or bulb syringe. *This maintains the tube's patency by removing excess formula, which could occlude the tube.*

▶ If the patient develops diarrhea, administer small, frequent, less concentrated feedings, or administer bolus feedings over a longer time. Also, make sure that the formula isn't cold and that proper storage and sanitation practices have been followed. The loose stools associated with tube feedings make extra perineal and skin care necessary. Giving paregoric, tincture of opium, or diphenoxylate hydrochloride may improve the condition. Changing to a formula with more fiber may eliminate liquid stools.

▶ If the patient becomes constipated, the doctor may increase the fruit, vegetable, or sugar content of the formula. Assess the patient's hydration status *because dehydration may produce constipation*. Increase fluid intake as necessary.

If the condition persists, administer an appropriate drug or enema as ordered.

▶ Drugs can be administered through the feeding tube. Except for enteric-coated drugs, time-released, or sustained-release medications, crush tablets or open and dilute capsules in water before administering them. Be sure to flush the tubing afterward *to ensure full instillation of medication.* Keep in mind that some drugs may change the osmolarity of the feeding formula and cause diarrhea.

▶ Small-bore feeding tubes may kink, making instillation impossible. If you suspect this problem, try changing the patient's position, or withdraw the tube a few inches and restart. Never use a guide wire to reposition the tube.

▶ Constantly monitor the flow rate of a blended or high-residue formula *to determine if the formula is clogging the tubing as it settles. To prevent such clogging,* squeeze the bag frequently to agitate the solution.

▶ Monitor blood glucose levels to assess glucose tolerance. (A patient with a serum glucose level of less than 200 mg/dl is considered stable.) Also monitor serum levels of electrolytes, blood urea nitrogen, and glucose as well as serum osmolality and other pertinent findings *to determine the patient's response to therapy and to assess his hydration status.*

▶ Check the flow rate hourly to ensure correct infusion. (With an improvised administration set, use a time tape to record the rate *because it's difficult to get precise readings from an irrigation container or enema bag.*)

▶ For duodenal or jejunal feeding, most patients tolerate a continuous drip better than bolus feedings. Bolus feed-

ings can cause such complications as hyperglycemia and diarrhea.

Home care

Patient education for home tube feeding includes instructions on an infusion control device to maintain accuracy, use of the syringe or bag and tubing, care of the tube and insertion site, and formula mixing. Formula may be mixed in an electric blender according to package directions. Formula not used within 24 hours must be discarded. If the formula must hang for more than 8 hours, advise the patient to use a gavage or pump administration set with an ice pouch to decrease the incidence of bacterial growth. Tell him to use a new bag daily.

Teach family members signs and symptoms to report to the doctor or home care nurse as well as measures to take in an emergency.

Complications

Erosion of esophageal, tracheal, nasal, and oropharyngeal mucosa can result if tubes are left in place for a long time. If possible, use smaller-lumen tubes to prevent such irritation. Check your facility's policy regarding the frequency of changing feeding tubes *to prevent complications.*

Using the gastric route, frequent or large-volume feedings can cause bloating and retention. Dehydration, diarrhea, and vomiting can cause metabolic disturbances. Cramping and abdominal distention usually indicate intolerance.

Using the duodenal or jejunal route, clogging of the feeding tube is common. The patient may experience metabolic, fluid, and electrolyte abnormalities, including hyperglycemia, hyperosmolar

Troubleshooting

Managing tube feeding problems

Complication	Interventions
Aspiration of gastric secretions	■ Discontinue feeding immediately. ■ Perform tracheal suction of aspirated contents, if possible. ■ Notify the doctor. Prophylactic antibiotics and chest physiotherapy may be ordered. ■ Check tube placement before feeding *to prevent complication.*
Hyperglycemia	■ Monitor blood glucose levels. ■ Notify the doctor of elevated levels. ■ Administer insulin if ordered. ■ Change the formula to one with a lower sugar content as ordered.
Tube obstruction	■ Flush the tube with warm water. If necessary, replace the tube. ■ Flush the tube with 50 ml of water after each feeding to remove excess sticky formula, *which could occlude the tube.*
Vomiting, bloating, diarrhea, or cramps	■ Reduce the flow rate. ■ Administer metoclopramide to increase GI motility. ■ Warm the formula to prevent GI distress. ■ For 30 minutes after feeding, position the patient on his right side with his head elevated to facilitate gastric emptying. ■ Notify the doctor. *He may want to reduce the amount of formula being given during each feeding.*

dehydration, coma, edema, hypernatremia, and essential fatty acid deficiency.

The patient also may experience dumping syndrome, in which a large amount of hyperosmotic solution in the duodenum causes excessive diffusion of fluid through the semipermeable membrane and results in diarrhea. In a patient with low serum albumin levels, these symptoms may result from low oncotic pressure in the duodenal mucosa. (See *Managing tube feeding problems.*)

Documentation
On the intake and output sheet, record the date, volume of formula, and volume of water. In your notes, document abdominal assessment findings (including tube exit site, if appropriate); amount of residual gastric contents; verification of tube placement; amount, type, and time of feeding; and tube patency. Discuss the patient's tolerance of the feeding, including nausea, vomiting, cramping, diarrhea, and distention.

Note the result of blood and urine tests, hydration status, and any drugs given through the tube. Include the date and time of administration set changes, oral and nasal hygiene, and results of specimen collections.

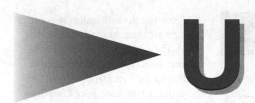

ULTRAVIOLET LIGHT THERAPY

Ultraviolet (UV) light causes profound biological changes, including temporary suppression of epidermal basal cell division followed by a later increase in cell turnover, and UV light–induced immune suppression. As a result, such skin conditions as psoriasis, mycosis fungoides, atopic dermatitis, and uremic pruritus may respond to therapy that uses timed exposure to UV light rays.

Emitted by the sun, the UV spectrum is subdivided into three bands—A, B, and C—each of which affects the skin differently. Ultraviolet A (UVA) radiation (with a relatively long wavelength of 320 to 400 nm) rapidly darkens preformed melanin pigment, may augment ultraviolet B (UVB) in causing sunburn and skin aging, and may induce phototoxicity in the presence of some drugs. UVB radiation (with a wavelength of 280 to 320 nm) causes sunburn and erythema. Ultraviolet C (UVC) radiation (with a wavelength of 200 to 280 nm) normally is absorbed by the earth's ozone layer and doesn't reach the ground. However, UVC kills bacteria and is used in operating-room germicidal lamps.

Contraindications to PUVA and UVB therapy include a history of photosensitivity diseases, skin cancer, arsenic ingestion, or cataracts or cataract surgery; current use of photosensitivity-inducing drugs; and previous skin irradiation (which can induce skin cancer). Ultraviolet light therapy is also contraindicated in patients who have undergone previous ionizing chemotherapy and in patients who are using photosensitizing or immunosuppressant drugs. PUVA is contraindicated in pregnant women.

Key nursing diagnoses and patient outcomes

Risk for fluid volume imbalance related to ultraviolet light therapy
The patient will:
▶ have normal skin color and temperature
▶ exhibit no signs of dehydration
▶ maintain urine output of at least (specify) ml/hour
▶ have bilirubin values within normal limits
▶ have intake equal output.

Risk for injury related to improper technique
The patient will:
▶ identify factors that increase risk for injury
▶ assist in identifying and applying safety measures to prevent injury.

Comparing skin types

Skin type	Sunburn and tanning history
I	Always burns; never tans; sensitive ("Celtic" skin)
II	Burns easily; tans minimally
III	Burns moderately; tans gradually to light brown (average Caucasian skin)
IV	Burns minimally; always tans well to moderately brown (olive skin)
V	Rarely burns; tans profusely to dark (brown skin)
VI	Never burns; deeply pigmented; not sensitive (black skin)

Equipment

For UVA radiation
Fluorescent black-light lamp • high-intensity UVA fluorescent bulbs

For UVB radiation
Fluorescent sunlamp or hot quartz lamp • sunlamp bulbs

For all UV treatments
Oral or topical phototherapeutic medications if necessary • body-sized light chamber or smaller light box • dark, polarized goggles • sunscreen if necessary • hospital gown • towels

Preparation of equipment
The patient can undergo UV light therapy in the hospital, in a doctor's office, or at home. Typically set into a reflective cabinet, the light source consists of a bank of high-intensity fluorescent bulbs. (At home, the patient may use a small fluorescent sunlamp.)

Check the doctor's orders to confirm the light treatment type and dose. For PUVA, the initial dose is based on the patient's skin type and is increased according to the treatment protocol and the patient's tolerance. (See *Comparing skin types*.) The doctor calculates the UVB dose based on skin type estimation or by determining a minimal erythema dose—the smallest amount of UV light needed to produce mild erythema.

Implementation
▶ Inform the patient that UV light treatments produce a mild sunburn that will help reduce or resolve skin lesions.
▶ Review the patient's health history for contraindications to UV light therapy. Also ask whether he's currently taking photosensitizing drugs, such as anticonvulsants, certain antihypertensives, phenothiazines, salicylates, sulfonamides, tetracyclines, tretinoin, and various cancer drugs.
▶ If the patient will have PUVA therapy, make sure he took methoxsalen (with food) 1½ hours before treatment. Methoxsalen photosensitizes the skin to enhance therapeutic effect.
▶ To begin therapy, instruct the patient to disrobe and put on a hospital gown. Have him remove the gown or expose just the treatment area once he's in the phototherapy unit. Make sure that he wears goggles *to protect his eyes* and a sunscreen, towels, or the hospital gown *to protect vulnerable skin areas*. All male patients receiving PUVA must wear protection over the groin area.
▶ If the patient is having local UVB treatment, position him at the correct distance from the light source. For instance, for facial treatment with a sunlamp, position the patient's face about 12″ (30.5 cm) from the lamp. For body treatment, position the patient's body

about 30″ (76 cm) from either the sun-lamp or the hot quartz lamp.

► During therapy, make sure the patient wears goggles at all times. If you're observing him through light-chamber windows, you should wear goggles too. If the patient must stand for the treatment, ask him to report any dizziness *to ensure his safety*.

► After delivering the prescribed UV dose, help the patient out of the unit and instruct him to shield exposed areas of skin from sunlight for 8 hours after therapy.

Special considerations

► Overexposure to UV light (sunburn) can result from prolonged treatment and an inadequate distance between the patient and light sources. It can also result from the use of photosensitizing drugs or from overly sensitive skin.

► Prevent eye damage by using gray or green polarized lenses during UVB therapy or UV-opaque sunglasses during PUVA therapy. The patient undergoing PUVA therapy should wear these glasses for 24 hours after treatment *because methoxsalen can cause photosensitivity*.

► Tell the patient to look for marked erythema, blistering, peeling, or other signs of overexposure 4 to 6 hours after UVB therapy and 24 to 48 hours after UVA therapy. In either case, the erythema should disappear within another 24 hours. Inform him that mild dryness and desquamation will occur in 1 to 2 days. Teach him appropriate skin care measures. (See *Skin care guidelines,* page 894.) Advise him to notify the doctor if overexposure occurs. Typically, the doctor recommends stopping treatment for a few days and then starting over at a lower exposure level.

► Before giving methoxsalen or etretinate, check to ensure that baseline liver function studies have been done. Keep in mind that both drugs are hepatotoxic agents and are never given together. Liver function and blood lipid studies are required before treatment with acitretin and at regular intervals during treatment. Liver function studies and a complete blood count are required before and during methotrexate treatment.

► If the doctor prescribes tar preparations with UVB treatment, watch for signs of sensitivity, such as erythema, pruritus, and eczematous reactions. If you apply carbonis detergens to the patient's skin before UV light therapy, be sure to remove it completely with mineral oil just before treatment begins *to let the light penetrate the skin.*

Complications

Erythema is the major adverse effect of UVB therapy. Minimal erythema without discomfort is acceptable, but treatments are suspended if marked edema, swelling, or blistering occurs.

Erythema, nausea, and pruritus are the three major short-term adverse effects of PUVA. Long-term adverse effects are similar to those caused by excessive exposure to sun — premature aging (xerosis, wrinkles, and mottled skin), lentigines, telangiectasia, increased risk of skin cancer, and ocular damage if eye protection isn't used. The patient can minimize effects by using emollients, sunscreens, and cover-ups.

Documentation

Record the date and time of initial and subsequent treatments, the UV wavelength used, and the name and dose of any oral or topical medications given. Record the exact duration of therapy, the distance between the light source and the skin, and the patient's tolerance. Note safety measures used such

Skin care guidelines

A patient who is receiving ultraviolet light treatments must know how to protect his skin from injury. Provide your patient with the following skin care tips:

- Encourage the patient to use emollients and drink plenty of fluids *to combat dry skin and maintain adequate hydration.* Warn him to avoid hot baths or showers and to use soap sparingly. *Heat and soap promote dry skin.*
- Instruct the patient to notify his doctor before taking any medication, including aspirin, *to prevent heightened photosensitivity.*
- If the patient is receiving PUVA therapy, review his methoxsalen dosage schedule. Explain that deviating from it could result in burns or ineffective treatment. Urge him to wear appropriate sunglasses outdoors for at least 24 hours after taking methoxsalen. Recommend yearly eye examinations *to detect cataract formation.*
- If the patient uses a sunlamp at home, advise him to let the lamp warm for 5 minutes before treatment. Stress the importance of exposing his skin to the light for the exact

amount of time prescribed by the doctor. Instruct the patient to protect his eyes with goggles and to use a dependable timer or have someone else time his therapy. Above all, urge him never to use the sunlamp when he's tired *to avoid falling asleep under the lamp and sustaining a burn.*

- Teach the patient first aid for localized burning: Tell him to apply cool water soaks for 20 minutes or until skin temperature cools. For more extensive burns, recommend tepid tap water baths after notifying the doctor about the burn. After the patient bathes, suggest using an oil-in-water moisturizing lotion (not a petroleum-jelly-based product, which can trap radiant heat).
- Tell the patient to limit natural-light exposure, to use a sunscreen when he's outdoors, and to notify his doctor immediately if he discovers any unusual skin lesions.
- Advise the patient to avoid harsh soaps and chemicals, such as paints and solvents, and to discuss ways to manage physical and psychological stress, which may exacerbate skin disorders.

as eye protection. Also describe the patient's skin condition before and after treatment. Note improvements and adverse reactions, such as increased pruritus, oozing, and scaling.

URINARY DIVERSION STOMA CARE

Urinary diversions provide an alternative route for urine flow when a disorder, such as an invasive bladder tumor, impedes normal drainage. A permanent urinary diversion is indicated in any

condition that requires a total cystectomy. In conditions requiring temporary urinary drainage or diversion, a suprapubic or urethral catheter is usually inserted to divert the flow of urine temporarily. The catheter remains in place until the incision heals.

Urinary diversions may also be indicated for patients with neurogenic bladder, congenital anomaly, traumatic injury to the lower urinary tract, or severe chronic urinary tract infection.

Ileal conduit and continent urinary diversion are the two types of permanent urinary diversions with stomas. (See *Types of permanent urinary diver-*

Types of permanent urinary diversion

The steps involved in creating an ileal conduit or a continent urinary diversion are described here.

Ileal conduit

A segment of the ileum is excised, and the two ends of the ileum that result from excision of the segment are sutured closed. Then the ureters are dissected from the bladder and anastomosed to the ileal segment. One end of the ileal segment is closed with sutures; the opposite end is brought through the abdominal wall, thereby forming a stoma.

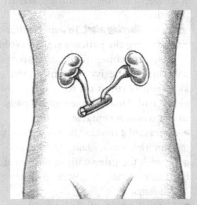

Continent urinary diversion

A tube is formed from part of the ascending colon and ileum. One end of the tube is brought to the skin to form the stoma. At the internal end of this tube, a nipple valve is constructed so urine won't drain out unless a catheter is inserted through the stoma into the newly formed bladder pouch. The urethral neck is sutured closed.

Another recently developed type of continent urinary diversion (not pictured here) is "hooked" back to the urethra, obviating the need for a stoma.

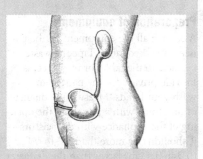

sion.) These procedures usually require the patient to wear a urine-collection appliance and to care for the stoma created during surgery.

Key nursing diagnoses and patient outcomes

Ineffective individual coping related to personal vulnerability
The patient will:
▶ become actively involved in planning own care
▶ identify effective and ineffective coping techniques.

Deficient knowledge related to lack of exposure to care of a urinary diversion stoma
The patient will:
▶ communicate a need to know about urinary diversion care
▶ state or demonstrate understanding of what has been taught.

Equipment

Soap and warm water • waste receptacle (such as an impervious or wax-coated bag) • linen-saver pad • hypoallergenic paper tape • povidone-iodine solution • urine collection container •

rubber catheter (usually #14 or #16 French) • ruler • scissors • urine-collection appliance (with or without antireflux valve) • graduated cylinder • cottonless gauze pads (some rolled, some flat) • washcloth • skin barrier in liquid, paste, wafer, or sheet form • appliance belt • stoma covering (nonadherent gauze pad or panty liner) • two pairs of gloves • optional: adhesive solvent, irrigating syringe, tampon, hair dryer, electric razor, regular gauze pads, vinegar, and deodorant tablets

Commercially packaged stoma care kits are available. In place of soap and water, you can use adhesive remover pads, if available, or cotton gauze saturated with adhesive solvent.

Preparation of equipment

Assemble all the equipment on the patient's overbed table. Tape the waste receptacle to the table for ready access. Provide privacy for the patient and wash your hands. Measure the diameter of the stoma with a ruler. Cut the opening of the appliance with the scissors — it shouldn't be more than $1/8''$ to $1/6''$ (0.3 to 0.4 cm) larger than the diameter of the stoma. Moisten the faceplate of the appliance with a small amount of solvent or water *to prepare it for adhesion*. Performing these preliminary steps at the bedside *allows you to demonstrate the procedure and show the patient that it isn't difficult, which will help him relax.*

Implementation

▶ Wash your hands again. Explain the procedure to the patient as you go along and offer constant reinforcement and reassurance *to counteract negative reactions that may be elicited by stoma care.*
▶ Place the bed in low Fowler's position so the patient's abdomen is flat. *This position eliminates skin folds that could cause the appliance to slip or irritate the skin and allows the patient to observe or participate.*
▶ Put on the gloves and place the linen-saver pad under the patient's side, near the stoma. Open the drain valve of the appliance being replaced *to empty the urine into the graduated cylinder.* Then, *to remove the appliance,* use a washcloth to apply soap and water or adhesive solvent as you gently push the skin back from the pouch. If the appliance is disposable, discard it into the waste receptacle. If it's reusable, clean it with soap and lukewarm water and let it air-dry.

Nursing alert *To avoid irritating the patient's stoma,* avoid touching it with adhesive solvent. If adhesive remains on the skin, gently rub it off with a dry gauze pad. Discard used gauze pads in the waste receptacle.

▶ *To prevent a constant flow of urine onto the skin while you're changing the appliance,* wick the urine with an absorbent, lint-free material. (See *Wicking urine from a stoma.*)
▶ Use water to carefully wash off any crystal deposits that may have formed around the stoma. If urine has stagnated and has a strong odor, use soap to wash it off. Be sure to rinse thoroughly *to remove any oily residue that could cause the appliance to slip.*
▶ Follow your facility's skin care protocol to treat any minor skin problems.
▶ Dry the peristomal area thoroughly with a gauze pad *because moisture will keep the appliance from sticking.* Use a hair dryer if you wish. Remove any hair from the area with scissors or an electric razor *to prevent hair follicles from becoming irritated when the pouch is removed, which can cause folliculitis.*

▶ Inspect the stoma *to see if it's healing properly and to detect complications.* Check the color and the appearance of the suture line and examine any moisture or effluent. Inspect the peristomal skin for redness, irritation, and intactness.

▶ Apply the skin barrier. If you apply a wafer or sheet, cut it to fit over the stoma. Remove any protective backing and set the barrier aside with the adhesive side up. If you apply a liquid barrier (such as Skin-Prep), saturate a gauze pad with it and coat the peristomal skin. Move in concentric circles outward from the stoma until you've covered an area 2″ (5.1 cm) larger than the wafer. Let the skin dry for several minutes — it should feel tacky. Gently press the wafer around the stoma, sticky side down, smoothing from the stoma outward.

▶ If you're using a barrier paste, open the tube, squeeze out a small amount, and then discard it. Then squeeze a ribbon of paste directly onto the peristomal skin about ½″ (1.5 cm) from the stoma, making a complete circle. Make several more concentric circles outward. Dip your fingers into lukewarm water and smooth the paste until the skin is completely covered from the edge of the stoma to 3″ to 4″ (7.5 to 10 cm) outward. The paste should be ¼″ to ½″ (0.5 to 1.5 cm) thick. Discard the gloves, wash your hands, and put on new gloves.

▶ Remove the material used for wicking urine and place it in the waste receptacle.

▶ Now place the appliance over the stoma, leaving only a small amount (³⁄₈″ to ³⁄₄″ [1 to 2 cm]) of skin exposed.

▶ Secure the faceplate of the appliance to the skin with paper tape, if recommended. To do this, place a piece of tape lengthwise on each edge of the

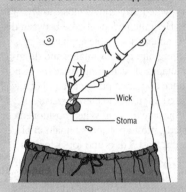

Wicking urine from a stoma

Use a piece of rolled, cottonless gauze or a tampon to wick urine from a stoma. Working by capillary action, wicking absorbs urine while you prepare the patient's skin to hold a urine-collection appliance.

Wick

Stoma

faceplate so that the tape overlaps onto the skin.

▶ Apply the appliance belt, making sure that it's on a level with the stoma. *If the belt is applied above or below the stoma, it could break the bag's seal or rub or injure the stoma.* The belt should be loose enough for you to insert two fingers between the skin and the belt. *If the belt is too tight, it could irritate the skin or cause internal damage.* Some devices don't require a belt. Instead, the pouch has a ridge that fits over the rim of barrier adhesive and snaps securely into place.

▶ Dispose of the used materials appropriately.

Special considerations

▶ The patient's attitude toward his urinary diversion stoma plays a big part in determining how well he'll adjust to it. *To encourage a positive attitude,* help him get used to the idea of caring for his stoma and the appliance as though they're natural extensions of himself. When teaching him to perform the procedure, give him written instructions and provide positive reinforcement after he completes each step. Suggest that he perform the procedure in the morning when urine flows most slowly.

▶ Help the patient choose between disposable and reusable appliances by telling him the advantages and disadvantages of each. Emphasize the importance of correct placement and of a well-fitted appliance *to prevent seepage of urine onto the skin.* When positioned correctly, most appliances remain in place for at least 3 days and for as long as 5 days if no leakage occurs. After 5 days, the appliance should be changed. With the improved adhesives and pouches available, belts aren't always necessary.

▶ Because urine flows constantly, it accumulates quickly, becoming even heavier than stools. *To prevent the weight of the urine from loosening the seal around the stoma and separating the appliance from the skin,* tell the patient to empty the appliance through the drain valve when it is one-third to one-half full.

▶ Instruct the patient to connect his appliance to a urine-collection container before he goes to sleep. *The continuous flow of urine into the container during the night prevents the urine from accumulating and stagnating in the appliance.*

▶ Teach the patient sanitary and dietary measures that can protect the peristomal skin and control the odor that commonly results from alkaline urine, infection, or poor hygiene. Reusable appliances should be washed with soap and lukewarm water, then air-dried thoroughly *to prevent brittleness.* Soaking the appliance in vinegar and water or placing deodorant tablets

in it can further dissipate stubborn odors. An acid-ash diet that includes ascorbic acid and cranberry juice may raise urine acidity, thereby reducing bacterial action and fermentation (the underlying causes of odor). Generous fluid intake also helps to reduce odors by diluting the urine.

▶ Tell the patient that mucus may be present in the urine.

▶ If the patient has a continent urinary diversion, make sure you know how to meet his special needs. (See *Caring for the patient with a continent urinary diversion.*)

▶ Inform the patient about support services provided by ostomy clubs and the American Cancer Society.

Home care
The patient or a family member can learn to care for a urinary diversion stoma at home. However, the patient's emotional adjustment to the stoma must be given special consideration before he can be expected to maintain it properly. Arrange for a visiting nurse or an enterostomal therapist to assist the patient at home.

Complications
Because intestinal mucosa is delicate, an ill-fitting appliance can cause bleeding. This is especially likely to occur with an ileal conduit, the most common type of urinary diversion stoma, *because a segment of the intestine forms the conduit.* Peristomal skin may become reddened or excoriated from too-frequent changing or improper placement of the appliance, poor skin care, or allergic reaction to the appliance or adhesive. Constant leakage around the appliance can result from improper placement of the appliance or from poor skin turgor.

Caring for the patient with a continent urinary diversion

In this procedure, an alternative to the traditional ileal conduit, a pouch created from the ascending colon and terminal ileum serves as a new bladder, which empties through a stoma. To drain urine continuously, several drains are inserted into this reconstructed bladder and left in place for 3 to 6 weeks until the new stoma heals. The patient will be discharged from the hospital with the drains in place. He'll return to have them removed and to learn to catheterize his stoma.

First hospitalization

- Immediately after surgery, monitor intake and output from each drain. Be alert for decreased output, *which may indicate that urine flow is obstructed.*
- Watch for common postoperative complications, such as infection or bleeding. Also watch for signs of urinary leakage, which include increased abdominal distention, and urine appearing around the drains or midline incision.
- Irrigate the drains as ordered.
- Clean the area around the drains daily—first with povidone-iodine solution and then with sterile water. Apply a dry, sterile dressing to the area. Use precut 4″ × 4″ drain dressings around the drain *to absorb leakage.*
- *To increase the patient's mobility and comfort,* connect the drains to a leg bag.

Second hospitalization or outpatient

- After the patient's drains are removed, teach the patient how to catheterize the stoma. Begin by gathering the following equipment on a clean towel rubber catheter (usually #14 or #16 French), water-soluble lubricant, washcloth, stoma covering (nonadherent gauze pad or panty liner), hypoallergenic adhesive tape, and an irrigating solution (optional).
- Apply water-soluble lubricant to the catheter tip *to facilitate insertion.*
- Remove and discard the stoma cover. Using the washcloth, clean the stoma and the area around it, starting at the stoma and working outward in a circular motion.

- Hold the urine-collection container under the catheter; then slowly insert the catheter into the stoma. Urine should then begin to flow into the container. If it doesn't, gently rotate the catheter or redirect its angle. If the catheter drains slowly, it may be plugged with mucus. Irrigate it with sterile saline solution or sterile water to clear it. When the flow stops, pinch the catheter closed and remove it.

Home care

- Teach the patient how to care for the drains and their insertion sites during the 3 to 6 weeks he'll be at home before their removal and teach him how to attach them to a leg bag. Also teach him how to recognize the signs of infection and obstruction.
- After the drains are removed, teach the patient how to empty the pouch and establish a schedule. Initially, he should catheterize the stoma and empty the pouch every 2 to 3 hours. Later, he should catheterize every 4 hours while awake and also irrigate the pouch each morning and evening, if ordered. Instruct him to empty the pouch whenever he feels a sensation of fullness.
- Tell the patient that the catheters are reusable, but only after they've been cleaned. He should clean the catheter thoroughly with warm, soapy water, rinse it thoroughly, and hang it to dry over a clean towel. He should store cleaned and dried catheters in plastic bags. Tell him he can reuse catheters for up to 1 month before discarding them. However, he should immediately discard any catheter that becomes discolored or cracked.

Documentation

Record the appearance and color of the stoma and whether it's inverted, flush with the skin, or protruding. If it protrudes, note how much it protrudes above the skin. (The normal range is ½" to ¾" [1.5 to 2 cm].) Record the appearance and condition of the peristomal skin, noting any redness or irritation or complaints by the patient of itching or burning.

URINE COLLECTION, ADULT

A random urine specimen, usually collected as part of the physical examination or at various times during hospitalization, permits laboratory screening for urinary and systemic disorders as well as for drug screening. A clean-catch midstream specimen is replacing random collection because it provides a virtually uncontaminated specimen without the need for catheterization.

An indwelling catheter specimen—obtained either by clamping the drainage tube and emptying the accumulated urine into a container or by aspirating a specimen with a syringe—requires sterile collection technique to prevent catheter contamination and urinary tract infection. This method is contraindicated after genitourinary surgery.

Key nursing diagnoses and patient outcomes

Impaired urinary elimination related to a medical condition
The patient will:
▶ voice understanding of treatment
▶ avoid or minimize complications.

Deficient knowledge related to lack of exposure to procedure
The patient will:
▶ verbalize understanding of need for procedure
▶ demonstrate correct procedure for obtaining urine specimen.

Equipment

For a random specimen

Bedpan or urinal with cover, if necessary • gloves • graduated container • specimen container with lid • label • laboratory request form

For a clean-catch midstream specimen

Soap and water • gloves • graduated container • three sterile 2" × 2" gauze pads • povidone-iodine solution • sterile specimen container with lid • label • bedpan or urinal, if necessary • laboratory request form

Commercial clean-catch kits containing antiseptic towelettes, sterile specimen container with lid and label, and instructions for use in several languages are widely used.

For an indwelling catheter specimen

Gloves • alcohol pad • 10-ml syringe • 21G or 22G 1½" needle • tube clamp • sterile specimen container with lid • label • laboratory request form

Implementation

▶ Tell the patient you need a urine specimen for laboratory analysis. Explain the procedure to him and his family, if necessary, *to promote cooperation and prevent accidental disposal of specimens.*

Collecting a random specimen

▶ Provide privacy. Instruct the patient on bed rest to void into a clean bedpan or urinal or ask the ambulatory patient to void into either one in the bathroom.

▶ Put on gloves. Pour at least 120 ml of urine into the specimen container and cap the container securely. If the patient's urine output must be measured and recorded, pour the remaining urine into the graduated container. Otherwise, discard the remaining urine. If you inadvertently spill urine on the outside of the container, clean and dry it *to prevent cross-contamination.*

▶ After you label the specimen container with the patient's name and room number and the date and time of collection, attach the request form and send it the laboratory immediately. *Delayed transport of the specimen may alter test results.*

▶ Clean the graduated container and urinal or bedpan and return them to their proper storage. Discard disposable items.

▶ Wash your hands thoroughly *to prevent cross-contamination.* Offer the patient a washcloth and soap and water to wash his hands.

Collecting a clean-catch midstream specimen

▶ Because the goal is a virtually uncontaminated specimen, explain the procedure to the patient carefully. Provide illustrations to emphasize the correct collection technique, if possible.

▶ Tell the patient to remove all clothing from the waist down and to stand in front of the toilet as for urination or, if female, to sit far back on the toilet seat and spread her legs. Then have the patient clean the periurethral area (tip of the penis or labial folds, vulva, and urinary meatus) with soap and water and wipe the area three times, each time with a fresh 2″ × 2″ gauze pad soaked in povidone-iodine solution or

with the wipes provided in a commercial kit. Instruct the female patient to separate her labial folds with the thumb and forefinger. Tell her to wipe down one side with the first pad and discard it, to wipe the other side with the second pad and discard it and, finally, to wipe down the center over the urinary meatus with the third pad and discard it. Stress the importance of cleaning from front to back *to avoid contaminating the genital area with fecal matter.* For the uncircumcised male patient, emphasize the need to retract his foreskin *to effectively clean the meatus* and to keep it retracted during voiding.

▶ Tell the female patient to straddle the bedpan or toilet to allow labial spreading and to keep her labia separated while voiding.

▶ Instruct the patient to begin voiding into the bedpan, urinal, or toilet. Then, without stopping the urine stream, the patient should move the collection container into the stream, collecting 30 to 50 ml at the midstream portion of the voiding. He can then finish voiding into the bedpan, urinal, or toilet.

▶ Put on gloves before discarding the first and last portions of the voiding and measure the remaining urine in a graduated container for intake and output records, if necessary. Be sure to include the amount in the specimen container when recording the total amount voided.

▶ Take the sterile container from the patient and cap it securely. Avoid touching the inside of the container or the lid. If the outside of the container is soiled, clean it and wipe it dry. Remove gloves and discard them properly.

▶ Wash your hands thoroughly. Tell the patient to wash his hands also.

▶ Label the container with the patient's name and room number, name of test,

Aspirating a urine specimen

If the patient has an indwelling urinary catheter in place, clamp the tube distal to the aspiration port for about 30 minutes. Wipe the port with an alcohol pad and insert a needle and a 20- or 30-ml syringe into the port perpendicular to the tube. Aspirate the required amount of urine and expel it into the specimen container. Remove the clamp on the drainage tube.

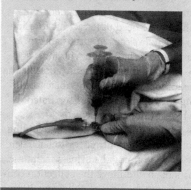

type of specimen, collection time, and suspected diagnosis, if known. If a urine culture has been ordered, note any current antibiotic therapy on the laboratory request form. Send the container to the laboratory immediately or place it on ice *to prevent specimen deterioration and altered test results.*

Collecting an indwelling catheter specimen

▶ About 30 minutes before collecting the specimen, clamp the drainage tube *to allow urine to accumulate.*
▶ Put on gloves. If the drainage tube has a built-in sampling port, wipe the port with an alcohol pad. Uncap the needle on the syringe and insert the needle into the sampling port at a 90-degree angle to the tubing. Aspirate the specimen into the syringe. (See *Aspirating a urine specimen.*)

▶ If the drainage tube doesn't have a sampling port and the catheter is made of rubber, obtain the specimen from the catheter. *Other types of catheters will leak after you withdraw the needle.* To withdraw the specimen from a rubber catheter, wipe it with an alcohol pad just above where it connects to the drainage tube. Insert the needle into the rubber catheter at a 45-degree angle and withdraw the specimen. Never insert the needle into the shaft of the catheter *because this may puncture the lumen leading to the catheter balloon.*

▶ Transfer the specimen to a sterile container, label it, and send it to the laboratory immediately or place it on ice. If a urine culture is to be performed, be sure to list any current antibiotic therapy on the laboratory request form.

▶ If the catheter isn't made of rubber or has no sampling port, wipe the area where the catheter joins the drainage tube with an alcohol pad. Disconnect the catheter and allow urine to drain into the sterile specimen container. Avoid touching the inside of the sterile container with the catheter and don't touch anything with the catheter drainage tube *to avoid contamination.* When you've collected the specimen, wipe both connection sites with an alcohol pad and join them. Cap the specimen container, label it, and send it to the laboratory immediately or place it on ice.

Nursing alert Make sure you unclamp the drainage tube after collecting the specimen *to prevent urine backflow, which may cause bladder distention and infection.*

Home care

Instruct the patient to collect the specimen in a clean container with a tight-fitting lid and to keep it on ice or in the refrigerator (separate from food items) for up to 24 hours.

Documentation

Record the times of specimen collection and transport to the laboratory. Specify the test as well as the appearance, odor, and color and any unusual characteristics of the specimen. If necessary, record the urine volume in the intake and output record.

URINE COLLECTION, PEDIATRIC

Collection of a urine specimen for laboratory analysis allows screening for urinary tract infection and renal disorders, evaluation of treatment, and detection of systemic and metabolic disorders.

Although a child without bladder control can't provide a clean-catch midstream urine specimen, the pediatric urine collection bag provides a simple, effective alternative. It offers minimal risk of specimen contamination without resorting to catheterization or suprapubic aspiration. Because the collection bag is secured with adhesive flaps, its use is contraindicated in a patient with extremely sensitive or excoriated perineal skin. Alternative methods of collecting urine from small children include the use of an inside-out disposable diaper.

Key nursing diagnoses and patient outcomes

Impaired urinary elimination related to a medical condition

The patient or caregiver will:
▶ voice understanding of treatment
▶ avoid or minimize complications.

Deficient knowledge related to lack of exposure to procedure
The patient or caregiver will:
▶ verbalize understanding of need for procedure
▶ demonstrate correct procedure for obtaining urine specimen.

Equipment
For a random specimen

Pediatric urine collection bag (individually packaged) • urine specimen container • label • laboratory request form • two disposable diapers of appropriate size • scissors • gloves • washcloth • soap • water • towel • bowl • linen-saver pad

For a culture and sensitivity specimen

Sterile pediatric urine collection bag • sterile urine specimen container • label • laboratory request form • two disposable diapers of appropriate size • scissors • gloves • sterile bowl • sterile or distilled water • sterile 4″ × 4″ gauze pads • antiseptic skin cleaner • alcohol pad • 3-ml syringe with needle • linen-saver pad

For a timed specimen

24-hour pediatric urine collection bag (individually packaged) with evacuation tubing • 24-hour urine specimen container • label • laboratory request form • scissors • two disposable diapers of appropriate size • gloves • washcloth • soap • water • bowl • towel • sterile 4″ × 4″ gauze pads • compound benzoin tincture • small medicine cup • 35-ml luer-lock syringe or urometer • tubing stopper • specimen preservative (such as formaldehyde solution) • linen-saver pad

Kits containing sterile supplies for clean-catch collections are commercially available and may be used to obtain a culture and sensitivity specimen.

Preparation of equipment

Check the doctor's order for the type of specimen needed and assemble the appropriate equipment. Check the patient's chart for allergies (for example, to iodineor latex). Complete the laboratory request form *to avoid delay in sending the specimen to the laboratory*. Wash your hands.

With scissors, make a 2″ (5.1-cm) slit in one diaper, cutting from the center point toward one of the shorter edges. Later, you'll pull the urine collection bag through this slit when you position the bag and diaper on the patient. Pour water into the bowl; use sterile water and a sterile bowl if you need to collect a specimen for culture and sensitivity.

If you need a culture and sensitivity specimen, check the expiration date on each sterile package and inspect for tears. Put on new gloves and open several packages of sterile 4″ × 4″ gauze pads.

If you need a timed specimen and will use benzoin in liquid form, pour it into the medicine cup. Cut the tubing on the urine collection bag so that only 6″ (15.2 cm) remain attached. Discard the excess. Place the stopper in the severed end of the tubing. If you're going to use a urinometer for the patient who voids large amounts, don't cut the tubing; simply attach the device.

Implementation

▶ Explain the procedure to the patient, if he's old enough, and his parents. Provide privacy, especially if the patient is beyond infancy.

Collecting a random specimen

▶ Wash your hands.
▶ Place the patient on a linen-saver pad.
▶ Clean the perineal area with soap, water, and a washcloth, working from the urinary meatus outward *to prevent contamination of the urine specimen*. Wipe gently *to prevent tissue trauma and stimulation of urination*. Separate the labia of the female patient and retract the foreskin of the uncircumcised male patient *to expose the urinary meatus*. Thoroughly rinse the area with clear water and dry with a towel. Don't use powders, lotions, or cream *because these counteract the adhesive*.
▶ Place the patient in the frog position, with his legs separated and knees flexed. If necessary, have the patient's parent hold him while you apply the collection bag.
▶ Remove the protective coverings from the collection bag's adhesive flaps. For the female patient, first separate the labia and gently press the bag's lower rim to the perineum. Then, working upward toward the pubis, attach the rest of the adhesive rim inside the labia majora. For the male patient, place the bag over the penis and scrotum and press the adhesive rim to the skin.
▶ Once the bag is attached, gently pull it through the slit in the diaper *to prevent compression of the bag by the diaper and to allow observation of the specimen immediately after the patient voids*. Fasten the diaper on the patient.
▶ When urine appears in the bag, put on gloves and gently remove the diaper and the bag. Hold the bag's bottom port over the collection container, remove the tab from the port, and let the urine flow into the container.
▶ Measure the output if necessary.
▶ Label the specimen and attach the laboratory request form to the contain-

er. Send it directly to the laboratory. Remove and discard gloves.

▶ Put the second diaper on the patient and make sure he's comfortable.

Collecting a culture and sensitivity specimen

Follow the procedure for collecting a random specimen, with these modifications:

▶ Use sterile or distilled water, an antiseptic skin cleaner, and sterile 4″ × 4″ gauze pads to clean the perineal area.

▶ After putting on gloves, clean the urinary meatus; then work outward. Wipe only once with each gauze pad; then discard it.

▶ After the patient urinates, remove the bag and use an alcohol pad to clean a small area of the bag's surface. Puncture the clean area with the needle, and aspirate urine into the syringe.

▶ Inject the urine into the sterile specimen container. Be careful to keep the needle from touching the container's sides *to maintain sterility*. Remember, a large volume of urine is unnecessary *because only about 1 ml of urine is needed to perform this test*. Remove and discard your gloves.

Collecting a timed specimen

▶ Check the doctor's order for the duration of the collection and the indication for the procedure. Prepare the patient, put on gloves, and clean the perineum as for random specimen collection.

▶ If getting the bag to adhere is difficult, apply compound benzoin tincture to the perineal area, if ordered, *so that the collection bag will adhere better and you won't have to reapply it during the collection period*. If using liquid benzoin, dip a gauze pad into the medicine cup containing it. If using benzoin spray,

cover the genitalia with a gauze pad before spraying *to prevent tissue trauma*.

▶ Allow the benzoin to dry. Then apply the collection bag, pull the bottom of the bag and the tubing through the slit in the diaper and fasten the diaper. Remove and discard your gloves.

▶ Check the collection bag and tubing every 30 minutes to ensure a proper seal *because any leakage prevents collection of a complete specimen*.

▶ When urine appears in the bag, put on gloves and remove the stopper in the bag's tubing. Then attach the syringe to the end of the tubing and aspirate the urine. Remove the syringe and insert the stopper into the tubing.

▶ Discard the specimen and begin timing the collection.

▶ When the next urine specimen is obtained, add the preservative to the 24-hour specimen container along with the specimen and refrigerate it, if ordered, *to keep the sample stable*.

▶ Periodically empty the collection bag *to prevent dislodgment of the collection bag*. Each time you remove urine, add it to the specimen container; then use the syringe to inject a small amount of air into the collection bag *to prevent a vacuum, which can block urine drainage*.

▶ When the prescribed collection period has elapsed (or as nearly as possible), stop the collection and send the total accumulated specimen to the laboratory.

▶ Put on gloves and wash the perineal area thoroughly with soap and water *to remove the benzoin;* then put the second diaper on the patient.

Special considerations

▶ Whatever the collection method used, avoid forcing fluids *to prevent dilution of the specimen, which can alter test results*. For a random collection or a culture and sensitivity collection, obtain a first-voided morning specimen, if possible.

▶ If the collection bag becomes dislodged during timed collection, immediately reapply benzoin and attach another collection bag *to prevent loss of the specimen and the need to restart the collection.*

Complications

Adhesive from the rim of the collection bag can cause skin excoriation.

Documentation

Record the date, time, and method of collection. Also record the name of the test, the amount of urine collected (if necessary), and the time of specimen transport to the laboratory. Document any use of restraints, any complications, and the patient's tolerance of the procedure. Note the patient's and family's responses to any teaching.

URINE COLLECTION, TIMED

Because hormones, proteins, and electrolytes are excreted in small, variable amounts in urine, specimens for measuring these substances must typically be collected over an extended period to yield quantities of diagnostic value.

A 24-hour specimen is used most commonly because it provides an average excretion rate for substances eliminated during this period. Timed specimens may also be collected for shorter periods, such as 2 or 12 hours, depending on the specific information needed.

A timed urine specimen may also be collected after administering a challenge dose of a chemical — inulin, for example — to detect various renal disorders.

Key nursing diagnoses and patient outcomes

Impaired urinary elimination related to (specify)
The patient will:
▶ voice understanding of treatment
▶ avoid or minimize complications.

Deficient knowledge related to lack of exposure to procedure
The patient will:
▶ verbalize understanding of the need for the procedure
▶ demonstrate correct procedure for obtaining urine specimen.

Equipment

Large collection container with a cap or stopper or a commercial plastic container • preservative, if necessary • gloves • bedpan or urinal if patient doesn't have an indwelling catheter • graduated container if patient is on intake and output measurement • ice-filled container if a refrigerator isn't available • label • laboratory request form • four patient-care reminders

Check with the laboratory to find out which preservatives may need to be added to the specimen or whether a dark collection container is required.

Implementation

▶ Explain the procedure to the patient and his family, as necessary, *to enlist their cooperation and prevent accidental disposal of urine during the collection period.* Emphasize that failure to collect even one specimen during the collection period invalidates the test and requires that it begin again.

▶ Place patient-care reminders over the patient's bed, in his bathroom, on the bedpan hopper in the utility room, and on the urinal or indwelling catheter collection bag. Include the patient's name and room number, the date, and the collection interval.

▶ Instruct the patient to save all urine during the collection period, to notify you after each voiding, and to avoid contaminating the urine with stool or toilet tissue. Explain any dietary or drug restrictions and make sure he understands and is willing to comply with them.

For 2-hour collection
▶ If possible, instruct the patient to drink two to four 8-oz (470- to 950-ml) glasses of water about 30 minutes before collection begins. After 30 minutes, tell him to void. Put on gloves and discard this specimen *so the patient starts the collection period with an empty bladder.*

▶ If ordered, administer a challenge dose of medication (such as glucose solution or corticotropin) and record the time.

▶ After each voiding, put on gloves and add the specimen to the collection container.

▶ Instruct the patient to void about 15 minutes before the end of the collection period, if possible, and add this specimen to the collection container.

▶ At the end of the collection period, remove and discard your gloves and send the appropriately labeled collection container to the laboratory immediately, along with a properly completed laboratory request form.

For 12- and 24-hour collection
▶ Put on gloves and ask the patient to void. Discard this urine *so the patient*

starts *the collection period with an empty bladder.* Record the time.

▶ After putting on gloves and pouring the first urine specimen into the collection container, add the required preservative. Refrigerate the bottle or keep it on ice until the next voiding, as appropriate.

▶ Collect all urine voided during the prescribed period. Just before the collection period ends, ask the patient to void again, if possible. Add this last specimen to the collection container, pack it in ice *to inhibit deterioration of the specimen* and remove and discard your gloves. Label the collection container and send it to the laboratory with a properly completed laboratory request form.

Special considerations
▶ Keep the patient well hydrated before and during the test *to ensure adequate urine flow.*

▶ Before collection of a timed specimen, make sure the laboratory will be open when the collection period ends *to help ensure prompt, accurate results.* Never store a specimen in a refrigerator that contains food or medication to avoid contamination. If the patient has an indwelling catheter in place, put the collection bag in an ice-filled container at his bedside.

▶ Instruct the patient to avoid exercise and ingestion of coffee, tea, or any drugs (unless directed otherwise by the doctor) before the test *to avoid altering test results.*

Home care
If the patient must continue collecting urine at home, provide written instructions for the appropriate method. Tell the patient that he can keep the collection container in a brown bag in his re-

frigerator at home, separate from other refrigerator contents.

Documentation

Record the date and intervals of specimen collection and when the collection container was sent to the laboratory.

URINE GLUCOSE AND KETONE TESTING

Reagent tablet and strip tests are used to monitor urine glucose and ketone levels and to screen for diabetes. Urine glucose tests are less accurate than blood glucose tests and are used less frequently because of the increasing convenience of blood self-testing. Urine ketone tests monitor fat metabolism, help diagnose carbohydrate deprivation and diabetic ketoacidosis, and help distinguish between diabetic and nondiabetic coma.

The copper reduction test (Clinitest tablet test) measures the concentration of reducing substances in the urine through the reactions of these substances with a tablet composed of sodium hydroxide, cupric sulfate, and other reagents. When the tablet is added to a test tube containing drops of water and urine, the reaction generates heat. Simultaneously, the reduction of cupric ions in the presence of glucose causes a color change. Comparison of the test color with a standardized color chart gives the approximate level of urine glucose. Similarly, the Acetest tablet test produces a color reaction that allows an estimate of urine ketone levels by comparing the color changes with a standardized color chart.

Glucose oxidase tests (such as Diastix, Tes-Tape, and Clinistix strips) pro-

duce color changes when patches of reagents implanted in handheld plastic strips react with glucose in the patient's urine; urine ketone strip tests (such as Keto-Diastix and Ketostix) are similar. All test results are read by comparing color changes with a standardized reference chart.

Key nursing diagnoses and patient outcomes

Anxiety related to lack of exposure to procedure
The patient will:
▶ communicate feelings of anxiety.

Deficient knowledge related to lack of exposure to procedure
The patient will:
▶ verbalize understanding of need for procedure
▶ demonstrate correct procedure for obtaining urine specimen.

Equipment

For reagent tablet test
Specimen container • 10-ml test tube • medicine dropper • gloves • Clinitest or Acetest tablet • Clinitest or Acetest color chart

For reagent strip test
Specimen container • gloves • glucose or ketone test strip • reference color chart

Implementation

▶ Explain the test to the patient and, if he's a newly diagnosed diabetic, teach him how to perform the test himself. Check his history for medications that may interfere with test results.
▶ Before each test, instruct the patient not to contaminate the urine specimen with stool or toilet tissue.

▶ Test the urine specimen immediately after the patient voids.

Clinitest tablet test
▶ Ask the patient to void and then ask him to drink a glass of water, if possible. Put on gloves and collect a second-voided urine specimen 30 to 45 minutes later.
▶ Perform the five-drop test: With the medicine dropper, transfer 5 drops of urine from the specimen container to the test tube. Rinse the dropper and add 10 drops of water to the test tube. Add one Clinitest tablet to the test tube.
▶ Hold the test tube near the top during the reaction *because the test solution will come to a boil.* Observe the color change that occurs during the reaction.
▶ Fifteen seconds after effervescence subsides, shake the tube gently. Observe the solution's color and compare it with the Clinitest color chart.
▶ Remove and discard gloves and record the test results. Ignore any changes that develop after 15 seconds.
▶ If the color changes rapidly in the five-drop test, record the result as "over 2%" glycosuria.
▶ Alternatively, perform the two-drop test: Transfer two drops of urine from the specimen container to the test tube and then add 10 drops of water and a Clinitest tablet. After the reaction, observe the color of the test solution and compare it with the Clinitest color chart.
▶ Remove and discard your gloves and record the test results.
▶ Rapid color change in the two-drop test indicates glycosuria up to 5%.

Acetest tablet test
▶ Put on gloves and collect a second-voided specimen, as for the Clinitest tablet test.

▶ Place the Acetest tablet on a piece of white paper and, using the medicine dropper, place one drop of urine on the tablet.
▶ After 30 seconds, compare the tablet's color (white, lavender, or purple) with the Acetest color chart. Remove and discard your gloves and record the test results.

Glucose oxidase strip tests
▶ Explain the test to the patient and, if he's diagnosed as diabetic, teach him to perform it himself. Check his history for medications that may interfere with test results. Put on gloves before collecting a specimen for the test and remove them to record test results.
▶ Instruct the patient to void. Ask him to drink a glass of water, if possible, and collect a second-voided specimen after 30 to 45 minutes.
▶ If you're using a *Clinistix* strip, dip the reagent end of the strip into the urine for 2 seconds. Remove excess urine by tapping the strip against the specimen container's rim, wait for exactly 10 seconds, and then compare its color with the color chart on the test strip container. Ignore color changes that occur after 10 seconds. Record the result.
▶ If you're using a *Diastix* strip, dip the reagent end of the strip into the urine for 2 seconds. Tap off excess urine from the strip, wait for exactly 30 seconds, and then compare the strip's color with the color chart on the test strip container. Ignore color changes that occur after 30 seconds. Record the result.
▶ If you're using a *Tes-Tape* strip, pull about $1\frac{1}{2}$" (4 cm) of the reagent strip from the dispenser and dip one end about $\frac{1}{4}$" (0.5 cm) into the specimen for 2 seconds. Tap off excess urine from the strip, wait exactly 60 seconds, and

then compare the darkest part of the tape with the color chart on the dispenser. If the test result exceeds 0.5%, wait an additional 60 seconds and make a final comparison. Record the result.

Ketone strip test

▶ Explain the test to the patient and, if he's diagnosed as diabetic, teach him to perform it himself. Check his medication history. If he's receiving phenazopyridine or levodopa, use an Acetest tablet instead *because a reagent strip will give inaccurate results.*
▶ Put on gloves and collect a second-voided midstream specimen.
▶ If you're using a *Ketostix* strip, dip the reagent end of the strip into the specimen and remove it immediately. Wait exactly 15 seconds and then compare the color of the strip with the color chart on the test strip container. Ignore color changes that occur after 15 seconds. Remove and discard your gloves and record the test result.
▶ If you're using a *Keto-Diastix* strip, dip the reagent end of the strip into the specimen and remove it immediately. Tap off excess urine from the strip and hold the strip horizontally *to prevent mixing of chemicals between the two reagent squares.* Wait exactly 15 seconds and then compare the color of the ketone part of the strip with the color chart on the test strip container. After 30 seconds, compare the color of the glucose part of the strip with the color chart. Remove and discard gloves and record the test results.

Special considerations

Keep reagent tablets and strips in a cool, dry place at a temperature below 86° F (30° C), but don't refrigerate them. Keep the container tightly closed.

Don't use discolored or outdated tablets or strips.

Wear gloves as barrier protection when performing all urine tests.

Nursing alert **Clinitest tablets contain caustic soda. If you must handle these tablets, keep your fingers dry *to prevent the tablet from leaving a deposit, which could then be accidentally ingested or brought into contact with the eyes, skin, mucous membranes, or clothing, causing caustic burns.***

Documentation

Record test results according to the information on the reagent containers, or use a flowchart designed to record this information. Indicate whether the doctor was notified of the test results. If you're teaching a patient how to perform the test, keep a record of his progress. Also, record any treatment given as a result of the testing.

URINE pH TESTING

The pH of urine — its alkalinity or acidity — reflects the kidneys' ability to maintain a normal hydrogen ion concentration in plasma and extracellular fluids. The normal hydrogen ion concentration in urine varies, ranging from pH 4.6 to 8.0, but it usually averages around pH 6.0.

The simplest procedure for testing the pH of urine consists of dipping a reagent strip (such as Combistix) into a fresh specimen of the patient's urine and comparing the resultant color change with a standardized color chart.

An alkaline pH (above 7.0), resulting from a diet low in meat but high in vegetables, dairy products, and citrus fruits, causes turbidity and the formation of phosphate, carbonate, and amorphous crystals. Alkaline urine may also result from urinary tract infection and from metabolic or respiratory alkalosis.

An acid pH (below 7.0), resulting from a high-protein diet, also causes turbidity as well as the formation of oxalate, cystine, amorphous urate, and uric acid crystals. Acid urine may also result from renal tuberculosis, phenylketonuria, alkaptonuria, pyrexia, diarrhea, starvation, and all forms of acidosis.

Measuring urine pH can also help monitor some medications, such as methenamine, that are active only at certain pH levels.

Key nursing diagnoses and patient outcomes

Anxiety related to lack of exposure to procedure
The patient will:
▶ communicate feelings of anxiety.

Deficient knowledge related to lack of exposure to procedure
The patient will:
▶ verbalize understanding of need for procedure
▶ demonstrate correct procedure for obtaining urine specimen.

Equipment

Clean-catch kit • urine specimen container • gloves • reagent strips (the reagent strip has a pH indicator as part of a battery of indicators)

Implementation

▶ Wash your hands thoroughly and put on gloves.
▶ Provide the patient with a specimen container and instruct him to collect a clean-catch midstream specimen. (See "Urine collection, adult," page 900.)

Dip the reagent strip into the urine, remove it, and tap off the excess urine from the strip.
▶ Hold the strip horizontally *to avoid mixing reagents from adjacent test areas on the strip.* Then compare the color on the strip with the standardized color chart on the strip package. This comparison can be made up to 60 seconds after immersing the strip.
▶ Discard the urine specimen. If you're monitoring the patient's intake and output, measure the amount of urine discarded.
▶ Remove and discard your gloves and wash your hands thoroughly *to prevent cross-contamination.*

Special considerations

▶ Use only a fresh urine specimen *because bacterial growth at room temperature changes urine pH.*
▶ Avoid letting a drop of urine run off the reagent strip onto adjacent reagent spots on the strip *because the other reagents can change the pH result.*
▶ Be aware that urine collected at night is usually more acidic than urine collected during the day.

Documentation

Record test results, time of voiding, and amount voided.

URINE SPECIFIC GRAVITY

The kidneys maintain homeostasis by varying urine output and urine concentration of dissolved salts. Urine specific gravity measures the concentration of urine solutes, which reflects the kidneys' capacity to concentrate urine. The capacity to concentrate urine is among the first functions lost when renal tubular damage occurs.

Using a urinometer

With the urinometer floating in a cylinder of urine, position your eye at a level even with the bottom of the meniscus and read the specific gravity from the scale printed on the urinometer.

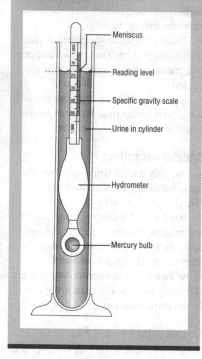

- Meniscus
- Reading level
- Specific gravity scale
- Urine in cylinder
- Hydrometer
- Mercury bulb

Urine specific gravity is determined by comparing the weight of a urine specimen with that of an equivalent volume of distilled water, which is 1.000. Because urine contains dissolved salts and other substances, it's heavier than 1.000. Urine specific gravity ranges from 1.003 (very dilute) to 1.035 (highly concentrated); normal values range from 1.010 to 1.025. Specific gravity is measured with a urinometer (a specially calibrated hydrometer designed to float

in a cylinder of urine), a refractometer, which measures the refraction of light as it passes through a urine specimen, or a reagent strip test.

Elevated specific gravity reflects an increased concentration of urine solutes, which occurs in conditions that cause renal hypoperfusion, and may indicate heart failure, dehydration, hepatic disorders, or nephrosis. Low specific gravity reflects failure to reabsorb water and concentrate urine; it may indicate hypercalcemia, hypokalemia, alkalosis, acute renal failure, pyelonephritis, glomerulonephritis, or diabetes insipidus.

Key nursing diagnoses and patient outcomes

Deficient knowledge related to lack of exposure to procedure
The patient will:
► verbalize understanding of need for procedure
► demonstrate correct procedure for obtaining urine specimen.

Equipment

Calibrated urinometer and cylinder, refractometer, or reagent strips (Multistix) • gloves • specimen container

Implementation

► Explain the procedure to the patient and tell him when you'll need the specimen. Explain why you're withholding fluids and for how long *to ensure his cooperation.*

Measuring with a urinometer

► Put on gloves and collect a random urine specimen. Let the specimen reach room temperature (71.6° F [22° C]) before testing *because this is the tempera-*

ture at which most urinometers are calibrated.

▶ Fill the cylinder about three-fourths full of urine. Then gently spin the urinometer and drop it into the cylinder.

▶ When the urinometer stops bobbing, read the specific gravity from the calibrated scale marked directly on the stem of the urinometer. Make sure the instrument floats freely and doesn't touch the sides of the cylinder. Read the scale at the lowest point of the meniscus to ensure an accurate reading. (For specific instructions, see Using a urinometer.)

▶ Discard the urine and rinse the cylinder and urinometer in cool water. Warm water coagulates proteins in urine, making them stick to the instrument.

▶ Remove your gloves and wash your hands thoroughly to prevent cross-contamination.

Measuring with a refractometer
▶ Put on gloves and collect a random or controlled urine specimen.

▶ Place a single drop of urine on the refractometer slide.

▶ Turn on the light and look through the eyepiece to see the specific gravity indicated on a scale. (Some instruments have a digital display.)

Measuring with a reagent strip
▶ Put on gloves and obtain a random or controlled urine specimen.

▶ Dip the reagent end of the test strip into the specimen for 2 seconds.

▶ Tap the strip on the rim of the specimen container to remove excess urine and compare the resultant color change with the color chart supplied with the kit.

Special considerations
Test the urinometer in distilled water at room temperature to ensure that its calibration is 1.000. If necessary, correct the urinometer reading for temperature effects; add 0.001 to your observed reading for every 5.4° F (3° C) above the calibration temperature of 71.6° F (22° C); subtract 0.001 for every 5.4° F below 71.6° F.

Documentation
Record the specific gravity, volume, color, odor, and appearance of the collected urine specimen. Indicate whether the doctor was made aware of the test results.

URINE STRAINING FOR CALCULI

Renal calculi, or kidney stones, may develop anywhere in the urinary tract. They may be excreted with the urine or become lodged in the urinary tract, causing hematuria, urine retention, renal colic and, possibly, hydronephrosis.

Testing for the presence of calculi requires careful straining of all the patient's urine through a gauze pad or fine-mesh sieve and, at times, quantitative laboratory analysis of questionable specimens. Such testing typically continues until the patient passes the calculi or until surgery, as ordered.

Key nursing diagnoses and patient outcomes
Impaired urinary elimination related to medical condition
The patient will:
▶ voice understanding of treatment
▶ avoid or minimize complications.

Deficient knowledge related to lack of exposure to procedure
The patient will:
▶ state or demonstrate what has been taught
▶ demonstrate ability to perform new health-related behaviors as taught.

Acute pain related to medical condition
The patient will:
▶ state feeling of comfort and relief from pain
▶ state and carry out appropriate interventions for pain relief.

Equipment

Fine-mesh sieve or 4" × 4" gauze pad • graduated container • urinal or bedpan • gloves • laboratory request form • three patient-care reminders • specimen container (for use if calculi are found)

Implementation

▶ Explain the procedure to the patient and his family, if possible, *to ensure cooperation and to stress the importance of straining all the patient's urine.*
▶ Post a patient-care reminder stating "STRAIN ALL URINE" over the patient's bed, in his bathroom, and on the collection container.
▶ Tell the patient to notify you after each voiding.
▶ If a commercial strainer isn't available, unfold a 4" × 4" gauze pad, place it over the top of a graduated measuring container and secure it with a rubber band.
▶ Put on gloves. With the strainer secured over the mouth of the collection container, pour the specimen from the urinal or bedpan into the container. If the patient has an indwelling catheter

in place, strain all urine from the collection bag before discarding it.
▶ Examine the strainer for calculi. If you detect calculi or if the filter looks questionable, notify the doctor, place the filtrate in a specimen container, and send it to the laboratory with a laboratory request form.
▶ If the strainer is intact, rinse it carefully and reuse it. If it has become damaged, discard it and replace it with a new strainer. Remove and discard your gloves.

Special considerations

▶ Save and send to the laboratory any small or suspicious-looking residue in the specimen container *because even tiny calculi can cause hematuria and pain.*
▶ Be aware that calculi may appear in various colors, each of which has diagnostic value.

Home care

If the patient will be straining his urine at home, teach him how to use a strainer and the importance of straining all his urine for the prescribed period.

Documentation

Chart the time of the specimen collection and transport to the laboratory, if necessary. Describe any filtrate passed and note any pain or hematuria that occurred during the voiding.

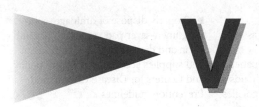

VACUUM-ASSISTED CLOSURE PRESSURE THERAPY

Vacuum-assisted closure pressure therapy, also known as negative pressure wound therapy, is used to enhance delayed or impaired wound healing. The vacuum-assisted closure device applies localized subatmospheric pressure to draw the edges of the wound toward the center. A special dressing is placed in the wound or over a graft or flap and vacuum-assisted closure therapy is applied. This wound packing removes fluids from the wound and stimulates growth of healthy granulation tissue.

Vacuum-assisted closure therapy is indicated for acute and traumatic wounds, pressure ulcers, and chronic open wounds, such as diabetic ulcers, meshed grafts, and skin flaps. It's contraindicated for fistulas that involve organs or body cavities, necrotic tissue with eschar, untreated osteomyelitis, and malignant wounds. This therapy should be used cautiously in patients with active bleeding, in those taking anticoagulants, and when achieving wound hemostasis has been difficult.

Key nursing diagnoses and patient outcomes

Risk for infection related to delayed wound healing

The patient will:
▶ have vital signs, temperature, and laboratory values remain within normal limits
▶ have wound site free from signs and symptoms of infection.

Impaired skin integrity related to delayed wound healing
The patient will:
▶ regain normal skin integrity (wound decreases in size by [specify])
▶ communicate an understanding of skin protection measures
▶ communicate feelings about change in body image.

Equipment

Waterproof trash bag • goggles • gown, if indicated • emesis basin • normal saline solution • clean gloves • sterile gloves • sterile scissors • linen-saver pad • 35-ml piston syringe with 19G catheter • reticulated foam • fenestrated tubing • evacuation tubing • skin protectant wipe • transparent occlusive air-permeable drape • evacuation canister • vacuum unit

Preparation of equipment

Assemble the vacuum-assisted closure device at the bedside per manufacturer's instructions. Set negative pressure according to the doctor's order (25 to 200 mm Hg).

Implementation

▶ Check the doctor's order and assess the patient's condition.

▶ Explain the procedure to the patient, provide privacy, and wash your hands. If necessary, put on a gown and goggles *to protect yourself from wound drainage and contamination.*

▶ Place a linen-saver pad under the patient *to catch any spills and avoid linen changes.* Position the patient to allow maximum wound exposure. Place the emesis basin under the wound *to collect any drainage.*

▶ Put on clean gloves. Remove the soiled dressing and discard it in the waterproof trash bag. Attach the 19G catheter to the 35-ml piston syringe and irrigate the wound thoroughly using the normal saline solution.

▶ Clean the area around the wound with normal saline solution; wipe intact skin with a skin protectant wipe and allow it to dry well. Remove and discard your gloves.

▶ Put on sterile gloves. Using sterile scissors cut the foam to the shape and measurement of the wound. More than one piece of foam may be necessary if the first piece is cut too small.

▶ Carefully place the foam in the wound. Next, place the fenestrated tubing into the center of the foam. *The fenestrated tubing embedded into the foam delivers negative pressure to the wound.*

▶ Place the transparent occlusive air permeable drape over the foam, enclosing the foam and the tubing together. Remove and discard your gloves.

▶ Connect the free end of the fenestrated tubing to the tubing that is connected to the evacuation canister.

▶ Turn on the vacuum unit.

▶ Make sure the patient is comfortable.

▶ Properly dispose of drainage, solution, linen-saver pad, and trash bag and clean and dispose of soiled equipment and supplies according to facility policy and Centers for Disease Control and Prevention guidelines.

Special considerations

▶ Change the dressing every 48 hours. Try to coordinate dressing change with the doctor's visit *so he can inspect the wound.*

▶ Measure the amount of drainage every shift.

▶ Audible and visual alarms alert you if the unit is tipped greater than 45 degrees, the canister is full, the dressing has an air leak, or the canister becomes dislodged.

Complications

Cleaning and care of wounds may temporarily increase the patient's pain and increases the risk for infection.

Documentation

Document the frequency and duration of therapy, the amount of negative pressure applied, the size and condition of the wound, and the patient's response to treatment.

VAGAL MANEUVERS

When a patient suffers sinus, atrial, or junctional tachyarrhythmias, vagal maneuvers — Valsalva's maneuver and carotid sinus massage — can slow his heart rate. These maneuvers work by stimulating nerve endings, which respond as they would to an increase in blood pressure. They send this message to the brain stem, which in turn stimulates the autonomic nervous system to increase vagal tone and decrease the heart rate.

Vagal maneuvers are contraindicated for patients with severe coronary artery disease, acute myocardial infarction, or hypovolemia. Carotid sinus massage is contraindicated for patients with digitalis toxicity or cerebrovascular disease and for patients who have had carotid surgery.

Although usually performed by a doctor, vagal maneuvers may also be done by a specially prepared nurse under a doctor's supervision.

Key nursing diagnoses and patient outcomes

Anxiety related to situational crisis
The patient will:
▶ state at least two ways to eliminate or minimize anxious behaviors
▶ report being able to cope with current situation without experiencing severe anxiety.

Deficient knowledge related to lack of exposure to vagal maneuvers
The patient will:
▶ communicate a need to know about the procedure
▶ state or demonstrate understanding of procedure.

Equipment

Crash cart with emergency medications and airway equipment • electrocardiogram (ECG) monitor and electrodes • I.V. catheter and tubing • tourniquet • dextrose 5% in water (D_5W) • optional: shaving supplies, if needed, and cardiotonic drugs

Implementation

▶ Explain the procedure to the patient *to ease his fears and promote cooperation.*

Ask him to let you know if he feels light-headed.
▶ Place the patient in a supine position. Insert an I.V. line, if necessary. Then administer D_5W at a keep-vein-open rate, as ordered. *This line will be used if emergency drugs become necessary.*
▶ Prepare the patient's skin, including shaving, if necessary, and attach ECG electrodes. Adjust the size of the ECG complexes on the monitor *so that you can see the arrhythmia clearly.*

Valsalva's maneuver

▶ Ask the patient to take a deep breath and bear down, as if he were trying to defecate. If he doesn't feel light-headed or dizzy, and if no new arrhythmias occur, have him hold his breath and bear down for 10 seconds.
▶ If he does feel dizzy or light-headed, or if you see a new arrhythmia on the monitor — asystole for more than 6 seconds, frequent premature ventricular contractions (PVCs), or ventricular tachycardia or ventricular fibrillation — allow him to exhale and stop bearing down.
▶ After 10 seconds, ask him to exhale and breathe quietly. If the maneuver was successful, the monitor will show his heart rate slowing before he exhales.

Carotid sinus massage

▶ Begin by obtaining a rhythm strip, using the lead that shows the strongest P waves.
▶ Auscultate both carotid sinuses. If you detect bruits, inform the doctor and don't perform carotid sinus massage. If you don't detect bruits, proceed as ordered. (See *Location and technique for carotid sinus massage,* page 918.)
▶ Monitor the ECG throughout the procedure. Stop massaging when the

Location and technique for carotid sinus massage

Before applying manual pressure to the patient's right carotid sinus, locate the bifurcation of the carotid artery on the right side of the neck. Turn the patient's head slightly to the left and hyperextend the neck. This brings the carotid artery closer to the skin and moves the sternocleidomastoid muscle away from the carotid artery.

Then, using a circular motion, gently massage the right carotid sinus between your fingers and the transverse processes of the spine for 3 to 5 seconds. Don't massage for more than 5 seconds to avoid risking life-threatening complications.

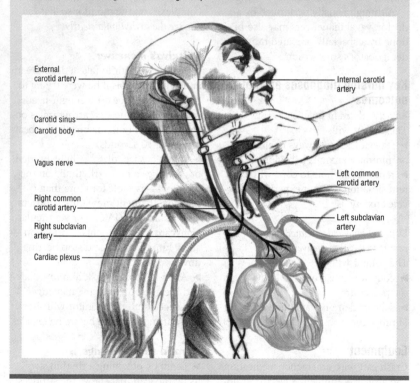

ventricular rate slows sufficiently to permit diagnosis of the rhythm. Or, stop as soon as any evidence of a rhythm change appears. Have the crash cart handy *to give emergency treatment if a dangerous arrhythmia occurs.*

▶ If the procedure has no effect within 5 seconds, stop massaging the right carotid sinus and begin to massage the left. If this also fails, administer cardiotonic drugs as ordered.

Special considerations

▶ Remember that a brief period of asystole — from 3 to 6 seconds — and

Adverse effects of vagal maneuvers

Both Valsalva's maneuver and carotid sinus massage are useful for slowing heart rate. However, they can cause complications, some of which are life-threatening.

Valsalva's maneuver

Valsalva's maneuver can cause bradycardia, accompanied by a decrease in cardiac output, possibly leading to syncope. The bradycardia will usually pass quickly; if it doesn't or if it advances to complete heart block or asystole, begin basic life support followed, if necessary, by advanced cardiac life support.

Valsalva's maneuver can mobilize venous thrombi and cause bleeding. Monitor the patient for signs and symptoms of vascular occlusion, including neurologic changes, chest discomfort, and dyspnea. Report such problems at once, and prepare the patient for diagnostic testing or transfer to the intensive care unit (ICU), as ordered.

Carotid sinus massage

Because carotid sinus massage can cause ventricular fibrillation, ventricular tachycardia, and standstill as well as worsening atrioventricular block that leads to junctional or ventricular escape rhythms, you'll need to monitor the patient's electrocardiogram (ECG) closely. If his ECG indicates complete heart block or asystole, start basic life support at once, followed by advanced cardiac life support. If emergency medications don't convert the complete heart block, the patient may need a temporary pacemaker.

Carotid sinus massage can cause cerebral damage from inadequate tissue perfusion, especially in elderly patients. It can also cause a cerebrovascular accident, either from decreased perfusion caused by total carotid artery blockage or from migrating endothelial plaque loosened by carotid sinus compression. Watch the patient carefully during and after the procedure for changes in neurologic status. If you note any, tell the doctor at once and prepare the patient for further diagnostic tests or transfer to the ICU, as ordered.

---

several PVCs may precede conversion to normal sinus rhythm.

▶ If the vagal maneuver succeeded in slowing the patient's heart rate and converting the arrhythmia, continue monitoring him for several hours.

Complications

Use caution when performing carotid sinus massage on elderly patients, patients receiving digoxin, and patients with heart block, hypertension, coronary artery disease, diabetes mellitus, or hyperkalemia. The procedure may cause arterial pressure to plummet in these patients, although it usually rises quickly afterward.

 Age alert Elderly patients with heart disease are especially susceptible to the adverse effects of vagal maneuvers.

Vagal maneuvers can occasionally cause bradycardia or complete heart block, so monitor the patient's cardiac rhythm closely. (See *Adverse effects of vagal maneuvers*.)

Documentation

Record the date and time of the procedure, who performed it, and why it was necessary. Note the patient's response, any complications, and the interventions taken. If possible, obtain a rhythm strip before, during, and after the procedure.

VENIPUNCTURE

Performed to obtain a venous blood sample, venipuncture involves piercing a vein with a needle and collecting blood in a syringe or evacuated tube. Typically, venipuncture is performed using the antecubital fossa. If necessary, however, it can be performed on a vein in the wrist, the dorsum of the hand or foot, or another accessible location.

Equipment

Tourniquet • gloves • syringe or evacuated tubes and needle holder • alcohol or povidone-iodine sponges • 20G or 21G needle for the forearm or 25G needle for the wrist, hand, and ankle, and for children • color-coded collection tubes containing appropriate additives • labels • laboratory request form • 2″ × 2″ gauze pads • adhesive bandage

Preparation of equipment

If you're using evacuated tubes, open the needle packet, attach the needle to its holder, and select the appropriate tubes. If you're using a syringe, attach the appropriate needle to it. Be sure to choose a syringe large enough to hold all the blood required for the test. Label all collection tubes clearly with the patient's name and room number, the doctor's name, and the date and time of collection.

Implementation

▶ Wash your hands thoroughly and put on gloves.
▶ Tell the patient that you're about to collect a blood sample and explain the procedure to ease his anxiety and ensure his cooperation. Ask him if he's ever felt faint, sweaty, or nauseated when having blood drawn.
▶ If the patient is on bed rest, ask him to lie supine, with his head slightly elevated and his arms at his sides. Ask the ambulatory patient to sit in a chair and support his arm securely on an armrest or a table.
▶ Assess the patient's veins to determine the best puncture site. (See *Common venipuncture sites.*) Observe the skin for the vein's blue color, or palpate the vein for a firm rebound sensation.
▶ Tie a tourniquet 2″ (5.1 cm) proximal to the area chosen. By impeding venous return to the heart while still allowing arterial flow, a tourniquet produces venous dilation. If arterial perfusion remains adequate, you'll be able to feel the radial pulse. (If the tourniquet fails to dilate the vein, have the patient open and close his fist repeatedly. Then ask him to close his fist as you insert the needle and to open it again when the needle is in place.)
▶ Clean the venipuncture site with an alcohol or a povidone-iodine pad. Don't wipe off the povidone-iodine with alcohol because alcohol cancels the effect of povidone-iodine. Wipe in a circular motion, spiraling outward from the site to avoid introducing potentially infectious skin flora into the vessel during the procedure. If you use alcohol, apply it with friction for 30 seconds or until the final pad comes away clean. Allow the skin to dry before performing venipuncture.
▶ Immobilize the vein by pressing just below the venipuncture site with your thumb and drawing the skin taut.
▶ Position the needle holder or syringe with the needle bevel up and the shaft parallel to the path of the vein and at a 30-degree angle to the arm. Insert the

Common venipuncture sites

The illustrations below show the anatomic locations of veins commonly used for venipuncture. The most commonly used sites are on the forearm, followed by those on the hand.

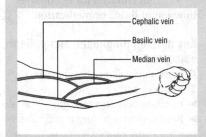

Cephalic vein
Basilic vein
Median vein

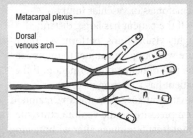

Metacarpal plexus
Dorsal venous arch

needle into the vein. If you're using a syringe, venous blood will appear in the hub; withdraw the blood slowly, pulling the plunger of the syringe gently to create steady suction until you obtain the required sample. *Pulling the plunger too forcibly may collapse the vein.* If you're using a needle holder and an evacuated tube, grasp the holder securely to stabilize it in the vein and push down on the collection tube until the needle punctures the rubber stopper. Blood will flow into the tube automatically.

▶ Remove the tourniquet as soon as blood flows adequately *to prevent stasis and hemoconcentration, which can impair test results.* If the flow is sluggish, leave the tourniquet in place longer, but always remove it before withdrawing the needle.

▶ Continue to fill the required tubes, removing one and inserting another. Gently rotate each tube as you remove it *to help mix the additive with the sample.*

▶ After you've drawn the sample, place a gauze pad over the puncture site and slowly and gently remove the needle from the vein. When using an evacuated tube, remove it from the needle holder to release the vacuum before withdrawing the needle from the vein.

▶ Apply gentle pressure to the puncture site for 2 to 3 minutes or until bleeding stops. *This prevents extravasation into the surrounding tissue, which can cause a hematoma.*

▶ After bleeding stops, apply an adhesive bandage.

▶ If you've used a syringe, transfer the sample to a collection tube. Detach the needle from the syringe, open the collection tube, and gently empty the sample into the tube, being careful to avoid foaming, which can cause hemolysis.

▶ Finally, check the venipuncture site to see if a hematoma has developed. If it has, apply warm soaks to the site.

▶ Discard syringes, needles, and used gloves in the appropriate containers.

Special considerations

▶ Never collect a venous sample from an arm or a leg that is already being used for I.V. therapy or blood administration because this may affect test results. Don't collect a venous sample from an infection site because this may introduce pathogens into the vascular system. Likewise, avoid collecting blood from edematous areas, arteriovenous shunts, and sites of previous hematomas or vascular injury.

▶ If the patient has large, distended, highly visible veins, perform venipuncture without a tourniquet to minimize the risk of hematoma formation. If the patient has a clotting disorder or is receiving anticoagulant therapy, maintain firm pressure on the venipuncture site for at least 5 minutes after withdrawing the needle to prevent hematoma formation.

▶ Avoid using veins in the patient's legs for venipuncture, if possible, because this increases the risk of thrombophlebitis.

Complications

A hematoma at the needle insertion site is the most common complication of venipuncture. Infection may result from poor technique.

Documentation

Record the date, time, and site of the venipuncture; the name of the test; the time the sample was sent to the laboratory; the amount of blood collected; the patient's temperature; and any adverse reactions to the procedure.

VOLUME-CONTROL SET USE

A volume-control set — an I.V. line with a graduated chamber — delivers precise amounts of fluid and shuts off when the fluid is exhausted, preventing air

from entering the I.V. line. It may be used as a secondary line in adults for intermittent infusion of medication.

 Age alert A volume-control set is used as a primary line in children for continuous infusion of fluids or medication.

Key nursing diagnoses and patient outcomes

Deficient fluid volume related to (specify)
The patient will:
▶ maintain normal vital signs
▶ have normal skin turgor and moist mucous membranes
▶ have adequate urine output
▶ maintain normal electrolyte levels.

Equipment

Volume-control set • I.V. pole (for setting up a primary I.V. line) • I.V. solution • 20G to 22G 1″ needle or needle-free adapter • alcohol pads • medication in labeled syringe • tape • label

Preparation of equipment

Ensure the sterility of all equipment and inspect it carefully *to ensure the absence of flaws.* Take the equipment to the patient's bedside.

Implementation

▶ Wash your hands and explain the procedure to the patient. If an I.V. line is already in place, observe its insertion site for signs of infiltration and infection.

▶ Remove the volume-control set from its box and close all the clamps.

▶ Remove the protective cap from the volume-control set spike, insert the spike into the I.V. solution container, and hang the container on the I.V. pole.

▶ Open the air vent clamp and close the upper slide clamp. Then open the lower clamp on the I.V. tubing, slide it upward until it's slightly below the drip chamber, and close the clamp (as shown below).

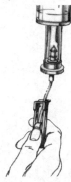

► If you're using a valve set, open the upper clamp until the fluid chamber fills with about 30 ml of solution. Then close the clamp and carefully squeeze the drip chamber until it is half full.

► If you're using a volume-control set with a membrane filter, open the upper clamp until the fluid chamber fills with about 30 ml of solution and then close the clamp.

► Open the lower clamp and squeeze the drip chamber flat with two fingers of your opposite hand. *If you squeeze the drip chamber with the lower clamp closed, you'll damage the membrane filter.*

► Keeping the drip chamber flat, close the lower clamp. Now release the drip chamber so that it fills halfway.

► Open the lower clamp, prime the tubing, and close the clamp. To use the set as a primary line, insert the distal end of the tubing into the catheter or needle hub. To use the set as a secondary line, attach a needle to the adapter on the volume-control set. Wipe the Y-port of the primary tubing with an alcohol pad and insert the needle. Then tape the connection.

► If you're using a needle-free system, attach the distal end of the tubing to the Y-port of the primary tubing, following the manufacturer's instructions.

► To add medication, wipe the injection port on the volume-control set with an alcohol pad and inject the medication. Place a label on the chamber, indicating the drug, dose, and date. Don't write directly on the chamber *because the plastic absorbs ink.*

► Open the upper clamp, fill the fluid chamber with the prescribed amount of solution, and close the clamp. Gently rotate the chamber (as shown below) *to mix the medication.*

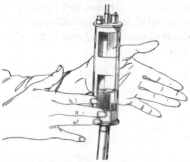

► Turn off the primary solution (if present) or lower the drip rate *to maintain an open line.*

► Open the lower clamp on the volume-control set and adjust the drip rate as ordered. After completion of the infusion, open the upper clamp and let 10 ml of I.V. solution flow into the chamber and through the tubing *to flush them.*

► If you're using the volume-control set as a secondary I.V. line, close the lower clamp and reset the flow rate of the primary line. If you're using the set as a primary I.V. line, close the lower clamp, refill the chamber to the prescribed amount, and begin the infusion again.

Special considerations

▶ Always check compatibility of the medication and the I.V. solution. If you're using a membrane-filter set, avoid administering suspensions, lipid emulsions, blood, or blood components through it.

▶ If the drip chamber of a floating-valve diaphragm set overfills, immediately close the upper clamp and air vent, invert the chamber, and squeeze the excess fluid from the drip chamber back into the graduated fluid chamber.

Documentation

If you add a drug to the volume-control set, record the amount and type of medication, amount of fluid used to dilute it, and date and time of the infusion.

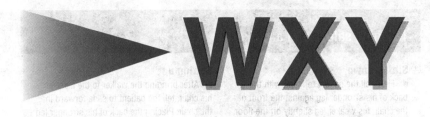

WALKER USE

A walker consists of a metal frame with handgrips and four legs that buttresses the patient on three sides. One side remains open. Because this device provides greater stability and security than other ambulatory aids, it's recommended for the patient with insufficient strength and balance to use crutches or a cane, or with weakness requiring frequent rest periods.

Attachments for standard walkers and modified walkers help meet special needs. For example, a walker may have a platform added to support an injured arm.

Key nursing diagnoses and patient outcomes

Deficient knowledge related to lack of exposure to walker procedure
The patient will:
▶ state or demonstrate understanding of what has been taught
▶ demonstrate ability to perform new health-related behaviors as they're taught.

Risk for injury related to improper technique
The patient will:
▶ identify factors that increase risk for injury

▶ assist in identifying and applying safety measures to prevent injury.

Equipment

Walker • platform or wheel attachments, as necessary

Various types of walkers are available. The standard walker is used by the patient with unilateral or bilateral weakness or an inability to bear weight on one leg. It requires arm strength and balance. Platform attachments may be added to a standard walker for the patient with arthritic arms or a casted arm, who can't bear weight directly on his hand, wrist, or forearm.

The stair walker, used by the patient who must negotiate stairs without bilateral hand-rails, requires good arm strength and balance. Its extra set of handles extends toward the patient on the open side. The rolling walker, used by the patient with very weak legs, has four wheels and a seat. The reciprocal walker, used by the patient with very weak arms, allows one side to be advanced ahead of the other.

Preparation of equipment

Obtain the appropriate walker with the advice of a physical therapist and adjust it to the patient's height: His elbows should be flexed at a 15-degree angle when standing comfortably within the walker with his hands on the grips. To

Teaching safe use of a walker

Sitting down

■ First, tell the patient to stand with the back of his stronger leg against the front of the chair, his weaker leg slightly off the floor, and the walker directly in front.

■ Tell him to grasp the armrests on the chair one arm at a time while supporting most of his weight on the stronger leg. (In the illustrations, the patient has left leg weakness.)

■ Tell the patient to lower himself into the chair and slide backward. After he is seated, he should place the walker beside the chair.

Getting up

■ After bringing the walker to the front of his chair, tell the patient to slide forward in the chair. Placing the back of his stronger leg against the seat, he should then advance the weaker leg.

■ Next, with both hands on the armrests, the patient can push himself to a standing position. Supporting himself with the stronger leg and the opposite hand, the patient should grasp the walker's handgrip with his free hand.

■ Then the patient should grasp the free handgrip with his other hand.

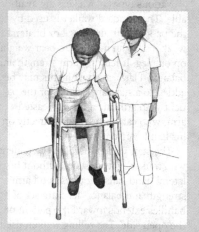
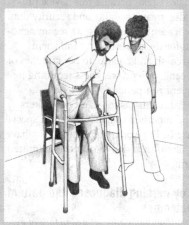

adjust the walker, turn it upside down and change the leg length by pushing in the button on each shaft and releasing it when the leg is in the correct position. Make sure the walker is level before the patient attempts to use it.

Implementation

▶ Help the patient stand within the walker and instruct him to hold the handgrips firmly and equally. Stand behind him, closer to the involved leg.

▶ If the patient has one-sided leg weakness, tell him to advance the walker 6″ to 8″ (15 to 20.5 cm) and step forward with the involved leg and follow with the uninvolved leg, supporting himself on his arms. Encourage him to take equal strides. If he has equal strength in both legs, instruct him to advance the walker 6″ to 8″ and step forward with either leg. If he can't use one leg, tell him to advance the walker 6" to 8" and to swing onto it, supporting his weight on his arms.

▶ If the patient is using a reciprocal walker, teach him the two-point gait. Instruct the patient to stand with his weight evenly distributed between his legs and the walker. Stand behind him, slightly to one side. Tell him to simultaneously advance the walker's right side and his left foot. Then have the patient advance the walker's left side and his right foot.

▶ If the patient is using a reciprocal walker, you may also teach him the four-point gait. Instruct the patient to evenly distribute his weight between his legs and the walker. Stand behind him and slightly to one side. Then have him move the right side of the walker forward. Then have the patient move his left foot forward. Next, instruct him to move the left side of the walker forward. Then have him move his right foot forward.

▶ If the patient is using a wheeled or stair walker, reinforce the physical therapist's instructions. Stress the need for caution when using a stair walker.

▶ Teach the patient how to use a chair safely. (See *Teaching safe use of a walker.*)

Special considerations
If the patient starts to fall, support his hips and shoulders to help him maintain an upright position if possible.

Documentation
Record the type of walker and attachments used, the degree of guarding required, the distance walked, and the patient's tolerance of ambulation.

WOUND DEHISCENCE AND EVISCERATION MANAGEMENT

Although surgical wounds typically heal without incident, occasionally the edges of a wound may fail to join or may separate even after they seem to be healing normally. This development, called wound dehiscence, may lead to an even more serious complication: evisceration, in which a portion of the viscera (usually a bowel loop) protrudes through the incision. Evisceration, in turn, can lead to peritonitis and septic shock. (See *Recognizing dehiscence and evisceration,* page 928.)

Key nursing diagnoses and patient outcomes
Deficient fluid volume related to active loss
The patient will:
▶ have vital signs remain stable
▶ have fluid and blood volume return to normal.

Ineffective tissue perfusion (specify type) related to decreased cellular exchange
The patient will:
▶ attain hemodynamic stability as evidenced by pulse not less than (specify) beats/minute and not more than (specify) beats/minute and blood pressure not less than (specify) mm Hg and not greater than (specify) mm Hg.

Equipment
Two sterile towels • 1 L of sterile normal saline solution • sterile irrigation set, including a basin, solution container, and 50-ml catheter-tip syringe • several large abdominal dressings • sterile, waterproof drape • linen-saver pads • sterile gloves

Recognizing dehiscence and evisceration

In wound dehiscence (top), the layers of the surgical wound separate. In evisceration (bottom), the viscera (in this case, a bowel loop) protrude through the surgical incision.

Wound dehiscence

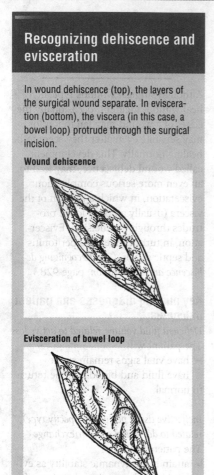

Evisceration of bowel loop

If the patient will return to the operating room, also gather the following equipment: I.V. administration set and I.V. fluids • equipment for nasogastric (NG) intubation • preoperative medications as ordered • suction apparatus.

Implementation

▶ Provide reassurance and support *to ease the patient's anxiety.* Tell him to stay

in bed. If possible, stay with him while someone else notifies the doctor and collects the necessary equipment.
▶ Place a linen-saver pad under the patient *to keep the sheets dry when you moisten the exposed viscera.*
▶ Using sterile technique, unfold a sterile towel to create a sterile field. Open the package containing the irrigation set and place the basin, solution container, and 50-ml syringe on the sterile field.
▶ Open the bottle of normal saline solution and pour about 400 ml into the solution container. Also pour about 200 ml into the sterile basin.
▶ Open several large abdominal dressings and place them on the sterile field.
▶ Put on the sterile gloves and place one or two of the large abdominal dressings into the basin *to saturate them with saline solution.*
▶ Place the moistened dressings over the exposed viscera. Then place a sterile, waterproof drape over the dressings *to prevent the sheets from getting wet.*
▶ Moisten the dressings every hour by withdrawing saline solution from the container through the syringe and then gently squirting the solution on the dressings.
▶ When you moisten the dressings, inspect the color of the viscera. If it appears dusky or black, notify the doctor immediately. *With its blood supply interrupted, a protruding organ may become ischemic and necrotic.*
▶ Keep the patient on absolute bed rest in low Fowler's position (elevated no more than 20 degrees) with his knees flexed. *This prevents injury and reduces stress on an abdominal incision.*
▶ Don't allow the patient to have anything by mouth *to decrease the risk of aspiration during surgery.*

▶ Monitor the patient's pulse, respirations, blood pressure, and temperature every 15 minutes *to detect shock.*

▶ If necessary, prepare the patient to return to the operating room.

▶ Continue to reassure the patient while you prepare him for surgery. Make sure that he has signed a consent form and that the operating room staff has been informed about the procedure.

Special considerations

▶ The best treatment is prevention. If you're caring for a postoperative patient who's at risk for poor healing, make sure he gets an adequate supply of protein, vitamins, and calories. Monitor his dietary deficiencies and discuss any problems with the doctor and the dietitian.

▶ When changing wound dressings, always use sterile technique. Inspect the incision with each dressing change and, if you recognize the early signs of infection, start treatment before dehiscence or evisceration can occur.

Complications

Infection, which can lead to peritonitis and, possibly, septic shock, is the most severe and most common complication of wound dehiscence and evisceration. Caused by bacterial contamination or by drying of normally moist abdominal contents, infection can impair circulation and lead to necrosis of the affected organ.

Documentation

Note when the problem occurred, the patient's activity preceding the problem, his condition, and the time the doctor was notified. Describe the appearance of the wound or eviscerated organ; amount, color, consistency, and odor of any drainage; and nursing actions taken. Record the patient's vital signs, his response to the incident, and the doctor's actions.

WOUND IRRIGATION

Irrigation cleans tissues and flushes cell debris and drainage from an open wound. Irrigation with a commercial wound cleaner helps the wound heal properly from the inside tissue layers outward to the skin surface; it also helps prevent premature surface healing over an abscess pocket or infected tract. Performed properly, wound irrigation requires strict sterile technique. After irrigation, open wounds usually are packed to absorb additional drainage. Always follow the standard precaution guidelines of the Centers for Disease Control and Prevention (CDC).

Key nursing diagnoses and patient outcomes

Risk for infection related to surgical incision
The patient will:

▶ have vital signs, temperature, and laboratory values remain within normal limits

▶ have incision site free from signs and symptoms of infections such as redness, malodor, and purulent drainage.

Anxiety related to situational crisis
The patient will:

▶ state at least two ways to eliminate or minimize anxious behaviors

▶ report being able to cope with current situation without experiencing severe anxiety.

Equipment

Waterproof trash bag • linen-saver pad • emesis basin • clean gloves • sterile gloves • goggles • gown, if indicated • prescribed irrigant such as sterile normal saline solution • sterile water or normal saline solution • soft rubber or plastic catheter • sterile container • materials as needed for wound care • sterile irrigation and dressing set • commercial wound cleaner • 35-ml piston syringe with 19G needle or catheter • skin protectant wipe

Preparation of equipment

Assemble all equipment in the patient's room. Check the expiration date on each sterile package and inspect for tears. Check the sterilization date and the date that each bottle of irrigating solution was opened; don't use any solution that has been open longer than 24 hours.

Using sterile technique, dilute the prescribed irrigant to the correct proportions with sterile water or normal saline solution, if necessary. Let the solution stand until it reaches room temperature, or warm it to 90° to 95° F (32.2° to 35° C).

Open the waterproof trash bag and place it near the patient's bed. Position the bag *to avoid reaching across the sterile field or the wound when disposing of soiled articles.* Form a cuff by turning down the top of the trash bag to provide a wide opening, *which will keep instruments or gloves from touching the bag's edge, thus preventing contamination.*

Implementation

▶ Check the doctor's order and assess the patient's condition. Identify the patient's allergies, especially to povidone-iodine or other topical solutions or medications.

▶ Explain the procedure to the patient, provide privacy, and position the patient correctly for the procedure. Place the linen-saver pad under the patient *to catch any spills and avoid linen changes.* Place the emesis basin below the wound *so that the irrigating solution flows from the wound into the basin.*

▶ Wash your hands thoroughly. If necessary, put on a gown to protect your clothing from wound drainage and contamination. Put on clean gloves.

▶ Remove the soiled dressing; then discard the dressing and gloves in the trash bag.

▶ Establish a sterile field with all the equipment and supplies you'll need for irrigation and wound care. Pour the prescribed amount of irrigating solution into a sterile container *so you won't contaminate your sterile gloves later by picking up unsterile containers.* Put on sterile gloves, gown, and goggles, if indicated.

▶ Fill the syringe with the irrigating solution; then connect the catheter to the syringe. Gently instill a slow, steady stream of irrigating solution into the wound until the syringe empties. (See *Irrigating a deep wound.*) Make sure the solution flows from the clean to the dirty area of the wound *to prevent contamination of clean tissue by exudate.* Also make sure the solution reaches all areas of the wound.

▶ Refill the syringe, reconnect it to the catheter, and repeat the irrigation.

▶ Continue to irrigate the wound until you've administered the prescribed amount of solution or until the solution returns clear. Note the amount of solution administered. Then remove and discard the catheter and syringe in the waterproof trash bag.

▶ Keep the patient positioned *to allow further wound drainage into the basin.*

▶ Clean the area around the wound with normal saline solution; wipe intact skin with a skin protectant wipe and allow it to dry well *to help prevent skin breakdown and infection.*

▶ Pack the wound, if ordered, and apply a sterile dressing. Remove and discard your gloves and gown.

▶ Make sure the patient is comfortable.

▶ Properly dispose of drainage, solutions, and trash bag and clean or dispose of soiled equipment and supplies according to facility policy and CDC guidelines. *To prevent contamination of other equipment,* don't return unopened sterile supplies to the sterile supply cabinet.

Special considerations

▶ Try to coordinate wound irrigation with the doctor's visit *so that he can inspect the wound.*

▶ Use only the irrigant specified by the doctor *because others may be erosive or otherwise harmful.* When using an irritating irrigant, such as Dakin's solution, spread sterile petroleum jelly around the wound site *to protect the patient's skin.*

▶ Remember to follow your facility's policy and CDC guidelines concerning wound and skin precautions.

▶ Irrigate with a bulb syringe if the wound is small or not particularly deep or if a piston syringe is unavailable. However, use a bulb syringe cautiously *because this type of syringe doesn't deliver enough pressure to adequately clean the wound.*

Irrigating a deep wound

When preparing to irrigate a wound, attach a 19G needle or catheter to a 35-ml piston syringe. This setup delivers an irrigation pressure of 8 psi, which is effective in cleaning the wound and reducing the risk of trauma and wound infection. To prevent tissue damage or, in an abdominal wound, intestinal perforation, avoid forcing the needle or catheter into the wound.

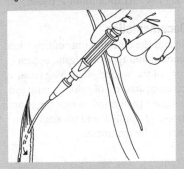

Irrigate the wound with gentle pressure until the solution returns clean. Then position the emesis basin under the wound to collect any remaining drainage.

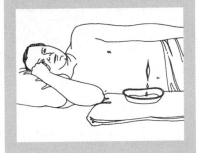

Home care

If the wound must be irrigated at home, teach the patient or a family member how to perform this procedure using strict aseptic technique. Ask for a return demonstration of the proper technique. Provide written instructions. Arrange for home health supplies and nursing visits, as appropriate. Urge the patient to call the doctor if he detects signs of infection.

Complications

Wound irrigation increases the risk of infection and may cause excoriation and increased pain. Pressure over 15 psi causes trauma to the wound and directs bacteria back into the tissue.

Documentation

Record the date and time of irrigation, amount and type of irrigant, appearance of the wound, sloughing tissue or exudate, amount of solution returned, skin care performed around the wound, dressings applied, and patient's tolerance of the treatment.

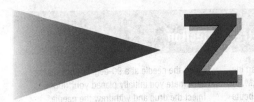

Z-TRACK INJECTION

The Z-track method of I.M. injection prevents leakage, or tracking, into the subcutaneous tissue. It's typically used to administer drugs that irritate and discolor subcutaneous tissue, primarily iron preparations such as iron dextran.

Key nursing diagnoses and patient outcomes

Deficient knowledge related to lack of exposure to procedure
The patient will:
▶ state or demonstrate understanding of what has been taught
▶ demonstrate ability to perform new health-related behaviors as they're taught.

Risk for injury related to improper technique
The patient will:
▶ identify factors that increase risk for injury
▶ assist in identifying and applying safety measures to prevent injury.

Equipment

Patient's medication record and chart • two 20G 1¼" to 2" needles • prescribed medication • gloves • 3- or 5-ml syringe • two alcohol pads

Preparation of equipment

Verify the order on the patient's medication record by checking it against the doctor's order. Wash your hands.

Make sure the needle you're using is long enough to reach the muscle. As a rule of thumb, a 200-lb (91-kg) patient requires a 2" needle; a 100-lb (45-kg) patient, a 1¼" to 1½".

Attach one needle to the syringe, and draw up the prescribed medication. Then draw 0.2 to 0.5 cc of air (depending on your facility's policy) into the syringe. Remove the first needle and attach the second *to prevent tracking the medication through the subcutaneous tissue as the needle is inserted.*

Implementation

▶ Confirm the patient's identity, explain the procedure, and provide privacy.
▶ Place the patient in the lateral position, exposing the gluteal muscle to be used as the injection site.
▶ Clean an area on the upper outer quadrant of the patient's buttock with an alcohol pad.
▶ Put on gloves. Then displace the skin laterally by pulling it away from the injection site. (See *Displacing the skin for Z-track injection,* page 934.)
▶ Insert the needle into the muscle at a 90-degree angle.

Displacing the skin for Z-track injection

By blocking the needle pathway after an injection, the Z-track technique allows I.M. injection while minimizing the risk of subcutaneous irritation and staining from such drugs as iron dextran. The illustrations here show how to perform a Z-track injection.

Before the procedure begins, the skin, subcutaneous fat, and muscle lie in their normal positions.

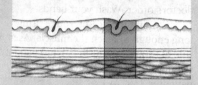

To begin, place your finger on the skin surface and pull the skin and subcutaneous layers out of alignment with the underlying muscle. You should move the skin about ½″ (1 cm).

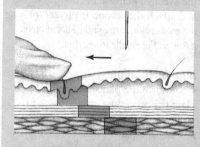

Insert the needle at a 90-degree angle at the site where you initially placed your finger. Inject the drug and withdraw the needle.

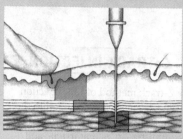

Finally, remove your finger from the skin surface, allowing the layers to return to their normal positions. The needle track (shown by the dotted line) is now broken at the junction of each tissue layer, trapping the drug in the muscle.

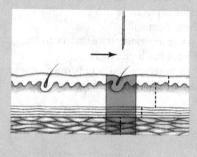

▶ Aspirate for blood return; if none appears, inject the drug slowly, followed by the air. *Injecting air after the drug helps clear the needle and prevents tracking the medication through subcutaneous tissues as the needle is withdrawn.*
▶ Wait 10 seconds before withdrawing the needle *to ensure dispersion of the medication.*

▶ Withdraw the needle slowly. Then release the displaced skin and subcutaneous tissue *to seal the needle track.* Don't massage the injection site or allow the patient to wear a tight-fitting garment over the site *because it could force the medication into subcutaneous tissue.*

► Encourage the patient to walk or move about in bed *to facilitate absorption of the drug from the injection site.*

► Discard the needles and syringe in an appropriate sharps container. Don't recap needles *to avoid needle-stick injuries.*

► Remove and discard your gloves.

Special considerations

► Never inject more than 5 ml of solution into a single site using the Z-track method. Alternate gluteal sites for repeat injections.

Complications

Discomfort and tissue irritation may result from drug leakage into subcutaneous tissue. Failure to rotate sites in patients who require repeated injections can interfere with the absorption of medication. Unabsorbed medications may build up in deposits. Such deposits can reduce the desired pharmacologic effect and may lead to abscess formation or tissue fibrosis.

Documentation

Record the medication, dosage, date, time, and site of injection on the patient's medication record. Include the patient's response to the injected drug.

APPENDIX

ALTERNATIVE AND COMPLEMENTARY THERAPIES

As the popularity of alternative and complementary therapies continues to grow, you'll need to become familiar with popular techniques. This appendix features some of the therapies you may see in everyday practice. The description of each therapy is followed by interventions and special considerations commonly associated with it.

AROMATHERAPY

Used since ancient times to heal the body, mind, and spirit, aromatherapy refers to the inhalation of essential oils distilled from various plants. Those who use aromatherapy today say it's effective in reducing stress, preventing disease, and treating certain illnesses — both physical and psychological. Aromatherapy is typically performed by a trained individual.

Implementation

For massage

▶ Dilute the essential oil in the appropriate carrier oil and apply it to the exposed body part or the entire body using massage techniques.

For inhalation

▶ Direct the patient to lean over a bowl of steaming water that contains a few drops of the essential oil. Instruct the

patient to keep his face far enough from the water's edge to prevent burn injury.

▶ To concentrate the steam, drape a towel over the patient's head and the bowl. Instruct the patient to inhale the vapors for a few minutes.

For a bath

▶ Add a few drops of essential oil to the surface of the bath water.

▶ Have the patient soak in the tub for 10 to 20 minutes, inhaling the vapors as he soaks.

Special considerations

▶ Aromatherapy is contraindicated during pregnancy because essential oils can pose a toxic risk to the mother and fetus or trigger spontaneous abortion (rare).

▶ Aromatherapy should be used with caution in infants and children under age 5 because essential oils are toxic to this age-group. Among these are oils with high levels of terpene, such as rosemary and eucalyptus.

▶ Advise patients to avoid applying cinnamon or clove oil to the skin and to stop using basil, fennel, lemon grass, rosemary, and verbena oils if skin irritations develop.

▶ Caution patients to keep essential oils away from the eyes and mucous membranes to avoid irritation. If contact occurs, the patient should flush copiously with water. If flushing doesn't relieve the irritation, the patient should seek medical attention.

ART THERAPY

Art therapy is the creative use of various expressive media to help a person deal with thoughts, emotions, life changes, personal issues, and conflicts commonly buried deep within his subconscious. If the patient can externalize his feelings for examination and reflection, he may discover meaning and insight, release, and transformation. Such discovery enhances integration of the whole person and supports growth, change, and the healing process.

Creative activities may include drawing, painting, sculpting, and making collages (using cuttings from recycled newspapers, magazines, catalogs, greeting cards, or calendars). Mask making is a powerful and popular form of expression commonly used in groups or as individual healing rituals. Puppetry is another form of artistic therapy. It requires fashioning a hand puppet, several puppets or marionettes, and perhaps even a stage, scenery, or puppet theater. Photography, videography, and computer-generated art are newer forms of art therapy.

Some conditions for which art therapy is useful are posttraumatic stress disorder, substance abuse or addiction, catastrophic illness (such as cancer and acquired immunodeficiency syndrome), chronic pain or disease, prolonged hospitalization or treatment, extensive surgery, loss of voice, aging and loss of roles, and chronic fatigue and immune dysfunction syndromes.

Implementation

▶ Explain the creative procedure to the patient and get his agreement. Assess the patient for special needs.
▶ Collect and prepare the necessary materials.
▶ Provide a quiet and comfortable environment and arrange a clean, flat surface on which the patient can work.
▶ Reassure the patient that he need not know how to draw or have any previous knowledge or training in art. Explain that stick figures can get his message across effectively.
▶ Praise all efforts and be careful not to make suggestions about colors or forms. Remain nonjudgmental and supportive.
▶ If the patient has certain signs and symptoms of a disease, encourage him to draw a picture representing himself in relation to them. You may suggest that the patient draw himself in the past, present, and future or before the disease, with the disease, and after treatment.
▶ Allow the patient time to complete the drawing to his satisfaction. Sometimes it's important for the patient to draw every small detail and search for just the right color.
▶ When the drawing is complete, allow the patient to show the drawing and tell you about it. Listen attentively. There may be a healing story involved, or the patient may discover new insights. You may want to point out certain details.
▶ Repeat to the patient what he has said to validate the meaning. Be supportive of the patient's efforts and summarize the experience for him.
▶ Notice how the patient represents his size in relation to other figures or objects. Is the entire body drawn? What are the dominant colors and shapes? Is there a smile or frown drawn on the face? What is the overall mood?

▶ Strong emotions may surface as a patient explores and connects with his underlying emotions. If the patient shows signs of agitation or uncontrolled emotion, end the session and reassure him that it's normal to have strong feelings and it's appropriate to express them. Refer the patient to other health care professionals as appropriate.

▶ If a patient is proud of an artwork, arrange to have it displayed so others may admire it, thereby adding a source of acknowledgment for the patient.

Special considerations

▶ Make sure the patient is physically capable of carrying out the artistic activity. Medications, a weakened condition, inflamed or painful joints in hands or fingers, or neurologic damage can impair the patient's ability. Someone who is physically unable to manipulate media may still be able to participate in making a collage, for example, by choosing pictures, words, or materials for someone else to cut and paste or by indicating the position of cutouts and colors. Also, computer programs may be available to create art with adapted controls.

▶ Some patients may not be open to participating in art therapy, either because they're shy and self-conscious or not interested. Don't insist; instead, work on building a trusting therapeutic relationship. The patient may be wiling to participate in the future.

BIOFEEDBACK

Biofeedback refers to any modality that measures and immediately reports information about the patient's physiologic processes. With biofeedback information, the patient can learn to consciously influence a measured body function, such as heart rate and blood pressure. The goal of biofeedback is to help him improve his overall health by consciously regulating bodily functions that are usually controlled unconsciously.

In this procedure, electrodes are attached to pertinent areas of the body to monitor such things as skeletal muscle activity, heart or brain wave activity, body temperature, and blood pressure. The electrodes feed information into a small monitoring box that reports the results by a sound or light, which varies in pitch or brightness as the body function increases or decreases (the "feedback"). A biofeedback therapist leads the patient in mental exercises to help him regulate functions, such as body temperature, blood pressure, bladder control, and muscle tension, and reach the desired result. The patient eventually learns to control the body's inner mechanisms through mental processes.

The most common forms of biofeedback involve the measurement of muscle tension, skin temperature, electrical conductance or resistance of the skin, brain waves, and respiration. As advances in technology have made measurement devices more sophisticated, the applications of biofeedback have expanded. Sensors can now measure the activity of the internal and external rectal sphincters, the activity of the bladder's detrusor muscle, esophageal motility, and stomach acidity.

Some biofeedback treatments are accepted in traditional medicine. The American Medical Association, for instance, has endorsed electromyelogram biofeedback training for the treatment of muscle contraction headaches.

Biofeedback has a vast range of applications for prevention and health restoration. It's most successful in cases where psychological factors play a role in the patient's health disturbance, such as in patients with sleep and stress-related disorders. Patients with disorders arising from poor muscle control, such as incontinence, postural problems, back pain, and temporomandibular joint syndrome, also benefit. Biofeedback training has also been shown to benefit patients who have lost control of function due to brain or nerve damage or chronic pain disorders.

Improvement has also been seen in patients with heart dysfunctions, GI disorders, swallowing difficulties, esophageal dysfunction, tinnitus, eyelid twitching, fatigue, and cerebral palsy. Biofeedback isn't recommended for severe structural problems, such as broken bones and slipped discs.

Implementation

▶ You'll probably work with a trained biofeedback practitioner when conducting the session.
▶ Provide the patient with a private environment that is free from noise and other distractions.
▶ Gather the necessary equipment and wash your hands.
▶ Explain the procedure to the patient and answer any questions he has. If relaxation techniques or imagery will also be used, review them with the patient.
▶ Depending on the body function that will be monitored, clean and prepare the skin and attach the electrodes according to the manufacturer's instructions. The patient may experience a local skin irritation from the electrodes used in the monitoring.
▶ Set the monitor where you and the patient can easily see the results.

▶ Set a goal for the session with the patient and review the information the patient will see on the monitor.
▶ Turn on the monitor and establish a baseline for the targeted body function.
▶ If goggles will be used, help the patient place them comfortably over his eyes.
▶ When the patient is ready, begin the session by starting the relaxation tapes or imagery sequence.
▶ At the close of the session, disconnect the monitor and remove the electrodes.
▶ Clean the patient's skin as needed.

DANCE THERAPY

Also known as dance movement therapy, dance therapy capitalizes on the direct relationship between body movement and the mind. Specific aspects of dance therapy, such as music, rhythm, and synchronous movement, can alter mood states, reawaken memories and feelings, and reduce isolation. Additionally, dance therapy organizes thoughts and actions and assists in establishing relationships. Used in a group setting, dance therapy is believed to create the emotional intensity necessary for behavioral change.

Dance therapy is used in a wide variety of settings. It's used to help emotionally disturbed patients express their feelings, gain insight, and develop relationships. With physically disabled people, dance therapy increases movement and self-esteem while providing an enjoyable, creative outlet. In groups of older people, dance therapy is used to maintain physical function, enhance self-worth, develop relationships, and help them express fear and grief.

A wide variety of disorders and disabilities can be treated using dance therapy. Typically, the target patient has social, emotional, cognitive, or physical problems. Dance therapy is even being used as a method of disease prevention and health promotion among healthy patients. Additionally, it's used for stress reduction by caregivers and patients with cancer, acquired immunodeficiency syndrome, and Alzheimer's disease. Dance therapy promotes flexibility, strengthens muscles, and improves cardiovascular and pulmonary functions. In addition, it provides socialization and a sense of connectedness.

Group dance, probably the most common form of dance therapy, allows people of different physical abilities to participate. By simply tapping their toes or patting their thighs in time to the music, patients can feel a part of the session. Dance routines range from simple clapping and swaying to intricate aerobic sessions.

The music should be appropriate to the group in its pace and aesthetic appeal. Fast-moving rock and roll music is probably less enjoyable for a group of agile senior citizens than a fast polka would be. Use faster music to stimulate the group and slower music for a calming effect.

Implementation

▶ Arrange the space to accommodate free movement of the participants.
▶ Arrange chairs around the periphery for those who can't stand or become tired during the session.
▶ Assess the group for risk factors. The presence of one or more risk factors doesn't preclude group members from participating but may influence the type of dance and length of the session. Risk factors to consider include poor cardiovascular status, a history of chronic obstructive pulmonary disease, or degenerative musculoskeletal problems.
▶ Explain the purpose of the session and encourage everyone to participate to the degree they feel able.
▶ When the group is ready, start the music and position yourself so you're facing the group.
▶ If a structured routine is being used, demonstrate the movements you're seeking and encourage the group to mimic your movements.
▶ If free expression is sought, circulate among the group, providing encouragement and motivation to those who are hesitant.
▶ After the session, praise the participants' efforts and encourage them to discuss the feelings they experienced while dancing. Also, document the type of activity and the group's response.

Special considerations

▶ Because dancing is an aerobic activity, watch for signs of cardiovascular compromise, such as dizziness, flushing, profuse sweating, and disorientation.
▶ Rapid motion may result in dizziness.
▶ Help a person who becomes dizzy to a seat as needed and check his vital signs.

MUSIC THERAPY

Music therapy uses the universal appeal of rhythmic sound to communicate, explore, and heal. It can take the form of creating music, singing, moving to music, or just listening.

Music therapy benefits patients with developmental disabilities, mental health disorders, substance addictions, and chronic pain. Studies have demonstrated the positive effects of music in reducing pain and procedural anxiety and in dental anesthesia.

Patients who listen to classical music before surgery and then again in the postanesthesia care unit reported minimal postoperative disorientation. Music has also been used to successfully communicate with patients with Alzheimer's disease or head trauma when other approaches failed. In one study on the effects of music on patients with Alzheimer's disease, those who listened to big band music during the day were more alert and happier and had better long-term recollection than members of the control group. Throughout the illness, music can reorient confused patients. In the final stages of the disease, music provides psychological comfort.

Implementation

▶ Arrange a comfortable environment.
▶ Choose music that is appropriate to the patients and the session objectives. The music should be meaningful to the participants.
▶ If your session will involve making music, collect instruments appropriate for the group.
▶ For sessions involving singing, choose music that is known to the group members. Provide words for the songs, either in writing or by repeating them to the group.
▶ Introduce the participants to one another. Explain the purpose of the session and encourage everyone to participate as they feel able.
▶ When the group is ready, start the music and position yourself so you're facing the group.
▶ If the group will be listening to music, watch the reactions of the partici-

pants. If they're making the music, circulate among them and offer individual support.
▶ After the session, encourage the participants to discuss the feelings they experienced while listening to the music and praise their efforts. Also, document the type of activity and the group's response.

Special considerations

▶ Music is especially effective as a means of reminiscence therapy for older people. For many of them, the music they enjoyed in their youth hasn't been part of their lives for decades.

PET THERAPY

Pets can combat loneliness in a patient and help bridge the gap between the patient and the health care provider. Commonly used in long-term care facilities, pet therapy helps the patient break through apathy and depression and improves interaction with others. Some facilities adopt a pet as a mascot for the facility and let the patients share the responsibility of caring for it. Sharing responsibility for the pet builds a sense of community.

Implementation

▶ Select a pet that is well-behaved and has a good temperament. Pets that have gone through obedience training are ideal.
▶ Make sure the pet is cleared by a veterinarian and is up-to-date on his immunizations.
▶ If the pet is chosen as a mascot for the facility, have a responsible person make a schedule for patients who are interested in caring for the pet.

▶ If the pet isn't a permanent resident of the facility, arrange for a volunteer from an animal shelter to accompany the pet to ensure the safety of the animal and the patients.

▶ Allow the patient to play with and hold the pet. Encourage him to talk to the pet and reminisce about pets he once had. Provide as much time as he needs with the pet, if possible.

Special considerations

▶ Ensure that the environment is appropriate for pet therapy. The facility should have an area where the pet can retreat and be kept out of the way of patients who are allergic to or afraid of animals and those who have no interest in pets.

YOGA THERAPY

Among the oldest known health practices, yoga (which means "union" in Sanskrit) is the integration of physical, mental, and spiritual energies to promote health and wellness. It's practiced by young and old alike, individually or in groups, and can be started at any age.

Based on the idea that a chronically restless or agitated mind causes poor health and decreased mental strength and clarity, yoga outlines specific regimens for lifestyle, hygiene, detoxification, physical activity, and psychological practices. By integrating these practices, yoga aims to raise the individual's physical vitality and spiritual awareness.

There are several styles of yoga. The most common in the West is Hatha yoga, which combines physical postures and exercises (called *asanas*), breathing techniques (called *pranayamas*), relaxation, diet, and "proper thinking."

Asanas fall into two categories, meditative and therapeutic. Meditative asanas promote proper blood flow through the body by bringing the spine and body into perfect alignment. The mind and body are brought into a state of relaxation and stillness, which facilitates concentration during meditation. Asanas also keep the heart, glands, and lungs properly energized. Therapeutic asanas are commonly prescribed for joint pain. The "cobra," "locust spinal twist," and "shoulder stand" are examples.

The goal of a properly executed asana is to create a balance between movement and stillness, which is the state of a healthy body. Very little movement is needed. Instead, the mind provides discipline, awareness, and a relaxed openness to maintain the posture and properly execute the asana. Using asanas, the individual learns to regulate autonomic functions, such as heartbeat and respirations, while relaxing physical tensions.

Pranayamas focus on disciplined breathing. They regulate the flow of *prana* (breath and electromagnetic force), keeping the individual healthy. Pranayamas have been shown to aid digestion, regulate cardiac function, and alleviate a variety of other physical ailments. They can also be especially effective in reducing the frequency of asthma attacks.

The goal of breathing in yoga is to make the process as smooth and regular as possible. The assumption is that the rhythm of the mind is mirrored in the rhythm of breathing. By keeping respirations steady and rhythmic, the mind will remain calm and focused.

Samadhi, or spiritual realization, is an additional component of Eastern yoga. Yoga practitioners compare samadhi to a fourth state of consciousness, separate from the normal states of waking, dreaming, and sleeping. A technique called *HongSau* uses meditation to develop the powers of concentration. Thought and energy are withdrawn from outer distractions and focused on any goal or problem the individual chooses. The *Aum* technique expands the individual's awareness beyond the limitations of the body and mind, allowing the user to experience what is called the "Divine Consciousness," which is believed to underlie and uphold all life.

Among yoga's measured benefits are improvement in the individual's health, vitality, and peace of mind. It's successfully used to alleviate stress and anxiety, lower blood pressure, relieve pain, improve motor skills, treat addictions, increase auditory and visual perception, and improve metabolic and respiratory function. Yoga has also been effective in the treatment of metabolic disorders and lung ailments. It can increase lung capacity and lower respiratory rates.

Yoga has been credited with decreasing serum cholesterol and increasing histamine levels to fight allergies. Its ability to help the user regulate blood flow is being studied in cancer therapy. Scientists are eager to see if restricted blood flow to the tumor region will slow growth.

Implementation

▶ Provide a private, quiet environment that is free from distractions.
▶ Participants should have enough room to move without touching or distracting other members.
▶ Each participant will need a small blanket or large towel to use in some of the postures.

▶ Explain the purpose of the session and describe the planned exercises and their benefits.
▶ Answer any questions and remind the participants that they shouldn't engage in any posture that may be uncomfortable.
▶ When the group is ready, talk them through the positions or breathing techniques, demonstrating each one.
▶ After they've all assumed the position, begin the breathing pattern; circulate among the patients to adjust their technique as needed.
▶ Offer praise for all their efforts.
▶ After you've led them through all the planned exercises, close the session by having everyone take slow, deep breaths.
▶ Document the session, the techniques used, and the patients' responses.

Special considerations

▶ Some of the more physical aspects of yoga can cause muscle injury if they aren't properly performed or if the patient tries to force his body into position.
▶ Caution patients to attempt the various techniques and postures cautiously and remind them that few people are able to perform all the techniques in the beginning.
▶ There are yoga techniques to fit the needs of all people regardless of their physical condition. Individuals who can't perform some of the more physically demanding postures can still benefit from the breathing or meditation techniques.

SELECTED REFERENCES

Auscultation Skills: Breath and Heart Sounds, Springhouse, Pa.: Springhouse Corp., 1999.

Bickley, L.S., and Hoekelman, R.A. Bates' Guide to Physical Examination and History Taking, 7th ed. Philadelphia: Lippincott Williams & Wilkins, 1999.

Braunwald, E., et al., eds. Heart Disease: A Textbook of Cardiovascular Medicine, 6th ed. Philadelphia: W.B. Saunders Co., 2001.

Carlson, K.K., and Lynn-McHale, D.J., eds. AACN Procedure Manual for Critical Care, 4th ed. Philadelphia: W.B. Saunders Co., 2000.

Carpenito, L.J. Handbook of Nursing Diagnosis, 8th ed. Philadelphia: Lippincott Williams & Wilkins, 1999.

Diagnostics: An A-to-Z Guide to Laboratory Tests and Diagnostic Procedures. Springhouse, Pa.: Springhouse Corp., 2001.

Elkin, M.K., et al. Nursing Interventions and Clinical Skills, 2nd ed. St. Louis: Mosby–Year Book, Inc., 2000.

Ellis, J.R., and Hartley, C.L. Managing and Coordinating Nursing Care, 3rd ed. Philadelphia: Lippincott Williams & Wilkins, 2000.

Fischbach, F.T. A Manual of Laboratory and Diagnostic Tests, 6th ed. Philadelphia: Lippincott Williams & Wilkins, 2000.

Fortunato, N.H. Berry & Kohn's Operating Room Technique, 9th ed. St. Louis: Mosby–Year Book, Inc., 2000.

Goldman, L., and Bennett, J.C. Cecil Textbook of Medicine, 21st ed. Philadelphia: W.B. Saunders Co., 2000.

Hadaway, L.C. "I.V. Infiltration: Not Just a Peripheral Problem," Nursing99 29(9):41-47, September 1999.

Hess, C.T. Clinical Guide to Wound Care, 3rd ed. Springhouse, Pa.: Springhouse Corp., 2000.

Horne, C., and Derrico, D. "Mastering ABGs. The Art of Arterial Blood Gas Measurement," AJN 99(8):26-33, August 1999.

Ignatavicius, D., et al. Medical-Surgical Nursing Across the Health Care Continuum, 3rd ed. Philadelphia: W.B. Saunders Co., 1999.

Jagger, J., and Perry, J. "Power in Numbers: Reducing Your Risk of Bloodborne Exposures," Nursing99 29(1):51-52, January 1999.

Joint Commission on Accreditation of Healthcare Organizations. Comprehensive Accreditation Manual for Hospitals, Oakbrook Terrace, Ill., 2000.

Kost, M. "Conscious Sedation: Guarding Your Patient Against Complications," Nursing99 29(4):34-39, April 1999.

Lanken, P.N. *The Intensive Care Unit Manual.* Philadelphia: W.B. Saunders Co., 2001.

Makelbust, J., and Sieggreen, M. *Pressure Ulcers: Guidelines for Prevention and Management,* 3rd ed. Springhouse, Pa.: Springhouse Corp., 2001.

Nicol, M., et al. *Essential Nursing Skills.* St. Louis: Mosby–Year Book, Inc., 2000.

Nursing Procedures, 3rd ed., Springhouse, Pa.: Springhouse Corp., 2000.

Phillips, L.D. *Manual of I.V. Therapeutics,* 3rd ed. Philadelphia: F.A. Davis Co., 2001.

Phippen, M.L., and Wells, M.P. *Patient Care During Operative and Invasive Procedures.* Philadelphia: W.B. Saunders Co., 2000.

Pierson, F.M. *Principles and Techniques of Patient Care,* 2nd ed. Philadelphia: W.B. Saunders Co., 1999.

Rakel, R., ed. *Conn's Current Therapy.* Philadelphia: W.B. Saunders Co., 2001.

Shoemaker, W., and Grenvik, A., et al. *Textbook of Critical Care,* 4th ed. Philadelphia: W.B. Saunders Co., 2000.

Smeltzer, S.C., and Bare, B.G. *Brunner and Suddarth's Textbook of Medical-Surgical Nursing,* 9th ed. Philadelphia: Lippincott Williams & Wilkins, 2000.

Sole, M.L., et al., eds. *Introduction to Critical Care Nursing,* 3rd ed. Philadelphia: W.B. Saunders Co., 2001.

Turjanica, M.A. "Anatomy of a Code: How Do You Feel at the Start of a Code Blue?" *Nursing Management* 30(11):44-49, November 1999.

INDEX

A

Aging, medication administration and, 235
Airborne precautions, 3-5
Airway clearance
  therapy vest and, 153
  tips on, 574
Allen's test, performing, 34i
Ambulation, progressive, 8-11
Ambulatory peritoneal dialysis, continuous,
      200-204
Amniocentesis, 11-15
Amnioinfusion, 16
Amniotomy, 15-17
Amputation, care associated with, 768
Anaerobic specimen, collection of, 789i
Analgesia, patient-controlled, 145
Analgesic administration, epidural, 296-300
Anesthesia induction, latex allergy and, 500
Angioplasty
  laser-enhanced, 620
  percutaneous transluminal coronary,
      618-623
Antiembolism stockings
  applying, 17-18, 19-21
  measuring for, 19i
Apgar scoring, 21-24
Apnea monitoring, 24-26
Arrhythmias, treating, 176
Arterial blood gas analysis, documenting
      blood withdrawal for, 37
Arterial pressure monitoring, 26-33
Arterial puncture
  blood gas analysis and, 33-38
  technique for, 36i
Arterial waveform
  abnormal, 32i
  understanding, 30i
Arteriovenous hemofiltration, continuous,
      204-207

Arteriovenous shunt care, 38-40
Arthroplasty care, 40-43
Automated external defibrillation, 43-46
Autotransfusion. See Transfusion of autolo-
      gous blood.

B

Back care, 47-49
Back massage, 48i
Bandaging techniques, 251i
Bed-making, 49-53
Bedpan and urinal use, 53-56
Bedside spirometry, 58-61
Biological dressings, 95t
Bladder
  irrigation, 207-209
  retraining, 420
  ultrasonography, 61-62
Blood culture, 62-63
Blood glucose and hemoglobin testing,
      bedside, 56-58
Blood glucose tests, 63-66
Blood pressure monitoring, 268
Body alignment and traction, maintain-
      ing, 81i
Body mechanics, 66-67
Bone marrow aspiration and biopsy, 67-70
Bottle-feeding, 70-72
Brachytherapy. See Radiation implant therapy.
Breast-feeding
  assistance with, 72-77
  breast care during, 75
  positions for, 74i
Breast pumps
  comparing, 78i
  using, 77-80
Bryant's traction, 80-82
Buccal drugs, 83-84

i refers to an illustration; t refers to a table.

Burn care, 84-94
    estimating burn surfaces and, 86-87i
    evaluating burn severity for, 88i
    preventing deformity in burn patient
        and, 89-90t
Burn dressing use, biological, 94, 96-97

C

Cane use, 98-100
Carbon dioxide
    levels, analyzing, 287
    waveform, 288i
Cardiac drugs, emergency, 173-175t
Cardiac monitoring, 100-101, 103-106
Cardiac output measurement, 106-110
Cardioversion, synchronized, 791-793
Cardioverter-defibrillator, implantable, 218i
Carotid sinus massage, location and tech-
        nique for, 918i
Cartridge-injection system, 1
Cast
    care, 392-395
    cylindrical, 111i
    petaling, 113i
    preparing, 110-115
Catheter, placement of epidural, 298i
Catheter irrigation, urinary, 115-117
Central venous catheter
    guide to, 120-123i
    pathways, 118i
Central venous dressing, steps in chang-
        ing, 128
Central venous line insertion and removal,
        117-119, 124-129
Central venous pressure monitoring,
        129-132, 135
Cerebral blood flow
    inserting sensor for, 137i
    monitoring, 135-139
Cerebrospinal fluid drainage, 139-142
Cervical collar application, 142-143
Chemotherapeutic drug
    administration, 144, 146-149
    preparation, 150-152
Chemotherapy, intraperitoneal, 146i
Chest electrodes, positioning, 258i
Chest physiotherapy, 153, 156-158
Chest tube
    insertion, 158-161
    removal, 160

Children
    drug administration in, 222-224, 227,
        229-230
    injection sites in, 228i
    restraints for, 704i
Chorionic villi sampling, 12
Circumcision, 161-163
Clavicle strap application, 163-166
Clinitron therapy bed use, 166-168
Closed-wound drain management, 168-170
Closure pressure therapy, vacuum-assisted,
        915-916
Code management, 170-172, 175, 177-178
Cold application, 178-182
Colostomy
    care, 182, 184-187
    irrigation, 187-190
Commode use, 55
Compliance aid use, 240i
Compression therapy, sequential, 723-726
Condom catheter, applying, 416i
Contact lens care and removal, 190-193
Contact precautions, infectious diseases
        and, 193, 195-196
Continent ileostomy care, 196-199
Controllers and infusion pumps, 476i
Coronary angioplasty, percutaneous trans-
        luminal, 618-623
Crash cart, organizing, 172i
Credé's maneuver, 209-211
Credé's treatment, 321-322
Cricothyrotomy, 211-213
Crutch use, 213-216
Cuff–pressure measurement, tracheal,
        817-819
Cystostomy tube care. See Nephrostomy and
        cystostomy tube care.

D

Debridement, mechanical, 511-512
Defibrillation, 217-219
    automated external, 43-46
Dehiscence, recognizing, 928i
Delivery (childbirth), emergency, 269-272
Dentures, dealing with, 526
Diabetic patients, foot care for, 356
Dialysis, peritoneal, 200-204, 642-649
Diseases
    airborne precautions and, 4t
    contact precautions and, 194-195t
    droplet precautions and, 221t

i refers to an illustration; t refers to a table.

Diseases (*continued*)
   neutropenic precautions and, 567t
   reportable, 701t
Disposable drainage systems, 800i
Donor graft site, care of, 732
Doppler use, 219-220
Drainage systems, disposable, 800i
Droplet precautions, 220-222
Drug administration
   buccal routes for, 84i
   cardiac, 173-175t
   chemotherapeutic, 144, 146-149
   in children, 222-224, 227, 229-230
   documenting, 774
   endotracheal, 273-274
   implantation and, 230-235
   intrapleural, 463-467
   liquid, 570i
   ocular, 317-321
   in older adults, 235-239, 241
   oral, 569-571
   skin, 733-736
   sublingual routes for, 84i
Dying patient care, 241-244

E

Eardrop instillation, 245-247
Ear irrigation, 247-249
ECG. *See* Electrocardiography.
Elastic bandage application, 249-252
Elderly patient
   compliance aids and, 240i
   drug therapy in, 235-239, 241
   recognizing adverse reactions in, 239
Electrical bone growth stimulation, 253-255
Electrocardiogram waveforms and compo-
      nents, 256i
Electrocardiography, 255-259
   posterior chest lead, 259-260
   right chest lead, 260-262
   signal-averaged, 262-264
Electrodes
   chest, positioning, 258i
   for signal-averaged electrocardiography,
      264i
Electrolyte testing with vascular intermittent
      access system, 264-267
Electronic vital signs monitor use, 267-269
Emergency delivery, 269-272
Endotracheal drug administration, 273-274

Endotracheal intubation, 274-278, 281-282
Endotracheal tube
   caring for, 282-285
   securing, 279-281i
End-tidal carbon dioxide monitoring,
      285-290
Enema administration, 290-296, 292i
Enemas, types of, 291t
Epidural analgesic administration, 296-300
Epidural catheter, placement of, 298i
Esophageal tube
   care of, 300-302
   insertion and removal of, 302-307
   securing, 305i
   types of, 303i
Evisceration, recognizing, 928i
External fixation, 307-309
External radiation therapy, 309-311
Extracorporeal membrane oxygenation, 585
Extravasation, managing, 149
Eye
   compress application, 311-312, 314
   irrigation, 314-317
   medication administration, 317-321
   prophylaxis, 321-322
Eye patch, applying, 313i

F

Face mask, applying, 470i
Falls
   medication associated with, 327t
   prevention and management of, 323-329
   risk assessment for, 324t
Fecal impaction removal (digital), 329-330
Fecal occult blood test, 330-332
Feeding, 332-333, 335-336
   devices, 334i
   gavage, 365-367
   syringe, 842i
   tube, insertion and removal of, 336-339
Fetal heart rate
   assessing, 339, 341, 343
   irregularities associated with, 350-353t
Fetal heart tones, instruments for, 340i
Fetal monitoring
   devices, 344i
   external, 343-346
   internal, 346-349, 352-355
   strip, 349i

Figure-eight strap. *See* Clavicle strap application.
Fixation devices
  external, 307-309
  internal, 440-442
Flow rates of I.V. solutions, calculating, 479i
Foot care, 355-357

G

Gastric lavage, 358-362
Gastric suction devices, 548i
Gastric tube use, 360i
Gastrostomy feeding button
  care of, 362-363
  reinsertion of, 364i
Gavage feeding, 365-367
Gloves
  applying, 778i
  removing, 471i
  selecting, 760
Glucose tolerance tests, oral and I.V., 65
Graft
  sheet, evacuating fluid from, 733
  site, donor, 732
  types of, 731

H

Hair removal, 737-739i
Halo-vest traction, 368-373
Handheld oropharyngeal inhalers, 373-376
Hand washing, 376-378
Heat application, 378-382
Hemodialysis, 383, 386-392
  access sites for, 384i
  process of, 385-386i
Hemodynamic pressure monitoring
  problems, 133-135t
Hemofiltration, continuous arterio-
    venous, 204-207
Hemoglobin testing, 56-58
Hip spica cast care, 392-395
Home I.V. therapy, 477
Hour of sleep care, 395-397
Humidifier therapy, 397-400
Hydrotherapy, 401-403
Hyperthermia-hypothermia therapy,
    403-407

I

Ice massage, reducing pain with, 179
Ileostomy care, 182, 184-187, 196-199

I.M. injection, 408-410, 412-413
  modification of, 236i
  sites for, 228i, 411i
Implantable cardioverter defibrillator, 218i
Incentive spirometry, 413-415
Incontinence device application and
    removal, 415-417
Incontinence management, 417, 419-423
Indwelling urinary catheter
  care and removal of, 423-427
  insertion of, 427-433
Infant, giving oral medication to, 224i
Infectious disease, standard precautions for
    protection against, 759-762
Informed consent, obtaining, 668
Inhalers, handheld oropharyngeal, 373-376
Injection
  I.M., 228i, 236i, 408-413
  intradermal, 459-460
  intrathecal, 297
  I.V. bolus, 472-474
  subcutaneous, 769-771, 773-774
  Z-track, 933-935
In-line filter, using, 488
Insulin infusion pumps, types of, 772
Intermittent infusion device
  inserting, 433-435
  I.V. therapy and, 434i
  needleless system for, 437i
  using, 435-437
Intermittent positive-pressure breathing,
    437-439
Intermittent pulmonary artery wedge pres-
    sure monitoring, 608-609, 611-616
Internal fixation, 440-442
Intra-aortic balloon
  counterpulsation, 442-450
  insertion sites, 448i
  pump, 444i
  waveforms, 446-447i
Intracranial pressure
  increased, managing, 458
  monitoring, 450, 452-455, 457-459
  understanding systems of, 451-452i
  waveforms, 456-457i
Intradermal injection, 459-460
Intraosseous infusion, 461-463
Intrapleural drug administration, 463-467
Intrathecal injection, 297
Iodine therapy, radioactive, 689-692

i refers to an illustration; t refers to a table.

Iontophoresis, 467-468
IPPB. *See* Intermittent positive-pressure breathing.
Irrigation
  bladder, 207-209
  colostomy, 187-190
  ear, 247-249
  eye, 314-317
  nose, 531-533
  urinary catheter, 115-117
Isolation equipment use, 469-472
Isometric exercises, 695-696
I.V. bolus injection, 472-474
I.V. clamp use, 478i
I.V. controllers and pumps, 474-477
I.V. flow rate
  calculation and control of, 478, 479i, 481
  deviations from, 480t
I.V. sites
  pediatric, 483i
  protecting, 485i
I.V. therapy
  home, 477
  intermittent infusion device and, 434i
  pediatric, 481-484, 486
  peripheral, 634-639t
  preparation of, 486-490
  secondary line for, 713-715
  teaching patient about, 489

J

Joint movements, glossary of, 694i

K

Ketone and urine glucose testing, 908-910
Knee extension therapy, 491-494
Kock ileostomy. *See* Continent ileostomy care.

L

Laser therapy, 495-497
Latex allergy protocol, 498-502
Leg bag, urinary drainage and, 426
Leopold's maneuver, performing, 342i
Lipid emulsion administration, 502-504
Lumbar puncture, 504-507

M

Manual ventilation, 508-511
Mechanical debridement, 511-512

Mechanical ventilation, 512-515, 518-519
Mechanical ventilator
  alarms, responding to, 517t
  weaning patient from, 516
Mist tent therapy, 519-521
Mixed venous oxygen saturation monitoring, 521-524
Monitoring leads, positioning, 102-103i
Montgomery straps, making, 781i
Mouth care, 524-525, 528
Mucus clearance, 528-530
Muscle sprain or spasm
  cold application for, 181i
  moist heat to relieve, 382

N

Nasal balloon catheters, 535i
Nasal irrigation, 531-533
Nasal packing, 533-534, 536-540
Nasoenteric-decompression tube
  care of, 540-543
  insertion and removal, 543, 545-547
  types of, 544i
Nasogastric tube
  care of, 547-551
  insertion and removal, 551-557
  types of, 552i
  use, at-home, 555
Nasopharyngeal airway insertion and care, 557-559
Nasopharyngeal specimen, obtaining, 788i
Nebulizer therapy, 559-562
Nephrostomy and cystostomy tube care, 562-566
Neutropenic precautions, 566-568
Nitroglycerin ointment, applying, 853i
Nosebleeds, preventing, 539

O

Open reduction. *See* Internal fixation.
Oral drug administration, 569-571
Oral irrigating device use, 527i
Organ donation, 244
Oronasopharyngeal suction, 571-575
Oropharyngeal airway insertion and care, 575-577
Oropharyngeal inhalers, handheld, 373-376
Ostomy pouching systems
  comparison of, 183i
  skin barrier application and, 185i

Oxygen administration
  in adults, 578-579, 583-584
  in neonates, 584-585, 587-590
Oxygen delivery systems
  comparison of, 586t
  guide to, 580-583i
Oxytocin administration, 590-593

PQ

Pacemaker, permanent
  codes for, 595t
  insertion and care of, 594-595, 597
  teaching patient about, 596
Pacemaker, temporary
  electrode placement for, 600i
  insertion and care of, 597-602, 604
  malfunction, 603-604i
Pain
  assessment of, 606
  ice massage for reducing, 179
  management of, 605-608
PAP monitoring. See Pulmonary artery
          pressure monitoring, continuous.
Papanicolaou testing, 616-618
Parenteral nutrition, total. See Total par-
          enteral nutrition.
PAWP monitoring. See Pulmonary artery
          wedge pressure monitoring, intermit-
          tent.
PCA. See Analgesia, patient-controlled.
PEEP valve. See Positive-end-expiratory
          pressure valve use.
Pelvic floor muscles, strengthening, 422
Percussion, 157i
Percutaneous endoscopic gastrostomy
          site care, 840i
Percutaneous endoscopic jejunostomy
          site care, 840i
Percutaneous transluminal coronary
          angioplasty, 618-623
Perineal care, 623-625
Peripheral I.V. line insertion, 625-633
Peripheral I.V. therapy, risks of, 634-639t
PICC. See Peripherally inserted central
          catheter insertion and removal.
Peritoneal dialysis, 200-204, 642-649
  catheters for, 644-645i
  principles of, 643i
Peritoneal lavage, 650-653, 651i
Phototherapy, 653-656

Peripherally inserted central catheter inser-
          tion and removal, 656-662
Piggyback set, assembling, 715i
Positive-end-expiratory pressure valve
          use, 509i
Postmortem care, 662-663
Postoperative care, 663-666
Postural drainage, positioning patient
          for, 154-156i
Pouch construction, 197i
Preoperative care, 666-668
Pressure dressing application, 668-669
Pressure ulcer
  assessment of, 670i
  care, 669-679
  topical agents for, 674t
Preventive devices, 6i
Prosthesis and stump care, 763-769
Protective precautions. See Neutropenic
          precautions.
PTCA. See Percutaneous transluminal coro-
          nary angioplasty.
Pulmonary artery
  catheter, 610i
  waveforms, normal, 613i
Pulmonary artery pressure monitoring,
          continuous, 608-609, 611-616
Pulmonary artery wedge pressure monitor-
          ing, intermittent, 608-609, 611-616
Pulse amplitude monitoring, 679-681
Pulse oximetry, 681-684

R

Radiation implant therapy, 685-689
Radiation therapy, external, 309-311
Radioactive iodine therapy, 689-692
Radioisotopes, uses of, 686-687t
Range-of-motion exercises, passive, 693-697
Rectal suppository and ointment administra-
          tion, 697-699
Rectal tube insertion and removal, 699-700
Reportable diseases, 701-702
Respirator seal check, 5i
Restraint application, 703-707
Resuscitation bag and mask, applying, 510i
Reverse isolation. See Neutropenic precau-
          tions.
Rotation bed use, 707-712
Roto rest bed, 708

i refers to an illustration; t refers to a table.

S

Safety
  at home, promotion of, 328
  walker use and, 926i
Seizure management, 715-720
Self-catheterization, 720-723
Semipermeable dressing, applying, 631i
Sequential compression therapy, 723-726
Shampoos, medicated, 735
Sheet graft, evacuating fluid from, 733
Shunt care, arteriovenous, 38-40
Sitz bath, 726-728
Skin
  biopsy, 728-730
  closures, adhesive, 744
  graft care, 730-733
  medication administration, 733-736
  preparation, preoperative, 736, 740-741
  staple and clip removal, 742-744, 743i
  types, comparing, 892
Skull tongs
  site care, 744-748
  types of, 746-747i
Sling, 881i
Soak application, 748-750
Spirometry, bedside, 58-61
Splint application, 750-753, 751i, 752i
Sponge bath, 753-755
Sputum collection, 755-759
Standard precautions, 759-762
Staple removal, 743i
Status epilepticus, 719
Stillbirth, handling, 23
Stockings, antiembolism, 17-21
Stool collection, 762-763
Stump and prosthesis care, 763-769
Subcutaneous injection, 769-774
  sites for, 770i
  technique for, 230i, 771i
Sublingual drugs, 83-84
Suction catheter, specimen trap and, 756-757i
Surgery, hair removal and, 737-739i
Surgical incision care, 782
Surgical reduction. See Internal fixation.
Surgical wound management, 774-783
Suture removal, 783-786
Swab specimen collection, 786-791
Swathe, applying, 882i
Synchronized cardioversion, 791-793
Syringe feeding, teaching patient about, 842i

T

Thermoregulation, neonatal, 794-797, 795i
Thoracentesis, 797-799
Thoracic drainage, 799-803
Thoracic electrical bioimpedance monitoring, 803-805
Tilt table use, 805-807
Tissue donation, 244
Total hip replacement, 40
Total parenteral nutrition, 807-817
  monitoring, 814-817
  problems associated with, 813t
  types of, 808-809t
Tracheal cuff–pressure measurement, 817-819
Tracheal suction, 819-825, 823i
Tracheostomy and ventilator speaking valve, 826-828
Tracheostomy care, 828-834
Tracheotomy, 834-838, 837i
Traction,
  Bryant's, 80-82
  halo-vest, 368-373
Traction bed, making, 50-51i
Transabdominal tube feeding and care, 838-843
Transcranial Doppler monitoring, 843-847
Transcutaneous electrical nerve stimulation, 847-850, 849i
Transcutaneous partial pressure of oxygen monitoring, 850-851
Transdermal drug therapy, 852-854
Transdermal medication patch, applying, 854
Transducer system setup, 854-857
Transfer
  from bed to stretcher, 857-859
  from bed to wheelchair, 859-860, 862
  with hydraulic lift, 862-864
  patient teaching and, 861i
Transfusion of autologous blood, 864-869
  managing problems of, 868t
Transfusion reaction, managing, 875, 877-878, 877t
Transfusion of whole blood and packed cells, 869-875, 872-873t
Translingual drugs, 83-84
Traumatic wound management, 878-880
Triangular sling application, 880, 882
T-tube care, 882-885, 883i
Tube feedings, 838-843, 885-889, 890t

i refers to an illustration; t refers to a table.

U

Ultraviolet light therapy, 891-894
Urinary catheter, indwelling
  care and removal of, 423-427
  insertion of, 427-433
Urinary diversion
  permanent, 895i
  stoma care for, 894-900
  techniques for, 563i
Urinary incontinence, 420
Urinary sphincter implant, 418i
Urine collection
  in adults, 900-903
  in children, 903-906
  timed, 906-908
Urine glucose and ketone testing, 908-910
Urine pH testing, 910-911
Urine specific gravity, 911-913
Urine specimen, aspirating, 902i
Urine straining for calculi, 913-914
Urinometer, using, 912i

V

Vacuum-assisted closure pressure therapy,
    915-916
Vagal maneuvers, 916-919
Valsalva's maneuver, 124
Vascular intermittent access system, 266i
Vascular stent, 622
Velocity waveforms, comparing, 846i
Venipuncture, 920-922, 921i
Venous access
  devices, comparing, 627
  site, methods of taping, 632-633i
Venous oxygen saturation, mixed
  equipment for, 523i
  monitoring, 521-522, 524
Ventilation
  manual, 508-511
  mechanical, 512-516, 517t, 518-519
Vertical suspension. See Bryant's traction.
Vibration, performing, 157i
Volume-control set use, 922-924

WXY

Walker use, 925-927
Warming system, using, 406i
Wound dehiscence and evisceration
    management, 927-929
Wound irrigation, 929-932, 931i

Z

Z-track injection, 933-935, 934i

i refers to an illustration; t refers to a table.